Visit our website

to find out about other books from Mosby and our sister companies in Harcourt Health Sciences

Register free at
www.harcourt-international.com

and you will get

- the latest information on new books, journals and electronic products in your chosen subject areas

- the choice of e-mail or post alerts or both, when there are any new books in your chosen areas

- news of special offers and promotions

- information about products from all Harcourt Health Sciences companies including W. B. Saunders, Churchill Livingstone, and Mosby

You will also find an easily searchable catalogue, online ordering, information on our extensive list of journals...and much more!

Visit the Harcourt Health Sciences website today!

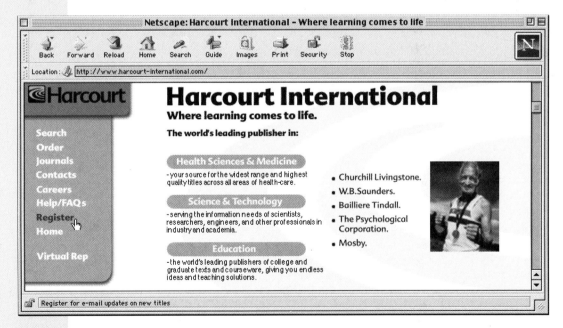

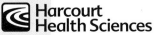

Commissioning Editor	Geoff Greenwood and Sue Hodgson
Project Development Manager	Jeremy Gross and Kim Benson
Project Manager	Hilary Hewitt
Production Manager	Mark Sanderson
Illustration Manager	Mick Ruddy
Design	Jayne Jones
Layout Artist	Alan Palfreyman

Comprehensive Urology

Robert M Weiss
Professor and Chief, Section of Urology
Yale University School of Medicine
New Haven
Connecticut, USA

Nicholas JR George
Senior Lecturer/Consultant in Urology
University Department of Urology
Withington Hospital
Manchester, UK

Patrick H O'Reilly
Consultant Urologist
Department of Urology
Stepping Hill Hospital
Stockport
Cheshire, UK

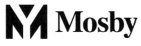 **Mosby**

London Edinburgh New York Philadelphia St Louis Sydney Toronto 2001

MOSBY
An imprint of Mosby International Limited

© Mosby International Limited 2001

M is a registered trademark of Mosby International Limited

The right of Robert M Weiss, Nicholas JR George, and Patrick H O'Reilly to be identified as the authors of this work has been asserted by them in accordance with the Copyright, Designs and Patents Act, 1988.

All figures in Chapter 3 (except Fig. 3.20) reproduced with permission from Gosling JA, Harris PF, Humpherson JR, Whitmore I, Willan PLT. Human anatomy, 2nd edn. London: Gower; 1990.

First Published 2001

ISBN: 0 7234 2949 9

British Library Cataloguing in Publication Data
A catalogue record for this book is available from the British Library

Library of Congress Cataloging in Publication Data
A catalog record for this book is available from the Library of Congress

Note
Medical knowledge is constantly changing. As new information becomes available, changes in treatment, procedures, equipment and the use of drugs become necessary. The editors, contributors, and the publishers have taken care to ensure that the information given in this text is accurate and up to date. However, readers are strongly advised to confirm that the information, especially with regard to drug usage, complies with the latest legislation and standards of practice.

The publisher's policy is to use **paper manufactured from sustainable forests**

Printed in England

Contents

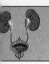

Contents

Contributors

John B Anderson
Consultant Urological Surgeon, Department of Urology, Royal Hallamshire Hospital, Sheffield, UK

Kevin R Anderson
Associate Professor of Surgery (Urology), Yale University School of Medicine, New Haven, Connecticut, USA

Demetrius H Bagley
Professor of Urology and Radiology, Department of Urology, Jefferson Medical College, Thomas Jefferson University, Philadelphia, Pennsylvania, USA

Linda A Baker
Assistant Professor of Pediatric Urology, Children's Medical Center, Pediatric Urology, Dallas, Texas, USA

Roy A Brandell
Assistant Professor of Urology, Section of Urologic Surgery, University of Kansas Medical Center, Kansas City, Kansas, USA

Stephen CW Brown
Consultant Urologist, Department of Urology, Stepping Hill Hospital, Stockport, Cheshire, UK

Janis M Brown
Associate Clinical Professor of Diagnostic Radiology, Department of Diagnostic Radiology, Yale University School of Medicine, New Haven, Connecticut, USA

Anthony A Caldamone
Professor of Surgery (Urology) and Pediatrics, Brown University School of Medicine and Chief of Pediatric Urology, Department of Urology, Hasbro Children's Hospital, Providence, Rhode Island, USA

Peter R Carroll
Professor and Chair of Urology, Department of Urology, University of California, San Francisco, California, USA

Noel W Clarke
Consultant Urologist, Hope Hospital, Salford, and The Christie Hospital, Manchester, UK

John W Colberg
Professor of Surgery, Section of Urology, Yale University School of Medicine, New Haven, Connecticut, USA

Christopher S Cooper
Associate Professor in Urology, University of Iowa, Division of Pediatric Urology, Children's Hospital of Iowa, Iowa City, Iowa, USA

Richard A Cowan
Consultant in Clinical Oncology, Department of Clinical Oncology, Christie Hospital, Manchester, UK

Neil Denbow
Assistant Professor of Diagnostic Radiology, Department of Diagnostic Radiology, Yale University School of Medicine, New Haven, Connecticut, USA

John S Dixon
Professor of Anatomy, Department of Anatomy, The Chinese University of Hong Kong, Hong Kong

Sven Dorph
Lecturer in Radiology, Department of Diagnostic Radiology, Copenhagen University Hospital at Herlev, Herlev, Denmark

Ahmed I El-Sakka
Lecturer of Urology, Suez Canal University and Consultant of Urology, Suez Canal University Hospital, Ismailia, Egypt

Andrew P Evans
Professor of Anatomy, Department of Anatomy and Cell Biology, Indiana University School of Medicine, Indianapolis, Indiana, USA

John M Fitzpatrick
Consultant Urologist, Professor and Chairman, Department of Surgery, Mater Misericordiae Hospital and University College Dublin, Dublin, Ireland

Robert C Flanigan
Albert J Sr and Claire R Spech Professor and Chairman of Urology, Department of Urology, Loyola University, Stritch School of Medicine, Maywood, Illinois, USA

Harris E Foster, Jr
Associate Professor of Surgery, Section of Urology, Yale University School of Medicine, New Haven, Connecticut, USA

Donald Fraser
Specialist Registrar in Nephrology, Institute of Nephrology, University Hospital of Wales, Cardiff, Wales, UK

John P Gearhart
Professor of Pediatric Urology, Johns Hopkins Hospital, Baltimore, Maryland, USA

Nicholas JR George
Senior Lecturer/Consultant in Urology, University Department of Urology, Withington Hospital, Manchester, UK

Morton G Glickman
Professor of Diagnostic Radiology and Surgery (Urology), Chief of Genitourinary Radiology, Department of Diagnostic Radiology, Yale University School of Medicine, New Haven, Connecticut, USA

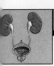

Margaret L Godley
Clinical and Research Scientist: Urology,
Institute of Child Health and Great
Ormond Street Hospital for Children
NHS Trust, University College London,
London, UK

John A Gosling
Professor of Surgery (Anatomy),
Department of Human Anatomy,
Stanford University School of Medicine,
Stanford, California, USA

David CS Gough
Consultant Paediatric Urologist, Royal
Manchester Children's Hospital,
Manchester, UK

Gary D Grossfeld
Assistant Professor of Urology,
Department of Urology, University of
California, San Francisco, California,
USA

Richard J Hale
Consultant Histopathologist,
Department of Pathology, Stockport
NHS Trust, Stepping Hill Hospital,
Stockport, Cheshire, UK

James Hall
Specialist Registrar in Urology,
Department of Urology, Royal
Hallamshire Hospital, Sheffield, UK

Stephen J Harland
Senior Lecturer in Medical Oncology and
Consultant Medical Oncologist,
Department of Oncology, University of
London Medical School, The Middlesex
Hospital, London, UK

Nicholas J Hegarty
Senior Registrar in Urology, Department
of Surgery, Mater Misericordiae Hospital
and University College Dublin, Dublin,
Ireland

D Andrew Jones
Consultant Urologist, Department of
Urology, Blackburn Royal Infirmary,
Blackburn, UK

Marc S Keller
Professor of Diagnostic Radiology and
Pediatrics, Yale University School of
Medicine, New Haven, Connecticut, USA

Fernando J Kim
Chief of Urology, Denver Health
Medical Center, and Assistant Professor
of Urology, Department of Surgery,
University of Colorado Health Sciences
Center, Denver, Colorado, USA

Roger Kirby
Consultant Urologist, Department of
Urology, St George's Hospital, London,
UK

Michael G Leahy
Senior Lecturer in Medical Oncology,
ICRF Cancer Medicine Research Unit,
Cancer Research Building, St James's
University Hospital, Leeds, UK

James E Lingeman
Clinical Professor of Urology, Indiana
University School of Medicine, and
Director of Research, Methodist
Hospital Institute for Kidney Stone
Disease, Indianapolis, Indiana, USA

R Wyndham Lloyd-Davies
Honorary Consultant Urologist,
St Thomas's Hospital, London, UK

Tom F Lue
Professor of Urology, Department of
Urology, University of California, San
Francisco, California, USA

Rex L Mahnensmith
Associate Professor of Internal Medicine,
Section of Nephrology, Yale University
School of Medicine, New Haven,
Connecticut, USA

Jack W McAninch
Professor of Urology, University of
California, San Francisco, and Chief of
Urology, San Francisco General Hospital,
San Francisco, California, USA

Thomas R McCauley
Associate Professor of Diagnostic
Radiology, Department of Diagnostic
Radiology, Yale University School of
Medicine, New Haven, Connecticut,
USA

Lorna J McWilliam
Consultant Histopathologist,
Department of Histopathology,
Withington Hospital of South
Manchester University Hospitals NHS
Trust, Manchester, UK

Charles S Modlin
Staff Transplant Surgeon, Urological
Institute, Section of Renal
Transplantation, Cleveland Clinic
Foundation, Cleveland, Ohio, USA

Jeffrey A Moody
Clinical Instructor, University of
Colorado, Colorado Springs, Colorado,
USA

Pierre DE Mouriquand
Professor of Pediatric Urology,
Department of Paediatric Urology,
Hôpital Debrousse, Lyon, France

Ravi Munver
Resident, Division of Urologic Surgery,
Department of Surgery, Duke University
Medical Center, Durham, North
Carolina, USA

Andrew C Novick
Chairman, Cleveland Clinic Foundation,
Cleveland, Ohio, USA

Kieran J O'Flynn
Consultant Urological Surgeon,
Department of Urology, Hope Hospital,
Salford, Manchester, UK

R Tim D Oliver
Sir Maxwell Joseph Professor in Medical
Oncology, Department of Medical
Oncology, St Bartholomew's and Royal
London School of Medicine, Queen
Mary and Westfield College, Smithfield,
London, UK

Patrick H O'Reilly
Consultant Urologist, Department of
Urology, Stepping Hill Hospital,
Stockport, Cheshire, UK

C Lowell Parsons
Professor of Surgery/Urology, Division of
Urology, University of California, San
Diego Medical Center, San Diego,
California, USA

Kent T Perry Jr
Chief Urology Resident, Department of
Urology, Northwestern University
Medical School, Chicago, Illinois, USA

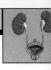

Glenn M Preminger
Professor, Division of Urologic Surgery, Department of Surgery, and Director, Duke Comprehensive Kidney Stone Center, Duke University Medical Center, Durham, North Carolina, USA

John P Pryor
Consultant Uro-andrologist, Emeritus Reader, London University, Institute of Urology, Lister Hospital, London, UK

David J Ralph
Consultant Urologist, Institute of Urology and Nephrology, University College London, London, UK

Norman L Reeve
Consultant Histopathologist, Department of Pathology, Stockport NHS Trust, Stepping Hill Hospital, Stockport, UK

Jerome P Richie
Elliot C Cutler Professor of Urologic Surgery, Harvard Medical School, and Chairman, Harvard Program in Urology (Longwood Area), and Chief of Urology, Brigham and Women's Hospital, Boston, Massachusetts, USA

Arthur T Rosenfield
Professor, Diagnostic Radiology and Urology, Department of Diagnostic Radiology, Yale University School of Medicine, New Haven, Connecticut, USA

Michael H Safir
Assistant Professor of Urology, New York Medical College, Valhalla, New York, USA

Anthony J Schaeffer
Professor and Chair of Urology, Northwestern University Medical School, Chicago, Illinois, USA

Peter N Schlegel
Associate Professor of Urology, Department of Urology, The James Buchanan Brady Foundation, The New York Presbyterian Hospital/Weill Medical College of Cornell University, New York, New York, USA

Leslie M Scoutt
Associate Professor, Department of Diagnostic Radiology, Yale University School of Medicine, New Haven, Connecticut, USA

Howard M Snyder III
Professor of Surgery in Urology, University of Pennsylvania School of Medicine, and Associate Chief, Division of Urology, Children's Hospital of Philadelphia, Philadelphia, USA

Graeme S Steele
Clinical Fellow in Surgery, Division of Urology, Harvard Medical School, Brigham and Women's Hospital, and Clinical Fellow in Surgery, Boston, Massachusetts, USA

David FM Thomas
Consultant Paediatric Urologist, Reader in Paediatric Surgery, Leeds Teaching Hospitals, Leeds, UK

Henrik S Thomsen
Professor of Radiology, Department of Diagnostic Radiology, Copenhagen Universtiy Hospital at Herlev, Herlev, Denmark

Mike Venning
Consultant Nephrologist, Withington Hospital, Manchester, UK

D Michael A Wallace
Consultant Urologist, Queen Elizabeth Hospital, Birmingham, UK

Graham M Watson
Consultant Urologist, Eastbourne District General Hospital, Eastbourne, UK

Robert M Weiss
Professor and Chief, Section of Urology, Yale University School of Medicine, New Haven, Connecticut, USA

Duncan T Wilcox
Consultant Paediatric Urologist, Great Ormond Street Children's Hospital and Guys Hospital, London, UK

Christopher RJ Woodhouse
Reader in Adolescent Urology, Institute of Urology and Nephrology, University College London, London, UK

Leonard M Zinman
Senior Staff, Department of Urology, Lahey Hitchcock Clinic Medical Center, Burlington, Massachusetts, USA

Foreword

The editors have successfully taken on the difficult task of creating a comprehensive urological text that incorporates precise clinical information concerning all aspects of the vast and expanding field of urology. The excellent group of internationally-renowned contributors present detailed clinical information in a crisp format which is not encyclopedic but contains carefully selected and nonbiased practical information backed by specific, relevant references. The standard format of tables of elegant illustrations throughout the book is user friendly and the illustrations are certainly one of the highlights of the text. The text is not heavily burdened by intricate basic scientific information; however, the first section concisely reviews basic anatomy, physiology, and molecular biology, which have relevance for the entire text. In addition, each chapter contains the basic science principles that lie behind the clinical entities being discussed.

The text is then divided into seven additional sections clearly arranged to comprehensively cover all the clinical aspects of the major domains of urology. The contributors have accomplished a difficult task and that is to write relatively short, concise, practical chapters distilling an immense amount of background material into its essence for the benefit of the reader rather than taking the easier route of simply compiling a compendium of information.

The text moves from an enjoyable history of urology to a look forward at the dramatic advances that will occur in the twenty-first century. The text will be of particular value to those entering urology and occupies a niche between the pocket handbooks introducing the field and the more comprehensive multi-volume definitive texts. However, it is likely that more established urologists, regardless of age or country of practice, will find this enjoyable to read, informative, and replete with useful old and new information. The editors owe a toast and a word of congratulations to the contributors who brought this text to fruition.

E. Darracott Vaughan, Jr, MD
James J. Colt Professor of Urology,
James Buchanan Brady Foundation,
Department of Urology,
New York Presbyterian Hospital/Weill Cornell Medical College,
New York, USA

Preface

Urology today is a vibrant speciality at once embracing the expanding horizons of molecular biology, the complexities of pathophysiology, and the solid bedrock of clinical observation and measurement. Within this single volume we have attempted to distil the information required from each of these essential spheres and present it in a rapidly and truly accessible form for both the trainee and established urological surgeon.

It is not our intention to compete head-to-head against presently available multi-volume conventional texts or highly specialised review literature in urology. Rather this volume is intended to be comprehensive in its coverage of all aspects of urology by virtue of the ability to link scientific and pathophysiologic background to clinical practice by means of the advanced techniques made available by modern print technology. Hence the extensive use of tables, diagrams, illustrations, and charts that permits a graphic and rapid understanding of subjects more usually covered by sterile blocks of plain text.

It is our hope that this simplified yet comprehensive approach will appeal equally to the urological trainee taking boards and the older physician facing reaccreditation,. The logical text and illustrative structure allows clinically relevant knowledge to be more easily accessed, digested and retained – surely an indispensable bonus in today's world of scientific information overload.

Finally, we are indebted to friends and colleagues worldwide who have helped conceive and project this unique approach to urological publishing. Their international reputation ensures that the content of this volume may truly be described as *Comprehensive Urology*.

RMW, NJRG, and PHO'R

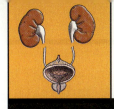

Chapter 1

Landmarks in the History of Urology

R Wyndham Lloyd-Davies

INTRODUCTION

Urology is as old as mankind: urinary calculi have been described dating back into pre-history, and a vesical calculus has been found within the pelvic skeleton of a young man from a prehistoric tomb that was approximately 7000 years old[1].

However, since we must rely on written records to know how urologic conditions were treated, one of the main themes presented in this introductory chapter is the management of stone disease over the past 3000 years. Professor Harold Ellis[2], in his monograph on stone disease, makes a telling point. 'Of the triad of 'elective' operations first performed by man – circumcision, trephination of the skull and cutting for bladder stone – the last was the only one free from religious or ritual conventions and may therefore be pronounced the most ancient operation undertaken for the relief of a specific surgical condition.'

It is remarkable that significant advances in the management of stone disease continue up to the present day, for it is only two decades ago that C H Chaussy[3] described in 1980 the first clinical use of extracorporeal lithotripsy.

Hand in hand with the management of stone disease has come the advent of, first, invasive surgical procedures and their special tools, leading in time to perurethral instruments and, over the last two centuries, the development of endoscopy has further refined stone manipulation and removal.

Other aspects of urology cannot be ignored, for circumcision dates back to Ancient Egypt and other urologic problems figure in the history of early medicine from all humankind's main ancient civilizations.

EGYPT, THE MIDDLE EAST, INDIA AND CHINA

Egypt

Stone disease can certainly be traced back to approximately 4800BC. A calculus obtained from the grave of a boy of some 16 years was found in a prehistoric cemetery at El Amrah in Upper Egypt and presented to the Royal College of Surgeons in London in 1901 by Professor G Elliott Smith. Found to be made of calcium phosphate and uric acid but with no oxalate present, it was thought possibly to be related to schistosomal disease, although no bilharzial ova were found within it. Sadly, this calculus was among the many specimens destroyed in the bombing of the Museum of the College in World War II. However, other calculi dating back to c.3000BC and 1000BC have been found in Egyptian tombs.

Circumcision also dates back to 3000BC and illustrations of the operation were found in ancient tombs at Saqqara in 1897.

The Ebers papyrus dating from 1550BC is one of the world's earliest medical compendia and mentions urology particularly in terms of retention of urine.

The Middle East

The Sumerians recognized parts of the urologic anatomy, including the kidneys and penis, as early as 4000BC. Persian medical references are found from around 1000BC and stone diseases and catheterization are mentioned in later treatises. However, even by the Middle Ages, little further progress had been made, and lithotomy does not appear to have been employed until relatively recent times.

In Hebrew medicine, circumcision, as in Egypt, was a religious procedure.

China and India

While a number of medical urology problems were recognized by the Chinese in ancient times, there was little said about stone disease and lithotomy was not practiced. However, in ancient Indian texts stone disease is well described and lithotomy, although regarded as hazardous even in expert hands, was undoubtedly practiced. These accounts, most notably one by the Hindu surgeon Susruta in the 6th century BC, probably refer to the origin of transperineal removal of bladder stones.

GREECE AND ROME

Medicine in Ancient Greece long predates Hippocrates. The worship of Aesculapius had led to the building of many temples, which later became medical schools, and on their teachings Hippocrates, born on the Greek island of Cos in 460BC, based his system of clinical medicine. In it he recognized and described stone disease, but stone surgery received a check, since in his original oath Hippocrates banned lithotomy, stating, 'I will not cut persons laboring under the stone but will leave this to be done by practitioners of this work.' Possibly this was the earliest recommendation for specialization!

Renal and bladder injuries and disorders were described by Hippocrates, and reference made to the drainage of renal abscesses. He regarded wounds of the bladder as carrying a very grave prognosis, and it may have been this view that held surgeons back from the transabdominal approach to the bladder and hence suprapubic lithotomy.

Aristotle, born in 384BC, pushed forward the understanding of anatomy and embryology from comparative studies of animal kidneys, though not human ones. From the city of Alexandria there came another milestone in the development of lithotomy when Ammonius, born in 276BC, improved lithotomy by introducing a technique to break up calculi in order to facilitate their removal.

The Greeks brought surgery to Rome and it was Celsus, living in Rome in the 1st century AD, who made the seminal description of lithotomy that was to hold good with little change through to the end of the 18th century. In Celsus's time catheters made of bronze were in use, and some of these, demonstrating the traditional double curve, would, centuries later, be found in the excavations of Pompeii.

The Greek physician Galen, living and traveling through Asia Minor in the 2nd century AD, brought together in his writings many of the theories of medicine that were current in his day. He described lower urinary tract obstruction and supported Celsus's technique of lithotomy.

THE TREATMENT OF THE STONE FROM THE MIDDLE AGES TO THE 18TH CENTURY

Perineal lithotomy

With its origins in the techniques of the Hindu surgeon Susruta and later that of Celsus, two types of perineal lithotomy developed.

The apparatus minor

In this simple operation, popular up till the 16th century, no special instruments were used other than a knife, forceps and a hook for extracting the calculus. It was particularly recommended for young boys of 9–14 years of age with small prostates and involved opening the bladder base just above the prostate. The German surgeon L Heister (1683–1758) gave a detailed description of the operation carried out with the patient in the lithotomy position, echoing the earlier reports of India and Rome.

The apparatus major

In the early 16th century a new technique developed that was ascribed to Franciscus de Romanis of Cremona but, published by a pupil of Marianus Sanctus in 1522, became known as the Marian procedure. Termed the Apparatus Major because of the extra instruments needed, it required a grooved staff to be passed via the urethra into the bladder. A midline perineal incision on to the staff gave access to the membranous urethra. A gorget followed by dilators opened up the wound, tearing through the prostate and bladder neck. The stone was removed by forceps, with initial crushing if it was too large for removal intact. Scoops and hooks then cleared the fragments. If the patient survived the primary hemorrhage, sinuses, incontinence and impotence frequently followed.

Two of the protagonists of this major surgery were the great French surgeon Ambroise Paré[4] (1510–90), who detailed in 1575 the preparation and positioning of the patient in lithotomy, and Frère Jacques, born Jacques Beaulieu in 1651, who was apprenticed to an itinerant lithotomist, became one himself, and developed the lateral approach, which was safe in adults and gained remarkable results (Fig. 1.1).

This work going on in France and across the continent was also widely practiced in England, and Thomas Hollyer (1609–90; Fig. 1.2) cut the diarist Samuel Pepys (Fig. 1.3) for the stone on

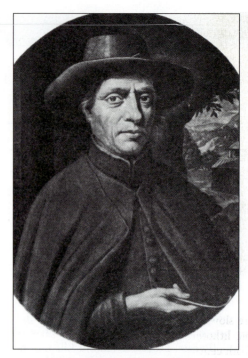

Fig. 1.1
Frère Jacques de Beaulieu (1651–1714).
(Courtesy of the Wellcome Library.)

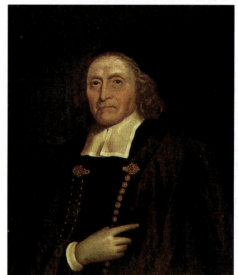

Fig. 1.2
Thomas Hollyer (1609–90).
(Reproduced by kind permission of the President and Council of the Royal College of Surgeons of England.)

March 26, 1658. The Hollyer family were accomplished lithotomists, Thomas Hollyer carrying out a series of 30 consecutive operations without a death up to 1661. His work was refined by William Cheselden[5] (1688–1752), appointed to the staff of St Thomas' Hospital in London in 1718. Not only one of the greatest English lithotomists, Cheselden was also an ophthalmic surgeon. He refined the lateral operation and published his results in 1778, with 20 deaths in 213 patients cut at St Thomas'. It is said that he could cut for the stone in 29 seconds.

High operation for the stone
Suprapubic lithotomy

Hippocrates had stated that wounds of the bladder were almost invariably fatal and, if not fatal, serious complications, with wound leakage, fistula formation, and herniation, could follow.

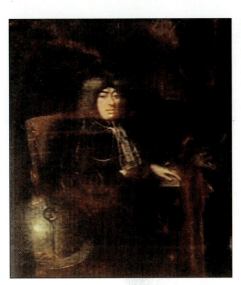

Fig. 1.3
**Samuel Pepys
(1633–1703).**
(Courtesy of the
Wellcome Library.)

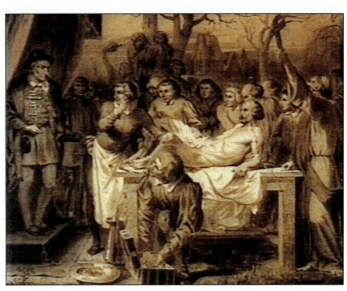

Fig. 1.4 Lithotomy in the 18th century. (Courtesy of the Wellcome Library.)

Hence surgeons were slow to take up this technique. The first successful suprapubic lithotomy was probably done by Pierre Franco in the early 16th century, removing a large calculus from a child's bladder by this approach. A few other sporadic reports followed until James Douglas, of 'pouch of Douglas' fame, described the surgical anatomy of the bladder in 1717. His brother John carried out the operation in 1719 and in his book commented on the considerably lower incidence of the problems accompanying perineal lithotomy. Cheselden then took up the procedure but later lost his initial enthusiasm for it, and even in 1825, Sir Astley Cooper at Guy's Hospital in London felt that this type of surgery should be reserved for patients with large stones and vast prostates. The suprapubic operation then had to wait for the advances of the mid-19th century before it became a safe and popular procedure.

Endourethral lithotomy

The 19th century saw the development of transurethral stone surgery. Undoubtedly, the origins of this technique go back to Ancient Egypt, with attempts to dilate the urethra and primitive procedures to fragment bladder calculi. In 1783 Colonel Martin, the educational pioneer who gave his name to the school he founded, the Martinière in Lucknow, immortalized as St Saviour's in Kipling's *Kim* and still functioning today, claimed to have disintegrated his own bladder stone with a curved roughened sound over a 9-month period. Several other pioneers developed ingenious instruments to destroy intravesical calculi, but it was not until 1824 that Jean Civiale[6] (1792–1867) carried out the first successful lithotomy at the Necker Hospital in Paris, where he was still a medical student. Using a trilabe, he seized the calculus, which was then broken up by a gimlet and the fragments passed naturally (Fig. 1.4).

These early attempts led to the development of the stone-crushing lithotrite apparatus, and the instrument that reposes as a souvenir on the present author's desk, which was still being used in the 1950s and 1960s, found its origins in L'Estrange's calculofractor of 1834, developed in Dublin.

Probably the most eminent lithotriptist of his day was the London surgeon Sir Henry Thompson, who successfully dealt with King Leopold I of Belgium's stone in 1863 after Civiale had carried out multiple lithotrities in 1862. Later Sir Henry operated on Napoleon III, under anesthesia given by a Dr Clover, when the French Emperor was in exile in England. Although after two procedures the calculus was successfully crushed, the Emperor, already a sick man, succumbed to infective complications and died on January 9, 1873.

Litholopaxy and the evacuating of the stone debris was then pioneered by Henry J Bigelow (1818–90) in the United States and Sir Peter Freyer in England. Further developments of stone management will be detailed later in this chapter.

UROLOGY FROM THE MIDDLE AGES TO THE 19TH CENTURY

In order to relate the advances that have gone to make up modern urology, which dates from the middle of the 19th century with the discovery of anesthesia and asepsis, it is necessary to consider earlier discoveries that laid the foundations of today's practice.

Galen founded the medical sciences with his anatomic discoveries, but it was not until the 15th century that the artists Michelangelo, Durer and especially Leonardo da Vinci carried out detailed scientific dissection of the human body and illustrated their findings with incomparable drawings. A succession of eminent Italian anatomists then continued their work.

Vesalius (1514–64) corrected their studies in 1543, and can certainly be considered to be the father of urologic anatomy. Gabriel Fallopius (1523–62) demonstrated intrarenal anatomy, Bartholomeus Eustachius (1520–74) took these studies further, and Lorenzo Bellini (1628–1704) and Marcello Malpighi (1628–94) refined them. The Frenchman Exupére Bertin in 1714 described his intrarenal columns, still beloved of uroradiologists to this day. These and many other anatomic discoveries laid the foundation for the advances in physiology and surgery that contributed to the development of modern urology.

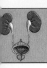

UROLOGIC INFECTIONS

Venereal infection has been described since ancient times and both gonorrhea and syphilis were recognized and differentiated by physicians from all the ancient cultures. The development of stricture as a result of gonorrheal infection was not realized until much later, but Paré noted in a patient who needed continuous catheterization that he had what appeared to be chronic retention and possibly pyocystis. Giovanni Morgagni (1682–1771) first used the term 'gonorrhea' in 1761, but by 1750 John Hunter (1728–93) in his London lectures had already described various forms of urethral inflammation resulting from the condition.

Perineal abscesses and other major infective incidents can be found described in all the ancient writings. As interventional techniques of stone treatment developed so did the recognition of infective urologic conditions, and by the end of the 19th century the frequently fatal onset of infective complications was noted. In a great breakthrough, Sir Henry Thompson realized that his new, and hence uninfected, instruments had avoided the usual postoperative fever when he operated on King Leopold.

Infections had been thought for centuries to be due to the miasmas emanating from poisons in the air, soil, rotting materials, and standing water, or from person-to-person contagion. In the 17th century came the great breakthrough. Hooke, Malpighi, and particularly Antoni van Leeuwenhoek (1632–1723) developed the microscope, and van Leeuwenhoek was the first to observe bacteria in various fluids. Another century was to pass, however, before Louis Pasteur (1822–96) proved the essential role of microorganisms in a wide series of biological experiments. Another giant in the same field was Robert Koch (1843–1910), who established the bacterial basis of disease and formalized this in his Postulates. These stated that the organism could be found in every instance of the disease, could be extracted and grown in pure culture, and that the disease could be produced in experimental animals, retrieved, and cultured again. Koch's great triumph came in 1882 with the discovery of *Mycobacterium tuberculosis*. From his further work on tuberculin came the development of an attenuated strain of tuberculosis leading to the vaccine developed in 1924 by the French researchers Albert Calmette and J-M Guerin – BCG.

The evolution of genitourinary tuberculosis

The remains of ancient skeletons have confirmed the characteristic changes of tuberculosis, indicating that the disease affected humans in about 4000BC. It is also known that it was a common disease in Egypt in about 1000BC, and in 375BC Hippocrates described phthisis as a lingering illness that was worse in winter, resulted in emaciation, caused diarrhea, and was terminal.

Galen in 180AD showed considerable interest in the disease, and his methods of treatment were followed for the next 1500 years. In 1696 an English physician called Wiseman wrote that he found scrofula, or the King's Evil, a difficult problem that confronted doctors frequently. During the 18th century in Europe, there were many epidemics of tuberculous infection, and 25% of all deaths then are thought to have been caused by consumption.

J-A Villemin established the infectious nature of the disease by carrying out experiments between 1865 and 1868. These proved that tuberculosis could be transferred from humans or cattle to rabbits. In 1879 Julius Cohnheim presented his elimination theory. According to his hypothesis, tubercle bacilli in the blood were eliminated in the urine, so that they became lodged as a focus somewhere in the urinary tract. Then in March 1982 came Koch's announcement that he had discovered the cause of tuberculosis, and 3 weeks later he published his first article describing the pathogenesis of the disease.

In 1882 Paul Ehrlich in Frankfurt discovered the acid-fast nature of the bacillus, and in 1908, 30 years after Cohnheim's hypothesis, G Ekehorn suggested his direct hematogenous theory, stating that the bacilli were transported like emboli to the renal capillaries, where they lodged and formed a tuberculous focus. According to this theory the kidneys and the urinary tract were secondarily infected through the urine, and it therefore formed the basis of the belief that renal tuberculosis could be treated by nephrectomy.

The pathogenesis of renal tuberculosis, however, remained uncertain until in 1926 the American E M Medlar[7] published his classic study of patients suffering from pulmonary tuberculosis. He reviewed 100,000 serial sections of the kidneys of these patients and found bilateral renal tuberculosis in 26%. He suggested that the changes should be called metastatic rather than secondary, because, in his view, it was clear that the lesions had been caused by infection in the bloodstream. He also revealed that the lesions in the kidney were nearly always bilateral.

In 1935 the Frenchman E Coulaud succeeded in inducing primary tuberculous lesions in the renal cortex in rabbits, and in 1937 Egon Wildboltz used the term 'genitourinary tuberculosis', emphasizing that renal and genital tuberculosis were not separate entities, but local manifestations of the same blood-borne infection.

Since then a major breakthrough has been the discovery of the antituberculous drugs, starting with streptomycin in 1943, paraaminosalicylic acid in 1946, isoniazid and pyrazinamide in 1952 and rifampicin in 1966. Following the introduction of these drugs, it was soon found that they had to be used in some combinations, otherwise resistant strains of organisms would develop, and, after the discovery of rifampicin, short courses of treatment were instituted after a thorough investigation, which has resulted in a great improvement in the management and treatment of genitourinary tuberculosis.

Bacterial infections

During the 19th century breakthroughs in the treatment of bacteria-induced infections came first with chemotherapy, pioneered by Paul Ehrlich (1854–1915) with his work on arsenical compounds. This culminated in '606', Salvarsan, the first cure for syphilis.

Gerard Domagh (1895–1964) then developed prontosil at IG Farben and subsequently the sulfonamide drugs. The field of antibiotic therapy, which was transforming the management of bacterial infection, was then entered by Alexander Fleming[8] (1888–1955), whose investigations into the byproducts of molds culminated in the development of penicillin by Howard Florey (1898–1968) and his team at Oxford in 1940. Subsequently, penicillin was manufactured in the USA.

Since World War II, with the increasing ability successfully to treat bacterial infections of the genitourinary tract, efforts have focused on precise bacteriologic diagnosis in terms of the organism and its antibiotic sensitivities, and the precise location of the infection within the urinary tract.

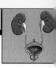

The work of E M Kass[9], F Hinman Jr[10] at ULCA, San Francisco and T A Stamey[11] at Stanford, among many others, highlighted our ability to localize accurately within the upper and lower urinary tract the site of bacterial infection, and the importance of residual bladder urine and the prostate as an infective reservoir.

Concomitant advances in hematology, including clotting defects and blood transfusion, together with the understanding of serum electrolyte disturbances and their treatment, have all helped to make possible the highly scientific management of patients before, during, and after surgery.

Imaging of the urinary tract has also developed along a number of lines and will be considered in a later section of this chapter.

CATHETERS AND URETHRAL INSTRUMENTATION

Catheters can be traced back into antiquity and were in common use in India and the Ancient Greece of Hippocrates. Early catheters were usually made of metal, often bronze, and later silver, copper, and brass, but other materials, including treated paper, cloth impregnated with wax, horn, or rushes, were also used. Both terminal and end-side orifices had their vogue. From an early time catheters were curved and by the Middle Ages the double curve had become established. The more flexible varieties had internal stilets.

In the 19th century a gum elastic catheter with its angled neck, the Coudé catheter of L A Mercier, became widely used, and the first attempts at a self-retaining catheter date from the same period of about 1840. With the advent of rubber, Auguste Nelaton (1807–73) developed the first catheter of this type, but it was not until 1927, with the invention of latex rubber, that F E B Foley[12] produced his 'bag catheter' and demonstrated it at the American Medical Association meeting in Atlantic City in 1935. Originally designed with a hemostatic bag to produce hemostasis within the prostatic cavity following prostatectomy, it became universally accepted as the ideal self-retaining catheter, replacing the flanged catheters of Malecôt and de Pezzer. With only the further advance of Silastic it has remained so to this day.

Suprapubic catheterization developed from suprapubic cystotomy. Suprapubic bladder puncture was multiply described at the end of the 16th century and subsequently. Initially a technique of last resort, it was used rarely as a long-term management of prostatic obstruction, and A M Valsalva in 1714 made the observation that the needles should be inserted obliquely downwards above the pubes.

It was refined in the 19th century along with the steady advance in urologic techniques. Up to recent times a Malecôt type of catheter was inserted through a metal cannula introduced with a trocar, but these have been superseded by the modern Silastic catheter with integral trocar and a retaining balloon such as the Bonano.

URETHRAL INSTRUMENTATION

As early as the second century AD Galen had described 'carnosities and caruncles' of the urethra. These were related to the urinary symptoms of dysuria and strangury.

Treatment with dilatation by primitive bougies followed and Marianus Sanctus of the Marian approach to the urethra for lithotomy introduced the concept of the stricture and noted that a severe stricture could prevent the passage of any instrument and lead to severe urinary retention and death.

John Hunter, one of the great British surgical pioneers, first studied the sites of urethral stricture formation and noted that they most frequently occurred at the urethral bulb. He thought gonorrhea to be the most frequent cause and advocated gradual dilatation followed by a more forcible approach, including sharp trocar-like instruments to bore through impassable strictures.

External urethrotomy goes back to post-Hippocratic Greek medicine, with perineal surgery to relieve urinary retention in extreme cases. In the 17th century reports of successful perineal urethrotomy appear, even with cure without the development of a urinary fistula in some cases.

Internal urethrotomy was first attempted in the 17th and 18th centuries, as noted above by Hunter, and a whole series of different blind instruments were developed during the 18th century, popularized by Civiale, who designed his second urethrotome in 1844, and improved by J G Maisonneuve in 1855 and F N Otis in 1876. However, complications, particularly hemorrhage, limited the use of this technique.

The great advance had to wait until 1974 when H Sachse developed the direct-viewing optical urethrotome with its non-electrified blade – the cold knife instrument that has revolutionized the modern management of urethral stricture.

THE EVOLUTION OF THE MODERN CYSTOSCOPE

For many centuries people's natural curiosity has led them to produce a variety of instruments to help investigate how the human body functions. Initially, though, these were crude and difficult to use, and it was only slowly in the 19th century that technical advances allowed development of more complex diagnostic systems.

At the beginning of the century, animal fats and waxes, fossil and vegetable oils, resin, and wood were the only sources of light available. The great stimulus to endoscopy came with the emergence of better light sources. First came electric filament lamps, especially the Mignon, and more recently fiberoptic noncoherent light cables.

The medical problems associated with the dark cavities of the urogenital tract formed a massive challenge that encouraged a young Italian, Phillipp Bozzini in Frankfurt, to design what he called the 'Lichtleiter' in about 1804. In 1806 he demonstrated his invention to the Vienna Academy of Medicine.

The instrument consisted of a large, barrel-shaped apparatus, holding a candle and on which several specula made of light-reflective material could be fixed. At the back there was a round opening through which the cavity could be inspected. The instrument was clearly designed for a multitude of functions: inspection of the nasopharynx, the vagina, the urethra, the anal canal, and rectum. It was made of silver covered in sharkskin, to prevent burns, and the light source was a beeswax candle, spring-loaded, the flame of which was in a constant position. However, Bozzini received scant encouragement for his invention, which was felt to be clumsy and, with its scant light, ineffective.

The same principle of light-conduction was applied by Pierre Segalas (1792–1874), who used a tubular conical mirror from which the light was projected into the cavity. Whereas Bozzini's invention was used mainly to inspect the vagina and rectum, Segalas demonstrated his *speculum urethrocystique* before the Royal French Academy as an instrument for the inspection of the bladder. However, once again, the light was judged insufficient for the purpose and the invention failed to interest surgeons.

Several attempts at endoscopy were made for a variety of conditions until Antoine Desormeaux (1815–82), the father of endoscopy, introduced his cystoscope in Paris in 1853. He was the first surgeon to succeed in designing an endoscopic instrument that had both diagnostic and therapeutic value for urology. As a light source he used a so-called gazogene lamp, which burnt a mixture of turpentine and alcohol. His endoscope was made of silver tubes, into which he projected light, using a combination of lenses and a mirror set at an angle of 45°. Francis Cruise[13], an Irish surgeon in Dublin, collaborated with Desormeaux and demonstrated his first instrument in 1865. He found that the brightest illumination available was the flat flame of a petroleum lamp with camphor dissolved in the petroleum and the intensity of the flame increased by a tall draught chimney. He also designed new sheaths for examination of the urethra, bladder, and other body cavities, and urologists using a bladder catheter filled with boracic solution were able to inspect the greater part of the bladder mucosa.

J Andrews improved the light intensity still further in 1867, using wire that burnt with a white light so intense that it could illuminate the interior of the urethra.

None of the techniques available attracted much attention until a young urologist in Berlin decided to reopen the whole question of endoscopy. Max Nitze (1848–1906; Fig. 1.5) had two new ideas. First, in 1876 he used lenses in the form of a miniature telescope to magnify the image down the endoscope, and secondly he illuminated the interior of the bladder by a water-cooled electric platinum filament. He combined the light source, the reflector, and the tube in one instrument and, again using a heated platinum filament at the end of the tube, was able to introduce the source of light into the bladder. The light still had to be cooled, which made the instrument clumsy, and to try to overcome the criticism of this, Nitze moved to Vienna. Here he was given every opportunity to develop his technique and could work with the well-known surgical instrument maker, Leiter, and a lampmaker, Heyman.

Heat from the white-hot filament remained a limiting factor until in 1878 Thomas Edison, using a carbon filament in a vacuum, produced an incandescent lamp. This discovery rapidly led to the Mignon lamp, a small vacuum lamp that would be inserted at the end of a cystoscope into a water-filled bladder. In 1880 the Mignon lamp was incorporated into the cystoscope, thanks to the ingenious work of Leiter, and to enlarge the visible area Nitze adopted the stereoscope principle of using two lenses, which gave a 90° image.

With cystoscopy it was necessary to catheterize repeatedly during inspection, a painful procedure for the patient. Nitze succeeded in producing the irrigating cystoscope, where the bladder could be inspected and drained at the same time. Furthermore he arranged for production of surgical cystoscopes, which made it possible to perform operations on the bladder.

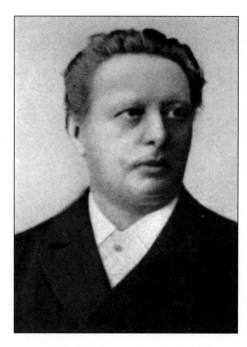

Fig. 1.5
Max Nitze
(1848–1906).
(Courtesy of the Wellcome Library.)

Towards the end of the 19th century two further developments had occurred. In 1887 the German Alexander Brenner designed a catheterizing cystoscope with a curved catheter that could be inserted into the ureter. In 1896 a French urologist, Joachim Albarran (1860–1912), developed a system by which the catheter could be elevated or lowered by a small lever that could be sunk into a slot near the tip of the instrument.

By the end of the 19th century cystoscopy was well established in urologic medical centers throughout the world. By then the main problem facing those who used the technique was the mirror image of the 90° optical system, which required great skill on the part of the urologist who performed intravesical operations. In 1907 opticians of the Swiss Zeiss Company succeeded in improving the optical system with a different type of prism, the Amici prism. The image was now vertical, much sharper, and much brighter, as less light was lost by dispersion. This Ringleb Optical System, named after the German urologist, soon found its way into all endoscopes.

There were a number of other developments. In 1887 the American H A Kelly used an aerocystoscope, a simple endoscopic tube, illuminated by means of a head mirror, for use in the air-filled bladder. Feisender Otis presented his aerourethrascope at the American Association of Genitourinary Surgeons in 1902. Instead of Kelly's mirror, he used the light of a condensing lens, and Antal's method of inflating the bladder with air through a rubber tube. This system was improved by F Tilden, who also modified his cystoscope by using a sheath fitted with a terminal lamp, admitting several telescopes.

During the next few years the lamp was brought back into the tube by means of removable optical telescopes. Jim Valentine in New York introduced use of the cold lamp for cystoscopy, and in France Georges Luys combined small cold lamps, which, inserted on a thin rod, could be introduced into a sheath to illuminate the mucous membrane of the urethra.

Nevertheless, the so-called dark area behind the neck of the bladder was still difficult to see, and in 1903 Felix Schlagintweit inserted a rotating prismatic mirror near the vertical end of the

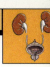

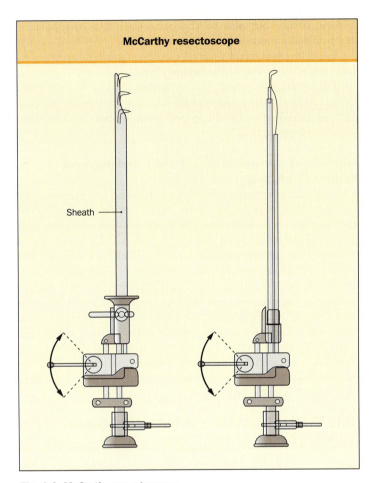

Fig. 1.6 McCarthy resectoscope.

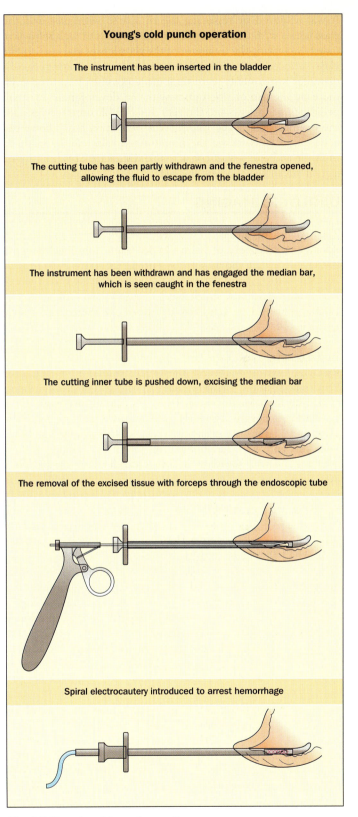

Fig. 1.7 Young's cold punch operation.

optical tube, and the same principle was tried by Hugh Hampton Young at Johns Hopkins. The improvements resulted in the so-called Universal Cystoscope, which provided efficient irrigation, direct vision, right-angle and retrograde optical systems, and the Albarran lever.

Electroresection of the prostatic gland was developed by Joseph F McCarthy[14] around 1930 (Fig. 1.6). The development of the resectoscope gave urology a special place in surgery. After Nitze contributed the lens to cystoscopy and solved many of the problems of illumination, many American urologists supported the transurethral procedure to a level at which urologists work at present.

In 1909 Young introduced the cold punch operation, which remained the preferred technique until about 1925, and in 1919 the cold punch operation was performed under direct vision, thanks to William F Braasch's work, refined by H C Bumpus[15] and Gershon Thompson at the Mayo Clinic (Fig. 1.7).

Maximilian Stern presented the first resectoscope in 1926, and Herman C Bumpus combined diathermy cutting and coagulation. The fore-oblique lens introduced by McCarthy, continuous irrigation, and the development of a flexible handle for resectoscopes, all represent refinements permitting improved diagnosis and treatment.

The most important advance since Nitze in 1876 has been the development of the Hopkins rod-lens system. In 1957 J G Gow of Liverpool asked Professor Harold Hopkins of Reading University to make improvements to the optical design of telescopes. This resulted in the publication of Hopkins's patent in 1977. It described how the total light transmission through the telescope was 80 times greater than the traditional system.

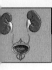

It was achieved by replacing the air spaces with glass and the glass lenses with thin lenses of air, using a glass of high refractive index, increasing the diameter of the glass lenses and coating the glass surfaces with a multilayer antireflection coating. Small-diameter instruments were then made possible, improved even more by the use of fiberoptics with the development of small pediatric instruments and the very slim flexible ureteroscopes for the examination of the upper tract. Television now allows the endoscopist to work via the monitor and relay can be made to multiple audiences over considerable distances. This has proved a great advantage as a teaching aid.

UROLOGIC IMAGING

The origins of urologic imaging are frequently related to Roentgen's discovery of X-rays in 1895 and the developments therefrom, but it should also be noted that the industrial production of ultrasound, based on the piezo-electric effect transforming electric into mechanical energy by way of synthetic crystal transducers, was first described by Pierre and Marie Curie in 1880.

Radiography
Radiology was undoubtedly the prime technique in early urologic investigation, being applied to the diagnosis of urinary calculi by John MacIntyre in 1896 in Glasgow, but requiring a 12-minute exposure. The use of radio-opaque ureteric catheters using metal stilets to outline the ureteric path followed in 1901. Voelcker and von Lichtenberg initiated retrograde studies, instilling a silver solution into the bladder and carrying out cystography with unexpected reflux outlining the whole of one pelviureteric system. Braasch, in his book *Pyelography* of 1915, described and illustrated this and other techniques. Voiding cystourethrography, the key investigation for vesicoureteric reflux, did not follow until 1953.

In 1923 Rowntree and his co-workers at the Mayo Clinic, using sodium iodide, achieved the first studies in excretion urography, using the agent both orally and by intravenous injection. The development of uroselectan by a young urologist, Moses Swick, reported by von Lichtenberg in 1929 produced the first safe and good quality images.

The use of air insufflation was employed to outline the kidneys and adrenals in 1921. Cystography also originally employed air to demonstrate calculi in 1902, and diverticula in 1904. Because of the dangers of air embolism, attention turned to radio-opaque media, and both bismuth and colloidal silver were successfully employed. Urethrography, first used in 1910, was not very successful until 1933 when Ruben Flocks produced a method of making the opaque medium more viscous with tragacanth, and seminal vesiculography followed with the development of endoscopic catheterization techniques by McCarthy in 1932.

R Dos Santos and his colleagues in Lisbon pioneered aortography in 1929 by the translumbar route, and, following the initial work by P L Farmas in 1941 in femoral artery puncture, it was refined by the Seldinger technique of selective renal artery catheterization. Venacavography was also developed at that time.

Urologic radiology has continued to develop. The modern nonionic contrast media have made safe intravenous urography, which was initially subject to many adverse reactions of an allergic nature but also to the occasional fatal anaphylactic reaction and a mortality rate of 1 in 40,000.

Ascending pyelography can now outline the whole ureter using bulb-ended catheters of the Braasch type.

Radiofluoroscopy and image intensification have further enhanced the quality and immediacy of radiographic imaging, and percutaneous antegrade procedures now allow studies of the obstructed upper tract.

Ultrasound, computed tomography, and magnetic resonance imaging
Ultrasound investigations, being both safe and noninvasive, have in many ways superseded some of the established radiologic techniques. Ultrasonography is now the first-line screening procedure for evaluation of the urinary tract. The technique is excellent for the assessment of a wide range of urinary tract disorders, and is the investigation of choice of fetal urinary tract abnormalities. Transrectal ultrasound, pioneered by W B Peeling and his colleagues in Newport, Wales, is now the essential investigative tool for the diagnosis and assessment of prostatic tumors.

Computed tomography (CT), pioneered by Godfrey Hounsfield in the UK, and magnetic resonance imaging (MRI) now give the clinician images of the body that hitherto could not even have been imagined by our predecessors; all these modern techniques are covered in detail below.

THE EVOLUTION OF MODERN UROLOGIC SURGERY

The remarkable strides surrounding surgery made in the mid and late 19th century made possible the development of modern surgery and the urology we practice today.

Anesthesia led the way. The early experiments were with carbon dioxide, nitrous oxide, and then ether, and the key pioneer was W T G Morton, a Boston dentist who first used his inhaler for anesthesia in 1846.

Chloroform, discovered by Marie Flourens in Paris in 1847, displaced ether and was promoted by Professor J Y Simpson in Edinburgh, its social acceptance greatly enhanced when Dr John Snow administered it to Queen Victoria during the birth of Prince Leopold in 1853.

However, although pain was conquered, patients were still at grave risk from sepsis. The initial breakthrough came in the 1840s when I Semmelweis noted the great difference in sepsis in his two maternity wards: medical students, who visited many other wards in the hospital in the course of their work, communicated sepsis through the ward they worked in, whereas midwifery pupils in the second ward, who worked nowhere else, did not. Changing them over was followed by the previous death rates in the two wards being reversed.

Joseph Lister, when Regius Professor of Surgery at Glasgow, learnt of Pasteur's work showing that putrefaction was caused by airborne bacteria. Lister used carbolic acid (phenol) to cleanse and produce a chemical barrier in open wounds. He developed an antiseptic ritual with careful wound debridement and carbolic lavage of the wound, and he operated under a carbolic spray. He reported this in *The Lancet* in 1867.

Antisepsis spread across Europe, with a concomitant and great diminution of death rates from sepsis. Asepsis followed,

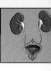

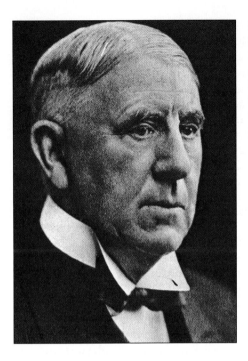

Fig. 1.8 Berkeley, Lord Moynihan (1835–96).

(With permission of Karger, Basel, from Clark P. Moynihan the urologist. Eur Urol. 1976;2:48–53.)

pioneered by Berkeley Moynihan (Fig. 1.8) who first used rubber gloves in Britain. In North America W Halsted had previously popularized rubber gloves, first introduced in the 1840s, and he persuaded the Goodyear company to manufacture them in a particularly thin rubber, although he did not operate in them himself.

Pasteur's and Koch's work had laid the basis of bacteriology, which led eventually to antibiotic therapy, but one more great advance was to come right at the outset of the 20th century with the discovery in Vienna by Karl Landsteiner (1868–1943) of the ABO blood antigen system in 1900. This he refined at the end of his life in the early 1940s by the discovery of the Rhesus factor.

Biochemistry, dating back to Richard Bright's finding of raised blood urea in renal diseases by a simple blood test in 1827, and A Becquerel's urinalysis studies of 1841, in due course led the way to the understanding of electrolyte disturbances and their treatment.

THE ADVENT OF MODERN UROLOGIC SURGERY

After the conquest of pain and the advent of sepsis the way was open for the development of modern surgery. Although sporadic reports of major urologic surgery had been made over the centuries, it was only in the mid-19th century that series of successful major urologic operations were regularly reported.

Renal surgery

Professor Gustav Simon at Heidelberg carried out the first successful planned nephrectomy in 1869. Nephropexy also came into vogue at this time. Nephrectomy for hydronephrosis was established by 1885 when S W Gross[16] reviewed 21 nephrectomies with a mortality of 38%. Nephrotomy to drain the hydronephrotic sac was performed at this time and had a lower mortality.

Plastic procedures date back to F Trendelenburg, who first operated on the renal pelvic outflow in 1886, and the first

successful pyeloplasty followed in 1891 by E Kuster. Albarran developed his lateral anastomosis between renal pelvis and ureter in 1888 and in 1898 devised dependent drainage by means of partial nephrectomy. Alberran's first operation was then further developed by A von Lichtenberg in Berlin in 1921 for the high implanted ureter.

Aberrant arteries causing hydronephrosis were noted in 1904 by F Legner, who divided them. Nephroplication, described by H Hamilton Stewart in 1947, dealt with the aberrant vessels by mobilizing them and remodeling the kidney to carry the vessels away from the pelviureteric function.

The modern techniques of pyeloplasty evolved, with the Y–V Foley pyeloplasty described in 1937, the intubated Davis ureterstomy in 1943, the dismembered Anderson–Hynes pyeloplasty in 1949, and the pelvic flap Culp operation in 1951.

Operations to remove renal calculi began around 1870. V Czerny in 1880 carried out one of the earliest successful nephrectomies for stone, but it was Sir Henry Morris[17] (1844–1926) who first removed a calculus from an otherwise normal kidney, naming the operation nephrolithotomy. He published a series of 34 cases with but one death in 1898.

Pyelolithotomy was first performed by W Heineke in 1879, and the first attempts to locate intrarenal calculi were suggested by A E Barker in 1880.

Incisions in the renal substance were initially made vertically through the convex border of the kidney. The work of J Hyrtl in 1882 and later Max Brodel[18] in 1902 then established that there was a relatively avascular plane posterior to the midline of the kidney – 'Brodel's bloodless line'. Czerny in 1887 first sutured a nephrotomy incision and partial nephrectomy followed in 1889 by Hermann Kummell. The full understanding of renal vasculature came with F T Graves's[19] work in 1971.

Intra-operative use of X-rays was attempted at the turn of the century, but was not successfully achieved until the work of J E Burns in 1917 produced radiographs of the exposed kidney. The development of flexible films by W C Quinby in 1925 further improved this technique.

Partial nephrectomy took time to gain acceptance and did not do so until 1930, though 222 reports were found in the literature. Hamilton Stewart in 1952 demonstrated that 75% of renal calculi were located and grew in size in the lowest calyces, which were often radiologically abnormal, and lower-pole partial nephrectomy, particularly by the transverse or guillotine technique, became popular for gaining access to staghorn calculi.

Open surgery for renal calculi reached its apogee in the 1970s with the work of J M Gil-Vernet in Barcelona and J P Blandy and J E A Wickham in London, but the advent of extracorporeal shockwave lithotripsy and percutaneous renal surgery has now superseded open renal work.

Renal tumors in adults were recognized in the early 19th century, and P Grawitz in 1883 described their histology, O Lubarsch giving them the name of hypernephroma in 1894, while Max Wilms described nephroblastoma of children in 1882.

Surgical treatment of these tumors began sporadically in the late 19th century, and in 1905 R Gregoire recommended radical surgery with removal of the perirenal fascia and fat together with the suprarenal and lymphatic glands. This technique took some time to gain acceptance but, with the thoracoabdominal approach, it remains the operation of choice today. Partial nephrectomy was first carried out for a renal tumor by Czerny in 1887 and on a solitary kidney by C Semb in 1954.

Solitary metastases have also been resected from several sites and in 1912 Sir John Bland-Sutton removed the lower end of a humerus for this condition. Spontaneous regression of metastases has also been occasionally described in this disease process. Nephrectomy for nephroblastoma started concurrently and was first achieved successfully in 1877, though a high proportion of the children operated upon died of their metastases. Only with the coming of combined therapy, with radiotherapy, surgery, and adjuvant chemotherapy using actinomycin D, did the prognosis improve in the 1950s and 1960s.

The diagnosis of epithelial tumors of the renal pelvis and ureter followed the development of cystoscopy and ascending pyelography, and they were rarely reported, only 47 cases being described up to 1922. The first nephroureterectomy was performed by A le Dentu and Albarran in 1898 and remains the standard procedure to this day, although epithelial polyps and low-grade transmitted cell tumors have been successfully resected locally and percutaneous techniques have been employed in recent times.

Ureteric surgery

Duplex ureters were recognized in the 16th and 17th centuries. Ureteroceles were noted and the term was coined by Lechler at a post mortem in 1835 reported by E Papin in 1914. There were also a number of reports suggesting ureteric calculi within ureteroceles during the 18th century. Blind opening and excision of a ureterocele was first performed by Hurry Fenwick, using scissors passed per urethram in 1900, and he later opened a ureterocele by endoscopic cautery. Suprapubic surgery for calculi within a ureterocele was carried out by Sir Peter Freyer in 1897.

The observation of the mechanism by which vesicoureteric reflux is prevented by the oblique transit of the ureter through the muscle coats of the bladder was made by Morgagni in 1671, but it did not gain universal acceptance. Reflux was recognized by John Sampson at Johns Hopkins Hospital in 1903 and was demonstrated by several workers over the next 30 years, during which time the view that ascending renal infection could originate in this way gained credence.

The introduction of micturating cystography in 1953 by Hamilton Stewart led to the full recognition of vesicoureteric reflux and subsequently the surgery of this condition developed. The work of J Hutch, V Politano, and W Leadbetter,[20] and A J Paquin, among others, developed antireflux procedures by ureteric orifice advancement, tunneling techniques, and the formation of a valve at the ureteral orifice to cure this condition, which eradicated upper tract infection and prevented renal functional deterioration. The recognition of the condition as a maturation defect and the conservative approach to reflux in prepubertal children by Dr Jean Smellie in London has again changed the modern approach to the problem, and endoscopic procedures such as the 'sting' injection of inert plastic has combined to reduce the number of children requiring antireflux surgery.

The treatment of ureteric stone disease mirrored that of its renal counterpart. Bilateral ureteric blockage by stone with subsequent anuria was first successfully treated surgically by B Bardenheuer in 1882, and in 1890 Sir Arbuthnot Lane first performed extraperitoneal ureterolithotomy with ureteric suture.

Sir Henry Morris in 1898 demonstrated that the whole of the pelvic ureter could be exposed by the extraperitoneal route, and an oblique muscle-splitting incision became that of choice.

Endoscopic ureteral calculus manipulation was achieved successfully by G Kolischer in 1898, who injected sterile oil through a ureteric catheter and the stone was subsequently successfully passed. Hugh Hampton Young disimpacted a calculus from the ureteric orifice with a catheter, and Hurry Fenwick in 1904 removed such a stone by suction. Treatment by leaving a ureteric catheter in situ for 24–48 hours was also employed, as was ureteric meatal dilatation and meatotomy. Stone extractors using a cage or loop were then designed in the 1930s by a number of urologists, and the Dormier retractable basket, together with the loop Davis catheters, became the type of instrument most frequently employed. While still useful in calculi lying in the lower third of the ureter, upper ureteric stones are now normally treated by extracorporeal lithotripsy or perureteral ultrasound, or electrohydraulic techniques.

The entity of idiopathic retroperitoneal fibrosis was not fully recognized until the classic description of the condition by J K Ormond in 1948. Several techniques of ureteric mobilization have been described and F Raper at Leeds added lateral displacement, which can be aided by placing the ureter in a psoas muscle trench. Reimplantation of the ureter to the bladder, together with uretero-ureteral reanastomosis techniques, was developed for the treatment of ureteric disease or iatrogenic damage during surgery. Nephrectomy and then ureteric ligation were the initial methods of treating the severed ureter. Gustave Simon in 1869 did this during the first nephrectomy, thus curing a ureteric fistula. Primary end-to-end anastomosis of a divided ureter was first successfully carried out by W Tauffer in Budapest in 1885, and in 1897 J W Boree cut the ureteric ends obliquely to lessen the chance of stenosis.

Transureteroureterostomy also stems from that time, as did ureterovesical anastomosis. A Boari[21] described his bladder flap operation in 1894, and it is still used to this day. Ureterointestinal anastomosis was first performed by Sir John Simon at St Thomas' Hospital, London, in 1852 on a boy of 13 with ectopia vesicae. The patient survived 8 months but died of a pyonephrosis. However, the contralateral kidney and ureter remained normal, with a patent ureterorectal anastomosis.

The development of ureterorectal implantation then progressed from the early work of H Stiles in 1907 with minimal tunneling through the bowel wall and no suturing of the ureter to rectal mucosa, via the tunneling techniques of R C Coffey from 1910 to 1930, and then the anatomic suture techniques with tunnels of R M Nesbit in 1948 and J M Cordonnier in 1950, culminating in W Leadbetter's[22] combined technique of both suture and tunnel in 1951, which avoided both stenosis and reflux.

Ectopia vesicae stimulated many surgeons to describe ingenious operations for this condition, and in time this led to reconstruction with vesicorectal anastomosis, as done by W Gregoire and C C Schulman in 1978 with a proximal colostomy. Urinary continence problems can be controlled with the use of an artificial urinary sphincter.

One of the major advances in the management of total incontinence, urinary fistulae, and where total cystectomy had been performed was the development of the ileal loop diversion by

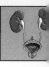
E Bricker[23] in 1950. As early as 1911 pioneers had tried to develop such surgery, but it was not for another 40 years that the technique was achieved satisfactorily and, of Bricker's series of 307 cases, only 3.4% mortality was attributable to the urinary diversion.

Bladder surgery

Surgery of the bladder mirrors that of stone disease, which has been considered previously, and that of bladder tumors.

Chronic irritation, infection, and chemical carcinogenesis have been recognized since Percivall Pott in 1775 described the scrotal cancer induced in young chimney sweeps. Bilharzial infection was thought to be a cause of bladder cancer as early as 1887, but it was L Rehn's description in 1895 of the increased incidence of bladder cancer in aniline dye workers that set the basis of chemical carcinogenesis. W C Hueper isolated β-naphthylamine in 1938, and R A M Case in 1954 studied workers in Birmingham in the rubber and associated industries. The use of exfoliative cytology pioneered by L Dudgeon and J Bamforth in 1927, and later popularized by G N Papanicolaou, allowed the noninvasive diagnosis of industrial bladder cancer.

Suprapubic cystotomy for the removal of bladder tumors was pioneered by T Billroth in Vienna in 1874 and partial cystectomy was first done in that year, with ureteric reimplantation in 1895.

Total cystectomy was first successfully carried out with vaginal implantation of the ureters by Bardenheuer in 1887. Cutaneous ureterostomy followed, and successful ureterointestinal anastomosis was achieved by F Krause in 1899.

Bladder reconstruction and continent diversion have evolved from cystectomy and diversion. Ileum, cecum, sigmoid colon, and even stomach have all had their proponents, and the low-pressure reservoir techniques were pioneered by K G Kock in 1969, M Ghoneim in Egypt in 1981 and R Hohenfellner at Mainz in 1991. P Mitrofanoff (1980) revived the flap-valve technique using the appendix as the cutaneous conduit.

Prostate surgery

Outflow obstruction due to prostatic enlargement has been recognized since ancient times, and by 1538 it was described in detail and illustrated by Vesalius. Enlargement was recognized by the mid-17th century and in 1788 John Hunter described the pathology of hyperplasia and its effect on the upper tracts. It was another century, however, before A F McGill (1830–90) at Leeds on March 18, 1887 carried out the first complete suprapubic transvesical prostatectomy. The author possesses a copy of the patient's notes written by the dresser, one Berkeley Moynihan (Fig. 1.9).

W J Belfield[24] (1856–1929) carried out the first planned procedure at Chicago in 1886 and the suprapubic approach was popularized by Sir Peter Freyer[25]. At the same time, at Johns Hopkins, Hugh Hampton Young[26] developed and promoted perineal prostatectomy, reporting his remarkable series in 1908 with only two deaths in 326 patients.

Many modifications of the conservative enucleation have been made. Professor S H Harris (1880–1936) at Sydney, Australia achieved complete hemostasis by trigonizing the cavity, and this was taken further by T Hryntschak (1889–1952), who removed a wedge from the posterior bladder neck and practiced direct

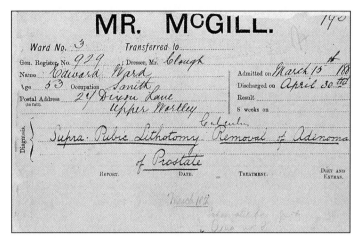

Fig. 1.9 Front case-sheet of McGill's first prostatectomy.
(With permission of Karger, Basel, from Clark P. Moynihan the urologist. Eur Urol. 1976;2:48–53.)

suture of the major prostatic vessels. Retropubic prostatectomy was reintroduced by Terrence Millin[27] in 1947. Although first performed in 1908, it had failed then to attract attention, and it has remained the operation of choice for open prostatectomy in the UK in the few cases of very large benign prostates that still warrant this approach.

Although surgery remains the gold standard treatment of benign prostatic hyperplasia, new medical approaches have been developed using α-blockers to relax the prostatic urethra and 5α-reductase inhibitors such as finasteride to decrease prostatic size.

The treatment of carcinoma of the prostate has led to a multidisciplinary approach in place of an essentially surgical one. The condition was first fully described by Benjamin Brodie in 1832. It was regarded as a rare condition then, but by 1908 Young was reporting a 21% incidence of carcinoma, and Freyer in 1913 a 13% occurrence in their series of prostatic resections. Radical suprapubic prostatectomy came in 1896, and by 1904 Young, aided by Halsted, carried out a radical perineal prostatectomy. Palliative cold punch resection, pioneered by Braasch, refined by Bumpus in 1926, and later by G Thompson in 1935, allowed resection of the obstructing tumor.

In 1941 came the first major breakthrough in the management of prostatic carcinoma with the work of Charles Huggins[28] on the androgen hormone sensitivity of this tumor, for which he gained a Nobel Prize in 1966.

Radical prostatectomy, although first performed around 1900, came again to the fore with the work of H J Jewett[29] in 1975, who reported survivals of up to 32 years in 27% of 103 patients with a discrete malignant nodule. P C Walsh has refined the radical operation with a nerve-sparing technique to preserve potency in these patients.

Radiotherapy has become one of the major adjuvant and in some cases primary therapies for urologic neoplasia. Radium was first used in the first decade of the 20th century and, while tumor regression was observed, damage to surrounding tissues limited its use. The early radiotherapy machines produced no significant advantage over control series, and it was not until 1952 that Ruben Flocks[30] introduced his new method of local injection of radioactive gold, [198]Au, as gold grains into the malignant prostate and a significant advance was achieved.

The use of interstitial radiotherapy sources into the bladder was also popularized initially with radium needles by B S Barringer in 1915, implanted into the base of a resected tumor, tantalum by Wallace et al. in 1952, and iridium wires by Botto et al. in 1980. External radiotherapy with the supervoltage machines largely superseded interstitial methods, although recently renewed interest in this technique for carcinoma of the prostate has been revived.

In 1965 M A Bagshawe[31] and his colleagues at Stanford, using the linear accelerator, reported excellent results in external radiation treatment of primary prostatic tumors.

Radiotherapy has also come to be one of the major therapeutic options in carcinoma of the bladder and testis.

Urethra and penis

Surgery of the urethra is principally reconstructive for both hypo- and epispadias, urethral stricture, injury, and the rare tumor of the urethra.

Hypospadias and its associated curvature (chordee) was described by Galen in the 2nd century AD, and epispadias by Morgagni in 1761. Morgagni at that time was operating on cases of hypospadias. During the 19th century skin-flap operations to close the urethral defect were developed by Moutet and S Duplay for hypospadias and K Thiersch for epispadias. L Ombrédanne, Denis Browne and B Johanson buried ventral penile skin, tubularized in the Denis Browne operation. Free grafts were used by A H McIndoe in 1937 and improved by C J Horton and C E Devine in 1961. More recent developments by R T Turner Warwick and J W Duckett in 1980 have led to single-stage repairs.

The development of urethroplasty mirrored the surgery for hypospadias established by Browne and Johanson. A Badenoch in 1954 then developed his pull-through operation and Turner Warwick in 1976 the scrotal flap procedure with the transpubic approach to severe strictures of the posterior urethra.

Injuries to the lower urinary tract were first managed by suprapubic cystostomy, introduced by R F Weir in 1897 and modified by urethral stenting by H Rutherford in 1904. Primary repair has had its advocates, but initial urinary diversion by suprapubic drainage and secondary repair has now returned as the treatment of choice.

Circumcision, along with lithotomy, shares the accolade of the earliest form of urologic surgery. Developing as both a religious ritual and a rite of early manhood, it is interesting that carcinoma of the penis rarely occurs after circumcision in infancy.

Penile cancer was recognized as early as the 7th century AD. Morgagni in 1761 appears to have performed the first planned partial amputation, with ligature of the vessels. He also mentioned the use of 'fire' to destroy the tumor. Proximal ligature above the tumor was condemned as too painful, and initially a guillotine amputation was performed, but by the latter part of the 19th century flaps were used to cover the site, with the urethra brought through a hole in one of them, as advocated by S D Gross in 1882. In 1878 Cabade carried out the first recorded radical excision of the penis, bringing out the urethra as a perineal urethrostomy.

Local excision or external and interstitial radiotherapy supplemented by systemic chemotherapy have now superseded radical surgery.

Peyronie's disease, causing penile curvature, deserves mention. Well known to Fallopius and Vesalius in 1561, it was described by Francois de la Peyronie, a surgeon to King Louis XV, in 1743. Described also by John Hunter, Sir James Paget (1814–99) noted its similarity to Dupuytren's contracture of the palmar fascia. Surgical excision of the plaque dates back to 1882. Excision and grafting were introduced by O S Lowsley in 1943 and Horton and Devine in 1974, while R M Nesbit in 1965 developed his technique of removing ellipses from the sheath of the corpus cavernosus opposite the plaque and closing them transversely, thus straightening the penis.

Modern developments in penile surgery included the introduction of rigid Small–Carrion prostheses by M P Small in 1978, the semirigid type by U Jonas in 1978, and the inflatable prosthesis by Brantley Scott in 1973.

Scrotum, testis, and penis

Hydroceles have been recognized since Roman times, and a terracotta votive figurine has been excavated that probably demonstrates the condition. Arculanus (1419–84) described the vaginal and congenital forms and recommended treatment by cautery. Tapping the hydrocele fluid became the preferred mode of treatment, but almost certainly led to the death of Edward Gibbon, the historian, in 1794. M Jaboulay (1860–1913) described his partial excision of the tunica, suturing it behind the epididymis, and P H Lord in 1964 his plication operation, while cysts of the epididymis and spermatoceles were recognized by Sir Robert Liston (1794–1847).

Scrotal cancer was the first occupational cancer to be recognized. The Industrial Revolution in the cotton industry brought a further form of industrial disease with mule (type of machine) spinners' scrotal tumors developing as a result of lubricating oil from spinning machinery soaking the workers' trousers. With the refining of oils and worker protection this has now become very rare.

Cryptorchidism was recognized in Ancient Greece, but orchidopexy was only described as late as 1899 by A D Bevan. Testicular descent was described by John Hunter, who first named the gubernaculum by which it was thought the testis was guided to the scrotum. The idea was later developed by an anatomist called Lockwood, whose 'gubernacular tails' attempted to explain the multiple end sites of ectopic testes. The importance of early orchidopexy was stressed by F Hinman Sr, and through the second half of the 20th century the early bringing down of the incompletely descended testis moved to infancy, as described by C G Scorer in 1967. F Torek, L Ombrédanne and Denis Browne developed their methods of mobilization and scrotal fixation of these testes, and the dartos pouch described by J K Lattimer in 1957 has become the maneuver of choice.

Ectopy has long been associated with the development of testicular cancer, and a rate of between 3.4% and 11.6% has been reported, of which one fifth may arise in the contralateral descended testis.

Germ cell tumors were fully classified by F H Dixon and R A Moore in 1952, refined by S K Mostofi[32] in 1973 and adopted by the WHO classification.

Inguinal orchiectomy, promoted by M W MacDonald in 1982, became the primary management. Treatment of type I disease – seminoma – has become based on its marked radiosensitivity, and orchiectomy with postoperative radiotherapy has become the primary therapy. Embryonal carcinoma, on the other hand, has led to diversity on either side of the Atlantic, and while lymphadenectomy has been the treatment favored in the USA, chemotherapy with lymphadenectomy only for large gland masses has been the approach in the UK.

The development of lymphangiography, described by J B Kinmonth in 1950, led to the ability to assess iliac and paraortic metastatic spread of tumor, overtaken now by CT scanning, and a combination of surgery, radiotherapy, and chemotherapy has evolved for the management of nonseminiferous germ cell tumors in both the USA and the UK.

IN CONCLUSION

The 20th century saw a remarkable plethora of methods of investigation and treatments that have revolutionized the management of urologic conditions. All this has been based on the understanding of anatomy, physiology, and pathology painstakingly observed, investigated, and pioneered in earlier times.

Surgery was well established by the beginning of the 20th century and has been refined in recent years, but the major advances of recent years have underpinned the broad basis of knowledge that has led urology to its present-day level of excellence.

Urodynamic studies pioneered by von Garrelts[33] in Stockholm in 1960 have formed the essential investigation of the neuropathic bladder and its management, and are applicable to a very wide range of urologic problems. Investigation of the urinary tract has been refined with the advent of spiral CT, MRI, isotopic, and positron emission tomography (PET) scans.

Chemotherapy has become a major adjunct to the management of all urologic cancers, and the author was himself involved in the early work on thiotepa reported by Burnand et al.[34] in 1976 in the reduction of superficial bladder recurrence.

Stone disease remains one of the most interesting aspects of urology, but noninvasive lithotripsy and endourology have replaced the open techniques for stone removal that dominated treatment from ancient times until very recently.

All these advances, set on the broad-based knowledge of the past, have determined the urology of today and tomorrow.

ACKNOWLEDGEMENTS

I am deeply endebted to Mr J G Gow of Liverpool, England, for his contributions on genitourinary tuberculosis and the development of endoscopic instruments.

No-one approaching a work on the history of urology can undertake this without the invaluable contribution of Leonard J T Murphy in his *History of Urology* published in 1972.

REFERENCES

1. Murphy LJT. The history of urology including L'Histoire de l'urologie, Desnos E 1914, trans. Leonard JT Murphy. Springfield, IL: Charles C Thomas; 1972.
2. Ellis H. A history of bladder stones. Oxford: Blackwell Scientific; 1969.
3. Chaussy CH, Brendel W, Schmiedt E. Extracorporeally induced destruction of kidney stones by shock waves. Lancet. 1980;2: 1265–8.
4. Paré A. The workes of that famous chirurgion Abrose Parey, trans Th. Johnson. London; 1634.
5. Cheselden WA. Treatise on the high operation for stone. London; 1723.
6. Civiale J. De la lithotritie ou broiement de la pierre dans la vessie. Paris: Bechet; 1827.
7. Medlar EM. Cases of renal infection in pulmonary tuberculosis; evidence of healed tuberculous lesions. Am J Pathol. 1926;2:401.
8. Fleming A. On the antibacterial action of cultures of a penicillium with special reference to their use of isolation of *B. influenzae*. Br J Exp Pathol. 1929;10:226–36.
9. Kass EH. Asymptomatic infections of the urinary tract. Trans Assoc Am Phys. 1956;69:56.
10. Hinman F Jr. Bacterial elimination. J Urol. 1968;99:811.
11. Stamey TA. Pathogenesis and treatment of urinary tract infections. Baltimore, MD: Williams & Wilkins; 1980.
12. Foley FEB. A self-retaining bag catheter. J Urol. 1937;38:140–3.
13. Cruise FR. The endoscope as an aid in the diagnosis and treatment of disease. Dublin Q J Med Sci. 1865;39:329.
14. McCarthy JF. A new apparatus for endoscopic plastic surgery of the prostate diathermia and excision of vesical growths. J Urol. 1931;26:695.
15. Bumpus HC. Punch operation for prostatic obstruction. Surg Clin North Am. 1927;7:1473.
16. Gross SW. Nephrectomy; its indications and contraindications. Am J Med Sci. 1885;90:79.
17. Morris H. The origin and progress of renal surgery. London: Cassell; 1898.
18. Brodel M. The intrinsic blood vessels of the kidney and their significance in nephrectomy. Bull Johns Hopkins Hosp. 1901;12:10.
19. Graves FT. The arterial anatomy of the kidney, the basis of surgical technique. Bristol: John Wright & Son; 1971.
20. Politano VA, Leadbetter WF. An operation for correction of vesicoureteral reflux. J Urol. 1958;79:932.
21. Boari A. La Uretero-cisto-neostomia. Rome: Societá Editrice Dante Alighieri; 1899.
22. Leadbetter WF. Consideration of problems incident to the performance of uretero-enterostomy. Report of a technique. J Urol. 1951;65:818.
23. Bricker EM. Bladder substitution after pelvic evisceration. Surg Clin North Am. 1950;30:1511.
24. Belfield WT. Prostatic myoma – a so-called 'middle lobe' of the hypertrophied prostate – removed by suprapubic prostatectomy. JAMA 1887;8:303.
25. Freyer PJ. Clinical lectures on disease of the prostate, 5th ed. London: Baillière Tindall & Cox; 1920.

26. Young HH. Studies on hypertrophy and cancer of the prostate. Bull Johns Hopkins Hosp. 1906;14:1–628.

27. Millin T. Retropubic prostatectomy: A new extravesical technique. Lancet. 1945;2:693.

28. Huggins C, Hodges CV. Studies of prostatic cancer 1. The effect of castration of oestrogen and of androgen injection on serum phosphatases in metastatic carcinoma of the prostate. Cancer Res. 1941;1:293.

29. Jewett HJ. The present status of radical prostatectomy in stages A and B prostatic cancer. Urol Clin North Am. 1975.;2:105.

30. Flocks RH, Kerr MD, Elkins HB, Culp D. Treatment of carcinoma of the prostate by interstitial radiation with radio-active gold, Au^{198}. J Urol. 1952;68:510.

31. Bagshawe MA, Kaplan HS, Sagerman RH, Linear accelerator super voltage radiotherapy VII. Carcinoma of the prostate. Radiology. 1965;85:121.

32. Mostofi SK. Testicular tumours: epidemiologic; etiologic and pathologic features. Cancer. 1973;32:1186.

33. Von Garrelts B. Analysis of micturition: a new method of recording the voiding of the bladder. Acta Chir Scand. 1956;112:328–40.

34. Burnand KG, Boyd PJR, Mayo ME et al. Single dose intravesical thiotepa as an adjuvant to cystodiathermy in the treatment of transitional cell bladder carcinoma. Br J Urol. 1976;48:55–9.

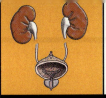

Chapter 2

Clinical Embryology of the Urinary Tract

Anthony A Caldamone

KEY POINTS

- Embryologic development of the genital and urinary tracts provides an understanding of the congenital disorders.
- The kidney evolves through three phases of development – pronephros, mesonephros, and metanephros.
- Close association occurs between the position of the ureteral bud on the mesonephric duct and renal dysplasia, vesicoureteral reflux, and ureteral ectopia.
- Exstrophy – epispadias complex results from an abnormality in the formation of the anterior cloacal membrane; hypospadias from failure of fusion of the urethral folds.
- Intersexuality results from excessive androgenization of the female or from deficient androgenization of the male, with abnormalities occurring at the chromosomal, gonadal, or phenotypic stages of development.

INTRODUCTION

The genitourinary tract is an integrated developmental complex, the result of a precise sequence of interrelated events. Understanding the embryology of the genital and urinary tracts provides an infrastructure on which to explain congenital disorders.

DEVELOPMENT OF THE KIDNEY

The kidney evolves through three phases of development: pronephros, mesonephros, and metanephros. This development occurs in a cranial to caudal sequence. Cells from the intermediate mesoderm aggregate and differentiate into the pronephric tubules, which are evident by the third week of fetal development. These same intermediate mesoderm cells give rise to cells of the gonads and wolffian ductal system (Fig. 2.1). The pronephric tubules appear between the second and sixth somites. These primitive tubules are nonsecretory; however, their caudal end becomes the mesonephric duct while the remainder of the pronephros involutes.

The mesonephros is formed from the descending mesonephric duct, which contains the intermediate mesoderm. This union induces the formation of the mesonephric nephron. By the fifth week of fetal life, 40 pairs of tubules are connected to the mesonephric duct. As more caudal pairs develop, more cranial units involute. The mesonephric ducts fuse caudally to enter the

urogenital sinus. The mesonephric tubules form an excretory complex, which secretes into the urogenital sinus from the sixth to the tenth weeks of gestation. In the female, the mesonephric duct involutes. In the male, however, the mesonephric duct (wolffian) develops under the influence of testosterone, produced by the Leydig cells, into the epididymis, vas deferens, and seminal vesicles.

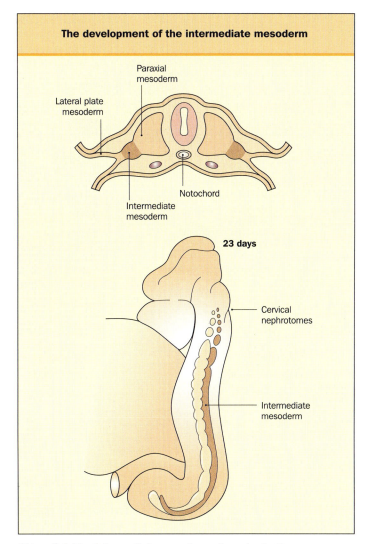

The development of the intermediate mesoderm

Figure 2.1 The intermediate mesoderm gives rise to the pronephros, somatic portion of the gonads and the internal male ductal system. (Adapted with permission from Larsen[1].)

The final, and renal, phase of development depends on the union of the ureteral bud and the metanephric blastema, derived from the intermediate mesoderm, in the sacral region of the developing fetus (Fig. 2.2). The metanephric blastema develops from the terminal portion of the nephrogenic cord, dissociating from the cord when it contacts the ureteral bud. The blastema develops into the nephrogenic structures and supporting tissues, and the bud becomes the ureter, calices, and collecting ducts. Union of the metanephric blastema and ureteral bud occurs in the upper sacral region (fourth week). As the ureteral bud elongates and the blastema ascends (within 4–6 weeks) to reach the lumbar segments, nephrogenic differentiation occurs (within 6–34 weeks).

The ureteral bud has its origin as an outpouching off the distal portion of the mesonephric duct. The development of the ureteral bud is divided into four phases, as it undergoes a series of intricate branchings that develop into the ureter, calices, and collecting ducts (Fig. 2.3)[2]. Potter divided ureteral bud development into four phases[2]. During phase 1 (weeks 5–14), the cranial ends of the ureteral bud dilate to form an ampulla as it advances the metanephric blastema cranially. Reciprocal induction of both components occurs, as both are necessary for further development of the kidney and collecting system. The ampulla of the ureteral bud undergoes a dichotomous branching, and each branch has at its tip an ampulla. The initial branch establishes the

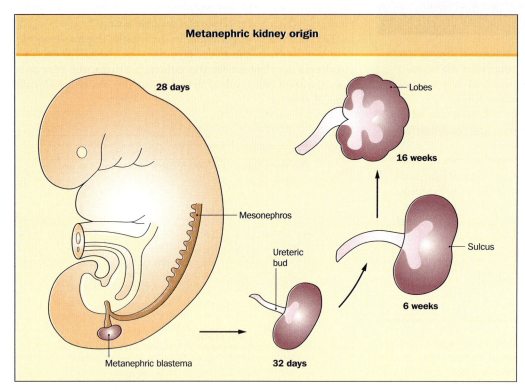

Figure 2.2 Metanephric kidney origin. At 28 days, the metanephric blastema develops from the intermediate mesoderm and at 32 days, the ureteral bud from the mesonephric duct contacts the metanephric blastema. By the sixth week, the metanephric bud bifurcates and induces superior and inferior lobes and at 16 weeks additional lobules develop from further branching of the ureteral bud. (Adapted with permission from Larsen[1].)

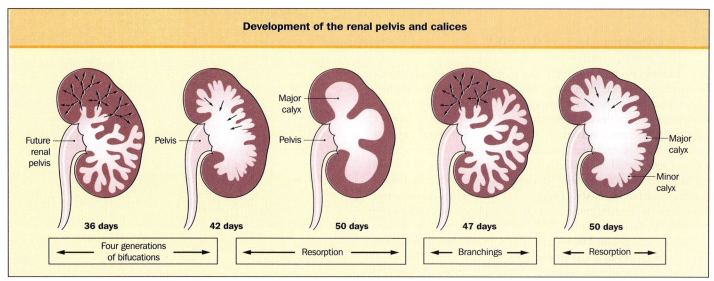

Figure 2.3 Development of the renal pelvis and calices. Between 36 and 50 days, bifurcation of the ureteral bud is followed by resorption to produce major calices. Between 47 and 50 days, the ampulla process forms the nephron and generations of bifurcation that result in minor calices. (Adapted with permission from Larsen[1].)

superior and inferior poles. The second branching is asymmetric with longer branches at the poles and shorter branches directed between the two poles. This asymmetric division leads to the characteristic reniform shape. The initial three to five generations form the renal pelvis and major calices, and subsequent generations form the minor calices and medullary collecting ducts. By the seventh week, the metanephric blastema is induced to form nephrons by the sixth division ampullae. After this point, at each branching one ampulla differentiates into a nephron, whereas the other continues to divide.

In phase 2, the ampulla grow peripherally while inducing arcades of 4–6 nephrons sequentially. The collecting tubules of these nephrons become linked together successively and linked to the advancing ampulla by a common duct. In phase 3 (weeks 26–36), the advancing ampulla extends farther into the outer zone or cortex. During this period, cortical nephrons are developed. The blastema forms discrete masses, each of which corresponds to an ampulla from which the definitive glomerulus and nephron form. In period 4 (weeks 36 to term), no further nephron induction occurs. The collecting tubules elongate, the proximal tubules convolute, and the loops of Henle extend deeper into the medulla[3].

Nephron development results from close interaction between the ampullae of the ureteral bud and the metanephric blastema. In the absence of the ureteral bud or other inductive tissue, or if the ureteral bud does not come into close contact with the blastema, nephron development does not occur[4]. Other tissues can be experimentally induced by the ureteral bud to form tubules (e.g. the thoracic spinal cord); however, only the metanephric blastema can form renal tubules[3]. Nephrogenesis begins by ureteral bud induction at the eighth week of gestation, with renal function beginning by the 12th week. However, nephrogenesis continues until the 34th week. Beyond this time, no new nephrons develop; however, tubular function continues to mature.

Renal agenesis

Renal agenesis results from abnormalities of either the ureteral bud, the metanephric blastema, or their union. There is a mutually dependent relationship between the ureteral bud and the metanephric blastema. If the ureteral bud is absent or abnormal, or if the ureteral bud does not contact the metanephric blastema, nephron differentiation does not arise, even in the presence of a normal blastema. Alternatively, if the metanephric blastema is absent, either primarily or because of failure of the nephrogenic cord or metanephric precursors (pronephros, mesonephros) to develop, the kidney does not develop. In this situation, the ureter may or may not be present. Most anephric patients have a rudimentary ureter, which indicates that the embryologic accident occurs after the ureteral bud outpouches from the mesonephric duct. In anephric patients with ureteral atresia, wolffian duct structures are normal. This indicates that the insult to the ureteral bud occurs after its formation. In 10% of patients, testicular agenesis is also found[5], which emphasizes the close association between the renal and gonadal anlage on the dorsal aspect of the coelomic cavity.

In contradistinction to bilateral renal agenesis, the embryologic insult in unilateral agenesis is most often to the ureteral bud. This theory is supported by the observation that the ipsilateral gonad is most often unaffected, and by the high occurrence

of abnormalities of the proximal wolffian duct structures in the male and of the müllerian structures in the female.

Renal dysplasia and hypoplasia

Renal dysplasia is associated with obstruction (ureteral, vesical, or urethral) in up to 50% of patients and is thought by some investigators to result from obstruction[6]. The work of Berman and Maizels[7] in the chick embryo and Tanagho in the mammalian fetus[8] demonstrates that simple ureteral ligation in the fetus results predominantly in hydronephrosis and not in dysplasia. It is likely that obstruction must be coupled with a quantitative deficiency of metanephric blastema if dysplasia is to occur. Maizels and Simpson demonstrated that dysplasia is more likely to occur after intrauterine ureteral ligation if the ureteral buds are depleted of condensed metanephrogenic mesenchyme[9].

An additional factor in the development of renal dysplasia and hypoplasia (hypodysplasia) is based on the clinical observation that a ureteral orifice that is abnormal in position is more likely to be associated with renal hypodysplasia. Ureters that terminate on the trigone generally have normal renal units, whereas those that are lateral or ectopic have a higher incidence of hypodysplasia. This is the theory of Mackie and Stephens, which explains the association of renal dysplasia with refluxing or ectopic ureters[10]. The embryologic basis is that the bud of the ectopic ureter originates from an abnormal position on the mesonephric duct and therefore meets only a small amount of metanephric blastema. The dysplasia seen with urethral obstruction (i.e. posterior urethral valves) is more often associated with reflux, which suggests that an abnormal ureteral orifice position is more likely to be the cause of the dysplasia rather than the result of the obstruction itself.

Multicystic kidney

Multicystic kidney is almost always associated with ureteral atresia or obstruction at the ureteropelvic junction. Attempts at induction of a multicystic kidney by *in utero* ligation of the ureter have not been universally successful[7,8]. This may indicate that the obstruction causing multicystic kidney occurs at a very early stage of renal development, or that some other factor is necessary (e.g. an abnormal metanephric blastema). Some investigators place multicystic kidney at the extreme end of the spectrum of hydronephrosis, a concept supported by clinical situations in which features of both hydronephrosis and multicystic kidney are apparent. Another theory proposes failure of union between the blastema and ureteral bud, which would explain the high incidence of ureteral atresia and agenesis. Whereas multicystic kidney is most commonly unilateral, often it is associated with contralateral renal abnormalities such as ureteropelvic junction obstruction or vesicoureteral reflux.

Simple renal ectopia and malrotation

The ureteral bud elongates to meet the metanephros in the region of the upper sacral somites at weeks 7–8. Factors responsible for renal ascent sequentially include[3]:

- caudal growth of the spine;
- active elongation of the ureter into the metanephros;
- elongation of the renal parenchyma with other architectural changes; and
- further elongation of the spine when the kidney is fixed to retroperitoneal structures.

The kidney adopts its blood supply from regional vessels during its ascent – the middle sacral, external, and common iliac arteries, and finally the aorta. During this ascent, the kidney rotates on its longitudinal axis from lateral to medial with respect to the renal pelvis, which accounts for the typical association of renal ectopia with malrotation or, rather, failure of rotation. Other factors that contribute to ascent failure include abnormalities of the ureteral bud (failure to elongate), defective metanephric blastema that fails to induce ascent, and genetic or teratogenic causes. Also, persistence of early vascular attachments has been proposed as a mechanism, but it is thought that this may be a result rather than a cause.

Crossed renal ectopia with and without fusion

Renal fusion is explained by one of two theories. The parenchyma of both nephrogenic cords may either fuse along with their respective ureters or by means of a wandering bud that crosses the midline and makes contact with the contralateral nephrogenic cord. In the former instance, a horseshoe kidney develops, whereas various forms of crossed renal ectopia result from the latter. Although the exact etiology of crossover is uncertain, several theories have been proposed. Wilmer explained the phenomenon by the presence of an abnormal umbilical artery that prevents ascent of one renal unit, and thus causes compression and fusion of the two abnormally juxtaposed renal anlage in the pelvis[11]. Cook and Stephens theorized that lateral flexion and rotation of the entire hind end of the fetus forces the ureteral bud and wolffian duct to cross the midline[12].

It is inferred that fusion most commonly occurs prior to or at the initial stages of renal ascent. It may also occur at later stages of ascent, which would explain unusual forms of fusion (e.g. the superior pole fused horseshoe kidney, or the superiorly and inferiorly fused horseshoe). Several variations of fusion anomalies have been described – the final morphology depends on the timing and extent of fusion, degree of renal rotation, and final location of the units. Malrotation is the rule, because little if any rotation is possible once fusion takes place. As pointed out by Perlmutter and coworkers, the orientation of each renal pelvis provides some evidence as to the embryologic timing of the fusion – the anteriorly placed pelvis indicates early fusion whereas the medially directed pelvis suggests fusion after rotation has been completed[13].

Fusion is involved in 90% of crossed ectopia. In crossed ectopia without fusion, the orthotopic unit is in its normal position and orientation, whereas the ectopic unit is usually caudal, incompletely rotated with an anteriorly directed pelvis, and assumes a horizontal or tangential lie. Anomalies, such as reflux, multicystic dysplasia, and ureteropelvic junction obstruction, most commonly arise in the crossed unit.

Ureteropelvic junction obstruction

Ureteropelvic junction obstruction is the most common congenital obstruction of the urinary tract. Its exact etiology is, however, obscure and may be multifactorial. Histologic evidence points to either a disorientation of muscle fibers (longitudinal fibers replacing the normal spiraling fibers) or excessive collagen and fibrous tissue[14,15]. This muscular disorientation may result from developmental arrest caused by compression of the ureter by fetal vessels or from ischemia to the ureteropelvic junction.

An alternative explanation is based on work by Ruano-Gil et al., who demonstrated that the developing ureter passes through a solid phase followed by recanalization[16]. Ureteropelvic junction obstruction, therefore, may be caused by failure of recanalization of the cephalic end of the ureter.

Other intrinsic lesions of the ureteropelvic junction include polyps, valves, and persistent ureteral folds. Congenital ureteral folds arise when the ureter lengthens out of proportion to renal ascent, which results in excess ureteral length. These folds rarely persist beyond infancy, because postnatally the growth rate of the infant exceeds that of the ureter. Persistence of these folds, which contain muscle, produces a valve-like obstruction at the ureteropelvic junction and at the ureterovesical junction (Fig. 2.4)[17].

DEVELOPMENT OF THE URETER AND TRIGONE

The ureteral bud appears as an outpouching from the caudal end of the mesonephric duct at the seventh week of gestation. Between days 37 and 40, the ureter goes through a stage of loss of lumen throughout most of its length, with sparing of the proximal and distal ends[16]. It then progressively recanalizes, beginning with the midsection (Fig. 2.5). Rapid elongation of the ureter may be the cause of loss of patency. When patency is established as a result of recanalization, it is the distal and proximal ureteral ends that are last to recanalize. This may explain why congenital obstructions of the ureter are most common at the ureteropelvic and ureterovesical junctions. It is thought that hydrostatic pressure from the mesonephric secretion of urine may contribute to the recanalization process.

The relationship between the ureteral bud and the mesonephric duct explains many of the congenital anomalies associated with the ureteral orifice[18]. The ureteral bud originates from the mesonephric duct at a relatively fixed site. The portion of the mesonephric duct between the ureteral bud and urogenital sinus is termed the common excretory duct. This segment, a precursor of the trigone and bladder neck, contributes to its muscularization as it becomes absorbed into the urogenital sinus. The orifice of the mesonephric duct migrates caudally and the ureteral bud cranially. While this opposed migration occurs, rotation takes place. Initially, the ureteral bud is located medial and distal with respect to the mesonephric duct, which becomes the seminal vesicles, vas deferens, and epididymis. As the ureteral bud migrates cephalad and laterally, the mesonephric duct crosses over the ureter, migrating medially and caudally. The final position of these structures is about equidistant from the bladder neck.

There is a close association between the position of the ureteral bud on the mesonephric duct and the development of renal hypodysplasia (Fig. 2.6). Mackie and Stephens proposed that the nephrogenic ridge contains blastema with varying potential for normal renal development[10]. The central zone, which corresponds to the area normally contacted by the ureteric bud, has the best potential for normal nephron induction; the potential is less on either side of this zone. The ureteral bud that initiates from an abnormal position on the mesonephric duct may strike the blastema away from the central zone, and therefore induce abnormal renal formation. This would explain the high incidence of dysplasia found in upper pole segments of duplicated systems, along with dysplasia associated with reflux from an abnormally placed lower pole ureteral orifice.

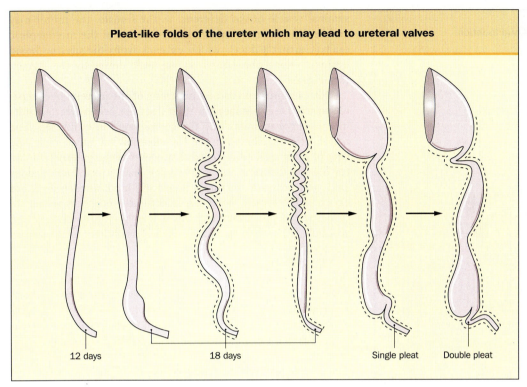

Pleat-like folds of the ureter which may lead to ureteral valves

12 days   18 days   Single pleat   Double pleat

Figure 2.4 Pleat-like folds of the ureter which may lead to ureteral valves. Around 18 days of gestation the ureter undergoes relative elongation resulting in redundancy which may lead to leaflets or valves. (Adapted with permission from Maizels and Stephens[17].)

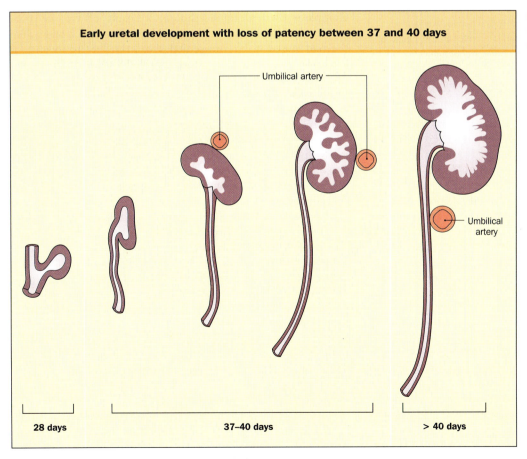

Early uretal development with loss of patency between 37 and 40 days

Umbilical artery

Umbilical artery

28 days   37–40 days   > 40 days

Figure 2.5 Early ureteral development with loss of patency between 37 and 40 days. (Adapted with permission from Maizels[3].)

Influence of ureteral bud location

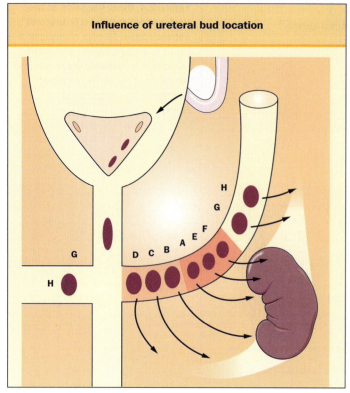

Figure 2.6 Influence of ureteral bud location on renal parenchymal development, as proposed by Mackie and Stephens. A–H represent different sites of budding of the ureter off the mesonephric (wolffian) duct. A, E and F are in a normal zone and will result in a ureter on the trigone of the bladder. (Adapted with permission from Mackie and Stephens[10].)

Vesicoureteral reflux

Primary vesicoureteral reflux results when a ureteral bud forms from a more caudal site on the mesonephric duct (i.e. closer to the urogenital sinus) and leads to a foreshortened common excretory duct. The shorter common excretory duct is absorbed sooner, which allows the ureter to migrate more cranially and laterally, and further separates it from the mesonephric duct. A wider trigone develops with deficient muscle, as less mesenchyme is contributed by the common excretory duct. The final product is a ureteral orifice that lies more lateral and superior than normal. It is poorly fixed to the trigone, which results in a shortened submucosal ureteral tunnel (see Fig. 2.6).

Ureteral ectopia

If the ureteral bud forms at a more cranial position on the mesonephric duct, a longer than normal common excretory duct results. The ureter then migrates for a longer time, attached to the mesonephric duct, before it separates as the longer common excretory duct is absorbed completely. This leaves little or no opportunity for the ureter to migrate separately from the mesonephric duct. When the ureteral bud arises only slightly higher than normal on the mesonephric duct, the ureteral orifice assumes its final position closer to the bladder neck. In a more cephalad outpouching of the ureteral bud, it may terminate in the urethra or, in the male, it may maintain its attachment to the mesonephric duct connecting with the

seminal vesicle or vas deferens. In the female, the ureter may end in the urethra or in the distal remnant of the mesonephric duct (Gartner's duct), which extends from the uterine broad ligament along the lateral vagina wall down to the hymen (see Fig. 2.6).

With a more cephalad outpouching of the ureteral bud, separation from the mesonephric duct does not occur, which results in a ureter that drains into the genital tract in either sex. The major difference between the two sexes is that, in the male, the sites of ectopia all lie cephalad to the level of the external sphincter (i.e. vas deferens, seminal vesicles, ejaculatory duct, bladder neck and prostatic urethra); therefore, incontinence does not occur. In the female, however, an ectopic ureter may terminate distal to the sphincter mechanism (i.e. bladder neck, urethra, vestibule, uterus, cervix and vagina) and result in constant urinary leakage.

With bilateral ureteral ectopia from single systems in which the ureters end distal to the bladder neck, the bladder is poorly developed and small in capacity. This is the result of two factors:

- urine does not fill the bladder; and
- the trigone and bladder neck do not develop because muscularization is dependent upon mesenchyme from the common excretory duct.

Thus, children tend to be incontinent when the ureters are simply reimplanted in the bladder.

Duplication anomalies of the ureter

Complete ureteral duplication as a result of two separate ureteral buds follows the Weigert–Meyer law, which states that the bud closest to the urogenital sinus, the first to migrate, is the lower pole ureter. The more cephalad bud, which maintains its contact with the mesonephric duct for a longer period of time, is the upper pole ureter. On the trigone, the lower pole orifice is more lateral and cephalad, and the upper pole ureter is more medial and caudal. Exceptions to the Weigert–Meyer law occur if, rather than two separate buds originating from the mesonephric duct, a single bud divides immediately and leads to complete duplication. If both buds are within the normal region for outpouching on the mesonephric duct, no pathologic consequences ensue.

If one ureteral bud arises in a normal location, but the other is in a more caudal position, complete duplication with reflux into the more caudal bud occurs. The caudal bud is carried more superior and lateral on the bladder wall, which accounts for reflux; because of its original position of outpouching on the ureteral bud, it corresponds to the lower pole ureter. However, if one bud is in a normal position and a second takes off cephalad to the normal zone (upper pole ureter), an ectopic ureter to the upper pole results. This accounts for the clinical observations in duplicated systems of a high incidence of reflux into the lower pole and ureteral ectopia of the upper pole.

Ureterocele

The exact embryologic events that lead to ureterocele formation are unclear. The traditional theory involves a delayed rupture of Chwalle's membrane, a two-cell ureteric membrane present at the time of budding of the ureter from the mesonephric duct[19]. Persistence of this membrane after urine excretion begins could lead to ureteral obstruction and dilatation.

This obstructive theory complies with the clinical observation that many ureteroceles have a stenotic orifice. In other ureteroceles, however, the orifice is patulous or the ureter is blind-ending: These developments are not easily explained by Chwalle's membrane theory. An intrinsic defect in the musculature of the terminal ureter that leads to dilatation of the distal segment is another plausible theory for the formation of ureteroceles[20].

Primary obstructive megaureter

A primary obstructive megaureter results from a derangement of the distal ureteral musculature that impedes the normal peristaltic wave from conveying a bolus of urine. This is often described physiologically as an adynamic segment. Early muscularization is predominantly of the circular type. Longitudinal musculature, however, is essential for proper peristalsis. A development arrest prior to formation of longitudinal musculature may lead to a nonperistaltic segment of ureter. Tanagho noted that the final segment of ureter to acquire its musculature is the distal segment[21]. Infrequently, an anatomic obstruction may be the cause of obstructive megaureter, and may be explained by the persistence of fetal ureteral folds with intrinsic musculature or by failure of recanalization of the ureter.

DEVELOPMENT OF THE BLADDER

The cloaca is divided by the urorectal septum into an anterior compartment (the primitive urogenital sinus) and a posterior compartment (the hindgut). The body of the bladder is derived principally from the primitive urogenital sinus this being in continuity superiorly with the allantois, which becomes the urachus. The cephalad portion is dilated and becomes the bladder, the midportion is narrowed and becomes the posterior urethra, and the inferior portion becomes the definitive urogenital sinus[1]. The base of the bladder and trigone are further derived from the distal ends of the wolffian duct – the common excretory duct.

The cloaca is a pouch that has a short extension to the caudal portion of the embryo, the tail gut; it receives in its cephalad portion the allantoic duct and the hindgut (Fig. 2.7). The cloacal membrane regresses as the mesoderm migrates from the medial and caudal directions, to leave only the lower two-thirds of the cloaca covered anteriorly by the cloacal membrane. Mesodermal migration proceeds to form the anterior abdominal wall. Any impediment to this migration results in lateral displacement of the musculoskeletal elements of the abdominal wall[22].

This mesenchymal plate migrates between the endodermal and ectodermal layers of the cloaca. The lateral ridges proliferate and fuse to form the genital tubercle. Enlargement of the genital tubercle is accompanied by outward migration of the cloacal membrane, which forms the floor of the phallus and later becomes the urethral groove (see Development of the urethra, below). As this process occurs, the cloaca becomes divided by the urorectal septum, which migrates in a cephalad to caudad direction. The anterior portion of the cloaca forms the bladder and the posterior portion the hindgut. The residual communication between the anterior and posterior portions of the cloaca is a narrow channel called the cloacal duct of Reichel. Persistence of this duct, as occurs in imperforate anus, results in a urethrorectal or vesicorectal fistula.

The urinary tract becomes separated from the hindgut when the advancing urorectal septum reaches the cloacal membrane. The anterior cloacal membrane, or urogenital membrane, perforates to establish the urogenital orifice. In the female, the urogenital canal shortens, which allows separate urethral and müllerian duct openings. In the male, the urogenital sinus progressively lengthens.

Agenesis of the bladder

Agenesis of the bladder is one of the rarest anomalies of the urinary tract. Only 37 patients have been reported in the literature, 29 of whom were stillborn; seven of the eight survivors were female[23]. The exact embryogenesis is not clear. If other

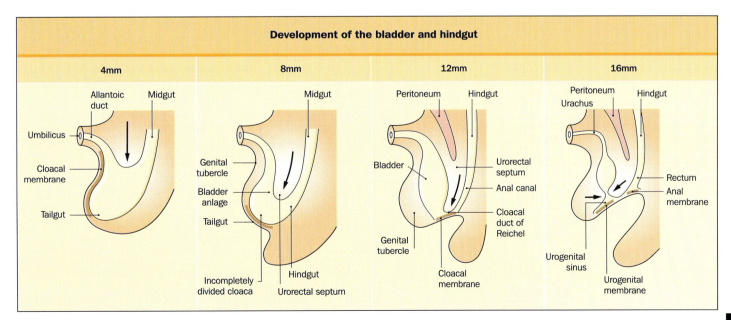

Figure 2.7 Development of the bladder and hindgut by division of the cloaca and cloacal membrane by the urorectal septum.
Lengths in mm refer to length of the fetus. (Adapted with permission from Muecke[22].)

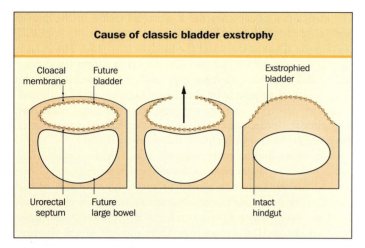

Cause of classic bladder exstrophy

Cloacal membrane · Future bladder · Exstrophied bladder · Urorectal septum · Future large bowel · Intact hindgut

Figure 2.8 Persistence of the cloacal membrane after urorectal septal division produces classic bladder exstrophy. (Adapted with permission from Muecke[22].)

associated anorectal malformations are present, persistence of the cloaca and failure of urogenital sinus development result in termination of the ureteric orifices in the rectum. Failure of the lower portions of the mesonephric ducts to form the trigone and proximal urethra is a likely sequence, which leads to bladder agenesis. In the female, because the müllerian duct structures are likely to develop normally, the ureteric orifices end in the uterus, anterior vaginal wall, or vestibule. The ureters may remain separate or form a common channel. The upper tracts are often hydronephrotic and dysplastic.

Exstrophy–epispadias complex

The embryologic basis for the development of bladder exstrophy is based on experimental work of Muecke in which exstrophy was produced in the chick embryo by inhibiting anterior cloacal membrane formation with a plastic wedge inserted above the cloacal membrane[24]. A persisting cloaca, or an abnormally large cloaca that does not retract normally toward the perineum, accounts for bladder exstrophy and its variants. This wedge effect prevents medial mesenchymal ingrowth, causing the future abdominal wall to remain lateral. With dehiscence of the cloacal membrane in the ninth week, the posterior surface

of the bladder becomes exposed to the exterior on the surface of the abdominal wall. The infraumbilical membrane is absent, and thus the umbilicus is adjacent to the bladder wall. The urogenital groove also fails to form, creating the associated epispadias. The corpora of the phallus assume a more widely divergent course proximally. The paired genital tubercles fuse inferiorly, to leave the urethral groove anteriorly.

If dehiscence of the cloacal membrane occurs after the urorectal septum has completed its partitioning of the cloaca, bladder exstrophy results (Fig. 2.8). However, if this dehiscence occurs prior to division of the cloaca, the hindgut becomes exposed as well, which separates the bladder into two halves with the hindgut between them, and leads to cloacal exstrophy (Fig. 2.9). Epispadias results if persistence of the cloacal membrane occurs only inferiorly, whereas a superior vesical fissure results if the persistence is superiorly only.

Mesodermal invasion of the infraumbilical membrane may be merely delayed rather than entirely absent, so that secondary closure of the parietes occurs before formation of the exstrophy. Such development produces covered exstrophy. Rarely, sequestration includes portions of viscera not ordinarily involved in exstrophy.

DEVELOPMENT OF THE URETHRA

Posterior urethra

The urorectal septum grows caudally to reach the cloacal membrane and, in so doing, divides the cloaca into anterior urogenital, sinus and posterior hindgut portions. During this process, the wolffian ducts, which entered the primitive cloaca, become incorporated into the ventral wall of the urorectal septum, to form Müller's tubercle. The portion of the urogenital sinus that is proximal to Müller's tubercle forms the entire urethra in the female and the prostatic urethra in the male. The more proximal portion of the urogenital sinus just distal to the tubercle develops longitudinal striations in its lateral walls, these striations extend from the tubercle to the site of origin of Cowper's glands in the male and to Bartholin's gland in the female. In the male, these folds persist as the plicae colliculi in the posterolateral urethral wall[19].

The embryologic basis for the four types of posterior urethral valves is variable. Type I valves consist of posterior mucosal leaflets

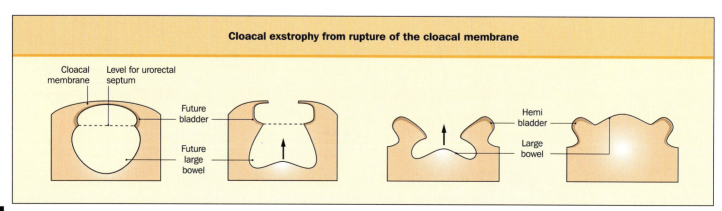

Cloacal exstrophy from rupture of the cloacal membrane

Cloacal membrane · Level for urorectal septum · Future bladder · Future large bowel · Hemi bladder · Large bowel

Figure 2.9 Cloacal exstrophy from rupture of the cloacal membrane prior to division of the cloaca by the urorectal septum. (Adapted with permission from Muecke[22].)

that originate distal to the verumontanum and fuse anteriorly to a variable extent, and thereby create an elliptical opening that is widest proximally. Tolmatschen proposed that these valves are an exaggeration of the normal urethrovaginal folds[25]. Stephens believes that they are an abnormal junction of the portion of the wolffian duct and the urogenital sinus[20]. Type II valves are urethral folds that originate at the verumontanum and diverge toward the bladder neck; they are not considered obstructive. Type III valves represent either a severe form of Type I valves with extensive anterior and posterior fusion or a congenital urethral membrane. They occur in either the membranous or proximal bulbous urethra (and may appear as a diaphragm with a central lumen) or as a redundant membrane that prolapses into the bulbous urethra ('windsock'). Type III valves may be caused by a persistence of the urogenital membrane, the anterior portion of the cloacal membrane[26]. Thickening of the urogenital membrane, because of an abnormal amount of mesoderm between the epithelial layers, impedes its dissolution and results in Type III valves.

Stephens described a Type IV urethral valve, characterized by a deep infold of the anterior and anterolateral urethral walls, that overrides the lumen of the membranous urethra[27]. These folds are noted on voiding cystourethrography in some children with prune-belly syndrome.

Anterior urethra
During the fourth week of gestation, paired swellings appear anterolateral to the cloacal membrane; these later fuse in the midline to form the genital tubercle. The phallic portion of the urogenital sinus (the anterior portion of the cloaca) remains undifferentiated between the fifth and tenth weeks of gestation. The urethral and genital folds are formed from the posterolateral anal tubercles and the lateral mesoderm. The mesodermal components convert testosterone into dihydrotestosterone (DHT) and allow external virilization. The phallic portion (bulbar and penile) of the urogenital sinus near the urogenital membrane and the proximal portion near the bladder become the posterior urethra. The primary urethral groove forms from elongation of the urogenital sinus outward onto the ventral phallic surface. The anterior walls of the urogenital sinus converge to form an endodermal urethral plate. The urogenital sinus then disintegrates, to expose the urethral groove. Under the influence of testosterone and DHT, the genital tubercle enlarges, which causes elongation of the phallus and extension of the urethral groove to the level of the corona. The penile urethra is tubularized by fusion of the endodermal edges of the urethral groove. The ectodermal edges fuse to create the median raphe (Fig. 2.10). External genital virilization is influenced by DHT.

The glandular urethra appears during the fourth month of gestation. The exact mechanism of its development remains unclear. It is thought by some investigators that the glandular urethra forms in the same manner as the bulbous and penile urethra[28], while others believe the glandular ectoderm forms a solid core of tissue that joins the penile urethra formed by closure of the urethral groove[29]. It has been proposed that canalization of this core by epithelial ingrowth forms the distal urethra. The point at which the penile and glandular portions of the urethra meet is the fossa navicularis. The coalescence of the mesenchyme dorsal to

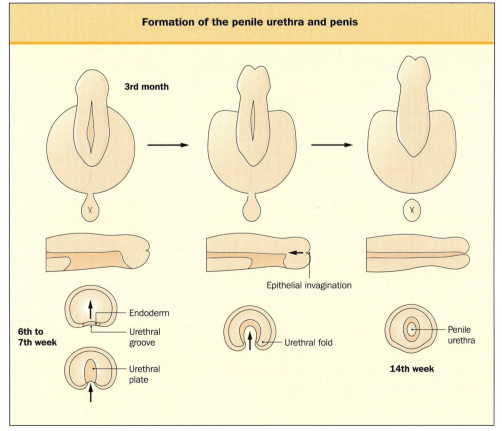

Formation of the penile urethra and penis

Figure 2.10 **Formation of the penile urethra and penis.** (Adapted with permission from Larsen[1].)

the urethra forms the corporal bodies and neurovascular channels. The mesenchyme is also responsible for the development of Buck's fascia, dartos fascia, and the corpus spongiosum. The labioscrotal swellings migrate medially and fuse at the base of the penis to form the scrotum.

Hypospadias mechanically results from failure of fusion of the endodermal edges of the urethral groove (urethral folds) at variable levels between the perineum and distal penile shaft. Distal shaft, coronal, and glandular hypospadias may be caused by anomalous canalization of the glans penis. Formation of the glandular urethra is a relatively late embryologic event compared to renal development, which accounts for the infrequent association of upper tract anomalies with distal hypospadias. Biochemically, any defect that results in inadequate androgen synthesis (testosterone or DHT) or defective androgen action (androgen-receptor deficiency) may lead to hypospadias. The deficiency need not be continuous; rather, it must be manifest at the gestational time that corresponds to genital differentiation. Attempts have been made to determine androgen receptor and 5α-reductase levels in penile tissue obtained from hypospadiac patients, but the results are conflicting. Progesterone administration during pregnancy can be associated with hypospadias.

SEXUAL DIFFERENTIATION

Normal and abnormal sexual differentiation demonstrate that an understanding of embryology is critical in the approach to and management of a group of complex and intriguing clinical disorders. Normal sexual differentiation is the result of an integrated sequence of events. When one or more of these steps are interrupted or interfered with, disorders of sexual differentiation result.

Sexual differentiation is a sequential process that can be divided into three stages; Jost established the sequence. Chromosomal sex is determined at fertilization and dictates the differentiation of the gonad (gonadal sex; Fig. 2.11), which in turn dictates the phenotype sex, or the differentiation of the internal ductal system and external genitalia. The gonadal blastema is undifferentiated until the sixth week of gestation, at which time differentiation occurs based on the chromosomal complement. The differentiated gonad (ovary or testis) directs the development of the internal ductal system and external genitalia, which is mediated by hormonal secretions.

Chromosomal sex is determined at the moment of conception by the sex chromosome complement of the fertilizing sperm.

If this sperm carries an X chromosome, a 46XX complement results (normal female); if the sex chromosome is Y, a 46XY (normal male genotype) results. The critical genes (SRY- on sex-determining region of Y chromosome) necessary for differentiation of the primordial gonad into a testis are located on the distal aspect of the short arm of the Y chromosome (Y_p). This gene is necessary but not sufficient for testicular development[30]. Testis-determining factor (SRY proteins), thought to be produced by this gene region, attaches to the surface of gonadal primordia to induce development into a testis. The SRY protein, or a transcription factor, is elaborated in the sex cord cells of the undifferentiated gonad. This protein causes the medullary region to develop into Sertoli cells and later into testis cords and seminiferous tubules. The cortical cells degenerate and later are separated from the developing testis by a connective tissue layer, the tunica albuginea. Two genes on the long arm of the Y chromosome (Y_q) are thought to be necessary for spermatogenesis, DAZ and Y-chromosome RNA-recognitive motive on YRRM[31].

In addition to the SRY gene region, genes on the X chromosome are thought to influence, actively or passively, sexual differentiation in so far as mutations to these genes result in disorders of sexual differentiation. Some of those genes include the Wilms' tumor I (WTI) gene (Denys–Drash syndrome, WAGR syndrome), and the sex reversal or adrenal hypoplasia gene (DAXI).

The gonad develops from both somatic and germ cells. The somatic cells are located in the ventral region of the mesonephros and arise from the mesonephric cells and the coelomic epithelium. Somatic cells become the Sertoli cells of the testis and the granulosa cells of the ovary. The germ cells migrate from a more inferior position on the yolk sac to the genital ridge, just medial to the mesonephros on each side. This occurs between the fourth and sixth week of gestation. Once the germ cells reach the gonadal ridge, they become surrounded by the somatic cells, which seem to regulate germ cell differentiation.

Prior to the seventh week of gestation, the gonad remains histologically undifferentiated; however, submicroscopic differentiation is occurring already. The predetermined testis grows at an accelerated rate compared to the predetermined ovary because the number of cell divisions is increased. In contrast, ovarian histologic differentiation occurs later in gestation, usually at about the 20th week. The primitive sex cords involute and secondary sex cords are formed from the mesenchyme of the gonadal ridges. It is these secondary sex cords that surround the germ cells to form the follicular cells. The initial event is that of a meiotic prophase,

Disorders of gonadal and chromosomal sex		
	Disorder	**Chromosome**
Gonadal sex	Pure gonadal dysgenesis	46XY or 46XX
	Gonadal agenesis (testicular regression)	46XY
Chromosomal sex	Klinefelter's syndrome	47XXY
	Sex reversal syndrome	46XX
	Turner's syndrome (gonadal dysgenesis)	45XO
	Mixed gonadal dysgenesis	46XY/45XO
	True hermaphroditism	46XY; 46XY mosaicisms

Figure 2.11 Disorders of gonadal and chromosomal sex.

Disorders of phenotypic sex		
Pseudohermaphroditism	Cause	Outcome
Female (46XX; virilized female)	Endogenous androgen production	Congenital adrenal hyperplasia Maternal virilizing tumor (arrhenoblastomas, luteomas)
	Exogenous androgen administration	
	Maternal progestin ingestion	
Male (46XY; inadequately virilized male)	Deficient müllerian inhibiting factor	Hernia uteri inguinali (persistent müllerian duct syndrome)
	Defective androgen synthesis	Congenital adrenal hyperplasia
	Androgen insensitivity	Primary amenorrhea
	Deficiency of 5α-reductase	Pseudovaginal perineoscrotal hypospadias

Figure 2.12 Disorders of phenotypic sex.

which is thought to be influenced by elevated gonadotropins, somatic cells, and/or as yet undetermined factors. Most of these primordial germ cells are lost, because of the absence of a surrounding protective layer of follicular cells and stroma. The development of this protective layer is controlled by ovarian-determining genes. The follicular cells are thought to inhibit further germ-cell divisions until puberty.

The gonadal sex is established by the seventh week of gestation. Differentiation of the internal ductal system and the external genitalia is determined by the gonadal sex. At this stage, the fetus contains two internal ductal systems (wolffian and müllerian), and undifferentiated external genital primordia that are recognized as protuberances anterolateral to the cloacal membrane. Both internal ductal systems are derived from the mesonephric system. The wolffian (or mesonephric) duct is a tubular structure that connects the capillary network of the mesonephros to the urogenital sinus. Evagination of the coelomic epithelium leads to formation of a second tubular structure adjacent to the mesonephric duct, the paramesonephric, or müllerian duct. The distal ends of these two ducts are joined. The wolffian duct is essential for müllerian duct development. That portion of the urogenital sinus distal to the termination of these ducts contributes to external genital development, whereas the proximal portion develops into the bladder, trigone, and posterior urethra.

Phenotypic sexual differentiation is predicated on the establishment of gonadal sex (Fig. 2.12). If an ovary develops, the wolffian duct involutes due to lack of testosterone, and only its terminal portion persists, as Gartner's duct. Some of the mesonephric excretory tubules and a portion of the wolffian duct form the epoöphoron in the mesovarium. The müllerian ducts develop into the proximal vagina, uterus, and fallopian tubes (Fig. 2.13).

The unfused cephalic portions of the müllerian ducts form the fallopian tubes, while the caudal ends fuse to form the uterovaginal canal. The union of the fused caudal ends of the müllerian ducts and urogenital sinus forms the vagina. The proximal two-thirds of the vagina is of müllerian duct origin and the distal one-third is of urogenital sinus origin. The exact roles that ovarian development and secretion play in female phenotypic differentiation is unclear. As ovarian development lags somewhat behind genital development and female phenotypic development occurs in cases of gonadal agenesis regardless of the chromosomal complement, the ovaries may not have a critical determining role

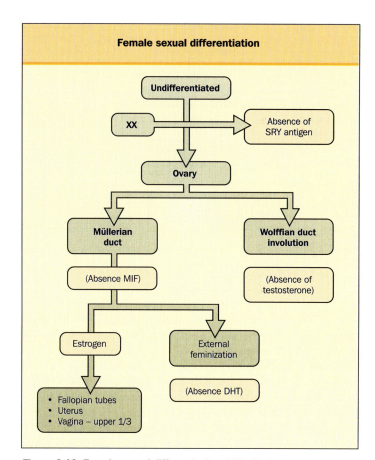

Figure 2.13 Female sexual differentiation. DHT, dihydrotestosterone; MIF, müllerian inhibiting factor; SRY, sex-determining region of Y chromosome.

in early female differentiation. It is possible that this process results from the high estrogen milieu from the placenta and maternal circulation. However, both estrogen and progestin secretion by the ovary are more active in the development of the secondary sexual structures later in fetal development.

Male phenotypic differentiation is the result of the elaboration of two distinct testicular hormones, testosterone and müllerian inhibiting factor (MIF; Fig. 2.14). These are produced and secreted by the 8th week of development, and are essential for normal male differentiation. Involution of the müllerian ducts is caused by MIF, which is a glycoprotein secreted by the fetal

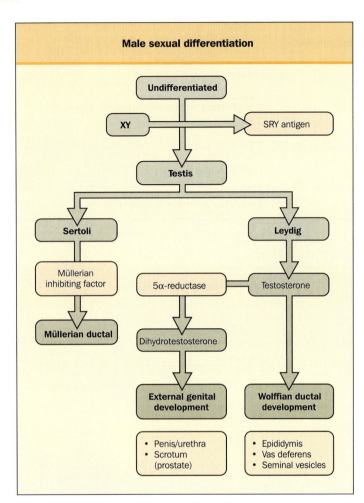

Figure 2.14 Male sexual differentiation. SRY, sex-determining region of Y chromosome.

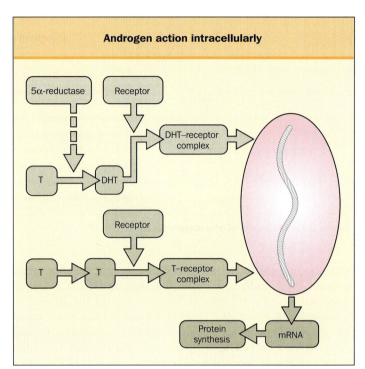

Figure 2.15 Androgen action intracellularly with its conversion into dihydrotestosterone (DHT) by 5α-reductase and the intracellular transport mediated by androgen binding protein. T, Testosterone. (Adapted with permission from Aaronson[32].)

Sertoli cells. The remnants of the müllerian ducts persist caudally as the prostatic utricle and cephalically as the appendix testis. The action of MIF is exerted unilaterally and locally (exocrine secretion) rather than bilaterally via the systemic circulation.

Immediately after müllerian duct regression, the wolffian ducts develop under the influence of testosterone secreted by the fetal Leydig cells. The Leydig cells, as do the Sertoli cells, differentiate from the mesenchymal cells within the gonadal ridges. This occurs at 9–10 weeks of gestation. Again under the influence of testosterone, the wolffian ducts evolve into the epididymis, vas deferens, and seminal vesicles. The mesonephric tubules develop into the ductuli efferentes, which provide continuity between the seminiferous tubules and rete testis to the vas deferens. This process occurs as a direct action of testosterone on the ductal structures. By the 12th week of gestation, virilization relies on the ability of the tissues involved to convert testosterone into a more potent androgen, DHT. The cytoplasm of the target cells possesses the enzyme 5α-reductase, which is necessary for this conversion (Fig. 2.15). Once bound to a cytoplasmic receptor, DHT is transported to the cell nucleus where it acts on deoxyribonucleic acid to direct the formation of various proteins necessary for virilization of the external genitalia (Fig. 2.16). It is unclear whether testosterone synthesis from the fetal testis is dependent on gonadotropins or whether it is an intrinsic function

of the fetal testis. The development of the prostate gland is influenced by DHT. This gland begins to evolve during the tenth week of gestation as a group of evaginations of the posterior portion of the urethra.

Disorders of sexual differentiation
Intersexuality results from excessive androgenization of the female or deficient androgenization of the male. These processes result from events that occur at the chromosomal, gonadal, or phenotypic stages of development. Not all intersex states result in ambiguous genitalia. Intersex conditions in which chromosomal, gonadal, or internal phenotypic disorders do not affect external phenotypic expression may be accompanied by external genitalia of normal appearance. In some disorders with normal external genitalia, the internal ductal system is either poorly developed or develops along lines inconsistent with external genital and sexual differentiation. Such patients may have infertility, delayed puberty, primary amenorrhea, inguinal hernia with müllerian contents in a phenotypic male, or an inguinal hernia with a gonad in a phenotypic female.

Disorders of chromosomal sex occur when either the number or structure of each of the sex chromosomes is abnormal. These include Klinefelter's syndrome, 46XX male (sex reversal syndrome), gonadal dysgenesis (Turner's syndrome), mixed gonadal dysgenesis, and true hermaphroditism. The common denominator in disorders of chromosomal sex is an abnormality of the structure or number of sex chromosomes or of the autosomal chromosomal components responsible for differentiation of the gonad into an ovary or testis. For example, in the 46XX male syndrome, a defect in production of antigens is responsible for

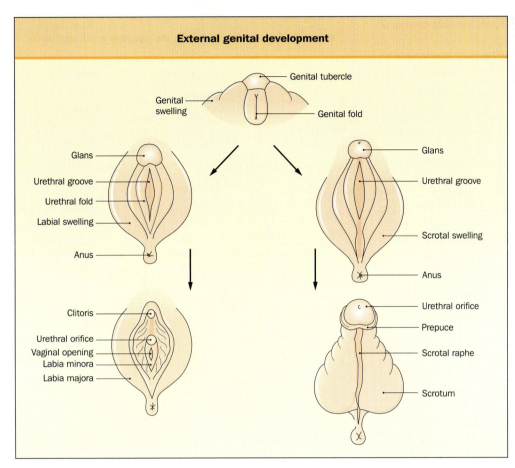

External genital development

Figure 2.16 External genital development. (From Rubenstein and Mandell[33], reprinted with permission from Contemporary Urology magazine, a Medical Economics Company publication.)

testis differentiation (Fig. 2.12). Gonadal dysgenesis (45XO), mixed gonadal dysgenesis (46XY/45XO), and Klinefelter's syndrome (47XXY) are all characterized by an abnormality in the sex chromosome number. The exact mechanism responsible for gonadal development in true hermaphroditism is poorly understood, because many dysgenic patterns have been described, including 46XX (most common), 46XY, and various mosaicisms. It is thought that testis development in true hermaphroditism in which no Y chromosome is present is probably derived from translocated genetic material from a Y chromosome. Alternatively, differential growth rates of the undifferentiated gonad may lead to development of a testis on one side and an ovary on the other. The gonad with accelerated growth forms a testis despite the presence or absence of testis-determining antigens.

Disorders of gonadal sex are caused by abnormalities of gonadal development in which the chromosomal sex does not correlate with the gonadal or phenotypic sex. These disorders include pure gonadal dysgenesis, either 46XY or 46XX, and gonadal agenesis (testicular regression). Pure gonadal dysgenesis occurs in phenotypic females with streak gonads who lack the somatic features of gonadal dysgenesis (Turner's syndrome) and who may have either a 46XX or 46XY complement. Regardless of the chromosomal complement, a female phenotype develops with a rudimentary internal müllerian ductal system as a result of failure of gonadal development.

Disorders of phenotypic sex are those syndromes in which a normal chromosomal complement and appropriate gonadal development are seen; however, the phenotypic expression is either incomplete or in contradistinction to the chromosomal and phenotypic sex. These syndromes are categorized into female and male pseudohermaphroditism.

Female pseudohermaphroditism, or virilization of a 46XX patient with ovaries, is caused by either endogenous androgen production (congenital adrenal hyperplasia, maternal virilizing tumor) or exogenous androgen administration. Congenital adrenal hyperplasia is an inherited disorder in which one of five enzymes responsible for the production of cortisol from cholesterol is deficient. Androgen synthesis shares the initial three steps of this pathway. A deficiency of the two enzymes responsible for glucocorticoid synthesis (21-hydroxylase and 11-β-hydroxylase) affects only hydrocortisol production. Lack of hydrocortisol induces increased production of adrenocorticotropin hormone, which in turn forces the steroid pathway toward increased production of adrenal androgens. Deficiencies of the proximal three enzymes in the pathway (20,22-desmolase, 3-β-hydroxysteroid dehydrogenase, 17-hydroxylase) affect both glucocorticoid and androgen production, which results in congenital adrenal hyperplasia and undervirilization of the male. In the female, normal ovaries, müllerian structures, and varying degrees of external virilization are found, depending on the severity of the enzyme deficiency.

Other causes of female pseudohermaphroditism are rare in comparison to congenital adrenal hyperplasia. Maternal ingestion of certain progestins used to maintain pregnancy may cause external virilization; however, it is usually not seen to the same degree as occurs in congenital adrenal hyperplasia. This is true also for maternal virilizing tumors, for example, arrhenoblastomas or luteomas.

Male pseudohermaphroditism, or inadequate virilization of the 46XY male with normal testes, is the result of one of:

- deficient MIF (hernia uteri inguinali);
- defective androgen synthesis;
- defective androgen action; or
- deficiency of 5α-reductase (pseudovaginal perineoscrotal hypospadias).

Deficiency of MIF leads to the persistent müllerian duct syndrome. These 46XY males are fully virilized because testosterone is produced normally; however, they have either unilateral or bilateral fallopian tubes, a uterus, and the upper third of the vagina. This is thought to occur because of deficient MIF production by the fetal testis or inability of the müllerian ducts to respond to MIF.

A defect in one of five enzymatic steps in the synthesis of testosterone from cholesterol leads to deficient androgen production. As noted, the initial three enzymatic steps are common to adrenal glucocorticoid synthesis as well; therefore, a deficiency in one of these initial enzymes results in congenital adrenal hyperplasia in an undervirilized male.

Androgen insensitivity or defective androgen action is a result of a deficiency of the cytoplasmic receptor protein needed to transport DHT into the cell nucleus to mediate virilization. The same, or a similar, protein is necessary to transport testosterone into the nucleus to stimulate spermatogenesis. The result is an undervirilized male with normal testes. The degree of undervirilization depends on the degree of deficiency of the androgen-binding protein. When severe deficiency is present, the external genitalia are completely feminized with a short vagina, no internal müllerian structures, and intra-abdominal testes (complete testicular feminization). These patients present with either a palpable inguinal testis in a hernia sac or primary amenorrhea. Incomplete forms of testicular feminization are also seen, although these are much less frequent. Incomplete forms may be seen as mild virilization of what appears to be female genitalia (Lubs syndrome) or infertility because of azoospermia (infertile male syndrome).

Lack of 5α-reductase in target cells results in a failure of conversion of testosterone into DHT, which causes undervirilization of the external genitalia. The wolffian ductal system, because of adequate testosterone production and action, develops normally. The syndrome is sometimes referred to descriptively as pseudovaginal perineoscrotal hypospadias. Such children appear feminized with a mild degree of clitoral hypertrophy. Most are assigned a female gender and may not be seen by a physician unless a testis is palpable inguinally or masculinization occurs at puberty because of the increased testosterone production.

TESTICULAR DESCENT

Chromosomal sex determines gonadal sex. Genes located on the distal portion of the short arm of the Y chromosomes produces SRY protein, which attaches to the undifferentiated gonadal primordia to induce testicular development. By the sixth week of gestation, the germ cells have migrated in a cephalad direction to the gonadal ridges, adjacent to the mesonephros. The gubernaculum is apparent at this stage as a mesenchymal

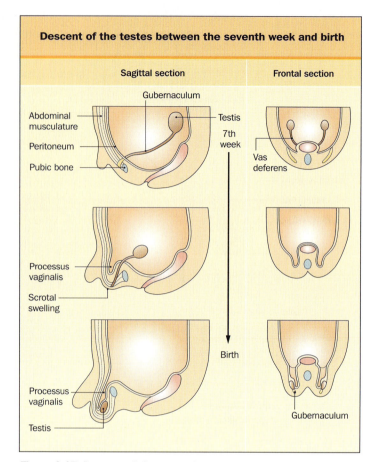

Figure 2.17 Descent of the testes between the seventh week and birth. (Adapted with permission from Larsen[1].)

ridge that extends from the genital swelling to the gonadal ridges[34,35]. The processus vaginalis develops ventral to the gubernaculum as an outpouching of the peritoneum.

Descent of the testis (Fig. 2.17) is thought to occur in two phases; intra-abdominal migration and inguinal migration. By the end of the first trimester, the testis lies just proximal to the internal inguinal ring. Whether this represents true migration of the testis from the gonadal ridges or results from differential body growth remains unclear. MIF may play an active role in the intra-abdominal phase of testicular descent.

The inguinal phase of testicular descent occurs early in the third trimester of gestation (Fig. 2.18). The gubernaculum, which attaches to the epididymis, swells while the processus vaginalis extends to the scrotum. Swelling and contraction of the gubernaculum results in descent of the epididymis, followed rapidly by descent of the testis. Once the testis reaches the scrotum, the proximal processus vaginalis obliterates while the distal end forms the tunica vaginalis.

Various theories have been proposed regarding testicular descent. Endocrine factors, supplemented by mechanical factors, probably play the major role in testicular descent[37–39]. In 1932, Engle demonstrated that premature testicular descent in monkeys could be induced by gonadotropins. The mediating agent is thought to be DHT, which may affect the gubernaculum either directly or through action on the genitofemoral nerve. Data indicate that cryptorchid infants have an abnormality of the

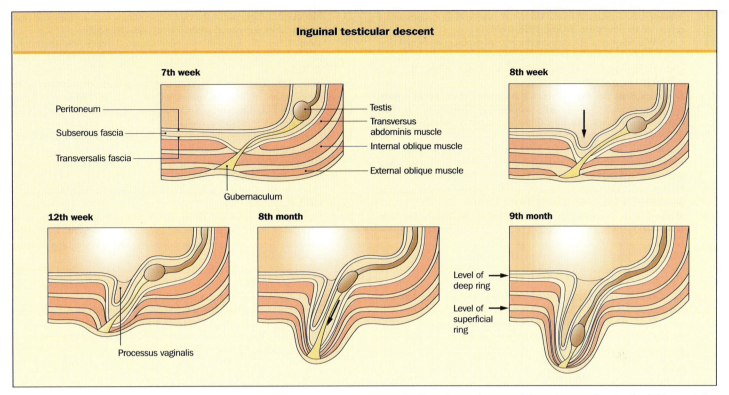

Figure 2.18 Inguinal testicular descent with development of the processus vaginalis and attachment of the gubernaculum to the labioscrotal folds. (Adapted with permission from Larsen[1].)

hypothalmic–pituitary–gonadal axis (decreased basal luteinizing hormone and testosterone and blunted response to gonadotropin-releasing hormone) that is not detectable before puberty.

Intra-abdominal pressure is thought to play a role in testicular descent. Evidence for this comes from experimental studies and observation of certain clinical states (such as prune-belly syndrome, abdominal wall defects, and diaphragmatic hernia) that are accompanied by an increased incidence of testicular maldescent. The traction theory proposes that the gubernaculum and/or cremasteric muscles pull the testis into the scrotum. This may be mediated by the genitofemoral nerve, which supplies the gubernaculum. The role of the cremasteric muscle has been

refuted. Since the gubernaculum is thought to attach to the epididymis, abnormal development or attachment of the ductal system to the testes could also lead to testicular maldescent. The ductal system develops abnormally in approximately one-third of males with undescended testes, a higher incidence than that of the case of more proximal undescended testes. The differential growth rate theory assumes a more passive role of the testis in descent; it proposes that the testis remains at an internal inguinal ring location, but rapid growth of the body wall causes the testis to find itself in the scrotum. The presence of active changes in gubernaculum development provides evidence against this theory.

REFERENCES

1. Larsen WJ. Essentials of human embryology. New York: Churchill Livingstone; 1998.
2. Potter EL. Normal and abnormal development of the kidney. Chicago: Year Book Medical Publishers; 1972.
3. Maizels M. Normal and anomalous development of the urinary tract. In Walsh PC, Retik AB, Vaughan ED Jr, Wein AJ, eds. Campbell's urology, 7th edn. Philadelphia: WB Saunders; 1998:1545–1600.
4. Grobstein C. Trans-filter induction of tubules in mouse metanephrogenic mesenchyme. Exp Cell Res. 1956;10:424.
5. Ashley DJB, Mostofi FK. Renal agenesis and dysgenesis. J Urol. 1960;83:211–30.
6. Rubenstein M, Meyer R, Bernstein J. Congenital abnormalities of the urinary system. I. A postmortem survey of the developmental

anomalies and acquired congenital lesions in a children's hospital. J Pediatr. 1961;58:356.
7. Berman DJ, Maizels M. The role of urinary obstruction in the genesis of renal dysplasia: a model in the chick embryo. J Urol. 1982;128:1091–6.
8. Tanagho EA. Surgically induced partial ureteral obstruction in the fetal lamb. III. Ureteral obstruction. Invest Urol. 1972;10:35–52.
9. Maizels M, Simpson SB Jr. Primitive ducts of renal dysplasia induced by culturing ureteral buds denuded of condensed renal mesenchyme. Science. 1983;219:509–10.
10. Mackie GG, Stephens FD. Duplex kidneys. A correlation of renal dysplasia with position of the ureteral orifice. J Urol. 1975; 114:274–80.

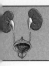

11. Wilmer HA. Unilateral fused kidney: A report of five cases and a review of the literature. J Urol. 1938;40:551.

12. Cook WA, Stephens FD. Fused kidneys: morphologic study and theory of embryogenesis. In Bergsma D, Duckett JW, eds. Urinary system malformations in children. New York: Allen R. Liss; 1977:327–40.

13. Bauer SB, Retik AB, Perlmutter AD. Anomalies of the upper urinary tract. In Walsh PC, Retik AB, Stamey TA, Vaughan ED Jr, eds. Campbell's urology, 6th edn. Philadelphia: WB Saunders; 1992: 1357–442.

14. Hanna MK, Jeffs RD, Sturgess JM, et al. Ureteral structure and ultrastructure. Part II. Congenital ureteropelvic obstruction and primary obstructive megaureter. J Urol. 1976;116:725–30.

15. Notley RG. Electron microscopy of the upper ureter and the pelviuretric junction. Br J Urol. 1968;40:37.

16. Ruano-Gil D, Coca-Payeras A, Tejedo-Maten A. Obstruction and normal re-canalization of the ureter in the human embryo: its relation to congenital ureteric obstruction. Eur Urol. 1975;1:287–93.

17. Maizels M, Stephens FD. Valves of the ureter as a cause of primary obstruction of the ureter: anatomic, embryologic and clinical aspects. J Urol. 1980;123:742–7.

18. Tanagho EA. Embryologic basis for lower ureteral anomalies: a hypothesis. Urology. 1976;7:451–64.

19. Chwalle R. The process of formation of cystic dilatations of the vesical end of the ureter and of diverticula at the ureteral ostium. Urol Cutan Rev. 1927;31:499.

20. Stephens FD. Congenital malformations of the rectum, anus and genitourinary tracts. London: E & S Livingstone; 1963.

21. Tanagho EA. Intrauterine fetal ureteral obstruction. J Urol. 1973; 109:196–203.

22. Muecke EC. Exstrophy, epispadias, and other anomalies of the bladder. In Walsh PC, et al., eds. Campbell's urology, 5th edn. Philadelphia: WB Saunders; 1986:1856.

23. Retik AB, Bauer SB. Bladder and urachus. In Kelalis PP, King LR, Belman AB, eds. Clinical pediatric urology. Philadelphia: WB Saunders; 1976:544.

24. Muecke EC. The role of the cloacal membrane in exstrophy: the first successful experimental study. J Urol. 1964;92:659–67.

25. Tolmatschen N. Ein fall von semilunaren klappen der harnrohre und von vergrosserter vasicula prostatica. Arch Pathol Anat. 1870;49:348.

26. Beck AD. The effect of intra-uterine urinary obstruction upon development of the fetal kidney. J Urol. 1971;105:784–9.

27. Stephens FD. Congenital malformations of the urinary tract. New York: Praeger Publishers; 1983.

28. Devine CJ Jr. Embryology of the male external genitalia. Clin Plast Surg. 1980;7:141–8.

29. Glenister TW. The origin and fate of the urethral plate in man. J Anat. 1954;288:413.

30. Hawkins JR. Cloning and mutational analysis of SRY. Horm Res. 1992;38:222–5.

31. Najmabadi H, Chai N, Kapali A, et al. Genomic structure of a Y-specific ribonucleic acid binding motif-containing gene: a putative candidate for a subset of male infertility. J Clin Endocrinol Metab. 1996;81:2159–64.

32. Aaronson IA. Sexual differentiation and intersexuality. In: Kelalis PP, King LR, Belman AB, eds. Clinical pediatric urology, 3rd edn. Philadelphia: WB Saunders; 1992:977–1014.

33. Rubenstein SD, Mandell J. The diagnostic approach to the newborn with ambiguous genitalia. Contemp Urol. 1994;14–15.

34. Heynes CF, Hutson JM. Historical review of theories on testicular descent. J Urol. 1995;153:754–67.

35. Heynes CF. The gubernaculum during testicular descent in the human fetus. J Anat. 1987;153:93.

36. Rajfer J. Hormonal regulation of testicular descent. Eur J Ped. 1987;146(Suppl 2):S6–S7.

37. Husmann DA, McPhaul MJ. Localization of the androgen receptor in the developing rat gubernaculum. Endocrinology. 1991; 128:383–7.

38. Rajfer J, Walsh PC. Hormonal regulation of testicular descent: experimental and clinical observations. J Urol. 1977;118:985–90.

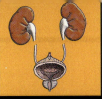

Chapter
3
Applied Anatomy of the Urinary Tract

JA Gosling and JS Dixon

KIDNEYS

The two kidneys lie behind the peritoneum on either side of the upper lumbar vertebrae. They are embedded in fat in the paravertebral gutters of the posterior abdominal wall and are placed obliquely with their anterior surfaces directed slightly laterally (Fig. 3.1). The left kidney usually lies at a higher level than the right.

Each kidney is bean-shaped, flattened anteroposteriorly, and approximately 11cm long. The anterior and posterior surfaces are gently convex and the superior and inferior poles are rounded. The lateral border is convex while the indented medial border bears an aperture, the hilum (Fig. 3.2), which is traversed by the renal pelvis or ureter, the renal vessels, lymphatics, and autonomic nerves. The hilum leads into a cavity within the kidney, the renal sinus, which is occupied by the calices and renal pelvis (Fig. 3.3), the renal blood vessels, and a quantity of fat.

Covered by a thin capsule, the kidney comprises an outer cortex and an inner medulla. The medulla contains numerous pyramids the apices of which project into the renal sinus as the renal papillae. Urine discharged from the papillae is collected by about ten trumpet-shaped chambers, the minor calices, which unite to form two or three major calices. These fuse into the

single, funnel-shaped renal pelvis, which lies posterior to most of the vessels and is continuous with the ureter (see Fig. 3.3).

Control of ureteric peristalsis

The minor calices are spontaneously active regions of pacemaker muscle cells that initiate and exert a controlling influence on the peristaltic activity of the ureter[1,2]. Since each minor calix possesses such cells (and is linked across the renal parenchyma to other calices by similar cells), the number of pacemaker sites within a given system is related to the number of minor calices. It is probable that the normal sequence of events begins with the initiation of a contraction wave at one of the several minor caliceal pacemaker sites. Once initiated, the contraction is propagated through the wall of the adjacent major calix and activates the smooth muscle of the renal pelvis. The proximal pacemaker site for successive contractions usually changes between the minor calices, although sometimes the same minor calix initiates consecutive contractions before the site changes. Functionally, the proximal location of these pacemaker sites ensures that, once initiated, contraction waves are propagated away from the kidney, which thereby avoids undesirable pressure

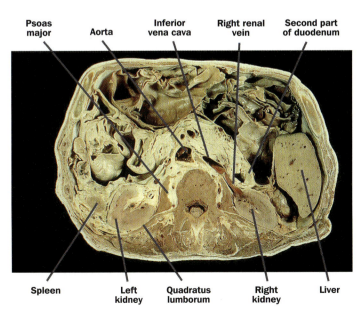

Figure 3.1 Transverse section at the level of the second lumbar vertebra showing the oblique position of the kidneys in the paravertebral gutters viewed from above.

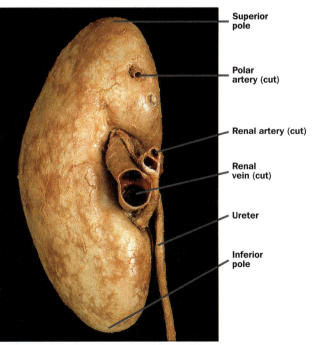

Figure 3.2 Medial aspect of the right kidney showing the renal vessels passing through the hilum.

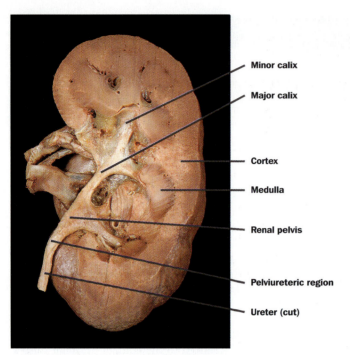

Figure 3.3 Right kidney dissected from behind to show the renal pelvis and calices located in the renal sinus.

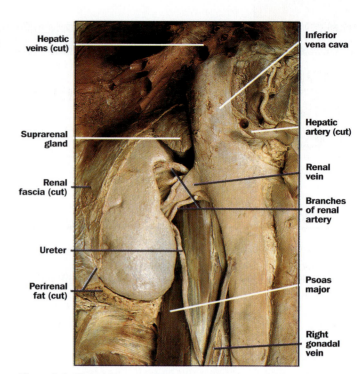

Figure 3.4 Right kidney and suprarenal gland seen within the renal fascia and perirenal fat, part of which has been removed.

rises directed against the renal parenchyma. In addition, since several potential pacemaker sites exist, the initiation of contraction waves is unimpaired by partial nephrectomy because the minor calices spared by the resection remain *in situ* and continue their pacemaker function.

Each contraction wave extends across the renal pelvis as far as the pelviureteric region; it seems likely that the onward transmission into the ureter is dependent upon the volume of fluid contained within the renal pelvis. At high urine flow rates, every contraction wave that reaches the pelviureteric region is propagated as a ureteric contraction wave. At low flow rates not all of the renal pelvic contractions are transmitted to the ureter. Only when a sufficient quantity of urine has accumulated in the renal pelvis does a pelvic contraction wave propagate distally beyond the pelviureteric region. Thus, the pelviureteric region acts as a 'gate' that allows ureteric peristalsis to occur only when the volume of each bolus of urine propelled from the renal pelvis is above a critical amount[2].

In summary, ureteric peristalsis is apparently dependent upon two mechanisms within the proximal part of the urinary tract:

- contraction waves in the renal pelvis are initiated by spontaneously active pacemaker sites located within the wall of each minor calix; and
- a regulating mechanism at the pelviureteric region determines whether a contraction of the renal pelvis is propagated into the ureter.

The latter event is related to urine flow and probably depends upon the stretching forces or tension generated in the wall of the pelviureteric region. It is unclear whether a malfunction of one or both of these mechanisms is involved in the etiology of functional obstruction of the upper urinary tract.

Contraction waves are thought to be propagated across the renal pelvis and along the ureter by means of myogenic conduction, which results from electronic coupling of one muscle cell to

its immediate neighbors. The direction of propagation is normally from the renal pelvis toward the bladder, as dictated by the pacemaker mechanism in the minor calices. Since muscle cells can conduct from one cell to the next in either direction, the direction of propagation is sometimes reversed, which results in retrograde contraction waves. See also detail in Chapter 5.

Perirenal tissues

Each kidney is surrounded by a layer of perirenal fat enveloped in a thin sheet of connective tissue, the renal fascia (Fig. 3.4). This fascia also encloses the suprarenal gland and the proximal part of the ureter. From the inferior pole of the kidney, the renal fascia tapers downward into the iliac fossa. Around the fascia is a further layer of fat (pararenal fat) that lies against the posterior abdominal muscles and is covered anteriorly by the peritoneum.

Renal blood vessels

The most usual vascular arrangement of each kidney consists of a single renal artery derived from the abdominal aorta, accompanied on its anterior aspect by a renal vein that terminates in the inferior vena cava (Fig. 3.5). As each artery approaches the kidney, it divides into approximately five branches, which enter the renal hilum. In the renal sinus the arteries are usually arranged anterior and posterior to the urinary tract. These arteries pierce the walls of the sinus between the attachments of the minor calices and are accompanied by renal veins similar in number and arrangement. The veins usually continue as far as the renal hilum before they unite anterior to the urinary tract to form a single renal vein.

Variations from the above-described pattern are common and are of particular importance in the case of the arteries. Both supernumerary and polar arteries (Fig. 3.6) are encountered

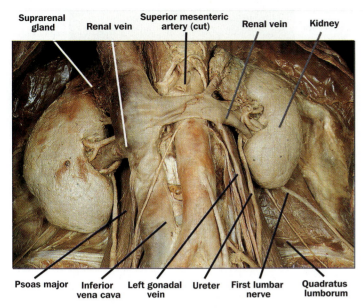

Suprarenal gland — Renal vein — Superior mesenteric artery (cut) — Renal vein — Kidney

Psoas major — Inferior vena cava — Left gonadal vein — Ureter — First lumbar nerve — Quadratus lumborum

Figure 3.5 Kidneys, suprarenal glands, and some of the vessels associated with them.

frequently. A supernumerary renal artery originates from the aorta at a level above or below that usually occupied by the renal artery. Alternatively, such vessels may arise from other sites, which include the common or internal iliac arteries or, more rarely, from the lumbar, gonadal, phrenic, median sacral, or external iliac vessels. Supernumerary renal arteries are present in approximately 20% of individuals. In some texts, such vessels are often described as 'anomalous', 'aberrant', or 'accessory' – terms that are inappropriate as these arteries are relatively common and form part of the essential blood supply to the kidney. Usually, supernumerary vessels traverse the renal hilum and pierce the renal substance from within the sinus, but they may occasionally enter the kidney directly by way of the medial border of the organ, either above or below the hilum. The latter vessels are examples of polar arteries, which provide the principal blood supply to the polar segments of renal parenchyma; ischemia and necrosis may follow their ligation. The latter events are explained by an important feature of intrarenal vascular anatomy – a kidney normally consists of five segments, each

supplied and drained by its own artery and vein. While effective anastomoses link adjacent segmental veins, the arteries are distributed exclusively to their own segments.

Relation of kidneys

The right and left kidneys have similar posterior relations. The superior poles lie against the diaphragm and the twelfth ribs, below which run the subcostal nerves and vessels. On the left the upper pole is also related, through the diaphragm, to the pleura and eleventh rib. The medial border of each kidney overlaps the psoas major, while the inferolateral portion is related to quadratus lumborum and transversus abdominis, and to the first lumbar nerve (Fig. 3.7).

The anterior relations of the kidneys are asymmetric. On the right, from above downward, they include the bare area of the liver, the second part of the duodenum, the right flexure of the colon, and the coils of jejunum. The medial border of the right kidney is related to the inferior vena cava, the renal vessels, and the upper part of the ureter.

On the left, from above downward, the anterior relations include the stomach and spleen, the splenic vessels, the tail of the pancreas, the left colic flexure, and the coils of jejunum. The medial border relates to the suprarenal gland, the renal and suprarenal vessels, the left gonadal vein, and the proximal part of the ureter.

SUPRARENAL GLANDS

The suprarenal glands lie adjacent to the superior poles of the kidneys, embedded in the perirenal fat. On the right the gland is tetrahedral and occupies the angle between the superior pole of the kidney and the inferior vena cava (Fig. 3.8). The left gland is crescentic and is applied to the medial border of the kidney above the hilum (Fig. 3.9).

The blood supply to the suprarenal glands is provided by branches of the renal and inferior phrenic arteries and the aorta. The right suprarenal vein is very short and enters the inferior vena cava directly, while that on the left descends to enter the left renal vein.

The medulla of each suprarenal gland is richly innervated by preganglionic sympathetic nerves from the adjacent part of the sympathetic trunk.

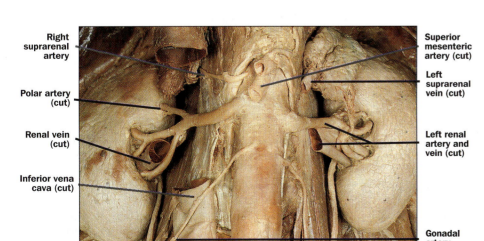

Right suprarenal artery — Polar artery (cut) — Renal vein (cut) — Inferior vena cava (cut)

Superior mesenteric artery (cut) — Left suprarenal vein (cut) — Left renal artery and vein (cut)

Gonadal artery

Figure 3.6 Renal arteries exposed by removal of the renal veins and a portion of the inferior vena cava. Note the polar artery that supplies the upper pole of the right kidney.

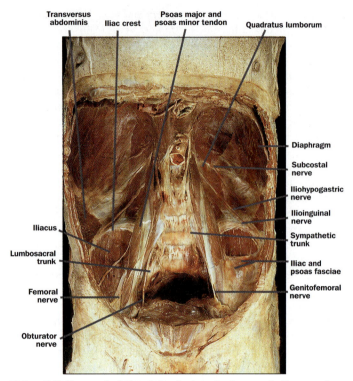

Figure 3.7 Removal of the abdominal contents reveals the muscles and nerves of the posterior abdominal wall. On one side some iliac and psoas fasciae have been preserved and the nerves that form the posterior relations of the kidneys are clearly evident.

URETERS

Relations of ureters

From the pelviureteric region each ureter descends through the retroperitoneal tissues of the posterior abdominal wall as far as the pelvic brim. Here it crosses in front of the external iliac vessels and continues down the lateral wall of the pelvis. Within the abdomen the ureter lies on psoas major, behind which are the lumbar transverse processes.

The right ureter commences behind the second part of the duodenum and is crossed by the root of the mesentery, the gonadal vessels (Fig. 3.10), and branches of the superior mesenteric artery and accompanying veins. This ureter is also related to coils of small intestine, and sometimes to the caecum and appendix. The left ureter is covered initially by the pancreas and is crossed subsequently by the gonadal vessels (Fig. 3.11), branches of the inferior mesenteric artery, and vein and coils of small intestine and sigmoid colon. At the pelvic brim, it passes behind the root of the sigmoid mesocolon. During retroperitoneal exploration for the ureter, the structure is almost invariably elevated with the peritoneum.

Each ureter enters the pelvis by crossing in front of the common iliac vessels or the commencement of the external iliac vessels, a particularly useful landmark for locating the tube at surgery (Fig. 3.12). The ureter passes downward and backward before it curves forward to reach the posterior surface of the bladder. The ureter crosses the medial aspect of the obturator nerve and vessels and the superior vesical vessels before it runs forward along the levator ani muscle. The pelvic peritoneum

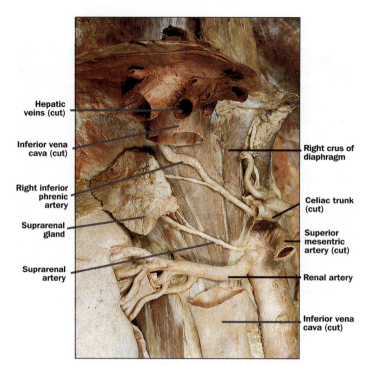

Figure 3.8 Right suprarenal gland and its arteries exposed by removal of the renal vein and a portion of the inferior vena cava.

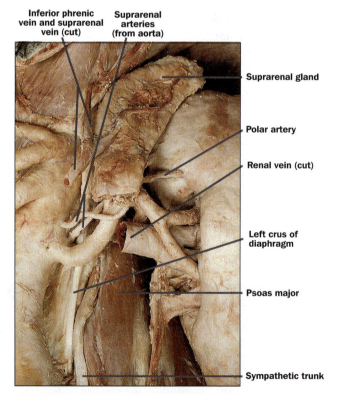

Figure 3.9 Left suprarenal gland and its vessels. The renal vein and inferior tip of the gland have been excised to reveal the suprarenal arteries.

covers the medial aspect of the ureter and separates it from the rectum, sigmoid colon, and coils of ileum.

In the male the ureter passes under the vas deferens and terminates near the seminal vesicle (Fig. 3.13). In the female the

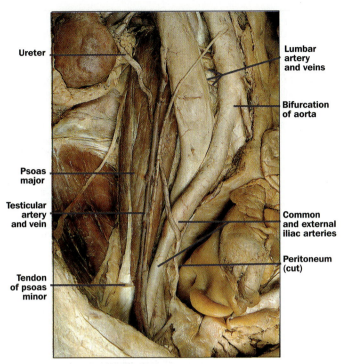

Figure 3.10 The right ureter lies on the psoas major and is crossed by the testicular vessels.

Labels: Ureter; Psoas major; Testicular artery and vein; Tendon of psoas minor; Lumbar artery and veins; Bifurcation of aorta; Common and external iliac arteries; Peritoneum (cut)

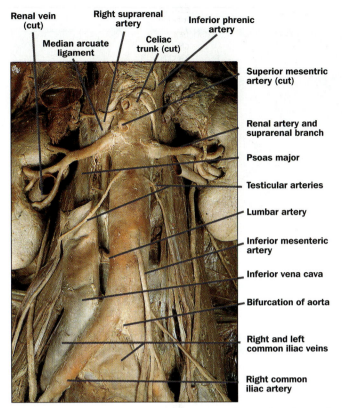

Figure 3.11 Both ureters cross the psoas major as they descend toward the pelvis. On the left, the ureter is crossed by the testicular artery and a branch from the inferior mesenteric artery.

Labels: Renal vein (cut); Median arcuate ligament; Right suprarenal artery; Celiac trunk (cut); Inferior phrenic artery; Superior mesentric artery (cut); Renal artery and suprarenal branch; Psoas major; Testicular arteries; Lumbar artery; Inferior mesenteric artery; Inferior vena cava; Bifurcation of aorta; Right and left common iliac veins; Right common iliac artery

ureter descends close to the posterior aspect of the ovary and is covered with peritoneum as far as the root of the broad ligament. Here the ureter crosses under the uterine artery and is closely related to the lateral aspect of the uterine cervix.

Blood supply and lymphatic drainage

The calices and the renal pelvis receive their blood supply via minute branches from the renal arteries within the renal sinus; the renal veins receive the venous drainage from these parts of the urinary tract. Each ureter obtains arterial branches – which are often quite long despite their small diameter – from several sources. Although the precise arrangement of vessels is very variable, the general pattern can be described by considering the ureter in three portions.

The uppermost third is supplied by branches that arise from the renal artery, supplemented by vessels from the gonadal and

colic arteries. The vascularization of the intermediate portion of the ureter is subject to considerable variation. Usually, this segment is supplied by one or more vessels that originate directly from the aorta, although the iliac and gonadal arteries are also potential sources of supply. In a small proportion of individuals, the blood supply may be provided solely by minute peritoneal vessels. The pelvic portion of the ureter receives arterial contributions from the vesical arteries, augmented by branches of the uterine or middle rectal arteries.

The small arteries that supply the ureter adhere to the overlying peritoneum and, on reaching the viscus, subdivide into ascending and descending branches, which form a plexus in the

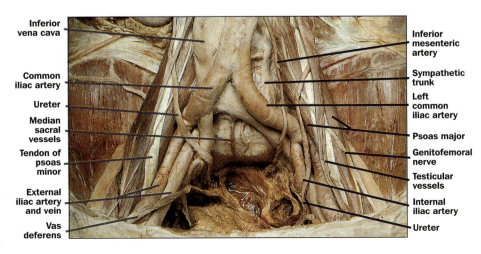

Labels: Inferior vena cava; Common iliac artery; Ureter; Median sacral vessels; Tendon of psoas minor; External iliac artery and vein; Vas deferens; Inferior mesenteric artery; Sympathetic trunk; Left common iliac artery; Psoas major; Genitofemoral nerve; Testicular vessels; Internal iliac artery; Ureter

Figure 3.12 In this specimen both ureters cross the commencement of the external iliac arteries and enter the pelvis anterior to the internal iliac arteries.

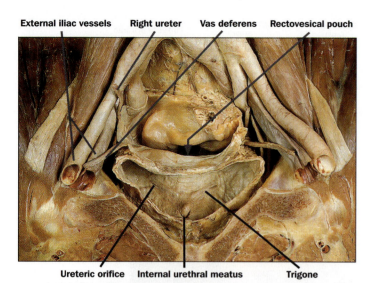

External iliac vessels | Right ureter | Vas deferens | Rectovesical pouch

Ureteric orifice | Internal urethral meatus | Trigone

Figure 3.13 Coronal section through the male pelvis to show the interior of the bladder and some of its relations.

ureteric adventitial coat. The venous plexus of the ureteric adventitia drains both proximally to the renal and gonadal veins and distally to the uterine veins and the vesical venous plexus.

The lymphatic channels of the ureter follow the course of the arteries and carry the lymph predominantly in proximal or distal directions to the lumbar and pelvic lymph nodes.

The ureteric muscle coat

The muscle coat of the ureter is fairly uniform in thickness throughout its length, with a width of about 800μm. The muscle bundles that constitute this musculature are frequently separated from one another by relatively large amounts of connective tissue. Branches that interconnect muscle bundles are common and result in frequent interchange of muscle fibers between adjacent bundles. As a result of this extensive branching, individual muscle bundles do not spiral around the ureter as has often been described, but rather form a complex meshwork of interweaved and interconnected smooth muscle bundles[3]. In addition, unlike those in the gut, the muscle bundles are so arranged that morphologically distinct longitudinal and circular layers cannot be distinguished. However, in the upper part of the ureter, the inner muscle bundles tend to lie longitudinally, while those on the outer aspect have a circular or oblique orientation. In the middle and lower parts of the ureter, additional outer fibers orientated longitudinally are also present. As the ureterovesical junction is approached, the ureteric muscle coat consists predominantly of muscle bundles orientated longitudinally.

Innervation of the upper urinary tract

The upper urinary tract receives efferent and afferent innervation from both the sympathetic and parasympathetic parts of the autonomic nervous system. The sympathetic contribution is derived from the lower thoracic and upper lumbar segments (T11 to L2) of the spinal cord and passes to the kidney and upper ureter by way of the thoracic and lumbar splanchnic nerves and then via the celiac, superior hypogastric, and renal plexuses. The parasympathetic nerves originate in the sacral portion of the spinal cord, from the second, third, and fourth

segments. These fibers travel by way of the pelvic splanchnic nerves via the pelvic plexuses to reach the juxtavesical parts of the ureters. Parasympathetic nerves that are destined for the proximal parts of the ureters and the calices ascend in the hypogastric (presacral) nerves. There is considerable intermingling of the different types of autonomic nerve so that it is impossible to separate them by gross dissection.

The muscle coat of the caliceal wall, the renal pelvis, and the ureter receive dual autonomic innervation by both noradrenergic and cholinergic nerve fibers. Some of these nerves directly innervate smooth muscle cells within the wall of the upper urinary tract, while others form dense perivascular nerve plexuses[4]. The density of innervation throughout the ureteric wall gradually increases in a proximodistal direction, so that the juxtavesical segment of each ureter is innervated relatively richly[5]. Ganglion cells do not occur in the wall of the upper urinary tract.

Autonomic nerves in the wall of the upper urinary tract presumably have a modulatory function on the contractile activity of the muscle coat. However, it is believed generally that they are not directly responsible for the propagation of contraction waves, since the electrical activity measured in the ureteric wall during peristalsis together with the rate of propagation of contraction waves are characteristic of smooth muscle and not nervous activity[6,7]. Furthermore, the ratio of axon terminals to smooth muscle cells is extremely low, and also the ureteric peristalsis continues *in vivo* in the presence of nerve-blocking agents, such as tetrodotoxin, and *in vitro* in denervated ureteric segments[8].

URINARY BLADDER

The urinary bladder lies in the anterior part of the pelvic cavity. When distended the organ has an approximately spheric shape, but when empty it assumes the form of a tetrahedron with four angles and four surfaces. The two posterolateral angles receive the ureters, while the inferior angle (the bladder neck) is continuous with the urethra. The anterior angle gives attachment to a fibrous cord, the urachus. This remnant of the fetal allantois ascends in the extraperitoneal tissues of the anterior abdominal wall to the umbilicus.

The superior surface and the two inferolateral surfaces expand considerably as urine accumulates, but the comparatively small posterior surface or base expands only a little. This surface lies between the entrances of the ureters and the bladder neck.

Although the interior of the distended bladder is smooth, the mucosa becomes rugose when the organ empties, except in the region of the trigone[9]. This is the triangular area between the ureteric orifices and the internal urethral meatus (Fig. 3.13).

The distal 1–2cm of each ureter is surrounded by an incomplete collar of detrusor smooth muscle, which forms a sheath (of Waldeyer) separated from the ureteric muscle coat by a connective tissue sleeve[10]. The ureters pierce the posterior aspect of the bladder and run obliquely through its wall for a distance of 1.5–2.0cm before terminating at the ureteric orifices. This arrangement is believed to assist in the prevention of ureteric reflux, since the intramural ureters are thought to be occluded during increases in bladder pressure. The longitudinally orientated muscle bundles of the terminal ureter continue into the bladder wall and at the ureteric orifices become continuous with the superficial trigonal muscle.

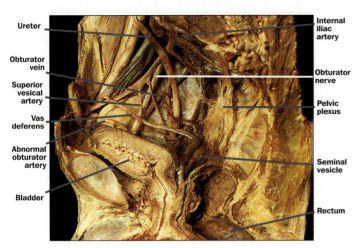

Figure 3.14 A dissection to demonstrate the relationships and blood supply of the male bladder. The pelvic plexus of autonomic nerves lies on the lateral aspect of the pelvic cavity.

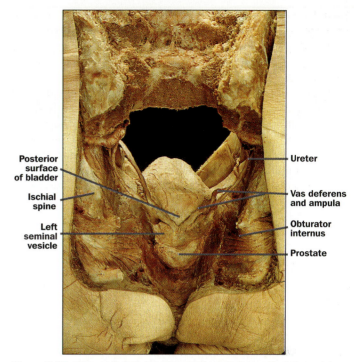

Figure 3.15 Removal of the rectum and posterior wall of the pelvis exposes the bladder, prostate, seminal vesicles, and vasa deferentia.

A recent histologic study of the ureterovesical junction in infants[11] demonstrated an incomplete intermediate muscle layer that lies between the intramural ureteric muscle coat and the surrounding detrusor muscle. It has been suggested that these clusters of tightly packed smooth muscle cells may represent a remnant of the mesonephric duct from which the ureter originates during fetal development[11,12].

Relations of the urinary bladder

The superior surface of the bladder is covered with peritoneum on which rests coils of ileum and sigmoid colon. In both sexes the inferolateral surfaces lie against the obturator internus and levator ani muscles and their associated fascial coverings. Between the bladder and these muscles run the obturator nerve and vessels and the superior vesical vessels (Fig. 3.14). Anterior to the bladder is the retropubic space, filled with adipose tissue and veins. The empty bladder lies behind the pubic bones, but as it fills it rises above the level of the pubic crests and comes into contact with the lower part of the anterior abdominal wall. The distended bladder intervenes between the parietal peritoneum and the abdominal wall; surgical access to the organ can be made through an abdominal incision without opening the peritoneum.

In the male the seminal vesicle and the ampulla of the vas deferens are applied to each side of the posterior surface (Fig. 3.15). Peritoneum descends a short distance on this surface before being reflected onto the anterior surface of the rectum to form the rectovesical pouch. Below the level of this pouch the bladder is related to the rectovesical septum and the ampulla of the rectum. Inferior to the male bladder lie the prostate gland (Fig. 3.16) and the prostatic plexus of veins.

In the female the posterior part of the superior surface of the bladder is related to the body of the uterus. Peritoneum passes from the superior surface of the bladder onto the uterine body, which forms the vesicouterine pouch. Against the posterior surface of the female bladder lie the cervix of the uterus and the anterior wall of the vagina. The inferior angle of the bladder in the female lies at a lower level than in the male and is closely related to the two levator ani muscles.

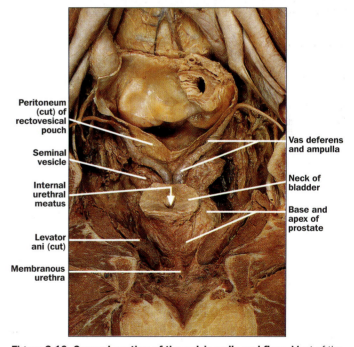

Figure 3.16 Coronal section of the pelvic walls and floor. Most of the bladder has been removed to reveal the prostate, the seminal vesicles, and the vasa deferentia.

Blood supply of the urinary bladder

In both sexes the arterial supply to the bladder is provided by branches of the internal iliac arteries. The largest branches are usually the superior vesical arteries, which run anteriorly along the lateral pelvic walls and then divide into two or more terminal vessels that extend medially to reach the bladder. Additional branches arise from the internal iliac arteries and all of these are involved in the supply of blood to the inferior aspects of the bladder wall. These vessels include the inferior vesical, the obturator, and the inferior gluteal arteries. In the female the uterine and vaginal arteries also contribute to the vascular supply of the bladder.

Venous blood from the bladder passes into the extensive plexuses of veins that lie within the pelvis in both sexes. The vesical venous plexus lies in the fascia close to the neck of the bladder and communicates with the prostatic or vaginal plexus of veins. Blood from these plexuses drains directly into the internal iliac veins, although anastomoses with the ovarian, superior rectal, and sacral veins provide alternative routes to the inferior vena cava.

Lymphatic drainage
Most of the lymph that originates in the wall of the urinary bladder is conveyed to the external iliac group of lymph nodes. In addition, lymph from the base and the inferolateral surfaces of the bladder may pass directly to lymph nodes alongside the internal iliac or common iliac vessels; lymph from the bladder neck may pass into sacral nodes situated posterior to the rectum.

Histology of the urinary bladder
The wall of the urinary bladder consists of three layers:
- outer adventitial layer of connective tissue, which possesses in some regions a serosal covering of peritoneum;
- smooth muscle layer (the detrusor muscle); and
- inner layer of mucous membrane that lines the interior of the bladder[13].

Detrusor muscle
The muscle coat of the bladder is composed of relatively large diameter interlacing bundles of smooth muscle cells arranged as a complex meshwork. Discrete layers of smooth muscle are not discernible, although muscle bundles orientated longitudinally tend to predominate on the inner and outer aspects of the detrusor muscle coat. Posteriorly, some of these outer longitudinal bundles extend over the bladder base and merge with the capsule of the prostate or with the anterior vaginal wall; other bundles extend on to the anterior aspect of the rectum to form the rectovesical muscle. Anteriorly, some outer longitudinal bundles continue into the pubovesical ligaments and contribute to the muscular component of these structures. Exchange of fibers between adjacent muscle bundles within the bladder wall frequently occurs so that, from a functional viewpoint, the detrusor comprises a single unit of interlacing smooth muscle that, on contraction, causes a reduction in all dimensions of the bladder lumen.

Nerve supply
The bladder receives an autonomic innervation derived from the left and right pelvic plexuses (see Fig. 3.14); these nerves usually accompany the principal vascular supply. That part of each pelvic plexus specifically related to the urinary bladder is sometimes designated the 'vesical plexus of autonomic nerves'. This plexus receives input from the pelvic splanchnic nerves derived from the second, third, and fourth sacral segments of the spinal cord. In addition, the inferior hypogastric (presacral) nerves carry fibers from the tenth thoracic to the second lumbar segments of the cord, which also contribute to the formation of the vesical plexus.

The vesical plexus lies adjacent to the posterior and lateral walls of the urinary bladder and includes many small autonomic ganglia that contain both sympathetic and parasympathetic neurons[14]. Similar mixed autonomic ganglia occur throughout all regions of the bladder wall, both within and on the outer surface of the detrusor muscle; occasional ganglia are found in the connective tissue of the mucosal lining[15].

Histochemical stain for acetylcholinesterase shows that the body of the human urinary bladder receives a profuse innervation by presumptive cholinergic nerves[16–18], which stimulate contraction of the bladder at the time of micturition. In contrast, the detrusor muscle is only very sparsely supplied with sympathetic (noradrenergic) nerves, those that do occur being mainly perivascular in location[19–21]. Thus, sympathetic nerves have little, if any, direct involvement in the control of bladder smooth muscle, although they do have an inhibitory influence on the parasympathetic neurons within the vesical plexus and intramural ganglia[22]. For further details see Chapter 6.

Bladder neck
The smooth muscle of this region is histologically, histochemically, and pharmacologically distinct from that which comprises the detrusor proper[23]. Hence the bladder neck should be considered as a separate functional unit. The arrangement of smooth muscle in this region is quite different in males and females and consequently each sex is described separately.

Male
At the male bladder neck, the smooth muscle cells form a complete circular collar, which extends distally; the location and orientation of its constituent fibers mean the terms internal, proximal, or preprostatic sphincter are suitable alternatives for this particular component of urinary tract smooth muscle. On stimulation the sympathetic nerves cause contraction of smooth muscle in the wall of the genital tract, which results in seminal emission. Concomitant sympathetic stimulation of the bladder neck muscle causes sphincteric closure of the region, and thereby prevents reflux of ejaculate into the bladder. Although this genital function of the male bladder neck is well established, it is not known whether the smooth muscle of this region plays an active role in maintaining urinary continence.

Female
Unlike the circularly orientated smooth muscle of the male bladder neck, the majority of muscle bundles in the female bladder neck extend obliquely or longitudinally into the urethral wall. The female does not therefore possess a smooth muscle sphincter at the bladder neck, and it is unlikely that active contraction of this region plays a significant part in the maintenance of female urinary continence.

THE FEMALE URETHRA

The female urethra is a fibromuscular tube 3–4cm long and begins at the internal urethral meatus of the bladder. Embedded in the anterior wall of the vagina, it inclines downward and forward through the pelvic floor and terminates in the vestibule at the external meatus between the clitoris and the vaginal opening.

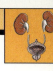

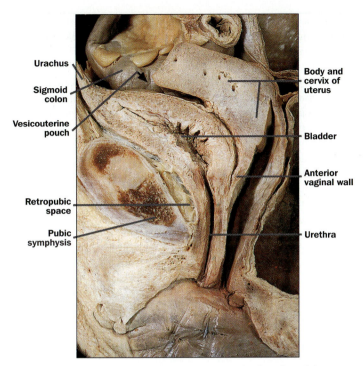

Figure 3.17 Median sagittal section through the female pelvis to show the bladder and urethra and some of their relationships.

The urethra passes close to the posterior aspect of the pubic symphysis (Fig. 3.17), to which it is attached by the pubourethral ligaments. The middle third of the urethra is encircled by striated muscle fibers of the external urethral sphincter, of which the tone is the principal factor to maintain continence of urine. Occlusive force on the urethra is also provided by contractions of the levator ani muscles. Micturition occurs when bladder pressure is higher than urethral pressure, and is produced by contraction of the detrusor muscle of the bladder wall accompanied by relaxation of the external urethral sphincter.

The arterial supply to the urethra is provided by the inferior vesical arteries, and venous drainage is to the vesical plexus of veins. The mucosa receives its sensory nerve supply from the pudendal nerve, derived from the second, third, and fourth sacral segments (which also innervate the external urethral sphincter by way of the pelvic splanchnic nerves).

THE PROSTATE GLAND

The prostate is shaped like an inverted pyramid and lies between the male urinary bladder and the pelvic floor. It has a base and an apex, and anterior, posterior, and inferolateral surfaces. The base is the upper surface adjacent to the bladder neck while the blunt apex is the lowest part. The anterior surface limits the retropubic space posteriorly and is connected inferiorly to the pubic bones by the puboprostatic ligaments. The inferolateral surfaces are clasped by the levator prostatae parts of the levator ani muscle[24], while the posterior surface lies in front of the lower rectum and is separated from it by the rectovesical fascia. The ejaculatory ducts pierce the posterior surface just below the bladder and pass obliquely through the gland for about 2cm, to open separately into the prostatic urethra about half way along its length on the verumontanum (Fig. 3.18).

A thin layer of connective tissue at the periphery of the prostate forms a 'true' capsule, outside of which is a condensation of pelvic fascia that forms the so-called 'false' capsule. A plexus of veins lies between these two capsules.

Blood supply and lymphatic drainage
The main arterial supply to the prostate is from the prostatic branch of the inferior vesical artery; some small branches from the middle rectal and internal pudendal vessels pass to the lower part. Occasionally, the middle rectal artery provides the major supply. The veins from the prostate form the prostatic venous plexus situated between the true capsule of the prostate and the outer fibrous sheath.

The lymph vessels from the prostate drain into the internal iliac nodes.

The prostatic urethra
The prostatic urethra is the widest and most dilatable part of the entire male urethra. It is about 3cm long and extends through the prostate from base to apex. The prostatic urethra is divided into proximal and distal segments of approximately equal length by an abrupt anterior angulation of its posterior wall at the midpoint between prostate apex and bladder neck. The angle of deviation is approximately 35°, but can be quite variable and tends to be greater in men with nodular hyperplasia. The prostatic urethra lies nearer the anterior than the posterior surface of the prostate. It is widest in the middle and

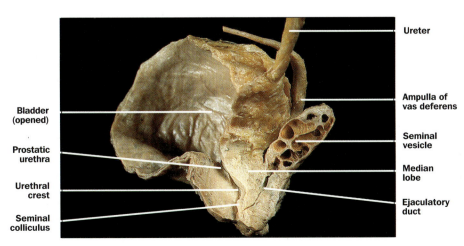

Figure 3.18 Dissection of prostate gland and left seminal vesicle.

narrowest below, and adjoins the membranous part. In cross-section it appears crescentic in outline, with the convex side facing ventrally.

The characteristic crescentic shape results from the presence on the posterior wall of a narrow median longitudinal ridge formed by an elevation of the mucous membrane and its subjacent tissue, called the urethral crest. On each side of the crest lies a shallow depression termed the prostatic sinus, the floor of which is pierced by the openings of the prostatic ducts. At about the middle of the length of the urethral crest, the colliculus seminalis (or verumontanum) forms an elevation on which the slit-like orifice of the prostatic utricle is situated. On each side of, or just within, this orifice are the openings of the two ejaculatory ducts (Fig. 3.19). The prostatic utricle is a blind-ending diverticulum about 6mm long, which extends upward and backward within the substance of the prostate. It develops from the paramesonephric ducts or urogenital sinus and as a consequence is a remnant of the system that forms the reproductive tract in the female.

The proximal urethral segment is surrounded by a sleeve of smooth muscle fibers, which form the preprostatic sphincter. Tiny ducts and abortive acinar systems are scattered along the length of the proximal urethral segment and arborize exclusively inside the confines of the preprostatic sphincter to form the periurethral gland region. The preprostatic sphincter is thought to function during ejaculation to prevent retrograde flow of seminal fluid from the distal urethral segment. It may also have resting tone that maintains closure of the proximal urethral segment and thereby aids urinary continence. The preprostatic sphincter is compact on the posterior aspect of the urethra; however, anteriorly its fibers do not form complete rings, but terminate within the tissue of the anterior fibromuscular stroma.

Slender bundles of smooth muscle cells also occur in the proximal part of the urethral crest, and extend as far as the prostatic utricle, where they become continuous with the muscle coat of the ejaculatory ducts[25]. Proximally, these muscle bundles are continuous with those that extend from the superficial trigone along the posterior wall of the preprostatic urethra.

Below the openings of the ejaculatory ducts the distal prostatic urethra possesses a thin coat of smooth muscle, which consists of both circularly and longitudinally orientated muscle bundles, which are themselves continuous with the strands of smooth muscle that pervade the prostate gland. The distal urethral segment is also surrounded by a sphincter formed of small-diameter, striated muscle fibers separated by connective tissue, which represent a proximal extension of the external sphincter located distal to the prostate apex. The sphincter within the prostate gland is incomplete posterolaterally where the striated fibers anchor into the prostatic stroma.

According to McNeal[26-28] the glandular prostate may be subdivided into three zones (Fig. 3.20):

- peripheral zone;
- central zone; and
- transitional zone.

Peripheral zone

The peripheral zone represents about 70% of the glandular part of the prostate. This zone forms the lateral and posterior or dorsal part of the organ. It may be regarded as a funnel that distally constitutes the apex of the prostate and cranially opens to receive the distal part of the wedge-shaped central zone. The ducts of the peripheral zone open into the distal prostatic urethra. They extend mainly laterally in the coronal plane, with major branches that curve anteriorly and minor branches that curve posteriorly.

Central zone

The central zone comprises about 25% of the glandular prostate. This zone is wedge-shaped and surrounds the ejaculatory ducts, with its apex at the verumontanum and its base against the

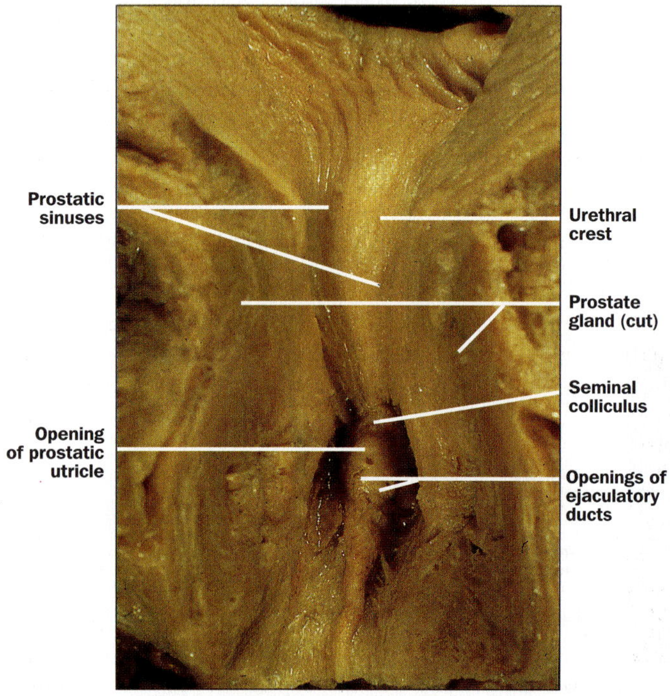

Figure 3.19 Prostatic urethra opened through its anterior wall to show the urethral crest and seminal colliculus.

Labels: Prostatic sinuses; Urethral crest; Prostate gland (cut); Seminal colliculus; Opening of prostatic utricle; Openings of ejaculatory ducts

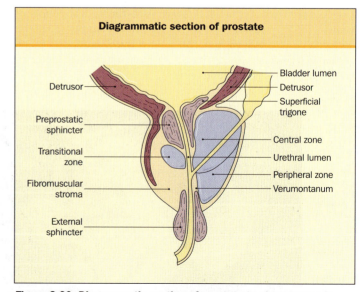

Diagrammatic section of prostate

Labels: Detrusor; Preprostatic sphincter; Transitional zone; Fibromuscular stroma; External sphincter; Bladder lumen; Detrusor; Superficial trigone; Central zone; Urethral lumen; Peripheral zone; Verumontanum

Figure 3.20 Diagrammatic section of prostate to show anatomic subdivisions. For simplicity, the 35% anterior angulation of the prostatic urethra has been omitted.

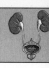

bladder neck. Thus, the central zone is, at least in its distal part, surrounded by the peripheral zone and its ducts open into the prostatic urethra, in close proximity to the ejaculatory ducts.

The central zone, like the peripheral zone, has a funnel shape to accommodate the proximal segment of the urethra. Both funnels are incomplete ventrally, where their borders are held together by the fibromuscular stroma.

Transitional zone

The smallest glandular part comprises only about 5–10% of the prostate and is called a transitional zone. This zone consists of two independent small lobes the ducts of which leave the posterolateral recesses of the urethral wall at a single point, just proximal to the point of urethral angulation and at the lower border of the preprostatic sphincter. The main ducts of the transitional zone extend laterally around the distal border of the sphincter and curve sharply anteriorly; they arborize toward the bladder neck immediately external to the preprostatic sphincter and fan out laterally. The most medial ducts and acini of the transitional zone curve medially to penetrate into the sphincter.

Innervation

The human prostate gland receives a dual autonomic innervation from both parasympathetic (cholinergic) and sympathetic (noradrenergic) nerves via the prostatic nerve plexus (i.e. that part of the pelvic autonomic plexus that lies adjacent to the prostate gland). The pelvic plexus (and hence the prostatic plexus) receives parasympathetic input from the sacral segments of the spinal cord (S2, S3, and S4) and sympathetic fibers from the hypogastric (presacral) nerves (T10 to L2). These nerves ramify within the prostatic plexus, which contains both cholinergic and noradrenergic nerve cell bodies[29]. The autonomic nerves that supply the prostate (and also the seminal vesicles, urethra, and corpora cavernosae) arise from the pelvic plexus and travel together with the vascular supply. These neurovascular bundles approach the base of the prostate on its posterior aspect and generally lie in the same coronal plane as its rectal surface. Most of the nerve branches to the prostate leave the neurovascular bundles at a level just above the prostate base and extend medially within a layer of fatty tissue. The nerve branches in these superior pedicles fan out over the prostatic capsule, which contains many autonomic ganglia embedded in a layer of fat. Some nerve branches continue medially over the prostate base to supply the central zone, while others fan out distally and penetrate the capsule at a very oblique angle. A few nerve branches leave the neurovascular bundles at the apex of the prostate via two small inferior pedicles and penetrate the capsule directly. Within the prostatic parenchyma small nerve branches lie immediately adjacent to the walls of the ducts and acini, while other nerves form branching plexuses among the smooth muscle bundles of the stroma.

Both cholinergic and noradrenergic nerves innervate the smooth muscle bundles of the prostatic stroma[30], while cholinergic nerves also innervate the smooth muscle of the capsule. In addition, at least some of the glandular acini within the prostate receive a cholinergic secretomotor innervation. It is well known that parasympathetic stimulation increases the rate of secretion and under sympathetic stimulation (such as occurs during ejaculation) prostatic fluid is expelled into the urethra[31].

SEMINAL VESICLE

Each seminal vesicle is a sacculated gland, approximately 3cm long, that lies lateral to the ampulla of the vas deferens (see Fig. 3.18). The seminal vesicles lie in front of the rectum and rectovesical pouch of peritoneum and extend up the posterior wall of the bladder as far as the terminal parts of the ureters.

VAS (DUCTUS) DEFERENS

Each vas (ductus) deferens begins at the tail of the epididymis in the scrotum, ascends within the spermatic cord, and traverses the inguinal canal. After it emerges from the deep inguinal ring, the vas runs along the lateral pelvic wall, covered by peritoneum, and passes medial to the superior vesical vessels and obturator nerve and vessels (see Fig. 3.14). The vas then crosses above the ureter and turns downward and medially posterior to the bladder. The terminal part of the vas is dilated to form the ampulla, which lies medial to the seminal vesicle. The ampulla is related posteriorly to the peritoneum of the rectovesical pouch and to the rectovesical septum and rectum.

EJACULATORY DUCT

The duct of each seminal vesicle joins the ampulla of the corresponding vas deferens to form the ejaculatory duct (see Fig. 3.18). The right and left ducts pierce the prostate gland and run downward, forward, and medially through its substance to open into the prostatic urethra at slit-like orifices on the summit of the seminal colliculus.

Blood supply

The artery to the vas deferens is usually a small vessel that arises from the superior vesical artery and accompanies the vas as far as the epididymis. The ampulla of the vas, the seminal vesicle, and prostate gland are supplied by the inferior vesical artery. From the internal reproductive organs, blood passes into the venous plexus that surrounds the prostate to drain into the internal iliac veins.

THE MALE URETHRA

The male urethra is a fibromuscular tube approximately 20cm long and is usually described in three parts – prostatic (already described), membranous, and spongy. The prostatic and membranous parts pass downwards while the spongy part turns forwards in the bulb of the penis. This abrupt angulation is of considerable importance when catheters or cystoscopes are being introduced. Furthermore, although the spongy and prostatic parts can be readily dilated, the external meatus and the membranous urethra are comparatively narrow.

Membranous urethra

On emergence from the anterior aspect of the apex of the prostate, the membranous urethra (Fig. 3.21) descends through the pelvic floor and pierces the perineal membrane. It is approximately 2cm long and its mucosa is folded, which gives the lumen a stellate appearance on cross-section. Encircling the membranous urethra is the striated muscle of the external urethral sphincter (the rhabdosphincter). Lateral to the sphincter are the medial borders of the levatores ani.

The striated muscle fibers that comprise the rhabdosphincter are unusually small in cross-section, with diameters of only 15–20µm. Most of the fibers are physiologically of the slow twitch type[32,33], unlike the pelvic floor musculature, which is a heterogeneous mixture of slow- and fast-twitch fibers of larger diameter[34]. Moreover, the rhabdosphincter is devoid of muscle spindles and is probably supplied by the pelvic splanchnic nerves, which further distinguishes it from the periurethral levator ani muscle. The slow-twitch fibers of the external sphincter are capable of sustained contraction over relatively long periods of time and actively contribute to the tone that closes the urethra and maintains urinary continence. See also description in Chapter 6.

Posterolateral to the membranous urethra are the paired bulbourethral glands, each about 1cm in diameter. Their ducts pierce the perineal membrane and open into the spongy urethra. An additional posterior relation of the membranous urethra is the ampulla of the rectum, while anteriorly lies the lower border of the pubic symphysis to which the urethra is anchored by the pubourethral ligaments.

Spongy urethra

The spongy (or penile) urethra (Fig. 3.21) is approximately 15cm in length; it commences in the bulb of the penis and traverses the erectile tissue of the corpus spongiosum and glans. The mucosa presents numerous small recesses or lacunae and most of its lumen forms a transverse slit. Within the bulb the urethra is wider, and forms the intrabulbar fossa. The lumen is also expanded within the glans to form the navicular fossa, which opens at the surface as a vertical slit, the external meatus.

Blood supply

The prostatic and membranous parts of the urethra receive blood from the inferior vesical arteries. The spongy part is supplied by the internal pudendal artery via the dorsal arteries of the penis and the arteries to the bulb. Venous blood passes into the prostatic venous plexus and the internal pudendal veins.

Nerve supply

The principal sensory innervation of the mucosa is provided by the pudendal nerve, a branch of the sacral plexus. The same spinal cord segments innervate the external sphincter via the pelvic splanchnic nerves (S2, S3, and S4).

PENIS

The erectile tissue of the shaft of the penis consists of the paired corpora cavernosa, which lie in apposition, and the midline corpus spongiosum (Fig. 3.22).

The corpus spongiosum is uniform in diameter, except at its extremity where it expands into the glans, the prominent margin of which forms the corona of the penis. Proximally, the corpus spongiosum continues into the root of the penis to form the bulb attached to the inferior surface of the perineal membrane. The urethra pierces the perineal membrane, enters the bulb from above, and curves downward and forward. It traverses the corpus spongiosum and glans, and terminates at the external urethral meatus near the apex of the glans.

Dorsal to the corpus spongiosum are the paired corpora cavernosa, which extend distally as far as the concave proximal surface of the glans. Proximally, the corpora cavernosa continue inferior to the pubic symphysis and diverge as the crura. Each crus tapers posteriorly and is attached to the inferior surface of the perineal membrane and the adjacent rami of the pubis and ischium.

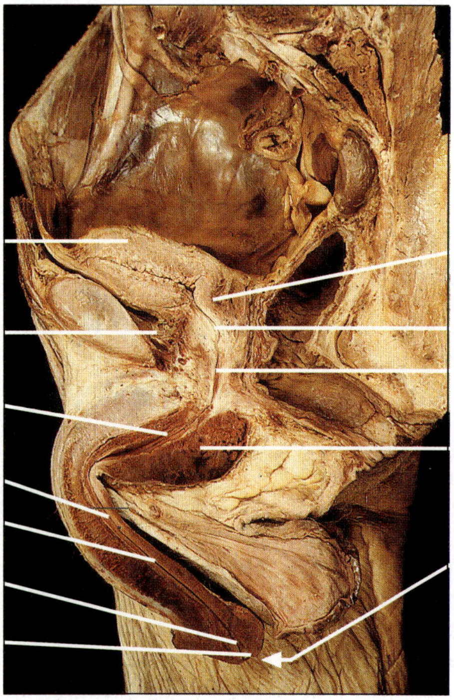

Bladder

Puboprostatic ligaments

Intrabulbar fossa

Corpus spongiosum

Spongy urethra

Glans penis

Navicular fossa

Prostate gland

Prostatic urethra

Membranous urethra

Bulb of penis

External urethral meatus

Figure 3.21 Male urethra in sagittal section.

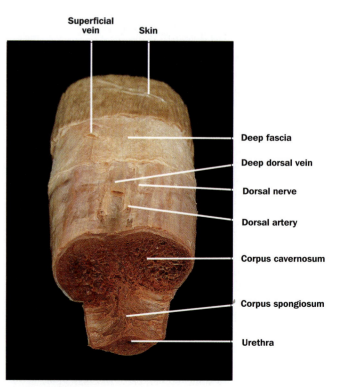

Superficial vein

Skin

Deep fascia

Deep dorsal vein

Dorsal nerve

Dorsal artery

Corpus cavernosum

Corpus spongiosum

Urethra

Figure 3.22 Dissection of the shaft of the penis to show the spongy urethra, the corpora, and the dorsal vessels.

SCROTUM

The scrotum is a pouch of skin and fascia derived from the anterior abdominal wall; it contains the testes, epididymides, and the lower parts of the spermatic cords.

Skin and superficial fascia

The skin of the scrotum is supplied anteriorly by the external pudendal vessels and innervated by the ilioinguinal nerve. The remainder of the scrotal skin is supplied by branches of the internal pudendal vessels, and by branches of the pudendal nerve and posterior cutaneous nerve of the thigh. Lymph drains to the superficial inguinal nodes.

Deep to the skin lies the superficial fascia, continuous superiorly with the superficial fascia of the abdominal wall. The scrotal superficial fascia, which contains smooth muscle called the dartos, but little fat, forms a median septum that divides the pouch into right and left sides and is anchored posteriorly to the perineal membrane.

Spermatic fasciae

Deep to the superficial fascia of each side of the scrotum lie three layers of spermatic fascia. Each layer takes the form of a sleeve derived from one of the layers of the abdominal wall:

- the outermost sleeve, the external spermatic fascia, begins at the superficial inguinal ring and is continuous with the external oblique aponeurosis;
- the intermediate sleeve is the cremasteric fascia and muscle, continuous within the inguinal canal with the internal oblique muscle; and
- the transversalis fascia of the abdominal wall provides the deepest sleeve, the internal spermatic fascia, which commences at the deep inguinal ring.

These three fascial layers surround the components of the spermatic cord and continue downward to enclose the testis and epididymis (Fig. 3.23). For derivation see also Fig. 2.19.

Spermatic cord

The spermatic cord runs from the superficial inguinal ring into the scrotum, and comprises the vas deferens and the vessels and nerves of the testis and epididymis together with the layers of spermatic fascia.

The principal artery of the spermatic cord is the testicular artery, a branch of the abdominal aorta. Also present is the artery to the vas, which often arises from the superior vesical artery within the pelvic cavity. The veins that drain the testis and epididymis form a network, the pampiniform plexus. From this plexus, one or two veins continue through the deep inguinal ring and ascend the posterior abdominal wall with the testicular artery. The testicular vessels are accompanied by a plexus of autonomic nerves and by lymph vessels that terminate in the aortic lymph nodes.

Tunica vaginalis

The tunica vaginalis is a closed serous sac that covers the medial, anterior, and lateral surfaces of the testis and the lateral aspect of the epididymis. Like the peritoneum from which it is derived, the tunica vaginalis has parietal and visceral layers separated by a small quantity of serous fluid. An excessive accumulation of fluid in the sac produces a swelling (hydrocele) anterior to the testis.

In the fetus the processus vaginalis links the tunica vaginalis with the peritoneal cavity. Usually the processus closes before birth, but occasionally it remains patent.

Testis

The testis is an ovoid organ approximately 5cm long in the adult (Fig. 3.24), suspended by the spermatic cord in the lower part

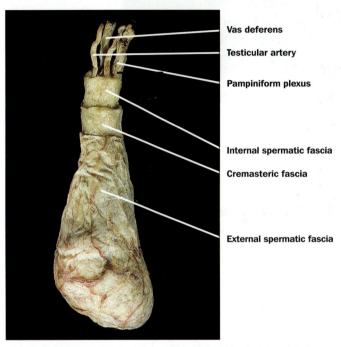

Figure 3.23 Left testis and spermatic cord within their fascial sleeves.

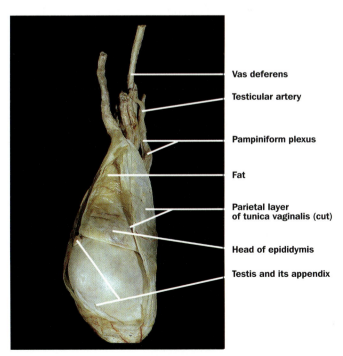

Figure 3.24 Anterolateral part of the parietal layer of the tunica vaginalis has been removed to reveal the testis and head of the epididymis. The testis bears a vestigial tag, the appendix of the testis.

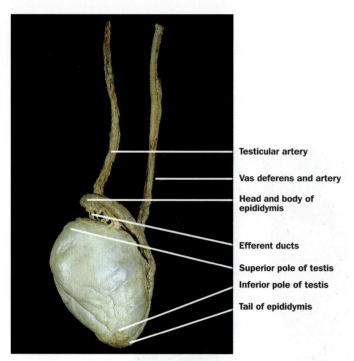

Figure 3.25 Lateral aspect of the testis and epididymis after removal of the tunica vaginalis and pampiniform plexus. The head of the epididymis has been lifted to display the efferent ducts.

Testicular artery
Vas deferens and artery
Head and body of epididymis
Efferent ducts
Superior pole of testis
Inferior pole of testis
Tail of epididymis

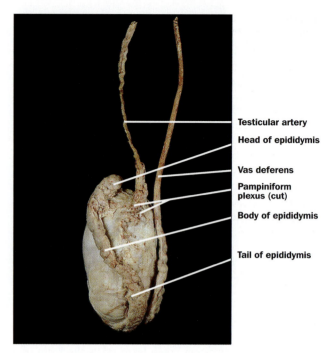

Figure 3.26 Posterior view of the testis, epididymis, and vas deferens.

Testicular artery
Head of epididymis
Vas deferens
Pampiniform plexus (cut)
Body of epididymis
Tail of epididymis

of the scrotum, with its superior pole tilted slightly forward. The testis has a thick fibrous capsule, the tunica albuginea, which is covered laterally, anteriorly, and medially by the visceral layer of the tunica vaginalis. The posterior surface of the organ, devoid of a covering of tunica vaginalis, is pierced by the efferent ducts, branches of the testicular artery, and numerous small veins that form the pampiniform plexus.

Epididymis

The epididymis consists of a narrow, highly convoluted duct applied to the posterior surface of the testis. Its broad superior part, the head, overhangs the upper pole of the testis from which it receives several efferent ducts (Fig. 3.25). The body of the epididymis tapers into the tail (Fig. 3.26), which is continuous with the vas deferens. The epididymis is supplied by branches of the testicular artery and drained by the pampiniform plexus.

REFERENCES

1. Dixon JS, Gosling JA. The musculature of the human renal calices, pelvis and upper ureter. J Anat. 1982;135:129–37.
2. Constantinou CE. Renal pelvic pacemaker control of ureteral peristaltic rate. Am J Physiol. 1974;226:1413–6.
3. Woodburne RT. The ureter, ureterovesical junction and vesical trigone. Anat Rec. 1965;151:243–9.
4. Duarte-Escalante O, Labay P, Boyarsky S. The neurohistochemistry of mammalian ureter: a new combination of histochemical procedures to demonstrate adrenergic, cholinergic and chromaffin structures in the ureter. J Urol. 1969;101:803–11.
5. Edvane KA, Trussell DC, Jonavicius J, Henwood A, Marshall VR. Presence and regional variation in peptide-containing nerves in the human ureter. J Auton Nerv Sys. 1992;39:127–38.
6. Deane RF. Transmural electrical stimulation of the ureter. Br J Urol. 1969;41:417–20.
7. Cole RS, Fry CH, Shuttleworth KED. The action of the prostaglandins on isolated human ureteric smooth muscle. Br J Urol. 1988;61:19–26.
8. Kiil F. The function of the ureter and renal pelvis. London: WB Saunders; 1957.
9. Tanagho EZ, Meyers FH, Smith RD. The trigone: anatomical and physiological considerations. 1. In relation to the ureterovesical junction. J Urol. 1968;100:623–2.
10. Elbadawi A. Anatomy and function of the ureteral sheath. J Urol. 1972;107:224–9.
11. Gearhart JP, Canning DA, Gilpin SA, Lam EE, Gosling JA. Histological and histochemical study of the vesicoureteric junction in infancy and childhood. Br J Urol. 1993;72:648–54.
12. Dixon JS, Canning DA, Gearhart JP, Gosling JA. An immunohistochemical study of the innervation of the ureterovesical junction in infancy and childhood. Br J Urol. 1994;73:292–7.
13. Woodburne RT. Structure and function of the urinary bladder. J Urol. 1960;84:79–85.
14. Lincoln J, Burnstock G. Autonomic innervation of the urinary bladder and urethra. In: Maggi CA, ed. Nervous control of the urogenital system, vol. 3. Harwood Academic Publishers; 1993:33–68.

15. Smet PJ, Edyvane KA, Jonavicius J, Marshall VR. Neuropeptides and neurotransmitter-synthesizing enzymes in intrinsic neurons of the human urinary bladder. J Neurocytol. 1996;25:112–24.

16. Ek A, Alm P, Andersson K-E, Persson CGA. Adrenergic and cholinergic nerves of the human urethra and urinary bladder. A histochemical study. Acta Physiol Scand. 1977;99:345–52.

17. Kluck P. The autonomic innervation of the human urinary bladder, bladder neck and urethra. A histochemical study. Anat Rec. 1980;198:439–47.

18. Elbadawi A. Functional anatomy of the organs of micturition. Urol Clin North Am. 1996;23:177–210.

19. Gosling JA, Dixon JS, Lendon RG. The autonomic innervation of the human male and female bladder and proximal urethra. J Urol. 1977;118:302–5.

20. Sundin T, Dahlstrom A, Norlen L, Svedmyr N. The sympathetic innervation and adrenoreceptor function of the human lower urinary tract in the normal state and after parasympathetic denervation. Invest Urol. 1977;14:322–8.

21. Benson GS, McConnell JA, Wood JG. Adrenergic innervation of the human bladder body. J Urol. 1979;122:189–91.

22. De Groat WC, Booth AM. Inhibition and facilitation in parasympathetic ganglia of the urinary bladder. Fed Proc. 1980;39:2990–6.

23. Gosling JA, Dixon JS. The structure and innervation of smooth muscle in the wall of the bladder neck and proximal urethra. Br J Urol. 1975;47:549–58.

24. Manley CB. The striated muscle of the prostate. J Urol. 1966;95:234–40.

25. Clegg E. The musculature of the human prostatic urethra. J Anat. 1959;91:345–51.

26. McNeal JE. Regional morphology and pathology of the prostate. Am J Clin Pathol. 1968;49:347–57.

27. McNeal JE. The prostate and prostatic urethra: a morphologic synthesis. J Urol. 1972;107;1008–16.

28. McNeal JE. Anatomy of the prostate: an historical survey of divergent views. Prostate. 1980;1:3–13.

29. Crowe R, Chapple CR, Burnstock G. The human prostate gland: a histochemical and immunohistochemical study of neuropeptides, serotonin, dopamine-β-hydroxylase and acetylcholinesterase in autonomic nerves and ganglia. Br J Urol. 1991;68:53–61

30. Gosling JA. Autonomic innervation of the prostate. In: Hinman F, ed. Benign prostatic hypertrophy. New York: Springer-Verlag; 1983:349–60.

31. Brushini H, Schmidt RA, Tanagho EA. Neurologic control of prostatic secretion in the dog. Invest Urol. 1978;15:288–91.

32. Shroder HD, Reske-Nielsen E. Fiber types in the striated urethral and anal sphincters. Acta Neuropathol (Berl). 1983;60:278–82.

33. Tokuna S, Murakami U, Fujii H, et al. Coexistence of fast and slow myosin isoenzymes in human external urethral sphincter. A preliminary report. J Urol. 1987;138:659–62.

34. Gosling JA, Dixon JS, Critchley HOD, Thompson SA. A comparative study of the human external sphincter and periurethral levator ani muscles. Br J Urol. 1981;53:35–41.

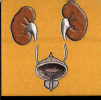

Chapter 4

Applied Physiology of the Urinary Tract: Kidney Function

Rex L Mahnensmith

KEY POINTS

- The kidney eliminates products of metabolism including organic and inorganic acids, nitrogenous wastes such as urea, end products of nucleic acid turnover such as uric acid and xanthines, and drugs and toxins.
- The kidney maintains extracellular fluid sodium and water content in response to hormonal and baroreceptor signals through the renin–angiotensin–aldosterone and autonomic nervous system.
- The kidney participates in vascular tone regulation through the renin–angiotensin system.
- The kidney maintains electrolyte content of the extracellular fluid and indirectly regulates ionic composition of the intracellular fluid.
- The kidney produces renin, which is involved in the production of angiotensin and aldosterone, erythropoietin, which stimulates the production of red blood cells, and 1,25-dihydrocholecalciferol, an active form of vitamin D that is involved in calcium–phosphorus homeostasis.

INTRODUCTION

Basic concepts regarding kidney functions

Each person is normally endowed with two kidneys. Each kidney weighs approximately 150g, spans 10–11cm in length, and is typically served with one main renal artery that originates from the lower abdominal aorta. Nearly 20% of the cardiac output, or 1,000–1,200mL/min of whole blood, flow through the kidneys[1]. Per gram of tissue, the blood flow rate through the kidneys is over 10 times the blood flow through other organs. This very high blood flow rate far exceeds metabolic requirements. Yet the high blood flow rate is necessary for the essential functions of the kidneys, namely the steady excretion of metabolic waste products and regulation of blood chemical composition and volume. As such, kidneys are vital organs essential to life. Without kidneys, we die. Yet humans can endure substantial loss of renal function with little threat to good health and wellbeing. This benefit exists because we are endowed with redundant renal mass and, when kidneys are diseased, remaining renal tissue will hypertrophy anatomically and functionally, leading to sustained body chemistry homeostasis.

The life-supporting functions of the kidney can be categorized as follows.

Excretion of metabolic endproducts

The kidney eliminates numerous products of metabolism, in particular organic and inorganic acids, nitrogenous waste such as urea, and endproducts of nucleic acid turnover, such as uric acid and other xanthine products. Metabolic waste and endproducts are generated constantly from metabolism of dietary intake and catabolic turnover of cells.

Excretion of toxins and drugs

Many drugs and toxins are eliminated through the urine. This task may be accomplished via glomerular filtration or tubular secretion. The mechanisms that secrete drugs and toxins are commonly those mechanisms which secrete organic acids and bases. Renal impairment requires medication dose adjustments by the clinician.

Maintenance of extracellular fluid volume

Blood volume is determined by its sodium and water content in relation to vascular tone and capacitance. The kidney maintains extracellular fluid sodium and water content in response to hormonal and baroreceptor signals through the renin–angiotensin–aldosterone and autonomic nervous systems. The kidney also participates in vascular tone regulation through the renin–angiotensin system.

Maintenance of body fluid composition

The kidney maintains electrolyte content and concentration of the extracellular fluid. Most important in this regard are sodium, potassium, chloride, bicarbonate, pH, magnesium, calcium, and phosphorus. The kidney also regulates the water content of plasma. Our body fluids are constantly impacted by our dietary variations. Yet the kidney governs and regulates plasma chemistry with perfect precision. The kidney indirectly regulates the ionic composition of intracellular fluid. Intracellular ionic compositions are regulated by distinct cellular and subcellular ion transport mechanisms.

Production of enzymes and hormones with systemic actions

Most important are renin, erythropoietin, and 1,25-dihydroxycholecalciferol. Renin is an enzyme that catalyzes production of angiotensinogen, a precursor to angiotensin. Angiotensin stimulates aldosterone production and is itself a potent vasoconstrictor. Erythropoietin stimulates bone marrow production of erythrocytes. 1,25-dihydroxycholecalciferol is the active form of vitamin D. It is essential for calcium–phosphorus homeostasis and bone health.

Filtration of the blood is the first step in waste excretion and body fluid chemical homeostasis. Filtration is simply the act of separating plasma water from the other components of whole blood – cells, proteins, fats. This filtrate travels through a long, convoluted epithelial tubule, wherein it is modified and concentrated into the final urine product. The functioning unit of the kidney that accomplishes filtration and excretion is the nephron, a complex structure composed at its proximal end of a convoluted capillary system (glomerulus) encompassed by a water-tight epithelial capsule (Bowman's capsule) that joins to the epithelial tubule (Fig. 4.1). Each kidney has approximately 1,000,000 nephrons[2].

Arterial blood flows into the renal parenchyma at physiologic arterial pressures and courses to the outer 1cm of the kidney, the renal cortex, where the glomeruli reside. There are few branches to the renal arteries as they direct blood to the cortex but once in the cortex, the arteries branch until each glomerulus is served by one tiny, muscular arteriole, the afferent arteriole. Arteriolar blood flows into its glomerulus under a forward head of pressure determined by systemic arterial pressure and the caliber of the afferent arteriole, which dilates or constricts to maintain a constant delivery of blood to the glomerulus it serves (Fig. 4.2). Incoming blood pressure is 60–80mmHg, held constant by variations in afferent arteriolar tone despite wide fluctuations of systemic blood pressure[3]. The glomerular capillary bed is suspended between the afferent arteriole and the efferent arteriole, the arteriole through which blood exits the glomerulus. Both arterioles are muscular and vasoactive. While afferent tone will vary to assure constant blood delivery and constant incoming blood pressure, efferent tone will vary too, providing outflow resistance that sustains necessary intraglomerular filtration pressures and glomerular filtration rate. This is unique. Synchronized vascular tone regulation of the afferent and efferent arterioles maintains glomerlular capillary blood pressure at 50–60mmHg, which is sufficient to sustain filtration of water and solute from plasma into Bowman's space[4].

Accordingly, as blood flows through a glomerulus, approximately 20–25% of plasma water and its non-protein-bound solutes are sieved into Bowman's capsule[4]. The rate of filtration, or glomerular filtration rate (GFR), refers to the volume of filtrate formed per minute. In healthy kidneys, filtration across the entire nephron population occurs at an average rate of 80–140mL/min. This means that plasma water is separated from whole blood and deposited in Bowman's space at a rate of 80–140mL/min. This filtrate flows continuously out of Bowman's capsule into the proximal epithelial tubule, while remnant blood exits the glomerulus through its efferent arteriole. The efferent arteriole soon breaks into a second capillary network, which surrounds the epithelial tubule of its nephron[5] (Fig. 4.1). As the filtrate trickles through the lumens of its epithelial tubules, water and solutes are selectively reabsorbed back into the peritubular capillary network. Through this process, the peritubular capillary blood becomes reconstituted in volume and chemical composition. It is essential to realize that nearly 6L of plasma filtrate will be formed per hour, but 97–98% of the volume of this filtrate is promptly returned to pericapillary blood through various reabsorptive mechanisms, leaving less than 3% as final urine[3]. This final urine serves as the fluid vehicle for the excretion of metabolic endproducts, minerals, acid, and water.

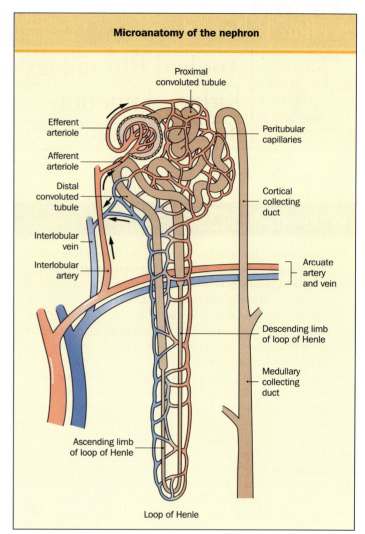

Microanatomy of the nephron

Proximal convoluted tubule

Efferent arteriole

Afferent arteriole

Distal convoluted tubule

Interlobular vein

Interlobular artery

Peritubular capillaries

Cortical collecting duct

Arcuate artery and vein

Descending limb of loop of Henle

Medullary collecting duct

Ascending limb of loop of Henle

Loop of Henle

Figure 4.1 Microanatomy of the nephron. The nephron consists of the glomerulus, the proximal tubule, the loop of Henle, the distal tubule, and the collecting duct. Blood flows into the glomerulus through the afferent arteriole, then exits through the efferent arteriole. The efferent arteriole leads to a peritubular capillary network.

Reabsorption from filtrate to pericapillary blood is selective by solute, which enables the tubular epithelium to govern the final composition of the urine solute by solute. Additionally, some solutes are highly reabsorbed and then secreted back into the urine further down the tubule. Potassium and uric acid are examples. Some solutes, such as acid and ammonium, gain entrance into the urine exclusively via secretion. Secretion enables the urine to contain much higher concentrations of solutes than would be possible with simple filtration. The epithelium of the nephron is differentiated into specialized transporting cells that differ from region to region of the tubule. Specialization of transport functions is what allows precise regulatory governance of individual solute concentrations in reconstituted, renal venous blood.

While 'making urine' is a cardinal operation of the kidney, a 'balanced urine' is not an ordained outcome. The most important 'product' of a healthy kidney is its venous blood, not its urine. The venous blood that returns to the central circulation is cleansed of metabolic waste, balanced in volume, ionic composition, and pH, and carries hormones and an enzyme that head to their respective targets. Filtration of whole blood in the glomeruli, formation of a plasma water filtrate, and then reabsorptive and secretory transport by epithelial tubules is the essence of this process. These steps require adequate blood delivery to the kidney, a patent arterial network, intact filtration structures, healthy and intact tubules, intact peritubular capillary systems, adequate tubular oxygen delivery, precisely operating transport systems, and unobstructed flow of urine out of the kidney. The unique microanatomy of the tubules and the tubular relationships to their adjacent capillary networks are essential to proper physiological functions[1,5].

GLOMERULAR FILTRATION

Glomerular filtration is a passive process of water ultrafiltration across the semipermeable glomerular capillary walls. The substance of these walls includes a flat, fenestrated capillary endothelial cell layer, a collagenous glomerular basement membrane,

and a squamous epithelial cell that resides on the external surface of the basement membrane. The squamous epithelial barrier is not continuous. Rather, it permits passage of water and solute by virtue of its discontinuous microvillous morphology[1] (Fig. 4.3). The entire filtration barrier is size and charge selective[4]. It poses a low resistance to water flow, as evidenced by the fact that filtration rate is normally greater than 80mL/min. However, neutral-charged molecules with pore radius greater than 60Å are not filterable[2]. Neutral molecules with lesser pore radii show increasing sieving coefficients such that those smaller than 26Å have little restriction to passage[2,3]. Molecules with net negative charge are less filterable, regardless of size, owing to a strong anionic nature of the squamous foot processes. In particular, albumin, which has a radius of 36Å, is highly restricted in its filtration owing to its polyanionic nature. It is effectively repelled from passage through the glomerular capillary fenestrations because of its charge[2,4].

Water and non-protein-bound low-molecular-weight substances exhibit high flux across the capillaries. The same Starling

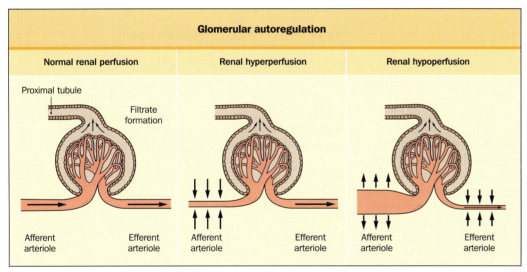

Figure 4.2 Glomerular autoregulation. (Left) Blood delivery to the glomerulus and glomerular filtration rate are maintained constant by variations in the caliber of the afferent and efferent arterioles. (Center) When renal hyperperfusion is threatened, the afferent arteriole constricts, protecting the glomerulus from hyperperfusion damage and precluding hyperfiltration. (Right) When renal hypoperfusion evolves, the afferent arteriole dilates, assuring adequate blood delivery to the glomerulus, and the efferent arteriole constricts, which maintains adequate glomerular filtration pressure.

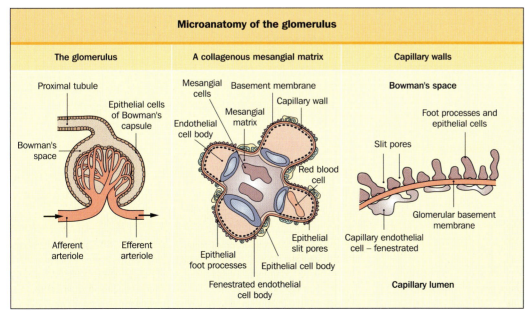

Figure 4.3 Microanatomy of the glomerulus. (Left) The glomerulus is a specialized capillary bed sandwiched between two vasoactive muscular arterioles. (Center) A collagenous mesangial matrix, secreted by mesangial cells, supports the glomerular capillaries. (Right) The capillary walls have three components: a flat, fenestrated endothelium; the basement membrane; epithelial cells, which possess microvillus foot processes. Filtration is selective according to solute charge and size.

forces that determine fluid movement across blood capillaries in general govern filtrate formation[3]:

- hydrostatic pressure in the glomerular capillaries, which tends to drive water out of the capillary;
- hydrostatic pressure in Bowman's space, which opposes water entry into the space;
- oncotic pressure in the capillaries, which tends to oppose water movement out of the capillary; and
- oncotic pressure in Bowman's space, which will favor movement of water into Bowman's space.

Hence, net ultrafiltration pressure is the difference between the hydrostatic and oncotic pressure differences in the glomerular capillaries and Bowman's space. The hydrostatic pressure in the glomerular capillary is high, owing to the incoming blood pressure, so it is principally this variable that drives ultrafiltration. However, plasma oncotic pressure, owing to albumin and other plasma proteins, opposes filtration partially. Although direct measurements from human kidneys have never been made, measurements extrapolated from other mammals suggest that intraglomerular capillary hydrostatic pressures are 50–60mmHg and proximal tubular hydrostatic pressures 17–20mmHg[2,3]. Plasma colloid pressure in humans is approximately 25mmHg, so the effective transcapillary filtration pressure in glomeruli can vary from 5mmHg to as high as 18mmHg. Hydrostatic pressure in Bowman's space effectively opposes filtration only when there is downstream obstruction of filtrate or urine flow, which can occur in various pathologic conditions.

Glomerular filtration rate may vary as a function of blood flow rate through the glomerulus, the hydrostatic pressure difference between the glomerular capillary lumen and Bowman's space, the surface area of the glomerular capillary bed, and permeability characteristics of the glomerular basement membrane barrier (Fig. 4.4). However, vasoactive mechanisms usually keep GFR relatively constant over a wide range of incoming perfusion pressures (Fig. 4.2). This is referred to as 'autoregulation of GFR'[6,7] (Fig. 4.5).

Two events are primary in the normal performance of GFR autoregulation when renal perfusion pressures are falling: dilation of the preglomerular afferent arteriole and constriction of the postglomerular efferent arteriole[6,7]. Afferent vasodilation preserves glomerular blood delivery in the context of falling perfusion pressures. Efferent vasoconstriction increases glomerular outflow resistance, which raises transcapillary hydraulic pressures within the glomerular capillary bed (Fig. 4.2). This action supports glomerular filtration pressure in the context of falling forward perfusion pressure.

Afferent arteriolar tone is governed by a balance of vasoactive forces[6,7]. Chief among these are locally produced histamine, prostaglandins and thromboxanes, myogenic reflexes activated by local wall tension signals, catecholamines, endothelin, and the endothelial production of nitric oxide[6,7]. Efferent arteriolar tone is governed chiefly by angiotensin II. The constrictor effects of angiotensin II and norepinephrine are exerted on both the afferent and efferent arterioles. However, it seems that afferent constriction is physiologically countervailed by vasodilator signals, while the efferent reaction is not[6,7].

Accordingly, when renal blood flow declines, afferent vasodilation is achieved along with efferent vasoconstriction, and GFR is preserved. Renal blood flow is similarly autoregulated. Below arterial pressures of 70mmHg, these autoregulatory mechanisms are insufficient to preserve GFR[1]. Conversely, if the kidney is subjected to high perfusion pressures, as occurs with systemic hypertension, the afferent arteriole will constrict, preventing a rise in GFR and protecting the delicate glomerular capillary bed from hyperperfusion injury.

PROXIMAL TUBULE FUNCTIONS

Plasma water resulting from glomerular filtration enters the proximal portion of the nephron, referred to as the proximal convoluted tubule. The proximal convoluted tubule possesses a large reabsorptive membrane surface area owing to its distinctive luminal brush border structure[1,5]. This plasma water filtrate contains low-molecular-weight solutes at the same concentrations as

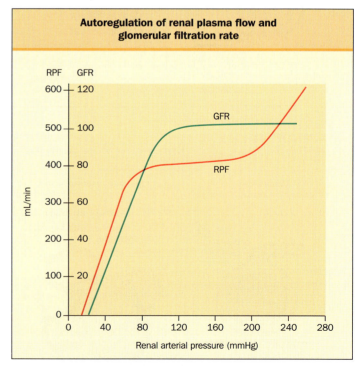

Figure 4.5 **Autoregulation of renal plasma flow (RPF) and glomerular filtration rate (GFR).** Glomerular filtration rate is maintained at a constant level over a wide range of renal perfusion pressures. Refer to Figure 4.2. (With permission from Mahnensmith RL. Acute and chronic renal failure. In Bone RC, ed. Pulmonary and critical care medicine. Chicago: Mosby; 1998.)

Physiologic determinants of glomerular filtration rate

*SNGFR = $K \times S([P_{gc} - P_T] - [\Pi_{gc} - \Pi_T])$

Permeability of the glomerular capillary wall = K

Total glomerular capillary surface area = S

Hydrostatic pressure in the glomerular capillary = P_{gc}

Hydrostatic pressure in Bowman's space = P_T

Oncotic pressure in the glomerular capillary = Π_{gc}

Oncotic pressure in Bowman's space = Π_T

Figure 4.4 Physiologic determinants of glomerular filtration rate. SNGFR, single nephron glomerular filtration rate.

in plasma, with the exception of those that are protein-bound. The chief function of the proximal tubule is to reclaim in bulk much of the water and solutes that have just been filtered, and its cells are differentiated to achieve high-volume transport of solute and water in the direction from filtrate to pericapillary blood. Approximately 65–70% of filtered sodium, chloride, calcium, and water are reabsorbed isosmotically here, along with 90% of filtered potassium and bicarbonate and virtually all amino acids and glucose. Phosphate is 85% reabsorbed under the control of parathyroid hormone. Uric acid is highly reabsorbed too, but then regains entrance into the tubular lumen via secretion further down the proximal tubule. This latter proximal tubular segment also secretes organic acids and bases. This pathway is the mechanism for drug and toxin elimination by the kidney. Proximal tubule cells also synthesize and secrete ammonium into the tubular urine, which is an essential for acid excretion by the kidney (Fig. 4.6).

Quantitatively, the major operation of the proximal tubule is the bulk reclamation of filtered substances. Since sodium is the dominant osmotic solute in the extracellular fluid and therefore the solute that tonically defines extracellular volume, regulated reabsorption of sodium and water in the proximal tubule is critically important for the regulation and preservation of extracellular fluid volume. Complete reclamation of HCO_3, glucose, and amino acids is essential so that these filtered species are not lost in the urine.

LOOP OF HENLE

The loop of Henle commences where the proximal tubule narrows and descends into the renal medulla. At its deepest point in the core of the kidney, Henle's loop makes a 180° turn and ascends back into the cortex[1] (Fig. 4.1). The morphology and function of the epithelial cells that constitute both the descending and ascending limbs of Henle's loop are different from proximal tubular cells, and the loop has a unique operation essential for salt and water homeostasis[1,5]. Filtrate leaving the proximal tubule is isosmotic to plasma. Water homeostasis demands that the nephron be able to excrete excess ingested water or conserve water from the filtrate, i.e. excrete a urine more dilute than plasma or more concentrated than plasma. The formation

of a dilute or concentrated urine is the function of the loops of Henle in concert with adjacent collecting ducts of the distal nephrons. The mechanism that achieves this nephron flexibility with regard to water is termed the 'countercurrent multiplier mechanism'[8,9] (Fig. 4.7). What the loop of Henle accomplishes is a medullary environment that is extremely hypertonic in relation to plasma.

The basic elements of this process are these[8,10]. The descending limb of Henle does not possess active transport mechanisms. However, it is passively permeable to NaCl and water. The ascending limb possesses active NaCl transport mechanisms that extrude sodium and chloride from the urine into the renal interstitium. Water stays in the tubule lumen, however, because this section of the tubule is water-impermeable. This transport of NaCl out of the lumen of the nephron here generates an osmotic difference between the tubular fluid and surrounding local interstitium, such that the interstitial fluid is kept hypertonic to intratubular fluid in the ascending limb. In essence, the ascending limb filtrate is made hypotonic by exporting NaCl solute from it, leaving behind water. The descending limb of Henle's loop is permeable to solute, so it receives sodium and chloride passively, equilibrating its solute content with the medullary interstitium. This process results in progressive medullary hypertonicity. Where the osmolality of the proximal tubular filtrate is approximately 300mOsm/L, the osmolality of the filtrate as it descends down the loop of Henle progressively rises until it reaches nearly 1200mOsm/L in its sharp upward turn at the actual loop of Henle. Hypertonicity is a result of NaCl plus urea accumulation. Urea contributes nearly 50% of the medullary hypertonicity, but this is not a result of water export from the loop of Henle[8]. Urea accumulates there from the adjacent medullary collecting duct. Urea leaves the collecting duct filtrate by passive diffusion through water channels and across the epithelium. The 180° loop juxtaposes and its distinctive transport and permeability characteristics create and sustain medullary hypertonicity through these countercurrent mechanisms[8,9].

This unique hypertonic microenvironment is essential for water transport out of the collecting duct[10,11]. The collecting ducts reside just parallel to the limbs of the loops of Henle in the medullary region[1]. The filtrate flowing through the collecting ducts has nearly completed its journey through the nephron and

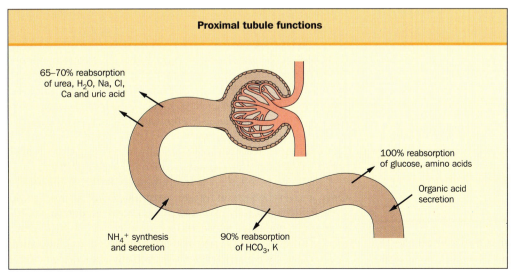

Proximal tubule functions

65–70% reabsorption of urea, H_2O, Na, Cl, Ca and uric acid

NH_4^+ synthesis and secretion

90% reabsorption of HCO_3, K

100% reabsorption of glucose, amino acids

Organic acid secretion

Figure 4.6 Proximal tubule functions.
The proximal tubule reclaims the bulk of the glomerular filtrate. It also possesses a mechanism for ammonium synthesis, which is essential for acid excretion and new bicarbonate generation, and pathways for organic acid secretion, which also serve as pathways for drug elimination by the kidney.

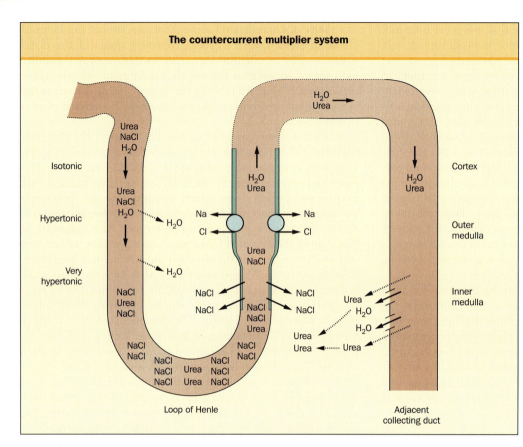

The countercurrent multiplier system

Figure 4.7 The countercurrent multiplier system. The loop of Henle is depicted with a juxtaposed collecting duct. NaCl is actively pumped out of the ascending limb of Henle's loop. Water remains in the lumen. The NaCl collects in the interstitium and permeates the descending limb of Henle's loop. The urine in the loop becomes hypertonic. These events plus the addition of urea from the adjacent collecting duct maintain medullary hypertonicity. Medullary hypertonicity is essential for water reabsorption from the collecting duct, which occurs when vasopressin is present and activates the formation of water channels across the collecting duct epithelium. Not shown is the vasa recta, a thin loop of venule that resides along the loop of Henle. The vasa recta provides oxygen and nutrients for these cells and carries away salt and water at a slow rate.

is about to become final urine. However, one last processing step is required – water balancing. So far, water has returned to the plasma only via the proximal nephron. Solute has returned to the plasma all along the nephron. The collecting duct is the final opportunity for water return to the plasma. This is provided by the action of vasopressin[11]. If present, vasopressin action will result in the synthesis of water pores, or channels, which cross the collecting duct epithelium. Water in the collecting duct then has an opportunity to leave the urine and return to plasma. This movement of water is passive, driven by the osmotic gradient that exists between the medullary interstitium and the collecting duct urine. That gradient exists because of medullary hypertonicity, created by the countercurrent multiplier mechanism of the loop of Henle[8]. Hence, if water channels open under the influence of vasopressin, water will leave the collecting duct urine, enter the medullary blood vessels, and be swept away into the renal venous capillary system. Under the influence of vasopressin, the final urine can reach an osmolality of 1200mOsm/L. In the absence of vasopressin, the collecting duct permeability to water remains very low, and the final urine will remain hypo-osmolar. The kidney will accomplish a net loss of water from the body.

In addition to transporting sodium and chloride out of the tubular fluid, the thick ascending limb is a major site for magnesium and calcium reabsorption[9]. The NaCl transport mechanism is the target for diuretic compounds such as furosemide and bumetanide.

DISTAL NEPHRON

The distal nephron includes the distal convoluted tubule, the connecting tubule, and the cortical and medullary collecting

ducts[1]. These portions of the nephron make the final and determining adjustments in urine acidity and tonicity, urine volume, and urine sodium and potassium content. As such, the distal nephron is responsible for the final composition of venous blood as it completes its passage through the renal parenchyma.

NITROGENOUS WASTE EXCRETION

The kidney is responsible for excretion of nitrogenous waste products formed from the metabolisms of our diet and tissue repair mechanisms. Filtration of blood at the glomerulus is the cardinal operation in nitrogenous waste excretion. Impairment in renal excretory function leads to accumulation of this nitrogenous substance, causing azotemia (nitrogen in the blood) or uremia, a life-threatening intoxication that occurs when nitrogenous waste accumulation is large[12]. Many substances fall into this category, but urea is the most abundant nitrogen waste in mammals. Creatinine, a byproduct of muscle creatine metabolism, is another nitrogen compound, which is virtually nontoxic but routinely measured as an indicator of glomerular filtration efficiency. There are other important nitrogen waste substances that the kidney continuously eliminates from our bodies, such as spermine, xanthine, guanidine, and indole compounds, but urea and creatinine are clinically measured as the chief representatives of this class of compounds in the blood.

Creatinine is soluble and freely filtered at the glomerulus[13]. Once in the tubular fluid filtrate, creatinine is not reabsorbed, so what is filtered is fully excreted. A very small amount of creatinine enters the urine via secretion also. Because of creatinine's ease of filtration and because it is not reabsorbed, its elimination or clearance from plasma depends principally upon the efficiency or rate of plasma filtration in the glomeruli. Hence, significant renal blood flow reductions, intrinsic glomerular disease, and any process that obstructs nephron passages or urine flow will impair filtration and will impair creatinine excretion. Accordingly, the concentration of creatinine in serum will rise in proportion to the degree of impairment in glomerular filtration[12,13] (Fig. 4.8).

Urea also is freely filtered at the glomeruli[14]. Like creatinine, the excretion of urea also will be impaired and its blood concentration will rise as glomerular filtration declines, as a result of any disease in the glomerular structures, compromise of blood delivery to the kidney, or obstruction of urine outflow. However, unlike creatinine, urea is a substance that is partially reabsorbed by the tubules[14]. Its reabsorption occurs passively with water, particularly in the proximal tubule and medullary collecting ducts, so urea's overall urinary excretion is considerable less than the amount filtered. Accordingly, its serum concentration depends upon filtration and its degree of tubular reabsorption. Normally, approximately 50% of filtered urea is passively reabsorbed along the nephron[14].

The serum creatinine concentration is our best marker of renal filtration efficiency and overall nitrogenous waste excretion because it is not reabsorbed once it is filtered[12,13]. The blood urea concentration also reflects filtration efficiency and will rise with filtration impairment. However, overall concentration of urea in plasma also reflects its extent of tubular reabsorption and

overall urea generation rate from nitrogen catabolism, so other variables affect its serum concentration.

Glomerular filtration rate is measured by determining the urinary excretion of a marker compound whose total urinary excretion per minute is equal to its filtration at the glomerulus[15]. Measurement of glomerular filtration rate can be accomplished by the injection of inulin, which is freely filtered and neither reabsorbed nor secreted, but inulin is not available for clinical use. Injectable radioisotope markers are available but not widely used. What is widely used is creatinine, since its release into the circulation is typically constant and its excretion is dependent upon glomerular filtration with only a very small contribution from tubular secretion. In comparison to inulin, creatinine excretion rates overestimates true GFR by about 10–15%[15]. Nevertheless, creatinine clearance is accepted as our best clinical measure of GFR. It can be computed simply from a 24-hour collection of urine, assaying total excretion of creatinine in that time period and plasma creatinine (Fig. 4.9).

REGULATION OF NaCl EXCRETION

Regulated excretion of sodium salts and water determines extracellular fluid volume because sodium salts are the most abundant tonically active extracellular solutes and hence govern plasma water content[16]. In the proximal tubule, the majority of sodium reabsorption is primarily energized by the Na–K–ATPase, which resides on the basolateral membranes of the tubular epithelial cells[16]. Active extrusion of sodium from cell into the interstitial fluid of the kidney leaves a low sodium concentration in the cell interior. Sodium then enters the cell across the luminal membrane via a Na–H countertransporter and Na–glucose, Na–amino-acid, and Na–phosphate cotransporters. A smaller portion of sodium is reabsorbed with chloride by gradient diffusion between the epithelial cells. In total, 65–70% of filtered sodium is reabsorbed in the proximal tubule. Nearly all filtered HCO_3 is reabsorbed here through the Na–H countertransport mechanism[17] (Fig. 4.10). Reabsorption in the

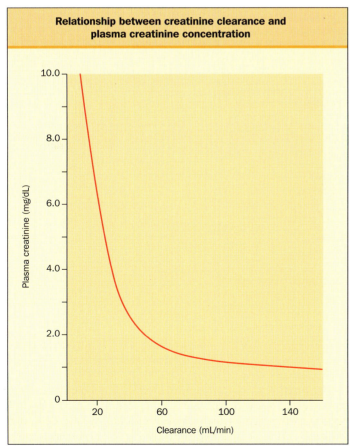

Figure 4.8 Relationship between creatinine clearance and plasma creatinine concentration. This relationship is not linear. (With permission from Mahnensmith RL. Acute and chronic renal failure. In Bone RC, ed. Pulmonary and critical care medicine. Chicago: Mosby; 1998.)

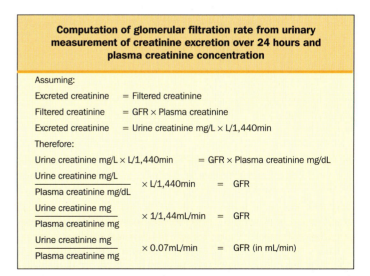

Relationship between creatinine clearance and plasma creatinine concentration

Computation of glomerular filtration rate from urinary measurement of creatinine excretion over 24 hours and plasma creatinine concentration

Assuming:

Excreted creatinine	= Filtered creatinine
Filtered creatinine	= GFR × Plasma creatinine
Excreted creatinine	= Urine creatinine mg/L × L/1,440min

Therefore:

Urine creatinine mg/L × L/1,440min = GFR × Plasma creatinine mg/dL

$$\frac{\text{Urine creatinine mg/L}}{\text{Plasma creatinine mg/dL}} \times \text{L/1,440min} = \text{GFR}$$

$$\frac{\text{Urine creatinine mg}}{\text{Plasma creatinine mg}} \times \text{1/1,44mL/min} = \text{GFR}$$

$$\frac{\text{Urine creatinine mg}}{\text{Plasma creatinine mg}} \times \text{0.07mL/min} = \text{GFR (in mL/min)}$$

Figure 4.9 Computation of glomerular filtration rate from urinary measurement of creatinine excretion over 24 hours and plasma creatinine concentration. GFR, glomerular filtration rate.

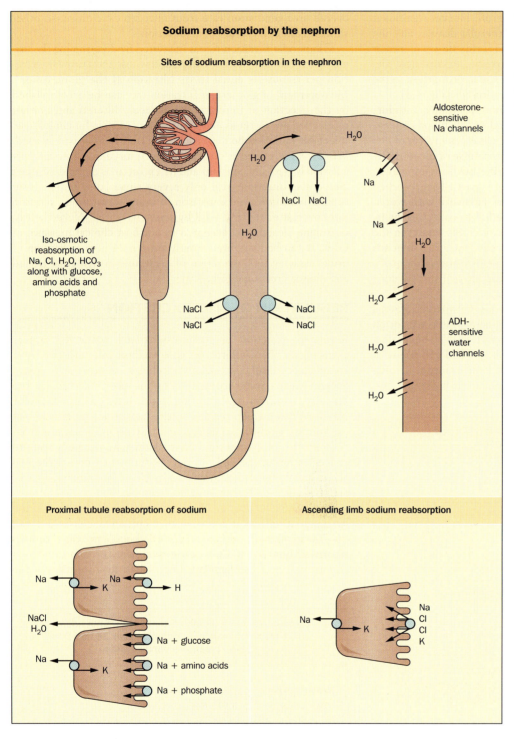

Figure 4.10 Sodium reabsorption by the nephron. (Top) The sites of sodium reabsorption in the nephron. Aldosterone regulates only distal nephron sodium reabsorption. (Bottom left) Proximal tubule reabsorption of sodium occurs by Na–H countertransport, Na–glucose, Na–amino-acid, and Na–phosphate cotransport, and NaCl paracellular diffusion. (Bottom right) Ascending limb sodium reabsorption occurs via the Na–K–2Cl cotransporter. ADH, antidiuretic hormone (vasopressin).

proximal tubule is isosmotic to plasma, which means that water travels across the epithelium in proportion to the sodium salts so that the osmolality of the filtrate does not change. Angiotensin, renal sympathetic nerve activity, local prostaglandins, atrial natriuretic peptide, and local hydrostatic factors all influence proximal tubule sodium reabsorption[16].

In the ascending loop of Henle, sodium is reabsorbed via a Na–K–2Cl cotransporter from lumen to cell and is then transported out of the cell into the renal interstitium by the basolateral Na–K–ATPase transporter[14]. The ascending limb reabsorbs 20% of filtered NaCl, and can increase its reabsorption under the influence of angiotensin. Reabsorption here is without water[6]. This act maintains medullary hypertonicity, which is essential for collecting duct water reabsorption.

The distal nephron possesses two additional sodium transport operations. In the distal convoluted tubule resides a Na–Cl cotransport system, which transports additional sodium and chloride from the lumen into the cell[16]. Further down the distal nephron are selective sodium channels, which permit gradient-driven movement of sodium from tubular fluid into the cell[18]. Both mechanisms ultimately depend upon the basolateral membrane sodium extrusion step, which is

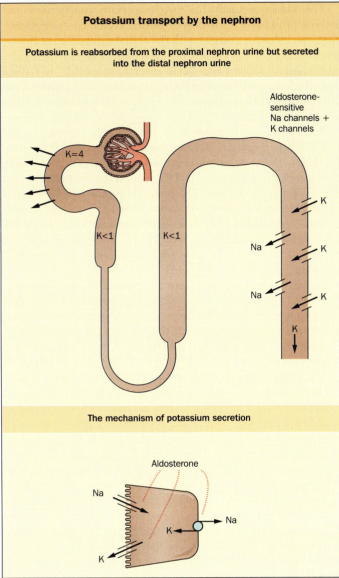

Potassium transport by the nephron

Potassium is reabsorbed from the proximal nephron urine but secreted into the distal nephron urine

Aldosterone-sensitive Na channels + K channels

K=4

K<1   K<1

Na

Na

K

K

K

K

The mechanism of potassium secretion

Aldosterone

Na

Na

K

K

Figure 4.11 Potassium transport by the nephron. (Top) Potassium is reabsorbed from the proximal nephron urine but secreted into the distal nephron urine. Aldosterone controls potassium transport only in the distal nephron. (Bottom) The mechanism of potassium secretion involves specialized potassium channels in the luminal membrane and the Na–K–ATPase in the basolateral membrane. Aldosterone regulates Na–K–ATPase activity in this region of the nephron and opens the potassium channels. Accordingly, aldosterone will stimulate potassium secretion from blood to urine.

accomplished by the Na–K–ATPase pump. Opening of the distal nephron sodium channels is regulated by aldosterone[18]. Aldosterone also stimulates activity of distal nephron Na–K–ATPase (Fig. 4.11).

While all transport processes are critical to sodium reabsorption, the final governance of extracellular fluid volume is achieved by the renin–angiotensin–aldosterone system[16]. This system is activated by sympathetic nervous tone, a baroreceptor apparatus in the afferent arteriole, and low flow states in the ascending limb of Henle, where renin synthesis occurs. Renin production is stimulated by high sympathetic tone, low flow in the afferent

arteriole, and low flow in the ascending limb of Henle's loop. Renin provokes production of angiotensin, which stimulates synthesis of aldosterone, influences sodium reabsorption in the proximal nephron and loop of Henle, and constricts blood vessels. Aldosterone activity influences distal sodium return to the plasma (Fig. 4.10).

WATER REGULATION

Over 65% of filtered water is returned to the circulation in the proximal nephron, along with sodium and other solutes. This transport conserves osmolality of the filtrate and rapidly returns a majority of the plasma filtrate to blood. Further water movement occurs out of the descending limb of Henle's loop. This movement commences the creation of filtrate hypertonicity as the filtrate descends through Henle's loop. However, further water movement out of the renal tubules is virtually prohibited until the filtrate reaches the collecting ducts, where water movement occurs through specialized water channels or pores independent of sodium, driven by osmotic gradients but governed by the presence or absence of vasopressin. This is an important point because this separation of operations allows the nephron to balance the body's need of water independently of sodium[8].

The governance of final water reabsorption independent from sodium in the collecting ducts serves to control body fluid osmolality. Vasopressin is the principal regulator. It is secreted from the hypothalamus when plasma osmolality rises above 285mOsm/kg[8]. Vasopressin's principal function is to increase the water permeability of the collecting duct. It accomplishes this by binding to membrane receptors and activating second messengers in the cytoplasm, which lead to the formation of water channels across the epithelial cell. Water permeability increases dramatically, and water will move according to osmotic gradients from tubular lumen into the interstitium. Medullary hypertonicity, generated by Henle's loop countercurrent multiplier mechanisms, pulls water out of the nephron and allows the water to return to the venous circulation of the kidney.

The hypothalamus–vasopressin–renal axis permits either retention of water independent of sodium or the excretion of water independent of sodium. The physiologic objective is protection of body fluid osmolality. Hence, excreted urine may be hyperosmolar in relation to plasma, meaning that the collecting duct is conserving water; or excreted urine may be hypoosmolar in relation to plasma, meaning that the collecting duct is not reabsorbing water presented to it.

The existence of a hypertonic medulla is essential to renal conservation of filtered water and the excretion of hyperosmolar urine[6]. The medullary interstitium is made hypertonic by the reabsorption of NaCl without water in the medullary ascending limb of Henle's loop. Urea presence in this region also contributes (Fig. 4.7). Tubular urine traveling through the distal nephron is hypotonic in relation to plasma. It has a water surplus. As distal nephron urine descends through the collecting duct, it will either be reabsorbed or excreted, depending upon the activity of vasopressin on the collecting duct. If vasopressin is present and active, collecting duct water channels will open and water will exit, drawn by the hypertonic medullary interstitium. The final urine will become hyperosmolar, or concentrated. The functional objective, however, was the return of water independent of solute to

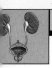
the plasma. If vasopressin is absent, then distal nephron urine will pass in its hypotonic state. The kidney will excrete a dilute urine, achieving net water loss from the body.

The hypothalamus is exquisitely sensitive to changes in osmolality[8]. Plasma tonicity higher than 284mOsm/L will promote vasopressin release, bringing about water conservation by the kidney aimed at returning plasma osmolality to 285mOsm/L. If the hypothalamus does not sense hypertonicity, it will not release vasopressin, and the kidney will excrete a final urine unaltered from its hypotonic condition as it descends the collecting ducts. However, vasopressin release from the hypothalamus will occur when vascular baroreceptors signal effective hypovolemia. In this setting, vasopressin and vasopressin-induced water reabsorption from the collecting ducts participate in extracellular volume homeostasis.

POTASSIUM REGULATION

Potassium is present in low concentrations in the circulating plasma, normally 4.0–4.4mEq/L. Filtered potassium is nearly completely reabsorbed from the filtrate in the proximal nephron and ascending loop of Henle[19]. Excretion of potassium, therefore, depends upon renal tubular secretion in the distal nephron. Potassium secretion occurs via two steps[19]. The first step is potassium uptake from plasma and interstitial fluid, driven by Na–K–ATPase. The second step is movement across the tubular lumen membrane through potassium channels, which are voltage-sensitive. Aldosterone influences both steps[21]. Aldosterone stimulates Na–K–ATPase, thereby increasing intracellular potassium concentrations and providing a gradient for potassium movement from cell into tubular lumen. Aldosterone also opens luminal membrane potassium channels and sodium channels[21]. By stimulating the basolateral Na–K–ATPase and opening both sodium and potassium channels in the luminal membrane, aldosterone sets a gradient for sodium transport from lumen to cell and a potassium gradient from cell to tubular lumen. The open channels provide the pathway. Sodium reabsorption from the urine also increases the lumen negativity, which amplifies the driving force for potassium to exit the cell through the open potassium channels (Fig. 4.11).

Variables in addition to aldosterone that influence potassium secretory rate are sodium delivery to the collecting duct, tubular water flow rate, and the intracellular potassium concentration, which is influenced by plasma potassium concentration and intracellular pH[19]. Disease states that preferentially damage tubules will impair potassium secretion without significant impairment in glomerular filtration rate. Examples include interstitial nephritis and analgesic nephropathy.

ACID–BASE REGULATION

Plasma pH is tightly defended by tissue-bound and circulating buffers, the lungs, and the kidneys. Maintenance of plasma pH at 7.38–7.42 depends upon readily available buffer systems that accept a hydrogen ion when it is produced, liberate hydrogen ions when necessary, and are readily renewable. Our bodies depend upon circulating HCO_3/CO_2 as a principal buffer system because it is renewable and flexible – the lungs can instantly change plasma PCO_2, and the kidneys can promptly generate new HCO_3.

The kidney actually has two important functions in the defense of pH and regulation of plasma HCO_3 concentration[22]. First, the kidney is charged with the actual elimination of hydrogen ions generated from diet and catabolism. Second, the kidney must conserve filtered HCO_3 and generate new HCO_3 to replace that which is consumed in buffering processes. Both proximal and distal regions of the nephron are operationally important in these activities (Fig. 4.12).

Reabsorption of filtered HCO_3 is absolutely essential for pH and HCO_3 homeostasis. Reabsorption of filtered HCO_3 is virtually 100% and is accomplished chiefly by the proximal tubule Na–H exchange mechanism[17]. This process does not result in net HCO_3 gain by the kidney. The proximal tubule simply reclaims filtered HCO_3, which otherwise would be lost from the plasma.

Frank excretion of liberated hydrogen ions from circulating acids and the generation of new HCO_3 is the other essential process of the kidney[22]. These are coupled, and two operations make the following contributions.

- Free hydrogen ions are secreted into the tubule lumen by specialized cells in the distal nephron that possess an H–ATPase transport system. This transport system is capable of extruding free hydrogen ions out of the cell into the tubular lumen, where the hydrogen ion can either exist freely and lower urinary pH or be picked up by urinary buffers, the most important being filtered phosphate (HPO_4). The cellular process that generates free hydrogen ions actually leads to the formation of HCO_3 ions. These HCO_3 ions then exit the cell across the basolateral membrane and return to the blood[22].
- Urinary excretion of hydrogen also occurs as ammonium (NH_4). Ammonium is generated in the proximal tubule from glutamine. Two NH_4 ions and two HCO_3 ions result from glutamine's metabolism. The NH_4 ions are secreted through specialized transport pathways into the lumen of the proximal tubule, and the new HCO_3 ions are transported across the basolateral membrane into the interstitial fluid and plasma[22].

Urinary excretion of hydrogen buffered by HPO_4 amounts to 40–50mmol per day. Urinary excretion of hydrogen in the form of NH_4 also amounts to 40–50mmol per day. In the setting of metabolic acidosis, however, renal production of NH_4 can be augmented to 300–500mmol per day. This renal response not only eliminates threatening hydrogen from the body, it generates abundant quantities of new HCO_3, which must replace circulating HCO_3 consumed in the systemic hydrogen ion buffering process. On a day-to-day basis, a typical adult will generate 70–100mmol of nonvolatile mineral acid. Liberated hydrogen ions will be buffered by circulating HCO_3. Ultimately, however, millimole for millimole, the renal epithelium will excrete these hydrogen ions and regenerate new HCO_3. Hydrogen ions will appear in the urine as NH_4 and H_2PO_4.

CALCIUM, MAGNESIUM AND PHOSPHORUS EXCRETION

Calcium circulates in plasma both as a free ion (~45%) and bound to carrier proteins (~55%), principally albumin. Only ionized calcium is filterable at the glomerulus. The kidney reabsorbs over 95% of filtered calcium, leading to a final urine calcium excretion of less than 200mg per day[23]. The proximal tubule reabsorbs 65% of filtered calcium in association with

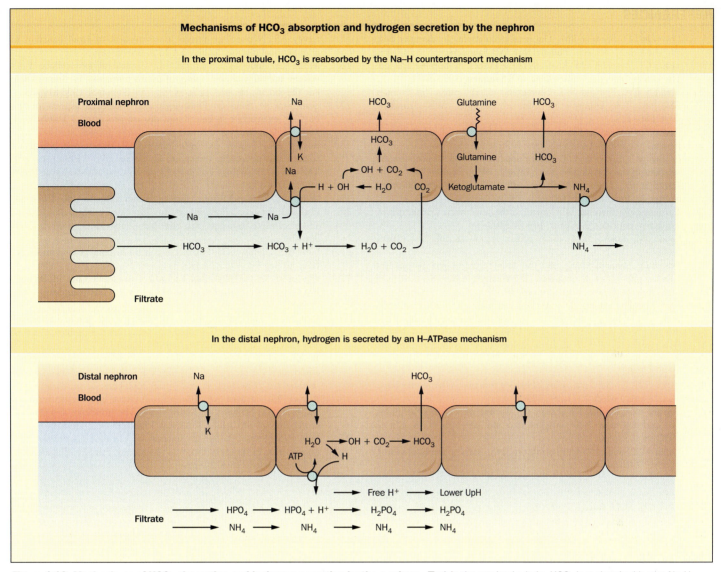

Figure 4.12 Mechanisms of HCO$_3$ absorption and hydrogen secretion by the nephron. (Top) In the proximal tubule, HCO$_3$ is reabsorbed by the Na-H countertransport mechanism. This action simply reclaims filtered HCO$_3$. The proximal tubule cells also synthesize NH$_4$ from glutamine. This biochemical sequence creates new HCO$_3$ ions, which enter the pericapillary blood and return to the general circulation of the body. NH$_4$ then carries hydrogen out in the urine. (Bottom) In the distal nephron, hydrogen is secreted by an H–ATPase mechanism. The free hydrogen will lower the pH of the urine to approximately 4.5 at most. Very little hydrogen is actually eliminated as free hydrogen ions. Most of this secreted hydrogen will be picked up by urinary HPO$_4$ floating downstream from filtration. HPO$_4$ serves as a urinary buffer and carrier of hydrogen out of the body. New HCO$_3$ is also generated by these cells. UpH, urinary pH.

sodium ions. There is no hormonal control in this segment. Approximately 25% of filtered calcium is reabsorbed in the loop of Henle. Transport here is driven electrically. The distal convoluted tubule reabsorbs the remaining 6–8% of calcium under the regulation of parathyroid hormone. The serum concentration of ionized calcium does not deviate much, despite large intrusions from diet. Tight regulation is accomplished by changes in its binding to its carrier proteins in plasma, principally albumin, and calcium movements between intestine, kidney, and bone, which are regulated by parathyroid hormone and 1,25-dihydroxycholecalciferol[24].

Phosphorus circulates as organic and inorganic forms. Only 30% of circulating phosphorus is inorganic, and 85% of this exists as monohydrogen or dihydrogen phosphate[25]. These phosphorus forms are filterable at the glomerulus. Phosphate is 80–85% reabsorbed in the proximal tubule. Reabsorption occurs in association with sodium and is regulated by parathyroid hormone and 1,25-dihydroxycholecalciferol[25]. As mentioned earlier, that portion of phosphate that escapes proximal reabsorption serves as a urinary buffer, receiving secreted hydrogen ions in the distal nephron[22]. Serum phosphorus concentrations vary widely during the day and are not tightly regulated.

Magnesium is 15% bound to carrier proteins in serum and 85% ionized. Ionized magnesium is freely filtered at the glomerulus and largely reabsorbed, principally in the ascending loop of Henle. There is no certain knowledge as to the mechanisms of magnesium regulation by the tubule but in states of hypomagnesemia, urinary excretion can decline to 0.5% of the filtered load of magnesium and in states of hypermagnesemia, excretion will rise to 40–60% of the filtered load[26].

REFERENCES

1. Dworkin LD, Brenner BM. The renal circulations. In: Brenner BM, ed. The kidney, 5th edn. Philadelphia: WB Saunders; 1996: 247–85.
2. Tisher CC, Madsen KM. Anatomy of the kidney. In: Brenner BM, ed. The kidney, 5th edn. Philadelphia: WB Saunders; 1996:3–71.
3. Maddox DA, Brenner BM. Glomerular ultrafiltration. In: Brenner BM, ed. The kidney, 5th edn. Philadelphia: WB Saunders; 1996:286–333.
4. Baylis C. Glomerular filtration dynamics. In: Lote CJ, ed. Advances in renal physiology. London: Grune & Stratton; 1986:33–83.
5. Beauwkes R, Bonventre JV. Tubular organization and vascular-tubular relations in the dog kidney. Am J Physiol. 1975;229:695–703.
6. Dworkin LK, Ichikawa I, Brenner BM. Hormonal modulation of glomerular function. Am J Physiol. 1983;224:F95–104.
7. Carmines PK, Fleming JT. Control of the renal microvasculature by vasoactive peptides. FASEB J. 1990;4:3300–9.
8. Sands JM, Kokko JP. Countercurrent system. Kidney Int. 1990; 38:695–9.
9. Rose BD. Loop of Henle and the countercurrent mechanism. In: Clinical physiology of acid–base and electrolyte disorders, 4th ed. New York: McGraw-Hill; 1994:116–38.
10. Rose BD. The total body water and the plasma sodium concentration. In: Clinical physiology of acid–base and electrolyte disorders, 4th edn. New York: McGraw-Hill; 1994:219–34.
11. Robertson GL, Berl T. Pathophysiology of water metabolism. In: Brenner BM, ed. The kidney, 5th edn. Philadelphia: WB Saunders; 1996:873–928.
12. Kassirer JP. Clinical evaluation of kidney function: Glomerular function. N Engl J Med. 1971;285:385–9.
13. Perrone RD, Madias NE, Levey AS. Serum creatinine as an index of renal function: new insights into old concepts. Clin Chem. 1992;38:1933–53.
14. Gillin AG, Sands JM. Urea transport in the kidney. Semin Nephrol. 1993;13:146–54.
15. Levey AS. Nephrology forum: measurement of renal function in chronic renal disease. Kidney Int.1990;38:167–84.
16. Miller JA, Tobe SW, Skorecki KL. Control of extracellular fluid volume and the pathophysiology of edema formation. In: Brenner BM, ed. The kidney, 5th edn. Philadelphia: WB Saunders; 1996:817–72.
17. Soleimani M, Sing G. Physiologic and molecular aspects of the Na^+/H^+ exchangers in health and disease processes. J Invest Med. 1995;43:419–30.
18. Rossier BC, Palmer LG. Mechanisms of aldosterone action on sodium and potassium transport. In: Seldin DW, Giebisch G, eds. The kidney: Physiology and pathophysiology. New York: Raven Press; 1992:1373–409.
19. Wright FS. Renal potassium handling. Semin Nephrol. 1987;7:174–84.
20. Rose BD. Potassium homeostasis. In: Clinical physiology of acid–base and electrolyte disorders, 4th edn. New York: McGraw-Hill; 1994: 346–78.
21. Field MJ, Giebisch GJ. Hormonal control of renal potassium excretion. Kidney Int. 1985;27:379–87.
22. Alpern RJ, Rector FC Jr. Renal acidification mechanisms. In: Brenner BM, ed. The kidney, 5th edn. Philadelphia: WB Saunders; 1996: 408–71.
23. Bushinsky DA. Homeostasis and disorders of calcium and phosphorus concentration. In: Greenberg A, ed. Primer on kidney diseases. San Diego, CA: Academic Press; 1994:406–13.
24. Bushinsky DA, Krieger NS. Integration of calcium metabolism in the adult. In: Coe FL, Fauus MJ, eds. Disorders of bone and mineral metabolism. New York: Raven Press; 1992:417–32.
25. Kovach KL, Hruska KA. Phosphate balance and metabolism. In: Jacobson HR, Striker GE, Klahr S, eds. The principles and practice of nephrology. St Louis: CV Mosby; 1995:986–92.
27. Suki WN, Rouse D. Renal transport of calcium, magnesium, and phosphorus. In: Brenner BM, ed. The kidney, 5th edn. Philadelphia: WB Saunders; 1996:472–515.

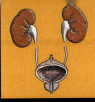

Chapter 5

Physiology and Pharmacology of the Ureter

Robert M Weiss

KEY POINTS

- Ureteral peristalsis begins with the origin of electrical activity at multiple functionally integrated pacemaker sites located in the proximal portion of the upper collecting system. The electrical activity propagates distally and gives rise to the mechanical contractile event that transports the urine in a distal direction.
- The electrical activity of the ureter depends on the distribution of ions across the cell membrane and the relative permeability of the cell membrane to these ions. The contractile activity of the ureter is related to the concentration of calcium in the region of the sarcoplasmic contractile proteins, actin and myosin.
- The ureter can efficiently transport a set maximum amount of fluid per unit time. Inadequate urine transport can result from too much urine entering the ureter per unit time or from too little urine exiting the ureter per unit time. Either process can lead to stasis of urine, increased intraluminal ureteral pressures, and urinary tract dilatation.
- The nervous system has a modulatory effect on ureteral function.

INTRODUCTION

In multicalyceal collecting systems, as are present in the human, urine transport from the kidneys to the bladder begins with the origin of electrical activity at multiple functionally integrated pacemaker sites located at the border of major and minor calyces[1–3]. As the electrical activity is propagated distally, from cell to cell, it gives rise to the mechanical propulsive event, i.e. the contraction wave, which under normal conditions completely coapts the ureteral walls and propels the urine distally in boluses[4]. Contraction waves occur at a frequency of approximately 6/min and are propagated at a velocity of 2–6cm/s[5]. The urine passes into the bladder through the ureterovesical junction (UVJ), which under normal conditions permits urine to pass in an antegrade direction from the ureter into the bladder but not in a retrograde direction from the bladder into the ureter.

ELECTRICAL ACTIVITY

Resting potential

The electrical properties of the ureter, like other excitable tissues, depend on the distribution of ions across the cell membrane and the relative permeability of the cell membrane to these ions. In the nonexcited or resting state, the electrical potential difference across the cell membrane, the resting membrane potential (RMP), is primarily determined by the distribution of potassium ions (K^+) across the cell membrane and the preferential permeability of the resting membrane to potassium[6] (Fig. 5.1). In the resting state the concentration of K^+ on the inside of the cell membrane is greater than that on the outside of the cell membrane and there is a tendency for the positively charged potassium ions to diffuse from the inside of the cell, where they are more concentrated, to the outside of the cell, where they are less concentrated. This leads to the development of an electrical gradient with the inside of the cell membrane being more negative than the outside. The electrical gradient that is formed tends to oppose the further outward movement of K^+ across the cell membrane along its concentration gradient. At equilibrium there is a greater concentration of K^+ on the inside of the cell membrane and the inside of the cell membrane is negatively charged with respect to the outside of the cell membrane. The RMP of the ureter ranges from –33mV to –70mV[7].

Action potential

When the ureteral cell is excited by an external stimulus, whether it be electrical, mechanical (stretch), or chemical, or by

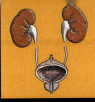

Nonpacemaker cell action potential

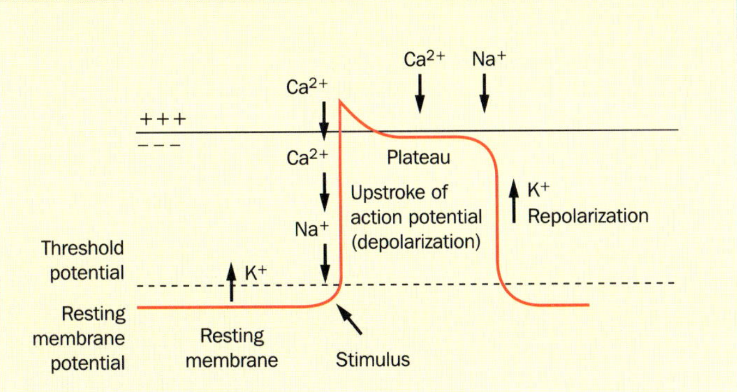

Figure 5.1 Nonpacemaker cell action potential. ↑ = outward current; ↓ = inward current.

conduction of electrical activity from an already excited adjacent cell, its membrane loses its preferential permeability to K^+ and becomes more permeable to calcium ions (Ca^{2+}) which move inward across the cell membrane[8] (Fig. 5.1). With the inward movement of the positively charged calcium ions the cell membrane depolarizes; the inside of the cell membrane becomes less negative than it was before stimulation and in fact may even become positive with respect to the outside of the cell membrane at the peak of the action potential, a state referred to as *overshoot*. If a sufficient area of the cell membrane is depolarized rapidly enough to reach a critical level, the *threshold potential*, a regenerative depolarization, or *action potential*, is initiated. The upstroke of the action potential, which is the primary event in conduction of electrical activity, is related to the inward movement of Ca^{2+} across the cell membrane, although there is some evidence that sodium ions (Na^+) also play a role in the upstroke of the action potential[9]. The rate of rise of the upstroke of the ureteral action potential is relatively slow, $1.2 \pm 0.06V/s$ in the cat[10].

After reaching the peak of its action potential, the ureteral cell membrane maintains its potential for a period of time (*plateau of the action potential*) before the transmembrane potential returns to its resting level (*repolarization*). The plateau phase is dependent on the persistence of an inward Ca^{2+} current and on Na^+ influx through a voltage-dependent Na^+ channel[11] (Fig. 5.1). The repolarization phase appears to depend on an outward Ca^{2+}-dependent K^+ current[11]. The action potential duration in the cat is in the range of $259-405ms$[12] and the configuration of the ureteral action potential more closely resembles a cardiac action potential than action potentials of other smooth muscles.

Pacemaker activity

Pacemaker cells are cells in which electrical activity develops spontaneously and do not require an external stimulus for excitation (Fig. 5.2). In contrast to the findings in nonpacemaker cells, the transmembrane potential does not remain constant in a resting phase but rather undergoes a slow spontaneous depolarization. When the membrane potential reaches the threshold potential, an action potential is generated that propagates distally from cell to cell across regions of close cellular contact, *intermediate junctions*[13]. Although the primary pacemakers for ureteral peristalsis are located in the proximal portion of the urinary collecting system, other regions such as the ureterovesical junction can serve as latent pacemakers. These latent pacemakers may become functional when freed from the domination of the primary pacemakers.

CONTRACTILE ACTIVITY

Contractile activity is related to the concentration of calcium in the region of the sarcoplasmic contractile proteins, actin and myosin. Any event that leads to an increase in the calcium concentration in the region of the contractile proteins favors contraction, and any event that leads to a decrease in the calcium concentration in the region of the contractile proteins favors relaxation (Fig. 5.3). During excitation the calcium involved in the contractile process is derived from two main sources. Inward movement of extracellular Ca^{2+} into the cell during the upstroke of the action potential provides a significant source of sarcoplasmic Ca^{2+}, and sarcoplasmic Ca^{2+} also can be derived from the release of Ca^{2+} from intracellular storage sites such as the endoplasmic (sarcoplasmic) reticulum, mitochondria, and membrane binding sites. The decrease in the concentration of free sarcoplasmic Ca^{2+} in the region of the contractile proteins that leads to relaxation results from the uptake of Ca^{2+} into intracellular storage sites and the extrusion of calcium across the cell membrane.

With excitation there is a transient increase in the concentration of free sarcoplasmic Ca^{2+} and this calcium binds to a calcium-binding protein, calmodulin (Fig. 5.4). The calcium–calmodulin

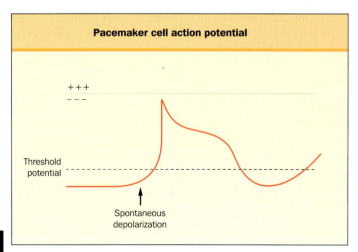

Figure 5.2 Pacemaker cell action potential.

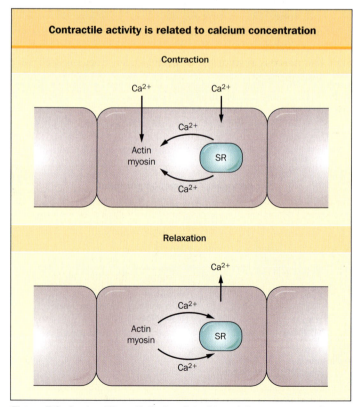

Figure 5.3 Contractile activity is related to calcium concentration.
SR, sarcoplasmic reticulum.

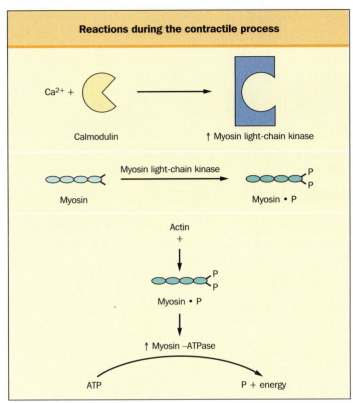

Figure 5.4 Reactions during the contractile process. Ca^{2+}, calcium; ATP, Adenosine triphosphate; P, phosphorous.

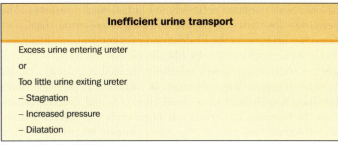

Figure 5.5 Inefficient urine transport.

complex in turn activates a calmodulin-dependent enzyme, myosin light-chain kinase, which phosphorylates the 20,000Da light chain of myosin. The phosphorylated myosin allows for activation by actin of myosin Mg^{2+}–ATPase activity, with resultant hydrolysis of adenosine triphosphate (ATP) and contraction of the smooth muscle. Relaxation is related to a decrease in free sarcoplasmic Ca^{2+} concentration, which hampers myosin phosphorylation, a process that is required for smooth muscle contraction. Myosin also may be dephosphorylated, i.e. inactivated by a phosphatase.

URINE TRANSPORT

Renal pelvis and ureteropelvic junction
With filling of the renal pelvis there is a rise in renal pelvic pressure and urine is extruded into the collapsed ureter[14]. At this stage the ureteropelvic junction (UPJ) is closed and may be protective to the kidney, since ureteral contractile pressures are higher than renal pelvic pressures. The frequency of calyceal and renal pelvic contractions is greater than that of the ureter, with a conduction block at the UPJ[15]. Since, at normal urine flow rates, the empty ureter is collapsed, urine transport in the ureter occurs in the form of boluses. As urine is transported from the renal pelvis into the upper ureter, renal pelvic pressure decreases to its baseline value and the process of filling and emptying is repeated.

Ureter
At normal flow rates contraction waves originating in the proximal ureter coapt the ureter and move the bolus of urine, which is located in front of it in a passive, noncontracting portion of

the ureter, distally toward the bladder. Resting ureteral pressure is approximately $0–5cmH_2O$ and contraction waves at a pressure of $20–60cmH_2O$ are generated at 10–30s intervals[16]. Conduction velocity is approximately 2–5cm/s.

Ureterovesical junction
In order for urine to pass across the ureterovesical junction (UVJ) into the bladder, intraluminal ureteral pressures must exceed intravesical pressures. During the process the UVJ does not relax, but telescoping and shortening of the distal ureter facilitates urine passage across the UVJ[17,18].

Inefficient urine transport
As with any tubular structure the ureter can efficiently transport a set maximum amount of fluid per unit time. Inefficient urine transport can result from too much urine entering the ureter per unit time or from too little urine exiting the ureter per unit time (Fig. 5.5). Either process can result in stasis of urine and urinary tract dilatation.

Changes in ureteral dimensions in themselves can result in inefficient urine transport. The Laplace equation expresses the relationship between the variables that affect intraluminal pressure:

Pressure = (Stress × Wall thickness) ÷ Radius.

Thus an increase in ureteral diameter in itself can decrease ureteral intraluminal pressure and result in inefficient urine transport[19].

Diuresis
With diuresis increased urine transport is initially dependent on an increase in peristaltic frequency. Once reaching a maximum, further increase in urine transport is dependent on increases in bolus volume. With further increases in diuresis the urine boluses coalesce and finally the ureter becomes filled with a column of urine. At high flow rates the ureteral walls do not coapt and urine is transported distally in a continuous column.

DISTENDED BLADDER AND NEUROGENIC VESICAL DYSFUNCTION

Increased intravesical pressure resulting from an overdistended bladder or from neurogenic vesical dysfunction may act as an obstructive factor and result in impaired urine transport. Intravesical pressures during the storage phase or phase of bladder filling are most important in determining the efficacy of urine transport into the bladder. With filling of the normal bladder, sympathetic impulses and the viscoelastic properties of the bladder wall maintain relatively low intravesical pressures. The relatively low intravesical pressures facilitate urine transport from the ureter into the bladder and prevent ureteral dilatation. In the noncompliant fibrotic bladder or in some forms of neurogenic vesical dysfunction, relatively small increases in bladder volume result in large increases in intravesical pressure, with resultant impairment of ureteral emptying and ureteral dilatation. In humans, the ureter has been shown to decompensate when intravesical storage pressures exceed $40 cmH_2O$[20]. To a lesser extent a greatly distended normal bladder can impair ureteral emptying even though intravesical pressures are low. This results from stretch of the UVJ and decreased retractability of the intravesical submucosal ureteral segment.

PATHOLOGIC PROCESSES AFFECTING URINE TRANSPORT

Obstruction

The deleterious effects of obstruction are dependent on the degree and duration of the obstruction, the rate of urine flow, the mechanical and anatomic properties of the urinary tract, the nature of the obstructing process, the presence or absence of infection, and the age of the individual in whom the obstructive process is present. In general, dilatation of the urinary tract occurs proximal to the site of obstruction, and a number of factors may influence the degree of dilatation or even determine whether dilatation occurs. A mildly or intermittently obstructed system may manifest dilatation at high but not at low flows; a normal system that is acutely obstructed with a stone may not necessarily dilate; an intrarenal pelvis may dilate less than an extrarenal pelvis; a nonfunctioning system may not dilate even when obstructed; and a noncompliant or encased system may manifest a decreased degree of dilatation at any given magnitude of obstruction. Furthermore, obstructed systems that develop a proximal leak may not manifest dilatation. This is classically seen with an acute high-grade obstruction resulting from a ureteral calculus and it also manifests itself as urinary ascites in utero or in the neonate resulting from urethral valves or ureteropelvic junction obstructions.

Dilatation proximal to the site of obstruction is the classic finding. With the onset of obstruction, urine is impeded at the obstructive site and there is an increase in ureteral intraluminal resting (basal) pressure. The increase in intraluminal pressure depends on the ability of the kidney to continue to produce urine and the dilatation results from the increase in intraluminal pressure and from the backup of urine in the urinary tract[21] (Fig. 5.6). Early in the obstructive process there is a transient increase in the amplitude and frequency of ureteral peristalsis[22] but, as the ureter fills with urine, the amplitude of the contractions decrease. With time intraluminal pressure reaches a peak and then begins to decline toward baseline levels. The decrease in intraluminal pressure in the obstructed system with time is attributed to a decrease in renal blood flow and resultant decrease in glomerular filtration rate (GFR) and to pyelovenous and pyelolymphatic backflow. Ureteral dilatation tends to persist during this period of decreasing intraluminal pressure, and this is attributed to the hysteretic properties of the viscoelastic ureteral structure[23]. The subsequent gradual increase in ureteral dimensions in the face of relatively low intraluminal pressures requires the production of

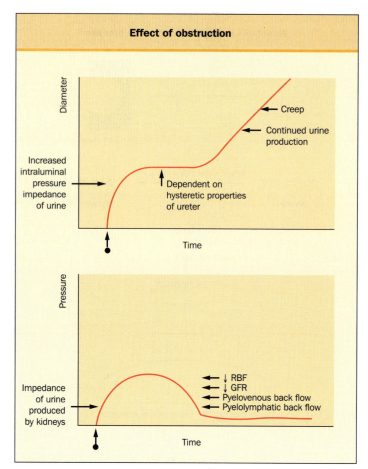

Figure 5.6 Effect of obstruction. ↕, time of onset of obstruction; RBF, renal blood flow; GFR, glomerular filtration rate.

at least a small amount of urine and is explained by creep of the viscoelastic ureteral structure[24]. The chronically obstructed upper urinary tract, although massively dilated, may have relatively low intraluminal pressures. In some instances the dimensions of the chronically obstructed ureter will subsequently decrease and this depends on the reabsorption of urine and the mechanical properties of the ureter.

Infection

Bacteria and endotoxins inhibit ureteral activity and pyelonephritis in the monkey, and in humans is associated with decreased ureteral peristaltic activity[25,26]. Furthermore, ureteral dilatation can occur with retroperitoneal inflammatory processes secondary to appendicitis, ulcerative colitis, regional enteritis, and peritonitis.

Aging

Clinically, more marked degrees of dilatation are observed in the neonate and young child than in the adult (Fig. 5.7). This may be a result of differences in pathologic processes that affect the ureter in the various age groups and/or to age-dependent differences in the ureteral response to a given pathologic process. In support of the latter hypothesis is the demonstration of a greater degree of deformation of the neonatal than the adult rabbit ureter in response to an applied intraluminal pressure load[27] and the decreased contractility of the neonatal compared

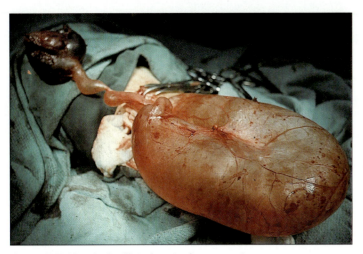

Figure 5.7 Massively dilated ureter in a neonate.

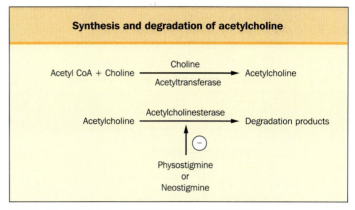

Figure 5.8 Synthesis and degradation of acetylcholine.
CoA, coenzyme A.

to the adult ureter[28]. There also are age-dependent differences in the response of the ureter to pharmacologic agents. The neonatal rabbit ureter is more sensitive to norepinephrine than the adult ureter[27] and the relaxant response of the ureter to beta-adrenergic agonists such as isoproterenol decreases with age[29]. The latter appears to be due to a decrease in adenylyl cyclase activity and an increase in inhibitory G-proteins, G_i, with age[30,31]. The excitatory responses to cholinergic agonists such as acetylcholine are more marked in ureters from younger than older guinea-pigs[32].

Pregnancy

Hydroureteronephrosis of pregnancy occurs more on the right side than on the left. It tends not to occur below the pelvic brim. Upper urinary tract dilatation begins in the second trimester and usually subsides within the first month after parturition. It would appear that both obstruction and hormonal changes are etiologic factors in ureteral dilatation of pregnancy[33,34].

NEUROPHYSIOLOGY

Multiunit smooth muscles have a specific innervation for each smooth muscle cell, whereas syncytial-type smooth muscles such as the ureter lack discrete neuromuscular junctions and depend on a diffuse release of neurotransmitter with spread of excitation from one muscle cell to another. Although ureteral peristalsis can occur without innervation, the nervous system has a modulatory effect on ureteral function[35].

Autonomic nervous system

Both catecholamines and acetylcholine (ACh) can be released from the ureter in response to electrical field stimulation indicating that the ureter is supplied by both the sympathetic and parasympathetic nervous systems[36,37]. The ureter contains adrenergic and muscarinic cholinergic receptors and catecholamine- and acetylcholinesterase-containing neurons have been demonstrated in the ureter[38-40]. The α-adrenergic and parasympathetic receptor mechanisms are excitatory and the β-adrenergic receptor mechanisms are inhibitory.

Acetylcholine is the prototype cholinergic agonist and serves as the neurotransmitter at neuromuscular junctions of somatic motor nerves, preganglionic parasympathetic and sympathetic neuroeffector junctions (nicotinic sites), and postganglionic parasympathetic neuroeffector junctions (muscarinic sites). ACh is synthesized in the nerve terminals from acetyl coenzyme A (CoA) and choline by the enzyme choline acetyltransferase (Fig. 5.8). ACh is degraded by acetylcholinesterase (AChE). The muscarinic effects of cholinergic agonists can be potentiated by anticholinesterases, such as physostigmine and neostigmine, which inhibit ACh degradation and can be inhibited by parasympatholytic agents such as atropine. Norepinephrine, the prototype adrenergic agonist, serves as the neurotransmitter at postganglionic sympathetic neuroeffector junctions. Norepinephrine (NE) is synthesized in the neuron from tyrosine (Fig. 5.9). Neuronal reuptake of NE limits the time that it is in contact with the neuroeffector junction and thus limits the magnitude and duration of its action. Agents such as cocaine, which inhibit neuronal reuptake, potentiate the stimulatory effects of norepinephrine. The enzymes monoamine oxidase (MAO) and catechol-O-methyltransferase (COMT) degrade NE.

Activation of α_1-adrenergic receptors leads to ureteral contraction via activation of an enzyme, phospholipase C (PLC), which results in the hydrolysis of polyphosphatidylinositol 4,5-biphosphate (PIP_2) with the formation of two second messengers, 1,4,5-inositol trisphosphate (IP_3) and diacylglycerol (DG)[41] (Fig. 5.10). Activation of PLC involves a guanine nucleotide regulatory protein, G protein. IP_3 is involved in calcium mobilization from intracellular storage sites such as the endoplasmic (sarcoplasmic) reticulum[42], and DG increases Ca^{2+} influx across the cell membrane via a process that involves activation of protein kinase C (PKC)[43]. α-Adrenergic antagonists such as phentolamine and phenoxybenzamine inhibit the excitatory effects of NE on the ureter.

Activation of β-adrenergic receptors, with agonists such as isoproterenol, results in the formation of cyclic adenosine 3′5′-monophosphate (cyclic AMP), with resultant ureteral relaxation (Fig. 5.11). The process involves activation of an enzyme, adenylyl cyclase[30]. A stimulatory, G-protein, Gs, functionally links the receptor-agonist complex and the active unit of the enzyme, adenylyl cyclase. The relaxant effects of cyclic AMP are in part related to its causing an uptake of Ca^{2+} in the sarcoplasmic reticulum (SR) with a resultant decrease in free sarcoplasmic Ca^{2+}. Cyclic AMP is degraded by an enzyme, phosphodiesterase. Inhibition of phosphodiesterase by agents such as theophylline also increases cyclic AMP levels and leads to ureteral relaxation.

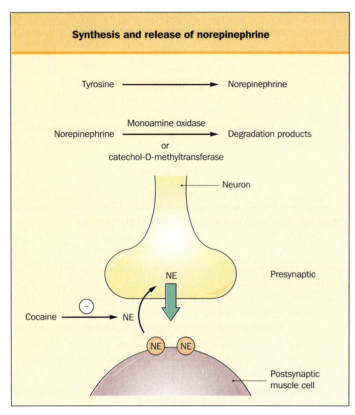

Figure 5.9 Synthesis and release of norepinephrine (NE).

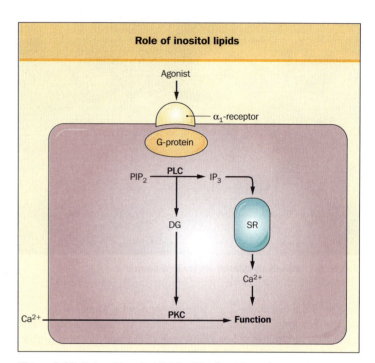

Figure 5.10 Role of inositol lipids. DG, diacylglycerol; IP_3, 1,4,5-inositol trisphosphate; PIP_2, polyphosphatidylinositol 4,5-biphosphate; PKC, protein kinase C; PLC, phospholipase C; SR, sarcoplasmic reticulum.

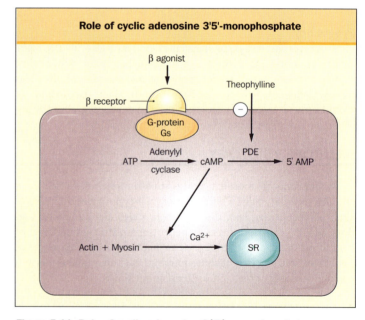

Figure 5.11 Role of cyclic adenosine 3′5′-monophosphate. AMP, adenosine monophosphate; ATP, adenosine triphosphate; cAMP; cyclic adenosine 3′5′-monophosphate; PDE, phosphodiesterase; SR, sarcoplasmic reticulum.

β-adrenergic antagonists such as propranolol block the inhibitory effects of β-adrenergic agonists on the ureter.

Activation of muscarinic cholinergic receptors increases the amplitude of ureteral contractions. Some of these actions are related to activation of phospholipase C (PLC) and an increase in inositol lipid metabolism with a resultant increase in sarcoplasmic Ca^{2+}, and other actions appear to be related to activation of an inhibitory G-protein, G_i, with resultant inhibition of adenylyl cyclase activity[44]. The excitatory effects of α_2-adrenergic agonists are also in part due to activation of an inhibitory G-protein.

NITRIC OXIDE TRANSDUCTION MECHANISMS

An enzyme, nitric oxide synthase (NOS), converts L-arginine to nitric oxide (NO) and citrulline (Fig. 5.12). NO activates an enzyme, guanylyl cyclase, which converts guanosine triphosphate (GTP) to cyclic GMP. NOS-containing nerves have been demonstrated in the ureter[45] and NOS has been demonstrated in the ureterovesical junction[46]. Cyclic GMP relaxes a number of smooth muscles, including the ureter[47], and NO inhibits ureteral contractility and relaxes the pig UVJ[48].

PEPTIDERGIC NERVOUS SYSTEM

The ureter contains capsaicin-sensitive sensory nerves[49]. Release of the tachykinins substance P (SP), neurokinin A (NKA), and neuropeptide K (NPK) from these nerves has an excitatory effect on ureteral peristalsis, whereas release of calcitonin-gene-related peptide (CGRP) has an inhibitory effect[50]. The inhibitory effects of CGRP are in part related to the opening of ATP-sensitive K^+ channels, which hyperpolarizes the membrane

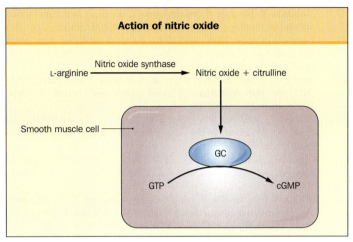

Figure 5.12 Action of nitric oxide. cGMP, cyclic guanosine monophosphate; GC, guanylyl cyclase; GTP, guanosine triphosphate;

and results in the blockage of voltage-sensitive Ca^{2+} channels. This blocks the inward movement of calcium that is involved in the upstroke of the action potential[51]. The inhibitory effects of CGRP also may be related to stimulation of adenylyl cyclase activity with resultant increase in cyclic AMP[52]. Peptidergic neurons containing neuropeptide Y (NPY) and vasoactive intestinal polypeptide (VIP), the latter of which is inhibitory to ureteral peristalsis, are present in the ureter[38]. NOS colocalizes with VIP and NPY in nerves supplying the human ureter[53].

Ureteral peristaltic activity begins with the origin of electrical activity in pacemaker sites located in the proximal portion of the upper urinary tract. The electrical activity propagates distally and leads to the mechanical contractile event of peristalsis, which pushes the bolus of urine distally into the bladder. Ureteral peristalsis is influenced and modulated by the nervous system.

REFERENCES

1. Bozler E. The activity of the pacemaker previous to the discharge of a muscular impulse. Am J Physiol. 1942;136:543.
2. Weiss RM, Wagner ML, Hoffman BF. Localization of pacemaker for peristalsis in the intact canine ureter. Invest Urol. 1967;5:42.
3. Constantinou CE, Silvert MA, Gosling JA. Pacemaker system in the control of ureteral peristaltic rate in the multicalyceal kidney of the pig. Invest Urol. 1977;14:440.
4. Woodburne RT, Lapides J. The ureteral lumen during peristalsis. Am J Anat. 1972;133:255.
5. Kobayashi M. Conduction velocity in various regions of the ureter. Tohoku J Exp Med. 1964;83:220.
6. Hendrickx H, Vereecken RL, Casteels R. The influence of potassium on the electrical and mechanical activity of the guinea pig ureter. Urol Res. 1975;3:155.
7. Kuriyama H, Osa T, Toida N. Membrane properties of the smooth muscle of guinea-pig ureter. J Physiol (Lond). 1967;191:225.
8. Kobayashi M. Effects of Na and Ca on the generation and conduction of excitation in the ureter. Am J Physiol. 1965;208:715.
9. Muraki K, Imuizumi Y, Watanabe M. Sodium currents in smooth muscle cells freshly isolated from stomach fundus of the rat and ureter of the guinea pig. J Physiol (Lond). 1991;442:351.
10. Kobayashi M. Effect of calcium on electrical activity in smooth muscle cells of cat ureter. Am J Physiol. 1969;216:1279.
11. Imaizumi Y, Muraki K, Watanabe M. Ionic currents in single smooth muscle cells from the ureter of the guinea pig. J Physiol (Lond). 1989;411:131.
12. Kobayashi M, Irisawa H. Effect of sodium deficiency on the action potential of the smooth muscle of the ureter. Am J Physiol. 1964;206:205.
13. Libertino JA, Weiss RM. Ultrastructure of human ureter. J Urol. 1972;108:71.
14. Griffiths DJ, Notschaele C. The mechanics of urine transport in the upper urinary tract: I. The dynamics of the isolated bolus. Neurourol Urodynam. 1983;2:155.
15. Morita T, Ishizuka G, Tsuchida S. Initiation and propagation of stimulus from the renal pelvic pacemaker in pig kidney. Invest Urol. 1981;19:157.
16. Edmond P, Ross JA, Kirkland IS. Human ureteral peristalsis. J Urol. 1970;104:670.

17. Weiss RM, Biancani P. Characteristics of normal and refluxing ureterovesical junctions. J Urol. 1983;129:858.
18. Blok C, van Venrooij GEPM, Coolsaet BLRA. Dynamics of the ureterovesical junction: a qualitative analysis of the ureterovesical pressure profile in the pig. J Urol. 1985;134:818.
19. Griffiths DJ. The mechanics of urine transport in the upper urinary tract. II. The discharge of the bolus of urine into the bladder and dynamics at high rates of flow. Neurourol Urodynam. 1983;2:167.
20. McGuire EJ, Woodside JR, Borden TA, Weiss RM. Prognostic value of urodynamic testing in myelodysplastic patients. J Urol. 1981;126:205.
21. Biancani P, Zabinski MP, Weiss RM. Time course of ureteral changes with acute and chronic obstruction. Am J Physiol. 1976;231:393.
22. Rose JG, Gillenwater JY. Effects of obstruction on ureteral function. Urology. 1978;12:139.
23. Weiss RM, Bassett AL, Hoffman BF. Dynamic length-tension curves of cat ureter. Am J Physiol. 1971;222:388.
24. Biancani P, Zabinski MP, Weiss RM. Bidimensional deformation of acutely obstructed in vitro rabbit ureter. Am J Physiol. 1973;225:671.
25. King WW, Cox CE. Bacterial inhibition of ureteral smooth muscle contractility. I. The effect of common urinary pathogens and endotoxin in an in vitro system. J Urol. 1972;108:700.
26. Roberts JA. Experimental pyelonephritis in the monkey. III. Pathophysiology of ureteral malfunction induced by bacteria. Invest Urol. 1975;13:117.
27. Akimoto M, Biancani P, Weiss RM. Comparative pressure-length-diameter relationships of neonatal and adult rabbit ureters. Invest Urol. 1977;14:297.
28. Hong KW, Biancani P, Weiss RM. Effect of age on contractility of guinea pig ureter. Invest Urol. 1980;17:459.
29. Wheeler MA, Cho YH, Hong KW, Weiss RM. Age-dependent alterations in beta-adrenergic receptor function in guinea pig ureter. In Sperelakis N, Wood J, eds. Frontiers in smooth muscle research. Progress in Clinical and Biological Research 327. New York: Alan R Liss; 1990:711–5.
30. Wheeler MA, Housman A, Cho YH, Weiss RM. Age dependence of adenylate cyclase activity in guinea pig ureter homogenate. J Pharmacol Exp Ther. 1986;239:99.

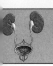

31. Derweesh IH, Wheeler MA, Weiss RM. Alterations of G proteins in rat bladder during aging. J Urol. 1998;159:17.

32. Weiss RM, Wheeler MA, Biancani P. Age related changes in the response of ureteral smooth muscle to autonomic agonists. Fed Proc. 1985;44:506.

33. Roberts JA. Hydronephrosis of pregnancy. Urology. 1976;8:1.

34. Van Wagenen G, Jenkins RH. An experimental examination of factors causing ureteral dilatation of pregnancy. J Urol. 1939;42:1010.

35. Morita T, Wada I, Saekai H, Tsuchida S, Weiss RM. Ureteral urine transport: changes in bolus volume, peristaltic frequency, intraluminal pressure and volume of flow resulting from autonomic drugs. J Urol. 1987;137:132.

36. Weiss RM, Bassett AL, Hoffman BF. Adrenergic innervation of the ureter. Invest Urol. 1978;16:123.

37. DelTacca M. Acetylcholine content of and release from isolated pelviureteral tract. Naunyn Schmiedebergs Arch Pharmacol. 1978;302:293.

38. Edyvane KA, Smet PJ, Trussell DC, Jonavicius J, Marshall VR. Patterns of neuronal colocalisation of tyrosine hydoxylase, neuropeptide Y, vasoactive intestinal polypeptide, calcitonin gene-related peptide and substance P in human ureter. J Auton Nerv Syst. 1994;48:241.

39. Latifpour J, Kondo S, O'Hollaren B, Morita T, Weiss RM. Autonomic receptors in urinary tract. Sex and age differences. J Pharmacol Ther. 1990;253:661.

40. Prieto D, Simonsen U, Martin J, et al. Histochemical and functional evidence for a cholinergic innervation of the equine ureter. J Auton Nerv Syst. 1994;47:159.

41. Berridge MJ. Inositol trisphosphate and diacylglycerol as second messengers. Biochem J. 1984;220:345.

42. Streb H, Irvine RF, Berridge MJ, Schulz I. Release of Ca^{++} from a non-mitochondrial store in pancreatic acinar cell by inositol 1,4,5-triphosphate. Nature. 1983;306:67.

43. Nishizuka Y. The role of protein kinase C in cell surface signal transduction and tumor production. Nature. 1984;308:693.

44. Londos C, Cooper DMF, Rodbell M. Receptor-mediated stimulation and inhibition of adenylate cyclases: the fat cell as a model system. Adv Cyclic Nucleotide Res. 1981;14:163.

45. Stief CG, Taher A, Meyer M, et al. A possible role of nitric oxide (NO) in the relaxation of renal pelvis and ureter. J Urol. 1993;149:492A.

46. Phillips JL, Wheeler MA, Weiss RM. Differential nitric oxide synthase (NOS) activity in developing fetal pig ureterovesical junction. FASEB J. 1995;9:A679.

47. Cho YH, Biancani P, Weiss RM. Adenyl and guanyl nucleotide induced relaxation of ureteral smooth muscle. Fed Proc. 1984;43:353.

48. Chiu AW, Babayan RK, Krane RJ, Saenz deTejada I. Effects of nitric oxide on ureteral contraction. J Urol. 1994;151:335A.

49. Maggi CA, Santicioli P, Guiliani S, Abelli L, Meli A. The motor effect of the capsaicin-sensitive inhibitory innervation of the rat ureter. Eur J Pharmacol. 1986;126:333.

50. Hua XY, Lundberg JM. Dual capsaicin effects on ureteric motility: low dose inhibition mediated by calcitonin gene-related peptide and high dose stimulation by tachykinins? Acta Physiol Scand. 1986;128:453.

51. Meini S, Santicioli P, Maggi CA. Propagation of impulses in the guinea-pig ureter and its blockade by calcitonin gene-related peptide (CGRP). Naunyn Schmiedebergs Arch Pharmacol. 1995;351:79.

52. Santicioli P, Morbidelli L, Parenti A, Ziche M, Maggi CA. Calcitonin gene-related peptide selectivey increases cAMP levels in the guinea-pig ureter. Eur J Pharmacol. 1995;289:17.

53. Smet PJ, Edyvane KA, Jonavicius J, Marshall VR. Colocalization of nitric oxide synthase with vasoactive intestinal peptide, neuropeptide Y, tyrosine hydroxylase in nerves supplying the human ureter. J Urol. 1994;152:1292.

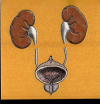

Chapter 6

Bladder and Urethra: Function and Dysfunction

Nicholas JR George

KEY POINTS

- A detailed knowledge of neuroanatomy does not fully explain the function of the lower urinary tract.
- Pathologic conditions affecting regions above the pons are usually associated with synchronous bladder/sphincter activity.
- Under normal circumstances high bladder compliance is maintained during filling by active neurologic processes.
- Urodynamic tests need to be specifically tailored to the needs of the individual patient.
- Obstructive renal failure is linked to abnormalities of the filling (not voiding) phase of the micturition cycle.
- Underactive detrusor function may or may not develop from pre-existing intravesical obstruction.

INTRODUCTION

In recent years significant advances have taken place relating to detailed knowledge of both macroscopic and microscopic anatomy of the human lower urinary tract. Such studies, together with observations from earlier animal work and necessarily limited experiments on humans, provide a reasonable starting point for hypotheses relating structure to function. Caution must, however, be exercised when extrapolating from nonphysiologic animal experiments which may additionally be subject to error due to species difference. Hence it will be recognized that present understanding of integrated lower urinary tract function in humans relies in considerable part on derived pharmacologic and neurologic principles thought to be important for both sensory and motor control but for which little direct experimental evidence is in existence. This chapter gives a brief overview of such understanding, relates it to the common dysfunctions of the bladder and urethra, and outlines the test procedures by which such abnormalities may be diagnosed.

GROSS ANATOMY

Bladder

The adventitia (peritoneum), smooth muscle (detrusor), and urothelium constitute the three layers of the bladder. Layers and folds of the external fascia covering the bladder pass laterally to the pelvic side walls and anteriorly to the anterior abdominal wall to locate and support the organ, which is further fixed by its attachment to the prostate and by fascial folds passing posteriorly to the rectum. The detrusor smooth muscle constitutes the bulk of the bladder dome, the fibers being arranged in no specific direction or layer; interlacing bundles form a complex meshwork of smooth muscle rather than discrete layers as was originally proposed[1]. In the normal healthy bladder connective tissue components constitute a small proportion of the wall structure (Fig. 6.1a), collagen being dispersed throughout the detrusor bundles while elastin is typically associated with vascular bundles. Aging and obstruction may dramatically alter the composition of the muscle mass leading to significant clinical bladder dysfunction (described below) typified by type III collagen infiltration (Figs 6.1b & c), compensatory smooth muscle hypertrophy[2], and decreased autonomic innervation[3].

The main body of the detrusor muscle passes behind the trigone, which is itself a thin superficial layer of alpha-adrenergic smooth muscle contiguous with the ureters, passing down to the veru montanum in the male and fading out in the proximal urethra in the female[1,4]. The trigone is of functional importance in the control of the vesicoureteric orifices.

In both sexes at the bladder neck the detrusor bundles loop and spiral around the urethra, fading away distally. The functional purpose of this relatively insignificant part of the detrusor remains open to debate; most agree that in the normal human this 'proximal' or 'internal' sphincter plays no convincing role in the maintenance of urinary continence, although relaxation of urethral fibers is known to occur during micturition.

In the male a circumferential collar of alpha-adrenergic smooth muscle surrounds the bladder neck and is described as the preprostatic sphincter (Fig. 6.2). This muscle merges distally with the prostate and prostatic capsule before thinning at the apex of the gland, and the entire morphologic unit may be regarded as having a genital function. The preprostatic sphincter prevents retrograde ejaculation while α-innervated periprostatic muscle assists drainage of ducts during sexual intercourse. In the neurologically normal human resection of the bladder neck muscle during transurethral resection of the prostate does not result in urinary incontinence, illustrating the functional distinction between urinary and genital sphincters at the base of the bladder.

In the female, bladder neck support is naturally much weaker than in the male. Nevertheless, urinary 'milk back' after a stop test is usually rapid and must be accomplished by a mixture of looping detrusor fibers as well as connective tissues including elastin, striated muscle, and vascular tissue.

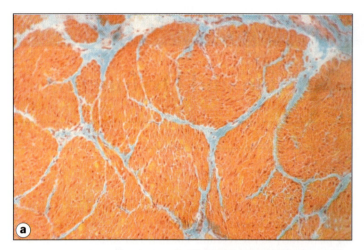

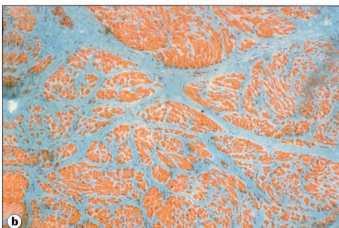

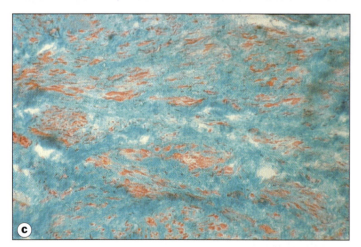

Figure 6.1 Progressive changes within detrusor muscle leading to poor compliance. (a) Normal bladder. (b) Muscle bundles progressivly replaced by collagen infiltration (staining green). (c) Almost total collagen infiltration, Masson's trichrome. (Courtesy of Professor JA Gosling.)

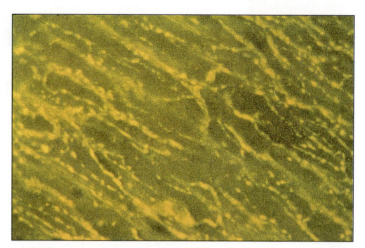

Figure 6.2 Vividly fluorescent nonadrenergic nerves present among muscle bundles of the preprostatic sphincter. (Courtesy of Professor JA Gosling.)

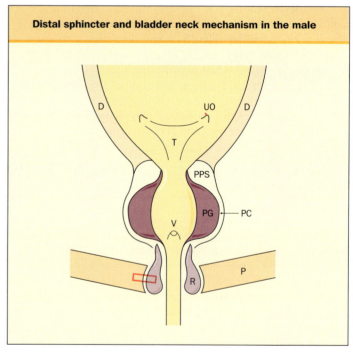

Figure 6.3 Distal sphincter and bladder neck mechanism in the male. P, periurethral striated muscle (levator ani); R, rhabdosphincter; V, verumontanum; PG, prostate gland; PC, prostatic capsule; PPS, preprostatic sphincter; T, trigone; UO, ureteric orifice; D, detrusor; Oblong box, section through periurethral striated muscle and rhabdosphincter illustrated in Figure 6.4.

Urethral sphincter mechanism
Terminology
In the past the terminology of the urethral sphincter has given rise to confusion. Clearly separate from the bladder neck mechanism (the 'proximal' sphincter), the functional distal sphincter mechanism has been variously associated with either the distal intrinsic sphincter (rhabdosphincter; Fig. 6.3) or the periurethral striated muscle, essentially the levator ani muscle of the pelvic floor (pubourethral sling). Most authorities now agree that the rhabdosphincter is the true sphincteric mechanism responsible for urinary continence, and the surrounding striated periurethral component is for emergency reinforcement of sphincter tone.

Morphology

Significant differences exist between the striated muscle of the periurethral pubourethral sling and that of the rhabdosphincter itself (Fig. 6.4). That of the levator ani is typically a mixture of fast- and slow-twitch fibers of relatively large diameter while fibers of the rhabdosphincter are usually small in cross section (15–20μm) and predominantly of the slow twitch type[5]. These cells are packed with mitochondria and lipid droplets, features known to be associated with fibers capable of maintaining tone over long periods of time; hence such fibers are ideally suited to the preservation of continence[6].

The disposition of the intrinsic rhabdosphincter is remarkable; rather than the expected circular fibers, most run either longitudinally or obliquely and the muscle is relatively deficient posteriorly, being seen in cross-section to be horseshoe- or signet-ring-shaped. The nerve supply (see below) to the intrinsic sphincter originates not from the motor cell nuclei of the anterior horn of the sacral cord, which supply the true pelvic floor (Fig. 6.5), but from a nucleus more medially placed in the ventral horn of S2 and S3 known as Onuf's nucleus X; fibers from this nucleus also supply the striated muscles of the anal sphincter[7].

AFFERENT INNERVATION FROM THE LOWER URINARY TRACT

Classic, specialized, sensory end organs are not to be found within the lower urinary tract. Nevertheless an extensive plexus of nerves may be found under the urothelium within the lamina propria as well as within the bulk of the covering muscle[8]. Such simple or free nerve endings may respond to mechanical, thermal, or painful (nociceptor) stimuli. It is considered that some such endings may respond to more than one

type of stimulus – polymodal receptors (see below) – interpretation is thought to be by frequency analysis of incoming neurologic signals.

The urothelial lining of the anterior urethra is sensitive to touch, thermal sensation, and pain[9]. 'Stretch' sensations from the level of the urethral sphincter zone are interpreted as 'imminent micturition,' although muscle spindles as observed within the periurethral pelvic floor cannot be found with the rhabdosphincter. Afferent activity from throughout the bladder

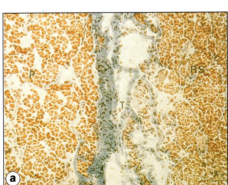
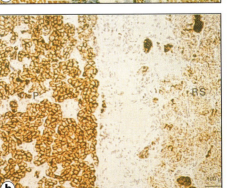

Figure 6.4 Adjacent sections through urethral wall identified in Figure 6.3. (a) Stained with Masson's trichome. (b) Stained to demonstrate tissue cholinesterase. A collagen sleeve (staining green in Masson's preparation) runs through both sections. To the right the relatively small cells of the rhabdosphincter are identified while to the left the larger-diameter cells are seen to be relatively rich in cholinesterase. (Courtesy of Professor JA Gosling.)

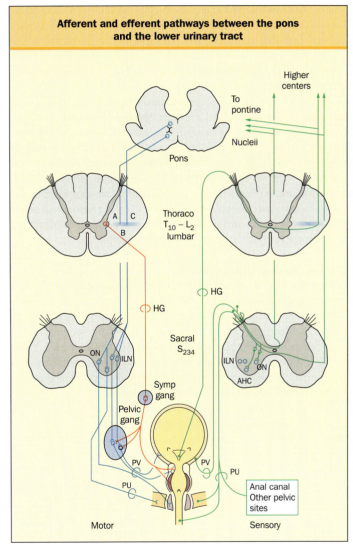

Afferent and efferent pathways between the pons and the lower urinary tract

Figure 6.5 Afferent and efferent pathways between the pons and the lower urinary tract[14]. Pu, pudendal nerve; Pv, pelvic nerve; T, trigone; Pelvic gang, pelvic ganglion; Symp gang, sympathetic ganglion; Hg, hypogastric nerve; ON, Onuf's nucleus; AHC, anterior horn cell nucleus; ILN, intermediolateral nucleus. A, B, C, tracts running in equatorial plane through central canal: A, autonomic efferent fibers; B, somatic efferent fibers; C, centripetal (afferent) fibers. Note that two pathways terminate at the bladder neck region: sympathetic fibers activate the reproductive preprostatic sphincter while postganglionic parasympathetic neurons relax (nitric oxide synthase) the looping smooth muscle fibers of the true bladder neck. Blue, parasympathetic efferent; Red, sympathetic efferent; Green, afferent.

probably responds to increases in pressure rather than volume, at least after the initial stages of bladder filling[10,11]. Over-distention or fullness and a sensation of vague pain originate from the trigonal area[12]. Other somatic sensory afferents that may play a role in micturition dysfunction originate from perineal skin, the anal canal, or associated pelvic structures. Afferent information that may be received from nonspecific areas such as the anterior abdominal wall, peritoneum, or pelvic floor, caused, for example, by the bulk of a distended bladder, remain unquantifiable at the present time.

The peripheral and spinal pathways transmitting sensory impulses are summarized in Figures 6.5 & 6.6. Pressure–volume fibers travel in the pelvic nerves to the sacral cord, where some local synapsing to preganglionic parasympathetic cell bodies occurs, but the majority cross the midline and ascend in the lateral funiculus to the pontine micturition center. Some fibers project upwards to the cortex to enable conscious awareness of bladder filling.

Impulses relating to overdistention or trigonal pain travel in the hypogastric nerve to T10–L2, where the majority again cross the midline to ascend to the pons in the lateral columns. Sensations of pain and temperature from the urethra travel via the pudendal nerve and also cross the midline to ascend in the lateral columns, whereas extroceptive sensation (touch, pressure) from the same origin passes from the pudendal nerve to ascend in the contralateral posterior columns. The location of these spinal tracts was deduced by careful observation on patients undergoing cordotomy for relief of pain of malignant origin[9].

Pontine micturition center

Integration of storage and voiding function takes place within the dorsolateral region of the pons, the pontine micturition center. Afferent inputs described above synapse on these nuclei, which are also served by suprapontine projections from the cerebral cortex, cerebellum, extrapyramidal system, and brainstem[13]. Such higher influences, the details of which are poorly understood in the human, explain well-described conscious, psychologic, and emotional influences over micturition behavior.

The pons represents the critical level of integration of storage and voiding function of the lower urinary tract. Lesions above this level allow synchronous, co-ordinated detrusor–sphincter activity to continue while lesions involving the basic afferent/pons/efferent reflex 'loop' invariably lead to dissociated dysfunction of detrusor, sphincter, and pelvic floor. Hence retention, urgency or hyper-reflexic disorder, which may frequently be observed in cases of suprapontine pathology (tumor, stroke), are not necessarily associated with unco-ordinated bladder and sphincter function.

EFFERENT INNERVATION TO THE LOWER URINARY TRACT

Descending axons from the pontine micturition center pass distally in the equatorial plane of the cord within the lateral columns[14] (Fig. 6.5) to synapse in regions containing sacral preganglionic neurons together with some projections from bladder afferent fibers (see above). The cell bodies of the preganglionic parasympathetic fibers are located in the intermediolateral column of S2, S3, and S4 and the nerves run as the nervi erigentes to synapse within ganglia on the cell bodies of postganglionic parasympathetic nerves, which themselves terminate within the detrusor muscle and urethra as well as other pelvic organs.

Descending fibers carrying impulses integrated in the pontine micturition center additionally project to Onuf's nucleus, the neurons of which pass with the nervi erigentes to the rhabdosphincter. More laterally placed in the anterior horn (Fig. 6.5), the cell bodies of the true pelvic floor (periurethral striated muscle) give rise to fibers that pass within the pudendal nerve. Some dispute arises as to whether the rhabdosphincter fibers pass within the pelvic or pudendal nerve; practical experience, however, shows that continence and urethral sphincter tone are maintained after pudendal blockade so at least some of the essential fibers must pass via the pelvic route[15,16].

The hypogastric nerves arise in the intermediolateral column of T10–L2 and postganglionic fibers pass down in the plexus to terminate on the smooth muscle of the genital sphincter (preprostatic sphincter), the muscle surrounding and infiltrating the prostate and the blood vessels of the bladder. Some postganglionic nerves are thought to terminate in extravesical parasympathetic ganglia (Fig. 6.5) where an inhibitory effect on parasympathetic ganglion transmission has been proposed[17,18].

CONTRACTILE AND RELAXANT MECHANISMS OF THE BLADDER

Bladder contraction is mediated by the actions of postganglionic parasympathetic nerves that lie adjacent to detrusor smooth muscle cells in a ratio of approximately 1:1[18]. Axonal varicosities contain numerous small (50nm diameter), clear, agranular vesicles, together with occasional large (80–160nm diameter)

Origin and course of sensory impulses from the lower urinary tract				
		To posterior column	**To anterolateral column**	
From pudendal nerve	Exteroception	– Urethral mucosa – Anal canal	Pain Temperature	– Urethral mucosa
	Proprioception	– Periurethral sphincter		
From pelvic nerve			Pressure/volume sensors (afferent arm micturition reflex)	
			Pain	– Bladder mucosa – Lower ureters
			Distension	– Rectum

Figure 6.6 Origin and course of sensory impulses from the lower urinary tract.

granulated vesicles. Histochemical analysis suggests that the agranular vesicles contain acetylcholine, which is thus the presumed neurotransmitter at the neuromuscular junction. Excitation spreads both through the neuronal plexus and within the detrusor muscle fibers themselves, which have 'regions of close approach' (not true gap junctions[18,19]), allowing spread of activity from muscle cell to muscle cell enabling the detrusor muscle mass to act as a functional syncytium, contracting synchronously to expel the contents of the bladder.

Neuromuscular transmission results in muscular contraction, the essential prerequisite being a rise in intracellular calcium, which is bound by and activates the calcium binding protein calmodulin, which in turn activates the cascade leading to shortening of actin and myosin filaments. Excitation at the neuromuscular junction by electromechanical means leads to an action potential, which is associated with membrane depolarization and opening of voltage sensitive channels that allow influx of calcium from outside the cell; pharmacomechanical coupling by contrast involves neurotransmitter binding to G-protein-linked receptors, which release second messenger and elevate intracellular calcium by release of the ion from intracellular stores within the endoplasmic reticulum. The G-protein receptor concerned is the muscarinic receptor, of which the M_2 subtype is thought to predominate by number[20] but the M_3 subtype is acknowledged to be of greater functional importance[21].

The precise functional relationship of neurotransmitter to ion channel and G-protein (muscarinic) receptors in the human is not known at the present time. Previously, pharmacologic studies in animals had suggested that, as a response to stimulation could not be completely abolished by the muscarinic blocking agent atropine, other forms of neurotransmitter [i.e. a nonadrenergic, noncholinergic (NANC) mechanism[22]] might be responsible for this phenomenon, known as atropine resistance. However, it has become clear that in normal human detrusor muscle this effect is not detectable and thus the neurotransmitter is indeed acetylcholine released from the clear, agranular vesicles of the postganglionic parasympathetic nerves. In other species, by contrast, reports of atropine resistance have been confirmed[22–25] and the alternative transmitter is thought to be adenosine triphosphate (ATP)[26]. It will be appreciated that in certain animals the bladder may subserve a dual function: storage and excretion of renal waste products and excretion for the purposes of territorial marking. It is proposed that, while urine evacuation is indeed under cholinergic control, the 'territorial reflex' is mediated by the 'NANC' atropine-resistant type of contraction, which leads to the ejection of a small volume of urine for marking purposes.

Traditionally, lack of contraction was regarded as the natural mechanism promoting relaxation in the lower urinary tract. Nitric oxide, known to be capable of initiating smooth muscle relaxation, has been found to play little part in altering detrusor contractility in the human. By contrast, nitric oxide synthase has been identified as important in neurologically mediated relaxation in the urethra[27] suggesting the possibility of further pharmacologic means by which urethral tone might be manipulated.

Gating theory and reflex control of the lower urinary tract

A number of reflexes have been described and reviewed relating to the neurologic control of micturition[28]. Having described the

pathways involved, it is helpful to summarize the mechanisms thought to be operative during the micturition cycle of normal humans.

Polymodal afferent mechanoreceptors sensitive to distention of the bladder (but not to contraction of the viscus) respond to bladder volume as well as the chemical composition of the contents, including pH, potassium concentration, or inflammatory mediators such as bradykinin[29]. In this way relatively low threshold mechanoreceptors may be sensitized by other stimuli, leading to accentuated reflex activity. Conversely, intravesical treatment with neurotoxic agents such as capsaicin may reduce afferent input under certain conditions and with this agent symptomatic improvement has been observed in patients with hypersensitive bladders or detrusor instability[30]. The majority of afferent impulses pass upwards in the pelvic nerve to enter the dorsal root of S2, S3, S4. Section of the cord between the sacral center and the thoracolumbar outflow results in retention and loss of all sensation except for a generalized overdistention pain, which passes upwards in the hypogastric nerves. Some afferents may pass in the pudendal nerve as it has been noted that after pudendal blockade a considerable reduction in the force of detrusor contraction may be observed[31]. Within the cord, interneurons (possibly inhibitory, see below) project on to preganglionic efferent nerves while the majority of impulses ascend in the long tracts to the pontine micturition center. Activity related to emotional, psychologic, and other higher functions passes downwards to synapse on the pontine nuclei, which in turn co-ordinate impulses passing down the long tracts (Fig. 6.5) to terminate on the cell bodies of preganglionic parasympathetic nerves in the intermediolateral column of S2, S3, and S4. Impulses pass out in the nervi erigentes to synapse in pelvic ganglia, postganglionic neurons supplying the smooth muscle of the bladder (contraction) and urethra (relaxation). Co-ordinated impulses pass synchronously from the pons to Onuf's nucleus, controlling the rhabdosphincter, and additionally to the anterior horn cells of S2, S3, and S4, passing via the pudendal nerve to control the tone of the pelvic floor (levator ani). Finally, the sympathetic outflow from T10–L2 (hypogastric nerves) passes to the trigone and prostatic smooth muscle, incorporating the reproductive sphincter. Postganglionic branches from this outflow project to parasympathetic ganglia, where an inhibitory effect on parasympathetic nerve transmission is postulated[17,18].

The work of de Groat has suggested that an extensive gating mechanism exists within this neurologic pathway whereby postganglionic parasympathetic nerves may be protected from afferent input until a certain activity threshold is reached[32,33]. Impulses reaching the cord may be initially nullified by inhibitory interneurons that restrict transmission to preganglionic parasympathetic cell bodies. Additionally, gating within the parasympathetic ganglia prevents onward transmission to postganglionic nerves and this inhibitory barrier is further reinforced by postganglionic sympathetic nerves projecting to the parasympathetic ganglia as described above.

As the frequency of afferent activity is increased, the threshold for onward transmission is breached and a volley of activity passes down the postganglionic parasympathetic nerves, leading to co-ordinated contraction (detrusor) and relaxation (urethra) of the smooth muscle elements of the lower urinary tract[33]. It seems reasonable to suppose that other gating mechanisms, as yet undetected, may operate at other levels within the primary spinobulbospinal reflex 'loop' or even within higher centers above the pons.

These repeated changes of neurologic activity associated with gradual bladder filling and micturition are known as the *fill–void cycle* of the urinary tract.

BLADDER COMPLIANCE

The pressure/volume relationship of the bladder is known as *compliance*, where $C = V/P_{det}$, P_{det} being the intrinsic detrusor pressure rise, measured in centimeters of water, observed during filling, measured in milliliters. Bladder compliance in the normal human is high, i.e. there is very little rise in intrinsic pressure ($<10cmH_2O$) during bladder filling to the physiologic adult capacity of 450–550mL.

The putative neurologic process whereby the intrinsic bladder pressure is kept low during filling has been outlined above. At low volumes ($<150mL$) the natural elasticity of the bladder wall structures allows filling without stimulation of afferent receptors; thereafter the gating theory of de Groat[33] is advanced to explain the lack of postganglionic parasympathetic activity (low intravesical pressure) until the threshold is reached.

Low or poor compliance is caused by an alteration to the viscoelastic properties of the bladder wall, which is chiefly composed of collagen, elastin, and smooth muscle[34]. Under these conditions the bladder wall may be thought of as 'too stiff' and it is not surprising that rate of filling during cystometry has been suggested as an artifactual reason for abnormal compliance[35]. Each component of the bladder wall may be responsible for the poor compliance, and the change may be reversible or irreversible. Acute inflammation and edematous change of the mucosa (acute cystitis) will result in reduced compliance that resolves on antibiotic medication. Extreme detrusor smooth muscle hypertrophy (Fig. 6.7), as seen in cases of high pressure chronic retention[36], causes marked loss of compliance associated with obstructive uropathy; surgery allows resolution of the upper tracts but bladder compliance rarely returns completely to normal[37]. Increased collagen content, whether resulting from disease, radiation treatment (Fig. 6.8), or severe, smooth muscle degeneration (Fig. 6.1c), is acknowledged to be the fundamental abnormality in most cases of reduced bladder compliance (Fig. 6.9). Such a pathologic abnormality usually leads to symptoms of severe frequency and nocturia but is not often associated with incontinence unless a sphincter abnormality is present, although females with relatively weak sphincteric mechanisms and males who have undergone transurethral resection of the prostate in the presence of unsuspected poor compliance may be significantly bothered by leakage.

URODYNAMIC INVESTIGATION OF BLADDER AND URETHRAL DYSFUNCTION

Uroflowmetry

Uroflowmetry is the only noninvasive urodynamic test of bladder and urethral dysfunction but the flow rate record itself represents only the resultant sum total of various forces and influences within the lower urinary tract. Setting aside technical aspects of the uroflowmeter design that may influence data

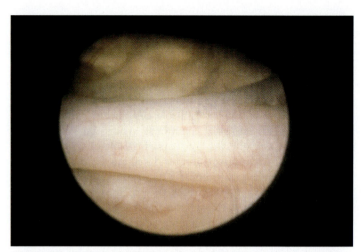

Figure 6.7 Endoscopic photograph of interior of poorly compliant bladder. Biopsies of heavily trabeculated muscle demonstrated moderate collagen infiltration as in Figure 6.1b.

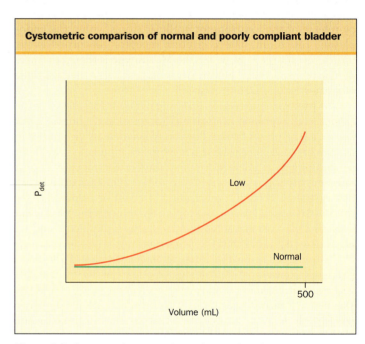

Cystometric comparison of normal and poorly compliant bladder

P_{det}

Low

Normal

500

Volume (mL)

Figure 6.8 Cystometric comparison of normal and poorly compliant bladder. P_{det}, intrinsic detrusor pressure rise.

presentation, the urine flow results from the opposing physiologic forces of detrusor contraction and sphincterourethral relaxation, to which may be added any 'mechanical' restriction of the outflow tract such as urethral stricture. Hence the measurement of this single index cannot with certainty indicate any specific pathophysiologic disorder of the lower urinary tract. Nevertheless when correctly performed after adequate instruction (Fig. 6.10) the flow rate is a cost-effective screening test that may give a strong indication of the direction in which further investigations should be pursued.

It is generally accepted that for a valid flow test in an adult the voided volume should exceed 150mL. Hence those unable to hold such volumes – such as patients with severe urge symptom complex – will tend to give unreliable recordings. Likewise, younger

Causes of low bladder compliance
Tuberculous cystitis
Interstitial cystitis
Radiation cystitis
Detrusor hypertrophy
Neurologic disease
• Cord injury
• Pelvic surgery
Long-term catheterization

Figure 6.9 Causes of low bladder compliance.

children with less natural bladder capacity will have 'normal' values less than those found in the adult. Nomograms making allowance for the effective voided volume have been constructed by a number of authors[38]. In the male an aging effect caused by the growth of prostatic tissue reduces the normal maximum flow rate (Q_{max}) to a significant degree. Most adolescents and younger men pass urine at between 22 and 35mL/s. This diminishes after the age of 40/50 until at age 70 a flow rate of 12mL/s may be regarded as normal. Appreciation of age-related values is clearly very important in the interpretation of an individual flow rate as inappropriate investigations or therapy may be advised on the basis of the test alone. The shorter urethral length and lower outflow resistance of the normal female leads in general to faster (often up to 50mL/s) flow rates, which for obvious anatomic reasons reduce less when compared to men as age progresses. Overall, the greater pathophysiologic importance of filling phase as opposed to voiding phase abnormalities in the female determines that the clinical utility of simple uroflowmetry is largely restricted to the diagnosis and assessment of the male lower urinary tract.

Electromyographic recordings

The diagnosis of dyssynergic sphincter dysfunction, usually present in patients with suprasacral neurologic disorder, remains difficult to achieve other than in centers with specialized equipment and trained personnel. Consideration of the detailed anatomy of the urethral sphincter apparatus (Fig. 6.3) illustrates the difficulty of ensuring that electrodes record precisely from the target muscle and hence observed effects – silence or recruitment – are commonly artifactual in nature. Such tests are commonly employed in an attempt to distinguish overtly neurologic from behavioral bladder dysfunction, an example of the latter being the inadequate relaxation of the pelvic floor sometimes observed during micturition in children. Sophisticated neurophysiologic studies to demonstrate either neuropathy or myopathy require even greater expertise and are unsuited to the routine urodynamic laboratory.

Urethral pressure profile

Measurement of the intraluminal urethral pressure along its functional length has been undertaken for many years in an attempt to understand the site and significance of resistive forces helping to maintain continence[39]. Defined by the

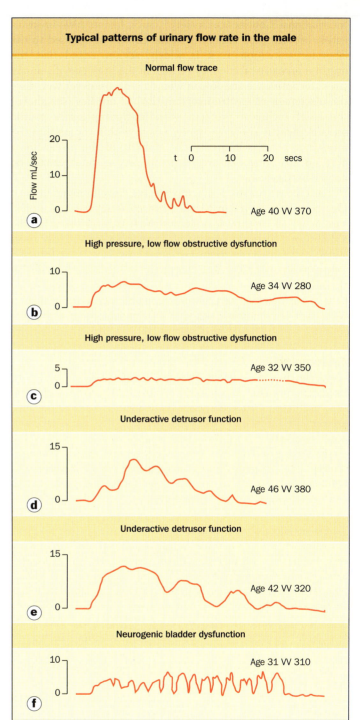

Figure 6.10 Typical patterns of urinary flow rate in the male.
(a) Normal flow trace. (b) High pressure, low flow obstructive dysfunction – benign prostatic hypertrophy. (c) High pressure, low flow obstructive dysfunction – urethral stricture. Note typical 'flat top' to trace. (d) Low pressure, low flow disorder – underactive detrusor function. (e) Low pressure, low flow disorder – underactive detrusor function. (f) Neurogenic bladder dysfunction – dyssynergic contraction of pelvic floor. The traces clearly demonstrate that it is not possible to make a confident urodynamic diagnosis on the basis of a simple flow rate test. VV, voided volume (mLs).

International Continence Society[40], such factors have unfortunately proved to be unhelpful in the clinical as opposed to the laboratory situation as it is widely acknowledged that the urethral pressure profile may be high in the presence of genuine stress incontinence and low in women who are never wet. Like the placement of electromyogram (EMG) needles (see above) the chief technical problem with urethral pressure profile measurement is knowing exactly where within the urethra the measuring point is located – the mobility of the pelvic floor/urethral mechanism ensures that this precise detail cannot be known with certainty[41].

Leak point pressure is a physiologic development of profileometry popularized by Maguire that measures the vesical pressure at which urethral leakage occurs. It is recorded using the Valsalva maneuver and reasonable correlation of low leak pressures with intrinsic sphincter weakness has been found[42]. Detrusor leak point pressure measurement may also be helpful in the assessment of poorly compliant bladders[43] but, as with other tests of the outflow tract, unforeseen contraction of the sphincter muscle or uninhibited detrusor activity may lead to artifactual results.

Cystometry

Cystometry is the fundamental urodynamic test and refers to the measurement of bladder pressure under various circumstances. Simple cystometry is the basic measurement of pressure against volume while videocystometry is the same measure combined with a video recording usually, but not always, of the outflow tract. Filling and voiding cystometry relate to events during the storage and micturition phase respectively. Cystometry may be performed using various media including gas, water, saline, or X-ray contrast media.

Technique and approach to cystometry

Cystometry is an expensive, time-consuming, and demanding test, the latter particularly so for the patient. Therefore, careful thought and planning will be required by the physician to define exactly the purpose of the test and to determine how best that purpose may be achieved. Subjectivity is recognized as the greatest weakness of the technique. The patient interprets afferent information as well as possible and attempts to transmit his/her feelings to the investigator, who in turn has to assess the meaning of this verbal report before recording the 'objective' results of the test. Typical inclusion and exclusion criteria for patients under consideration for urodynamic tests are shown in Figure 6.11. In general, where a complex clinical situation exists or surgery is contemplated, urodynamic tests give invaluable information on which to form a rational plan of management.

With regard to filling phase studies, a literature review reveals two contrasting philosophies as to the purpose and function of the inflow test; at one end of the spectrum low levels of filling rate are used to mimic as nearly as possible the physiologic state[44] while the opposite view suggests that a normal bladder and urethra should be able to handle very abnormal filling rates and that such a 'stress test' is the best way of provoking abnormalities that may be of relevance to the patient's symptom complex[45]. Physiologic filling rates[44] may be up to 10mL/min, 'medium' fill is defined as between 10 and 99mL/min (commonly 60mL/min) while fast fill is defined as rates over 100mL/min – usually found

Indications, contraindications, and advisable technique for cystometric tests		
Indication	**Condition**	**Technique**
Abandon	Undue anxiety, phobia	
	Urinary tract infection	
	Sore urethra (postcystoscopy catheter trauma)	
	Patient in retention	
	Patient catheterized	
Absolute	Neurogenic patients	Video mandatory
	Women with complex incontinence	Video mandatory
	Men <55 years, outflow tract symptoms	Simple or video
	Men, all ages, prior to redo surgery	Video ideal
Relative	Older men, 'simple' outflow symptoms	Simple adequate
	Women, simple history stress incontinence	Simple adequate
	(prior to surgery)	Video preferred
	Children	Simple practical

Figure 6.11 Indications, contraindications, and advisable technique for cystometric tests.

during tests where infusions are gravity-fed through tubing into the bladder catheter. A full description of the various test procedures will be found in specialized urodynamic texts, but cystometric technique is important whichever particular method of investigation is chosen. Sympathetic handling of the patient is vital, as is careful and atraumatic placement of the pressure lines both for the intravesical and intra-abdominal pressure measurements. Clearly it is important that the subject understands the various stressors to be employed during the test such as coughing, jumping, standing, or handwashing.

Gas cystometry

Gas cystometry is usually confined to office-based tests, being quick and simple to perform[46]. Rapid fill rates (up to 300mL/min), the compressibility of the gas, and the acidity generated when carbon dioxide dissolves in water are disadvantages of its use. Additionally, no voiding studies are possible with the medium, which is thus almost invariably used to provoke and detect possible bladder instability during the filling phase.

Simple inflow cystometry

Simple (i.e. nonvideo) filling cystometry using normal saline warmed to body temperature is the most basic urodynamic technique, which, if carefully performed, will reveal most disorders of the bladder during the storage phase. Bladder capacity (cystometric capacity) may be misleading if diverticulae or free reflux into the upper tracts are present. Bladder instability is a detrusor contraction that may be spontaneous or provoked (Fig. 6.12) and occurs despite the patient attempting to inhibit micturition. For this reason contractions occurring near the termination of filling are extremely difficult to distinguish from a premature (i.e. poor patient understanding of instructions) attempt at micturition. An identical contraction in the presence of confirmed neurologic disease is termed detrusor

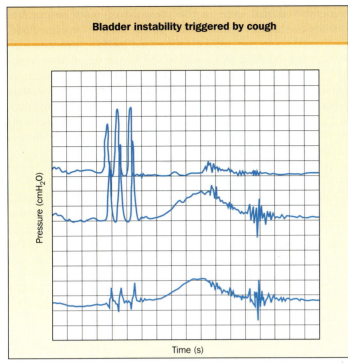

Bladder instability triggered by cough

Figure 6.12 Bladder instability triggered by cough. Top trace, rectal pressure; middle trace, bladder pressure; bottom trace, subtracted detrusor pressure. Three coughs during inflow cystometry (medium fill, 60mL/min) have induced an unstable wave. (Courtesy of Bristol Urodynamic Unit.)

hyper-reflexia. Poor compliance has been discussed above. Classically, certain tests have been described that may be performed during inflow cystometry in an attempt to identify neurologic disorder. Denervation hypersensitivity, which may be seen in some cases of 'acontractile' bladder caused by peripheral neuropathy, may be identified by the bethanechol supersensitivity test[47], while the ice water test was introduced by Bors to determine the level of neurologic injury[48]. Almost invariably, measurements taken during simple cystometry are recorded by remote pressure transducers connected to the patient by fluid-filled lines; electronic catheter tip transducers may be used but differences in recording technique may be required, particularly with respect to the establishment of 'zero' or atmospheric pressure levels.

Simple voiding cystometry

The synchronous measurement of bladder pressure during voiding together with the urine flow rate determines the pressure–flow relationship of micturition. For men, a sensitively and well performed pressure–flow study (i.e. subject seated, no Valsalva assistance, alone in a quiet room) is one of the most accurate and reproducible urodynamic measures, which can be of great assistance in patient management. Typical examples of urodynamic traces, their relationship to 'prostatism', and problems of interpretation are discussed below. In women the voiding study is not generally so helpful; frequently urethral/pelvic floor relaxation allows urine to leave the bladder at rates so high that little if any detrusor pressure rise may be registered before the bladder is completely empty (colloquially described as

'bombs-away' micturition). A stop test (P_{detIso}, the isometric rise in intrinsic detrusor pressure) may be attempted so as to reveal detrusor contractility but often by definition fails in the presence of stress incontinence. It is recognized that emotion and anxiety often prevent initiation of micturition in females who are not used to voiding 'in public'. As emphasized under Uroflowmetry above, filling phase studies are generally of overriding importance in the investigation of female patients, particularly those who have not had previous incontinence or gynecologic surgery (Fig. 6.11).

Videocystometry

Performance of a good-quality synchronous videocystometrogram investigation is the mainstay of most large urodynamic units. The technique was originally pioneered by a collaboration between Enhorning and Hinman[49]. In addition to pressure measurement and electronic recording capability, expensive X-ray screening units in appropriately shielded facilities are required. X-ray dosimetry to the pelvic and lumbar area is high and considerable expertise is required to obtain the crucial video information in the shortest possible exposure time. For certain disorders and patient groups (Fig. 6.11), video studies are mandatory as anatomic localization combined with measurement of the observed abnormality (pelvic floor descent, reflux) is essential for accurate urodynamic diagnosis and treatment. For others, such as males with 'simple' symptoms of outflow tract obstruction, physician choice can be exercised between simple and video studies. As noted above, many women find passing urine 'in public' an inhibitory experience, particularly so in the presence of extra X-ray personnel and equipment; in the author's experience no more than 50% of otherwise neurologically normal women can void to completion under such circumstances. The ability of videocystometric recordings to be played back at the physician's convenience during conference is a particular advantage that enables the necessary level of teaching and management experience to review and focus on the problems in question.

Ambulatory studies

Development and miniaturization of electronic recording devices has allowed the production of fully portable pressure measurement modules, which of necessity are linked to pressure tip transducers for the measurement of abdominal and intravesical pressure. By definition, ambulatory studies follow the 'physiologic' approach[44] to cystometry referred to earlier with natural bladder filling rates of around 1ml/min. Studies under a variety of conditions with different patient groups have demonstrated significant differences between ambulatory and artificial (usually medium fill) cystometry, including a lesser rise in pressure during filling (higher compliance) and a greater incidence of spontaneous phasic unstable contractions[50]. The technique may be used to study voiding dysfunction but the chief utility is the ability of the test to prove the presence of bladder instability – often suggested by a strong history of frequency and urgency – when conventional cystometrogram studies have recorded a normal inflow limb. Such confirmation may be particularly helpful if surgery for genuine stress incontinence is contemplated (Fig. 6.13). In general however this expensive and time-consuming technique has not gained wide acceptance

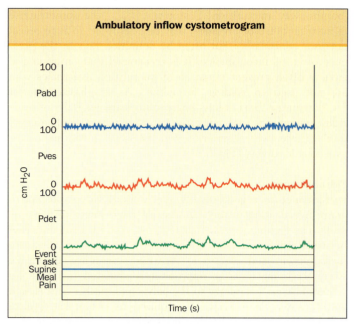

Figure 6.13 Ambulatory inflow cystometrogram. A 45-year-old woman with urgency but normal medium fill (60mL/min) conventional videocystometry. Clear evidence of bladder instability occurring towards the end of the ambulatory study.

outside the specialist urodynamic laboratory, as clinical suspicion based on the patient's history may indicate the need for, for example, a trial of anticholinergic therapy and under such circumstances the ambulatory study does not provide data that significantly alters patient management.

CLINICAL SPECTRUM OF DETRUSOR/URETHRAL DYSFUNCTION AS CLASSIFIED BY URODYNAMIC MEASUREMENT

The range of lower urinary tract dysfunction in the neurologically normal human is broad and it is not surprising that urodynamic observations on such patients demonstrate equally wide variations of pressure and flow measurement. To classify these disorders or dysfunctions of bladder and urethra, either studies must be undertaken on each and every patient and an attempt made to rationalize the findings or – the author's preferred choice – the pure forms of dysfunction should first be studied and faithfully recorded in the literature, following which the area between these uncontrovertible extremes may be analyzed in detail. Subsequently, if possible, agreement may be reached on the clinical and urodynamic features of patients occupying this middle ground or 'gray zone'. The following examples therefore reflect the consensus view of defined abnormalities during both filling and voiding cystometry with a subsequent note on the diagnosis of patients who fall into the gray zone.

Filling phase abnormalities

Intrinsic detrusor pressure rise (P_{det}) during filling to physiologic volumes (450–550mL) in normal humans is low, usually less than 10cmH$_2$O. Poor compliance (Figs 6.8 & 6.9) and phasic instability (Fig. 6.12) have been described above. It must be

remembered that even in the presence of quite severe frequency the bladder spends nearly all the time in 'storage mode' so alterations in compliance with raised intrinsic pressure may effect ureteral fluid transmission and hence upper tract function. Normally under these circumstances either pain or extreme urge cause the patient to release bladder volume, thus protecting the upper tract; nevertheless, studies in patients with acute painful retention (raised intrinsic bladder pressure) demonstrate that ureterohydronephrosis may occur if catheterization is delayed[51,52].

In high pressure retention, however, absent sensation of the raised pressure within the chronically retained bladder almost invariably leads to obstructive uropathy[36]. Experimental urodynamic and renographic studies[53,54] show conclusively that the critical intravesical pressure for development of upper tract changes is approximately 25cmH$_2$O, a level slightly less than the detrusor leak point pressure described by Maguire, although this data referred to myelodysplastic patients[43]. It is noteworthy that the much lower urethral resistance in women determines that chronically raised filling pressures cannot easily be maintained and urinary voiding or leakage thus protects the upper tracts from dilatation.

Voiding phase abnormalities

Disturbances in micturition are usually confined to male patients. Although urethral stenosis and detrusor voiding dysfunction may affect females it has been noted above that almost all symptom complexes in women are likely to relate to abnormalities of the filling phase. In men two unequivocal disorders of the lower urinary tract relate to obstruction and underactive detrusor function.

Bladder neck obstruction

It is generally agreed that it is not possible to offer a precise definition of outflow tract obstruction in terms of intrinsic detrusor pressure and urine flow rate. It is, however, possible to reach consensus about the more extreme forms of this dysfunction, the most typical example being bladder neck obstruction in younger men (Fig. 6.14 top panel). Classic cases of this disorder generate very high detrusor pressures associated with low flow rates, the findings being related to a thickened raised muscular bladder neck in the absence of significant prostatic enlargement. Occasionally, detrusor power may be great enough to raise the flow rate into the nonobstructed range – high pressure, high flow disorder[55] – although such cases are rare in the author's experience. Bladder neck obstruction has been accurately described since the mid-19th century but in recent times careful studies have suggested that prolonged obstruction (>10 years) may lead to poor compliance in the filling phase and consequent obstructive uropathy[56]. The spectrum of bladder neck dysfunction is further discussed below in terms of the underactive detrusor.

High pressure, low flow voiding

Infravesical prostatic obstruction leads to high pressure, low flow voiding and, while values in such older men rarely attain those seen in bladder neck obstruction in younger men, levels are usually such that there is little disagreement about the diagnosis of 'obstruction' (Fig. 6.14 center panel).

Low pressure, low flow voiding

At the other end of the pressure–flow spectrum lie patients with low flow rates because of poor bladder contractility – underactive detrusor function. Often seen in younger men before prostatic enlargement, detrusor pressure rise is typically undulating and poorly maintained (Fig. 6.14 bottom panel). Hesitancy may be marked, together with daytime frequency, and certain patients have been associated with psychologic overlay – the 'anxious bladder'[57]. Endoscopically the bladder neck may be mildly elevated (made prominent by the lack of prostatic tissue) but incision rarely makes a significant difference to voiding performance, in contrast to the spectacular results obtained after incision of genuine bladder neck obstruction. Whether detrusor failure may supervene with the addition of increasing prostatic outflow resistance in old age is a matter for conjecture[58].

The development of residual urine is now understood to be a complex process related to detrusor contractility rather than mechanical concepts of outflow tract 'obstruction'. It is acknowledged that markedly obstructed patients may empty the bladder to completion[45] (Fig. 6.14 top panel) while those with underactive dysfunction often leave postmicturition residual urine[57,58]. This concept was first popularized by the work of Griffiths, who emphasized that the lower urinary tract could not be analyzed in terms of rigid flow physics[59]. Overall, failure to empty the bladder would appear to be related more to detrusor dysfunction than to outflow tract resistance per se.

Equivocal obstruction – the gray zone

Between the extremes of high and low pressure voiding, where agreement may be reached on the urodynamic diagnosis, lies an equivocal zone of variable size according to differing authorities. No absolute consensus can be reached within this gray zone (obstructed, underactive, neither, or both?) and in an attempt to overcome these difficulties complex methods of pressure flow analysis have been developed by a number of authors, of which the simplest and most functional is probably the Abrams–Griffiths nomogram (Fig. 6.15). Using a plot of pressure against flow, a pressure flow loop is drawn and the slope of the plot, together with other parameters, indicates the presence or otherwise of obstruction. Nevertheless, in a significant number of cases doubt persists and this longstanding and complex urodynamic debate demonstrates that that for the clinical urologist there is no simple answer to the dilemma of results that fall into the 'gray zone'. The situation has been recently reviewed and developed in a discussion paper[60].

The development of underactive detrusor function

Classically, poorly contracting bladders were considered to result from the process of obstruction and subsequent decompensation giving a large, thin-walled viscus with hydroureteronephrosis and residual urine[61]. Close examination of this hypothesis suggests that the chain of events is unlikely to be valid. Severely obstructed bladders may not develop residual urine[45] and such bladders with residual urine and poor compliance develop terminal obstructive renal failure if untreated[36]. Undoubtedly, older patients with prostatic obstruction may develop a degree of detrusor decompensation with residual urine but it is noticeable that patients with underactive dysfunction (Fig. 6.14 bottom panel) are frequently younger than

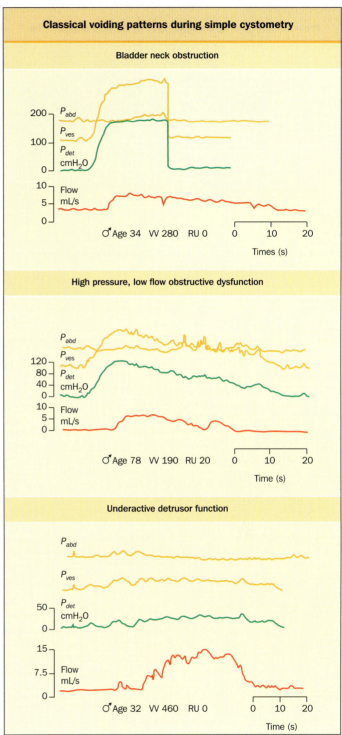

Figure 6.14 Classical voiding patterns during simple cystometry. Top trace, rectal pressure; middle trace, intravesical pressure. Green trace, subtracted detrusor pressure; red trace, flow rate. (Top) Bladder neck obstruction. Very high voiding pressures in a younger man with lifelong poor stream and hesitancy. Bladder pressure line expelled half-way through voiding – note dyssynergic twitch of discomfort. (Center) High pressure, low flow obstructive dysfunction caused by prostatic hypertrophy. Note that residual urine is minimal despite significant intrinsic detrusor pressure rise and clinical history extending for at least 5 years. (Bottom) Underactive detrusor function. Note relatively poorly maintained and undulating flow rate. VV, voided volume; RU, residual urine; P_{abd}, abdominal pressure; P_{ves}, vesicle pressure; P_{det}, detrusor pressure.

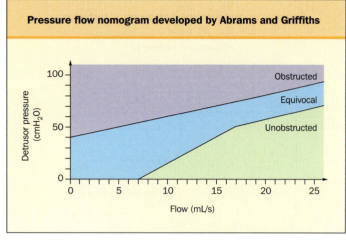

Pressure flow nomogram developed by Abrams and Griffiths

Figure 6.15 Pressure flow nomogram developed by Abrams and Griffiths. (Original data from Abrams and Griffiths[59].)

patients with prostatic enlargement and analysis of their history often suggests that this might have been a lifelong disorder[57,58], although longitudinal studies have yet to show the expected emergence of residual urine. Other authors have suggested defective neuromuscular transmission as a cause of the poor detrusor contractility[62]. These findings raise the possibility that underactive dysfunction is an inherited or developmental pathophysiologic abnormality of the detrusor or its nerve supply rather than a simple failed reaction to obstruction of the outflow tract.

REFERENCES

1. Gosling J. The structure of the bladder and urethra in relation to function. Urol Clin North Am. 1979;6:31–8.
2. Gilpin SA, Gosling JA, Barnard RJ. Morphological and morphometric studies of the human obstructive, trabeculated urinary bladder. Br J Urol. 1985;57:525–9.
3. Gosling J, Gilpin SA, Dixon JS, Gilpin CJ. Decrease in the autonomic innovation of human detrusor muscle in outflow obstruction. J. Urol. 1986;136:501–4.
4. Gosling JA. Structure of the female lower urinary tract and pelvic floor. Urol Clin North Am. 1985;12:207–14.
5. Crichley HOD, Dixon JS, Gosling JA. A comparative study of periurethral and perianal parts of the human levator ani muscle. Urol Int. 1980;35:226–32.
6. Gosling JA, Dixon JS, Crichley HOD, Thompson SA. The comparative study of the human external sphincter and periurethral levator ani muscles. Br J Urol. 1981;53:35–41.
7. Schroder HD. Onuf's nucleus X: a morphological study of a human spinal nucleus. Anat Embryol. 1981;162:443–53.
8. Gabella G. The structural relations between nerve fibres and muscle cells in the urinary bladder of the rat. J Neurocytol. 1995;24:159–87.
9. Nathan PW, Smith MC. The centripetal pathway from the bladder and urethra within the spinal cord. J Neurol Neurosurg Psychiat. 1951;14:262–80.
10. Iggo A. Tension receptors in stomach and urinary bladder. J Physiol. 1955;128:593–607.
11. Janig W, Morrison JFB. Functional properties of spinal visceral afferents supplying abdominal and pelvic organs with special emphasis on visceral nociception. In: Cervero F, Morrison JFB, eds. Visceral sensation. Amsterdam: Elsevier; 1986:87–114.
12. Learmonth JR. A contribution to the neurophysiology of the urinary bladder in man. Brain. 1931;54:147–76.
13. Morrison JFB. Bladder control: role of higher levels of the central nervous system. In: Torrens M, Morrison JFB, eds. The physiology of the lower urinary tract. Berlin: Springer-Verlag; 1987:237–74.
14. Nathan PW, Smith MC. Centrifugal pathway for micturition within the spinal cord. J Neurol Neurosurg Psychiat. 1958;21:177–9.
15. Zrara P, Carrier S, Kour NW, Tanagho EA. The detailed neuroanatomy of the human striated urethral sphincter. Br J Urol. 1994;74:182–7.
16. Emmett JL, Dant RV, Dunn JH. Role of the external urethral sphincter in the normal and cord bladder. J Urol. 1948;59:439–54.
17. Dixon J, Gosling JA. Structure and innervation in the human. In: Torrens M, Morrison JFB, eds. The physiology of the lower urinary tract. Berlin: Springer-Verlag; 1987:3–22.
18. Daniel EEL, Cowan W, Daniel VP. Structural basis for neural and myogenic control of human detrusor muscle. J Physiol Pharmacol. 1983;61:1247–73.
19. Gabella G. Structure of smooth muscles. In: Bülbring E, Brading AF, Jones AW, Tomita T, eds. Smooth muscle: an assessment of current knowledge. London: Edward Arnold; 1981:1–46.
20. Wang P, Luthin GR, Ruggierie MR. Muscarinic acetylcholine receptor substypes mediating urinary bladder contractility and binding to GTP binding proteins. J Pharmacol Exp Ther. 1995;272:959–66.
21. Kondo S, Morita T. A study of muscarinic cholinergic receptor subtypes in human detrusor muscle. Jpn J Urol. 1993;84:1255–61.
22. Ambache N, Zar MA. Non cholinergic transmission by postganglionic motor neurones in the mammalian bladder. J Physiol. 1970;210:761–83.
23. Henderson VE, Roepke MH. The role of aceylcholine in bladder contractile mechanisms and in parasympathetic ganglia. J Pharmacol Exp Ther. 1934;51:97–111.
24. Ursillo RC, Clark B. The action of atropine on the urinary bladder of the dog and on an isolated nerve–bladder strip preparation of the rabbit. J Pharmacol Exp Ther. 1956;118:338–47.
25. Brindley GS, Craggs MD. The effect of atropine in the urinary bladder of the baboon and of man. J Physiol. 1995;255:55.
26. Burnstock G. The changing face of autonomic transmission. Acta Physiol Scand. 1986;126:67–91.
27. Andersson KE, Persson K. Nitric oxide synthase and nitric oxide mediated effffects in lower urinary tract smooth muscles. World J Urol. 1994;12:274–80.
28. Kuru M. Nervous control of micturition. Physiol Rev. 1965;45:425–94.
29. Floyd K, Hick VE, Koley J, et al. The effects of bradykinin on afferent units in intraabdominal sympathetic nerve trunks. Q J Exp Physiol. 1977;62:19–25.
30. Fowler C, Beck RO, Gerrard S, et al. Intravescial capsaicin for treatment of detrusor hyperreflexia. J Neurol Neurosurg Psychiat. 1994;57:169–73.
31. Brindley GS, Craggs MD. The pressure exerted by the external sphincter of the urethra when its motor nerve fibres are stimulated electrically. Br J Urol. 1994;46:453–62.

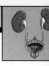
32. De Groat WC. Nervous control of the urinary bladder in the cat. Brain Res. 1975;87:201–11.

33. De Groat WC. Physiology of urinary bladder and urethra. Ann Intern Med. 1980;92:312–5.

34. McGuire EJ. Bladder compliance. J Urol. 1994;151:965–6.

35. Webb RJ, Styles RA, Griffiths CJ, et al. Ambulatory monitoring of bladder pressures in patients with low compliance as a result of neurogenic bladder dysfunction. Br J Urol. 1989;64:150–5.

36. George N J R, O'Reilly PH, Barnard RJ. High pressure chronic retention. Br Med J. 1983;282:1780–3.

37. Jones DA, Gilpin SA, Holden D, et al. Relationship between bladder morphology and long-term outcome of treatment in patients with high pressure chronic retention. Br J Urol. 1991;67:265–285.

38. Siroky BM, Olsson CA, Krane RJ. The flow rate nomogram: development. J Urol. 1979;122:665–8.

39. Brown M, Wickham JEA. The urethral pressure profile. Br J Urol. 1969;41:211–7.

40. Abrams PH, Blaivas JG, Stanton SL, et al. The standardisation of terminology of lower urinary tract function. Neurol Urodyn. 1988;7:403–27.

41. Bunne G, Obrink A. Urethral closure pressure with stress: a comparison betewwen stress incontinent and continent women. Urol Res. 1978;6:127–34.

42. Maguire EJ, Fitzpatrick CC, Wan J, et al. Clinical assessment of urethral sphincter function. J Urol. 1993;150:1452–4.

43. Maguire EJ, Woodside JR, Borden TA, et al. Prognostic value of urodynamic testing in myelodysplastic patients. J Urol. 1981;126:205–9.

44. Klevmark B. Natural pressure–volume curves and conventional cystometry. Scand J Urol. Nephrol Suppl. 1999;201:1–4.

45. Turner-Warwick R. Observations on the function and dysfunction of the sphincter and detrusor mechanisms. Urol Clin North Am. 1979;6:13–30.

46. Merrill DC. Air cystometer: new instrument for evaluating bladder function. J Urol. 1971;122:210–214.

47. Lapides J, Friend CR, Ajemian EP, et al. A new test for neurogenic bladder. J Urol. 1962;88:245–247.

48. Bors EH, Blinn KA. Spinal reflex activity from the vesical mucosa in paraplegic patients. Arch Neurol Psychiat. 1957;78:339–354.

49. Enhorning G, Miller ER, Hinman F. Urethral closure studied with cine roentgenography and simultaneous bladder–urethral pressure recording. Surg Gynaecol Obstet. 1964;118:507–16.

50. Robertson AS. Behaviour of the human bladder during natural filling. Scand J Urol Nephrol Suppl. 1999;201:19–24.

51. George NJR. Obstructive and functional abnormalities 1. In: O'Reilly PH, ed. Obstructive uropathy. Berlin: Springer-Verlag; 1986:235–75.

52. Pierce JM, Braun E. Ureteral response to elevated intravesical pressure in humans. Surg Forum. 1960;11:482–4.

53. Jones DA, Holden D, George NJR. Mechanism of upper tract dilatation in patients with thick walled bladder, chronic retention of urine and hydroureteronephrosis. J Urol. 1988;140:326–9.

54. Jones DA, George NJR. Interactive obstructive uropathy in man. Br J Urol. 1992;69:337–45.

55. Gerstenberg TC, Andersson JT, Klarskov P, et al. High flow intravesical obstruction in men: symptomatology, urodynamics and the results of surgery. J Urol. 1982;127:943–5.

56. Badenoch AW. Congenital obstruction of the bladder neck. Ann R Coll Surg Engl. 1949;4:295–307.

57. George NJR, Slade N. Hesitancy and poor stream in neurologically younger men without outflow tract obstruction – the anxious bladder. Br J Urol. 1979;51:506–10.

58. George NJR, Feneley RCL, Roberts JBM. Identification of the patient with 'prostatism' and detrusor failure. Br J Urol. 1986;58:290–5.

59. Abrams PH, Griffiths DJ. The assessment of prostatic obstruction from urodynamic measurements and from residual urine. Br J Urol. 1979;51:129–34.

60. Abrams P. Bladder outlet obstruction index, bladder contractility index and bladder voiding efficiency: three simple indices to define bladder voiding function. Br J Urol. 1999;84:14–5.

61. Lutzeyer W, Hannappel J, Schafer W. Sequential effects in prostatic obstruction. In: Hinman F Jr, ed. Benign prostatic hypertrophy. Berlin: Springer; 1983:693–700.

62. Kinn AC. The lazy bladder – appraisal of surgical intervention. Scand J Urol Nephrol. 1985;19:93–9.

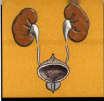

Chapter 7

Radiologic Imaging: Contrast Studies

Henrik S Thomsen and Sven Dorph

KEY POINTS

- Conventional uroradiology encompasses intravenous urography, direct pyelography, cystography, urethrography, cavernosography, arteriography and venography.
- Conventional radiography still has an important role in urologic disease.
- A plain radiograph of the kidneys and bladder is useful for the diagnosis of calculi, soft-tissue calcifications, and gas, and to assess various stents and devices. Contrast studies should be tailored to the clinical problem.
- The risk of nephropathy induced by contrast media in patients without risk factors is limited (<1%), whereas that in high-risk patients varies between 5 and 90%, depending on the study population.
- Users of contrast media should regularly review their protocols for the treatment of adverse reactions.

INTRODUCTION

Only a few months after the introduction of radiography, a role for plain radiographs of the abdomen in the diagnosis of urologic diseases was recognized. For the first time, calcification could be seen, and flexible metal wires placed in the bladder and the ureters demonstrated the location of these structures and their relation to such calcification[1]. Following the introduction of modern iodinated contrast media in the 1950s, intravenous urography (IVU) became the corner stone in the work-up of nearly all patients with signs and symptoms of urologic disease. The vessels were well visualized at angiography, the Seldinger technique was introduced, and the quality of urethrography and cystography also improved considerably after the new contrast media had been introduced. In recent years the role of these conventional examinations has diminished because of the increased availability of cross-sectional radiologic techniques – magnetic resonance imaging (MRI), computed tomography (CT) scanning, and ultrasonography – which also show the surrounding structures. For example, in some institutions the number of urographic tests has decreased by 75% during the past 10 years. Diagnostic angiography may also decline in the next decade; magnetic resonance angiography (MRA) seems to be at a stage where it could replace conventional angiography and thereby avoid radiation and an invasive procedure. Within the European Union a new treaty (EURATOM 97/43) that requires a reduction in medical radiation

came into effect in May 2000. It may cause a further shift from the radiating procedures to ultrasonography and MRI within the field of urogenital radiology.

EXAMINATIONS

Kidney, ureter, and bladder

A plain radiograph of the kidneys, ureters, and bladder (KUB) may be used for the diagnosis of calculi, soft-tissue calcifications, and gas. It is an integral part of all conventional radiographic examinations of the urinary tract; it should always be performed prior to contrast-medium injection (Fig. 7.1). A single radiograph of the abdomen that includes the pubic bone may suffice in some patients, whereas in others an additional radiograph coned to the kidneys is needed.

The identification of stones can be difficult when an excessive amount of gas and feces are in the bowel. Therefore, the bowel should be cleaned prior to plain radiographs taken to follow stones. For optimal stone detection, the kilovoltage should be kept below 70. The presence of some amount of calcium is also necessary to see a stone on a plain radiograph. Compared with CT, the plain radiograph overlooks about one-third of the stones[2]. If CT is not available, a full set of linear tomograms may be of value in a patient in whom small stones are suspected[3]. An

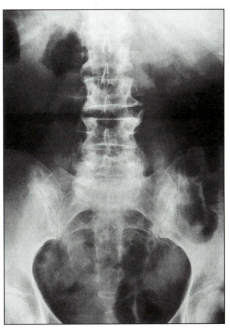

Figure 7.1 Normal plain film from the upper pole of the right kidney to just above the symphysis.

oblique preliminary radiograph may be useful to localize radio-dense structures that overlie the kidney. All exposures should be made after the patient has fully exhaled, to minimize the geometric distortion of the renal image that occurs when deep inspiration causes descent and ventral rotation of the lower poles of the kidneys.

On plain radiographs of the upper tract, calcification other than stones is often easy to recognize as renal or extrarenal vascular calcification, pancreatic calcification, calcified lymph nodes and gallstones (Fig. 7.2). Intrarenal calcification can be quite characteristic, such as that seen in medullary sponge kidney or the very dense calcification that fills out cavities after renal tuberculosis. Renal masses can also contain calcium; in particular renal cell carcinoma can have quite typical calcification – amorphous and irregular – while cysts often have a fine calcified rim. Thick calcified rims are suspicious of carcinoma in the wall of the cyst. After vigorous instrumentation ureteral stones may occur in the wall or outside the ureter. Bladder stones are often opaque, but may be completely nonopaque. Stones are extremely frequent in bladder substitutes with reservoir, often with a central nidus represented by an exposed metallic clip (Fig. 7.3). Calcification in the bladder wall can be seen in schistosomiasis or tuberculosis. Calcification below the bladder in women is rare, but most often localized to an urethral diverticulum. Calcification is frequent in the prostate, sometimes as a result of prostatitis, and calcification of vasa deferentia or seminal vesicles is seen in diabetic patients.

Soft-tissue masses in the pelvis may be tumor or bladder urine. Pelvic lipomatosis may be seen as radiolucency. Air in the

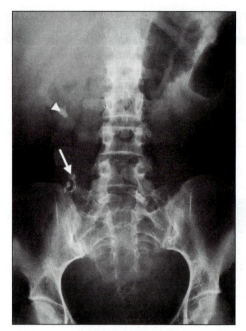

Figure 7.3 Plain radiography of the kidneys, ureter, and bladder demonstrating two stones (arrow, arrowhead) in an ileal bladder substitute (Koch bladder). Both stones formed at a nidus of an exposed metallic clip; one (arrowhead) of the stones has migrated up into a lower calix on the right side.

bladder or bladder wall is also seen on the plain radiograph. Emphysematous cystitis is almost exclusively seen in diabetic patients. Gas in the ureter or pelvis often results from fistula in the bowel, and more rarely from gas-forming bacteria (which can cause life-threatening infection).

Finally, plain radiographs may also be used to monitor stents in the ureter (Fig. 7.4) or urethra, or other foreign bodies and

Figure 7.2 Etiology of calcification within or close to the genitourinary tract found on plain radiography of the kidneys, ureter, and bladder.

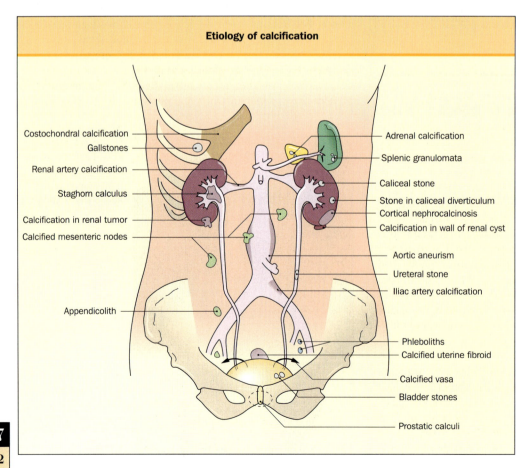

Etiology of calcification

Costochondral calcification
Gallstones
Renal artery calcification
Staghorn calculus
Calcification in renal tumor
Calcified mesenteric nodes
Appendicolith

Adrenal calcification
Splenic granulomata
Caliceal stone
Stone in caliceal diverticulum
Cortical nephrocalcinosis
Calcification in wall of renal cyst
Aortic aneurism
Ureteral stone
Iliac artery calcification
Phleboliths
Calcified uterine fibroid
Calcified vasa
Bladder stones
Prostatic calculi

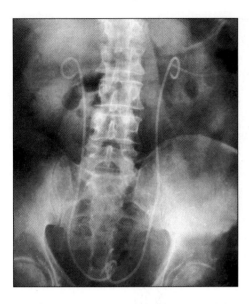

Figure 7.4 Plain film demonstrating a double J-stent in both ureters.

devices like penile prosthesis and artificial urethral sphincters. For the latter, the radiographs are useful to control the integrity of contrast-filled cuff, reservoir, tubings, and connections.

Intravenous urography

The goal of IVU, sometimes called intravenous pyelography (IVP), is to obtain clinically useful information about the upper urinary tract and its related structures. This requires that each examination be designed to meet unique needs. The elements that contribute to a successful study include[4]:

- adequate dose of contrast medium;
- radiograph to record the nephrogram;
- sequence of radiographs to assess the dynamics of urine formation and propulsion;
- adequate distention of the opacified caliceal system;
- use of oblique, prone, and upright positions;
- use of tomography;
- reinjection of contrast material if needed; and
- minimization of the risks to the patients.

Unnecessary radiography should be avoided; for example, films of the nephrographic phase can be avoided if ultrasonography of the kidneys is carried out during or in relation to the examination. The number and sequence of films in IVU, following injection of the contrast medium, should be individualized to each patient.

For many years it has been recommended fluid intake be restricted for 4, 6, or 8 hours before the examination. Bowel cleansing has also been recommended. Fluid restriction is a remnant of the use of high osmolar contrast media. The diuretic properties of such contrast media resulted in a good urinary output lowering the iodine concentration in the upper urinary tract (i.e. produce a poorer urogram). The lower diuretic properties of iso- and low osmotic contrast media make fluid restriction unnecessary. In our experience free fluid intake improves the comfort of the patient in relation to the examination. The usefulness of bowel cleansing remains unclear. Food intake in the community may affect whether bowel cleansing should be used routinely.

After the KUB has been taken, contrast medium [e.g. 1mL per kg body weight of a 300mg iodine (I) per milliliter of solution independent of the kidney function] is injected into a vein. Within the first 60 seconds one exposure over the kidney may be made

to visualize the renal parenchyma during the nephrographic phase of the contrast passage (Fig. 7.5a). Some radiologists still take up to three exposures or obtain these exposures with a tomographic technique. Another film over the kidney region is taken 5 minutes post contrast passage (Fig. 7.5b). If there are no contraindications (e.g. hydronephrosis, aortic aneurysm, recent surgery, large abdominal tumor), ureteral compression is applied to retain the contrast and/or urine in the pelvis and ureter (Fig. 7.5c). Adequate distention of the pelvicaliceal system is an essential component of the well-performed IVU.

Modern low osmolality contrast materials do not induce the same diuresis and distention as the old high osmolar contrast media. External compression of the ureters by two small inflatable rubber balloons is a simple and effective way to produce distention. The balloon(s) are held in place by a plastic foam block and a band that passes around the patient. The ureters are compressed at the point at which they pass over sacral prominence. A new exposure of the kidneys is appropriate 5 minutes after application of compression; oblique views may also be taken. The compression is then removed and a kidney-bladder exposure is obtained. When the bladder is well filled a coned exposure is taken (Fig. 7.6). Linear tomograms of the kidneys, late radiographs, erect or prone views, and bladder views after voiding are taken as needed.

Optimum bladder filling is reached at 30 minutes in patients with normal glomerular filtration rate (GFR) and no obstruction. Oblique or lateral views of the bladder can be useful for suspected filling defects and other bladder pathology. Only two-thirds of bladder tumors are revealed, but a postvoid film can disclose a few of the missed tumors. Leakage is sometimes better seen on a postvoid film.

The strengths and weaknesses of urography are given in Figure 7.7. Inadequate visualization of the pelvis and ureter does not necessarily indicate poor renal function (Fig. 7.8). The GFR, however, can be determined by drawing a blood sample 3–4 hours after the contrast medium injection and measuring the iodine content in the sample (see later).

Currently, the ability of IVU to show detailed caliceal anatomy and the overlying parenchyma is probably the strongest argument for referring a patient for this examination (Fig. 7.9). Before CT became available, it was thought that a plain radiograph followed by subsequent radiographs after administration of contrast medium was ideal to demonstrate stones in the upper urinary tract. However, comparative studies have shown that plain radiographs only reveal 47–76% of the calcifications within the upper urinary tract seen at unenhanced CT[2]. Small stones may only cause intermittent obstruction (i.e. pain); such stones may be overlooked at IVU if they are not causing obstruction at the time of urography, but they are seen on unenhanced CT. Dilatation and stranding at CT is identical with the presence of acute obstruction; the sensitivity of obstruction at CT is similar to that of urography[5]. Forcing the diuresis with application of contrast media may cause pyelosinous backflow (rupture of a caliceal fornix), if the rupture has not yet occurred (Fig. 7.10). A combination of KUB and Doppler ultrasonography is an alternative to enhanced CT. This combination can reduce the number of acute urographies by 60% in patients with renal colic[6].

Small mucosal abnormalities in the pelvicaliceal system and the ureter are best diagnosed at IVU, which is therefore important in

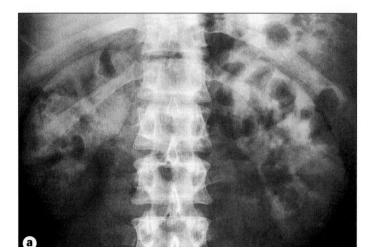

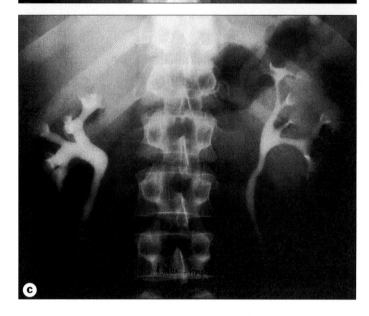

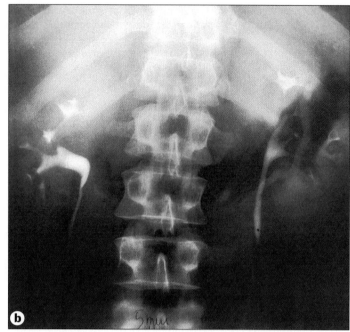

Figure 7.5 Normal urograms. (a) Nephrogram (30 seconds after injection) demonstrating the size and surface of the kidney. (b) An exposure after 5 minutes demonstrating the excretion of the contrast medium into a nonobstructed upper urinary tract. (c) Exposure taken 5 minutes later than that shown in (b), after abdominal compression had been applied for 4 minutes.

institution we do not carry out IVU for patients with stable serum creatinine levels above 400–500µmol/L (4.52–5.67mg/dL).

Direct pyelography

Direct pyelography means the direct injection of contrast medium into the upper urinary tract. It may be carried out either through a catheter placed in the ureter during cystoscopy (retrograde) or through a needle or a nephrostomy tube (antegrade). Antibiotic cover should be instituted before instrumentation takes place. A meticulous technique (e.g. sterile conditions, low injection pressure, diluted contrast medium solution with a low viscosity, fluoroscopic surveillance) is necessary[8].

the diagnosis of early transitional cell carcinoma in the upper urinary tract. Congenital anomalies, such as fusions, rotation anomalies, caliceal variants and duplications, are well demonstrated by IVU.

When the renal injury was thought to be minor, IVU was considered a quick and effective screen in traumatized patients, but this is unclear[7]. If there is time carry out urography, then is there a need for it at all? When the injury is thought to be more than minor, CT is the imaging method of choice.

In the 1970s high-dose urography was recommended for patients with renal failure – the dose of contrast medium was doubled or tripled according to the GFR. At that time this was an important advance, as knowledge of the kidney size gives information about whether renal failure is chronic or acute. Visualization of caliceal distention is, in many cases, enough to determine whether the renal failure is primary and nonobstructive or postrenal and obstructive. However, the increased risk of contrast medium nephropathy in patients with abnormal serum creatinine levels (see below) requires that IVU should generally be avoided and only performed in selected cases for which visualization of the upper tract is important and cannot be obtained by other modalities. The poorer the renal function, the poorer is the visualization of the upper urinary tract. At our

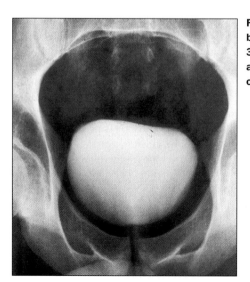

Figure 7.6 Coned bladder view taken 30 minutes after the administration of the contrast medium.

Figure 7.7 Strengths and weaknesses of intravenous urography.

Strengths and weaknesses of intravenous urography	
Strengths	**Weaknesses**
Rapid overview of the entire urinary tract	Depends on kidney function
Detailed anatomy of the collecting system	Provides little assessment on parenchymal structure (e.g. cystic versus solid)
Demonstration of major calcification	Does not show the whole renal contour and may miss masses that arise from the anterior or posterior part of kidney
Sensitive for acute obstruction	Perinephric space is not demonstrated
Low cost	Necessitates the use of radiation and contrast medium
	Provides no assessment of glomerular filtration rate

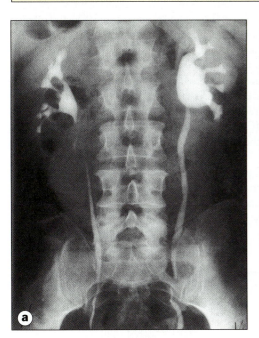
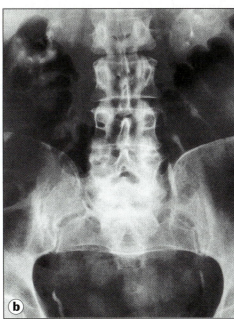

Figure 7.8 Upper urinary tract on 15 minute exposures in two different patients with exactly the same glomerular filtration rate (85mL/min). (a) Good visualization; (b) poor visualization.

Indications for intravenous urography	
Renal diseases	**Urinary tract disease**
Papillary necrosis with destruction and/or loosening of the tip of the papilla	Stone disease, if CT is not available
Medullary sponge kidney	Obstruction, if CT or MR urography are not available or ultrasonography is insufficient; radionuclide studies give the best information about functional aspects
Tuberculosis	Subtle mucosal changes (early transitional cell carcinoma, pyeloureteritis cystica, malacoplakia, fungi and schistosomiasis)

Focal scarring:
  with caliceal abnormalities: reflux nephropathy
  without caliceal abnormalities: renal infarction
	Congenital anomalies

Figure 7.9 **Indications for intravenous urography.** CT, computed tomography; MR, magnetic resonance.

Once the catheter is in place, the radiographic investigation should be carried out as soon as possible in the radiology department. A preliminary view is fundamental to know the position of the catheter tip, which may occasionally have perforated the kidney or ureter or dropped down into the bladder. If possible, the outer end of the catheter is disinfected and urine aspirated before contrast medium is injected. A dilute and heated contrast medium (75–100mg I/mL or less; body temperature) is used to ensure that subtle lesions are not obscured. To avoid overfill the contrast medium is injected slowly under fluoroscopic control. To use as little contrast medium as possible and to keep the pelvic pressure as low as possible, gravity is used to move the contrast medium by turning and tilting the patient.

Visualization of the calices, pelvis, and ureter is independent of renal function, unlike in IVU. Backflow (extravasation) into the renal parenchyma and surroundings [pyelosinous backflow, intrarenal backflow (Fig. 7.11), pyelovenous backflow and pyelolymphatic backflow] should be avoided by a low injection pressure, since backflow may not only cause complications (e.g. pain, infection) but also obscure the disease (Fig. 7.12). The indications for direct pyelography are given in Figure 7.13.

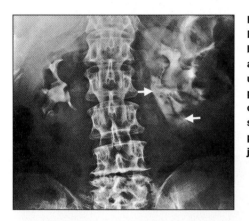

Figure 7.10 Pyelosinous backflow (arrows) at intravenous urography in a patient with an obstructing ureteral stone and pelviureteral junction.

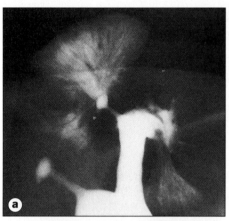

Figure 7.11 Retrograde pyelography demonstrating intrarenal backflow of contrast medium. (a) Into the collecting ducts and nephrons; (b) into sloughed papillae in papillary necrosis.

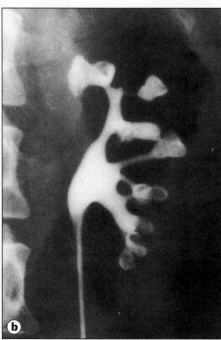

Cystography

Cystography means specific examination of the bladder with contrast medium. It can be carried out following intravenous injection of contrast media (in conjunction with IVU) or following direct instillation of contrast medium (75–100mg I/mL) heated to body temperature either through a urethral or a suprapubic catheter. To avoid leakage, ruptures, and reflux, infusion pressure must not exceed 40mmHg (5.3kPa) when the bladder reaches its maximal capacity and/or extension. The bladder is examined in several views and exposures are often also taken during voiding. A postvoid film is essential.

Cystography is mainly used for the diagnosis of post-traumatic (intra- or extraperitoneal rupture[9]; Fig. 7.14) or postoperative urinary extravasation, to evaluate diverticula, and to seek vesicoureteral reflux. The investigation of leakage from pouch bladders is also an indication for cystography.

If vesicoureteric reflux is suspected the field of view should include both ureters and kidneys, and fluoroscopic surveillance should be performed both during the filling (low pressure) and voiding (high pressure) phase, but with fluoroscopy time kept to a minimum. It is recommended to take images with the patient sitting bent over (Chassard-Lapine view). To secure the highest degree of reflux the patient should be dehydrated (low urinary output)[10].

For the investigation of female incontinence the vagina is marked with barium sulfate (colpocystourethrography), but the clinical relevance of this indication is unclear. Pelvic floor examinations by MRI may be more useful in these patients.

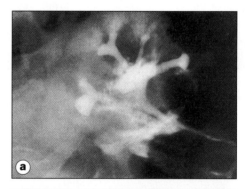

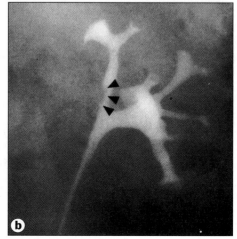

Figure 7.12 Retrograde pyelography carried out a few days apart with (a) high and (b) low pressure, respectively. A small tumor, shown by arrowheads on (b), is obscured by backflow at the first examination.

Indications for direct pyelography

- Nonvisualization of the upper urinary tract on intravenous urography (if there is an obvious cause, such as a large tumor, CT is preferred)

- Inconclusive or suspicious appearance of a segment of the upper urinary tract that may be better visualized with direct pyelography

- Unexplained hematuria (erythrocytes) in which intravenous urography did not completely delineate the entire ureter and/or renal pelvic cavity

- Previous severe contrast material reaction (the examination may be performed with carbon dioxide or gadolinium contrast media)

- As an aid in the diagnosis of renal failure, such as renal papillary necrosis and the possibility of upper urinary tract obstruction (stricture, calculus, papilla)

- As an aid to brush biopsy

- With endourologic procedures (e.g. percutaneous nephrolithotomy)

Figure 7.13 Indications for direct pyelography. CT, computed tomography.

Urethrography

Urethrography may be antegrade (micturition, voiding) or retrograde. In males an obturating cannula system or a small balloon catheter is placed with the tip in the fossa navicularis and contrast medium (75–100mg I/mL) is injected retrogradely through the urethra and up into the bladder[11]. The patient should be lying in the oblique dorsal recumbent position. The penis is stretched by mild traction on the instrument (Fig. 7.15a). Usually some resistance occurs at the urogenital diaphragm, which needs to be overcome by gentle pressure applied on the 50-mL syringe before the contrast will flow into the bladder. In females the short urethra is difficult to examine, but special catheters with two balloons (one for the internal orifice and one for the external orifice) have been developed[12]. Examination during voiding is best for the posterior urethra, but nearly always results in inferior visualization of the anterior urethra. Retrograde studies are excellent for the anterior urethra, but inferior for the posterior urethra.

Urethrography is used for the diagnosis of urethral strictures (Fig. 7.15b), diverticula, and tumors, as well as in trauma. It may also be helpful in certain postoperative conditions.

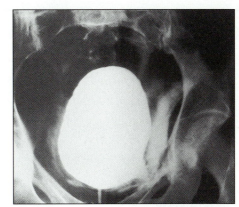

Figure 7.14 Cystogram demonstrating extraperitoneal bladder rupture caused by pelvic trauma.

Cavernosography

The corpora cavernosa can be visualized by cavernosography (Fig. 7.16a). A 21G butterfly is inserted into one corporal body by puncture in the dorsolateral aspect of the sulcus coronalis, after local anesthetic, with the needle directed cranially and the oblique cut of the needle directed downward. Dilute contrast medium is infused or injected under fluoroscopic guidance to fill the corpus cavernosum. Injection into one corpus cavernosum fills both. Indications include penile deformities caused by Peyronie's disease or penile fracture (Fig. 7.16b) and assessment of priapism[13].

Vasculogenic insufficiency has attracted increasing interest as cause of organic impotence. It may be caused by inadequate inflow or by deficient veno-occlusion that prevents erection from occurring or being maintained despite adequate inflow. Cavernosography is combined with cavernosometry, which determines the cavernosal pressure response to standardized infusion of fluid and thus quantitates venous leakage. This requires a needle in the other corpus for pressure recording.

Simple cavernosography only demonstrates the venous penile anatomy; it does not reliably demonstrate venous leaks. After intracorporeal injection of certain vasoconstrictive drugs (papaverine 30–60mg, often supplemented with a few milligrams of phentolamine) regions of insufficient venous occlusion can be identified (Fig. 7.17). This can help guide an operation or percutaneous venoablation[14].

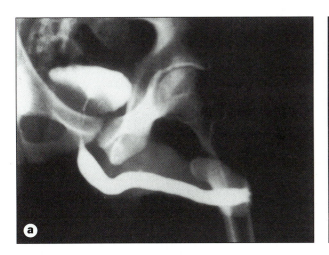

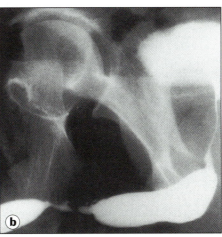

Figure 7.15 Retrograde urethrography. (a) Normal; (b) showing a stricture in the penile urethra.

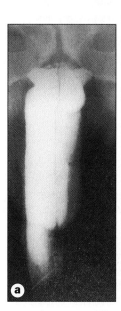

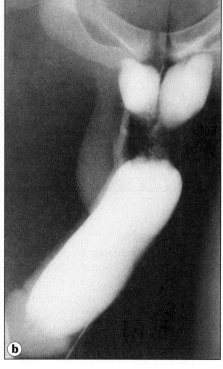

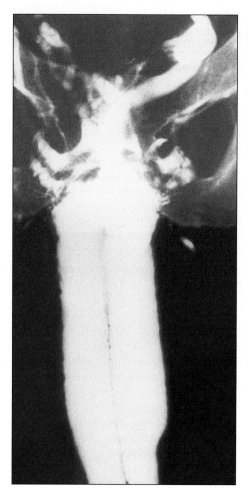

Figure 7.17 Cavernosography in a patient with venous leakage. No rigidity is obtained after papaverine followed by contrast medium. The open veins drain to the pelvis.

Figure 7.16 Cavernosography. (a) In a normal patient. The contrast medium is injected into the right corpus, which results in rigidity; the left corpus is less filled because of the high pressure. The venous outflow is almost closed. (b) A filling defect in the corpora cavernosa after a penile fracture.

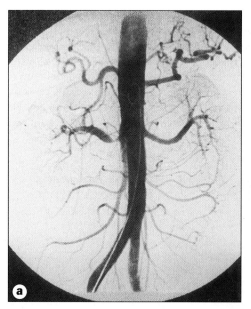

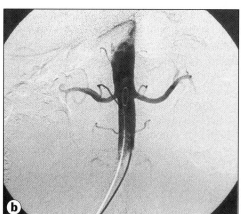

Figure 7.18 Renal aortogram with the pigtail catheter placed (a) too high in the aorta, which results in overlying celiac and superior mesenteric vessels, and (b) after correct placement. In (a) there is a right arterial stenosis; (b) is a control after percutaneous angioplasty.

Angiography

Angiography of the genitourinary system does not differ from angiography of other organ systems. A catheter is introduced into the venous or arterial system using the Seldinger technique.

A complete examination of the arterial supply to the kidney includes an aortogram and selective renal arteriograms of all the renal arteries. For aortography, the catheter should have a distal curve and side holes to promote mixture of contrast material with the blood and to minimize the amount of contrast material that flows into the celiac and superior mesenteric arteries (Fig. 7.18). A J-shaped, or preferably pigtail, catheter with three or four side holes closely grouped 2–3cm from the

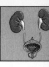

straight limb meets this requirement. The position can be verified by a test injection of 5–10mL of contrast material. To perform the aortogram contrast material is injected at 20mL/s for 2 seconds. A typical sequence comprises three images per second over a 3 second period and one image per second over a 4 second period. Usually the initial study is carried out using an anteroposterior projection, but 20–30° posterior oblique sequences may be used, particularly when searching for stenotic lesions of the proximal arteries. Careful coning of the recorded image to the margins of the kidneys greatly enhances diagnostic quality.

Selective renal arteriography is carried out with a catheter shaped to conform to the renal artery. The orifice of the desired renal artery is sought at the level of origin identified in an initial aortogram. If an aortogram is not available, most arteries can be located by moving the catheter up and down a segment of the aorta from the upper margin of L1 to the lower margin of L2. Often, continuous clockwise or counterclockwise torque must be applied to the catheter to keep its tip in a lateral direction. A sudden lateral movement of the catheter signals insertion into the renal artery. Injection of 2–3mL of contrast material under fluoroscopic control verifies accurate positioning and ensures that the tip is not pointed into the arterial wall. This procedure may have to be repeated in kidneys with more than one renal artery. The amount of contrast material used in selective renal arteriography depends on the size of the kidney and the renal blood flow. An average total dose is 10mL administered over 1.5 seconds. This should be decreased in patients with low flow status, as in chronic renal failure, and increased in those with high flow states, as in vascular renal carcinoma and conditions with arteriovenous shunting. The rate of image for average flow is four images per second over a 2 second period, two images per second over a 6 second period. Usually, anteroposterior and posterior oblique projections are obtained for each kidney, but the actual approach is determined by individual circumstances. Again, the value of careful collimation to achieve images of superior quality cannot the overemphasized.

The tip of the catheter is placed with fluoroscopic guidance in a vessel that leads to or comes from the region of interest. Injection of vasoconstrictive drugs may be useful when the veins are examined through retrograde injection, but with the modern digital equipment visualization of the venous tree is often possible after intra-arterial injection of contrast material.

Renal arteriography to diagnose and differentiate renal masses is rarely performed now because of the development of both ultrasonography and, especially, CT. Angiography may be carried out when planning surgery on an anomaly (e.g. horseshoe kidney) or partial nephrectomy. Other residual indications for renal arteriography include suspected renal artery stenosis, aneurysms, and arteriovenous fistulae in relation to intervention (see Chapter 11). The diagnosis of vasculitis (e.g. polyarteritis nodosa) is specific (Fig. 7.19).

Renal venography is still carried out at some institutions to secure the correct placement of a catheter for renin sampling in patients with renovascular hypertension.

With the considerable improvement of MRA, diagnostic renal angiography is very rarely carried out at institutions with adequate access to this modern cross-sectional imaging.

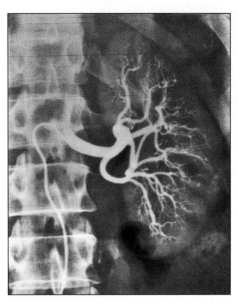

Figure 7.19 Selective renal arteriogram demonstrating multiple microaneurysms in the small arteries in a patient with polyarteritis nodosa.

CONTRAST MEDIA

Since the 1950s contrast media have been based on the benzene ring. Three iodine atoms are attached to each benzene ring. At the three other positions various radicals are attached. Currently, four different classes of contrast media are available (Fig. 7.20). High osmolar ionic contrast media are no longer used intravascularly in many countries because of the high frequency of side-effects.

Nonrenal side-effects

Although contrast media are relatively well tolerated, adverse effects and reactions can be expected:

- minor – nausea, limited vomiting, limited urticaria, pruritus, and diaphoresis;
- moderate – faintness, severe vomiting, profound urticaria, facial edema, laryngeal edema, and bronchospasm; and
- severe – hypotensive shock, pulmonary edema, respiratory arrest, cardiac arrest, and convulsions.

The overall frequency of these adverse reactions is 7–54% with ionic high osmolar contrast media and 2–17% with nonionic low-osmolar contrast media[15]. A moderate reaction that is not life-threatening and requires some treatment occurs in 1–2% of patients who receive ionic high osmolar contrast media and in 0.2–0.4% of those who receive nonionic low osmolar contrast media. Severe, life-threatening reactions can be expected in about 0.2% of patients after ionic high osmolar and 0.04% after nonionic low-osmolar contrast media.

Adverse reactions (Fig. 7.21) to intravascular contrast media are generally classified as either systemic (idiosyncratic) or chemotoxic. Idiosyncratic (i.e. anaphylactoid) reactions occur unpredictably and independently of the dose or concentration of the agent. Most anaphylactoid reactions relate to release of active mediators. Conversely, chemotoxic effects relate to dose, the molecular toxicity of each agent and the physiologic characteristics of the contrast agents (i.e. osmolality, viscosity, hydrophilicity, calcium binding properties, and sodium content). Some reactions to the injection of contrast media (e.g. sudden cardiopulmonary arrest) are difficult to categorize specifically in either of the two major reaction types.

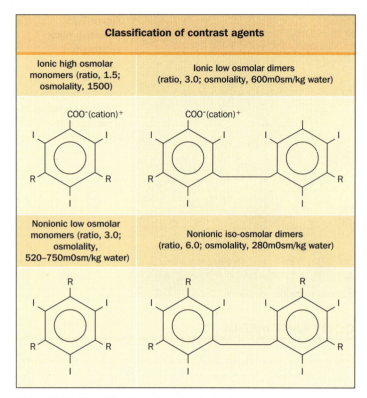

Figure 7.20 Classification of contrast agents.

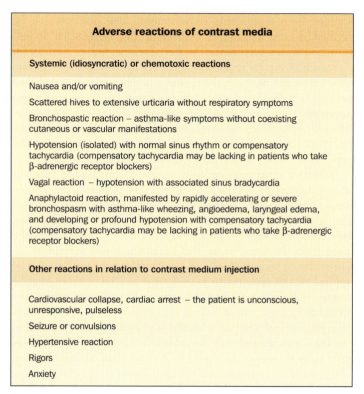

Figure 7.21 Adverse reactions of contrast media.

Chemotoxic effects of contrast media are more likely in patients who are debilitated or medically unstable. Hence, patients should be screened for conditions such as renal dysfunction, renovascular disease, severe cardiovascular disease or recent seizures. Alternative diagnostic procedures that do not require contrast media should be considered.

The use of corticosteroids as premedication is unclear. Some groups favor premedicating patients with methylprednisolone (32 mg) 12 and 2 hours before contrast media administration[16]. Other investigators believe that the small advantage of corticosteroid prophylaxis and the more certain gain from nonionic media may be combined and use both[17].

Prompt recognition and treatment can be invaluable in blunting an adverse response of a patient to radiologic contrast media and may prevent a reaction from becoming severe or even life threatening. Users of contrast media and their staff should review treatment protocols regularly so that all participants can accomplish their role efficiently. Excellent protocols that cover all aspects from nausea or urticaria to anaphylactic shock are available in the literature[15]. Knowledge, training, and preparation are crucial to guarantee appropriate and effective therapy in the event of an adverse event related to contrast media.

The kidney and contrast media

When contrast media molecules reach the systemic circulation, they quickly equilibrate across capillary membranes (except an intact blood–brain barrier). During the first phase of distribution, the increase in intravascular osmolality for hypertonic agents as well as the low osmolar contrast media causes a rapid fluid shift across capillary membranes toward the intravascular compartment. At the same time the contrast medium molecules move rapidly through capillary pores into the interstitial, extracellular space; they also move into the renal tubules by glomerular filtration.

The plasma concentration of iodine follows a biexponential decay curve similar to that of drugs that are freely distributed in the extracellular phase and excreted by pure glomerular filtration (e.g. ^{99m}Tc-diethylenetriamine pentaacetic acid). The first exponential term represents the mixing of the contrast media in the plasma volume and its distribution into the interstitial space. After 120–150 minutes the concentration of contrast medium decreases monoexponentially in patients with normal renal function (Fig. 7.22); in patients with severely reduced renal function this phase is delayed[18].

Since the molecular weights of currently used iodinated intravascular media are below 2000 Da and since protein binding of modern urographic contrast media is negligible, the contrast media molecules are freely filtered without hindrance. The concentration of contrast medium within the tubule depends on the concentration in the glomerular filtrate and on the amount of water reabsorbed as the filtrate passes down the tubule. The concentration in the initial filtrate is the same as that in the plasma. However, the concentration in mature urine is 50–100 times that in the plasma[19], since 75% of the filtered water is reabsorbed in proximal tubule, 5% in the loop of Henle, 15% in the distal tubule, and nearly 5% in the collecting ducts.

As molecules of contrast material, like those of mannitol, are not reabsorbed, they continue to exert an osmotic force, which markedly reduces reabsorption of water from the tubules. This increases pressure in the Bowman capsule and creates an acute internal hydronephrosis associated with individual nephron dilation; this leads to global renal enlargement. The main resistance

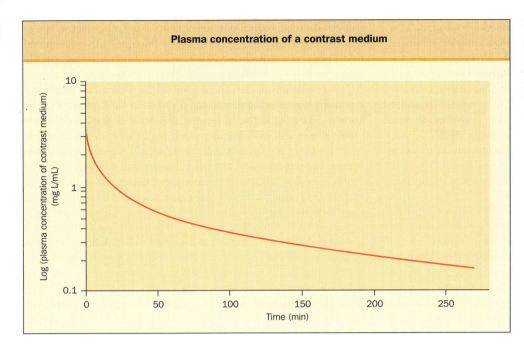

Plasma concentration of a contrast medium

Figure 7.22 Plasma concentration of a contrast medium after an intravenous bolus injection in patients with glomerular filtration rates within the normal range. After 120–150 minutes the concentration decreases monoexponentially.

Figure 7.22 Plasma concentration of a contrast medium after an intravenous bolus injection in patients with glomerular filtration rates within the normal range. After 120–150 minutes the concentration decreases monoexponentially.

to urine flow in the kidney occurs in the collecting ducts, which have a total cross-sectional intraluminal area smaller than the total cross-sectional intraluminal area of the tubules of the nephrons. The contrast-induced reductions in GFR, filtration fraction, and renal perfusion are explained by these intratubular and intracapsular pressure changes caused by the hypertonic solution. On the basis of Sterling's law, the increase in proximal tubular hydrostatic pressure decreases the gradient for filtration from the glomerular capillary. These effects are markedly attenuated when low osmolar contrast media and isotonic contrast media are used.

Within minutes after an intravascular osmotic diuretic is injected, water and sodium excretion from the kidney increases markedly. Much of the diuretic action can be accounted for by the inhibition of sodium and water reabsorption in the proximal tubule, along with inhibition of sodium and water transport in the loop of Henle[20]. During brisk osmotic diuresis, the distal tubule and collecting duct fail to recapture any notable portion of the increased sodium and water load delivered into the early distal tubule. Increases in the rate of perfusion of the distal portion of the loop lead to decrease in whole kidney GFR, which is a function of the so-called tubuloglomerular feedback (TGF) mechanism. This is, in part, related to the marked increase in proximal tubular pressure with increased flow rates within the nephron.

Features of contrast-medium nephropathy

The most important features of nephropathy induced by contrast medium are a decrease in creatinine clearance, increase in serum creatinine that peaks within 3–4 days of the administration of contrast medium, oliguria, and reduction in renal function, which often resolves within 1–2 weeks. Whether a persistent nephrogram on a plain radiograph or CT is an important feature of nephropathy induced by contrast medium is unclear, since its presence is not always associated with a subsequent reduction in renal function[21]. Nevertheless, if this sign is detected renal function should be assessed and further administration of contrast media avoided if the results are abnormal.

As many patients have more than one risk factor, determining the independent contribution of each factor to the development of renal failure is not possible. It is generally accepted that the coexistence of several or many of the factors increases the risk of contrast medium considerably.

Incidence of contrast medium-nephropathy

Intravascular administration of contrast media was claimed in the 1980s to be a common cause of hospital-acquired acute renal failure. However, the frequency data provided by these studies may be overestimated because of the bias limitations inherent in retrospective analysis. Furthermore, the awareness of nephropathy induced by contrast medium is much higher in the 1990s than it was in the 1980s, and so a lower incidence would be expected for the 1990s. However, neither a drop nor an unchanged level have been reported. Finally, the reported incidence of contrast-medium nephropathy can, both in retrospective and prospective studies, vary significantly as a result of several factors, which include reporting criteria, type of radiologic procedure, use of high, low or iso-osmolar contrast media, other prophylactic measures like hydration, and the presence or absence of risk factors, such renal insufficiency, diabetes mellitus, and volume of contrast medium. Another important factor that impacts the incidence of contrast medium nephrotoxicity is the coadministration of nephroprotective as well as nephrotoxic drugs. Also, the insensitivity of serum creatinine as a correct measure of GFR affects the figures.

Patient selection is critical, since the relative risk of the patients included predictably influences the number of cases identified[22]. For example, a 0–5% incidence was reported for studies of consecutive prospectively enrolled patients undergoing similar imaging procedures[23]. Conversely, retrospectively analyzed consecutive cases that involved patients undergoing similar imaging procedures yielded an incidence rate of 11–12%[24]. Since the definition of contrast-medium nephropathy was similar for the prospective and the retrospective studies, it seems that the

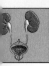
expected rate of change in serum creatinine of >44mmol/L or 50% for an unselected population undergoing a contrast-enhanced imaging procedure lies between 2 and 7%. However, when the population is stratified for a preprocedure serum creatinine value >120mmol/L, a five-fold increase in the incidence rate is found.

Serum creatinine has become a practical parameter by which to diagnose contrast-medium nephropathy. However, several expressions of serum creatinine change are being used:

- percent change from baseline with the usual range being from 20 to 50%; and
- absolute change from baseline with a range from 44mmol/L to 200mmol/L.

When five different serum creatinine definitions were applied to the same database, Lautin et al.[25] found a variation in the incidence of contrast medium nephrotoxicity from 2.8 to 21.2%, with the lower values reported for definition based on absolute changes (mmol/L) and the higher for percent change expressions. It is possible that these underestimates of toxic results are not severe enough to affect such insensitive markers of renal function[26]. The serum creatinine concentration, the measure most often used to indicate renal dysfunction, depends on muscle mass and may not become elevated above the normal range until GFR falls to 50% of normal because its relationship with GFR is nonlinear. Creatinine clearance as a measure of GFR is also inaccurate, especially when renal function is low, because the compensatory increase in tubular secretion limits its validity as a glomerular filtration marker.

The patients at highest risk for developing acute renal failure induced by contrast media are those who have both diabetes mellitus and also preexisting renal insufficiency or diabetic nephropathy. Given equal states of hydration neither diabetes alone nor renal insufficiency alone results in a statistically significantly greater incidence of renal dysfunction after contrast medium administration, although patients with these conditions are at a somewhat higher risk for renal failure than the healthy population.

Reductions in creatinine clearance levels are less after coronary angiography with low osmolar contrast media than with high osmolar contrast media. In one study[27] creatinine clearance levels at 24 hours decreased by 19% in patients who received low osmolar contrast medium, but decreased by 40% in those who received high osmolar contrast medium. In the patients who received the high osmolar contrast medium, creatinine clearance remained depressed by 47% at 48 hours, at which time it was normal in the low osmolar contrast medium group. In another study[28] nephrotoxicity occurred almost entirely in high-risk patients with underlying renal insufficiency [baseline serum creatinine >132mmol/L (1.49mg/dL)] and diabetes, the frequency of contrast-induced acute renal failure was 27% in the diatrizoate group versus 12% in the iohexol group. In this study the frequencies were based on patients who demonstrated a postcontrast increase in serum creatinine level to 88mmol/L (0.99mg/dL) or more. In both contrast groups the frequency of contrast-induced nephropathy was significantly higher among patients with renal insufficiency caused by diabetes mellitus (diabetic nephropathy; 33% in the iohexol group and 48% in the diatrizoate group) than that from other causes (12% in the iohexol group and 27% in the diatrizoate group). In a third study[29] acute renal failure was found to be important disorder in its own right, noting that even apparently minor perturbations in renal function

conferred excess mortality independent of any other factor. It was emphasized that only recently has it become fully recognized that apparently small decreases in renal function may greatly exacerbate the mortality caused by the underlying condition. A 25% rise in serum creatinine level may appear to be small, but it actually represents a substantial decrease in GFR because of the known exponential rise in serum creatinine level with declining GFR. These authors also identified major new events that are more frequent in patients with acute renal failure and that contribute to morbidity and mortality; these events include acquired sepsis, bleeding, coma, and respiratory failure. Among the more than 16,000 patients undergoing contrast-enhanced examinations the mortality was 0.4%, and 0.1% of the subjects required renal replacement therapy. The mortality in patients with renal failure was 34%, but it was 7% for those without renal failure.

It seems appropriate to conclude that in patients with diabetic nephropathy the incidence averages between 15 and 35%. In other renal diseases the incidence averages between 5 and 15%. In patients with no history, signs or symptoms of renal disease the risk is below 1%. The incidence of acute nephrotoxicity in high-risk patients is significantly less with nonionic low osmolar contrast media compared to the conventional, high osmolality ionic contrast media. Inadequate information is available for ionic low osmolar and nonionic iso-osmolar contrast media; no definite evidence has been presented that these are more nephrotoxic than the nonionic low-osmolar contrast media.

Patient-related factors in the development of contrast medium nephropathy

Diabetic nephropathy (insulin and noninsulin dependent) and dehydration are important patient-related factors in the development of contrast-medium nephropathy. Other risk factors include old age, renal insufficiency from causes other than diabetes mellitus, congestive heart failure, and concurrent administration of nephrotoxic drugs, such as gentamicin and cisplatin. The importance of a well-documented history of nephropathy induced by contrast medium is unknown[30]; the same applies to gender.

Concurrent administration of nonsteroidal anti-inflammatory drugs (NSAIDs) is a risk factor for the development of contrast-medium nephropathy[31]. These drugs are widely used and can enhance the ischemic insult of contrast media in the kidney. Also, concurrent administration of gentamicin and chemotherapeutic agents (e.g. cisplatin) increases the risk of contrast-medium nephropathy. Therefore it is recommended that these drugs are withdrawn for at least 24 hours before contrast-medium administration in patients at risk of contrast-medium nephropathy.

Contrast media are often used in the investigation of obstruction (e.g. renal colic). It is not clear if obstruction in itself is a risk factor. However, in animals contrast-medium administration may enhance the renal medullary ischemia associated with obstructive nephropathy[32].

Contrast-media factors in the development of contrast-medium nephropathy

The dose of contrast medium is an important risk factor, particularly in patients with abnormal serum creatinine levels. Good renal tolerance in patients with normal renal function has been demonstrated in spite of the administration of very large doses of contrast medium. There is probably a positive correlation between the dose of contrast medium and the rise in serum creatinine. The threshold nephrotoxic dose of contrast medium in patients with various levels of renal function remains unclear. The type of contrast media is important – administration of high osmolar contrast media should be avoided. No difference in renal tolerance has been shown between low osmolality agents (dimers and nonionic monomers). Previous contrast injection may also increase the risk in patients with abnormal renal function, particularly when the repeat administration occurs within 24 hours of the previous injection. Finally, the route of administration may be important; there is evidence that the intra-arterial route has an increased risk.

Pathophysiology of contrast-medium nephropathy

A reduction in renal perfusion, caused by a direct effect of contrast media on the kidney, and toxic effects on the tubular cells are generally accepted as the main factors in the pathophysiology of contrast-medium nephropathy. However, the importance of direct effects of contrast media on tubular cells is unclear. The mechanisms responsible for reduction in renal perfusion involve tubular and vascular events. High osmolality contrast media produce marked natriuresis and diuresis, which can activate the TGF response. This leads to vasoconstriction of the glomerular afferent arterioles, which causes a decrease in GFR and an increase in renal vascular resistance (RVR). The TGF may be responsible for almost 50% of the increase in RVR induced by ionic high osmolar contrast media. In contrast, iso-osmolar dimers, which induce only a mild diuresis and natriuresis, do not activate this mechanism. The activation of the TGF is osmolality dependent and low osmolar contrast media, which are still hypertonic solutions compared to blood, may also stimulate this mechanism. Possible other tubular events in the pathogenesis of nephropathy induced by contrast medium include an increase in the intratubular pressure, and tubular obstruction by Tamm–Horsfall protein and abnormal proteins. However, no strong evidence indicates these tubular effects are important in the pathophysiology of contrast-medium nephropathy.

The structural effects of contrast media on the renal tubules include vacuolization of the epithelial cells of the proximal tubules, DNA fragmentation (abnormal activation of apoptosis or 'programmed' cell death), and necrosis of the cells of the thick ascending limbs of loops of Henle in the renal medulla. Active engulfing of contrast media in tubular cells causes vacuolar responses in the tubular cells, which cause lysosomal changes. The vacuolization is reversible and resolves within a few days of contrast-medium administration. There is no correlation between the degree of vacuolization in the tubular cells and the reduction in renal function. The structural effect of contrast medium in the renal medulla results from ischemia and is less with low osmolar contrast media. Activation of apoptosis may play an important role in nephron injury and renal failure induced by contrast media.

The vascular events that follow contrast-media administration are mainly secondary to the direct renal effects of contrast media, which modulate the synthesis and release of vasoactive mediators within the kidney. The endogenous vasodilators prostaglandins and nitric oxide are not directly involved in the renal hemodynamic effects of contrast media. Nevertheless, the intrarenal production of these vasodilators is important to maintain the perfusion and oxygen supply of the medulla, a tissue that is poorly perfused and inadequately supplied with oxygen. In situations in which the synthesis of these mediators is hampered, the renal insult produced by contrast media is enhanced.

The vasoactive substances endothelin (ET) and adenosine are important in mediation of the renal hemodynamic effects of contrast media. Contrast agents stimulate the release of ET by endothelial cells in culture and increase both the plasma ET concentration and the urinary ET excretion after intravascular administration. The fall in GFR and reduction in renal perfusion induced by contrast media may be prevented by ET receptor antagonists. In addition, after contrast media administration the increase in plasma ET is greater in patients whose renal function declines when compared with those whose renal function remains unchanged[33].

Adenosine is an important mediator of the reduction in GFR and renal blood flow induced by contrast media. The biologic interaction between adenosine and ET is unknown.

Long-term effects of contrast media

There is extremely limited knowledge regarding the long-term effects of contrast media on renal function in humans. High osmolar contrast medium can enhance the progression of glomerulosclerosis and renal failure in old spontaneously hypertensive male rats[34]. Whether this is also the case in human is not known.

Prevention of contrast-medium nephrotoxicity

Several measures have been recommended to prevent nephropathy induced by contrast medium, which include:

- hydration with NaCl 0.9%, NaCl 0.45%;
- infusion of mannitol, or atrial natriuretic factor;
- administration of loop diuretics, calcium antagonists, theophylline, and dopamine;
- use of nonionic low osmolar contrast media instead of ionic high osmolar contrast media;
- rapid hemodialysis after contrast administration;
- minimization of the volume of contrast medium; and
- prolongation of the interval between procedures in which contrast media are used.

Of all these many measures, extracellular volume expansion has been shown repeatedly to be effective and is the most widely recommended[22].

Patients with pre-existing renal failure, independent of cause, should not undergo radiologic procedures in which contrast medium is administered unless they have been hydrated. The only exception is patients with congestive heart failure. An adequate hydration procedure includes the administration of 100mL/h of 0.9% saline from 4 hours before contrast-medium administration until 24 hours after, for patients who are not allowed to drink or eat because they are undergoing an interventional or surgical procedure. Patients who can and may drink should have at least the same volume: 500mL of water or soft drinks before and 2500mL during the following 24 hours. This volume should cover insensible perspiration and secure a diuresis of at least 1mL/minute. Furthermore, nonionic low osmolar contrast media should always be used. The interval between two examinations in which contrast media are administered should

European Society of Urogenital Radiology simple guidelines to avoid contrast medium nephrotoxicity		
Definition		Contrast-medium nephrotoxicity is a condition in which an impairment in renal function [an increase in serum creatinine by more than 25% or 44mmol/L (0.5mg/dL)] occurs within 3 days following the intravascular administration of a contrast medium in the absence of an alternative etiology
Risk factors	Look for	Serum creatinine levels, particularly secondary to diabetic nephropathy
		Dehydration
		Congestive heart failure
		Age over 70 years
		Concurrent administration of nephrotoxic drugs (e.g. nonsteroidal anti-inflammatory drugs)
In patients with risk factor(s)	Do	Make sure that the patient is well hydrated – give at least 100mL [oral (e.g. soft drinks) or intravenous (normal saline) depending on the clinical situation] per hour starting 4 hours before to 24 hours after contrast administration (in warm areas increase the fluid volume)]
		Use low- or iso-osmolar contrast media
		Stop administration of nephrotoxic drugs for at least 24 hours
		Consider alternative imaging techniques that do not require the administration of iodinated contrast media
	Do not	Give high osmolar contrast media
		Administer large doses of contrast media
		Administer mannitol and diuretics, particularly loop diuretics
		Perform multiple studies with contrast media within a short period of time

Figure 7.23 European Society of Urogenital Radiology simple guidelines to avoid contrast-medium nephrotoxicity.

be at least 48 hours. Concomitant use of nephrotoxic drugs (e.g. gentamicin, NSAIDs) should be avoided. Recently, the Contrast Media Safety Committee of the European Society of Urogenital Radiology[30] proposed guidelines to diminish the risk of nephropathy induced by contrast medium (Fig. 7.23).

The efficacy of the other measures, particularly the use of renal vasodilators, theophylline, and calcium antagonists, remains unclear, but the administration of frusemide (furosemide) and mannitol is no longer recommended in the literature.

The presence of multiple myeloma has, for many years, been considered a contraindication for the administration of contrast media, since some patients developed anuria (caused by dehydration). Although the administration of contrast media to myeloma patients is not totally risk free (about 1%), it may be performed if the clinical need arises and the patient is well hydrated[35].

Treatment of contrast-medium nephropathy

The finding of increased serum creatinine and/or lack of urinary output within the first days following contrast medium administration, in the presence of no other cause for the change in renal function, indicates contrast-induced nephrotoxicity. There is no specific treatment. Hemodialysis has been tried, but this should only be carried out if clinically necessary. The patient should not be reexposed to contrast media before kidney function has returned to its previous level. If contrast medium is to be given again, the patient must be adequately hydrated.

Lactic acidosis and contrast media

The use of contrast media in patients who receive metformin is currently very unclear. The potential danger of lactic acidosis arises because if renal excretion is reduced, metformin accumulates. There is no evidence of interaction between contrast

media and metformin. In a review of metformin-associated lactic acidosis[36] only seven of the 110 cases reported in the world literature from 1968 to 1991 had received iodinated contrast material before developing lactic acidosis. Dachman[37] was able to find 13 documented cases of lactic acidosis after the administration of iodinated contrast material in patients who received metformin. Most patients either had renal dysfunction before the procedure or continued to use metformin despite the development of contrast-medium nephropathy. In 12 of the 13 cases, patients had elevated creatinine levels or decreased creatinine clearance before the administration of contrast medium.

Patients at risk are those who may develop renal insufficiency induced by contrast medium. Patients with diabetic nephropathy – insulin and noninsulin dependent – have the highest risk of developing contrast-medium nephropathy[15,30]. The poorer the renal function the higher the risk, and dehydration increases the risk even more. Despite the short half-life of metformin (from 1.5 hours, dependent on renal function), it is still present in the body when the renal effects of contrast media occur. These develop instantly after the administration of contrast media, but may not be detected until 24–48 hours later[30].

In Europe it is currently advised that metformin be stopped 48 hours before and for 48 hours subsequent to the administration of contrast media. Renal function (e.g. serum creatinine) should be checked to assure that it has remained at the precontrast level before metformin is resumed. In the USA it is recommended that metformin administration be stopped and serum creatinine level checked before the intravascular administration of contrast media. If the serum creatinine level is normal, contrast medium is injected and metformin administration can be restarted 48 hours later if the renal function remains normal (i.e. normal serum creatinine level)[15]. In the USA the use of

European Society of Urogenital Radiology guidelines for the administration of contrast media to diabetics taking metformin		
Patient type	Criteria	Action
Diabetics	On biguanides	Check serum creatinine Use low osmolar contrast media
Elective studies	Serum creatinine normal	Stop metformin and carry out study Recommence metformin after about 48 hours if creatinine normal
	Renal function abnormal	Stop metformin Carry out study 48 hours later Recommence metformin after about 48 hours if renal function normal

Emergency studies	Serum creatinine normal
	Renal function abnormal
		Proceed as for elective studies
		Weigh risks versus benefits
		Consider alternative imaging techniques
		If contrast is essential:
		   stop metformin
		   hydrate patient
		   monitor renal function, serum lactic acid, and serum pH
		   observe for signs of lactic acidosis

Figure 7.24 European Society of Urogenital Radiology guidelines for the administration of contrast media to diabetics taking metformin

metformin or phenformin is contraindicated in patients with renal insufficiency. Normal renal function, defined as a normal serum creatinine level, does not exclude totally the possible occurrence of lactic acidosis, but lactic acidosis is more frequent in patients with abnormal renal function (defined as patients who have abnormal serum creatinine levels). Recently, the Contrast Media Safety Committee of the European Society of Urogenital Radiology has agreed on guidelines (Fig. 7.24)[38].

REFERENCES

1. Pollack HM. History of iodinated contrast media. In: Thomsen HS, Muller RN, Mattrey RF, eds. Trends in contrast media. Berlin: Springer Verlag; 1999:3–19.
2. Levine JA, Neitlich J, Verga M, et al. Ureteral calculi in patients with flank pain: correlation of plain radiography with unenchanced helical CT. Radiology. 1997;204:27–31.
3. Goldwasser B, Cohan RH, Dunnick NR, Andriani RT, Carson CG, Weinert JL. The role of linear tomography in evaluation of patients with nephrolithiasis. Urology. 1989;23:253–6.
4. Davidson AJ, Hartman DS. Diagnostic uroradiologic techniques. In: Davidson AJ, Hartman DS, eds. Radiology of the kidney and urinary tract. Philadelphia: WB Saunders; 1994:3–32.
5. Talner LB. Non-contrast helical CT for acute flank pain (the CT 'KUB'): reflections after 500 cases. In: Grenier N, ed. 6th European Symposium on Radiology, European Society of Urogenital Radiology (ESUR): Strasbourg, 1998:42–4.
6. Dalla Palma L, Stacul F, Bazzochi M, Pagnan L, Festini G, Marega D. Ultrasonography and plain film versus intravenous urography in renal colic. Clin Radiol. 1993;47:333–6.
7. Goldman SM. Upper tract trauma. In: Willi UV, Kenney PJ, Thomsen HS, eds. International uroradiology '96. Copenhagen: FADL Publishers; 1996:21–5.
8. Thomsen HS. Pyelorenal backflow. Clinical and experimental investigations. Radiologic, nuclear medical and pathoanatomic studies. Dan Med Bull. 1984;31:438–57.
9. Gyanes SM, Hollander JB, Jafri SZH. Trauma of the lower genitourinarty tract. In: Jafri SZH, Diokino AC, Amendola MA, eds. Lower genitourinary radiology. New York: Springer Verlag; 1998.
10. Thomsen HS, Rygaard H, Strandberg C. Micturating cystourethrography and vesicoureteral reflux. Variations in technique. Eur J Radiol. 1985;5:318–20.
11. McCallum RW. The adult male urethra: normal anatomy, pathology and method of urethrography. Radiol Clin North Am. 1979;17:227–44.
12. Greenberg M, Stone D, Cochran ST, et al. Female urethral diverticula: double-balloon catheter study. AJR. 1981;136:259–64.
13. Velcek D, Evans JA. Cavernosography. Radiology. 1982;144:781–5.
14. Bookstein JJ. Cavernosal venooclusive insufficiency in male impotence: evaluation of degree and location. Radiology. 1987;164:175–8.
15. Thomsen HS, Bush WH Jr. Adverse effects of contrast media. Incidence, prevention and management. Drug Safety. 1998;19:313–24.
16. Lasser EC, Berry CC, Talner LB, et al. Pretreatment with corticosteroids to alleviate reactions to intravascular contrast media. N Engl J Med. 1987;317:845–9.
17. Dawson P, Sidhu PS. Is there a role for corticosteroid prophylaxis in patients at increased risk of adverse reactions to intravascular contrast agents? Clin Radiol. 1993;48:225–6.
18. Almén T, Frennby B, Sterner G. Determination of glomerular filtration rate (GFR) with contrast media. In: Thomsen HS, Muller RN, Mattrey RF, eds. Trends in contrast media. Berlin: Springer Verlag; 1999: 81–94.
19. Thomsen HS, Golman K, Hemmingsen L, Larsen S, Skaarup P, Svendsen O. Contrast medium induced nephropathy: animal experiments. Frontiers Eur Radiol. 1993;9:83–108.
20. Gennari FJ, Kassires JP. Osmotic diuresis. N Engl J Med. 1974; 291:714–20.
21. Yamazaki H, Matsushita M, Inoue T, et al. Renal cortical retention on delayed CT after angiography and contrast associated nephropathy. Br J Radiol. 1997;70:897–902.
22. Thomsen HS. Contrast nephropathy. In: Thomsen HS, Muller RN, Mattrey RF, eds. Trends in contrast media. Berlin: Springer Verlag; 1999;103–16.
23. Parfrey PS, Griffiths SM, Barrett BJ, et al. Contrast material-induced renal failure in patients with diabetes mellitus, renal insufficiency, or both. N Engl J Med. 1989;320;143–9.

24. Martin-Paredero V, Dixon SM, Baker D, et al. Risk of renal failure after major angiography. Arch Surg. 1098;118:1417–20.

25. Lautin EM, Freeman NJ, Schoenfeld AH, et al. Radiocontrast-associated renal dysfunction: a comparison of lower osmolality and conventional high-osmolality contrast media. AJR 1991;157:59–65.

26. Blaufox MD, Aurell M, Bubeck B, et al. 1996 Report of the radionuclides in nephrourology committee on renal clearance. J Nucl Med. 1996;37:1883–90.

27. Katholi RE, Taylor GJ, Woods WT, et al. Nephrotoxicity of nonionic low osmolality contrast media: a prospective double-blind randomized comparison in human beings. Radiology. 1993;186: 183–7.

28. Rudnick MR, Goldfarb S, Wexler L, et al. Nephrotoxicity of ionic and nonionic contrast media in 1196 patients. A randomized trial. Kidney Int. 1995;47:254–61.

29. Levy EM, Viscoli CM, Horwitz RI. The effect of acute renal failure on mortality: a cohort analysis. JAMA 1996;275:1489–94.

30. Morcos SK, Thomsen HS, Webb JAW and Members of the Contrast Media Safety Committee of the European Society of Urogenital Radiology (ESUR). Contrast media induced nephrotoxicity: A consensus report. Eur Radiol. 1999;9:1602–13.

31. Heyman SN, Rosen S, Brezis M. Radiocontrast nephropathy: a paradigm for synergism between toxic and hypoxic insults in the kidney. Exp Nephrol. 1994;2:153–7.

32. Heyman SN, Fuch S, Jaffe R, et al. Renal microcirculation and tissue damage during acute ureteral obstruction in the rat: effect of saline infusion, indomethacin and radiocontrast. Kidney Int. 1997;51:653–63.

33. Clark BA, Kim D, Epstein FH. Endothelin and arterial natriuretic peptide levels following radiocontrast exposure in humans. Am J Kidney Dis. 1997;30:82–6.

34. Duarte CG, Zhang J, Ellis S. The SHR as a small animal model for radiocontrast renal failure. Relation of nephrotoxicity to animal's age, gender, strain and dose of radiocontrast. Renal Failure. 1997;19:723–43.

35. McCarthy CS, Becker JA. Multiple myeloma and contrast media. Radiology. 1992;183:519–21.

36. Sirtori CR, Pasik C. Re-evaluation of biguanide, metformin. Mechanisms of action and tolerability. Pharmacol Res. 1994;30:187–228.

37. Dachman AH. Answer. Radiology. 1996;290:289.

38. Thomsen HS, Morcos SK and Members of the Contrast Media Safety Committee of the European Society of Urogenital Radiology. Lactic acidosis in non-insulin dependent diabetics after administration of contrast media. Guidelines to diminish the risk. Eur Radiol. 1999;9:738–40.

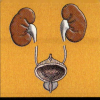

Section 2 Investigative Urology

Chapter 8

Radiologic Imaging: Computed Tomography, Ultrasound, and Magnetic Resonance Imaging

Leslie M Scoutt, Thomas R McCauley, and Arthur T Rosenfield

KEY POINTS

- Ultrasound is a safe, inexpensive, rapid, readily available imaging method.
- Doppler imaging has added physiologic hemodynamic information to the test.
- Computed tomography (CT) provides multiorgan information rapidly and accurately. Helical CT, three-dimensional studies, and virtual imaging are exciting new developments.
- Magnetic resonance imaging (MRI) has the potential to combine the safety of ultrasound with the wealth of information of CT and is becoming more widely used in urology.

INTRODUCTION

The past 25 years have witnessed a revolution in uroradiologic imaging that is not only remarkable in the reliability and complexity of the new techniques but is also ongoing and constantly changing. Every newly developed diagnostic imaging modality has had immediate and lasting application to the urinary tract. The intravenous urogram (IVU), the backbone of urologic imaging until the 1970s, when effective cross-sectional techniques were introduced, remains a useful way to evaluate the urothelium but is rarely able to stand alone. The IVU in its new role is discussed in this chapter in conjunction with computed tomography (CT) scanning.

Computed tomography has been very important in uroradiologic imaging because it provides multiorgan information rapidly and accurately. Many renal disorders are incidentally discovered on CT studies performed to evaluate other organ systems; conversely, many urinary tract examinations demonstrate major unexpected disease processes in other organs. Thus, while CT has greatly improved our ability to define renal and other urinary tract disease, it also has led to a blurring of the distinctions between imaging of the gastrointestinal, urinary, and gynecologic systems. Noncontrast CT in flank pain is a major example. CT has profited from changes in hardware and software leading to more rapid data acquisition (such as helical CT) and new ways to display acquired data such as three-dimensional (3D) studies (e.g. CT angiography) and virtual imaging (e.g. virtual cystoscopy). This chapter will attempt to merge the past in CT with the new techniques that are rapidly becoming standard parts of urologic practice.

Ultrasound (US) provides a safe, inexpensive, rapid, and readily available (it is portable) method of imaging. The introduction

of Doppler imaging, which depicts blood flow hemodynamics, has added physiologic information to the gray-scale ultrasound image. Hence, ultrasound is used as the initial imaging technique whenever appropriate. In areas such as the scrotum where there is no barrier from intervening tissue, sonography is the standard approach and can be definitive. In other situations, such as the evaluation of a renal mass, it is one of many techniques that may be applied. Modern ultrasonography differs substantially from ultrasonography as it was initially introduced. In this chapter we examine current applications of sonography.

Magnetic resonance imaging (MRI) has the potential to combine the safety of ultrasonography with the wealth of information of CT. It can do this while also providing new information unique to MRI. MRI has not yet become extensively used in urology, but this is now changing. This chapter demonstrates the utility of current MRI imaging.

As we enter the 21st century, we have an opportunity to alter the way in which diagnoses of urinary tract disease are made by using the latest techniques. In this section, modern imaging in urology is defined.

COMPUTED TOMOGRAPHY OF THE KIDNEY AND URINARY TRACT

Noncontrast computed tomography

This rapid technique requires no contrast medium and is able to identify ureteral stones with an accuracy greater than that of the IVU[1-5]. In addition, other nonstone causes of flank pain are readily identified with noncontrast CT and not with the IVU[2,6,7].

If a stone is identified within the ureter (Fig. 8.1), then the study is definitive. If a calcification is seen that is thought possibly to be in the ureter, reconstruction of the images between the slices,

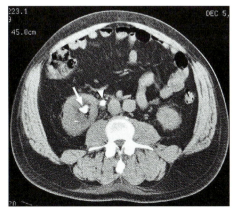

Figure 8.1 Classic ureteropelvic junction stone. A stone is seen at the right ureteropelvic junction (arrowhead). There is also nephrolithiasis (arrow).

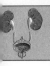

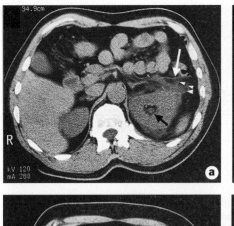

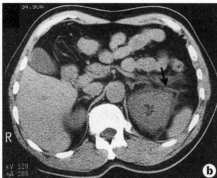

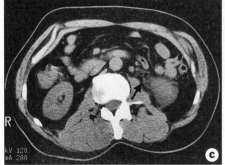

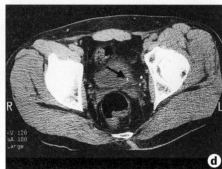

Figure 8.2 Secondary signs in the patient with a stone which has passed into the bladder.
(a) A scan through the upper pole of the left kidney demonstrates thickening of fascial planes as well as a small amount of extravasated urine (large arrowhead). The white arrow points to thickened Gerota's fascia and the small arrowheads to thickened fascial planes (bridging septa). Note the presence of hydronephrosis (black arrow). Hydronephrosis should be searched for in the region of the calices rather than the renal pelvis which has more variable normal appearance. (b) Scan at a lower level demonstrates more extensive thickening of the fascial planes. Arrow points to thickened Gerota's fascia. (c) Scan through the lower pole of the left kidney again demonstrates extensive stranding about the kidney. The lower pole of the kidney is the optimal place to search for perinephric stranding. There is ureterectasis (arrow). (d) Scan through the pelvis demonstrates a small stone within the bladder (arrow). When a question exists whether a stone is in the bladder or in the hemitrigone, the patient can be placed prone to see if the stone moves to the dependent portion of the bladder. That was done in this case and the stone moved to the more dependent portion with the patient prone. The presence of ureteral stranding and ureterectasis in a patient without clinical signs of pyelonephritis is considered characteristic of ureterolithiasis even if a stone is not identified.

which is possible with helical or multislice CT, can demonstrate whether or not a stone is present. In patients in whom a stone is not seen within the ureter (Fig. 8.2), secondary signs are important in diagnosis. The two most useful secondary signs are unilateral ureteral dilatation and unilateral or asymmetric perinephric stranding. In a series at our institution, the presence of both ureterectasis and perinephric stranding had a positive predictive value of 99%, while absence of both perinephric stranding and ureteral dilatation had a negative predictive value of 95%[3]. Thus, the combination of unilateral ureteral dilatation and asymmetric perinephric stranding is considered to be indicative of ureterolithiasis in the proper clinical setting. Using the following criteria on noncontrast CT as diagnostic of a ureteral stone, either identification of the stone in the ureter or a combination of ureteral dilatation and asymmetric perinephric stranding, excellent results were obtained: a sensitivity of 97%, a specificity of 96%, and an accuracy of 97% for diagnosing ureteral stone disease.[2]

The rim sign[8,9], the presence of an edematous cuff of tissue about the stone, is helpful in cases in which the ureter is difficult to trace (Fig. 8.3), with an accuracy of approximately 94% for ureterolithiasis[9]. A phlebolith can be distinguished from a stone if the 'comet tail' sign is identified[10]. This is a linear structure extending from the phlebolith and thought to represent the thrombosed vein itself. The major criteria for noncontrast computed tomography diagnosis of ureterolithiasis are:

• visualization of an opacity in the ureter;
• secondary signs: perinephric stranding and ureterectasis
• the 'rim sign'; and
• anatomic criteria (i.e. 'water under the bridge').

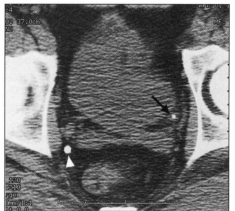

Figure 8.3 'Rim sign'.
A small stone in the distal left ureter (arrow) is surrounded by the edematous wall of the ureter. The rim sign is typically seen with stones 4mm or less in diameter. Note that the phlebolith present on the right (arrowhead) posterior to the seminal vesicle does not have a rim sign.

All stones are radioopaque on CT except for indinavir stones in HIV-infected patients undergoing therapy[11]. Since uric acid stones are opaque on CT but not IVU, and since smaller stones can be identified on CT than IVU, CT is a more specific technique for stone disease when ureteric obstruction is present. A good correlation has been shown in vivo between stone size on CT and actual stone size[12]. The density of the stone on CT is inversely related to slice thickness[12]. Scanning the patients prone permits distinction between ureterovesical junction stone and a stone that has passed into the bladder.

When a pregnant woman presents with flank pain without a clearcut cause or diagnosis identified by ultrasonography combined with a plain radiograph of the abdomen (kidneys, ureter,

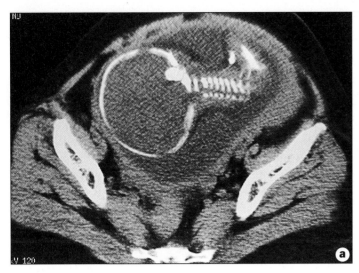

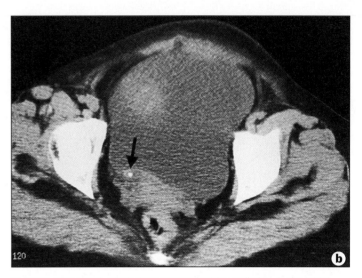

Figure 8.4 Flank pain protocol in pregnancy. This patient was in the third trimester of pregnancy. Right flank pain was present that was thought to be due to appendicitis. (a) Flank pain protocol was performed, demonstrating the fetus. A more caudad scan (b) shows a stone (arrow) in the region of the right hemitrigone with a rim sign. Surgery was avoided by using the flank pain protocol. This approach may be safely used if necessary during the second and third trimesters of pregnancy.

However, ultrasound, which does not use ionizing radiation, is the initial imaging modality of choice in pregnancy. When flank pain occurs, a low-dose, digital plain film should be obtained in conjunction with the ultrasound study. Computed tomography should be reserved for cases where the ultrasound is not diagnostic and a significant abnormality is clinically suspected that may mimic the symptoms of ureteral stone disease.

and bladder; KUB), a limited IVU is the technique of choice. However, if a serious abdominal problem such as appendicitis is in the differential diagnosis, noncontrast computed tomography can be safely used in the second and third trimester of pregnancy (Fig. 8.4) to diagnose or exclude major diseases as well as ureterolithiasis.

Of equal importance is the identification of nonstone disease by CT in patients presenting with flank pain. In 417 patients with flank pain, CT findings were positive for diagnoses unrelated to stone disease in 65 patients in one series[2]. These diagnoses were confirmed by a variety of methods. The most common nonurinary tract abnormality was an adnexal mass. Appendicitis (Fig. 8.5) and diverticulitis were the next most common entities and a large variety of other pathological entities were identified[2] (Fig. 8.6). Therefore, when evaluating a patient for flank pain, the initial search should be for calcifications in the course of the urinary tract as well as for nonstone disease such as leaking aortic aneurysm, appendicitis, or ovarian mass with torsion. If a stone within the ureter is identified or if nonstone disease is present, diagnostic workup is complete. However, even if a stone is identified within the ureter, a careful search must be made for nonstone disease.

Add-on computed tomography urography

The IVU remains an established technique for the evaluation of the urinary tract in several situations, such as the evaluation of hematuria. Compared to cross-sectional imaging studies, urography offers superior visualization of the collecting system and ureter. It also offers physiologic information about the handling of contrast media that is complementary to the information obtained on other studies. When add-on delayed computed tomography of the kidneys is used as the tomographic technique for the kidneys after the excretory urogram, optimal information can be obtained. Two situations exist for this usage: if an IVU is performed for a specific problem and a question arises,

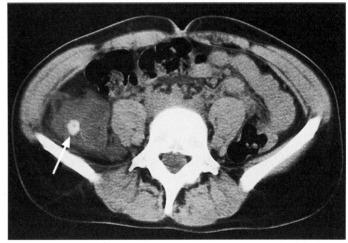

Figure 8.5 Appendicitis. Flank pain protocol, performed in a patient presenting with right lower quadrant pain thought to be either ureterolithiasis or appendicitis, demonstrates an appendiceal abscess containing an appendicolith (arrow). Noncontrast computed tomography using the identical technique to that for urinary tract stones has been used in the evaluation of appendicitis with excellent results. The flank pain protocol simultaneously evaluates the patient for ureterolithiasis as well as for extra-urinary-tract diseases, particularly ovarian masses with torsion, appendicitis, and diverticulitis.

then computed tomography[13] can be used to define whether an abnormality is present or not. Computed tomographic sections can be limited to the area of suspected abnormality. The CT study can be performed as long as 90 minutes after the IVU and at times longer (Figs 8.7 & 8.8). The computed tomographic study can also be used as a replacement for standard nephrotomography in patients with hematuria (Fig. 8.8). The IVU remains the best technique for the evaluation of the collecting

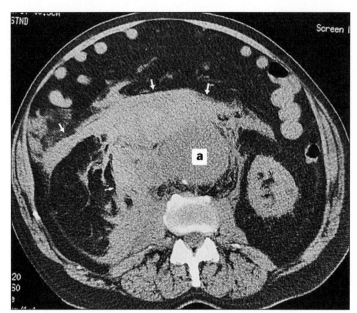

Figure 8.6 Ruptured abdominal aortic aneurysm. This patient presenting with right flank pain had a flank pain protocol that took under 3 minutes. A leaking aortic aneurysm (a) was readily apparent, leading to immediate surgery. The high attenuation of the extensive soft tissue stranding (arrows) in the retroperitoneum is consistent with hemorrhage. Noncontrast computed tomography is extremely accurate and rapid in the diagnosis of leaking aortic aneurysm, which is the most feared entity in the differential diagnosis of ureterolithiasis.

system, while computed tomography is optimal for evaluating the renal parenchyma. By using add-on CT, a complete IVU is obtained, supplemented by delayed CT scan so that minimal time on the CT scanner is required.

Contrast computed tomography

Renal masses are the most common indication for formal renal CT. CT and MRI are the most sensitive techniques for screening for renal masses (Fig. 8.9). CT, which is less expensive and more readily available, is the standard approach unless the patient has a contrast medium allergy or has had a prior suboptimal contrast CT or a previous CT with equivocal findings[14]. Helical scanning permits an arterial phase to be obtained before the standard imaging in the portal venous phase[15,16]. This can be useful in selected renal tumors, both for the kidney and for its liver metastases. The best phase for imaging the renal parenchyma with respect to identifying renal masses is after the corticomedullary phase has faded, which tends to take place at approximately 2 minutes. The standard renal mass protocol is comprised of four phases: (1) noncontrast CT; (2) arterial phase CT (approximately 20 seconds after injection); (3) standard portal venous phase imaging of the liver and kidneys (approximately 70 seconds after injection); and (4) delayed scans of the kidneys which can be performed at 2 minutes for optimal parenchymal definition or at 3 minutes and beyond for parenchyma and collecting system definition (Fig. 8.10)[17–20]. Post-processing using different 'windows' (by changing the level of interest and the number of shades of gray included in the image) may be required on any phase to best demonstrate abnormalities.

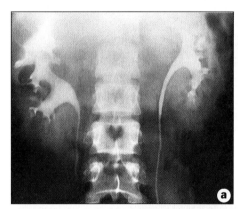

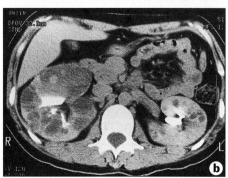

Figure 8.7 Add-on computed tomography urography/adult polycystic kidney disease. (a) Excretory urography in a 23-year-old female with hematuria demonstrates bilateral distortion of the collecting systems and nephromegaly. (b) Add-on computed tomography demonstrates multiple cysts of varying size in both kidneys – typical of adult (dominant) polycystic kidney disease. Using add-on computed tomography urography, additional studies are not needed. An immediate, definitive answer is obtained without the use of additional contrast medium.

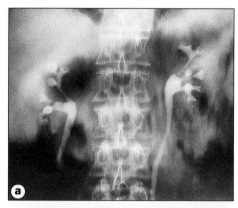

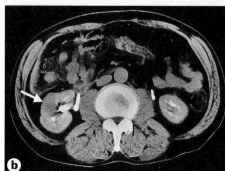

Figure 8.8 Add-on computed tomography demonstrating a tumor not seen on intravenous urogram. (a) Excretory urography with nephrotomography demonstrated no abnormality in this middle-aged man with hematuria. (b) Add-on computed tomography urography demonstrated a 2cm mass (arrow) in the right kidney, which was solid and proved to be renal cell carcinoma. Add-on computed tomography urography is capable of demonstrating masses not seen on excretory urography.

Methods of screening for renal masses (in order of sensitivity)
1. CT* ⎫ Equivalent
2. MRI* ⎭
3. Nuclear medicine (parenchymal study)
4. Ultrasound
5. IVU
* Contrast-enhanced (add-on or primary CT)

Figure 8.9 Methods of screening for renal masses (in order of sensitivity). CT, computed tomography; IVU, intravenous urogram; MRI, magnetic resonance imaging.

Phases of helical renal CT	
1. Non-contrast	
2. Arterial (corticomedullary)	20s
3. Portal venous for liver (corticomedullary)	70s
or	
Nephrogram	approximately 2min*
4. Excretory	about 3min
*If liver evaluation is not being performed	

Figure 8.10 Phases of helical renal computed tomography (CT).

Bosniak has described a classification of renal masses based on their CT appearance and other imaging studies[21,22]. Masses with the classic findings for cysts on imaging studies are characterized as Bosniak type I and need no further evaluation. Masses with the classic findings for a cyst and a minor additional finding such as fine, thin calcification are described as Bosniak type II and generally need no followup. In some situations, followup may be desirable for lesions in this class. Bosniak type III masses are cystic lesions with major findings that make it likely that they are neoplastic, such as extensive, coarse calcification. These generally require surgery. Bosniak type IV masses are cystic lesions that clearly appear malignant and definitely require surgical treatment. Modern helical CT with multiphase imaging has made this distinction easier but requires meticulous technique involving multiple phases of imaging for greatest accuracy.

The noncontrast phase of the abdominal CT is important to demonstrate findings that may be missed on the contrast phase. A baseline Hounsfield unit (HU) number for comparison with the postcontrast studies to evaluate for enhancement is crucial. Enhancement of greater than 10HU at any contrast phase compared to the noncontrast phase is indicative of a solid mass, presumably a malignancy.

Angiomyolipomas are benign lesions which have gross fat within them[23,24]. The demonstration of gross fat should lead one to treat the lesion as benign. The gross fat will often be missed on a contrast-enhanced study since angiomyolipomas are vascular. An exception to the rule concerning fat is when a malignancy has engulfed the renal sinus and has fat in it for that reason[25]. Therefore, any mass involving the renal sinus cannot be considered benign simply because it contains fat.

Calcium is also an important finding, which may be missed on contrast-enhanced studies. Coarse calcification within a mass,

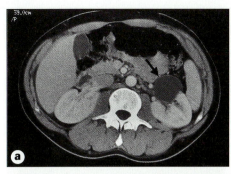
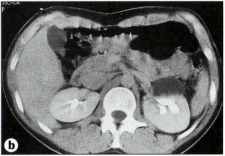

Figure 8.11 Standard contrast computed tomography scan: value of the delayed scan for the excretory (and nephrogram) phase. (a) Computed tomography scan performed at 70s during the standard portal phase demonstrates a fluid-filled mass (arrow) related to the anterior portion of the left kidney. (b) Delayed excretory phase demonstrates that this is the renal pelvis, which is anterior in this kidney with nonrotation. The pelvis fills readily with contrast, identifying it as such.

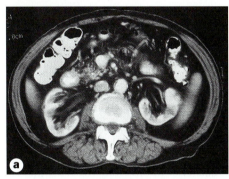
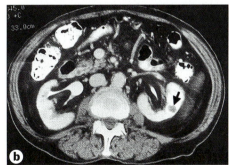

Figure 8.12 Standard computed tomography: value of delayed scan (nephrogram phase) to demonstrate masses. (a) Scan performed at 70s during the portal venous phase, which is the corticomedullary phase, demonstrates no definite mass. (b) Delayed scan demonstrates a 1cm mass (arrow) in the left kidney, which is nearly impossible to distinguish from a pyramid on the portal venous phase (a) although in retrospect it is faintly visualized.

even if the mass is cystic, is typical of malignancy. Linear fine calcification in a cystic mass is not. Identifying fat and calcium, both of which may be obscured on studies after injection of intravenous contrast medium, and obtaining base-line HU measurements for subsequent determination of the presence or absence of contrast enhancement within a mass all require a noncontrast study of the kidneys.

The nephrographic phase (delayed images) is generally superior to the corticomedullary phase whether viewed on the arterial or portal venous phase (Figs 8.11 & 8.12). More false-positive lesions with normal anatomy mimicking tumor and more false negative lesions with the tumors being missed are described on the corticomedullary phases compared to the nephrographic

CT in the characterization of renal masses

1. Malignant tumor

   Enhancement from noncontrast on any contrast phase*

   Cystic tumor: Enhancing septa and/or thick wall†

   Malignant tumor: chunky calcification†

   Malignant tumor: ill defined margin with renal parenchyma†

   Malignant tumor: fluid greater than water density† (must be distinguished from hyperdense cyst)

2. Angiomyolipoma

   Gross fat (excluding engulfment)

3. Cyst

   Paper-thin wall

   Smooth margin with renal parenchyma

   Thin, nonenhancing septa, if present

   Calcification thin and linear if present

   Water density (0–20HU)

4. Abscess

   Enhancing rim

   Low-density center with no enhancement

   Center water density or slightly higher

5. Focal pyelonephritis

   Mass that eventually enhances on delayed images

* Definitive
† Requires further evaluation

Figure 8.13 Computed tomography (CT) in the characterization of renal masses. HU, Hounsfield unit.

phase. The portal venous phase is more reliable than the arterial phase in demonstrating enhancement and the nephrographic phase tends to be the most reliable.

The main technical concepts in screening for renal masses using CT are therefore as follows:
- noncontrast images for calcium, fat, baseline HU;
- nephrographic phase superior to corticomedullary phases; and
- arterial phase may be useful in vascular tumors.

Cysts have a paper-thin wall, a smooth margin with the renal parenchyma, thin nonenhancing septa (if septa are present), calcification that is thin and linear if present, and water density (0–20HU). Malignancies are solid (Fig. 8.8) and may exhibit contrast enhancement, usually from the noncontrast phase to a later phase. Cystic tumors may have an enhancing septa and/or a thick wall. Malignant tumors may have chunky calcifications. An ill-defined margin with the renal parenchyma is also a finding typical of tumors. When greater than water density is present in a mass, the differential diagnosis is hyperdense cyst and a renal cell carcinoma[26]. Ultrasound can be of aid in distinguishing between these two possibilities, as can contrast-enhanced CT since hyperdense cysts will not enhance[27]. Hyperdense cysts contain blood or protein. Figure 8.13 summarizes the CT criteria used to characterize renal masses.

The other roles of urinary tract CT are legion. The phases to be performed must be chosen depending upon the clinical indication. Renal lymphoma can present as a diffusely enlarged abnormal kidney, bilateral renal masses, or a solitary renal mass. CT is extremely useful since renal lymphoma is frequently accompanied by extrarenal manifestations, which can readily be seen on CT[28].

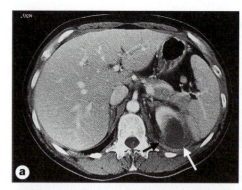

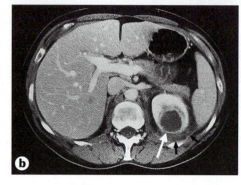

Figure 8.14 Renal abscess. (a) Sections through the left kidney demonstrate a fluid-filled mass in the upper pole (white arrow) with a surrounding halo of renal parenchyma that is less dense than normal parenchyma. (b) This finding of a halo of less dense parenchyma (caused by inflammation) surrounding a liquid center is typical of an abscess. There is inflammation posterior and lateral to the left kidney in the perinephric space (black arrows), but no fluid collection is seen outside the kidney. Thus the abscess can be both identified and staged.

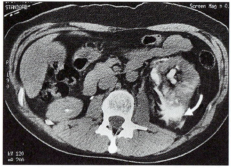

Figure 8.15 Post-traumatic extravasation of contrast medium from the left renal pelvis. A delayed computed tomography scan demonstrates extravasation of contrast medium (arrow) from the left renal pelvis into the perinephric space posteriorly. Note also the patchy nephrogram in the left kidney consistent with trauma (the appearance of the nephogram could be representative of infarction in other clinical settings). Delayed scans can be of great aid in trauma patients; initial scans are typically performed in the portal venous phase in order to optimally evaluate the liver. However, at this time there is no contrast medium in the collecting system.

Renal infection can also be associated with masses. 'Lobar nephronia' or focal renal parenchymal infection can lead to a mass effect on the CT scan[29]. Since this is composed of functioning parenchyma, delayed scans may demonstrate filling in of the parenchyma. Wedge-shaped defects in the nephrogram are also frequently seen with pyelonephritis[30]. Abscesses are fluid collections whose walls are typically less dense than the surrounding parenchyma (Fig. 8.14)[31]. In the proper clinical setting these findings are characteristic of the lesion.

Renal trauma is readily evaluated in the proper clinical setting (Fig. 8.15). An example of renal trauma is following treatment with extracorporeal shock-wave lithotripsy (ESWL).[32]

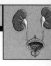

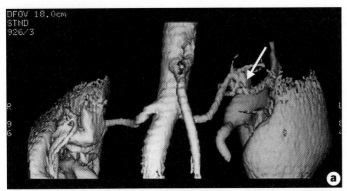

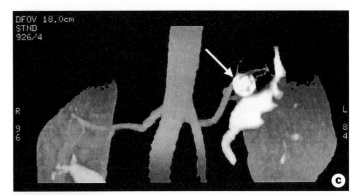

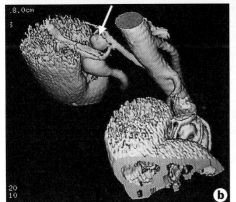

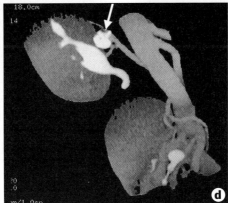

Figure 8.16 Three-dimensional imaging: renal artery aneurysm. (a) Surface-shaded display (of a three-dimensional computed tomography study of the renal arteries demonstrates single renal arteries bilaterally. A left renal artery aneurysm (arrow) is difficult to appreciate using this display format. (c) Rotating the image so that it is viewed from a more posterior and cranial position than in the top left image demonstrates the surface of the left renal artery aneurysm (arrow) to better advantage. (b) Maximum intensity projection: same image as above. The calcification in the renal artery aneurysm (arrow) is now visible. Note also that contrast medium in the collecting system and ureters is also visible and that the lumens of the aorta, renal arteries and superior mesenteric artery are seen instead of their surfaces. Surface-shaded display and maximum intensity projection displays provide complimentary information. (d) Maximum intensity projection display of same image as above.

Congenital abnormalities such as absent kidney, horseshoe kidney, duplication, and pelvic kidney can be identified and characterized. Perinephric disease and retroperitoneal and pelvic nodes are readily seen.

When obstruction to the urinary tract is present, CT generally can identify the point of obstruction and characterize the abnormality.

Acute problems such as renal infarction are readily identified, for instance in the patient with abdominal pain. The retroperitoneum is routinely evaluated for pathology such as retroperitoneal fibrosis or perianeurysmal fibrosis or masses. While evaluation of the bladder on standard CT is limited, protrusions from the bladder such as bladder diverticula are easily seen. Evaluation for neoplasm arising within the diverticula can be performed.

Three-dimensional imaging

Three-dimensional imaging (3D) using computed tomography has evolved over the past decade, becoming both more useful and less expensive. The earlier imaging of the urinary tract using 3D required expensive computers, while today's computer workstation is much less expensive and much more useful. A variety of techniques permit one to look at the surface and/or inside of structures such as vessels. In CT angiography, helical CT combined with an accurately timed peripheral intravenous injection of contrast medium permits rapid volumetric acquisition[33–35]. The actual images that are obtained on the CT study

can be rendered into 3D images of the vasculature by use of the computer. Among the methods of displaying the data are surface-shaded display (SSD; Fig. 8.16), maximum intensity projection (MIP; Fig. 8.16) and volume rendering[36]. Volume rendering has become the display technique of choice[17.] It is important that the source data, the actual images, be evaluated as carefully as the 3D ones, since some findings are only seen on the axial two-dimensional (2D) images.

While three-dimensional imaging can be used for any purpose, such as volumetric analysis of the kidneys or staging of renal tumors, it is in fact the renal vasculature that has proved to be its most important application. CT angiography, with its noninvasive advantage over standard arteriography, has become the technique of choice in the evaluation of potential renal transplant donors[33–35]. A second major application of CT angiography is prior to percutaneous endopyelotomy of ureteropelvic junction obstruction to identify the position of the ipsilateral renal artery. The three-dimensional model has proved to give highly reliable information about the relationship of the renal artery and its branches to the ureteropelvic junction itself[36–38]. Finally, 3D imaging has proved very useful in planning partial nephrectomies[39].

Virtual cystoscopy

Virtual cystoscopy uses 3D CT data to permit a 'fly through' of the organ being examined, in this case the bladder, so that the lumen of the bladder is viewed as if one were at a point in space inside the bladder looking at its inside surface. By data manipulation, movement in the bladder is simulated and computer graphics permit a light source to be mimicked[40,41]. Volume rendering, which, as noted earlier, is a powerful three-dimensional technique for the display of CT data, differs from other approaches in that it uses information from all voxels in a volume and thus avoids the loss of information associated with the other techniques. Because volume-rendered images are 'data rich' and use all the available CT data for 3D reconstruction, great anatomic detail and few artifacts are present. A sense of distance and depth, as well as motion, is achieved by using a perspective algorithm (perspective volume rendering)[40,41]. The algorithm is generated by a computer graphics program that causes the object to grow larger as the observer comes closer. Real-time viewing using this technique gives the effect of moving through the bladder lumen in vivo.

Sessile bladder lesions are readily identified. They can be examined in great detail both within the lumen and also using the conventional source CT data (Fig. 8.17). The region outside the bladder can be looked at with the latter as well. While virtual cystoscopy has not matched conventional cystoscopy when the two have been compared, they have been very close[40]. Virtual cystoscopy does not permit therapy, as conventional cystoscopy does. Nonetheless, virtual cystoscopy may decrease the number of conventional cystoscopies needed to follow patients with known bladder cancer and for evaluation or followup of lesions with a low suspicion of abnormality in patients with hematuria.

Conclusion

Helical computed tomography, which is likely to be the only CT used for most of the 21st century, has led to a much more rapid acquisition of data and to many applications ranging from non-contrast CT in patients with flank pain to virtual cystoscopy. Newer generations of scanners using multislice imaging will have even greater speed and greater resolution. Improvements in equipment should lead to improvements in all the techniques currently described and very probably new additional techniques and applications. Three-dimensional and virtual reality CT studies of the urinary tract will also improve, resulting in an even greater role for urinary tract imaging in diagnosis and exclusion of disease.

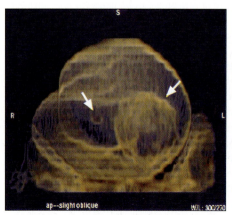

Figure 8.17 Virtual cystoscopy: three-dimensional imaging preliminary transparency. An image from a computed tomography scan of the bladder following an intravenous urogram demonstrates how a three-dimensional image can be processed to eliminate the opaque contrast medium. The bladder is viewed from outside of the structure. Two bladder tumors (arrows) are seen.

ULTRASOUND

Because of the ready accessibility of ultrasound (US) as well as its safety and relatively low cost, ultrasonography is the most commonly performed initial imaging procedure for evaluation of the urinary tract at most institutions. US provides exquisite morphological detail of the urinary tract. In fact, parenchymal anatomy is frequently visualized in finer detail on US than on CT. In addition, Doppler techniques provide physiologic information as well as a unique depiction of the renovascular tree. Moreover, the examination is not limited by renal failure and does not employ ionizing radiation or potentially nephrotoxic intravenous iodinated contrast agents. However, the US examination is operator-dependent, requiring meticulous attention to technique. US examination is also restricted by body habitus, overlying bowel gas and inability of the patient to cooperate.

Current accepted uses for US evaluation of the urinary tract include evaluation of patients with acute or worsening renal failure to exclude hydronephrosis, assessment and followup of children with vesicoureteral reflux, evaluation of complex or hyperdense masses seen on CT (to discriminate between proteinaceous or hemorrhagic cysts and neoplasms), evaluation of renal infection, bladder masses, and bladder outlet obstruction. Doppler US can be effectively used to assess patients for renal artery stenosis, renal vein thrombosis, renal infarcts, arteriovenous fistulae, and pseudoaneurysms (particularly in the renal transplant patient), and to document the integrity of the renal vascular pedicle in the trauma patient. US also provides an efficient guide for interventional procedures such as percutaneous nephrostomy and cyst or abscess aspiration.

The kidney

Ultrasound examination of the adult kidney generally requires a 2.5–5MHz transducer. No patient preparation is required for the real-time examination, although fasting for 6–8 hours is helpful for Doppler evaluation of the main renal arteries. Images are obtained in both the sagittal and axial planes. The maximum sagittal renal length is reported. The normal kidneys are symmetric in length, ranging from 9cm to 13cm depending on body habitus[42]. A difference in length greater than 1.5cm should raise suspicion of unilateral disease such as renovascular disease or an infiltrative process. The cortical echogenicity of the normal adult kidney is homogeneous and should be equal to or slightly less than that of the normal hepatic or splenic parenchyma (Fig. 8.18). Renal cortical echogenicity in adults is normally slightly greater than the echogenicity of the renal pyramids, which can be recognized as relatively hypoechoic triangular structures at the base of the renal cortex pointing into the brightly echogenic central renal hilum. The renal pyramids are separated by indentations of the renal cortex, the septa of Bertin. Corticomedullary differentiation is more pronounced in children, dehydrated patients, and patients with medical renal disease, because of increased cortical echogenicity (Fig. 8.19). The outer margin of the kidney may be smooth or lobular (termed fetal lobulation). The echogenic central renal hilum contains fibrous, fatty tissue as well as the segmental renal vessels, lymphatics, and portions of the intrarenal collecting system. With high-resolution US equipment, both the segmental vessels and small amounts of fluid within the intrarenal collecting system

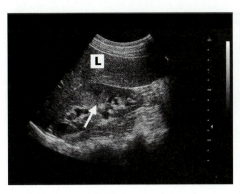

Figure 8.18 Sagittal image of the normal kidney: the echogenicity of the renal cortex is slightly less than that of the liver (L). Anechoic linear structures within the echogenic renal sinus represent the segmental vessels. Note prominence or bulging of the renal cortex directly opposite the renal pelvis (arrow), termed the hypertrophied septum of Bertin.

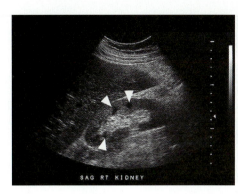

Figure 8.19 Medical renal disease. Note diffusely increased renal cortical echogenicity. The renal cortex is also more echogenic than the adjacent liver parenchyma. The triangular renal pyramids (arrowheads) appear relatively hypoechoic, i.e. there is increased corticomedullary differentiation.

may be seen on real-time examination as anechoic, linear branching structures converging on the renal pelvis. Color Doppler examination may be helpful in differentiating prominent vessels from a dilated collecting system.

The uroepithelium of the intrarenal collecting system is brightly echogenic and is therefore only visualized when the collecting system is distended as it otherwise blends into the echogenic renal sinus. When visualized, the uroepithelium should be thin and smooth. Thickening or a hypoechoic/striated appearance should suggest obstruction, edema, or infection. Ischemia or rejection may have a similar appearance in the transplant recipient[43]. The perinephric and pararenal spaces are very difficult to evaluate sonographically. The echogenicity of the perinephric fat is quite variable. In general the more perinephric fat, the less echogenic it is. Decreased echogenicity has also been shown to correlate with lower insulin resistance[44]. Since focal hypoechoic perinephric fat can mimic an abscess or hematoma and since complex fluid collections may mimic a normal structure sonographically, these spaces are best evaluated with CT.

The origins of the main renal arteries are best identified on transverse midline images of the aorta just below the level of the superior mesenteric artery (Fig. 8.20a). In some patients the main renal artery can be imaged all the way to the renal hilum (Fig. 8.20b). The main renal veins run parallel to the main renal arteries in the renal hilum (Fig. 8.20c). With color power Doppler, several further generations of vessels may be identified branching almost all the way to the renal cortex (Fig. 8.21). Doppler examination of the intraparenchymal vessels can be adequately performed in virtually all patients except those who are hypotensive or are unable to hold their breath. However, the Doppler examination of the main renal artery is technically difficult and it may be impossible to fully visualize both main renal arteries in up to 30% of adult patients because of overlying bowel gas, obesity, inability to breath-hold, or aortic calcifications. Furthermore, as many as 20% of patients will have accessory renal arteries, which are almost impossible to see on Doppler US examination.

Ultrasound examination of the kidneys is frequently requested in the setting of acute or worsening renal failure to exclude hydronephrosis. Prompt, accurate diagnosis of hydronephrosis is extremely important for patient management as decompression of the collecting system may reverse renal failure and salvage renal function. However, the incidence of bilateral hydronephrosis in the general population of patients presenting with acute renal failure is extremely low, approximately 1–2%[45,46]. The incidence is much higher, perhaps 30%, in patients with a history suggesting obstruction such as older men (secondary to an enlarged prostate) or women with pelvic masses, or in patients with a history of renal calculi or renal colic[46].

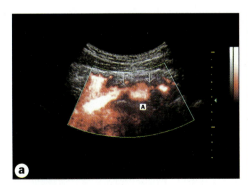

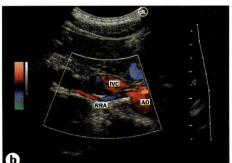

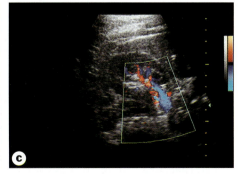

Figure 8.20 Main renal artery. (a) Transverse color power Doppler image of the aorta (A) demonstrating the origins of the main renal arteries (arrows). (b) Transverse color Doppler image of the right renal artery (RRA) from its origin off the aorta (AO) as it courses under the inferior vena cava (IVC) of the right kidney. (c) Color Doppler image of the renal hilum demonstrating the main renal artery and vein. By convention arterial flow leading towards the renal capsule is color-coded red and venous flow directed away from the kidney is color-coded blue.

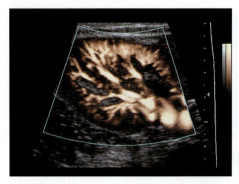

Figure 8.21 Color power Doppler image of the kidney. This image demonstrates numerous further generations of vessels branching beyond the arcuate arteries almost to the renal capsule. (Courtesy of Advanced Technology Laboratories, Bothel, Washington).

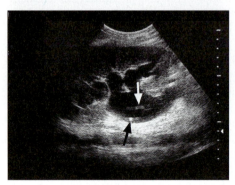

Figure 8.22 Dilatation of the intrarenal collecting system. Sagittal real-time image of the left kidney demonstrating moderate dilatation of the intrarenal collecting system, renal pelvis, and proximal ureter which has persisted despite placement of a drainage catheter (parallel echogenic lines) (arrows) which can be seen coiled in the renal pelvis.

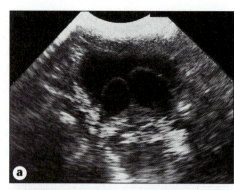

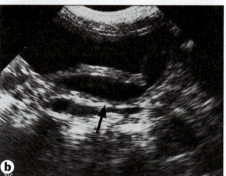

Figure 8.23 Bilateral ureteroceles. Transverse (a) and sagittal (b) views of the bladder in a patient with bilateral ureteroceles. Note that the ureteral wall prolapsing into the bladder is thin and smooth. The distal ureter (arrow), seen on the sagittal image, is dilated. (Courtesy of Dr Marc S Keller, Yale University School of Medicine.)

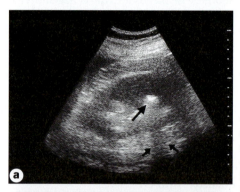

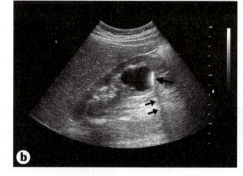

Figure 8.24 Renal calculi. (a) Sagittal image of the right kidney demonstrates an echogenic focus, a renal calculus, at the lower pole (straight arrow) with distal acoustic (black) shadowing (small arrows). (b) Sagittal image of the right kidney in another patient demonstrates numerous small, echogenic foci consistent with numerous small renal calculi layering within a dilated calyx to the lower pole (large arrow). Note distal acoustic shadowing (small arrows).

Dilatation of the intrarenal collecting system is recognized on US by separation of the central sinus echoes by anechoic branching structures representing the dilated calyces (Fig. 8.22). Since a distended bladder may cause mild dilatation of the intrarenal collecting system, scanning following voiding is always performed to determine if the hydronephrosis persists. Hydronephrosis is graded as mild, moderate, or severe and the extent (e.g., primary renal pelvis, single calyx, ureter) is determined by scanning the ureter distally as far as possible. If the dilated ureter cannot be followed into the pelvis because of shadowing from bowel gas, the distal ureter at the ureterovesical junction (UVJ) should always be evaluated either via a transabdominal approach through the distended urinary bladder or endovaginally to look for calculi as well as ureteral jets. Absence of the ureteral jet suggests complete obstruction (see below).

One should also carefully search for a cause of obstruction. Common causes of obstruction identifiable by US examination include calculus, mass, ureterocele (Fig. 8.23), or bladder outlet obstruction. If bilateral hydronephrosis is observed, careful examination of the pelvis, especially the prostate in males, is performed to search for a pelvic mass. If no cause is identified, further evaluation with CT or IVU is warranted.

Renal or ureteral calculi are a common cause of obstruction of the collecting system. Typically, calculi are echogenic with distal acoustic shadowing when imaged within the focal zone of the transducer (Fig. 8.24). The sonographic appearance of calculi depends on size. Even noncalcified calculi may be identified sonographically. Sonography is estimated to detect 80–90% of calculi located within the kidney and nearly 100% at the UVJ, but is nowhere near as sensitive in detecting ureteral calculi, yielding an overall detection rate for urinary tract calculi of only 65%[47,48]. Noncontrast enhanced helical CT is the most sensitive method of detecting renal and ureteral calculi[49] (see above). Echoes within a dilated collecting system suggest pyonephrosis, hemorrhage or debris and may require immediate intervention (Fig. 8.25). However, US is not very sensitive for detecting pyonephrosis. Therefore, pyonephrosis should be suspected in the clinical setting of hydronephrosis and signs of urinary tract infection.

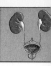

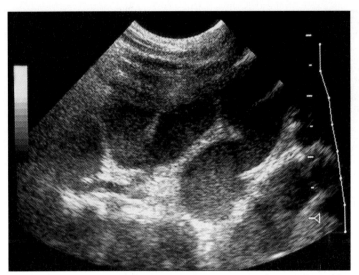

Figure 8.25 Pyonephrosis. Oblique US image through the lower abdomen of a child with abdominal pain and fever reveals a dilated tubular structure containing diffuse low-level echoes consistent with pyonephrosis. In this clinical setting, these findings require immediate drainage of the collecting system. (Courtesy of Dr Marc S Keller, Yale University School of Medicine.)

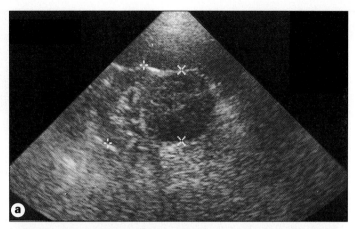

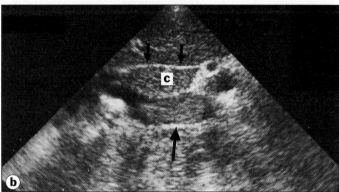

Figure 8.26 Renal cell carcinoma with vascular invasion.
(a) Transverse real-time ultrasound image demonstrating a homogenous, well-circumscribed solid mass (X-shaped calipers) arising posterolaterally from the left kidney (cross-shaped calipers). (b) Midline longitudinal image demonstrates tumor thrombus (long arrow) within the inferior vena cava as it passes underneath the caudate lobe (c) of the liver. The short arrows indicate the ligamentum venosum.

Ultrasound is estimated to be at least 90% accurate in the diagnosis of hydronephrosis. However, numerous pitfalls exist. Parapelvic cysts, papillary necrosis, or a dilated extrarenal pelvis may be confused by the inexperienced sonographer with hydronephrosis. Conversely, dilatation of the collecting system is not always due to obstruction. Elevation of the resistive index (RI) (>0.7) has been reported to help differentiate between obstructed and nonobstructed dilatation of the intrarenal collecting system, but not all authors agree[50]. Rarely, hydronephrosis will not be observed sonographically despite obstruction to the collecting system. This occurs primarily in the setting of severe dehydration or if the patient is imaged too quickly (<4 hours) after the onset of symptoms, such that urine within the collecting system has not had time to accumulate, or if pyelosinus extravasation has occurred, thereby decompressing the distended collecting system.

Magnetic resonance imaging and contrast-enhanced CT (CE-CT) are the most sensitive means of screening patients for solid renal masses. While US is less sensitive than CE-CT for the detection of small solid masses, it avoids repeated exposure to ionizing radiation and potentially nephrotoxic iodinated intravenous contrast. In addition, US or MRI is very helpful in further evaluating the indeterminate mass seen on CT. Angiomyolipomas are the most common benign solid renal neoplasm and are composed of varying amounts of blood vessels, muscles, and fat. These lesions tend to occur in middle-aged women and there is an increased incidence of both angiomyolipomas and renal cysts in patients with tuberous sclerosis. Bleeding is the most common complication. On US examination most angiomyolipomas are well-defined, homogeneous, brightly echogenic masses. Larger lesions, or those complicated by hemorrhage, may contain cystic areas. Posterior attenuation or shadowing may be noted[51]. However, the US findings are nonspecific and may be mimicked by liposarcomas or renal cell carcinomas[52,53]. As many as 12% of renal cell carcinomas (RCCs), especially small carcinomas, may also be echogenic[53]. Thus, any echogenic renal lesion larger than 1cm should be evaluated by CT or MRI to confirm that fat is indeed present. It is

reasonable to follow smaller echogenic renal lesions with serial ultrasound examinations, as the risk of developing metastatic disease from a small RCC is low. However, some may prefer to obtain a CT or MRI.

While RCCs are usually staged by CT or MRI, US can be helpful especially in documenting venous extension or contralateral tumors when CT or MRI cannot be performed or when those examinations are indeterminate. While venous invasion does not worsen prognosis, intravascular thrombus is resistant to chemotherapy and, therefore, should be resected if the lesion is considered operable. Hence, accurate determination of the extent of venous invasion is critical for patient management, specifically the surgical approach. Tumor extending into the renal vein, inferior vena cava (IVC) or even right atrium will appear as a color void on color Doppler examination. The vein on real-time examination will be distended by a mass similar in echogenicity to the primary tumor (Fig. 8.26). Tumor thrombosis may be differentiated from bland thrombosis by the presence of vascularity within the thrombus, which may be detected by Doppler examination. The contralateral kidney should be carefully examined as approximately 1% of RCCs will be bilateral at presentation. Multifocal RCCs also occur. One recent series reported that real-time US examination with Doppler was nearly as sensitive as CT and MRI for assessing vascular invasion[54]. Others suggest that, while US

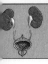

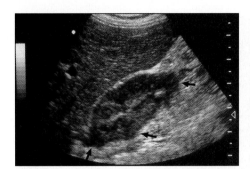

Figure 8.27 Non-Hodgkin's lymphoma.
Sagittal image of the kidney reveals several of the ultrasound patterns of lymphomatous involvement of the kidney: decrease in renal cortical echogenicity with loss of corticomedullary differentiation and decreased prominence and echogenicity of the renal sinus – due to diffuse lymphomatous infiltration. In addition, several focal cortical masses (arrows) are seen.

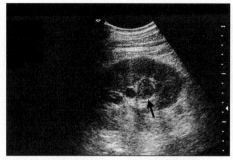

Figure 8.28 Transitional cell carcinoma.
Sagittal ultrasound image of the kidney reveals a hypoechoic mass (arrow) within a calyx at the lower pole. Mild dilation of the intrarenal collecting system is also noted. The patient presented with hematuria and had a transitional cell carcinoma of the collecting system. An intravenous urogram was subsequently performed to exclude multifocal disease.

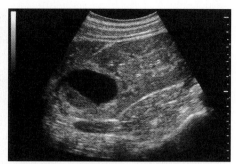

Figure 8.29 Renal abscess. Sagittal image reveals an upper-pole thin-walled cystic structure with a fluid/debris layer at the upper pole of the kidney. The patient had a renal abscess and aspiration yielded pus. Hemorrhagic cysts may have a similar appearance.

may have a sensitivity of 96% and specificity of 100% in detecting venous invasion when the renal vein and IVC are well visualized, the overall sensitivity of US may be as low as 18–33% because of inadequate visualization of the renal vein and IVC in many patients[55,56] It should be noted that all three imaging modalities are less sensitive for the detection of vascular invasion if extensive local disease (renal hilar or retroperitoneal lymphadenopathy) is present.

The US findings for RCCs are not specific, and not all solid masses detected on US represent RCCs. Oncocytomas may be indistinguishable although these lesions are rarer and tend to be sharply marginated. Larger lesions may have a central scar. However, imaging features are not always distinctive and surgery is often required[57]. Lymphoma or leukemia may involve the kidney either by direct invasion or by hematogenous spread, producing single or multiple hypoechoic masses, diffuse enlargement with loss of the normal corticomedullary differentiation (Fig. 8.27), or encapsulation of the kidney by tumor within the perinephric space. Focal lesions may appear to be nearly anechoic and may be differentiated from renal cysts only by the lack of posterior acoustic enhancement[58,59]. Metastatic disease may also cause multiple bilateral solid renal masses with the most common primaries being lung, colon, breast, melanoma, stomach, and pancreas.

Ultrasound is not as sensitive as CT/IVU for the detection of transitional cell carcinoma as many are small and multifocal. In particular, the nondistended ureter is poorly visualized by US examination. Thus, US alone is not an adequate or complete workup for a patient presenting with hematuria. When seen on US, however, transitional cell carcinomas appear as relatively hypoechoic, polypoid masses within the renal sinus (Fig. 8.28), collecting system, or bladder. Such masses may cause hydronephrosis[60]. US findings are nonspecific and can be mimicked by blood clots, fungus balls, debris, pus, polyps, malacoplakia, or even sloughed renal pyramids.

The primary role of ultrasound in evaluating patients with suspected renal infection is to exclude complications requiring intervention such as pyonephrosis (Fig. 8.25), renal abscess (Fig. 8.29), or perinephric abscess (see above)[61]. US may also be helpful in distinguishing focal bacterial pyelonephritis, which will be vascular, from an avascular renal infarct[62]. In particular, these two entities may be confused on CT examination. In patients with uncomplicated diffuse pyelonephritis, US examination may be normal. Occasionally, uroepithelial thickening or enlargement of the kidney with decreased vascularity and decreased renal cortical echogenicity will be observed. Scarring or thinning of the renal cortex may occur following severe infection. This is also commonly seen in patients with reflux, when the calyx will appear to extend to the renal capsule.

In the setting of abdominal or renal trauma, ultrasound demonstration of cortical blood flow is a safe, portable, and rapid means of documenting the integrity of the renal vascular pedicle. However, CT remains the gold standard for full evaluation of injuries to the kidney and collecting system as well as their retroperitoneal and intra-abdominal extent. Nonetheless, perinephric and renal hematomas and even pseudoaneurysms may be observed.

US examination is also an important imaging modality to assess for congenital renal anomalies. The junctional parenchymal defect, a common variant, appears on US as a wedge-shaped echogenic area (similar to a scar) located anteriorly at the junction of the upper and middle thirds of the kidney. The hypertrophied septum of Bertin can mimic a solid renal neoplasm, but should have echotexture and vascularity identical to the rest of the renal cortex. The hypertrophied septum of Bertin is classically located directly opposite the renal pelvis[63] (Fig. 8.18). Congenital ureteropelvic junction obstruction or a duplicated collecting system with obstruction of the upper pole (with or without reflux into the lower pole) may be easily identified as the ultrasound appearance is similar to hydronephrosis. Congenital malformations or ectopia such as multicystic dysplasia, crossed, fused renal ectopia, the horseshoe kidney (Fig. 8.30), or pelvic kidneys may also be easily identified. If renal agenesis is diagnosed, evaluation of the pelvis to exclude uterine malformation should also be performed.

While renovascular hypertension is estimated to occur in only 0.5–5% of the general hypertensive population[64], the prevalence is much higher in the subset of hypertensive patients with

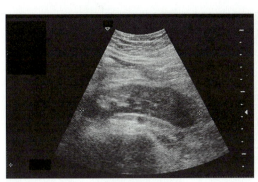

Figure 8.30 Horseshoe kidney. Transverse midline image of the abdomen reveals a U-shaped structure (calipers) crossing the midline in this patient with a horseshoe kidney.

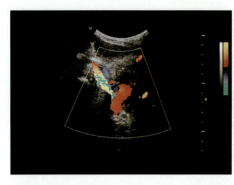

Figure 8.32 Renal artery stenosis. Note focal color aliasing, i.e. yellow and blue disorganized color at the origin of the right renal artery indicating high-velocity flow at the site of stenosis in this patient with renovascular hypertension.

early or late onset of hypertension (HT), rapidly progressive HT (especially with diastolic blood pressure >110mmHg), or HT associated with flank bruits, renal failure, or grade III–IV retinopathy[65].

Criteria for documenting significant (>60%) renal artery stenosis (RAS) by Doppler examination include demonstration of an increase in peak systolic velocity (PSV) to over 180–200cm/s at a site of color aliasing in the main renal artery[66,67]; or a renal-to-aortic peak systolic ratio (RAR) ratio (PSV renal artery/PSV aorta) greater than 2–3.5:1[66–68] (Figs 8.31 & 8.32). The sensitivity and specificity of these criteria have been reported to range from 84–91% and 73–97% respectively[66–68]. However, evaluation of the main renal artery from aorta to renal hilum is technically difficult and visualization of potentially significant stenoses in accessory renal arteries or in smaller branch vessels is unlikely because of limitations in resolution. The use of new intravenous contrast agents has been reported to increase both the sensitivity and success rate of Doppler examination of the renal arteries for RAS[69,70].

Acute renal vein thrombosis (RVT) is most often questioned in adults in the setting of flank pain, microscopic hematuria, and deteriorating renal function characterized by proteinuria. Risk factors include dehydration, hypercoagulopathies, malignancy, trauma, and membranous glomerulonephropathy. On color Doppler examination the renal vein will be enlarged, containing a color void representing the clot. The echogenicity of the

thrombus as well as the renal cortex depends upon the time course[71]. Acute thrombus may be nearly anechoic[72]. Particularly in renal transplant recipients, patients may also demonstrate decreased diastolic flow (increased RI) in the intraparenchymal or main renal arteries[73]. It is also important to note that documentation of parenchymal venous flow does not exclude RVT as collaterals may develop quickly, especially in children. Doppler US examination can not accurately diagnose RVT in intraparenchymal veins, which may nonetheless contribute to deteriorating renal function.

Arteriovenous fistulae are easily diagnosed on color and pulse Doppler examination by demonstration of an enlarged afferent feeding artery with increased PSV and diastolic flow (decreased RI), and a draining vein with pulsatile flow. Focal color aliasing and a color bruit may also be seen. Pseudoaneurysms may be indistinguishable from simple cysts on real-time examination. Doppler examination will reveal swirling blood flow and a characteristic 'to and fro' flow pattern within the neck of the pseudoaneurysm.

Color Doppler examination also provides a quick means of documenting cortical perfusion and can be extremely helpful in differentiating flank pain due to renal infarct or embolization from renal colic. When segmental embolization occurs, Doppler examination will demonstrate absence of renal blood flow in a wedge-shaped area in the renal cortex. Cortical perfusion will be completely absent in the case of embolization/occlusion of the main renal artery.

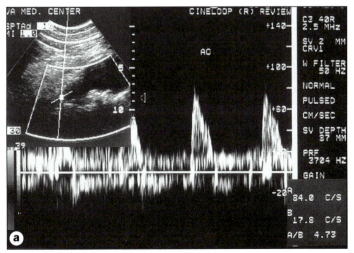

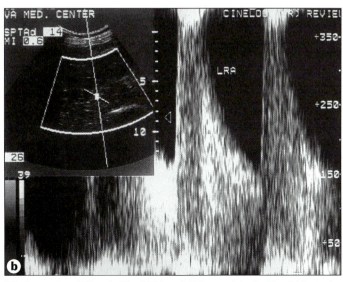

Figure 8.31 Renal artery stenosis. (a) Peak systolic velocity in the aorta is 84cm/s, while peak systolic velocity in the left main renal artery

(b) aliases over 350cm/s. The RAR is >4.5:1, consistent with a high-grade renal artery stenosis.

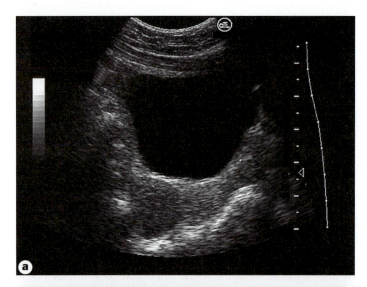

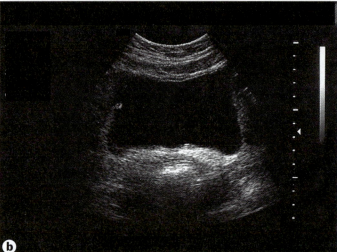

Figure 8.33 Normal bladder. (a) Sagittal and (b) transverse images. The bladder wall is thin, smooth, and symmetric. Fluid within the bladder is completely anechoic.

The bladder

The urinary bladder is best examined using the transabdominal approach, although endovaginal, endorectal, and even transurethral intracavitary scanning may be performed. The bladder must be fully distended for accurate evaluation of the wall. Both sagittal and transverse images should be obtained (Fig. 8.33).

Bladder volume is calculated using the formula: (height × width × depth)/2, although US measurements are not highly precise because of variations in bladder geometry. Nonetheless, US examination is frequently requested to determine bladder capacity or postvoid residual (PVR).

Fluid within the bladder should be completely anechoic. Internal echoes suggest hemorrhage, infection, or debris. Bladder stones are typically echogenic and mobile, causing a strong distal acoustic shadow. Fungal balls and blood clot may be mobile or adherent and are of variable echotexture without distal shadowing.

Ureteral jets are identified by color Doppler imaging as urine enters the base of the bladder through the ureterovesical orifice (Fig. 8.34). Ureteral jets are noted at regular intervals, but not

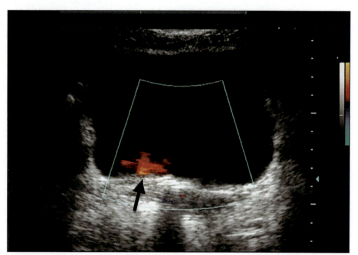

Figure 8.34 Ureteric jet. Color Doppler image of the bladder demonstrating a ureteric jet (arrow).

necessarily synchronously. Nonvisualization of the ureteral jet in a well hydrated patient after 5–15 minutes of observation suggests complete obstruction of the ureter[74]. This phenomenon can be very helpful in evaluating patients presenting with flank pain and clinical concern for obstructing ureteral calculi, particularly in children and pregnant women, where it is preferable to avoid the ionizing radiation associated with a noncontrast helical CT examination.

Several pitfalls may be encountered in the US examination of the bladder. Artifactual internal echoes caused by reverberation artifact, poor penetration, or inappropriate gain settings may mimic true internal echoes due to infection or hemorrhage. Large pelvic fluid collections may mimic or obscure the bladder. Conversely, a massively distended bladder may be mistaken for a pelvic cystic mass. Asking the patient to void or visualization of the ureteral jets or Foley catheter balloon within the bladder may help to clarify the examination if uncertainty exists.

MAGNETIC RESONANCE IMAGING

Over the last decade several important advances in magnetic resonance imaging (MRI) have vastly increased its clinical utility in imaging of the urinary tract. Ultrafast breath-hold scanning sequences have significantly decreased image degradation from motion artifact, resulting in markedly improved spatial resolution. In addition, the recent availability of gadolinium-based intravenous contrast agents allows for high-resolution evaluation of the renovascular tree, assessment of soft tissue vascularity, and possibly assessment of renal function[75]. Gadolinium-based intravenous contrast agents have minimal nephrotoxicity and rarely cause allergic reaction. Thus, gadolinium contrast enhancement may be safely performed in patients with renal failure or in preoperative patients without concern for renal damage and in patients allergic to iodinated contrast medium. MRI also offers multiplanar imaging capability and remarkable inherent soft tissue contrast, allowing differentiation of soft tissue, fat, and blood products. Hence, the role of MRI in the urinary tract has evolved as both a problem solver when CT or US imaging is inconclusive and as a substitute for CT,

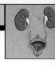

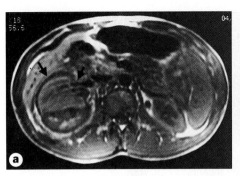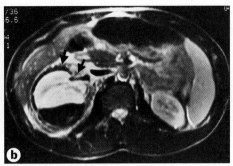

Figure 8.35 Perinephric hematoma. This patient presented with right flank pain following trauma during a basketball game. Axial T_1-weighted (a) and T_2-weighted (b) images demonstrate a perinephric fluid collection (arrows) displacing the right kidney posteriorly and deforming the renal cortex. The signal behavior, intermediate signal intensity on T_1- and high signal intensity on T_2-weighted images, is consistent with hemorrhage.

particularly in patients with renal failure[76] or allergies to iodinated contrast material, or in patients for whom it is desirous to limit radiation exposure (i.e. children or when multiple, serial studies are anticipated). Current indications for MRI of the urinary tract include the assessment of renal masses, staging of renal cell carcinoma, workup of renal artery stenosis and renal vein thrombosis, evaluation of the renal arteries in renal transplant donors, magnetic resonance (MR) urography, evaluation of bladder masses, and the detection of the undescended testis.

Magnetic resonance imaging of the kidneys and bladder is performed at our institution using the phased array torso coil. Both T_1- and T_2-weighted images are obtained in two orthogonal imaging planes. The pattern of signal intensity within lesions on these sequences is helpful for accurately identifying areas of fat, blood products, and fluid (Fig. 8.35). Internal architecture is best seen on T_2-weighted images, whereas optimal soft tissue contrast between lymph nodes and/or retroperitoneal structures and fat is obtained on T_1-weighted images. When scan parameters are kept constant, contrast enhancement of soft tissue masses can be assessed on pre- and post-gadolinium-enhanced images. Evaluation of the main renal artery, aorta, and main renal vein can be accomplished either by time of flight (TOF) imaging or by dynamic imaging following intravenous (IV) gadolinium enhancement.

Magnetic resonance imaging can be very helpful in the evaluation of renal masses that are indeterminate on either CT or US[77]

(Fig. 8.36). By keeping scan parameters the same on both pre- and postcontrast images, the presence of contrast enhancement indicates solid tissue within a mass, thereby differentiating complex proteinaceous or hemorrhagic cysts from either solid neoplasms or cysts with mural nodularity. Intravenous gadolinium may be used even in the setting of renal failure, which precludes evaluation by contrast-enhanced CT (Fig. 8.36).

Simple cysts are typically of low signal intensity on T_1-weighted images and high signal intensity on T_2-weighted images, although proteinaceous or hemorrhagic cysts may have higher (variable) signal intensity on T_1-weighted images (Fig. 8.36). However, neither simple nor complex cysts will demonstrate contrast enhancement. Morphologically, renal cysts should have a thin, regular wall. Angiomyolipomas, benign neoplasms containing a variable amount of fat, blood vessels, and smooth muscle, can be confidently diagnosed on MRI when fat is identified within a solid renal mass. Typically, angiomyolipomas will be isointense to fat on all pulse sequences, specifically of high signal intensity on T_1-weighted images and intermediate signal intensity on T_2-weighted images (Fig. 8.37). The observation of a decrease in signal intensity in a renal mass on fat suppression imaging sequences will unconditionally confirm the presence of fat within the lesion and is thus diagnostic of angiomyolipoma. Most commonly, angiomyolipomas demonstrate relatively little contrast enhancement. However, the MR appearance is variable, depending upon both the size and

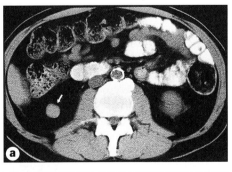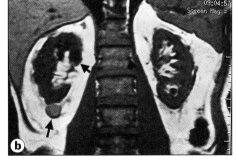
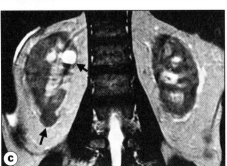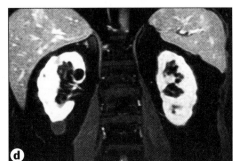

Figure 8.36 Renal cysts. (a) Noncontrast computed tomography scan reveals a high-attenuation lesion (arrow) at the lower pole of the right kidney. The differential diagnosis is renal cell carcinoma versus hyperdense (proteinaceous or hemorrhage) cyst. Iodinated intravenous contrast could not be given as the patient was in renal failure. (b) T_1-weighted and (c) T_2-weighted coronal images demonstrate a round structure (long arrow) at the lower pole of the right kidney, which demonstrates intermediate signal on the T_1-weighted image and drops in signal intensity on the T_2-weighted image, consistent with it being hemorrhage or proteinaceous fluid. Another lesion (short arrow) at the upper pole of the right kidney has signal behavior consistent with simple fluid, i.e. low signal on the T_1-weighted image and high signal on the T_2-weighted image. (d) Post intravenous gadolinium fat suppressed images demonstrate no enhancement of either lesion, confirming that they represent cysts. The lesion at the lower pole is slightly higher in signal intensity on the gadolinium enhanced image because of hemorrhage.

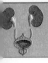

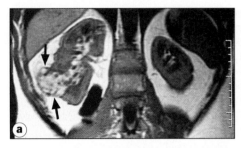

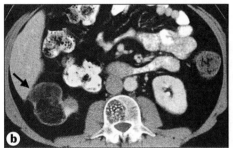

Figure 8.37 Angiomyolipoma. (a) T_1-weighted coronal magnetic resonance image demonstrates a heterogeneous exophytic mass (arrows) arising from the lower pole of the right kidney. Large areas of the mass are of high signal intensity – isointense to the surrounding perinephric fat – suggesting that the mass contains fat and thus represents an angiomyolipoma. (b) Computed tomography scan demonstrating low attenuation within the mass (arrow) indicates that fat is present, confirming the diagnosis.

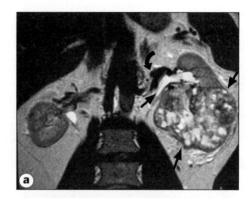

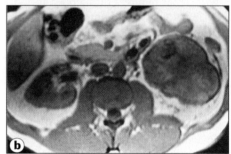

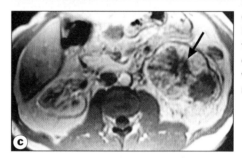

Figure 8.38 Renal cell carcinoma. (a) T_2-weighted coronal image demonstrates a large, heterogeneous lobular mass arising from the lower pole of the left kidney (large arrows). Serpiginous tubular structures in the surrounding perinephric fat represent prominent vessels. No evidence of perinephric invasion or hilar lymphadenopathy is seen. Urine within the renal pelvis and proximal ureter (short arrow) is of high signal intensity. The left renal artery is indicated by the curved arrow. (b, c) Pre- and post-intravenous gadolinium contrast-enhanced images demonstrate that this solid mass enhances peripherally with a nonenhancing or necrotic center (arrow).

the amount of fat present within the lesion. The less fat present, the greater the contrast enhancement observed. Larger lesions have a tendency to hemorrhage, which is easily identified on MR examination because of the characteristic pattern of signal behavior of hemorrhage[78].

Renal cell carcinomas arise from the proximal convoluted tubular epithelial cells. MRI may be performed to screen patients at risk, to work up patients presenting with pain or hematuria, or to further characterize an indeterminate lesion noted on US or CT. MRI is particularly helpful in patients in renal failure or with iodinated contrast allergy in whom contrast-enhanced CT cannot be performed. Once the diagnosis of renal cell carcinoma is suspected, imaging is performed to accurately stage the tumor. MRI is considered nearly equivalent to CT for the evaluation of intra-abdominal spread of disease (lymph nodes, liver metastases and contralateral renal lesions) as well as for brain lesions. CT is required to screen for metastases to lung or mediastinum.

Renal cell carcinomas (RCCs) have a variable, nonspecific MR appearance. Most often RCCs are lower in signal intensity on T_1-weighted images than the normal renal parenchyma[79], unless hemorrhage has occurred, in which case high-signal-intensity areas will be noted. On T_2-weighted images, RCCs are typically higher in signal intensity than the surrounding normal renal parenchyma although hemorrhagic areas may be lower in signal intensity. The lesions usually demonstrate marked heterogeneous contrast enhancement, but contrast enhancement is less than that of the normal parenchyma[78,80] (Fig. 8.38). Cystic or necrotic nonenhancing components may be observed. Oncocytomas reportedly enhance more homogeneously than RCCs and a central nonenhancing stellate scar may be seen in larger lesions[81]. However, the MR appearance is nonspecific and oncocytomas may be indistinguishable from renal cell carcinomas. Renal lymphoma or metastases, most commonly from lung, breast, colon, and malignant melanoma, may also present as a solid, enhancing

renal mass. However, these lesions are most often multiple. Diffuse renal enlargement or direct invasion by retroperitoneal adenopathy may also be seen with renal lymphoma. Because of the nonspecific appearance of these solid renal neoplasms, any non-fat-containing solid renal lesion or complex renal cyst with enhancing mural nodularity or thick septations is considered to be a RCC until proved otherwise.

T_1, T_2-weighted and fast short inversion-recovery images are obtained in the abdomen to assess for intra-abdominal spread of disease with particular attention to the liver, perinephric fat, and retroperitoneal adenopathy. One should note that while soft tissue stranding in the perinephric fat may represent tumor infiltration, inflammatory changes or lymphatic/venous edema may have a similar MR appearance[82]. Size is the only criterion used on MR to diagnose malignant lymphadenopathy. Neither shape, signal intensity, nor enhancement pattern can be used to accurately differentiate malignant from reactive lymph nodes.

Magnetic resonance is reportedly nearly 100% accurate for diagnosing tumor thrombus, which is as accurate or more so than CT or US[83,84]. The presence of bulky renal hilar adenopathy decreases the accuracy of all noninvasive imaging modalities for the detection of venous invasion[54,85].

Magnetic resonance angiography (MRA) has become an important imaging modality for the evaluation of patients with suspected renal artery stenosis (RAS) as well as for the preoperative evaluation of potential living related renal transplant

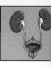

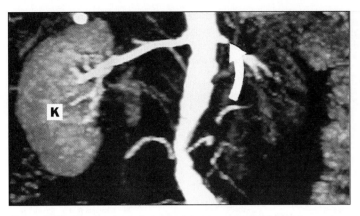

Figure 8.39 Renal artery stenosis. Intravenous gadolinium-enhanced magnetic resonance angiography of the renal arteries demonstrates complete occlusion of the left renal artery (arrow) approximately 5mm from the origin. The right renal artery is widely patent. No accessory renal arteries are seen. A stenosis is present of the distal infrarenal aorta. K, right kidney.

donors. MRA is usually performed with both 2D TOF imaging sequences and 3D dynamic contrast-enhanced images.

Dynamic contrast-enhanced MRA is reportedly 87–100% sensitive and 93–98% specific for detecting renal artery stenosis (≥ 50%) in the main renal artery[86,87] (Fig. 8.39). Phase-contrast MRA is reportedly helpful in determining the hemodynamic significance of a stenosis. On this type of sequence, signal dropout will occur at a hemodynamically significant stenosis as a result of spin dephasing caused by swirling or jet-like blood flow. Nonetheless, stenoses may be overestimated on MRA and the spatial resolution of MRA (even with the highest resolution sequences available) is not adequate for accurate assessment of stenoses in small accessory renal arteries or branch vessels.

Magnetic resonance urography is a new technique that provides remarkable anatomic detail of the collecting system. In particular, the course of the ureters from renal pelvis to bladder can be easily mapped out for the surgeons on a single coronal sequence (Fig. 8.40). MR urography can be performed either by

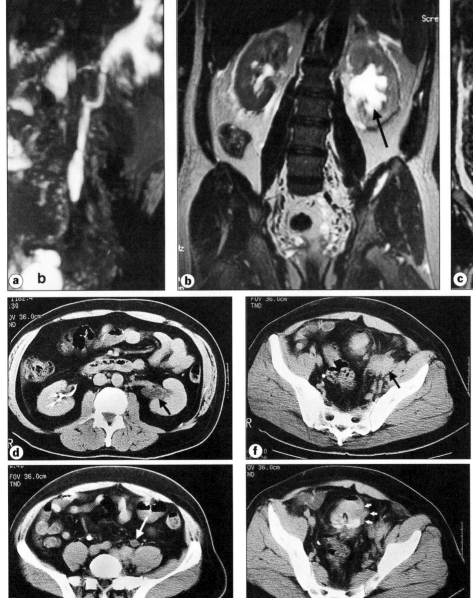

Figure 8.40 Hydronephrosis. Magnetic resonance urogram (a) demonstrating left hydronephrosis. The urine within the dilated collecting system is of high signal intensity. The dilated ureter stops abruptly several centimeters above the bladder. The exact cause of the obstruction can not be determined on this heavily T_2-weighted image. Coronal source images (b, c) demonstrate dilation of the left intrarenal collecting system (arrow, b) and of the distal left ureter (black arrow, c), which terminates abruptly at a low signal mass (curved white arrow) representing a conglomeration of enlarged lymph nodes. Note also thickening of the bladder wall (straight white arrow), consistent with a bladder cancer. Computed tomography scan confirms left hydronephrosis (arrow, d), dilated left ureter (arrow, e), lymphadenopathy (arrow, f) and thickening of the bladder wall on the left (arrows, g), consistent with a transitional cell carcinoma of the bladder.

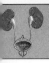

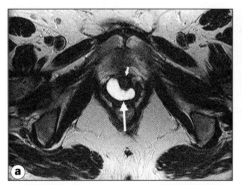

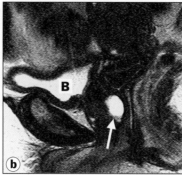

Figure 8.41 Urethral diverticulum. Axial (a) and sagittal (b) T$_2$-weighted images demonstrate a high-signal-intensity, fluid-filled structure (long arrow) posterolateral to the urethra (short arrow), consistent with a urethral diverticulum. B, bladder.

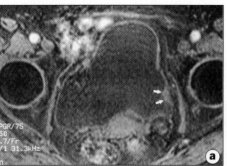

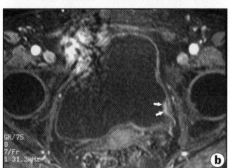

Figure 8.42 Carcinoma of the bladder. (a) Axial T$_1$-weighted fat-suppressed image of the bladder demonstrates minimal focal thickening of the bladder wall on the left (arrows). (b) Following the administration of intravenous gadolinium, the mass enhances (arrows). Findings are consistent with a small transitional cell carcinoma of the bladder. There is no evidence of invasion through the bladder wall into the perivesical fat.

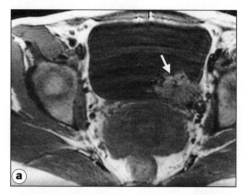

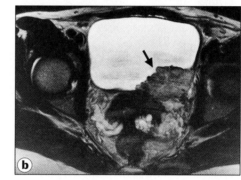

Figure 8.43 Bladder tumor. This patient presented with severe hypertension, elevated urinary catecholamines and flushing on urination. Axial T$_1$-weighted (a) and T$_2$-weighted (b) images of the pelvis demonstrate an irregular mass (arrow) arising from the left bladder wall near the ureterovesical junction. Given the patient's history, the findings are consistent with pheochromocytoma of the bladder. However, by magnetic resonance imaging characteristics alone, the appearance is indistinguishable from a transitional cell carcinoma of the bladder.

using a heavily T$_2$-weighted breath-hold fast spin echo sequence with a large field of view or by using a gadolinium-enhanced 3D gradient echo sequence. A low dose of gadolinium is used because too high a concentration of gadolinium in the collecting system can result in paradoxical loss of signal. Contrast-enhanced images are improved by first administering a small dose of furosemide (frusemide)[78,88]. Although motion artifact may still significantly degrade images of MR urography in some patients, it is a useful alternative for mapping the ureters or evaluating the collecting system in patients in whom it may be beneficial to avoid IVU, such as those with IV contrast allergy, children, and pregnant women. The technique is also useful for diagnosing urethral diverticula[89,90] (Fig. 8.41).

Magnetic resonance imaging of the bladder is useful as a complementary tool to CT for staging patients with bladder carcinoma, particularly when attempting to differentiate between T2, T3a and T3b disease. Contrast-enhanced MRI (CE-MRI) provides somewhat better differentiation between tumor and bladder wall. Bladder carcinomas are typically isointense or hyperintense to urine, bladder wall, and muscle (but hypointense to fat) on T$_1$-weighted images, which provide the highest sensitivity or conspicuity of bladder masses[91] (Figs 8.42 & 8.43). T$_1$-weighted images are also the most sensitive for detection of tumor extension into the perivesical fat[91,93]. Bladder wall invasion is best evaluated on T$_2$-weighted images, where the tumors are of higher signal intensity than the bladder wall. T2 (or lower) disease is suggested if the hypointense linear bladder wall is intact. Disruption of the bladder wall by tumor mass with preservation of the normal signal intensity of the perivesical fat suggests stage T3a disease, i.e. deep muscle invasion, and stage T3b is diagnosed when signal abnormality or tumor mass extends into the perivesical fat[91–93]. As bladder cancers tend to enhance before the bladder wall, dynamic contrast-enhanced imaging has been reported to improve tumor staging[94,95]. However, MR findings are nonspecific and may be indistinguishable from inflammation, scarring, or edema. Thus, MRI is of limited use in evaluating the postoperative or radiated patient[91]. Although the reported number of cases is small, the reported staging accuracy of CE-MRI for bladder cancer ranges from 74% to 93%[94,95]. Overstaging is reported more often than understaging.

While sonography remains the imaging modality of choice for the evaluation of most scrotal disease, MRI may be helpful in selected cases, particularly in differentiating a mass from hemorrhage or hematoma. MRI has a reported accuracy of 93–94% in locating the undescended testis[96]. Accuracy is lowest for the intra-abdominal testis.

REFERENCES

1. Smith RC, Verga M, McCarthy S, Rosenfield AT. Diagnosis of acute flank pain: value of unenhanced helical CT. AJR. 1996;166:97–101.

2. Fielding JR, Fox LA, Heller H, et al. Spiral CT in the evaluation of flank pain: overall accuracy and feature analysis. J Comput Assist Tomogr. 1997;21:635–8.

3. Preminger GM, Vieweg J, Leder RA, Nelson RC. Urolithiasis: detection and management with unenhanced spiral CT – a urologic perspective. Radiology. 1998. 207:308–9.

4. Bell TV, Fenlon HM, Davison BD, Ahari HK, Hussain S. Unenhanced helical CT criteria to differentiate distal ureteral calculi from pelvic phleboliths. Radiology. 1998;207:363–7.

5. Smith RC, Levine J, Rosenfield AT. Helical CT of urinary tract stones: epidemiology, origin, pathophysiology, diagnosis and management. Radiol Clin North Am. 1999;37;5:911–52.

6. Dalrymple NC, Verga M, Anderson KR, et al. The value of unenhanced helical CT in the management of acute flank pain. J Urol. 1998;159:735–40.

7. Katz DS, Lane MJ, Sommer FG. Unenhanced helical CT of ureteral stones: incidence of associated urinary tract findings. AJR. 1996;166:1319–22.

8. Henehan JP, Dalrymple NC, Verga M, Rosenfield AT, Smith RC. Soft tissue 'rim' sign in the diagnosis of ureteral calculi with the use of unenhanced helical CT. Radiology. 1997;202:709–11.

9. Kawashima A, Sandler CM, Boridy IC, et al. Unenhanced helical CT of ureterolithiasis: value of the tissue rim sign. AJR. 1997;168:997–1000.

10. Bell TV, Fenlon HM, Davison BD, et al. Unenhanced helical CT criteria to differentiate distal ureteral calculi from pelvic phleboliths. Radiology. 1998;207:363–7.

11. Blake SP, McNicholas MMJ, Raptopoulos V. Nonopaque crystal deposition causing ureteric obstruction in patients with HIV undergoing indinavir therapy. AJR. 1998;171:717–20.

12. Dobbins JM, Novelline RA, Rhea JT, et al. Helical computed tomography of urinary tract stones: accuracy and diagnostic value of stone size and density measurements. Emerg Radiol. 1997;4:303–8.

13. Perlman ES, Rosenfield AT, Wexler JS, Glickman MG. CT urography in the evaluation of urinary tract disease. J Comput Assist Tomogr. 1996;20:620–6.

14. Fein AB, Lee JKT, Balfe DM, et al. Diagnosis and staging of renal cell carcinoma: a comparison of MR imaging and CT. AJR. 148:749–53.

15. Yuh BI, Cohan RH. Helical CT for detection and characterization of renal masses. Semin Ultrasound CT MRI. 1997;18:82–90.

16. Herts BR, Coll DM, Lieber ML, Streem SB, Novick AC. Triphasic helical CT of the kidneys: contribution of vascular phase scanning in patients before urologic surgery. AJR. 1999;173:1273–7.

17. Smith RH, Baumgartner BR, Nelson RC, et al. Comparison of arterial phase and excretory phase contrast-enhanced spiral CT of the kidneys for the detection of focal abnormalities. Presented at the 14th annual meeting of the Society of Uroradiology, Palm Beach, FL, January 14, 1995.

18. Yuh BI, Cohan RH. Different phases of renal enhancement: role in detecting and characterizing renal masses during helical CT. AJR. 1999;173:747–55.

19. Glazer GM, Callen PW, Parker JJ. CT diagnosis of tumor thrombosis in the inferior vena cava: avoiding the false-positive diagnosis. AJR. 1981;137:1265–7.

20. Cohan RH, Sherman LS, Korobkin M, Bass JC, Francis IR. Renal masses: assessment of corticomedullary-phase and nephrographic-phase CT scans. Radiology. 1995;196:445–51.

21. Bosniak MA. The current radiological approach to renal cysts. Radiology. 1986;158:1–10.

22. Bosniak, MA. Re: cystic masses-a reevaluation of the usefulness of the Bosniak classification system (letter). Acad Radiol. 1996;3:981–3.

23. Bosniak MA, Megibow AJ, Hulnick DH, Horii S, Rgahavendra BN. CT diagnosis of renal angiomyolipoma: the importance of detecting small amounts of fat. AJR. 1988;151:497–501.

24. Steiner MS, Goldman SM, Fishman EK, Marshall FF. The natural history of renal angiomyolipoma. J Urol. 1993;150:1782–6.

25. Helenon O, Chretien Y, Paraf F, Melki P, Denys A, Moreau JF. Renal cell carcinoma containing fat: demonstration with CT. Radiology. 1993;188:429–30.

26. Coleman BG, Arger PH, Mintz MC, Pollack HM, Banner MP. Hyperdense renal masses: a computed tomographic dilemma. AJR. 1984;143:291–4.

27. Davidson AJ, Hartman DS, Choyke PL, Wagner BJ. Radiologic assessment of renal masses: implications for patient care. Radiology. 1997;202:297–305.

28. Hartman DS, Davis CJ Jr, Goldman SM, Friedman AC, Fritzsche P. Renal lymphoma: radiologic-pathologic correlation of 21 cases. Radiology 1982; 144:759–66.

29. Rosenfield AT, Glickman MG, Taylor KJ, Crade M, Hodson J. Acute focal bacterial nephritis (acute lobar nephronia). Radiology. 1979;132:553–61.

30. Hoddick W, Jeffrey RB, Goldberg HI, et al. CT and sonography of severe renal and perirenal infections. AJR. 1983;140:517–20.

31. Kawashima A, Sandler CM, Goldman SM, et al. CT of renal inflammatory disease. RadioGraphics. 1997;17:651–66.

32. Roberts JL, Dalen K, Bosanko, et al. CT in abdominal and pelvic trauma. RadioGraphics. 1993;13:735–52.

33. Dorffner R, Thumbar S, Prokesch R, et al. Spiral CT during selective accessory renal artery angiography: assessment of vascular territory before aortic stent grafting. Cardiovasc Intervent Radiol. 1998;21:179–82.

34. Pozniak MA, Balison DJ, Lee FT Jr, et al. CT angiography of potential renal transplant donors. Radiographics. 1998 18:565–87.

35. Beregi JP, Louvegny S, Gautier C, et al. Fibromuscular dysplasia of the renal arteries: comparison of helical CT angiography and arteriography. AJR. 1999;172:27–34.

36. Sommer FG, Olcott EW, Ch'en I, Beaulieu CF. Volume rendering of CT data: applications to the genitourinary tract. AJR. 1997;168:1223–6.

37. Quillin, SP, Brink JA, Heiken JP, et al. Spiral CT angiography: identification of crossing vessels at the utero pelvic junction. AJR. 1996;166:1125–30.

38. Siegel CL, McDougall EM, Middleton WO, et al. Preoperative assessment of uteropelvic junction obstruction with endoluminal sonography and helical CT. AJR. 1997;168:623–6.

39. Coll DM, Uzzo RG, Herts BR, et al. 3-Dimensional volume rendered computed tomography for preoperative evaluation an intraoperative treatment of patients undergoing nephron sparing surgery. J Urol. 1999;161:1097–102.

40. Fenlon HM, Bell TV, Ahari HK, Hussain S. Virtual cystoscopy: early clinical experience. Radiology. 1997;205:272–5.

41. Stenzl A, Frank R, Eder R, et al. 3-Dimensional computed tomography and virtual reality endoscopy of the reconstructed lower urinary tract. J Urol. 1998;159:741–6.

42. Kurtz AB, Middleton, WD. Kidney. In: Kurtz AB, Middleton WD, eds. US requisites. St. Louis, MO:Mosby-Year Book; 1996:73–121.

43. Nicolet V, Carignan L, Dubuc G, et al. Thickening of the renal collecting system: a nonspecific finding at US. Radiology. 1988;168:411–3.

44. Rosenfield AT, Black H, Camp A, Lange R. Correlation of CT and ultrasound with insulin resistance. Scientific session, Proceedings of the Society of Uroradiology, 1992.

45. Stuck KJ, White GM, Granke DS, et al. Urinary obstruction in azotemic patients: detection by sonography. AJR. 1987;149:1191–3.

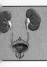

46. Ritchie WW, Vick CW, Glocheski SK, Cook, DE. Evaluation of azotemic patients: diagnostic yield of initial US examination. Radiology. 1988;167:245–7.

47. Hill MC, Rich JI, Mardiat JF, Finder CA. Sonography vs. excretory urography in acute flank pain. AJR. 1985;144:1235–8.

48. Lerner RM, Rubens D. Distal ureteral calculi: diagnosis by transrectal sonography. AJR. 1986;147:1189–91.

49. Smith RC, Verga M, McCarthy SM, Rosenfield AT. Diagnosis of acute flank pain: value of unenhanced helical CT. AJR. 1996;166:97–101.

50. Tublin ME, Dodd GD, Verdile VP. Acute renal colic: diagnosis with duplex Doppler US. Radiology. 1994;193:697–701.

51. Hartman DS, Goldman SM, Friedman AC, et al. Angiomyolipoma: ultrasound–pathologic correlation. Radiology. 1981;139:451–8.

52. Khan AN, Gould, DA, Shah SM, Mouasher YK. Primary renal liposarcoma mimicking angiomyolipoma on ultrasonography and conventional radiology. J Clin Ultrasound. 1985;13:58–9.

53. Yamashita Y, Mutsumasa T, Watanabe O, et al. Small renal cell carcinoma: pathologic and radiologic correlation. Radiology. 1992;184:493.

54. Habboub HK, Abu-Yousef MM, Williams RD, et al. Accuracy of color Doppler sonography in assessing venous thrombus extension in renal cell carcinoma. AJR 1997;168:267–71.

55. London NJM, Messios N, Kinder RB, et al. A prospective study of the value of conventional CT, dynamic CT, ultrasonography, and arteriography for staging renal carcinoma. Br J Urol. 1989;64:209–17.

56. Schwerk WB, Schwerk WN, Rodeck G. Venous renal tumor extension: a prospective US evaluation. Radiology. 1985;156:491–5.

57. Quinn MJ, Hartman DS, Friedman AC, et al. Renal oncocytoma: new observations. Radiology. 1984;153:49–53.

58. Weinberger E, Rosenbaum DM, Pendergrass TW. Renal involvement in children with lymphoma: comparison of CT with sonography. AJR. 1990;155:347–9.

59. Kumari-Subaiya S, Lee WJ, Festa R, et al. Sonographic findings in leukemic renal disease. J Clin Ultrasound. 1984;12:465–72.

60. Leder RA, Dunnick NR. Transitional cell carcinoma of the pelvicalices and ureter. AJR. 1990;155:713–22.

61. Goldman SM, Fishman EK. Upper urinary tract infection: the current role of CT, ultrasound, and MRI. Semin Ultrasound CT MR 1991;12:335–61.

62. Rosenfield AT, Glickman MG, Taylor KJW, et al. Acute focal bacterial nephritis (acute lobar nephronia). Radiology. 1979;132:553–61.

63. Prando A, Pereira RM, Marins JLC. Sonographic evaluation of hypertrophy of septum of Bertin. Urology. 1984;24:505–10.

64. Mann SJ, Pickering TG. Detection of renovascular hypertension. Ann Intern Med. 1992;117:845–53.

65. Pickering TG. Diagnosis and evaluation of renovascular hypertension: Indications for therapy. Circulation. 1991;83(suppl. 1):147–54.

66. Stavros S, Harshfield D. Renal Doppler, renal artery stenosis, and renovascular hypertension: direct and indirect duplex sonographic abnormalities in patients with renal artery stenosis. Ultrasound Q. 1994;12(4):217–63.

67. Strandness DE Jr. Duplex imaging for the detection of renal artery stenosis. Am J Kidney Dis. 1994;24(4):674–8.

68. Hansen KJ, Tribble RW, Reavis SW, et al. Renal duplex sonography: Evaluation of clinical utility. J Vasc Surg. 1990;12:227–36.

69. Melany ML, Grand EG, Duerinckx AJ, et al. Ability of a phase shift US contrast agent to improve imaging of the main renal arteries. Radiology. 1997;205:147–52.

70. Balen FG, Allen CM, Lees WR. Ultrasound contrast agents. Clin Radiol. 1994;49:77–82.

71. Rosenfield AT, Zeman RK, Cronan JJ, Taylor KJW. Ultrasound in experimental and clinical renal vein thrombosis. Radiology. 1980;137:735–41.

72. Avasthi PS, Greene ER, Scholler C, et al. Noninvasive diagnosis of renal vein thrombosis by ultrasound echo-Doppler flowmetry. Kidney Int. 1983;23:882–7.

73. Platt JF, Ellis JH, Rubin JM. Intrarenal arterial Doppler sonography in the detection of renal vein thrombosis of the native kidney. AJR. 1994;162:1367.

74. Burge HJ, Middleton WD, McClennan BL, et al. Ureteral jets in healthy subjects and in patients with unilateral ureteral calculi: comparison with color Doppler US. Radiology. 1991;180:437.

75. Choyke PL, Austin HA, Frank JA, et al. Hydrated clearance of gadolinium-DPTA as a measurement of glomerular filtration rate. Kidney Int. 1992;41:1595–8.

76. Terens WL, Gluck R, Golimbu M, Rofsky NM. Use of gadolinium-DPTA-enhanced MRI to characterize renal insufficiency. Urology. 1992;40:152–4.

77. Semelka RC, Hricak H, Stevens SK, et al. Combined gadolinium enhanced and fat saturation MR imaging of renal masses. Radiology. 1991;176:803–9.

78. Choyke PL. MR imaging of the kidneys and adrenal glands. In: McCarthy SM, Reinhold C, Palmer WE, eds. Categorical course in diagnostic radiology: body MR. Oak Brook; Radiological Society of America, Inc; 1999:67–71.

79. Hricak H, Williams RD, Moon KL, et al. Nuclear magnetic imaging of the kidneys: renal masses. Radiology. 1983;147:765–72.

80. Semelka RC, Hricak H, Stevens SK, et al: Combined gadolinium-enhanced and fat saturation MR imaging of renal masses. Radiology. 1991;178:803–809.

81. Sohn HK, Kim SY, Seo HS. MR imaging of a renal oncocytoma. J Comp Assist Tomogr. 1987;11:1085–7.

82. Krestin GP. Magnetic resonance imaging of the kidneys: current status. MR Q. 1994;10:2.

83. Roubidouz MA, Dunnick NR, Sostman HD, et al. Renal carcinoma: detection of venous extension with gradient-echo MR imaging. Radiology.1992; 182:269–72.

84. Kallman DA, King BF, Hattery RR, et al. Renal vein and inferior vena cava tumor thrombus in renal cell carcinoma: CT, US, MRI and venacavography. J Comp Assist Tomogr. 1992;16:240–7.

85. Horan JJ, Robertson CN, Choyke PL, et al. The detection of renal cell carcinoma extension into the renal vein and the inferior vena cava: a prospective comparison of venacavography and magnetic resonance imaging. J Urol. 1989;142:943–7.

86. Prince MR, Schoenberg SO, Ward JS, et al. Hemodynamically significant atherosclerotic renal artery stenosis: MR angiographic features. Radiology. 1997;205:128–36.

87. Hany TF, Debatin JF, Leung DA, et al. Evaluation of the aortoiliac and renal arteries: comparison of breath-hold, contrast-enhanced, three-dimensional MR angiography with conventional catheter angiography. Radiology. 1997;204:357–62.

88. Schad LR, Semmler W, Knopp MV, et al. Preliminary evaluation: magnetic resonance of urography using a saturation inversion projection spin-echo sequence. MR Imaging. 1993;11:319–27.

89. Neitlich JD, Foster HE Jr, Glickman MG, Smith RC. Detection of urethral diverticula in women: comparison of a high resolution fast spin echo technique with double balloon urethrography. J Urol. 1998;159(2):408–10.

90. Klein LT, Frager D, Subramanium A, Lowe FC. Use of magnetic resonance urography. Urology. 1998;52(4).602–8.

91. Barentsz JO, Jager GJ, Mugler JP III, et al. Staging of urinary bladder cancer: value of T1-weighted 3-D MP-RAGE and 2-D SE sequences. AJR. 1995;164: 109–15.

92. Buy JN, Moss A, Guinet C, et al. MR staging of bladder carcinoma: correlation with pathologic findings. Radiology. 1988;169:695–700.

93. Rholl KS, Lee JKT, Heiken JP, et al. Primary bladder carcinoma: evaluation with MR imaging. Radiology. 1987;163:117–21.

94. Narumi Y, Kadota T, Inoue E, et al. Bladder tumors: staging with gadolinium-enhanced oblique MR imaging. Radiology. 1993;187:145–50.

95. Sohn M, Neuerberg J, Teufl F, et al. Gadolinium-enhanced magnetic resonance imaging in the staging of urinary bladder neoplasms. Urol Int. 1990;45:142–7.

96. Fritzsche PJ, Hricak H, Kogan BA, et al. Undescended testis: value of MRI. Radiology. 1987;164:169–73.

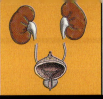

Chapter 9
Radiologic Imaging: Pediatric Uroradiology

Marc S Keller

KEY POINTS

- The imaging needs of young children place unique demands on uroradiologist and clinician
- Ultrasound scanning is the cornerstone of pediatric imaging
- Contrast studies such as urography and voiding cystography still have important roles
- Radionuclide studies reflect accurately renal function and upper tract urodynamics
- Computed tomography scanning has well-defined indications and is a powerful tool in oncologic imaging

INTRODUCTION

While other chapters in this text describe urologic imaging of adults, both the urologic conditions of childhood and the imaging needs of children are sufficiently different to create the need for a separate pediatric chapter. Some diagnostic evaluations, such as those performed for upper urinary tract trauma, are nearly identical to those in adults and need not be re-emphasized or repeated here. But others, such as the evaluation of urinary tract infections, postnatal evaluation of prenatally detected hydronephrosis, congenital anomalies, collecting system dilatation, neoplasms, and conditions of the inguinal canal and scrotum, have distinctly different uroradiology needs and patterns in children.

IMAGING MODALITIES

Ultrasound

Considerably greater emphasis nowadays is placed upon ultrasound (US) as the cornerstone of pediatric uroradiologic imaging than upon the other modalities. The examination is harmless, painless, fast, provides morphologic and dynamic information, and has the capacity to imply functional data indirectly at times. Furthermore, since the resolution of US is greater using higher-frequency transducers at shorter imaging distances, children are truly ideal targets for the ultrasound beam. Within the group of uroradiologic imaging modalities, perhaps none is more operator- and knowledge-dependent than US. Just as a pediatric urologist has a particular familiarity and expertise with the pediatric urinary tract, an analogy can be made to the individuals performing and interpreting the pediatric US examination as well. Merely making a set of standard screening images will not use the

modality to its fullest without an understanding of the anatomy and physiology special to children. Information can be captured concerning thickness and echo pattern of the renal parenchyma, status of the collecting systems, ureteral peristalsis, patterns of bladder wall thickening, posterior urethral dilatation, degree of bladder filling and efficiency of emptying, and Doppler evaluation of interlobar artery spectra, the combination of which can provide a very detailed and specific assessment of urinary tract pathophysiology for diagnosis.

Normal kidneys

The sonographic pattern of the normal kidney in children is, in general, quite similar to adults (Fig. 9.1) with the exception of the premature and neonates. In these smallest of children, the echogenicity of the normal renal cortex can be equal to or more intense than that of the adjacent liver or spleen, a finding that is abnormal in adults and older children. The youngest infants exhibit the most pronounced corticomedullary differentiation, as seen in Figure 9.2. Inexperienced observers may

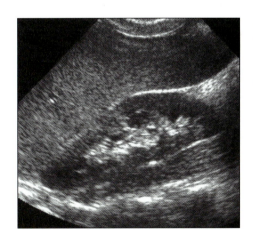

Figure 9.1 Right upper quadrant sagittal sonogram of a normal kidney in an older child.

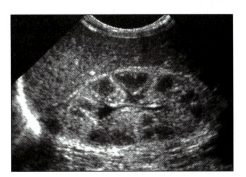

Figure 9.2 Right upper quadrant sagittal sonogram of a normal neonatal kidney. The image shows the intense cortical echogenicity adjacent to the relatively larger hypoechoic renal pyramids.

mistake the normal contrast between the neonatal renal cortex and medulla for hydronephrosis. The renal sinus contains fat and vessels, creating a plethora of acoustic interfaces, sound reflections, and its characteristic echogenic appearance. In general, the renal collecting system is inapparent; however, the excellent spatial resolution afforded by the high-frequency transducers used in the smallest of children will allow the imaging of small amounts of urine in a normal renal pelvis, a finding that when seen in adults leads to suspicions of abnormal collecting system dilatation.

Size and growth of kidneys in children is important to observe and plays a role in diagnosis. Standards are well established and are extremely useful[1].

Normal ureters
Most of the time in children, normal ureters are not directly imaged by sonography. Their imaging absence is taken for granted as a sign of normality. Normal ureters can be imaged most often proximally at the pelviureteric junction and distally at the ureterovesical junction (UVJ) with diameters of 3mm or less and regular waves of peristalsis every 10–20 seconds[2].

Normal bladder
From birth to adolescence, a remarkable consistency exists in the sonographic appearance of the bladder wall in the full and empty states. The inner lining of the bladder consisting of the mucosa and submucosa is echogenic, while the muscular wall is hypoechoic. By sonography, each of these layers has about the same thickness. When the bladder is full, the entire wall thickness usually ranges from 2 to 3mm. A normal bladder when empty or nearly empty in a child has a wall thickness equal to or less than 5mm[3].

Normal testes
From birth to adulthood, despite the changes in size, a uniform parenchymal echogenicity characterizes the testis. Beyond infancy, the linear longitudinal echo of the mediastinum testis can usually be identified.

Normal Doppler sonography
Doppler sonography of the kidney in the neonate, infant, and small child is remarkably different from in the older child and adult. Not only are the images much more challenging to obtain in uncooperative subjects who do not hold their breath, but the vascular resistances are different owing to the different renal physiology. Unlike the adult population, in whom the interlobar artery resistive index (RI) is normally 0.7 or less, higher resistances are routinely found in smaller children. In prematures and neonates, RI may range as high as 0.8–1.0. In infants and toddlers, RI values as high as 0.7–0.8 can be seen normally[4]. Studies have shown that the adult values of RI appear sometime in the 2–4-year-old range[5].

When examining the testis for arterial pulsations, the most sensitive Doppler US scanners can currently detect flow even in the smallest of testes in most instances. Absolute velocity and RI do not play a key role. Comparison of perfusion patterns of the clinically abnormal side with the normal one is much more helpful for interpretation of findings and diagnosis.

Radiography
Plain radiographs
Not much enthusiasm continues for the specific use of plain radiographs to answer urologic questions in children. In the search for calculi, other imaging will be more helpful. Sonography can find nephrocalcinosis and many instances of urolithiasis, but the most sensitive modality for the diagnosis of urinary tract calculi has been shown to be helical CT scanning, originally reported in adults but with applicability shown to extend to children[6].

Voiding cystourethrography
The voiding study remains important as the standard in the diagnosis of vesicoureteral reflux (VUR) and its grades 1–5. While a single-void voiding cystourethrogram (VCU) is an accurate study and the accepted norm for screening, at times a second or third cycle of voiding during the same study may improve diagnostic accuracy[7]. Modern fluoroscopy and spot filming with digital imaging and video capture have reduced considerably the radiation exposure when compared to the old screen film radiography method. While almost no pediatric female urethral abnormalities are seen[8], the VCU offers a detailed diagnostic image of the urethra and its abnormalities in boys.

In instances of vesicoureteral reflux to the upper tracts, radiography affords an excellent look at calyceal morphology, assessment of renal scars, and the seldom seen but important finding of intrarenal reflux (Fig. 9.3).

Excretory urography
Whether it is called intravenous pyelography (IVP), intravenous urography (IVU), or excretory urography (EU), this former cornerstone of morphology and function in the investigation of the pediatric urinary tract has been steadily diminishing in its use and utility over the last decade. Its findings have never been invalidated, but the frequent use of sonography for renal morphology and measurement, the performance of the VCU

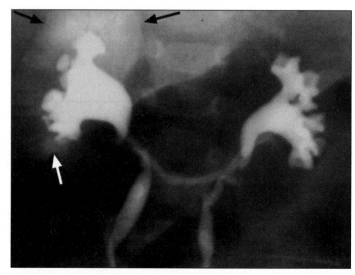

Figure 9.3 Frontal view of the upper abdomen following voiding during a voiding cystourethrography. There is a small amount of right lower pole intrarenal reflux (white arrow), with much greater opacification of the right upper pole (black arrows). Refluxed contrast opacifies the left collecting system but not the parenchyma.

to evaluate for reflux, and the selective use of radionuclide renography for quantitative evaluation of renal function and detection of renal scars have proved to yield a more helpful set of data for most evaluation and treatment decisions.

Radionuclide imaging

Properly done in children, the use of radioisotopes in imaging the urinary tract can be very elegant and extremely helpful. Main purposes include evaluation for obstructive uropathy, calculation of relative renal function, imaging of renal scars, and follow-up of vesicoureteral reflux. Quantification of function using computer-assisted methods is the positive trade-off for the lesser anatomic detail of nuclear imaging. The radio-nuclides used in urinary tract imaging are radiopharmaceuticals bound to ^{99m}Tc. Two principal agents are used for evaluation of obstructive uropathy. ^{99m}Tc-diethylenetriamine pentaacetic acid (^{99m}Tc-DTPA) is a glomerular-filtered radionuclide that depicts the collecting system well but the parenchyma only fairly. With a slightly higher radiation dose to the child, ^{99m}Tc-mercaptoacetyltriglycine (^{99m}Tc-MAG3) shows both the parenchyma and the collecting system well, giving excellent imaging and function quantification. Both can be used for diuretic radionuclide renography (Fig. 9.4).

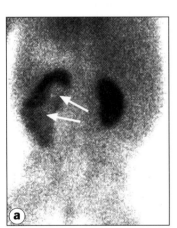
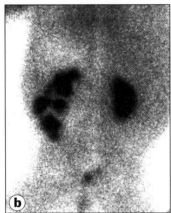

Figure 9.4 Radionuclide renogram with ^{99m}Tc-DTPA. (a) Early image shows photopenic areas (arrows) in the hydronephrotic kidney before concentrated tracer is excreted into dilated calyces. (b) Some minutes later activity has appeared in the same area.

For the depiction of parenchymal perfusion defects from pyelonephritis or scars, the renal tubular deposition of ^{99m}Tc-DMSA affords excellent imaging and relative function quantification. Furthermore, the study need not be hurried as the imaging is not time-dependent as in the more rapidly excreted agents.

In the follow-up of VUR, intravesical installation of ^{99m}Tc-sulfur colloid as a simple tracer can be used for radionuclide voiding cystograms (Fig. 9.5). Grading of VUR is necessarily less accurate but still useful. Not imaged by this method is the urethral anatomy, renal scars, and VUR from an everted extra-vesical diverticulum containing the ureteral insertion (Fig. 9.6).

Computed tomography

The use of computed tomography (CT) in the pediatric urinary tract has well-defined indications. No other modality in trauma has the capability for such rapid and accurate evaluation following injuries to the urinary tract. CT also has a pivotal role in evaluating renal and other retroperitoneal neoplasms, for not only can CT quickly and accurately perform local tumor imaging but it also is the single best way to evaluate the lungs for nodules. The ability of CT to evaluate both chest and abdominal disease in a single short examination makes it a powerful tool in oncologic imaging. Severe suppurative and opportunistic renal infections and their extrarenal extension are also well evaluated by CT. Recently, the applicability of helical CT scanning as the primary imaging study to evaluate for the possibility of urolithiasis in flank pain has been reported to be successful in children[6]. The use of three-dimensional CT reconstruction of the unenhanced urinary tract has been used and advocated for some children with myelodysplasia in order to visualize the urinary tract reliably in its entirety in this group with a high incidence of scoliosis and kyphosis that can confound sonographers.

Magnetic resonance imaging

While magnetic resonance imaging (MRI) is capable of diagnosing and evaluating the anatomy of many of the urologic conditions of childhood, its use in routine practice is not widespread. The higher cost and the longer imaging times play a significant role here. In certain instances, MRI is used fairly routinely when available to radiologists with pediatric expertise, such as in the evaluation of retroperitoneal neoplasms and adjacent

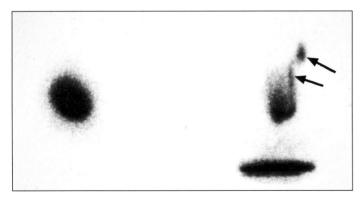

Figure 9.5 Isotope cystogram. The image on the left before voiding shows only the activity in the bladder. The image on the right during voiding shows unilateral reflux into the ureter and renal collecting system (arrows) and excretion into the bedpan below.

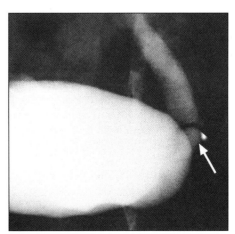

Figure 9.6 Voiding cystourethrography showing vesicoureteral reflux from a diverticulum (arrow) containing the ureterovesical junction. This unusual but relevant finding would not be imaged by an isotope cystogram.

vasculature. Current MRI research into parenchymal changes of pyelonephritis appears quite promising. At times, the anatomy of some of the more unusual congenital urinary tract abnormalities can be elucidated by MRI and its multiplanar capabilities when other imaging leaves doubt.

IMAGING OF UROLOGIC CONDITIONS IN CHILDHOOD

Congenital anomalies

Renal agenesis and ectopia

The number and location of kidneys in children is well detected by careful sonography with the examiner remembering to scan down the flanks and into the pelvis when a kidney is not found in the expected location. At times, one may wonder whether an absent kidney has been truly agenetic or has involuted prior to examination. A very helpful finding is the configuration of the adjacent adrenal gland. When a kidney has at some time formed in Gerota's fascia, the adrenal gland will assume its characteristic A shape in cross-section and retain it even if the kidney subsequently involutes. In cases of renal agenesis, the adrenal gland retains a disc shape so that in a longitudinal section, such as one sees by US, the appearance is much like that of a cigar (Fig. 9.7)[9]. To some prenatal sonographers and to some inexperienced neonatal examiners, this finding can be misinterpreted as an atrophic or a diminutive kidney. Obviously, in fetuses with bilateral renal agenesis, this will be a bilateral finding.

Pelvic kidneys, pan-cake kidneys, and cross-fused ectopic kidneys generally present no challenge in diagnosis when an orderly search of the abdomen is carried out. On the other hand, the horseshoe kidney frequently seems to baffle observers, probably because its upper ends are normal in location. The key to detecting horseshoe kidneys by US is that no one seems to be able to make a good image of their lower ends. As their lower poles course medially and toward the midline instead of going laterally along the psoas muscles, they hide behind intestinal gas. Once the horseshoe kidney is suspected, anterior compression scans can readily show the juxtaposed lower poles or even a parenchymal isthmus. Color Doppler images in the midline sagittal plane can depict the inferior mesenteric artery arching anteriorly over the isthmus. Horseshoe kidneys imaged by almost all other functional methods are easy to diagnose (Fig. 9.8).

Multicystic dysplastic kidney

The result of a proximally atretic ureter in the formation of the fetal kidney, multicystic dysplastic kidney (MCDK) has a characteristic sonographic appearance (Fig. 9.9). The variably sized noncommunicating cysts form a reniform but disorganized cluster with strands of echogenic parenchyma interspersed among them. The morphologic appearance is diagnostic, but if one also examines for blood flow by Doppler methods it is difficult to find. Formerly, radionuclide imaging was employed to confirm the diagnosis and poor function but nowadays this seems seldom done except in instances where MCDK has to be differentiated from a severe or unusual hydronephrotic kidney.

Renal duplication

During a screening US examination, the most obvious finding leading to suspicion of a renal duplication anomaly is renal

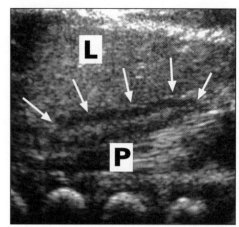

Figure 9.7 Right upper quadrant sagittal sonogram in a neonate with right renal agenesis. This shows the typical cigar-shaped adrenal gland (arrows) between the liver (L) and the psoas muscle (P).

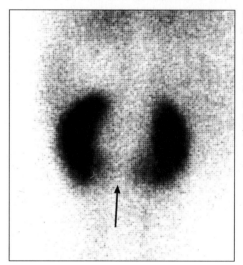

Figure 9.8 Horseshoe kidney. Radionuclide renogram early phase shows the abnormal renal axes with the lower poles meeting in the midline (arrow).

enlargement. Even kidneys with none of the obstructive or refluxing conditions will usually measure well above normal when they are duplex. In cases of complete duplication with obstructed upper poles (Fig. 9.10), US examination will readily show the collecting system dilatation, ureterectasis, and type of obstruction, whether it is the ectopic ureterocele at the outlet of the bladder (Fig. 9.11) or the ectopic insertion of the upper pole dilated ureter that courses below the trigone.

If excretory urography is performed, duplication is quite apparent when no obstruction exists. Ureters can be followed by plain radiographs or fluoroscopic spot films to elucidate whether they join above the bladder or not. When the upper pole is obstructed, the inferior displacement of the lower pole assumes a configuration most often likened to a drooping lily flower (Fig. 9.12). Because the obstructed upper pole generally concentrates poorly, the appearance of the bladder is key to determining the type of obstruction. The presence of an ectopic ureterocele makes an obvious filling defect, while a simple ectopic insertion of the upper pole creates no visible bladder finding at urography.

In some girls, complete duplication with mild upper moiety obstruction from an ectopic insertion of its ureter into the urethra or the vagina may present with years of constant urinary dribbling. Careful sonography or urography can be used to detect this anomaly, which is readily curable and gratifying to all involved (Fig. 9.13).

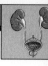

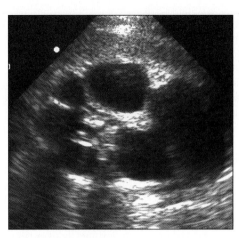

Figure 9.9 Multicystic dysplastic kidney. Sagittal sonogram shows multiple noncommunicating cysts without any normal renal parenchyma.

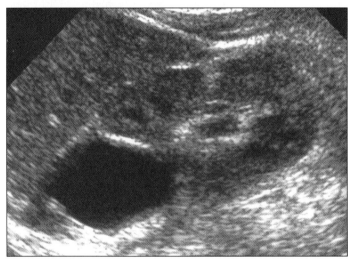

Figure 9.10 Complete renal duplication with upper pole obstruction. Coronal sonogram directly images the hydronephrotic upper pole and the normal-appearing lower pole.

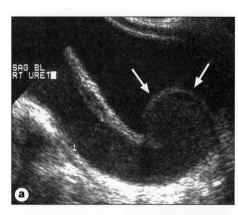

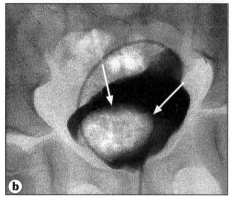

Figure 9.11 Renal duplication with upper pole obstruction by ectopic ureterocele. (a) Sagittal sonogram of the distal dilated ureter terminating in the ectopic ureterocele (arrows). The echoes in the obstructed upper moiety system are from infection. (b) Early filling phase of a voiding cystourethrography outlines the filling defect of the ureterocele (arrows) at the right bladder base.

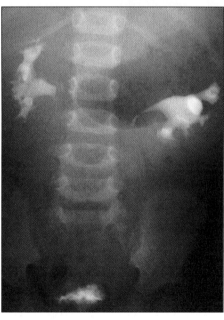

Figure 9.12 Renal duplication with upper pole obstruction by ectopic ureteral insertion. Excretory urogram shows the inferolateral displacement of the left lower pole with its 'drooping lily' appearance as a result of the obstructed, enlarged, poorly functioning upper pole. The bladder is empty and has no filling defect.

It is well known that the lower poles of completely duplicated kidneys often show VUR and, once duplication is diagnosed, assessing for VUR is fairly routine. At other times, a VCU may be performed before a diagnosis has been made. In these instances, careful observation will show that the refluxed contrast has filled only a lower-pole collecting system, allowing the diagnosis of complete duplication from a voiding study alone (Fig. 9.14).

Ureteropelvic junction obstruction

While abnormalities of urinary flow at the ureteropelvic junction (UPJ) may be lumped by some into a single diagnosis, in fact a spectrum of conditions exists that have different intrinsic and extrinsic anatomic etiologies, described elsewhere in this textbook. The role of imaging is to make an anatomically correct level of diagnosis and to attempt to gauge how much obstruction or impedance exists at the UPJ. This assessment can be accomplished with a number of imaging studies, although not all need to be used in caring for any particular child. Anatomic diagnosis by US is straightforward, but analyzing the sonogram for functional implications is more involved[10]. Helpful signs that lean toward significant obstruction include loss of corticomedullary differentiation and increased parenchymal echogenicity, thinned parenchymal rims of 5mm or less around all the dilated calyces, contralateral hypertrophy, interlobar RI in the hydronephrotic kidney of 10% or higher than the normal one, and an increase in the interlobar RI of 7% or more in the hydronephrotic kidney after intravenous hydration and furosemide diuresis[11,12]. Kidneys that show only collecting system dilatation without any of these other findings are only rarely found to have significant obstruction. The shape of the renal pelvis can also be a guide, since those that retain a funnel or conical shape are very infrequently obstructed. A dilated pelvis that is flattened against the adjacent psoas muscle, the so-called block pelvis, is more suspicious than the cone-shaped pelvis, but the most worrisome of all is when the renal pelvis assumes a rounded shape like a balloon and its tenseness is depicted by a tangential relationship with the adjacent psoas muscle (Fig. 9.15).

Excretory urography will show delayed excretion and hydronephrosis of the renal collecting system to the UPJ. It is more difficult to determine how obstructed the kidney is and whether its function is significantly diminished.

The current standard to assess the combination of obstruction and function is the diuretic radionuclide renogram. Preparation includes establishment of an intravenous line for hydration and drug injections along with the placement of a bladder catheter to remove the potential effects of VUR or elevated bladder pressure upon the examination of the upper tracts. Computer-assisted calculations of relative and absolute glomerular filtration rate (GFR) can be combined with nuclear imaging of the urinary tract. When the tracer fills the dilated collecting system, furosemide is administered to capture the performance of the urinary tract in a high flow state and portray it graphically over time (Fig. 9.16). While a collecting system proximal to a UPJ lesion that will not wash out and maintains or increases its activity is obviously obstructed, controversy exists as to whether a prolonged declining washout curve indicates obstruction. Some observers believe that a washout time for half the activity of more than 20 minutes implies obstruction; others disagree. Some authorities maintain that observing the relative function is key, for, unless the function of the affected kidney has significantly declined, surgery may not help the child[13].

In a UPJ obstruction, the dominant part of the collecting system is always the renal pelvis, in contrast to congenital megacalyces, in which the caliectectasis is quite florid but the renal pelvis retains normal size and shape (Fig. 9.17).

Primary megaureter

Abnormalities of the muscular wall of the distal ureter can result in a spectrum of varying degrees of impedance or obstruction showing ureterectasis with a narrowed juxtavesical segment as the common finding[14]. The mildest forms have dilatation only of the distal part of the ureter, while higher gradients across the narrowed distal portion may result in proximal ureterectasis and ultimately renal effects. Sonography of megaureters or ureterovesical obstructions can not only yield morphologic information but also allow some functional implications. The aforementioned

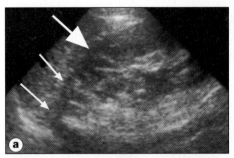

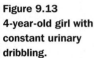

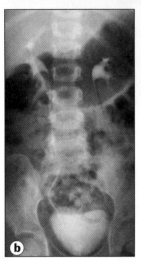

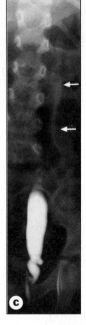

Figure 9.13
4-year-old girl with constant urinary dribbling.
(a) Coronal sonogram of the left kidney reveals a subtle cleft separating the very small upper pole moiety (small arrows) from the larger lower pole moiety (large arrow). (b) Excretory urogram shows bilateral excellent renal collecting system opacification, but note that the left kidney is missing the expected upper pole infundibulum and calyx. (c) Retrograde study of the ectopic vaginal urinary orifice opacifies the abnormal ureter and shows its course (arrows) from the upper pole moiety.

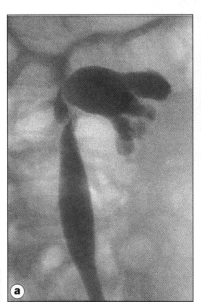

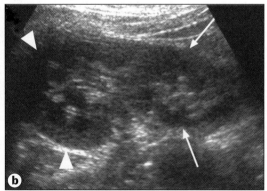

Figure 9.14 Diagnosis of complete duplication.
(a) Voiding cystourethrography image shows reflux into a left lower pole collecting system with blunted, crowded calyces from reflux nephropathy. (b) Coronal sonogram demonstrates the intact parenchyma of the upper moiety (arrowheads) contrasted against the thinner abnormal lower pole moiety (arrows).

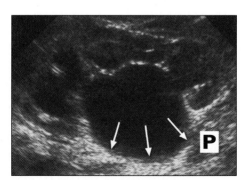

Figure 9.15 Balloon-shaped pelvis. Coronal sonogram of a toddler with a ureteropelvic junction obstruction depicts the relative tenseness of the renal pelvis retaining its round shape (arrows) and a tangential relationship against the psoas muscle (P) medially.

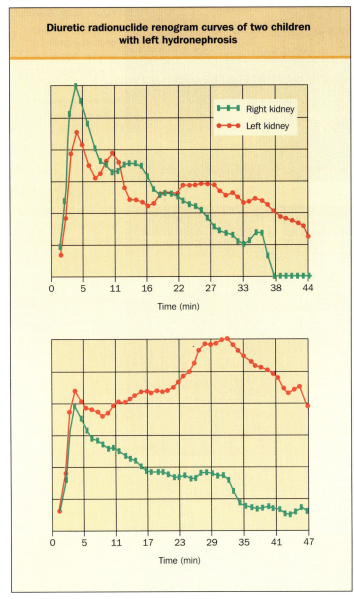

Diuretic radionuclide renogram curves of two children with left hydronephrosis

Right kidney

Left kidney

Time (min)

Time (min)

Figure 9.16 Diuretic radionuclide renogram curves of two children with left hydronephrosis. Diuretic is administered at 20 minutes. Time–activity curves show (top) nonobstructive washout of tracer from both collecting systems in a parallel manner and (bottom) postdiuretic increase and retention of activity in the obstructed left kidney.

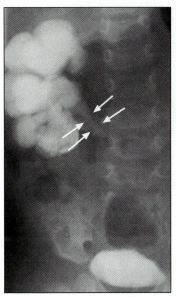

Figure 9.17 Congenital megacalyces. Huge right renal calyces are apparent but, in contrast to ureteropelvic junction obstruction, the renal pelvis is of normal size and configuration (arrows) in this excretory urogram.

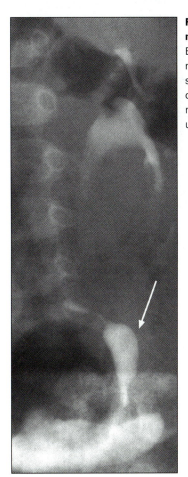

Figure 9.18 Primary nonobstructive megaureter. Excretory urogram depicts a mild form with characteristic segmental dilatation of the distal third of the ureter and narrowing just above the ureterovesical junction.

signs of obstruction can all be employed and, additionally, two other observations are useful in cases of megaureter. Abnormally slow, ineffective, or absent ureteral peristalsis correlates with higher degrees of obstruction, as does a ureteral diameter of 10mm or greater.[2]

The ability to identify confidently primary nonobstructed megaureters by sonography can reduce a great number of unnecessary studies and allow periodic non-invasive observation of this condition, which tends to remit over time in early childhood[15].

By excretory urography, the anatomy is apparent (Fig. 9.18). As in the UPJ conditions, the challenge is in determining the degree of obstruction and its effect upon renal function. The diuretic radionuclide renogram can be effectively employed to answer these questions in a quantitative manner.

Orthotopic ureterocele

Frequently called adult-type ureterocele, these lesions are of course present in childhood, as they are congenital, but they almost never create symptoms in young people. The ureterocele at the distal end of a single renal collecting system is located at the normal area of the trigone (Fig. 9.19) and, while it shows some impedance to flow, it seldom reveals significant obstruction. The kidney above it tends to have mild hydroureteronephrosis.

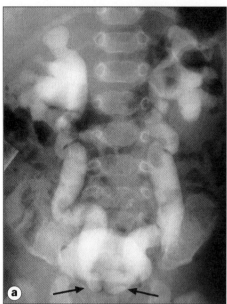

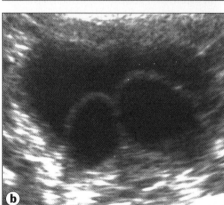

Figure 9.19 Bilateral orthotopic ureteroceles in an infant. Mild symmetric hydroureteronephrosis terminates at the ureteroceles (arrows) seen (a) at excretory urography and (b) during a transverse sonogram of the bladder.

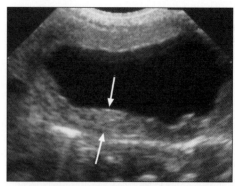

Figure 9.20 Bladder wall thickening in posterior urethral valves. Sagittal view of a neonatal bladder showing the wall thickening (arrows) seen in all boys with this condition.

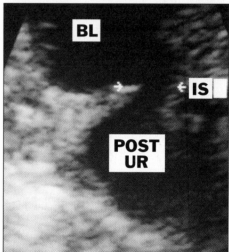

Figure 9.21 Dilated posterior urethra from valves. Caudally angled sagittal sonogram of the bladder outlet (BL) in a neonate captures the open internal sphincter (IS) and the dilated posterior urethra (POST UR).

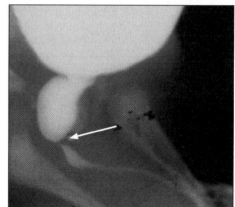

Figure 9.22 Posterior urethral valves. Voiding film demonstrates the dilated posterior urethra and the abrupt transition in urethral caliber (arrow) owing to the obstructing valve leaflets.

Sonography of the bladder can show the dynamic changes as the peristaltic ureter transports urine into the ureterocele, which can be seen to fill, empty, and even show a jet effect at color Doppler mapping.

Posterior urethral valves

Nowadays the widespread use of prenatal sonography finds infants with bilateral hydronephrosis or poor bladder emptying who are suspected of having bladder outlet obstruction from posterior urethral valves. A frequently helpful neonatal sign by sonography has been bladder-wall thickening (Fig. 9.20) reflecting bladder hypertrophy even when the upper tracts are not very dilated owing to the diminished renal function characteristic of newborns. Fortuitous US imaging of a filled bladder can at times show the dilated posterior urethra (Fig. 9.21). VCU is needed for definitive diagnosis (Fig. 9.22) as some other conditions may also show similar US findings. Prune belly syndrome (Eagle–Barrett syndrome) often results in bilateral hydroureteronephrosis, a large, thick-walled bladder, and a dilated posterior urethra from prostatic hypoplasia and not obstruction (Fig. 9.23). Some infants with spasm of the external urinary sphincter may also show some similar findings at US imaging. Well-performed voiding radiographs of the neonatal male urethra enable accurate diagnosis and differentiation of these conditions.

Reflux and trapping

The coexistence of VUR with upper tract impedance or obstruction may lead to an important and interesting pathophysiology in urodynamics[16]. While a UPJ or UVJ lesion may not by itself have a particularly deleterious effect upon renal function over time, the addition of a refluxed volume of urine several times a day into the already dilated system may effectively create repetitive episodes of intermittent acute obstructive uropathy that can threaten renal function even in the absence of infection. When upper tract dilatation occurs during a VCU, its pattern and time of drainage needs to be observed in order to detect reflux and trapping (Fig. 9.24). The presence of reflux and trapping also invalidates the use of the accepted grading system for reflux. If reflux and trapping is diagnosed as causing renal deterioration

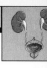

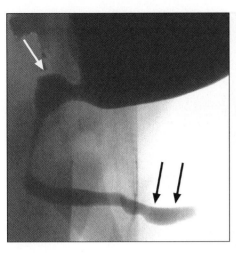

Figure 9.23 Prune belly syndrome (Eagle–Barrett syndrome). Voiding film shows a dilated posterior urethra from prostatic hypoplasia (white arrow) that gradually changes caliber and funnels down to the urogenital diaphragm. Another finding occasionally seen in this syndrome is megalourethra, demonstrated in the anterior urethra in this baby (black arrows).

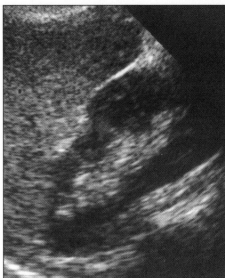

Figure 9.25 Reflux nephropathy in a girl with repetitive urinary tract infections and vesicoureteral reflux. Coronal sonogram of the left kidney portrays the thinned, scarred upper pole parenchyma, different in appearance from the normal lower pole.

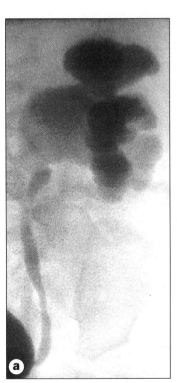 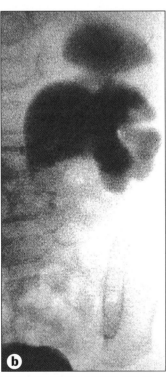

Figure 9.24 Reflux and trapping. (a) Spot film obtained at the end of voiding finds left vesicoureteral reflux into a dilated collecting system above a ureteropelvic junction kink. (b) Another image taken 20 minutes later shows that most of the reflux remains trapped above the ureteropelvic junction and is draining only very slowly.

and creating the need for surgical intervention, careful thought must be directed toward addressing whether the obstruction or the VUR is the more dominant lesion.

Urinary tract infection

Exactly how to image children with urinary tract infection (UTI) continues to create controversy and study, but in general, the younger the child, the more agreement exists on the need for both morphologic imaging, usually by US, and the evaluation of VUR by a voiding study[17]. The imaging of pyelonephritis is

favored by some but ignored by others. Some believe that finding, mapping, and counting the renal lesions of acute pyelonephritis in children through the use of ^{99m}Tc-DMSA scans helps them care for and treat these children with greater confidence. Others claim that clinical decisions are not influenced by these images, which add only radiation and cost. In routine screening studies, sonography seldom allows detection of signs of acute UTI. Rarely, some focal or diffuse renal swelling can be seen. The relative regional ischemia of pyelonephritis is difficult to see with color Doppler mapping, especially in small children with constantly moving kidneys because they cannot hold their breath. Contrast-enhanced CT is able to map pyelonephritis, but the radiation, expense, and little effect upon clinical decisions make it a seldom used tool except for infections unresponsive to initial treatment or those that are suspected of focal suppuration or extrarenal extension.

In follow-up, determination of the size, shape and growth of the kidneys is important. For many reasons, sonography is ideal for this purpose (Fig. 9.25). No doubt some small scars may be missed, but this does not usually make an important clinical difference. While lengths of kidneys are routinely followed, examining and recording the cross-sectional measurements brings a third dimension to light and allows a more accurate size estimation at times.

As stated above, radiographic or isotope VCUs play a key role in determining the presence and severity of VUR in children with UTI.

In children imaged during acute UTI episodes, sonography almost never shows any bladder abnormality. But, interestingly, the finding of measurable bladder wall thickening characterized by a prominent echogenic mucosal and submucosal layer and the ability to empty well almost always correlates with chronic symptoms of lower tract infection and urgency incontinence (Fig. 9.26).

Opportunistic infection of the urinary tract in immunocompromised children or in those who have been treated with a series of antibiotics may occur. Fever with neutropenia, oliguria, or funguria may all be presenting signs. Sonography offers a simple way to search for fungal debris in the collecting systems or bladder, which can accumulate and lead to obstructive uropathy (Fig. 9.27).

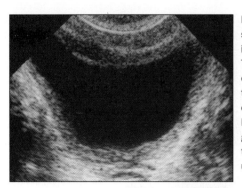

Figure 9.26 Bladder sonogram in chronic cystitis. Transverse view of the bladder shows the smooth thickened echogenic bladder lining seen in many girls with chronic lower tract symptoms and urgency incontinence.

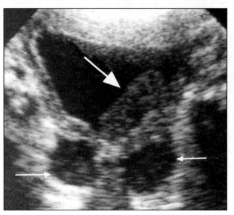

Figure 9.27 A septic oliguric neonate, treated with several antibiotics, who was found to have hyphae and mycelia in his urine. Transverse sonogram of the pelvis finds echogenic fungal debris in the bladder (large arrow) and similar material in the enlarged, obstructed distal ureters (small arrows). Cultures grew *Candida*.

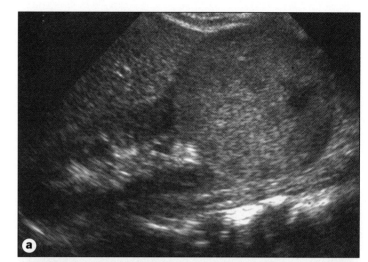

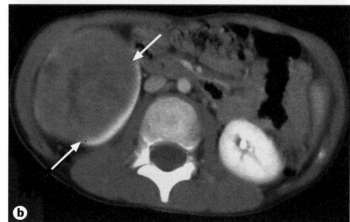

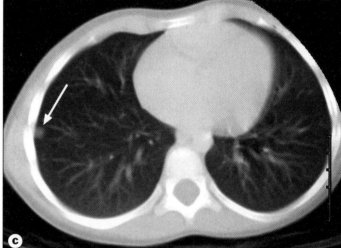

Neoplasia

Most of the neoplasms of the pediatric urinary tract are renal. The major role of imaging is staging and delineation in treatment planning. Attempting to make a histologic diagnosis from the images is not realistic in most instances but can be done at certain times.

One of the conditions that lends itself to a confident diagnosis by imaging is nephroblastomatosis in which the nodules are peripheral and cortical with typical low echogenicity at sonography and low attenuation on contrast CT. Almost all other renal neoplasms in children have similar mixed echogenicity at sonography and have much less enhancement by CT than the surrounding normal kidney. In neonates, one considers mesoblastic nephroma more because of the child's age than because of any imaging findings. With most renal tumors occurring in the 1–4-year-old group, Wilms tumor is the dominant diagnosis. Imaging is geared to assess the local disease in the involved kidney and adjacent retroperitoneum, the possibility of a contralateral renal lesion, and any evidence of venous invasion with extension into the renal vein or even up the inferior vena cava into the heart. A necessary part of the imaging evaluation is assessment of the lungs for nodules, best done by CT (Figs 9.28 & 9.29). Other renal neoplasms that may appear similar include the anaplastic variant of Wilms tumor, clear cell sarcoma, with its propensity for osseous metastases instead of pulmonary spread, rhabdoid tumor with frequent intracranial tumors that may be either metastatic or metachronous primitive neuroectodermal tumors. Occasionally, in the older child or teenager, renal cell carcinoma may be an unexpected diagnosis at pathology.

Figure 9.28 4-year-old boy with an asymptomatic right upper quadrant mass discovered during a routine physical examination. (a) Sagittal sonogram shows a mass arising from the lower pole of the right kidney. (b) Abdominal computed tomography depicts the interface (arrows) between the lower attenuation mass and the surrounding rim of enhancing kidney. (c) Computed tomography of the lung reveals a peripheral pulmonary metastatic nodule (arrow).

Involvement of the kidney by lymphoma in children occurs and is found usually as part of a staging evaluation and not through a presenting urinary tract symptom. By sonography, renal

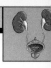

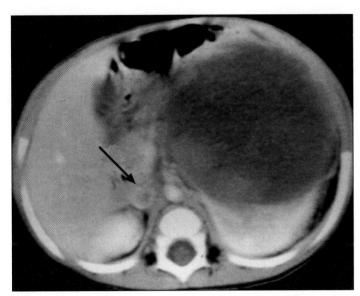

Figure 9.29 Computed tomography scan from a toddler with Wilms tumor. This shows the large left primary renal mass and a filling defect within the opacified inferior vena cava (arrow) from a tumor thrombus.

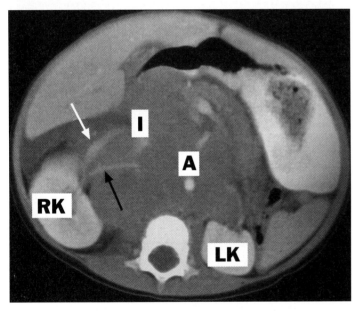

Figure 9.30 Infant with neuroblastoma. Right adrenal primary tumor displaces the right kidney (RK) inferolaterally. Local nodal spread fills the upper retroperitoneum, encases the right renal artery (black arrow) and vein (white arrow), and displaces the inferior vena cava (I) and aorta (A) anteriorly. Adenopathy extends across the midline to the hilum of the left kidney (LK).

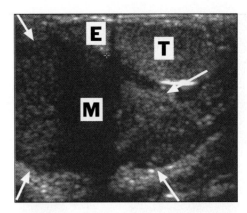

Figure 9.31 Paratesticular rhabdomyosarcoma in a 2-year-old. A large hard mass was discovered, and sonography shows that the tumor mass (M, arrows) is separate from and adjacent to the epididymis (E) and testis (T).

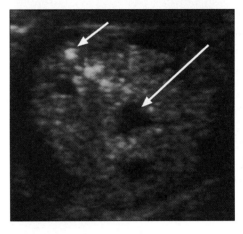

Figure 9.32 8-month-old boy with a hard, enlarged testis. Sonogram shows the testis replaced by an inhomogeneous mass composed of soft tissue, cysts (larger arrow), and calcifications (smaller arrow) that proved to be a benign teratoma.

lymphoma can be so hypoechoic as to mimic cystic lesions. On contrast CT, the nodules do not enhance. Leukemia involving the kidneys most often shows profound smooth, diffuse nephromegaly.

Most neuroblastomas occur in the adrenal glands, although some may arise in the pararenal areas or rarely even in the presacral pelvis. Generally, adrenal neuroblastomas extrinsically displace the adjacent kidney; however, at times they aggressively invade it. At imaging, calcification is frequent in neuroblastomas.

So is the tendency for local nodal spread and a particular characteristic encasement of the abdominal aorta and its branches that is not seen in the renal tumors (Fig. 9.30). Imaging of neuroblastoma must evaluate for potential invasion into adjacent neural foramina as well as for retrocrural paraspinal nodal spread into the adjacent upper abdomen or chest.

Rhabdomyosarcoma occurs in the pelvis of children either within the bladder base at the trigone or in the upper vagina or uterus. Its lobular appearance in this area has led to the long-used clinical designation of sarcoma botryoides. Whether imaging is by cystography, sonography, CT, or MRI, the grape-like fronds of tumor are quite typical. Contiguous local and nodal spread must be sought, and the lungs need examination for nodules during staging. In boys, paratesticular rhabdomyosarcomas occur (Fig. 9.31) and the staging imaging is similar.

Small boys with testicular masses often exhibit tumors with sonographic characteristics showing solid tissue, cystic areas, and shadowing calcifications that usually turn out to be benign germ cell tumors at orchiectomy (Fig. 9.32). In teenagers with testicular tumors, the imaging sequences, findings, and diagnoses essentially are those of young adults (Fig. 9.33).

In boys under treatment for leukemia, the testes have a peculiar propensity to be a site for recurrent disease. Usually, sonography is used to clarify clinical findings and justify the need for biopsy. Leukemia in the testis exhibits nodules that are hypoechoic.

Testis and spermatic cord

While imaging of the painful scrotum for torsion is the same as is done in adults, several points need to be mentioned that apply

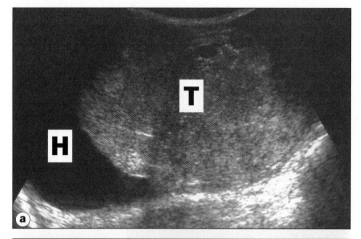

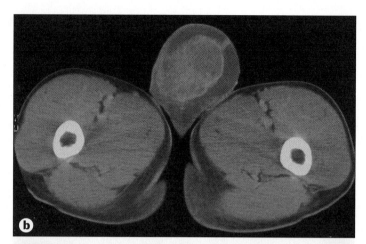

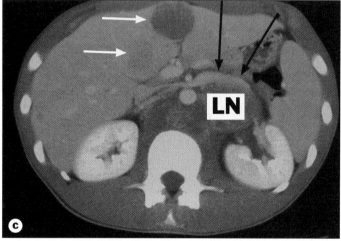

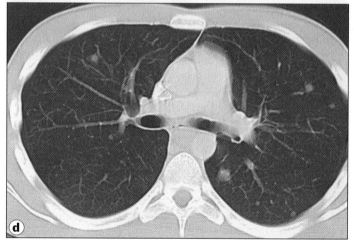

Figure 9.33 18-year-old with a large testicular mass. (a) Sonogram shows part of the enlarged left hemiscrotum with an inhomogeneous tumor (T) and some surrounding hydrocele (H). (b) Computed tomography scan of the primary tumor and (c) at the level of the left renal hilum finds not only metastatic pararenal adenopathy (LN) between the aorta and the left kidney, bowing the left renal vein anteriorly (black arrows), but also two hepatic metastases (white arrows). (d) Metastatic lung nodules are noted on this computed tomography scan of the chest. The diagnosis proved to be teratocarcinoma.

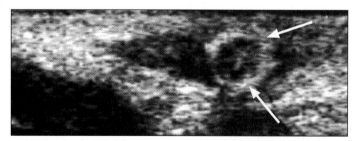

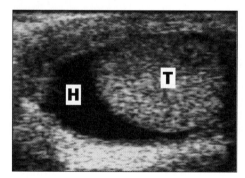

Figure 9.35 Simple hydrocele. Sagittal sonogram of the hemiscrotum shows the anechoic hydrocele fluid (H) adjacent to the normal testis (T).

Figure 9.34 Prenatal testicular torsion. An atrophic, pea-sized testis with an echogenic calcific rim is depicted on this sonogram.

to children. In neonates, the result of prenatal torsion is an infarcted testis that may present as an atrophic indurated nodule with a typical US appearance (Fig. 9.34). Also, a testis that is at a borderline level of rotation for intermittent torsion and detorsion may exhibit reactive hyperemia when detorsed that can mimic epididymo-orchitis[18]. The imaging of simple hydroceles is straightforward by US (Fig. 9.35). With inguino-scrotal masses, sonography can be useful to differentiate hydroceles of the cord from hernias (Fig. 9.36). As stated above, delineating testicular from paratesticular masses is also readily accomplished.

Imaging searches for undescended testes are generally un-rewarding unless the testis is located at or below the inguinal ring. The use of CT and MRI for this purpose can find nodules that may or may not be the testis. Laparoscopy seems to be a better choice to search for intra-abdominal testes.

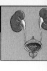

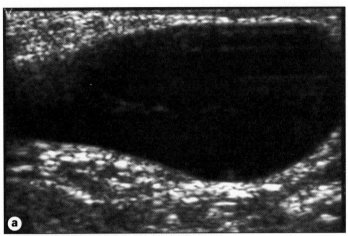

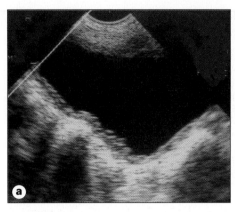

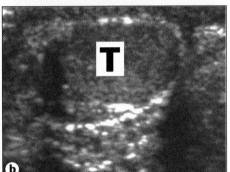

Figure 9.36
Hydrocele of the cord. In the inguinal area, examination of this fluctuant mass shows a fluid collection along the spermatic cord (a). At the caudal end in the scrotum (b) is a normal testis (T).

Figure 9.37
Neuropathic bladder. The sagittal sonogram (a) and the lateral view from the cystogram (b) both depict the bladder thickening and trabeculations. The thickening is from detrusor hypertrophy, which is hypoechoic by ultrasonography and is covered by normal-thickness mucosa and submucosa.

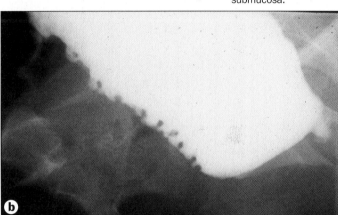

Bladder

Much of the evaluation of diseases of the bladder is done directly by urologists with cystoscopy and studies of bladder dynamics. Imaging is very helpful in selected instances. While acute cystitis tends not to have imaging findings, girls with chronic lower tract infections and urgency incontinence often show at sonography a particular pattern of bladder mucosal and submucosal thickening that is distinctive (Fig. 9.26). This appearance is different from the bladder wall thickening in a neuropathic bladder (Fig. 9.37).

When rhabdomyosarcoma arises in the bladder, cross-sectional images are needed for staging of local and distant disease as noted above. Occasionally, a child with Foley catheter drainage for some days will show hematuria and will acquire a focal inflammatory mass from irritation by the tip of the catheter of the collapsed bladder wall. The US imaging of this lesion can be very similar to sarcoma. Knowledge of this condition will allow removal of the catheter and a period of waiting to show regression of the lesion.

REFERENCES

1. Han BK, Babcock DS. Sonographic measurements and appearance of normal kidneys in children. AJR. 1985;154:611–16.
2. Keller MS, Weiss RM, Rosenfield NS. Sonographic evaluation of ureterectasis in children: the significance of peristalsis. J Urol. 1993;149:553–5.
3. Jequier S, Rousseau O. Sonographic measurements of the normal bladder wall in children. AJR. 1987;149:563–6.
4. Keller MS. Renal Doppler sonography in infants and children. Radiology. 1989;172:603–4.
5. Bude RO, DiPietro MA, Platt JF, et al. Age dependency of the renal resistive index in children. Radiology. 1992;184:469–73.
6. Traubici J, Fields J, Neitlich J, et al. Unenhanced helical CT in the evaluation of acute flank pain in children. Pediatr Radiol (in press).
7. Paltiel HJ, Rupich RC, Kiraluta HG. Enhanced detection of vesico-ureteral reflux in infants and children with use of cyclic voiding cystourethrography. Radiology. 1992;184:753–5.
8. Bisset GS III, Strife JL, Dunbar JS. Urography and voiding cystography: findings in girls with urinary tract infection. AJR. 1987;148:479–82.
9. McGahan JP, Myracle MR. Adrenal hypertrophy: possible pitfall in the sonographic diagnosis of renal agenesis. J Ultrasound Med. 1986;5:265–8.
10. Garcia-Pena BM, Keller MS, Schwartz DS, et al. The ultrasonographic differentiation of obstructive versus nonobstructive hydronephrosis in children: a multivariate scoring system. J Urol. 1997;158:560–5.
11. Bude RO, DiPietro MA, Platt JF, Rubin JM. Effect of furosemide and intravenous normal saline fluid load upon the renal resistive index in nonobstructed kidneys in children. J Urol. 1994;151:438–41.
12. Palmer JM, DiSandro M. Diuretic enhanced duplex Doppler sonography in 33 children presenting with hydronephrosis: a study of test sensitivity, specificity, and precision. J Urol. 1995;154:1885–8.

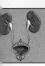

13. Ransley PG, Dhillon HK, Gordon I, et al. The postnatal management of hydronephrosis diagnosed by prenatal ultrasound. J Urol. 1990;144:584–7.

14. Belman AB. Megaureter. Classification, etiology, and management. Urol Clin North Am. 1974;1:497–513.

15. Baskin LS, Zderic SA, Snyder HM, Duckett JW. Primary dilated megaureter: long term followup. J Urol. 1994;152:618–21

16. Weiss RM, Schiff M Jr, Lytton B. Reflux and trapping. Radiology. 1976;118:129–31.

17. Bergman DA, Baltz RD, Cooley JR, et al. Practice parameter: the diagnosis, treatment, and evaluation of the initial urinary tract infection in febrile infants and young children. Pediatrics. 1999; 103:843–52.

18. Patriquin HB, Yazbeck S, Trinh B, et al. Testicular torsion in infants and children: diagnosis with Doppler sonography. Radiology. 1993; 188:781–5.

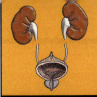

Chapter 10

Nuclear Medicine Techniques

Stephen CW Brown

KEY POINTS

- Modern nuclear medicine techniques utilize gamma-ray camera technology and radiopharmacy.
- Radiopharmaceuticals comprise the combination of radionuclide and a molecule or carrier that determines its biologic fate.
- Radionuclide techniques include clearance studies, renography, renal imaging, bladder imaging, and bone scanning.
- Diuresis renography is the investigation of choice to distinguish between obstructive and nonobstructive hydronephrosis.

INTRODUCTION

The potential use of radionuclides as 'tracers' in the study of biologic systems was realized early in the development of nuclear science. It was not, however, until the arrival of artificially produced radioactivity within reactors and cyclotrons in the 1940s that nuclides suited to medical applications became available.

At the same time, detection systems were evolving. Study of radiation-induced scintillations within detector crystals and their coupling to photomultiplier tubes led to the development of sensitive and directional scanners – the rectilinear scanner in 1949 and the 'gamma' camera in 1957[1]. Subsequent developments focused on radiopharmaceutical design and the inclusion of computer and digital technology to improve image processing.

Modern nuclear medicine embraces all applications of radioactive materials in diagnosis, treatment, and medical research, with the exception of the sealed radiation sources used in radiotherapy[2]. The ability to label molecules with a known physiologic course or destination in the body provides nuclear medicine with a unique potential in the study of the function and dynamics of biomedical systems. In urology it plays an important role in the investigation of kidney function, upper urinary tract dynamics, and the management of advanced prostate cancer.

To appreciate the role of nuclear medicine in urology and to ensure its safe and appropriate application, it is necessary to have some knowledge of the basic science, nomenclature, and principles involved.

The Bohr model of the atom

Figure 10.1 The Bohr model of the atom.

SCIENTIFIC BASIS

Atomic structure

Bohr described an atom as electrons orbiting in discrete energy levels or 'shells' around a nucleus (Fig. 10.1). This comprised two particles or nucleons – protons and neutrons. The mass number (A) is the total number of nucleons in the nucleus, and the atomic number (Z) is the number or protons; the standard notation used is ^{A}X and $_{Z}X$, respectively. A nuclide describes any combination of nucleons. The term isotopes is used to denote nuclides that share the same number of protons (e.g. ^{131}I, ^{123}I, and ^{125}I).

Radioactive decay

Different combinations of protons and neutrons can be artificially produced. In a nuclear reactor bombardment with neutrons forms nuclides with extra neutrons; in a cyclotron collision with other particles produces nuclides deficient in neutrons. Some nuclides formed may be at the ground state or stable; some may be unstable and release energy as they achieve the ground state. This change may be almost instantaneous; for others it may take time and a transitory metastable state may be

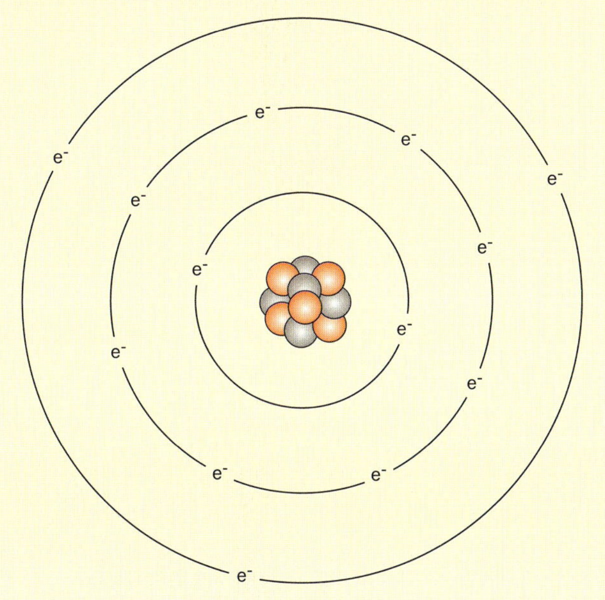

formed. This process is radioactive decay, of which a number of forms are recognized.

Alpha decay

The decay of some heavy radionuclides involves the emission of alpha particles that comprise two neutrons and two protons (a helium nucleus). This particulate radiation results in too much ionization for medical imaging and penetrates no more than 0.05mm in tissue.

Beta-minus decay

Beta-minus decay may occur from a nuclide with an additional neutron. The extra neutron decays to a beta-minus particle, which is a proton and electron, and a noncharged particle termed a neutrino. Subsequent gamma radiation may be released, as the daughter radionuclide achieves a stable state through gamma radiation alone, a process known as isomeric transition. An example is the parent nucleus ^{99}Mo, a beta emitter that decays to the daughter nucleus ^{99m}Tc. This metastable radionuclide (hence the 'm' after the mass number) decays to the stable state with a half-life of 6 hours and emits gamma-rays only. These properties are ideal for nuclear medicine studies of no more than a few hours duration.

Beta-plus decay (positron)

Positron decay arises from neutron-deficient nuclei. The excess proton decays to a neutron, neutrino, and positron. The mass of the latter, once its kinetic energy has been expended, is converted into two gamma rays 180° apart. This radiation forms the basis of positron emission tomography, a method for cross-sectional imaging.

Electron capture

If the nucleus does not have enough energy to decay by positron emission, the excess protons may be reduced by electron capture of an orbital electron. This leaves a vacancy in an inner electron shell. As this is replaced, characteristic X-rays are emitted. Gamma rays may also be released. Electron capture is typical of ^{51}Cr used in renal function studies.

Units

Decay of a single radionuclide is a random process. In a given mass, however, it is possible to determine the probable rate of decay, which is proportional to the number of atoms present. The mode of decay, energy level, and half-life of the emission are characteristic for a given radionuclide.

In SI units 1 Becquerel (Bq) equals 1 disintegration per second. For diagnostic purposes, a typical dose is 1MBq (10^6Bq), and for therapy it is 1GBq (10^9Bq)

X-Rays and gamma rays

Excitation of an atom occurs if an electron is moved from an inner to an outer electron shell as a result of collision with a photon or particle. If the electron is ejected altogether, the atom becomes ionized. If an electron ejected from an inner shell is replaced by one from an outer shell (higher energy), the energy released is equal to the difference in the binding energy of the two electrons. The emission is in the form of characteristic X-rays, which have properties identical to those of gamma

rays. They differ only in their source – the former arises from excitation and ionization of the electron shells, and the latter from an excited nucleus.

DETECTORS

Gamma rays interact with matter in two main ways, the photoelectric effect and Compton scatter (Fig. 10.2). The photoelectric effect describes the ejection of an inner shell electron by the incident ray (Eγ). The resultant photoelectron is

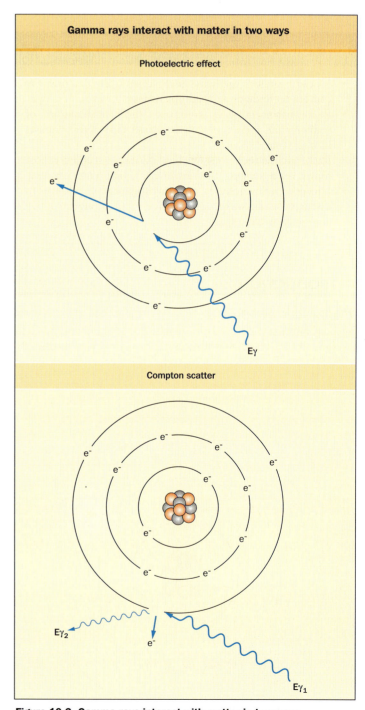

Figure 10.2 Gamma rays interact with matter in two ways.

e, electron; Eγ, incident ray; Eγ$_1$, incident gamma ray energy; Eγ$_2$, reduced-energy gamma ray.

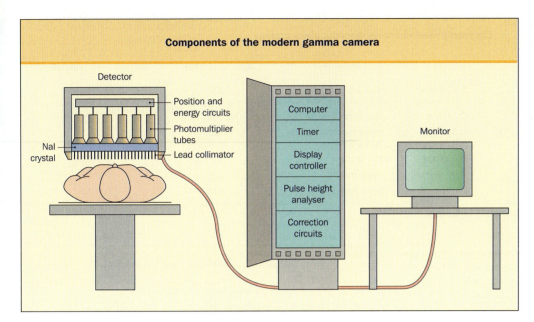

Components of the modern gamma camera

Detector

Position and energy circuits

Photomultiplier tubes

NaI crystal

Lead collimator

Computer

Timer

Display controller

Pulse height analyser

Correction circuits

Monitor

Figure 10.3 Components of the modern gamma camera.

the main radiation detected by a gamma camera. Compton scatter occurs when the incident gamma ray collides with an outer shell electron. Only a portion of the incident gamma ray energy ($E\gamma_1$) is passed onto the 'recoil electron' and the rest is emitted as a reduced-energy gamma ray ($E\gamma_2$). If the energy of the incident gamma ray is about 100–200keV, the majority of the rays pass through the patient and reach the detector without absorption and unnecessary patient radiation. Most of the tissue interaction is by Compton scatter.

The gamma camera
The components of the gamma camera are shown in Figure 10.3. Gamma rays that fall onto a NaI detector crystal are converted into light – photoelectric absorption. The position and intensity of the photons are detected by an array of photomultiplier tubes. The resultant signal is digitally processed to minimize distortion and permit pulse height analysis. The output is subjected to further computer processing. The rays that fall on the detector are controlled by a collimator, which comprises a lead shield with a honeycomb of holes, the diameter and solid angle of acceptance of which permit photons from only one direction (Fig. 10.4). The result is a linear image or scan. Collimators represent a compromise between resolution and sensitivity. Typically, around 0.02% of gamma rays emitted from a patient reach the detector crystal. Different types of crystal are used depending on the radiation and size of object to be scanned.

The scintillation well counter
For clearance studies, the measurement of test-tube samples of plasma or urine can be carried out using a scintillation well counter. This contains a NaI detector crystal with an appropriately drilled hole into which a test-tube can be placed. Accurate measurement can be made by comparison with a standard sample.

Dose calibrator
Accurate measurement of dose is essential before a radiopharmaceutical can be administered. The dose calibrator measures

the electric current across an ionization chamber into which has been placed the radionuclide dose. The ion pairs produced are proportional to the radioactivity present.

RADIOPHARMACEUTICALS

A radiopharmaceutical comprises the combination of the radionuclide and the molecule that determines its biologic fate. Figure 10.5 lists radiopharmaceuticals commonly used in urology.

Production and supply
The stages in production are summarized in Figure 10.6. ^{51}Cr is produced from ^{50}Cr by fission within a reactor. ^{123}I is cyclotron produced from ^{124}Xe and, as its half-life is short, it must be used

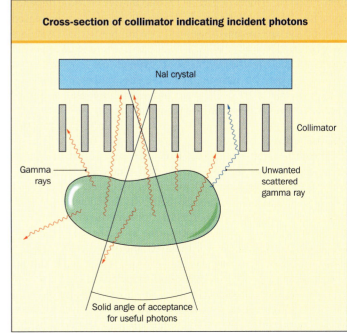

Cross-section of collimator indicating incident photons

NaI crystal

Collimator

Gamma rays

Unwanted scattered gamma ray

Solid angle of acceptance for useful photons

Figure 10.4 Cross-section of collimator indicating incident photons.

Commonly used radiopharmaceuticals in urology				
Radiopharmaceutical	Half-life	Application	Adult dose (MBq)	Effective dose (mSv/MBq)
^{123}I-Orthoiodohippurate (^{123}I-Hippuran)	13.2 hours	Renography Effective renal plasma flow	75	0.0120
^{51}Cr-Ethylenediaminetetraacetic acid (^{51}Cr-EDTA)	27.7 days	Glomerular filtration rate	0.0021	
^{99m}Tc-Diethylenetriamine pentaacetic acid (^{99m}Tc-DTPA)	6.02 hours	Glomerular filtration rate Renography	200	0.0052
^{99m}Tc-Mercaptoacetyltriglycine (^{99m}Tc-MAG3)	6.02 hours	Renography	70	0.0072
^{99m}Tc-Dimercaptosuccinic acid (^{99m}Tc-DMSA)	6.02 hours	Renal imaging	100	0.0087
^{99m}Tc-Methylene diphosphonate (^{99m}Tc-medronate)	6.02 hours	Bone imaging	800	0.0048

Figure 10.5 Commonly used radiopharmaceuticals in urology.

almost immediately. The need for rapid transportation therefore reduces the number of centers able to use ^{123}I-hippuran. However, although ^{99m}Tc also has a short half-life it is widely available by virtue of its production from a 'generator'.

Generators

^{99m}Tc is transported in the form of the parent radionuclide, the fission product ^{99}Mo. This decays at a much slower rate of 66 hours, which enables the daughter ^{99m}Tc to be extractable for up to a week following a single delivery. In this 'generator' form, ^{99m}Tc can be distributed widely and freely. Extraction from the generator is by simple column chromatography. The ^{99m}Tc in the form of pertechnetate is added to a cold-kit that contains the biologic ligand and freeze-dried reagents necessary to produce the required radiopharmaceutical. Technetium can exist in up to seven different oxidation states, which enables very stable binding with a variety of chelates and other molecules.

Safety and handling
Effects of radiation
Radiation effects are of two types – deterministic or stochastic. Deterministic effects (e.g. direct tissue injury) are dose dependent with a short latent period. Stochastic events (e.g. increased cancer risk) are so-called because they are predictable within a population, but not on an individual basis. There is no apparent threshold and the effects can occur even at low levels of exposure. They may be somatic, affecting the irradiated individual (e.g. leukemia after 2–10 years and solid tumors after 10–40 years), or genetic (affecting future generations).

Quantification
To establish safety standards, it is first necessary to quantify radiation exposure and its effects. For X-rays and gamma-rays this relates to the amount of ionization produced by the radiation source. Exposure rate is proportional to the activity of the source and is inversely proportional to the square of the distance from the source – the inverse square law. The dose (energy) absorbed per unit mass of tissue is measured in joules per kilogram [1J/kg = 1Gray (Gy)].

The tissue effects of a given dose of radiation vary with the type of radiation. To allow for this, the dose is multiplied by a radiation weighting factor (W_R) to obtain the equivalent dose. When considering radiation to the human body, allowance is also made for the relative sensitivities of different tissue types by

Stages of radiopharmaceutical production
1. Extraction of radionuclide from target substance
2. Purification of the radionuclide
3. Conversion of pure radionuclide into the biologically specific form
4. Addition of excipients to make suitable for medical administration
5. Testing of dose and quality

Figure 10.6 Stages of radiopharmaceutical production.

including a tissue weighting factor (W_T) for each tissue type. For example, gonads, bone marrow, and the lens have a high W_T. The effective dose of radiation to a body is therefore calculated from the range of equivalent doses for the different tissues involved. It is measured in Sieverts.

Radiation protection guidelines
The International Commission on Radiological Protection (ICRP)[3] issues guidelines that dictate that exposure to patients and staff should be kept as low as reasonably achievable (ALARA principle). Exposure of an individual should be no more than an effective dose of 20mSv/year averaged over 5 years for an occupational worker, and 1mSv/year for a member of the public.

A concept of 'dose constraint' is also suggested by the ICRP. It is the level of radiation that should be achievable in a well-managed operation, typically 5mSv/year for a hospital nuclear medicine department. Figure 10.7 shows typical radiation doses for a variety of common procedures.

By way of comparison, an average member of the population can expect 2.8mSv/year from the natural background, and an additional 0.4mSv/year from manufactured sources.

Additional care must be taken in children, whose tissues are more susceptible than those of adults and therefore doses must be reduced to a minimum. Specific additional risks must be taken into account, for example the concentration of ^{99m}Tc-medronate methylene diphosphonate (^{99m}Tc-MDP) in the epiphyses of long bones[4].

RENAL STUDIES

The ability to incorporate radionuclides into molecules with specific renal handling properties has given nuclear medicine a central role in the investigation of kidney function.

Effective radiation dose for common procedures	
Investigation	**Effective dose (mSv)**
Renogram	3
Bone scan	8
Intravenous urography	4
Chest radiograph	0.05

Figure 10.7 Effective radiation dose for common procedures.

Radiopharmaceuticals

The commonly used radiopharmaceuticals are shown in relation to nephron function in Figure 10.8.

Filtered agents

The metal chelate ^{51}Cr-ethylenediaminetetraacetic acid (^{51}Cr-EDTA) gained acceptance as a suitable marker for glomerular filtration in the late 1960s[5]. It is radiochemically pure, stable, and clearance studies demonstrated a high correlation with inulin[6]. The tracer doses used for glomerular filtration rate (GFR) measurement produce low radiation, which make it ideal for use in children. The only drawback is its lack of availability in some centers.

^{99m}Tc-Diethylenetriamine pentaacetic acid (^{99m}Tc-DTPA), however, is readily available and therefore widely used[7], but care must be taken with the cold kit used and its preparation, as protein-binding can be a problem. Extrarenal clearance can be demonstrated at lower levels of function. Good correlation with inulin is, however, reported.

Secreted agents

Some substances are effectively cleared on a single pass through the kidney by a combination of partial filtration and active tubular secretion. The resultant clearance equates to the total renal plasma flow rather than the fraction filtered. One such substance is ^{123}I-hippuran, a derivative of the traditional marker for effective renal plasma flow (ERPF), para-aminohippuric acid. The high extraction fraction leads to excellent target-to-background ratios during renography[8]. Maximum renal concentration is reached after only 5 minutes. As it is a cyclotron-produced radionuclide, its distribution is expensive and limited. It has therefore been largely replaced by the alternative radiopharmaceutical ^{99m}Tc-mercaptoacetyltriglycine (^{99m}Tc-MAG3), an analog of ortho-iodohippuran, introduced in 1986. Tubular secretion with ^{99m}Tc-MAG3 is not as active – it produces a clearance only 60% of that given by ^{123}I-hippuran. Studies of the renographic use of both hippuran and ^{99m}Tc-MAG3 show comparable results[9–11] and ^{99m}Tc-MAG3 is now the radiopharmaceutical of choice for renography.

Cellular uptake

^{99m}Tc-Dimercaptosuccinic acid (^{99m}Tc-DMSA), originally introduced as a chelating agent for heavy metal poisoning, accumulates in the cytoplasm of proximal tubule cells. As it is largely protein bound, little is filtered, but it is actively extracted from the blood by the tubule cells. This process is relatively slow, with only 50% of the injected bolus retained in the kidney at 1 hour. The resultant distribution makes ^{99m}Tc-DMSA the drug of choice for high-quality renal cortical imaging.

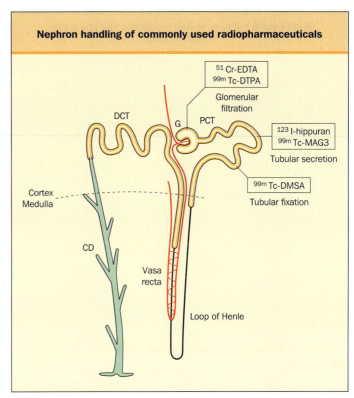

Nephron handling of commonly used radiopharmaceuticals

Figure 10.8 Nephron handling of commonly used radiopharmaceuticals. CD, collecting duct; DCT, distal convoluted tubule; ^{99m}Tc-DMSA, dimercaptosuccinic acid; ^{99m}Tc-DTPA, diethylenetriamine pentaacetic acid; ^{51}Cr-EDTA, ethylenediaminetetraacetic acid; G, glomerulus; ^{99m}Tc-MAG3, mercaptoacetyltriglycine; PCT, proximal convoluted tubule.

CLEARANCE STUDIES

In clinical practice different indications for measuring renal function have different requirements for accuracy and reproducibility. Measurement of the plasma concentration of endogenous creatinine provides an approximate assessment of glomerular filtration suitable for day-to-day management. A significant rise in plasma creatinine may not be apparent until the GFR is as low as 30% of normal[12] (Fig. 10.9). In patients who require more long-term monitoring of renal function, irreversible kidney damage may pass unrecognized if a more accurate assessment of GFR is not obtained[13].

For accurate and reproducible GFR estimation in clinical practice, the plasma clearance should be measured by a marker that behaves as plasma (i.e. is inert, freely filtered at the glomerulus, passes through the tubules without reabsorption or active secretion and is excreted by the renal route alone). Both ^{51}Cr-EDTA and ^{99m}Tc-DTPA have been shown to be satisfactory for this purpose, and have replaced the more difficult to handle fructose polymer inulin, widely regarded as the gold standard.

Classic clearance

The classic method for clearance measurement involves the establishment and measurement of a constant plasma concentration (P) by continuous infusion followed by accurate urine volume (V) and urine concentration measurements (U) over a time interval (t; Fig. 10.10). Clearance is then equal to

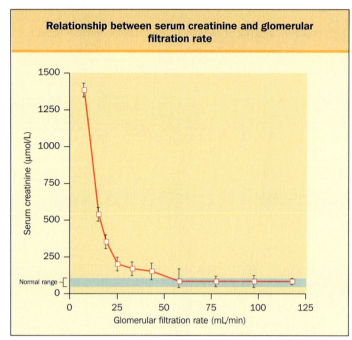

Figure 10.9 Relationship between serum creatinine and glomerular filtration rate.

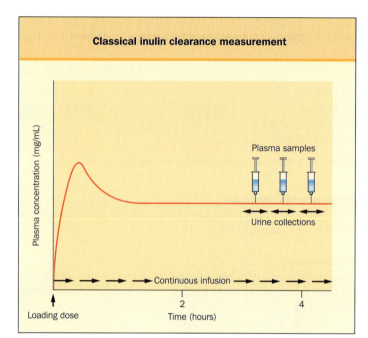

Figure 10.10 Classical inulin clearance measurement.

UV/P (mL/min). To take account of patient size, the clearance measurement is standardized for surface area using equation (10.1)[14].

$$\text{Surface area} = 0.024265 \times (\text{height})^{0.3964} \times (\text{weight})^{0.5378} \quad (10.1)$$

Single injection clearance techniques

The classic methodology is impractical for routine medical practice, although it remains the only accurate method for very low renal clearances. It has largely been replaced by single injection techniques[15]. Under these circumstances, equilibrium is not reached as the plasma level declines steadily. Figure 10.11 shows a typical plasma concentration decay curve. The amount excreted becomes the area under the curve and is equal to the product of the clearance (Cl) and the plasma concentration C, over time 'dt', equation (10.2).

$$\text{Plasma excreted} = \frac{(\text{Cl} \times \text{C})}{\text{dt}} \quad (10.2)$$

The curve can be obtained by taking a large number of plasma samples, or more realistically by applying a pharmacokinetic model to describe it mathematically. In this way the number of samples and the time period for measurement can be reduced. When the log of the plasma concentration is plotted (Fig. 10.12), it is seen that the final part of the decay curve approximates to a straight line. Using this monoexponential model a value for clearance (Cl_1) can be calculated from the injected dose (Q_0), the gradient 'λ', and the intercept C_0, equation (10.3).

$$Cl_1 = \frac{(Q_0 \times \lambda)}{C_0} \quad (10.3)$$

A minimum of two plasma samples is required for this method. This model does not, however, take into account the shaded area in Figure 10.12, which corresponds to early incomplete

mixing. From empiric studies with ^{51}Cr-EDTA, Brochner-Mortensen demonstrated that the shaded area remains virtually constant over a wide range of clearance values, but that the total area under the curve decreases as the clearance increases[16]. He proposed an empiric correction factor, equation (10.4), which is now widely adopted.

$$Cl = 0.990778Cl_1 - 0.001218(Cl_1)^2 \quad (10.4)$$

The investigation requires a bolus injection of a carefully calibrated dose followed by plasma samples taken at carefully noted times approximately 3 and 4 hours after the injection.

Alternative multiexponential models may also be adopted, but require more blood samples and offer little advantage in terms of accuracy[17]. Other investigators have proposed a single injection, single sample technique that estimates apparent volume of distribution (V) at time (t) 3–6 hours after injection of the initial dose (Q_0), and uses this to calculate clearance, equation (10.5)[18].

$$Cl = \frac{1}{(t/V) + 0.0016} \ln \frac{-Q_0}{VC_t} \quad (10.5)$$

Correction factors are also required for nonuniform distribution and early incomplete mixing.

RENAL IMAGING

Renography

Renography is the study of the uptake, transit, and elimination by the kidney of an intravenous dose of radiopharmaceutical. The kidney and bladder regions are scanned using a gamma camera and consecutive time frames analyzed to produce time–activity curves for chosen regions of interest (ROI). The best radiopharmaceuticals for this purpose are the actively secreted agents, which have maximal uptake by the kidney and produce the optimal target-to-background ratio. The radiopharmaceutical of choice is now ^{99m}Tc-MAG3.

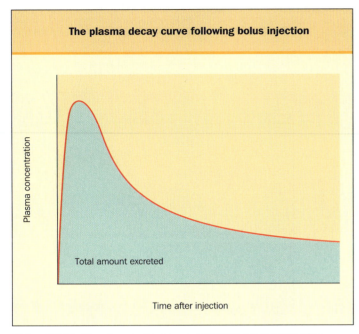

Figure 10.11 The plasma decay curve following bolus injection.

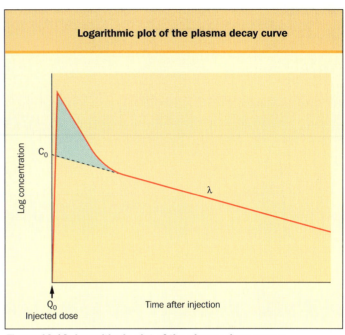

Figure 10.12 Logarithmic plot of the plasma decay curve.

Protocol

At the start of the test, the patient should be well hydrated, given 500mL of water to drink, and asked to empty his or her bladder. The investigation is usually conducted with the patient sitting in front of the camera (Fig. 10.13). The gamma camera field must include both kidneys and the bladder. The patient should adopt a comfortable position that can be maintained for at least 40 minutes. Very small infants may be lain on the camera.

The typical adult dose of 50–70MBq ^{99m}Tc-MAG3 is injected intravenously, with care taken to avoid extravasation or contamination. Frame rates of 10–20 seconds are utilized, although in many centers digital archiving and display systems are now available for storage. Scanning proceeds from the moment of injection until 20–40 minutes into the study, and at least 15 minutes after the injection of diuretic in the case of diuresis renography. Analog images are produced every 5 minutes. At the end of the procedure, the patient again empties the bladder. This reduces the radiation dose to the bladder and enables a check on the rate of urine production, which helps with interpretation.

To analyze the data collected ROIs are defined over both kidneys and the bladder. A further ROI is obtained for blood and/or tissue background, usually chosen as a C-shaped elliptic area around the kidneys (Fig. 10.14). The number of counts that occur in each ROI is computed for each time frame and the counts are plotted against time. The background count is subtracted from the other three. The resultant time–activity curves constitute the renogram (Fig. 10.14).

Interpretation

Curve analysis

Each point on a curve represents the number of counts (minus background) over a ROI at a given time. It follows that a positive gradient occurs when more radiopharmaceutical arrives within a ROI than leaves. If the curve is negative, there is an overall egress of tracer.

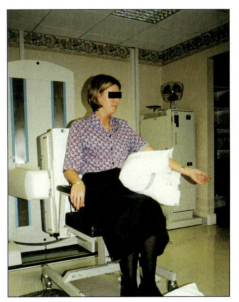

Figure 10.13 Patient position in renography.

The normal kidney curves have three classic phases (Fig. 10.15). The first is a rapid rise in counts immediately following intravenous injection; it reflects the speed of injection and the blood supply to the kidney. The second phase has a slightly more gradual slope. It represents the renal handling of the radiopharmaceutical, and transfer across tubular cell or glomerular membrane into the lumen of the nephrons. Consequently, it is liable to be affected by poor uptake and impaired renal handling. This part of the curve continues to rise as long as more radiopharmaceutical is being extracted from the plasma than leaves the region of interest in the urine. In the normal kidney, the curve peaks between 2 and 5 minutes. This marks the beginning of the third phase and coincides with the time that activity starts to become distinguishable in the bladder. During the third phase, although tracer continues to arrive in the kidney, the characteristics of this part of the curve reflect mainly

10

137

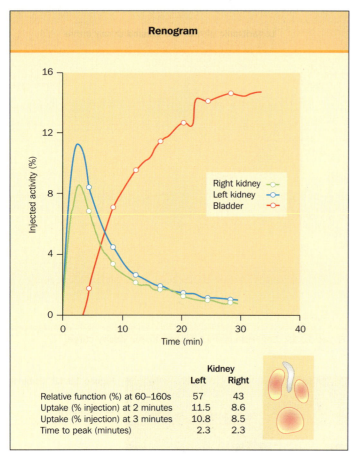

Figure 10.14 Renogram.

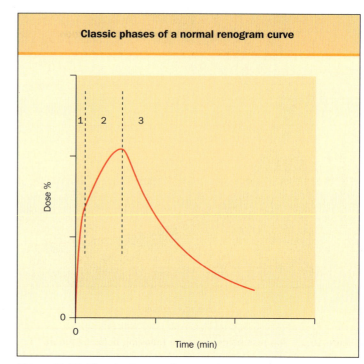

Figure 10.15 Classic phases of a normal renogram curve. 1, uptake phase; 2, renal handling phase; 3, drainage phase

the efficiency of excretion of tracer in the urine. A normal pattern virtually excludes any degree of obstruction.

Renal function and relative function

Evaluation of the early rising part of the renogram curve provides an estimate of renal function[19]. It is also possible to calculate the relative or 'split' function of each kidney. Assuming both kidneys are placed equidistant to the detector, relative function can be calculated by counting the activity under each background-corrected curve between 1 and 2 or 1 and 2.5 minutes after injection. Individual relative function is then expressed in percentage terms as the ratio of the mean uptake for each kidney to the sum of the two[20]. Obstruction depresses the slope of the second phase to a degree dependent on its duration and extent and therefore it affects relative function.

Obstruction

The earliest effect of obstruction on the third phase is to flatten the usual upper concavity of the curve (Fig. 10.16). Even if both kidneys exhibit equal percentage function, such patients should be followed carefully and further investigations made. Increasing levels of obstruction lead to a persisting phase 2 with a more upward curve (Fig. 10.16, curves b and c). As obstruction proceeds, function is depressed, and uptake is reduced until it becomes difficult to comment on the excretory pattern. Uptake is finally little more than the background count and the appearances are those of a nonfunctioning kidney.

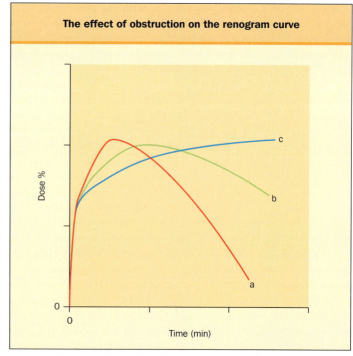

Figure 10.16 The effect of obstruction on the renogram curve. a, mild obstruction; b, moderate obstruction; c, high-grade obstruction.

If an obstructive curve is obtained without apparent cause, one of a number of explanations must be sought. It may result from inadequate hydration (Fig. 10.17). Although the kidney continues to extract tracer from the renal artery, the urine flow is too slow to wash the 'hot' urine out from the region of interest. It may also simply be the result of a dilated pelvicaliceal system. As

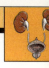

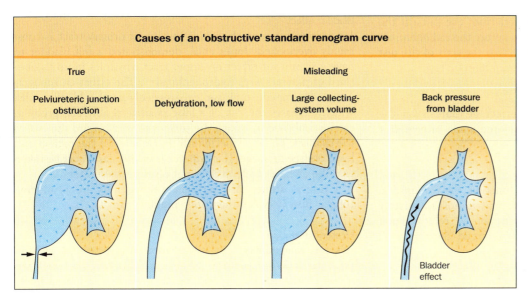

Causes of an 'obstructive' standard renogram curve

True	Misleading		
Pelviureteric junction obstruction	Dehydration, low flow	Large collecting-system volume	Back pressure from bladder

Bladder effect

Figure 10.17 True and misleading causes of an 'obstructive' standard renogram curve.

the flow at the pelviureteric junction equals the rate of urine production, dilution of the tracer in the urine in the collecting system results in only small diluted quantities of the tracer leaving the ROI. The continued net increase in the amount of tracer leads to a persistent rising curve. Finally, it may be the result of a bladder effect.

It is clinically essential to be able to distinguish genuine obstruction from these nonpathologic effects. Two modifications to standard renography have been developed to address this problem, namely diuresis renography and parenchymal transit-time analysis. The latter is technically demanding and rarely used clinically[21].

Diuresis renography

The principle of diuresis renography was first described in the late 1960s[22] and popularized by O'Reilly as a simple method to differentiate patients with equivocal obstruction of the upper urinary tract[23].

The basic principle of diuresis renography is simple. If a system is genuinely obstructed, flow is impaired at high and low urinary flow rates (Fig. 10.18). In contrast, slow elimination caused by urinary stasis alone responds to an increase in the urinary flow rate with a rapid washout of tracer. An increased flow at the time of renography is produced by the intravenous administration of a diuretic.

Practice and protocol

The diuretic universally chosen is the sulfonamide 'loop' diuretic frusemide (furosemide) in a dose of 0.5mg/kg (40mg in adults). In a well-hydrated patient with moderate-to-normal renal function an increase in flow from 1–3mL/minute to 20–40mL/minute may be expected[24]. It is essential that diuresis renography is conducted in a standardized manner with meticulous attention to detail. Protocols and investigation strategies have been set out in the 1996 Consensus on Diuresis Renography[25]. Patient preparation and choice of radiopharmaceutical is identical to that for standard renography.

The original description proposed injection of the diuretic 20 minutes after the radiopharmaceutical, referred to as 'F+20'

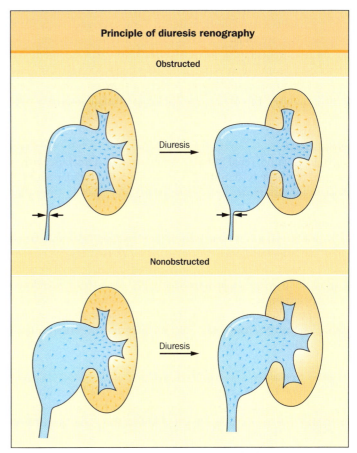

Principle of diuresis renography

Obstructed

Diuresis

Nonobstructed

Diuresis

Figure 10.18 Principle of diuresis renography. (Top) Increased urine production leads to an accumulation of tracer. (Bottom) Increased urine production leads to a corresponding increased washout.

diuresis renography. This enables the urodynamics through the upper tract to be studied without modification or manipulation. If rapid washout is observed, diuretic injection may be considered unnecessary, thus reducing the small but not insignificant inconvenience to the patient that results from diuretic injection.

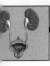

If the maximum flow rate is required from the outset, the diuretic should be injected 15 minutes before the radiopharmaceutical (F–15 diuresis renography), so that the start of the test coincides with the maximum effect of the diuretic[26].

Interpretation

A number of factors influence the effect of diuresis on the renogram curve and must all be considered when interpreting results, as discussed below.

Hydration

Even in the presence of normal renal function, the response to diuretic may by suboptimal if the patient is not adequately hydrated. Some authors have chosen not to rely on oral hydration alone, and have suggested a forced diuresis with intravenous hypotonic saline prior to the study[27].

Renal function

The level of renal function is a major determinant of the diuretic-induced flow rate. A linear relationship has been observed between diuretic-induced flow rate and both GFR and ERPF. Care must therefore be taken in the interpretation of diuresis renography in renal units with expected reduced function. From regression data, a single kidney GFR of <16mL/minute is unlikely to achieve a flow rate greater than 10mL/minute, the value chosen for perfusion pressure flow studies[24].

Renal disease

Certain isolated renal tubular disorders may interfere with a normal response to diuretic, for example acute tubular necrosis or Fanconi syndrome.

Collecting system volume

The primary application of diuresis renography is to determine whether a dilated upper urinary tract represents obstruction or merely stasis. Normally, the increased flow after a diuretic is sufficient to wash out the tracer that accumulates in a dilated renal pelvis and confirms the absence of obstruction. If, however, the collecting system is massively dilated, the increased flow may still be insufficient despite a normal diuretic response and the absence of obstruction[28].

System compliance

The volume of the collecting system is not fixed, but changes with alterations in intrapelvic pressure and tone in the pelvic and ureteric wall. The degree to which volume changes is a reflection of the compliance of the system. Compliance is variable and can influence interpretation of the diuresis renogram. A compliant renal pelvis dilates in response to diuresis, while the pressure needed to overcome the resistance remains low. In a rigid system such as an intrarenal pelvis, in which hydronephrosis is minimal, intrapelvic pressures in the presence of good function may build to overcome obstruction and the resultant diuresis renogram appears normal even though obstruction is present. Conversely, in a very compliant system, distention may occur without elevation of intrapelvic pressures, and an obstructed renogram may be obtained in the absence of significant obstruction.

Bladder effect

Interaction between the lower and upper urinary tract is commonly overlooked. Jones et al. demonstrated a full bladder to have a significant effect on upper tract dynamics in up to one-third of patients with hydronephrosis[29]. The effect on renography is to impede drainage progressively as the bladder fills, which increases the risk of a false positive result. The problem can be abolished by asking the patient to void toward the end of the drainage phase, or better still to catheterize the patient and leave on free drainage. If a catheter is *in situ*, care must be taken that the catheter balloon does not obstruct the ureters.

Ureteric stents also influence renography by producing tubular flow between the upper and lower tracts.

Ureteric dilatation

Diuresis renography is usually used to investigate the dilated renal pelvis. When performing a renographic study in which the ureter is also dilated, consideration must be given to a likely point of obstruction. If the region of interest is drawn around the kidney and pelvis alone, there is the danger that diuresis flushes the radioactive urine out of the region of interest and into the capacious ureter, without causing a true washout through the suspected point of obstruction. A false negative result may follow. It is therefore important to include in the region of interest the whole collecting system proximal to the suspected level of obstruction.

Tandem obstruction

A note of caution must be added regarding diuresis renography. It is unable to demonstrate easily obstructing lesions at multiple levels – its results reflect the tightest obstruction only. Radiographs must be used in conjunction to help with diagnosis in this rare and complex situation.

Curve analysis

Three classic responses (normal, obstructive, and nonobstructive or equivocal) were described in the original account of (F+20) diuresis renography (Fig. 10.19)[23]; a fourth (delayed compensation) was added recently[30]. Application to types of obstructive uropathy are described in Chapter 23.

Normal response, Type I

A normal washout is obtained at resting flow rates before the diuretic is given (Fig. 10.14). If the renogram is repeated after a diuretic injection it is possible that the system may decompensate and obstruct at diuretic flow rates. This is rare, as it is unusual to have significant obstruction without dilatation, and the latter should be detectable on the standard curve.

Obstructive response, Type II

The rising curve continues to rise despite injection of the diuretic, indicating obstruction (Fig. 10.20). Experimental evidence suggests that anything but an exponential clearance curve should be considered as evidence of obstruction[28]. Before accepting the conclusion of a definite obstructive response, the clinician must consider all possible reasons why it may be falsely positive, as discussed previously – unrecognized dehydration, poor renal function, massive dilatation, or a bladder effect. Hydration and bladder effects can be controlled. A volume

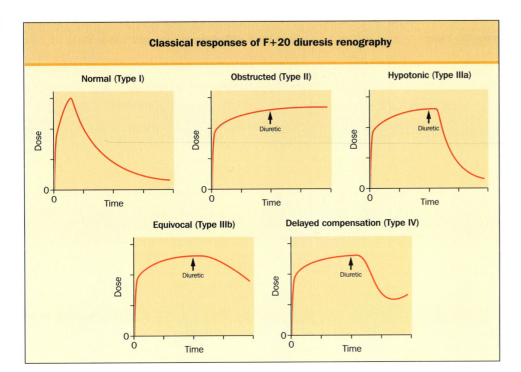

Figure 10.19 Responses of diuresis renography.

effect can be predicted from imaging studies and the analog images. If the available information suggests that function may be markedly reduced (e.g. single kidney GFR <16mL/minute), the result must be scrutinized. Obstruction may be present, but the increase in flow may not have been sufficient to wash out the tracer. Under these circumstances an F–15 study may be considered, but the increase in flow compared with the F+20 study is likely to be minimal when function is poor.

Nonobstructive response, Type IIIa

An initially obstructive rising curve falls on injection of the diuretic (Fig. 10.21). It indicates that at the diuretic flow rate achieved, the collecting system drains freely. Dilatation is the result of stasis rather than obstruction.

Equivocal response, Type IIIb

The initial obstructive rising curve on injection of diuretic neither washes out briskly nor continues to rise. The response is said to be equivocal (Fig. 10.22). It must be established whether the result reflects a good diuretic response and a partially obstructed outlet, or a suboptimal diuretic response and normal nonobstructed outlet. It may also represent a massively dilated system that an optimal diuretic response still cannot wash out.

Delayed decompensation, Type IV

The 'fourth' response was first described by Homsy et al. as a 'delayed double-peak pattern'[31]. The initial wash out in response to the diuretic is good, but then the curve flattens or even starts to rise (Fig. 10.23). The explanation rests with the steady increase in diuretic-induced urinary flow rate that does not peak until 15 minutes after the injection. During the resting and early diuretic phases, the pertaining flow can be transported by the pelviureteric junction. Eventually, the flow rate reaches a level at which the system under stress can no longer transmit the urine load. It decompensates and further dilatation occurs.

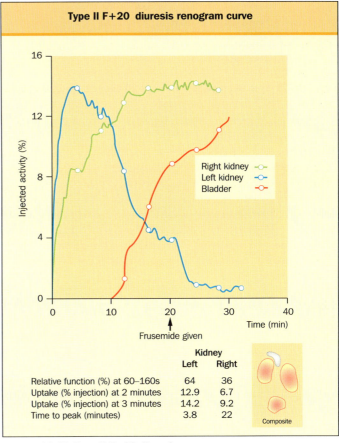

Figure 10.20 Type II F+20 diuresis renogram curve.

	Kidney	
	Left	Right
Relative function (%) at 60–160s	64	36
Uptake (% injection) at 2 minutes	12.9	6.7
Uptake (% injection) at 3 minutes	14.2	9.2
Time to peak (minutes)	3.8	22

Outflow obstruction may even increase as a result. The balance is tipped and the amount of tracer that enters the ROI drawn around the kidney exceeds the amount eliminated. The curve starts to rise once more.

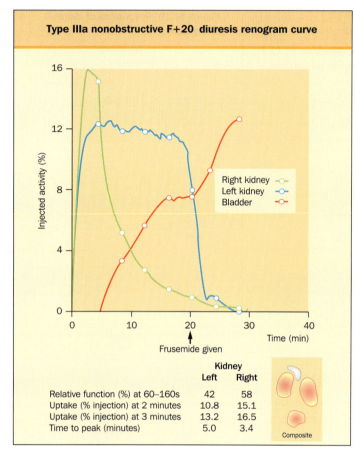

Figure 10.21 Type IIIa nonobstructive F+20 diuresis renogram curve.

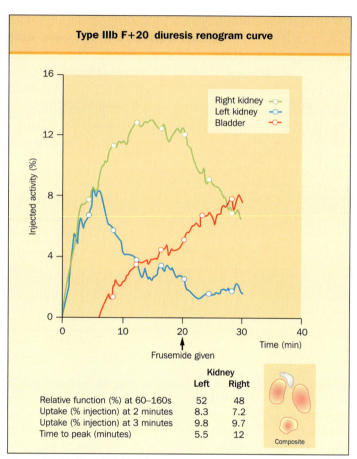

Figure 10.22 Type IIIb F+20 equivocal diuresis renogram curve.

F–15 diuresis renography

Type IIIb equivocal and the Type IV delayed decompensation curves may reflect subtotal obstruction. Injection of the diuretic 15 minutes before the radiopharmaceutical coincides the maximum diuresis with the onset of the study. The increased flow rate of the F–15 renogram is sufficient to convert the majority of equivocal results into 'obstructed or nonobstructed'. The three responses of the F–15 renogram are shown in Figure 10.24. Relative function estimation is unaffected by the earlier injection of frusemide[32].

Radionuclide clearance half-times

Some investigators prefer a more quantitative assessment of the derived renogram curves than that based on curve pattern alone. Radionuclide clearance half times, which measure the time taken to clear half of the activity present in the kidneys after the injection of frusemide, are the most popular. At least seven different methodologies for quantitating $T\frac{1}{2}$ have been described[33]. Unfortunately, these methods suffer from problems in defining the normal and obstructed ranges and such indices have a considerable range of equivocal results. The author's favored approach is to study the curve pattern as a whole and therefore use all the information available in reaching a diagnosis.

Diuresis renography and renal pelvic pressure measurement

Diuresis renography is interpreted in the absence of knowledge of intrapelvic pressure changes. Normal flow is equated with no

obstruction, and reduced flow with obstruction. The possibility exists that in the presence of partial obstruction, a 'normal' flow, and therefore normal diuresis renogram, may still be achieved providing the pressure gradient across the obstruction is increased. This has not, however, been noted when pelvic pressure measurements have been made at the time of diuresis renography[34]. Poulsen et al. found no correlation between the renographic response and pelvic pressures[35].

Comparison with perfusion pressure flow studies

An alternative method to assess obstruction, the perfusion pressure flow study (PPFS), was proposed by Whitaker in 1973 and gained popularity at about the same time as diuresis renography[36]. Saline or contrast medium is perfused across the obstruction at a fixed flow rate, usually 10mL/minute. Obstruction is assumed if the pressure in the infusate rises above $22cmH_2O$ (2.16kPa), whereas a rise $<15cmH_2O$ (1.47kPa) excludes obstruction.

When assessing both methods, the important question is not whether the urinary tract can deal with a high urine flow rate, but whether the urinary tract can, under normal physiologic circumstances, handle the volume presented to it without an adverse effect on renal function or without producing symptoms. Every system has its maximal transmission rate above which it decompensates. If physiologic flow rates do not exceed this, it is of little significance. In a poorly functioning kidney, this maximum may be <10 mL/minute; a PPFS would prove positive, but would

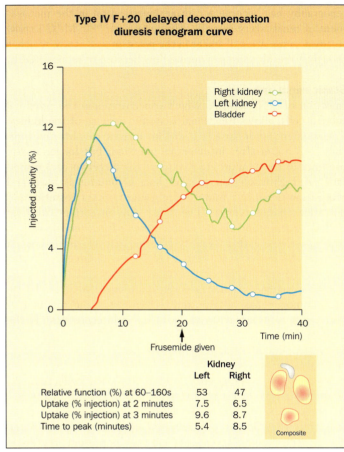

Figure 10.23 Type IV F+20 delayed decompensation diuresis renogram curve.

conditions of, for example, a forced alcoholic diuresis. The result would be the pain of intermittent obstruction. Under these circumstances a positive diuresis renogram may be obtained, but pressure rises during PPFS would not be encountered unless the flow rate is increased to 18mL/minute or more. Clearly, all factors must be considered when interpreting both types of investigation.

Transplantation

Radionuclide studies that help to quantify perfusion and function of a renal graft have assumed an important role. In the early days after transplantation, the graft may have to be monitored as frequently as three times a week until the patient is discharged or the graft is removed. Radionuclide studies may anticipate biochemical changes of rejection by as much as 48 hours. Monitoring should comprise a good early baseline study followed by reproducible and consistent repeat testing. In this way the confident recognition of lack of rejection can lead to a minimal use of immunosuppressive therapy.

Perfusion studies

Passage of a rapidly administered intravenous bolus of ^{99m}Tc-pertechnetate across the graft provides an assessment of renal perfusion. Pertechnetate is ideally suited as it produces low radiation and has a low renal uptake (and therefore high vascular transit). The gamma camera is positioned over the graft with the aorta also in view. As soon as the bolus reaches the lower aorta, 0.5 second frames are collected for 60 seconds. ROIs are drawn around the graft (excluding the underlying vessels) and the iliac artery (Fig. 10.25), and time–activity curves are produced (Fig. 10.25). Figure 10.26 illustrates typical perfusion changes.

Renography

The radiopharmaceutical of choice is ^{99m}Tc-MAG3. Acute rejection is indicated by reduced uptake, prolonged accumulation, and delayed excretion. By the addition of a 45 minute blood

be meaningless clinically. The converse may be true. A narrowed pelviureteric outlet in a healthy young adult may decompensate at 18 mL/minute, a flow rate that might well be exceeded during

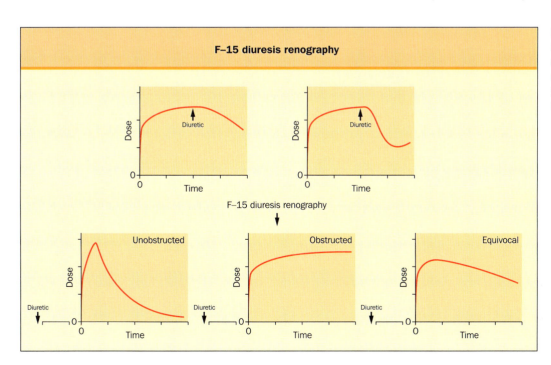

Figure 10.24 F–15 diuresis renography. (Top) Type IIIb equivocal and the Type IV delayed decompensation curves can be resolved by (bottom) F–15 diuresis renography.

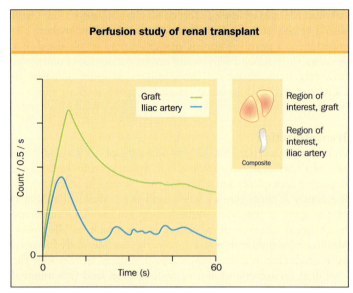

Figure 10.25 Perfusion study of renal transplant. Angioscintigraphy with 99mTc-pertechnetate. (Left) Curves and (right) analog image demonstrating regions of interest.

sample, the clearance of 99mTc-MAG3 can also be measured, which provides additional information to monitor function.

Renovascular hypertension

In 1983, Majd et al. noted a drastic unilateral reduction in 99mTc-DTPA uptake on renography in a patient with renal artery stenosis who was taking the angiotensin-converting enzyme inhibitor captopril[37]. Withdrawal of the drug led to normal bilateral 99mTc-DTPA uptake on a repeat renogram performed several days later[37]. The explanation of this phenomenon is the high level of angiotensin II found in patients with renovascular hypertension. This causes efferent arteriolar vasoconstriction, which preserves transglomerular filtration pressure and GFR. If angiotensin II is blocked by an angiotensin-converting enzyme inhibitor, the vasoconstriction is relieved and the GFR falls (Fig. 10.27). Captopril

renography has become a routine investigation in the management of renal artery stenosis. Hippuran and 99mTc-MAG3 show steady accumulation of tracer in the postcaptopril study, which is thought to result from slow urine flow because of reduced GFR.

Static renal imaging

Injection of 99mTc-DMSA, which concentrates in the proximal tubular cells, allows functional anatomic imaging of the kidney. The standard adult dose is 100MBq. Images are obtained typically 2–3 hours after intravenous injection, but longer in the presence of renal failure, to maximize the target-to-background ratio. A high-resolution parallel hole collimator is used and acquisition times of 5 minutes are used to obtain posterior and posterior–oblique views. The latter are important to help exclude scarring and also to enable relative function calculation. Anterior views with an empty bladder may be needed when scanning for an ectopic kidney. Use of a pinhole collimator enables higher resolution views of each kidney.

The appearances of normal kidneys are shown in Figure 10.28, with homogeneous distribution in the cortex and medulla. A number of factors may cause confusion in interpretation of the images:
- overlapping of left splenic margin;
- fetal lobulation; and
- obstruction or reflux may leave urine in the collecting systems, which may cause overestimation of relative function.

An abnormal scan is characterized by a change in relative function and/or an absent or decreased uptake over part of the cortex. Alternatively, an indentation may be present. If cortical thickness is maintained, the changes are more likely to be acute; with cortical loss, chronic scarring is more likely (Fig. 10.29).

BLADDER IMAGING

The importance of radionuclide cystography is found in pediatric urology in the investigation and management of vesicoureteric reflux. It has the advantage over conventional micturating cystography of a low radiation dose.

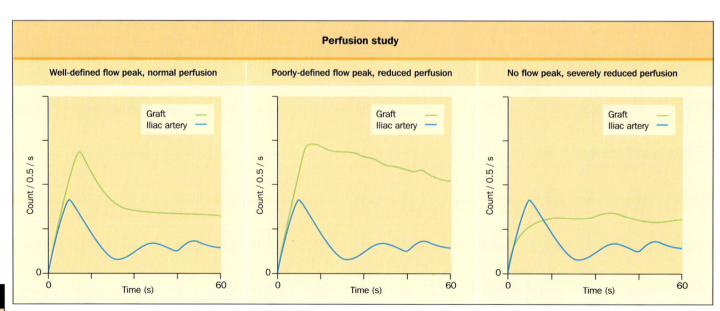

Figure 10.26 Perfusion study.

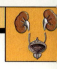

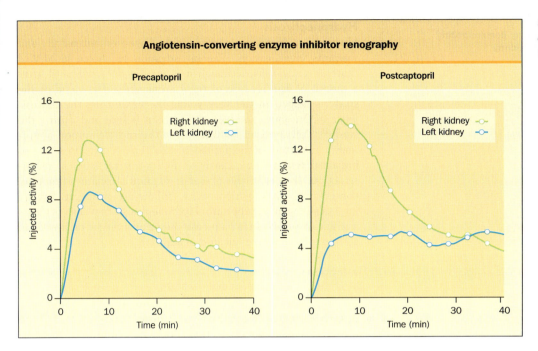

Angiotensin-converting enzyme inhibitor renography

Precaptopril

Postcaptopril

Figure 10.27 Angiotensin-converting enzyme inhibitor renography. The left kidney has the hypertension etiology.

Direct radionuclide cystography

Direct radionuclide cystography requires instillation of a radio-pharmaceutical into the bladder directly via a catheter. It is indicated in children who are not yet toilet-trained. Following catheterization and drainage, ^{99m}Tc-pertechnetate (20MBq) in saline is instilled until the bladder is full. The procedure is conducted on the gamma camera with the bladder region and both kidneys in view. Its main advantage is the low radiation dose, 20th that of a conventional micturating cystogram. The disadvantages are the need for a catheter and the lack of imaging of the urethra in the male child.

Indirect radionuclide cystography

Indirect radionuclide cystography is a more physiologic study, but only possible in children who are toilet-trained. At 30–60 minutes after an injection of ^{99m}Tc-MAG3, the well-hydrated child is asked to void in front of the gamma camera (a quiet room with as few personnel as possible is essential for good cooperation). The bladder and kidney regions are scanned and 1 second frames obtained, from which time–activity curves and cine replay views can be obtained. If the voided volume is measured and its activity counted, bladder volume, residual, and flow rate can all be quantified. A typical study that indicates reflux is shown in Figure 10.30. Indirect radionuclide cystography is the only technique that allows the assessment of both renal reflux and bladder function under physiologic conditions, as well as the effect of micturition on upper tract drainage and the difference between a true postmicturition residue and a false residue caused by secondary filling from dilated upper tracts.

PEDIATRIC CONSIDERATIONS

Nuclear medicine studies require a happy, relaxed cooperative child. The attitude and expertise of the staff is therefore of

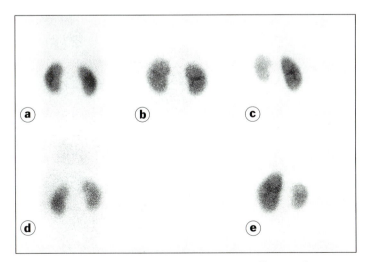

Figure 10.28 Appearances of normal kidneys on ^{99m}Tc-DMSA scan.
(a) Posterior; (b) anterior; (c) posterior pinhole (showing the column of Bertin); (d) right posterior–oblique; (e) left posterior–oblique.

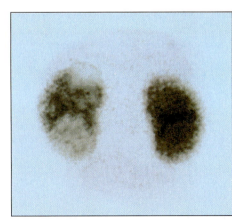

Figure 10.29 Pinhole posterior views of ^{99m}Tc-DMSA scan in a 2-year-old child showing defects in both poles in acute urinary tract infection.

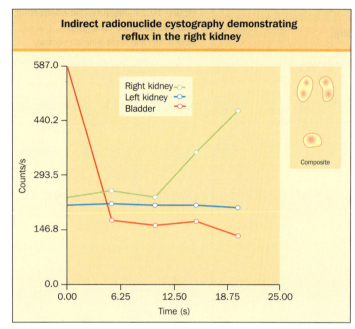

Figure 10.30 Indirect radionuclide cystography demonstrating reflux in the right kidney.

paramount importance. It should only be the toddler age group in which sedation, usually in the form of midazolam, need be considered.

Small children may be placed supine on the gamma camera. A vacuum extractor mattress to help maintain a constant position is extremely useful. Children are more susceptible to the stochastic effects of radiation, so doses should be scaled down on the basis of weight or surface area to ensure the minimum effective dose is used.

Renal immaturity must be taken into account when considering renal scanning. Tubular function is poor in the early months, but rises to 80–90% of adult levels at 1 year. For this reason, ^{99m}Tc-DMSA scans should not be performed before 12 weeks. In the neonate GFR and ERPF are low and then rise steadily to reach adult levels at 2 years. The diuretic response is also unpredictable in the first 4–6 weeks of life and must be considered when performing diuresis renography in the first year of life.

Hydronephrosis

Upper tract dilatation is increasingly diagnosed antenatally and warrants investigation. The investigation of choice is MAG3 diuresis renography, although it is usually deferred until after 1 month of age because of renal immaturity. The value of the study is helped in the very young by maximizing the diuresis with a 30 minute intravenous infusion before and during the study[11]. Pelviureteric obstruction is the most common abnormality detected. Renographic obstruction in the presence of impaired relative function is an indication for surgical reconstruction. If it is in the presence of normal relative function, conservative management with follow-up scans at regular intervals may be appropriate. Hydronephrosis may also occur as a result of reflux, in which case direct or indirect radionuclide cystography may be indicated in addition.

Infection

The ultimate goal of managing children with urinary tract infection is to prevent progressive renal damage. Diagnosis of any underlying treatable pathology is therefore vital. Any child with a proved urinary tract infection should therefore have an ultrasound of the urinary tract. If the ultrasound is normal, girls >5 years of age need have no further investigation. If <5 years of age, all children require a ^{99m}Tc-DMSA scan to exclude scarring. Figure 10.31 outlines a scheme for subsequent investigation[38].

In acute pyelonephritis, a ^{99m}Tc-DMSA scan is the most sensitive investigation for confirming renal parenchymal involvement. The majority of defects have disappeared by a follow-up scan at 3–6 months. Any that remain are suggestive of scarring. Investigation should proceed as above.

BONE SCINTIGRAPHY

High phosphate uptake by immature bone provides the basis for bone imaging. Subramanian and McAfee in the early 1970s investigated a number of ^{99m}Tc-labeled phosphate compounds, for their application in bone imaging[39]. The diphosphonates were found to be the most promising, of which methyl diphosphonate (medronate) is now the most widely used. Previous radiopharmaceuticals that used nuclides such as ^{85}Sr and ^{18}F produced too high a radiation dose and took too long to clear from the body. Medronate, on the other hand, has a much higher skeletal affinity and a much more rapid blood clearance.

Figure 10.31 Investigation of infection in children.

Investigation of infection in children			
^{99m}Tc-DTPA scan	Group	Age (years)	Investigation
Normal	Girls	<1	Direct radionuclide cystography
		1–5	No further investigation
	Boys	0–5	Micturating cystourethrogram
Abnormal	Girls	<3	Direct radionuclide cystography
		>3	Indirect radionuclide cystography
	Boys	0–5	Micturating cystourethrogram
		<3	Direct radionuclide cystography
		>3	Indirect radionuclide cystography

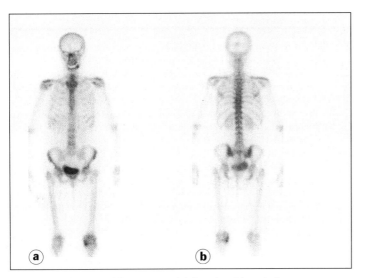

Figure 10.32 Normal bone scan. (a) Anterior; (b) posterior.

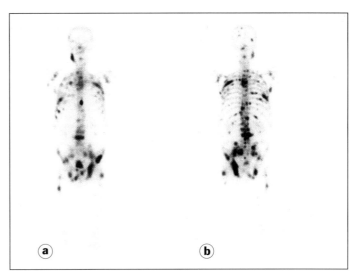

Figure 10.33 Bone scan – prostatic adenocarcinoma. (a) Anterior; (b) posterior.

Technique

A typical dose of 400–800 MBq dose of ^{99m}Tc-medronate is injected into a peripheral vein. Rapid distribution throughout the body occurs with maximal bone uptake after approximately 2 hours. Imaging is delayed a little longer to allow more time for unbound tracer to be removed. Of the tracer, 60% is eliminated via the kidneys. To increase soft-tissue elimination and reduce radiation to the bladder the patient is therefore asked to drink plenty in the interval between the injection and imaging, and to empty the bladder immediately prior to the commencement of imaging. This also minimizes obscuring of the bony pelvis by the bladder.

At 3–4 hours, image collection begins. Whole-body images are obtained using sweeps with a high-resolution collimator of both anterior and posterior projections (Fig. 10.32). Spot images of regions of particular interest may also be obtained.

Interpretation

Bone uptake is determined in part by local blood flow, but mainly by the level of osteoblastic activity of immature bone. In the normal skeleton increased activity is seen in weight-bearing areas and at points of muscle insertion. In children there is obviously high uptake in the metaphyseal–epiphyseal growth areas. Image density is affected by distance from the camera. The resultant artifacts must be appreciated and allowed for – the lumbar spine may be more prominent on the anterior views because of a marked lumbar lordosis.

Abnormally high activity is seen at the site of an injury, such as a fracture or metastasis, where there has been an attempt at a reparative process. Identification of an abnormal area of increased or decreased uptake is most readily appreciated by noting any lack of symmetry around the axial line. It is therefore important that the patient be carefully aligned for scanning to ensure no artifacts from malpositioning.

The staging of prostate adenocarcinoma is the most common indication for bone scintigraphy in urology (Fig. 10.33). The rich plexus of vertebral veins of Batson, which form valveless communications with the pelvic viscera, are thought to explain the predilection for the axial skeleton[40]. Lesions are typically seen as an irregular distribution of 'hot spots'. A solitary defect must be distinguished from a fracture, Paget's disease, or degenerative bone disease. The history and a plain radiograph help in further evaluation. Paget's extensive involvement of the whole bone or the less intense uptake around a degenerative joint can usually be differentiated from the more compact asymmetric appearance of a metastasis. A false-negative scan can occasionally result from a particularly aggressive tumor that induces little osteoblastic attempt at repair. Conversely, widespread metastases can result in a 'superscan' more typical of metabolic bone disease.

Resolution of a lesion on repeat scanning usually indicates healing; however, a hot spot can disappear or be replaced by a photopenic area as a result of complete bone destruction in advancing disease.

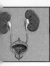

REFERENCES

1. Anger HO. Scintillation camera. Rev Sci Instrum. 1958;29;27–33.

2. World Health Organization. The medical uses of ionizing radiation. Technical Report Series No. 492. Geneva: WHO; 1972.

3. International Commission on Radiological Protection. Recommendations of the International Commission on Radiological Protection (Publication 60). Ann ICRP. 1991;21–6.

4. Administration of Radioactive Substances Advisory Committee (ARSAC). Notes for guidance on the administration of radioactive substances to persons for purposes of diagnosis, treatment or research. London: Department of Health and Social Security; 1993.

5. Stacy BD, Thorburn GD. Chromium-51 ethylenediaminetetraacetate for estimation of glomerular filtration rate. Science. 1966;152:1076–8.

6. Hagstam KE, Nordenfelt I, Svensson L, Svensson SE. Comparison of different methods for determination of glomerular filtration rate in renal disease. Scan J Clin Lab Inv. 1974:34;31–6.

7. Klopper JF, Hauser W, Watkins HL, et al. Evaluation of ⁹⁹ᵐTc-DTPA for the measurement of glomerular filtration rate. J Nucl Med. 1972;13:107–10.

8. Jewkes RF, Jayasingh K. Comparison of ¹²³I-hippuran and ⁹⁹ᵐTc-DTPA. Nucl Med Commun. 1981;2;.278–88.

9. Taylor AJR, Esh D, Fritzberg AR, et al. Comparison of ¹³¹Iodine OIH and ⁹⁹ᵐTechnetium-MAG3 renal imaging in volunteers. J Nucl Med. 1986;27:795–803.

10. Jaffre RA, Britton KE, Nimmon CC. Technetium-99m MAG3, a comparison with ¹²³Iodine and ¹³¹Iodine orthoiodohippurate in patients with renal disorders. J Nucl Med. 1988;29:147–58.

11. Hvid-Jacobsen K, Thomsen HS, Nielsen SL. Diuresis renography. A simultaneous comparison between ¹³¹I-hippuran and ⁹⁹ᵐTc-MAG3. Acta Radiol. 1990;31:83–6.

12. Gabriel R. Time to scrap creatinine clearance? Br Med J. 1986;293:1119–20.

13. Brown SCW, O'Reilly PH. Glomerular filtration rate: a neglected measurement in urological practice. Br J Urol. 1995;75:296–300.

14. Du Bois D, Du Bois EF. A formula to estimate the approximate surface area if height and weight be known. Arch Int Med. 1916;17:863.

15. Barnett HL. Renal physiology in infants and children. 1. Method for estimation of glomerular filtration rate. Proc Soc Exp Biol (NY). 1940;44:654–8.

16. Brochner-Mortensen J. A simple method for the determination of glomerular filtration rate. Scand J Clin Lab Inv. 1972;30:271–4.

17. Sapirstein LA, Vidt DG, Mandel MJ, Hanusek G. Volumes of distribution and clearances of intravenously injected creatinine in the dog. Am J Physiol. 1955;181:330–6.

18. Jacobsson L. A method for the calculation of renal clearance based on a single sample. Clin Physiol. 1983;3:297–305.

19. Gates GF. Split renal function testing using Tc-99m DTPA: a rapid technique for determining differential glomerular filtration. Clin Nucl Med. 1983;8:400–7.

20. O'Reilly PH, Shields RA, Testa HJ. Nuclear medicine in urology and nephrology, 2nd edn. London: Butterworth; 1986.

21. Whitfield HN, Britton KE, Hendry WF, et al. The distinction between obstructive uropathy and nephropathy by radioisotope transit times. Br J Urol. 1978;39:433–6.

22. Rado JP, Bano C, Tako J. Radioisotope renography during furosemide (Lasix) diuresis. Nucl Med Commun. 1968;7:212–21.

23. O'Reilly PH, Testa HJ, Lawson RS, Farrar DJ, Edwards EC. Diuresis renography in equivocal urinary tract obstruction. Br J Urol. 1978;50:76–80.

24. Brown SC, Upsdell SM, O'Reilly PH. The importance of renal function in the interpretation of diuresis renography. Br J Urol. 1992;69:121–5.

25. O'Reilly PH, Aurell M, Britton K, Kletter K, Rosenthal L, Testa T. Consensus on diuresis renography for investigating the dilated upper urinary tract. J Nucl Med. 1996;37:1872–6.

26. English PJ, Testa HJ, Lawson RS, et al. Modified method of diuresis renography for the assessment of equivocal pelviureteric obstruction. Br J Urol. 1987;59:10–14.

27. Sukhai RN, Kooy PP, Wolff ED, Scholtmeijer R.J Predictive value of ⁹⁹ᵐTc-DTPA renography studies under conditions of maximal diuresis for the functional outcome of reconstructive surgery in children with obstructive uropathy. Br J Urol. 1986;58:596–600.

28. Zechmann W. An experimental approach to explain some misinterpretations of diuresis renography. Nucl Med Commun. 1988;9:283–94.

29. Jones DA, Lupton EW, George NJR. Effect of bladder filling on upper tract urodynamics in man. Br J Urol. 1990;65:492–6.

30. O'Reilly PH. Diuresis renography. Recent advances and recommended protocols. Br J Urol. 1992;69:113–20.

31. Homsy YL, Mehta PH, Huot D, Danais S. Intermittent hydronephrosis: a diagnostic challenge. J Urol. 1988;140;1222–6.

32. Upsdell SM, Testa HJ, Lawson RS, Carroll RN, Edwards EC. The uses and interpretation of modified diuresis renography. Contrib Nephrol. ed: Blaufox MD, Hollenberg NK, Raynaud C. 1990;79:103–7. Radionuclides in Nephro-Urology. Basel; Karger.

33. Conway JJ. 'Well-tempered' diuresis renography: its historical development, physiological and technical pitfalls, and standardized technique protocol. Semin Nucl Med. 1992;22:74–84.

34. Israel AR, Mininberg D. Personal communication. In: Diagnostic techniques in urology. O'Reilly PH, George NJR, Weiss RM, eds. London: WB Saunders; 1982:420.

35. Poulsen EU, Frokjaer J, Taagehoj-Jensen F, et al. Diuresis renography and simultaneous renal pelvic pressure in hydronephrosis. J Urol. 1987;138:272–5.

36. Whitaker RH. Methods of assessing obstruction in dilated ureters. Br J Urol. 1973;45:15–22.

37. Majd M, Potter BM, Guzzetta PC, et al. Effect of captopril on efficacy of renal scintigraphy in detection of renal artery stenosis. J Nucl Med. 1983;24:23 (Abstract).

38. Gordon I. Urinary tract infection in paediatrics: the role of diagnostic imaging. Br J Radiol. 1990;63:507–11.

39. Subramanian G, McAfee JG. A new complex for ⁹⁹ᵐTc for skeletal imaging. Radiology. 1971;99:192–6.

40. Batson OV. The function of the vertebral veins and their role in the spread of metastases. Ann Surg. 1940;112:138–49.

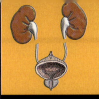

Chapter 11 Interventional Uroradiology

Janis M Brown, Neil Denbow, and Morton G Glickman

KEY POINTS

KEY POINTS

- Uroradiologists now carry out many techniques that replace surgical intervention.
- Percutaneous nephrostomy is the most commonly performed uroradiologic intervention, and is the first step in many other interventions.
- Fluoroscopy is the most versatile guidance system, although many radiologists prefer ultrasound.
- Radiologists have been developing techniques and equipment to make simpler and less invasive some of the problems of urologic diagnosis and therapy that formerly required surgery. Urologists have been adapting radiologic equipment and techniques to the advancing surgical technology to make urologic surgery simpler and less invasive. This chapter describes the radiologic side of this interface.

PERCUTANEOUS NEPHROSTOMY

Percutaneous nephrostomy is the most commonly performed uroradiologic intervention and is the first step in many other urologic interventions. When the urinary collecting system is distended, the procedure can be guided by ultrasound (US), computed tomography (CT), magnetic resonance imaging (MRI), or fluoroscopy.

Imaging systems
Fluoroscopy
Fluoroscopy is the most versatile guidance system. After opacification of the collecting system by intravenous contrast medium, the optimum location for puncture can be determined and the puncture needle guided under direct vision. Following puncture, fluoroscopy permits catheter manipulation and additional diagnostic or therapeutic maneuvers without moving the patient.

Ultrasound
No contrast medium is required for US guidance, which can be carried out rapidly in the US suite or, when necessary, at the bedside. It allows multiplanar imaging to identify an approach that avoids nearby organs, such as bowel, spleen, or liver, and in conjunction with color flow imaging it demonstrates major vessels. In most patients, high frequency transducers (5–7.5MHz) can be used and provide excellent resolution of even minimally dilated collecting systems. In large patients, lower frequency probes may be required to visualize the kidney.

A variety of guidance devices can be attached to the US transducer in order to direct the puncture needle. The needle, guidewire, and catheters are monitored in real time as they are advanced into the collecting system. Gupta et al. reported a success rate of 98.5% for needle puncture and 91% for catheter placement in a series of 273 percutaneous nephrostomies that used US for guidance[1].

According to the preference and experience of the physician, US may be used anytime, but should be considered particularly for patients at risk for contrast-medium reaction and for pregnant women. Also, US can be used to puncture and drain renal cysts. Procedures that require manipulation of catheters within the collecting system are best carried out with the patient in a fluoroscopy suite.

Computed tomography
The needle can also be guided by CT. During puncture, the position of the needle can be determined precisely. Unlike US, images are not degraded by air in the bowel. Oral or rectal contrast medium may be helpful, although retroperitoneal structures can be safely punctured from a posterior or oblique approach without the need for bowel opacification.

The primary disadvantage of CT guidance is the time required, as CT does not provide dynamic real-time images. The site and path of puncture is mapped on the machine's monitor. The needle, or trochar, is advanced in small increments. With each increment an image is obtained and the needle's direction is modified as required prior to further advancement. The length of the needle can be limited by the size of the gantry, and sterility is uncertain if the patient is less than fully cooperative.

The images available with CT guidance are comprehensive, showing in exquisite detail the tissue planes and the location of needles and catheters. In anatomically difficult or high-risk patients, CT may be the most precise, safest guidance method.

The most common indications for percutaneous nephrostomy are given in Figure 11.1.

Complications
The location of the puncture should be chosen to minimize the likelihood of causing harm (Fig. 11.2) and to facilitate the accomplishment of the diagnostic or therapeutic goal. Relative contraindications include any anatomic or physiologic abnormality that increases the likelihood of complication. The only absolute contraindication is uncontrolled coagulopathy.

Puncture of the lung and pleura along the percutaneous entry track allows air, or infused or draining fluid, access to the pleural space. The pleura may extend as low as the twelfth rib. When

Indications for percutaneous nephrostomy

Drainage

Acute ureteral obstruction

Diversion from a fistula

Access for diagnostic evaluation

Antegrade injection for anatomic display

Pelviureteral manometry

Biopsy

Access for therapy

Stone removal

Dilation of stricture

Figure 11.1 Indications for percutaneous nephrostomy.

Complications of percutaneous nephrostomy

Blood loss that requires transfusion

Pneumothorax and/or hemothorax

Sepsis

Injury to other organs

Figure 11.2 Complications of percutaneous nephrostomy.

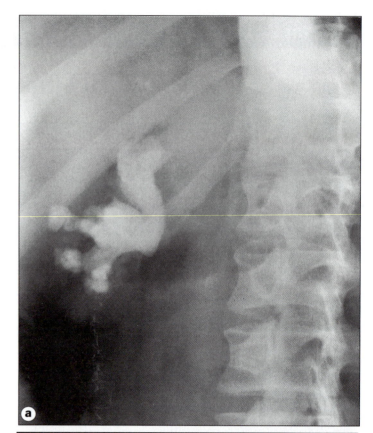

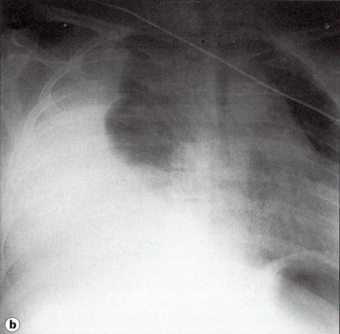

Figure 11.3 Hydrothorax following intercostal needle puncture.
(a) Staghorn calculus with its lowest edge above the 12th rib. Attempts to puncture from below the 12th rib angling cephalad were unsuccessful.
(b) A needle was advanced between the 11th and 12th ribs, but during stone removal the patient became dyspneic. The large hydrothorax was treated with a chest tube. The patient was discharged 3 days later.

the puncture needle is advanced from a position below the 12th rib, puncture of pleura, lung, or diaphragm can be avoided. When the puncture is made between ribs, pneumothorax becomes possible, but the frequency in experienced hands is low[2,3]. Precautions include advancing the needle only during expiration – puncture of the diaphragm occurs often and may cause pain, but is otherwise harmless[4,5].

Pneumothorax and hydrothorax can be managed with a chest tube. It is prudent to advise patients with high-riding kidneys that an intercostal puncture and subsequent chest tube drainage may occur (Fig. 11.3).

In approximately 2% of patients the retroperitoneal portion of the colon may move posterolateral to the kidney[6]. This particularly occurs in patients over 60 years old, those with a thin body habitus, or those who have recently lost weight. Colon puncture has been reported without incident[7], but serious complications that require exploratory surgery and even nephrectomy have occurred. It is likely that colon puncture often goes unnoticed, since most that have come to attention have been found incidentally. If discovered, prudence dictates immediate cessation of the procedure and careful follow-up, usually by CT scan. If the collecting system requires continued drainage, the percutaneous nephrostomy can be replaced using a new route for puncture.

Some degree of hemorrhage always occurs during percutaneous nephrostomy. Hematuria continues for 1–3 days after the procedure, but blood loss is rarely clinically significant unless an artery has been damaged. Arterial hemorrhage may require arteriography and embolization (Fig. 11.4).

To avoid serious hemorrhage, a posterolateral puncture has been recommended[8,9]. The aim of this approach is to puncture the renal parenchyma as close as possible to Brodel's avascular junction, between the anterior and posterior divisions of the

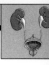

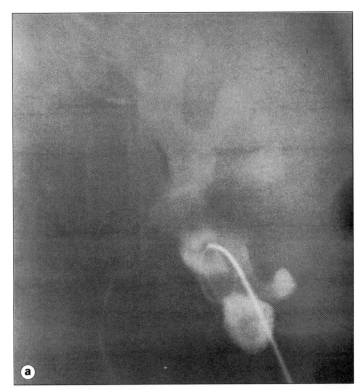

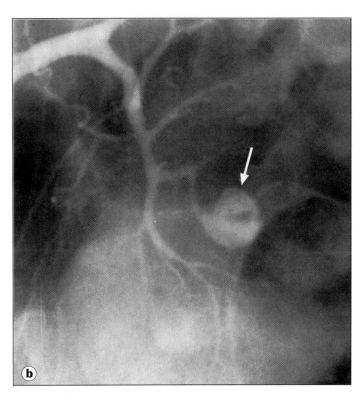

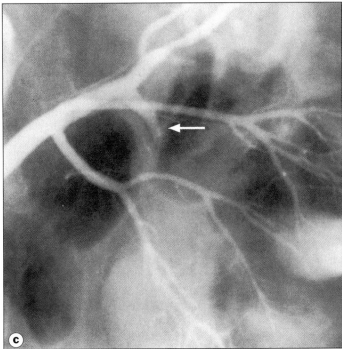

Figure 11.4 Patient referred for severe hemorrhage after percutaneous nephrolithotomy. (a) After puncture of a posterior calix with a 20-gauge needle, a guidewire was coiled in the lower infundibulum. (b) Arteriography shows contrast medium (arrow) extravasating from an interlobar artery. (c) After injection of a single surgical foam pledget, the vessel that had been bleeding became obstructed near its origin (arrow). Contrast medium in the parenchyma had accumulated from a prior injection. Bleeding stopped, there was no further hemorrhage, and the patient was discharged 2 days later.

kidney, and to enter the collecting system peripherally, through a calix (Fig. 11.5).

An alternative approach that acknowledges the difficulty of identifying Brodel's line simplifies the puncture by aiming at a calix from a direct posterior puncture (Fig. 11.5). Using either approach, the catheter traverses a plane between the paraspinal muscle groups. Catheter movement during muscular contraction and respiratory motion is considered less likely to cause discomfort than catheter movement along a percutaneous track lateral to the paraspinous muscle bellies. While these approaches are intended to keep the puncture needle away from the vulnerable central renal arteries, published reports show arterial hemorrhage in about 1% of patients[10,11].

We have used a straight posterior puncture of the renal pelvis adjacent to an infundibulum. This is the shortest route to the largest part of the collecting system (Fig. 11.5). In our recent review of 166 consecutive percutaneous nephrolithotomies the rate of arterial injury that required embolization was zero[12]. We attribute the absence of serious hemorrhage to exclusive use of a 22-gauge, flexible needle that is unlikely to puncture the muscular wall of a central artery.

Direct renal pelvic puncture offers access by catheter or nephroscope to the ureter and to all of the infundibula and calices. The medial location avoids colon puncture.

Although this approach pierces the paraspinal muscles, our patients have not described pain along the percutaneous track, perhaps because of the absence of sensory nerves in the granulation tissue that lines such tracks.

ANTEGRADE PYELOGRAPHY AND URETEROGRAPHY

The renal pelvis is punctured with a 22-gauge needle, using the technique described below for percutaneous nephrostomy.

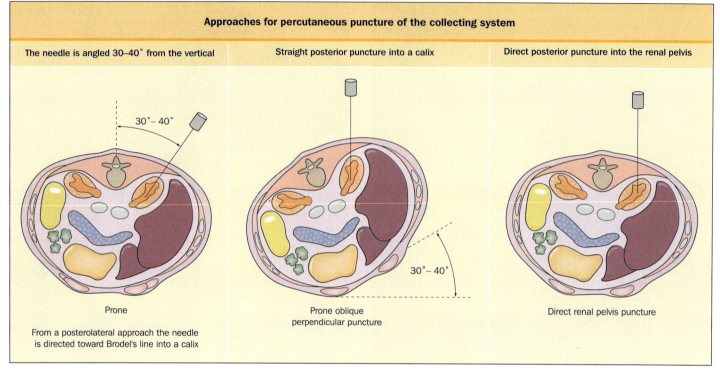

Figure 11.5 Approaches for percutaneous puncture of the collecting system.

When urine is aspirated, contrast medium is injected. Directly injected contrast medium offers considerably better resolution on fluoroscopy and radiographs than does excreted contrast medium following intravenous administration.

Since contrast medium has a higher specific gravity than urine, it can be moved within the collecting system by changing the patient's position. Injection of relatively small amounts of contrast and maneuvering the medium by moving the patient avoids overinjection. Elevation of pressure within a colonized collecting system may cause sepsis.

Accurate diagnosis of intraluminal lesions may be difficult on CT, MRI, and US, which show renal parenchyma much better than they show the collecting system. A well-executed excretory urogram (EU), with the patient dehydrated and with ureteric compression, shows collecting system abnormalities well, but a suboptimal EU does not. Masses (such as polyps) and mural lesions (such as leukoplakia) occasionally require antegrade examination or ureteroscopy. Urodynamic studies (e.g. the Whitaker test) can be carried out using a modification of this technique (see Chapter 23).

PERCUTANEOUS PUNCTURE

When the ureter is abruptly obstructed, the collecting system may not dilate. If percutaneous nephrostomy is required, intravenous contrast medium should be given about 30 minutes before the puncture. The more severe the obstruction, the longer the kidney and its contents remain opacified, and contrast medium given for a preceding diagnostic EU or CT scan may still offer a satisfactory target.

After the needle enters the collecting system and urine is aspirated, a guidewire is advanced into the collecting system to a

sufficient depth that respiratory movement or movement of the instruments during manipulation does not compromise catheter placement. An 8 French (8F) pigtail or Malecot-style catheter is usually sufficient to drain the collecting system.

Whereas the location of the puncture site is not important when a percutaneous nephrostomy is placed for antegrade study or drainage, when a nephrostomy is placed for a complex problem thoughtful selection of the puncture site may make the difference between simple or difficult catheter manipulation, and occasionally between a simple and impossible procedure.

For procedures that require instrumentation of the lower ureter, a more cephalad puncture allows easier manipulation of large instruments such as a ureteroscope. For procedures within the intrarenal collecting system, such as biopsy of tumors and percutaneous nephrolithotomy, puncture at the junction of the renal pelvis with the lower pole infundibulum is often preferable, since the direction of puncture guides the instruments cephalad. This site allows manipulation of the guidewire and catheter into the ureter to ease track dilation, while providing easy nephroscopic visualization of the pelvis and calices.

Intravenous contrast medium is administered and, once the collecting system is opacified, a skin puncture site is chosen and the C-arm fluoroscope is angled to superimpose the skin entrance site on the proposed collecting system puncture site. If the needle tip remains superimposed on the image of the collecting system throughout its course, the only remaining variable in needle placement is the depth.

Dilation of percutaneous track

Instruments such as a nephroscope or balloon catheter are advanced into the collecting system through a sheath that

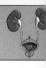

traverses and maintains the percutaneous track. The sheath is inserted over a dilating catheter. The size of the sheath varies with the size of the instruments to be used. The smaller the sheath, the easier its placement and the less the likelihood of complications.

The wire used to guide the dilator and sheath should be stiff enough to be unlikely to kink outside the kidney, and its tip should be placed in a location that minimizes the chance of dislodging it. The most secure location is the bladder. The best wire currently available for dilation is made of an alloy called 'nitinol', which is virtually impossible to kink.

A track that requires a caliber larger than 14F should be dilated with a balloon rather than with serial dilators. During inflation of a balloon the force is directed radially, which spreads tissue. Serial dilators are larger than the percutaneous track. As they advance they push tissues ahead of them and are much more likely to cause injury or dislodge the guidewire and catheter.

Ureteral strictures

After puncture and placement of a 7F or 8F sheath, a guidewire is advanced to the site of stricture. A 5F angiographic catheter with a bend near the tip is advanced to the site of narrowing. Injection of contrast medium with magnified fluoroscopy either opacifies the lumen of the stenotic segment or identifies the point of obstruction. A straight guidewire may traverse the track; if not, an angled wire with a hydrophilic coating should be used. After the wire crosses the stenosis, the catheter is advanced into the bladder.

Once the track through the stricture has allowed a 5F catheter to pass, a balloon catheter can be inserted (Fig. 11.6). The ureter can be safely dilated to a diameter of 10mm. Very narrow or very long strictures may require a nitinol wire to guide the balloon catheter. A 12F stent, placed for a period of 4–6 weeks, maintains a wide lumen during healing[13,14].

Nephrostomy access should be maintained during this period, even with an internal stent present. After removal of the stent, a week or more of external drainage may be necessary for resolution of spasm and edema. After ureteral integrity is restored, the nephrostomy catheter should be capped for a few days to test the ability of the ureter to transport urine in all states of hydration. If the patient remains asymptomatic and the collecting system does not distend, the nephrostomy catheter can be removed.

The likelihood of success of balloon dilation of ureteral strictures depends upon the cause. Causes can be divided into structural and functional. Dilation of ureters obstructed by malignant tumor is rarely successful, even for a short time[13]. If an anastomotic stricture is not a result of malignancy, the prognosis is good with success rates of 50–76% reported in series of patients followed for up to 5 years[13–16]. Short, nonanastomotic strictures of <3 months duration respond best (Fig. 11.7).

During balloon inflation a waist should appear. Inflation should continue until the waist disappears. If no waist appears during dilation, the obstruction is presumed to be functional, and the likelihood of successful balloon dilation is small.

Strictures that do not respond to balloon dilation can still be treated through a nephroscope using a cold knife or a cautery wire affixed to a balloon catheter. This procedure is most successful at the ureteropelvic junction; in the ureter, it is associated with greater morbidity[17].

If balloon dilation is unsuccessful and open or percutaneous surgical repair is not indicated, long-term stenting may be necessary. Permanent stents made of metal mesh have proved very useful in the treatment of arterial stenosis, but have been largely unsuccessful in the ureter[18,19]. Granulation tissue grows through the interstices of the stent and compromises the lumen. Metal stents that are covered with a plastic sheath, which closes the interstices, are now in clinical trial. Covered stents may provide the best solution for patients with functional ureteral strictures.

Percutaneous nephrolithotomy

Extracorporeal shock-wave lithotripsy (ESWL) remains the first line of treatment for renal and ureteral stones, but percutaneous nephrolithotomy finds frequent use in patients who are not appropriate for ESWL or who fail ESWL (Fig. 11.8). The puncture site is carefully chosen to offer access to the maximum amount of stone. The puncture is made with a 22-gauge needle using the percutaneous nephrostomy technique. A guidewire and catheter are manipulated down the ureter into the bladder. The percutaneous track is dilated to receive a 26–30F sheath. At least two guidewires are advanced to the bladder, one to lead a balloon dilator and the other to remain in place throughout the procedure as a safety wire. The safety wire serves two functions:

- it ensures access to the collecting system if the sheath should become dislodged during the procedure; and
- it guides a drainage catheter into the collecting system at the end of the procedure.

If a large volume of stone needs removal, it is useful to inflate a low-pressure latex balloon at the ureteropelvic junction to prevent stone fragments from reaching the ureter. A third wire, introduced through the sheath, can provide access for this balloon catheter if required.

A balloon catheter capable of withstanding up to 1.9kPa and capable of expanding to 1cm in diameter is used to dilate the track and the sheath is inserted. The sheath extends from the skin surface to the collecting system. A nephroscope is advanced through the sheath to the stone. Small stones can be removed with grasping forceps; larger stones can be broken with laser or ultrasonic energy, or with electrohydraulic shocks. The fragments can then be removed with suction and grasping forceps.

After the procedure, drainage catheters may be placed through the sheath or over the wires. A number of catheter drainage systems and follow-up regimens are in use. Our preference is a 16F or 18F latex Malecot catheter placed through the sheath to the renal pelvis, and an 8F pigtail catheter coiled in the renal pelvis or an 8F straight ureteral catheter with a side hole in the renal pelvis. We follow the procedure with a nephrostogram before discharge to determine whether any stones remain and to document the anatomic and functional status of the collecting system and ureter. Both catheters may be removed or one may be left for another week or two if edema or stone fragments in the ureter suggest that continued external drainage may be useful.

The procedure usually requires a 2–4 day hospital admission. Epidural anesthetic, used until about 1990 at our institution, has been replaced by general anesthetic. The procedure is well tolerated by most patients. With proper antibiotic coverage, use of an infracostal puncture, and exclusive use of a 22-gauge needle for puncture, complications occur rarely. The most common complication in our hands is hemorrhage sufficient to require

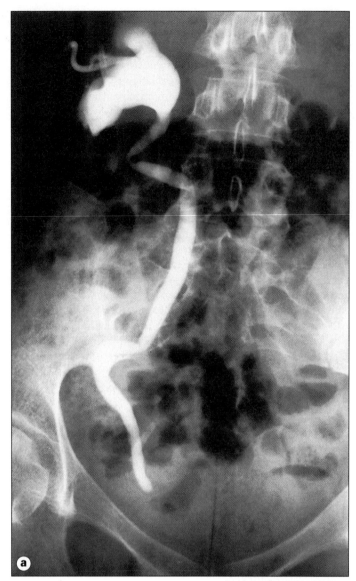

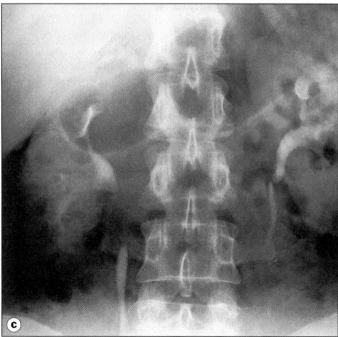

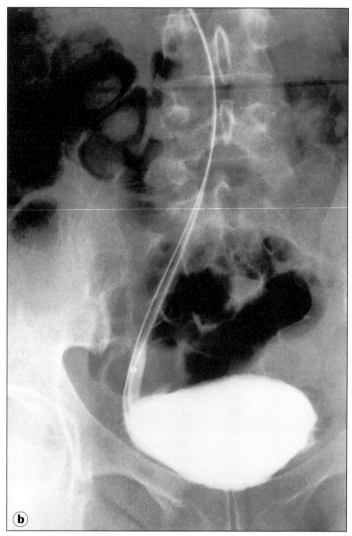

Figure 11.6 Obstruction of the distal right ureter shown by excretory urogram 3 days after hysterectomy. (a) Antegrade injection following percutaneous nephrostomy shows obstruction of the distal ureter at the location of the broad ligament. (b) After a guidewire was advanced through the obstruction into the bladder, an 8mm diameter balloon was inflated across the site of ligature. A safety wire traverses the ureter. (c) A 12F stent was left for 6 weeks and removed. Excretory urogram 3 months later shows symmetric excretion from nondistended collecting systems.

transfusion – between 1990 and 1997 transfusion was necessary in 4.3% of the patients undergoing percutaneous nephrolithotomy. No patient required embolization for arterial hemorrhage, even though the puncture was made into the renal pelvis[10].

Renal cyst puncture

Large renal cysts that cause pain or obstruction of the collecting system may be aspirated percutaneously. Since a cyst is a closed sac with no internal blood supply, the introduction of bacteria may lead to an abscess. A strict sterile technique must be observed – prophylactic antibiotic administration seems prudent.

The optimal imaging guidance system is US, since it is simple, rapid, and accurate. As only very large cysts require this form of therapy and precise guidance is not necessary, fluoroscopy (after intravenous contrast medium administration) may also be used.

Factors that decrease success rate in balloon dilation of ureteral strictures

Length >1.5cm

Duration >3 months

Malignant cause

Proximal location of stricture

Lesion previously treated

Total ureteral occlusion

Ureteroenteric anastomotic location

Figure 11.7 Factors that decrease success rate in balloon dilation of ureteral strictures.

Indications for percutaneous stone therapy (versus extracorporeal shock-wave lithotripsy)

Failed extracorporeal shock-wave lithotripsy

Unfavorable stone composition:

cysteine

some oxalate monohydrate

some uric acid

Abnormal body habitus or morbid obesity

Fragments may not pass:

large and/or staghorn calculi

ureteropelvic junction stenosis

caliceal diverticulum

atrophic lower calix

Figure 11.8 Indications for percutaneous stone therapy (versus extracorporeal shock-wave lithotripsy).

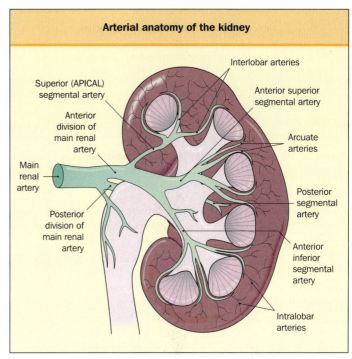

Arterial anatomy of the kidney

Figure 11.9 Arterial anatomy of the kidney.

Once cyst fluid is aspirated, a guidewire should be advanced and the needle replaced with a pigtail catheter. Adequate treatment requires aspiration of as much cyst fluid as possible, for which a pigtail catheter with side holes is more effective than a needle as the cyst begins to empty and its walls collapse. After complete aspiration the catheter is removed.

Recurrence is common after simple aspiration, although the recurrence may not be as large and may not reproduce the symptoms. Injection of a sclerosing agent slightly increases the potential morbidity, but reduces the likelihood of recurrence. Sclerosing agents may produce inflammation, and occasionally patients experience pain after the procedure.

For sclerosis, an agent such as absolute alcohol, sotradecol or tetracycline is injected after complete fluid aspiration. The volume of sclerosing agent should be 0.25–0.5 times the volume of cyst fluid to provide enough sclerosing agent to contact the entire endothelial surface of the cyst, but not enough to raise the internal pressure and cause leakage. Careful attention must be directed to insuring that all of the side holes of the catheter remain within the cyst cavity. The function of the sclerosing agent is cytotoxicity; none must be allowed to escape beyond the cyst. After about 15 minutes the sclerosing agent is aspirated and the catheter is removed.

Renal artery anatomy

Approximately 33% of the population has some form of renal arterial or venous variation from the described norm, most commonly multiple renal arteries or veins[20]. The right renal artery usually arises from the anterior and/or lateral aspect of the aorta at the L1/L2 level. The left arises at the same level and is more laterally oriented along the aorta.

The main renal artery divides into anterior and posterior divisions at the renal hilus, after giving off adrenal, renal pelvic, and capsular branches (Fig. 11.9). The anterior division divides into the superior, anterior, and posterior segmental arteries, while the posterior division gives rise to the middle segmental artery. The segmental branches terminate as interlobar arteries, which give rise to arcuate arteries, which in turn give rise to intralobar arteries. Divisional and interlobar arteries may communicate with capsular and renal pelvic arteries. Vessels smaller than these are not individually visible on arteriograms.

Renal venous anatomy

The right renal vein enters the inferior vena cava at or about the L1/L2 level. The left venal vein is somewhat less predictable. Most (about 85%) are solitary and pass anterior to the aorta and inferior to the proximal portion of the superior mesenteric artery. In the next most common form a circumferential renal venous system encircles the aorta and inserts as two branches at the L1/L2 level and at the L3 level. A solitary left retroaortic renal vein is present in approximately 5% of the population[20].

Embolization

'Embolization' is now used to describe interventional radiologic procedures that obstruct flow in the circulatory system. Renal artery embolization is useful in treating arterial injuries, in selected patients with tumors, and in ablating failed kidneys (Fig. 11.10). Materials used for embolization include balloons, stainless steel coils, particles of plastic foam, of surgical gelatin foam, histoacryl glue, and absolute alcohol[21].

Indications for renal artery embolization
Renal injury, needle biopsy, or nephrostomy trauma
Renal cell carcinoma:
prenephrectomy
palliation
Angiomyolipomas >4cm
Nonfunctioning kidneys

Figure 11.10 Indications for renal artery embolization.

Clinical factors that suggest renin-dependent hypertension
Patient <40 years of age
Uncontrolled on two or more drugs
Acute change in response to therapy

Figure 11.11 Clinical factors that suggest renin-dependent hypertension.

Trauma

In trauma patients the underlying principle is to control bleeding while preserving as much uninvolved renal parenchyma as possible. Selective renal arteriography is carried out first to demonstrate the intrarenal vascular anatomy and to identify which artery to occlude to best resolve the clinical problem. The catheter is advanced into that artery and embolic material is injected. For hemorrhage caused by trauma, solid thrombogenic materials (such as surgical gelatin foam or stainless steel coils) should be used. Published series report immediate resolution of bleeding and no recurrence for up to 1 year[22,23].

Tumor

Preoperative embolization of large renal carcinomas devascularizes the tumor and simplifies en bloc resection. An easy method, while in the operating room after induction of anesthesia, is to place an occlusion balloon at the origin of the main renal artery. As the surgical dissection approaches, the balloon is inflated to stop flow. The inflated balloon is palpable and allows identification of the renal artery for clamping and ligation[24].

Inoperative renal carcinomas may require embolization for palliation of symptoms such as pain or bleeding. Particulate emboli are the most effective agents.

Angiomyolipoma is a benign tumor, but has the potential for catastrophic hemorrhage because it contains poorly supported tumor arteries. The likelihood of bleeding increases with increasing tumor size. Angiomyolipomas in patients with tuberous sclerosis or lymphangiomyomatosis should be treated if they reach 3cm in diameter[25,26]. In patients with no underlying disease, tumors 4cm or more in diameter should be treated[25].

Treatment by embolization ablates the vascular part of the tumor and spares renal parenchyma outside the tumor. Since the diagnosis can be established and malignancy excluded if fat is recognized on CT examination, biopsy diagnosis is not necessary. Surgical gelatin foam or plastic foam particles are the embolic agents of choice.

The procedure causes infarction of a large volume of tissue, so severe pain, nausea, leukocytosis, and low-grade fever can be anticipated. This response begins within a few hours of treatment and usually resolves within 48 hours. Treatment consists of analgesics and antiemetics. Prophylactic antibiotic therapy prior to embolization and for the following few days seems reasonable to minimize the risk of infection.

Renal failure

In patients who receive hemodialysis or who have a transplanted kidney, the surviving native kidneys may be a liability.

Uncontrollable hypertension may require removal of the renin-secreting native kidneys. Renal ablation by embolization is a less invasive alternative to bilateral nephrectomy. Absolute alcohol is the best arteriographic material for complete destruction of an organ. Alcohol closes the lumina of the arteries it reaches, functioning as a cytotoxin to vascular endothelial cells. It is mixed with a small volume of contrast medium and injected through an occlusion balloon catheter placed at the orifice of the main renal artery. The inflated balloon obstructs blood flow, which allows slow, fluoroscopically monitored injection until the entire renal arterial system (main renal artery to intralobar arteries) is opacified, but also prevents reflux into the aorta. The injection is then stopped, and the alcohol is permitted to remain in contact with the arterial intima for 5–15 minutes[24].

Renin-dependent hypertension

In response to decreased renal perfusion from any cause, renin secretion by cells of the juxtaglomerular apparatus that surrounds the afferent and efferent arterioles is stimulated. Renin is metabolized to angiotensin I and then to the active vasoconstrictor, angiotensin II. Angiotensin II constricts efferent arterioles in the kidney, which increases perfusion pressure in the glomerulus. This homeostatic system effectively maintains renal perfusion during hypotensive events, but the system functions inappropriately when renal perfusion is reduced by renal artery stenosis rather than systemic hypertension. The elevated renin production in renal artery stenosis raises systemic blood pressure. In very young patients or in elderly patients who fail pharmacotherapy, restoration of renal perfusion is the rational therapy (Fig. 11.11).

No direct relationship occurs between renal artery anatomy and hypertension. Arteriographic and autopsy studies in normal and hypertensive individuals show that neither the presence nor severity of stenosis in a renal artery predicts improvement of hypertension after repair[27,28]. Diagnosis of renin-dependent hypertension requires investigation of the function of the renin–angiotensin system or demonstration of abnormal hemodynamics. Radioisotope renal scans or Doppler US arterial flow studies carried out while an inhibitor of angiotensin-converting enzyme (ACE) is given are the most common screening examinations. If either of these suggests a vascular cause of hypertension, diagnostic arteriography, carried out with the expectation of angioplasty or placement of a stent if it is abnormal, is recommended (Fig. 11.12).

In experienced hands the success rates of renal angioplasty and stent placement are similar to those obtained by surgery, but with less morbidity and mortality[29]. Prior to arteriography it is essential that the patient be well hydrated to minimize the likelihood of contrast-medium toxicity. After the procedure, blood pressure may be labile and requires close monitoring for the first 24–48 hours.

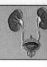

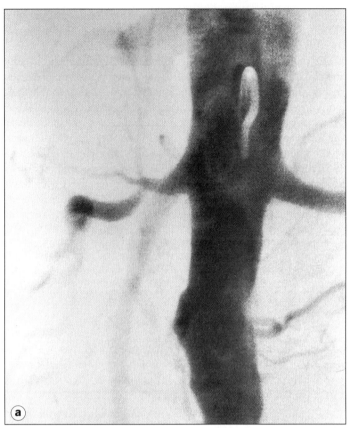

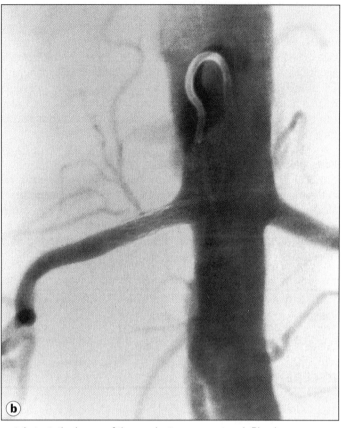

Figure 11.12 A 58-year-old man with medically uncontrollable hypertension. (a) Aortogram shows severe stenosis of the right renal artery about 1cm distal to its origin. (b) After placement of an expandable metal stent, the lumen of the renal artery was restored. Blood pressure has been normal without medication for a follow-up period of 2 years.

Renal transplant

Arteriography has been the standard for preoperative evaluation of possible living donors. The arterial, venous, and ureteric anatomy is demonstrated to assist surgical planning. Recently, CT and magnetic resonance angiography have been offered as less invasive alternatives. As their technology has evolved, they have become as accurate as conventional angiography in demonstrating the vascular and ureteric anatomy[30]. After transplantation, poor renal function, hypertension, or electrolyte imbalance in the perioperative period should be investigated with US, MRI, or radioisotope imaging. If rejection appears likely, needle biopsy of the allograft is the best diagnostic procedure. Biopsy is most expeditiously performed using US to guide an 18-gauge biopsy needle. The biopsy sample should extend from the capsule toward, but not into, the hilus.

Renal artery thrombosis usually occurs within 1 month of transplantation. Patients present with abrupt anuria. If quickly recognized, intra-arterial fibrinolytic therapy is recommended. If successful, diagnostic arteriography should be carried out immediately to identify any anatomic abnormality that may have induced thrombosis.

Renal artery stenosis most often occurs at the anastomosis, but may also occur proximally or distally. Reports describe a widely varying frequency (0.6–25.0%)[30,31,32]. Arterial stenosis at a pre-anastomotic site results from a cross-clamping injury. Stenoses beyond the anastomosis are more common after end-to-side anastomosis than after the end-to-end type. Postoperative renal artery stenosis responds to balloon angioplasty or stent placement.

Intrarenal aneurysm, periarterial hematoma, and arteriovenous fistula occur after renal biopsy or infection and have been associated with rejection. Treatment of choice for any of these results of arterial injury is selective embolization. The preferred embolic agent is a detachable balloon or stainless steel coils, since the injured artery must be closed as near to the site of injury as possible.

Extrarenal aneurysms occur at the anastomotic site and result from incomplete healing or from infection. Extrarenal aneurysms require surgical repair.

Ureteric complications may occur early or late. Perioperative obstruction may result from edema and may require no more than a few days of drainage with a double 'J' stent. Retrograde stent placement during cystoscopy is usually simpler and better tolerated than antegrade placement, which requires percutaneous nephrostomy. Fixed stenoses, which usually come to attention several months or more after surgery, require operative repair or nephrostomy and balloon dilation, with several weeks healing time over a large stent (see Ureteral strictures above).

Urinoma occurs in the perioperative period and results from leakage through the ureteral anastomosis. An internal stent is usually sufficient for treatment. With free passage of urine through the stent, the anastomosis can heal and the extravasated urine usually absorbs spontaneously. Persistent urinomas may be drained separately, usually under US guidance.

Lymphoceles may be asymptomatic (discovered by US or CT incidentally) or they may cause pain or a palpable mass. They are usually found 3–6 weeks after surgery and are treated by percutaneous drainage using US guidance. Injection of a sclerosing agent, such as absolute alcohol, sotradecol, or tetracycline, for 15 minutes after aspiration of the contents usually prevents recurrence (see Renal cyst puncture above). The lymphocele also can be treated laparoscopically with drainage of the lymphocele into the peritoneal cavity.

Varicocele

Surgical treatment may not be definitive, as retroperitoneal collateral circulation often reconstitutes the ligated veins after surgery and the varicocele may recur[33]. Percutaneous intravascular therapy allows obstruction of the entire length of the gonadal vein and its collaterals, and so decreases the likelihood of recurrence.

The gonadal vein is catheterized after percutaneous puncture of one of the femoral veins. Contrast-medium injection shows the full length of the gonadal vein and its branches. The vessel is obstructed, either with a detachable balloon or a coil, below and above the varicocele, at the entrance site of major collaterals, and at the termination of the gonadal vein. If detachable balloons are used, a sclerosant such as hypertonic glucose is injected between the balloon above the varicocele and the balloon at the termination of the gonadal vein. In this way the entire length of the gonadal vein is obstructed to minimize the likelihood of recurrence[34]. This is an outpatient procedure that requires no more than a local anesthetic[35]. Patients may return to work the following day. Cost analyses report that this technique is less costly and results in less morbidity than the surgical approach[36].

REFERENCES

1. Gupta S, Gulati M, Uday K, Shankar U, Runtga U, Suri S. Percutaneous nephrostomy with real-time sonographic guidance. Acta Radiol. 1997;38:454–7.
2. Dyer RB, Assimos DG, Regan JD. Update on interventional radiology. Urol Clin North Am. 1997;24:625–51.
3. Bjarnason H, Ferral H, Stackhouse DJ, et al. Complications related to percutaneous nephrolithotomy. Semin Intervent Radiol. 1994;11:213–25.
4. Young AT, Hunter DW, Castaneda-Zuniga WR, et al. Percutaneous extraction of urinary calculi: use of an intercostal approach. Radiology. 1985;154:633–8.
5. Picus D, Wenman PH, Clayman RV, McClennan BL. Intercostal space nephrostomy for percutaneous stone removal. AJR. 1986;147:393–7.
6. Hopper KD, Sherman JL, Williams MD, Ghaed N. The variable anteroposterior position of the retroperitoneal colon to the kidneys. Invest Radiol. 1987;22:298–302.
7. LeRoy AJ, Williams HJ, Segura JW, et al. Colon perforation following percutaneous nephrostomy and renal calculus removal. Radiology. 1985;155:83–5.
8. Coleman CC. Percutaneous nephrostomy: renal anatomy. In: Amplatz K, Lange PH, eds. Atlas of endourology. Chicago: Yearbook Medical Publishers; 1986:33–9.
9. Kandarpa K, Aruny JE. Handbook of interventional procedures. 2nd ed. New York: Little, Brown and Company; 1996:201–22.
10. Kessaris DN, Bellman GC, Nikolaos PP, Smith AG. Management of hemorrhage after percutaneous renal surgery. J Urol. 1995;153:604–8.
11. Lee WJ, Smith AD, Cubelli V, et al. Complications of percutaneous nephrolithotomy. AJR. 1987;148:177–80.
12. Brown JM, Hodges L, Kain T, Anderson KR, Glickman MG. Renal pelvis puncture for percutaneous nephrostomy. AJR. 1998;170(Suppl.):98.
13. Beckman CF, Roth RA, Behrle W III. Dilatation of benign ureteral strictures. Radiology 1989;172:437–41.
14. Chang R, Marshall FF, Mitchell S. Percutaneous management of benign ureteral strictures and fistulae. J Urol. 1987;137:1126–31.
15. Smith AD. Management of iatrogenic ureteral strictures after urological procedures. J Urol. 1988;140 (6):1372–4.
16. Lang EK, Glorioso LW III. Antegrade transluminal dilatation of benign ureteral ureteral strictures: long term results. AJR. 1988;150:131–4.
17. Goldfischer ER, Gerber GS. Endoscopic management of ureteral strictures. J Urol. 1997;157:770–5.
18. Pollack JS, Rosenblatt MM, Eglin TK, Dickey KW, Glickman M. Treatment of ureteral obstructions with Wallstent endoprosthesis: preliminary results. J Vasc Intervent Radiol. 1995;6:417–25.
19. Millward SF, Thijssen AM, Marriner JR, Moors DE, Mia KT. Effect of a metallic balloon-expanded stent on normal rabbit ureter. J Vasc Intervent Radiol. 1991;2 (5):557–60.
20. Kadir S: Kidneys. Atlas of normal and variant angiographic anatomy. Philadelphia: WB Saunders; 1991:387–428.
21. DiSegni R, Young AT, Qian Z, Castaneda-Zuniga WR. Embolotherapy: agents, equipment, and techniques. In: Casteneda-Zuniga WR, ed. Intervent Radiol. Baltimore: Williams and Wilkins; 1997:29–103.
22. Heyns CF, van Vollenhoven P. Increasing role of angiography and segmental artery embolization in the management of renal stab wounds. J Urol. 1992;147(5):1231–4.
23. Tzortzs G, Kolomodi D, Stathopoulou S, et al. Hyperselective renal artery embolisation in the treatment of post-traumatic iatrogenic haematuria. Intervent Angiology. 1998;17:58–61.
24. Glickman M. Urinary tract angiography. In: O'Reilly P, George NJR, Weiss RM, eds. Diagnostic techniques in urology. Philadelphia: WB Saunders; 1990:23–49.
25. Steiner MS, Goldman SM, Fishman EK, Marshall, EK. The natural history of renal angiomyolipoma. J Urol. 1993;150:1782–6.
26. Oesterling JE, Fishman EK, Goldman, SM, Marshall FF. The management of renal angiomyolypoma. J Urol. 1986;135:1121–4.
27. Eyler WR, Clark MD, Gorman JE, et al. Angiography of the renal areas including comparative study of renal artery stenoses in patients with and without hypertension. Radiology. 1962;78:879–92.
28. Haley KE, Hunt JC, Brown AL Jr, et al. Renal artery stenosis a clinical pathologic study in normotensive and hypertensive patients. Am J Med. 1964;37:14–22.

29. Weibull H, Berquist D, Bergent SE, Johnson K, Hulthen L, Manheim P. Percutaneous transluminal renal angioplasty versus surgical reconstruction of atherosclerotic renal artery stenosis: a prospective randomized study. J Vasc Surg. 1993;18:841–52.

30. Hany TF, Debatin JF, Leung DA, Pfammatter T. Evaluation of the aortoiliac and renal arteries: comparison of breath-hold, contrast-enhanced, three-dimensional MR angiography with conventional catheter angiography. Radiology. 1997;204:357–62.

31. Fervanza FC, Lafayette RA, Alfrey EJ, Petersen J. Renal artery stenosis in kidney transplants [Review]. Am J Kidney Dis. 1998;31:142–8.

32. Wong W, Flynn SP, Higgins RM, et al. Transplant renal artery stenosis in 77 patients – does it have an immunological cause? Transplantation. 1996;61:215–9.

33. Murray RR Jr, Mitchell SE, Kadir S. Comparison of recurrent varicocele anatomy following surgery and percutaneous balloon occlusion. J Urol. 1986;135:286–9.

34. White RI Jr, Radiologic management of varicoceles using embolization. In: Whitehead D, Harris N, eds. Management of impotence and infertility. Philadelphia: JB Lippincott; 1994:228–40.

35. Halden W, White RI Jr. Outpatient embolotherapy of varicocele. Urol Clin North Am. 1987;14:137–44.

36. Dewire DM, Thomas AJ Jr, Falk RM, Geisinger MA, Lammert GK. Clinical outcome and cost comparison of percutaneous embolization and surgical ligation of varicocele. J Andrology. 1994;15(Suppl.):38–42.

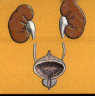

Chapter 12

Endoscopy: Upper Tract

Demetrius H Bagley

KEY POINTS

- Endoscopic access to the upper urinary tract can be percutaneous or transureteral.
- Effective endoscopic lithotriptors can treat almost any renal calculi.
- Ureteroscopy is best for biopsy of upper tract tumors.
- Treatment of upper tract transitional cell carcinoma is possible but surveillance is necessary.
- Ureteroscopy and percutaneous nephroscopy are effective for endopyelotomy.
- Ureteral strictures are most effectively treated ureteroscopically.
- Diverticuli in the upper pole are approached ureteroscopically and in the lower pole percutaneously.

INTRODUCTION

Endoscopy of the kidney has opened the entire intrarenal collecting system to visual inspection and manipulation. The diagnostic and therapeutic applications of endoscopy have widened with the development of appropriate endoscopes and effective working instruments. Percutaneous nephroscopy and flexible ureteroscopy constitute the major techniques used for interventional renal procedures. The relative applications of these two procedures continue to shift as instrumentation changes. Further refinements in procedures can be expected with miniaturization of the endoscopes and improved working devices.

Development of renal endoscopy

Endoscopy of the intrarenal collecting system has been termed nephroscopy or pyeloscopy. When approached transureterally, it has been called ureteropyeloscopy or ureteronephroscopy.

Nephroscopy has been performed as an adjunct to open surgical procedures in the kidney. This technique reached its maximal application with the use of a specific rigid nephroscope. This device consisted of a rigid rod lens optical system with the shaft angled at 90° approximately 8cm from the tip. Irrigation was carried to the tip in order to clear the field for visualization. The working instruments included forceps and graspers, which were attached to the rigid shaft of the endoscope, bringing the device into the visual field.

The surgical nephroscope could be employed after the kidney was surgically exposed. The angled tip of the endoscope could

then be placed through a pyelotomy into the renal collecting system. Most intrarenal regions could be accessed with the straight rigid device. The instrument was widely applied to retrieve calculi and to identify and potentially treat lesions responsible for chronic unilateral hematuria[1,2].

Flexible endoscopes were later applied for intraoperative use. In comparison to the rigid instrument, however, the flexible device lacked adequate irrigation and effective working instruments for use in that setting. Working instruments developed only later as other anatomic approaches developed and required the use of flexible instruments.

Percutaneous nephroscopy developed with techniques for percutaneous access. The endoscopes used for viewing and working within the kidney were initially those already available, cystourethroscopes. As experience grew with nephroscopy, the specific needs of renal endoscopy resulted in the design of specific nephroscopes, both rigid and flexible. Specific design features have been incorporated to maximize the effective application of the instruments. For example, rigid nephroscopes typically have an offset eyepiece to allow a straight channel that can accept a rigid ultrasound probe. More recently, there has been a tendency to downsize the nephroscopes with the need for smaller nephrostomy tracts and also for more effective lithotriptor devices.

Flexible nephroscopes have developed along with flexible cystoscopes and incorporate the same designs. There has recently been a great improvement in the applicability of flexible nephroscopes with the development of more effective retrieval devices and effective endoscopic lithotriptors.

Access through the ureter to the kidney can be gained with appropriately sized endoscopes. The rigid endoscopes initially designed for ureteroscopy are inadequate both to reach the renal pelvis routinely and to extend into the intrarenal collecting system. Such access depends upon the development of flexible ureteroscopes with a channel adequate for working instruments. Currently available instruments can reach the entire intrarenal collecting system from a transureteral approach and can sample tissue, fragment calculi and ablate tissue in any area (Fig. 12.1).

Intraoperative nephroscopy during open surgery has been almost entirely replaced by the other two endoscopic techniques for renal endoscopy. The relationship between percutaneous nephroscopy and ureteropyeloscopy is constantly shifting with the development of different instruments with different capabilities. The complementary nature of the procedures and the changes in the first choice in approach can be seen to vary with each application. In each instance, the goal remains the same, to achieve the purpose of the procedure with minimal intervention and discomfort to the patient and with a maximal effect.

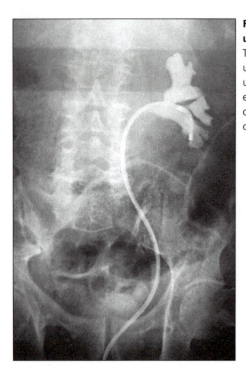

Figure 12.1 Flexible ureteroscope *in situ*. The flexible ureteroscope can be used to inspect the entire intrarenal collecting system in over 90% of patients.

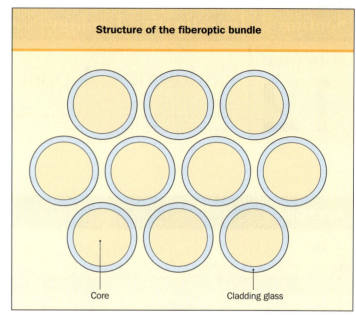

Structure of the fiberoptic bundle

Core   Cladding glass

Figure 12.2 Structure of the fiberoptic bundle. The fiberoptic bundle consists of glass fibers in two layers.

ENDOSCOPES

Optics

Urologic endoscopes usually contain one of two optical designs, either a rod lens system or fiberoptic imaging bundles. While the rod lens system is limited to rigid endoscopes, the fiberoptic version can be used in either flexible or rigid endoscopes and has been seen more frequently in smaller-diameter rigid instruments.

The rod lens system, patented by Harold Hopkins in 1960, consists of a series of glass rods with polished ends where the air interface functions as a lens[3]. The light is efficiently carried along the rod itself. This design proved to be more stable, with higher light carrying capacity, than the previously standard system of thin glass lenses placed at intervals along the length of the telescope.

In comparison, the fiberoptic optical bundle is composed of individual two-layer glass fibers capable of carrying light from one end to the other (Fig. 12.2). In order to provide an accurate optical image, the fibers must be coherent, that is, oriented identically at each end of the bundle. The fiberoptic bundle can be made in a flexible design and also can be made much smaller than a rod lens system. By the very nature of a fiberoptic bundle, with round fibers packed together with space between them, optical information is lost. Thus, the image seen with a rod lens is comparably clearer and brighter than the fiberoptic image.

Nephroscopes

Both rigid and flexible nephroscopes are available. The rigid instrument used for adult applications consists of a metal sheath with a removable telescope assembly, usually containing a rod lens optical system. Recent designs have incorporated a fiberoptic imaging system, which has made it possible to reduce the outer dimension of the endoscope by 2–4F size while maintaining the same 4–5 mm working channel with adequate irrigation (Fig. 12.3). With either optical design, the ocular is offset from the direct axis of the endoscope to leave a straight working

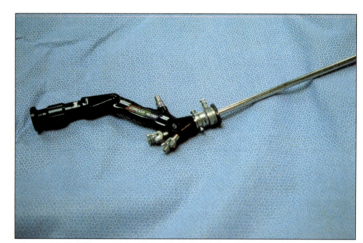

Figure 12.3 Fiberoptic imaging bundles have permitted the downsizing of ureteroscopes and nephroscopes. A rigid offset nephroscope of less than 20F can be designed with a 4mm working channel. The straight channel allows placement of a rigid working instrument.

channel, which can admit the ultrasonic lithotriptor probe and other rigid working instruments. Flexible nephroscopes are available from several manufacturers with an approximate outer dimension of 15–16F. Each endoscope consists of a flexible shaft containing fiberoptic imaging and illuminating bundles, a single channel and the mechanism for active deflection of the tip. The working channel is generally 5–7F to accept correspondingly sized flexible working instruments.

Ureteroscopes

Rigid ureteroscopes have been available in a wide range of sizes. The earliest designs were similar to a long pediatric cystoscope with a sheath containing interchangeable telescopes attached through a bridge apparatus. As these instruments have evolved, a smaller-diameter endoscope of approximately 7F with a

Actively deflectable flexible ureteroscopes			
Company	Outer Size (F)	Channel	Deflection
Circon-ACMI	9.8	3.6	160°
	8.5	2.5	160°
	8.4	3.6	120° and 180°
	7.4	3.6	120° and 170°
Mitsubishi	7.9	3.6	134° and 170°
Olympus	9.9	3.6	100° and 180°
	8.4	3.6	180° and 180°
Storz	7.5/8.4	3.6	120° and 170°
Wolf	9.0	4.5	130° and 160°
	7.5	3.6	130° and 160°
	5.0	2.0	90°

Figure 12.4 Actively deflectable flexible ureteroscopes.

Comparison of endoscopic lithotriptors				
	Effective fragmentation	Safety	Stone removal	Cost
EHL	+++	+	0	+
US	++	+++	++++	+
Impact	++++	+++	0	+
Lasers				
Pulsed dye	++	+++	0	++++
Holmium	++++	++	++	+++

Figure 12.5 Comparison of endoscopic lithotriptors. EHL, electrohydraulic lithotripsy; US, ultrasound.

fiberoptic imaging system and, usually, multiple working channels no larger than 4F has become standard. Although these endoscopes are available in lengths up to 43cm, which can reach the renal pelvis, the rigid ureteroscope is generally not considered an appropriate instrument for intrarenal procedures.

The flexible ureteroscope has made transureteral and intrarenal procedures a viable option. These endoscopes have evolved into a smaller design with a standard version of approximately 7–9F (Fig. 12.4). It contains a working channel of 3.6F with fiberoptic imaging and illumination systems and a mechanism for active deflection of the tip.

Working instruments

The treatment of calculi remains the most common use of intrarenal endoscopy. Therefore, endoscopic lithotriptors are among the most commonly employed working instruments. Several devices are presently available, each with advantages and disadvantages. Endoscopic lithotriptors are summarized in Figure 12.5. Ultrasonic and impact lithotripsy are the most common techniques used percutaneously while laser lithotripsy with the pulsed dye laser, the holmium laser, or electrohydraulic lithotripsy are used ureteroscopically. The most effective lithotriptor for use through a small-diameter flexible ureteroscope has been the holmium laser. Its use has changed the approach to many calculi and has made ureteroscopic lithotripsy the equivalent of or superior to percutaneous approaches in many patients.

Numerous working devices are available for other applications. The design and size often depends upon the endoscope through which it will be placed. Newer materials have vastly expanded the properties that make small working devices useful.

Working instruments for the rigid nephroscope can be up to 3–4mm in diameter and because of the straight channel within the endoscope can be rigid. Thus, very strong metal three-pronged graspers and forceps can be employed for retrieving calculi. Rigid knives with or without a metal sheath can be used for incisional procedures.

For flexible endoscopes, the size of the working instrument is necessarily limited by the size of working channel and flexibility becomes an important feature. For the flexible nephroscope,

instruments up to 4–5F can be used but the smaller channel within the flexible ureteroscope requires instruments of 3F or less.

There are numerous baskets designed for removal of calculi or fragments. The different designs available have different advantages and different purposes (Fig. 12.6). For example, one of the earlier designs, the helical, or Dormia basket is designed for retrieving stones within the ureter. Even impacted calculi can be engaged within the basket by rotating the basket to 'screw' the wires on to the stone. Another design that has been quite popular is the flat wire or Segura basket (Fig. 12.6a), which is composed of two, flat wire loops fitting a basket with a short tip and a wider opening between the wires. This was originally designed for nephroscopic use within the calyces. The flat wire basket opens more efficiently in a large space but, because of the balance of the wires, it cannot be rotated. There is a risk of kinking the wire and losing the shape of the basket.

A more recent introduction is a truly tipless basket made of nitinol (Fig. 12.6b)[4]. This metal is very springy and does not kink. Although it does not have the radial opening force or stability of the other stainless steel baskets, its characteristic to return to its original shape results in a basket very effective in engaging stones. Some of these baskets are available in sizes as small as 2F and can be used through ureteroscopes and nephroscopes.

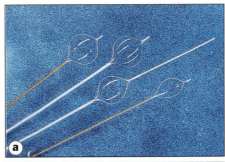

Figure 12.6 Types of stone-retrieval basket. The different basket designs have advantages and disadvantages which can be used for specific purposes in stone retrieval. (a) Segura basket. (b) Tipless or flat wire zero tip basket.

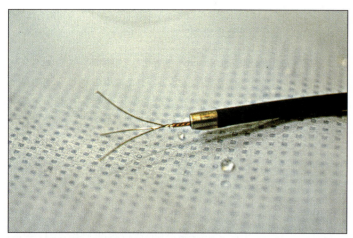

Figure 12.7 Three pronged wire grasper. This is a very safe and effective instrument to use for retrieval of calculi and fragments of calculi from the kidney. Its grasp is not as strong as that of a basket but it is reversible.

Endoscopic lasers		
Laser	Neodymium:YAG	Holmium:YAG
Wavelength	1060nm	2100nm
Penetration	Several millimeters	<0.5mm
Forward scatter	Yes	No
Tissue effect	Coagulation	Ablation and coagulation
Stone effect	None	Fragmentation

Figure 12.8 Endoscopic lasers.

Another retrieval device, which has been overlooked because of the difficulty in using it, is the wire-pronged grasper. The three-wire version is the most effective. The flexible versions are available in sizes from 2F to 4.5F (Fig. 12.7).

Incisional devices used through the flexible instrument can be electrosurgical or laser. The devices can be used for incisions and for coagulation of tissue. Insulated wires of 2–3F designed with a rounded, straight, or angled tip can be placed ureteroscopically for electrosurgical procedures.

The two lasers most commonly used for tissue treatment are the neodymium:YAG and the holmium:YAG lasers (Fig. 12.8). The neodymium laser produces a coagulative effect. The holmium:YAG gives some coagulative effect but also has an ablative effect. The latter can be used for ablating neoplasms or, by applying it in a linear fashion, it can be used to incise tissue. The laser energy is applied through a small flexible quartz fiber, which can be used through small endoscopes or stabilized with a catheter to use through endoscopes with a larger channel.

Tissue can be sampled for biopsy with forceps or retrieval devices. Cup forceps take an actual bite of tissue and are very effective for sampling flat or sessile lesions. Baskets such as the flat wire design may be more effective for sampling papillary lesions, such as typical low-grade transitional cell carcinomas. Other retrieval devices, including wire-pronged graspers, may be effective for sampling tissue in specific locations and circumstances.

Technique for endoscopic access

The major distinction between percutaneous procedures and ureteroscopic procedures is the need for a specific percutaneous access into the intrarenal collecting system for the former while access through the lumen of the ureter is available for uretero-scopic procedures. Ureteral access specifically limits the size of the endoscope that can be used. As noted above, the rigid endoscope has very limited use in the kidney when using the transureteral route but the rigid nephroscope is the major design for percutaneous use.

Percutaneous access is achieved in general by positioning a needle percutaneously into the collecting system, through which a guidewire is placed. The collecting system is visualized by fluoroscopy, sonography, or, in very specific circumstances, computerized tomography. Once the initial access has been gained with a guidewire, the tract is dilated with sequential dilators or a balloon catheter to the diameter required for the endoscope to be employed. Thus, for placement of a rigid nephroscope, the tract must be 7–10mm in diameter. In the acute situation with a fresh tract, a sheath is usually placed from the skin to the collecting system. Once the tract is established, the endoscope of choice can be passed directly into the intrarenal collecting system.

Access to the ureter for endoscopy is initiated by placing a guidewire into the ureter cystoscopically. The ureteral orifice must be dilated only when it will not accept the endoscope being employed. With use of the small-diameter flexible endoscope (7.5F), it is usually not necessary to dilate.

Irrigation must be maintained with any endoscopic technique to distend the lumen and to clear any blood within the visual field. Saline is the standard irrigant for all of these procedures. Rarely, a nonionic medium such as water or glycine can be used with electrosurgical procedures.

ENDOSCOPIC TREATMENT OF RENAL CALCULI

Applications

Nearly all urinary calculi are treated with either extracorporeal shock-wave lithotripsy or endoscopy. Endoscopic stone therapy is usually more likely to clear a comparable stone in a single procedure than extracorporeal shock-wave lithotripsy (EWSL). The choice between endoscopic techniques, percutaneous or ureteroscopic, is made on an individual basis depending on the size, location, and composition of the stone as well as the patient's body habitus and general health. The patient can be assured that there is treatment for almost any urinary calculus.

Open surgery

Open surgical removal was the mainstay of renal stone therapy until the advent of percutaneous nephrostolithotomy and extra-corporeal shock-wave lithotripsy. Surgical therapy was highly successful for solitary renal pelvic calculi but less so for multiple stones, those located within calyces, and the problematic staghorn calculus. It was in these more difficult stones that intrarenal endoscopy proved useful. For example, after surgical removal of the central portion of a staghorn calculus, the angled rigid nephroscope could be placed through the pyelotomy to inspect the infundibula and calyces and retrieve the residual calyceal extensions or calculi[1]. Endoscopic lithotriptors were not available and retrieval was the only option. The rigid

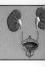

nephroscope gave excellent visibility with active irrigation, which could generally clear blood from the visual field. However, the rigid design allowed movement only in a straight line. As flexible endoscopes became available, these were also used as operative nephroscopes. However, the well-known limitations of flexible endoscopes, which continue, became evident. These limitations include the loss of quality with the fiberoptic image, a smaller channel with limited irrigating capacity and instability of the flexible design. Despite these limitations, the introduction of renal endoscopy into the surgical field demonstrated its value and laid the groundwork for other less invasive endoscopic approaches.

Percutaneous nephroscopy

Percutaneous nephrostolithotomy developed after the introduction of percutaneous renal drainage techniques. Percutaneous access was originally developed for drainage of obstructed kidneys[5]. It became evident that dilation of the nephrostomy tract produced a lumen adequate for introduction of an endoscope into the collecting system. The addition of endoscopic lithotripsy techniques with removal of the fragments completed the technique for percutaneous stone removal[6,7]. Percutaneous nephrostolithotomy remains the major application of percutaneous nephroscopy.

Recent modifications to the techniques of percutaneous nephrostolithotomy have made this a very efficient procedure for removing most large renal calculi. The nephrostomy tract can usually be placed and dilated acutely for immediate endoscopy. The field is usually bloodier than with a previously established nephrostomy, but can be managed. The nephrostomy site should be chosen carefully to give the best access to the entire renal calculus. This is especially important for large branched stones. The rigid nephroscope is placed through a sheath on to the calculus. The chosen lithotriptor is then employed to fragment and remove the calculus. The ultrasonic lithotriptor with a hollow probe is an excellent choice since fragments can be aspirated through the probe to remove stone efficiently. Very hard stones can be broken with an impact device, which is rapid and effective. However, the fragments must be removed as a second step. They can be retrieved through the nephroscope or through the Amplatz sheath by removing the entire nephroscope with the grasper and fragment in place. Nevertheless, it requires multiple passes of the endoscope and, except for extremely hard stones, is less efficient than ultrasonic lithotripsy. Similarly, electrohydraulic lithotripsy fragments the stone without removing the fragments formed. The holmium laser is also a powerful lithotriptor technique but it fragments the calculus into small pieces and is slower than the other lithotriptors.

Calculi extending into or located within infundibula or calyces not accessible to the rigid scope through the existing nephrostomy tract must be accessed by placing another nephrostomy directly on to the calculus or with the flexible nephroscope passed through the original nephrostomy. With the flexible instrument, the stone must be retrieved into the pelvis and through the tract or, in the case of a larger fragment, it can be left in the pelvis for fragmentation through the rigid nephroscope. Alternatively, the larger calyceal stones can be fragmented in situ by delivering one of the flexible lithotriptors to the stone and breaking them in place. The fragments can then be removed or, if they are small enough, allowed to pass.

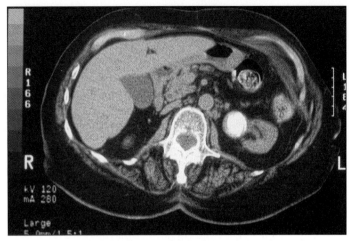

Figure 12.9 Large calculus in the left kidney. Large calculi such as this are best removed with a percutaneous approach. Shock-wave lithotripsy may require multiple treatments and ureteroscopic laser lithotripsy can be a very time-consuming procedure for very large stones.

Percutaneous nephrostolithotomy is a very successful procedure that can remove a large volume of stone. In this way, it is the first choice for the treatment of stones over 2.5cm in diameter (Fig. 12.9). At that size, shock-wave lithotripsy is plagued by failures, with residual fragments and the need for secondary and auxiliary procedures[8]. Percutaneous nephrostolithotomy is also the technique of choice as the first step in treatment of staghorn calculi[9]. It is more frequently successful in removing the entire volume of stone than ESWL when used as the initial treatment.

Percutaneous nephrostolithotomy is more prone to complications and has a higher morbidity than shock-wave lithotripsy or ureteroscopic lithotripsy. The patient must bear the burden of morbidity induced by the presence of the nephrostomy tube. There is a risk of bleeding in addition to the discomfort of the nephrostomy itself. These complications increase with an increasing number of nephrostomy tracts in the same kidney[10].

Ureteroscopic renal lithotripsy

Ureteroscopy has been employed for the treatment of ureteral calculi since its earliest introduction and remains the most frequent application of the procedure. Improvements in the successful completion of ureteroscopy with the addition of small- diameter rigid and flexible endoscopes and more effective endoscopic lithotriptors have expanded the range of ureteroscopy and the indications for its use.

Ureteroscopic lithotripsy of distal ureteral calculi has been uniformly successful at rates greater than 90%[11]. The addition of small-diameter rigid and flexible ureteroscopes and more effective endoscopic lithotriptors such as the small electrohydraulic lithotriptor, the pulsed dye laser, and the holmium laser have markedly improved the success in treating mid and proximal ureteral calculi ureteroscopically (Fig. 12.10).

The next logical step was to extend ureteroscopic lithotripsy techniques to the renal pelvis and intrarenal collecting system. Smaller calculi can be retrieved intact using graspers or baskets while larger stones can be fragmented. The holmium laser has been the most efficient endoscopic lithotriptor. Since small fragments of stone are removed during the lithotripsy procedure and

Ureteroscopic treatment of calculi: effect of instruments				
Year	→1990	1990→	1996	1999
Endoscopes	Rigid	10F flexible	7F rigid	7F rigid
			7.5F flexible	7.5F flexible
Lithotriptors	US, 5F EHL	3F EHL	1.6–1.9F EHL	
		60mJ pulsed dye laser	140μJ pulsed dye laser	Holmium laser
Stones removed ureteroscopically (%)				
Renal	–	96	–	76–91
Ureteral				
Proximal	50	95	96	98
Mid	62	69	91	99
Distal	95	61	93	98

Figure 12.10 Ureteroscopic treatment of calculi: effect of instruments. EHL, electrohydraulic lithotripsy; US, ultrasound.

Ureteroscopic treatment of intrarenal calculi	
	No. of patients
Total	100
≥ 2 calculi	68
>6mm	67
Stone free	77
<3mm fragment	12
≥ 3mm fragment	11
Success	89
Targeted stone removed or fragmented	98

Figure 12.11 Ureteroscopic treatment of intrarenal calculi[12].

washed away in the irrigant, large calculi can be treated effectively without the need to retrieve each fragment. This effect has expanded the application of ureteroscopic laser lithotripsy.

The initial reports on ureteroscopic treatment of renal calculi have shown a success rate of 89%[12] (Fig. 12.11). These data include incidental stones treated during ureteroscopic procedures for ureteral stones and specific targeting of renal stones. The stone-free rate increased from 64% to 77% when patients were followed postoperatively from 1–3 months and an additional 12% of patients had fragments less than 3mm in diameter, thus giving an 89% success rate. It was noted that 98% of targeted stones were fragmented or removed while no ureteral stones remained postoperatively. The success for lower-pole calculi was 87%.

Large stones, meaning those over 2cm in diameter, have also been effectively treated ureteroscopically[13]. Although the large stones are technically more difficult, even branched renal stones can be treated effectively with flexible ureteroscopy and holmium laser lithotripsy. For example, the stone shown in Figure 12.12 was treated in this way. The overall operative time was 135 minutes with an endoscopy time of 115 minutes and the laser was available for 100 minutes. One week postoperatively, at the time of the stent removal, the small fragments initially left in the upper pole had fallen into the lower pole or cleared.

Selection of treatment modality

Selection of the appropriate technique for treatment of calculi within the kidney depends upon several factors related to the stone, including the size, location, composition, and configuration. The patient factors include the configuration of the

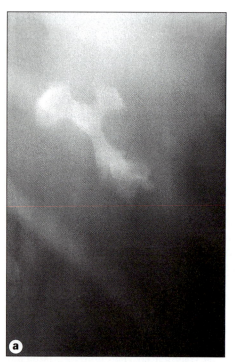
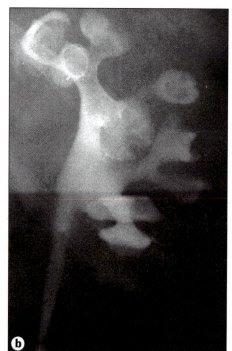
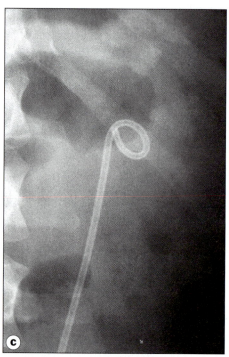

Figure 12.12 Branched upper renal calculus treated with ureteroscopic holmium laser lithotripsy. (a, b) The stone was considered to be too large for shock-wave lithotripsy and percutaneous removal would have required supracostal positioning of the nephrostomy tract. (c) There is excellent fragmentation clearance of most of the stone after a single procedure.

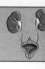

collecting system and other anatomic factors. The patient's general health status, pulmonary function, hematologic function, and body habitus are other major factors determining the approach to a calculus.

Shock-wave lithotripsy is often the first choice for treatment of calculi, when the result can be expected to be comparable to that which can be achieved endoscopically without undue morbidity. For many calculi, this is not the case and endoscopy becomes the first choice. For example, larger ureteral and renal calculi respond poorly to shock-wave lithotripsy, with more frequent repeat and secondary procedures. Renal stones over 2–2.5cm should be treated endoscopically, usually percutaneously. However, some large stones, which may not be easily accessible percutaneously or in patients who can poorly tolerate a percutaneous procedure can be treated better ureteroscopically. Stones that have been impacted in the ureter for long periods are also less amenable to shock-wave lithotripsy. These can respond better to endoscopic therapy. Cystine stones are also more resistant to ESWL. Branched stones are another major indication for a percutaneous approach since there is a greater success for removing these stones percutaneously than with shock-wave lithotripsy.

When selecting between ureteroscopic lithotripsy or percutaneous nephrostolithotomy, the balance of morbidity is generally in favor of the ureteroscopic procedure unless the calculi are too large or too numerous. When a ureteral stone is the major problem it is often better to approach it ureteroscopically and then treat the incidental renal stones as necessary. Often the renal calculi can be treated ureteroscopically during the same procedure. The ureteroscopic approach may be preferred in patients with pulmonary compromise in whom endotracheal intubation or the prone position could present pulmonary compromise. With the ureteroscopic approach, the patient can be maintained in the lithotomy position with the anesthesia of choice.

Thus, it is clear that the various techniques for treatment of calculi, ESWL, percutaneous nephrostolithotomy, and ureteroscopic lithotripsy are complementary, with considerable overlap among optimal applications. There are benefits of each and, in general, there is an increasing application of these endoscopic techniques.

Endoscopic treatment of neoplasms

Percutaneous nephroscopy and endoscopy of the upper tract has been employed for diagnosis and treatment of neoplasms and conditions suspicious for the presence of neoplasm. Just as in the bladder, visualization in the upper tract with endoscopy can provide a diagnosis and with adequate instrumentation can be used to treat lesions discovered. Both percutaneous nephroscopy and transurethral ureteroscopy have been employed for diagnosis while ureteroscopy has become the dominant technique. Both techniques have also been used for treating neoplasms with benefits accruing to either technique in specific circumstances.

Endoscopy has been of value in examining patients with symptoms suggesting the presence of a neoplasm, including gross or microscopic hematuria, abnormal cytology, or pain. Endoscopic surveillance after previous treatment of an upper tract lesion can also be valuable.

Radiologic studies are the first line in evaluation of suspicion of a neoplasm. One of the most common findings is a filling defect, which may give some suggestion of the nature of the lesion. Filling defects that do not change position with movement of the patient are more likely to be neoplasms than those that move freely within the collecting system. Mass lesions of the kidney can be either a cause of hematuria or can appear as filling defects.

Cytology from voided urine has been relatively ineffective in providing a diagnosis in the presence of hematuria or a filling defect. Only high-grade tumors shed individually malignant-appearing cells in sufficient quantity to give a diagnosis in a large fraction of patients.

Endoscopic diagnosis by inspection can be a very valuable technique. For example, direct inspection of a filling defect can distinguish the papillary structure typical of a low-grade transitional cell carcinoma from a lucent calculus or often from edema (Fig. 12.13). Similarly, a filling defect formed by external compression by a blood vessel can be distinguished from an intraluminal lesion. Actively bleeding lesions can occasionally be detected. Hemangiomas have been seen by direct inspection in the presence of hematuria or after it has cleared[14].

Inspection is clearly improved in a clear visual field without traumatic inflammatory changes. Therefore, ureteroscopy without previous stenting has become the most sensitive of endoscopic techniques for visual diagnosis. The percutaneous approach suffers from the need for creation of a nephrostomy tract or for maintenance of the tract's patency with a catheter.

Biopsy

Endoscopic biopsy forms the basis for many diagnoses. The small-diameter rigid and flexible ureteroscopes can deliver instruments adequate to biopsy lesions within the intrarenal collecting system. Cup forceps, baskets, graspers, and brushes are available. A flat wire basket has been most successful in some series to provide an adequate sample of papillary tumor for diagnosis[15]. Cup forceps obtain a smaller sample but can be beneficial for more solid, sessile, or flat lesions. The percutaneous approach presents the risks of dissemination of a lesion before its nature is known. Therefore, when possible, a ureteroscopic approach is preferred for biopsy within the upper urinary tract.

The technique for ureteroscopic biopsy has become quite successful in retrieving a sample that can provide an accurate diagnosis. Samples retrieved by any technique are best handled by cytopathologic techniques[16,17]. Cytologic examination can also give information regarding the grade of some transitional cell carcinomas. Higher grade tumors are composed of individually malignant-appearing cells. The presence of such cells in the cytologic specimen can therefore indicate the presence of a higher-grade tumor. In comparison, low-grade tumors are composed only of atypical cells arranged in a papillary structure. This combination then of atypical cells in a papillary structure can be diagnostic of a low-grade transitional cell carcinoma (Fig. 12.14).

Information can be gained by ureteroscopic biopsy regarding the grade and the stage of the neoplasm as well as its initial diagnosis. The grade reported from ureteroscopic cytology specimens after biopsy has correlated well with the grade seen on a final surgical pathologic specimen after nephroureterectomy or partial ureterectomy[18]. There was undergrading in 3 and overgrading in 3. This grade also correlated to some extent with the final pathologic stage. In one series, the stage was T1 or less in all lesions diagnosed as low grade on the ureteroscopic biopsy and was T2

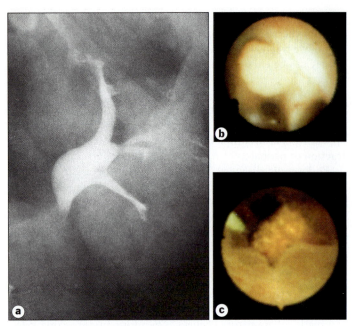

Figure 12.13 Endoscopic diagnosis. The filling defect (a) in a patient who had previously undergone a right nephroureterectomy for transitional cell carcinoma was recognized as a low-grade papillary tumor (b). (c) This could be distinguished from a calculus or ureteral edema.

or greater in 8 out of 12 specimens with a ureteroscopic biopsy indicating a high-grade tumor (Fig. 12.15). Thus, the very tiny biopsies obtained by ureteroscopic biopsy prepared and read by cytopathologic techniques give information on both the actual grade and stage of the upper tract tumor.

The risks of biopsy have been considered, one report suggesting that tumor can be spread beyond the confines of the intrarenal collecting system by ureteroscopic biopsy alone[19]. In this single case report, the transitional cell carcinoma of the renal pelvis was found in peripelvic tissue and not in lymph nodes. A subsequent series of 13 patients biopsied ureteroscopically for transitional cell carcinoma of the ureter or renal pelvis found no unusual pattern of spread[20]. However, a more comprehensive prospective study has been reported[21]. Two groups of 48 patients were compared and followed long term after nephroureterectomy for transitional cell carcinoma. One group had ureteroscopic biopsy prior to treatment and the other did not. There was no difference in the occurrence of metastases or in the rate of patients dying from their malignancy. Therefore, the authors concluded that there was no detrimental long-term effect of ureteroscopic biopsy.

Treatment

Since the upper urinary tract can be accessed endoscopically, either transureterally with ureteroscopy or percutaneously, treatment of lesions in these areas is also possible. There have been several series demonstrating the success of these approaches. In general, smaller tumors have been treated ureteroscopically while larger lesions have been approached percutaneously. There has been considerable crossover between the two approaches.

Ureteroscopy can reach the intrarenal collecting system and deliver devices for tissue ablation. Therefore, it is possible to treat neoplasms within the intrarenal collecting system. Usually,

treatment is combined with the initial biopsy procedure. When there is a papillary tumor, it may be more efficient to remove most of the volume of the tumor with a basket. This provides a large sample for pathologic study and simultaneously removes the mass of the tumor.

If the volume of the tumor has been removed sufficiently, then the base can be fulgurated with a small electrode. A larger volume is treated better with a laser[22]. The neodymium:YAG laser alone can coagulate tissue. This tissue remains in place and must be mechanically removed in order to evaluate the adequacy of treatment. The holmium laser can both coagulate and ablate tissue. It can be used alone or in conjunction with the neodymium:YAG laser to coagulate and then ablate tumors within the intrarenal collecting system. With use of the lasers, a large volume of tumor can be removed through a small flexible ureteroscope.

Ureteroscopic removal of upper urinary tumors has been quite successful using these techniques. It is a very efficient and effective technique for small tumors (less than 1cm). Larger tumors can also be treated but become technically more difficult (Fig. 12.16).

The percutaneous approach for the treatment of upper tract tumors has been effective and safe in several series. One of the major series has included standard percutaneous access to the tumor-containing kidney with an attempt to resect the lesion completely[23]. This is followed within a few days by second-look nephroscopy with biopsy, resection, and fulguration of the tumor base as necessary. If treatment was necessary during the second procedure, then a third procedure was performed to confirm the absence of any tumor. High-grade or invasive lesions and those that were technically impossible to resect were treated by immediate nephroureterectomy with removal of a cuff of bladder in those patients medically acceptable. The complications seen from percutaneous tumor resection have been similar to those of other percutaneous procedures and include bleeding or rarely injury to adjacent organs. The complications have been seen to increase with tumor grade and stage because of the more extensive resection required.

In a 9-year follow-up of 30 patients with upper tract transitional cell carcinoma, Jarrett et al. found 10 recurrences. Two of the 11 grade I tumors, treated percutaneously, recurred while five of the 10 grade III tumors recurred. The only cancer-related deaths were observed in grade III lesions. When compared to open nephroureterectomy, the survival was similar for patients with grade II lesions (53.8 ± 7.2 months with open resection versus 53.3 ± 9.7 months after percutaneous removal)[24]. Lesions of grades I and III also showed no significant difference in disease specific survival between the two treatment techniques.

Post-treatment surveillance

Surveillance after endoscopic treatment differs from that usually employed after open surgical treatment by nephroureterectomy. In the latter case, the search is for recurrence within the bladder or the renal fossa or as distant metastases. After endoscopic resection with preservation of the renal unit, there is the additional concern of local recurrence. The protocols employed have varied but some similarities remain. Frequencies have been roughly similar with cystoscopy every 3 months for at least 1–2 years, decreasing to every 6 months for the next 4 years and yearly after that.

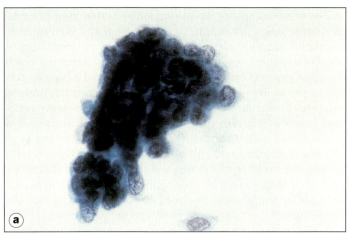

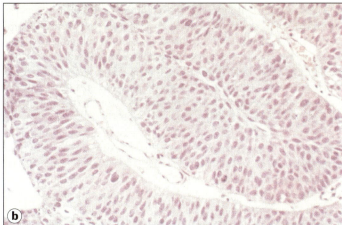

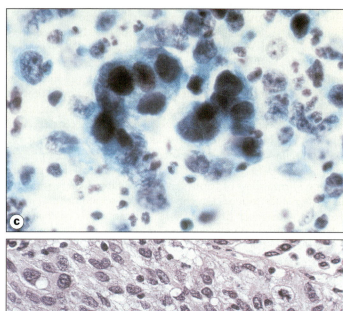

Figure 12.14 Cytologic appearance of transitional cell carcinoma. (a, b) Low-grade papillary transitional cell carcinoma consists of atypical cells in a papillary structure. These can be recognized on cytologic smear as well as a cell block. (c, d) High-grade tumor is characterized by individually malignant-appearing cells on the cytology smear of the cell block.

Accuracy of ureteroscopic biopsy (no. of patients)				
		Grade from surgical specimen		
		1	2	3
	Low grade	5		
Grade from	1–2	1	6	1
ureteroscopic biopsy	2	2	6	2
	High grade		1	11

Figure 12.15 Accuracy of ureteroscopic biopsy.

The optimal technique to locate local intraluminal recurrences has been controversial. In one series, radiographic study with retrograde ureteropyelography was seen to be considerably inferior to ureteropyeloscopy but superior to urinalysis or cytology of voided or cystoscopically drained bladder urine[25]. In a series of 49 patients with endoscopically proven recurrences, urinalysis showed hematuria by chemical dipstick or microscopic examination in only 37% while cytology was positive or suggestive of malignancy in 50%. The retrograde ureteropyelogram suggested an abnormality in 72% of patients when read immediately in the endoscopy room and only 27% with the final radiologist's reading. Thus, it appears that ureteropyeloscopy is more sensitive in

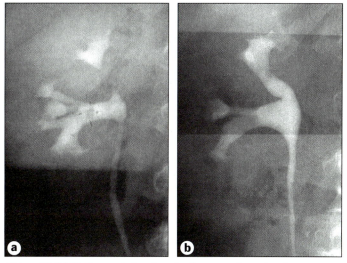

Figure 12.16 Endoscopic treatment of upper urinary tract carcinoma. (a) A renal pelvic filling defect discovered after an episode of hematuria was found to be a grade I–II transitional cell carcinoma and was treated endoscopically. (b) There was no evidence of recurrence by either retrograde pyelogram or ureteroscopy after 9 months follow-up.

detecting recurrent lesions than the other noninvasive or less invasive studies.

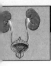

Endoscopic treatment of upper tract transitional cell carcinoma is becoming an accepted mode of therapy. It has been recommended as the treatment of choice for Grade I disease in some papers. Grade II lesions have been the basis for more controversial discussion. Although many of these lesions do well and appear to have statistically equivalent disease-specific survival rates, at least after percutaneous treatment, with acceptable rates seen after ureteroscopic therapy, such treatment must be considered an option. The value of sparing the kidney and the morbidity of nephroureterectomy must be balanced against the need for future surveillance and the risk of recurrence. Grade III lesions tend to do poorly regardless of treatment and are more likely to present as higher-stage lesions. On this basis, the recommendation for patients with grade III transitional cell carcinoma has been for nephroureterectomy.

Endoscopic incisional procedures

Endoscopic incision has assumed a major role in the treatment of obstruction within the upper urinary tract. Endopyelotomy for the treatment of ureteropelvic junction obstruction has become first-line therapy. An endoscopic approach is similarly the major option for ureteral strictures. Symptomatic calyceal diverticula with or without calculi can also be treated best by endoscopic approaches.

Endopyelotomy

Endopyelotomy has assumed a predominant role as the treatment of choice for ureteropelvic junction obstruction. There is more controversy regarding the preoperative evaluation of these patients and any need for definition of periureteral vasculature in a search for crossing vessels.

The diagnosis of ureteropelvic junction obstruction remains dependent upon the patient's presentation with symptoms or radiographic findings of obstruction. Studies with the Lasix washout renogram to demonstrate obstruction have been extremely useful to provide a quantitative indication of split renal function and to quantify drainage. It has been extremely useful to follow patients after endoscopic treatment. The decision to treat is then based on the patient's symptoms, renal function, and the extent of obstruction. Once a decision has been made to treat, the options can be presented to the patient. These include open or laparoscopic pyeloplasty, in addition to one of the techniques for endopyelotomy, including percutaneous nephroscopy ureteroscopy or balloon electroincision.

The techniques for endopyelotomy differ mainly in their endoscopic approach to the ureteropelvic junction. The nephroscopic technique necessarily entails the establishment of a nephrostomy tract while the ureteroscopic approach is transluminal. The percutaneous approach was first used for endopyelotomy[26,27]. It provides an excellent view of the ureteropelvic junction with appropriate nephrostomy placement and can be used for essentially any type of obstruction. The complications are those of nephrostomy placement, in addition to the potential for bleeding from the incision and for recurrent obstruction. The incision can be performed with any cutting device. Both electrosurgical instruments and cold knives have been employed. A stent is placed for internal drainage for varying periods but usually for approximately 6 weeks. Success has been determined by the absence of symptoms and improvement in radiologic studies. Success has generally been approximately 85%.

The ureteroscopic approach was initially attempted as a simpler endoscopic approach to the same site at the ureteropelvic junction. The technique was initially limited by the availability of suitably sized instruments and cutting devices. After the initial report of two successful cases,[28] one series noted a high success rate at the ureteropelvic junction but also found distal ureteral strictures in over 20% of the patients treated[29]. This was considered unacceptably high and was probably related to the use of larger-diameter (greater than 12F) rigid endoscopes and large introducer sheaths for the flexible ureteroscopes. Thomas tried to avoid the problem of stricture and the difficulty of endoscopy with these instruments by prestenting the patient for at least 2 weeks prior to the ureteroscopic procedure[30]. This dilated the ureter and also was suggested to realign the ureteropelvic junction. Endoscopy with a rigid ureteroresectoscope was then possible and endopyelotomy with this technique resulted in a success rate of 81%, increasing to over 90% with a single postprocedural dilation. The advent of small-diameter rigid and flexible ureteroscopes allowed ureteroscopic endopyelotomy without prior stenting. This has the benefit of endopyelotomy in a single endoscopic procedure with the patient in a single position without the morbidity of a nephrostomy tube. The success with this technique has been 85%[31,32] (Fig. 12.17).

Several variables seem to affect the success of endopyelotomies. Van Cangh first showed that the presence of hydronephrosis and, more significantly, the presence of crossing arterial vessels decrease the success of percutaneous endopyelotomy[33]. In the ureteroscopic series, the success of endopyelotomy was 72% when a vessel present was demonstrated by endoluminal ultrasound, while the success was 100% in the absence of a vessel. Others have suggested that the presence of crossing vessels is significant in only 4% of patients with failed endopyelotomies requiring operative intervention[34].

Bleeding during endopyelotomy is an ever-present risk. The rate in reported series has varied from less than 1% to over 14%.

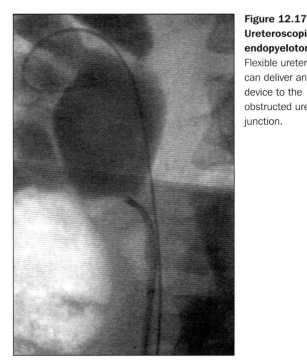

**Figure 12.17
Ureteroscopic
endopyelotomy.**
Flexible ureteroscopy
can deliver an incisional
device to the
obstructed ureteropelvic
junction.

Anatomy of the obstructed ureteropelvic junction							
Series	No. of kidneys	Kidney with vessels		No. of vessels		Septum	
		CT	US	CT	US	CT	US
Keeley	20	7	14	9	19	0	7
Siegel	13	9	10	13	15	Not stated	
Total	**33**	**16**	**24**	**22**	**34**		

Figure 12.18 Anatomy of the obstructed ureteropelvic junction on endoluminal sonography and helical computed tomography (CT). US, ultrasound.

Bleeding has not been noted in those series using endoluminal ultrasound to detect crossing vessels prior to the incision.

The best technique for detecting vessels at the obstructed ureteropelvic junction (UPJ) has been controversial. Relying upon the normal anatomy, which indicates the absence of vessels located directly laterally, may not be appropriate in the abnormal ureteropelvic junction with obstruction. Computerized tomographic scanning of the UPJ has been compared with intraoperative endoluminal ultrasound. The ultrasound technique has been more accurate in both series (Fig. 12.18)[35,36].

There is considerable interest in the appropriate selection of patients for endopyelotomy. Possibly, by eliminating those patients with factors associated with the risk of failure, such as an involved crossing vessel, greater success for the procedure may result from treating high-risk patients with a pyeloplasty, either open or laparoscopic.

Ureteral strictures

Ureteral strictures often present similarly with flank pain or hydronephrosis diagnosed radiographically. Further diagnosis is by radiographic means with Lasix washout renogram playing a major role in defining the presence and extent of obstruction. A retrograde ureteropyelogram is particularly valuable to define the caliber and extent of the ureteral stricture.

An endoscopic approach can usually be ureteroscopic. Rarely, if a nephrostomy is already in place or if, for some reason, it is impossible to access the ureteral orifice, a percutaneous approach may be used. In that case, it is also necessary to pass a ureteroscope but in an antegrade fashion. An incision can then be made with a ureteral resectoscope fitted with a cold knife if that instrument can be delivered to the site of obstruction. More commonly, a narrow-diameter endoscope has been employed and an incision is made either with an electrosurgical device or with a holmium laser. An internal stent is placed and left for several weeks.

Success has been measured as clearance of symptoms and an improvement in radiographic findings. Success has been reported in up to 85% of strictures[37]. Shorter strictures appear to respond better than longer strictures. It is difficult to compare series because of the great variability in ureteral strictures by etiology, length, and location.

Calyceal diverticula

Endoscopic treatment has become the primary mode of therapy for calyceal diverticula. These lesions may be symptomatic, usually presenting with flank pain. Hematuria or passage of stones

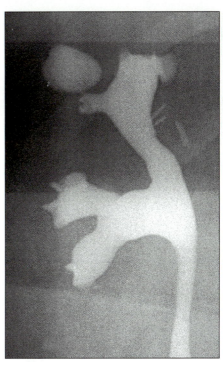

Figure 12.19 Ureteroscopic treatment of diverticulum. A symptomatic diverticulum located in the mid to upper portion of the kidney can be reached ureteroscopically.

can also be observed and occasionally diverticula are totally asymptomatic. The goal in treatment is to remove any calculus, provide better drainage from the diverticulum, or eradicate it totally. Both percutaneous and ureteroscopic procedures have been used in treatment.

Shock-wave lithotripsy has also been applied in the treatment of diverticula containing stones. Usually, the stone can be fragmented but these fragments do not always pass. Many of the patients with adequate fragmentation have been relieved of symptoms although fragments remain. Shock-wave lithotripsy does nothing to treat the basic problem, which is the diverticulum itself.

Treatment with nephroscopy or ureteroscopy

Again these procedures may be complementary in the treatment of diverticula. The percutaneous approach can be most direct and easier in the lower pole. The ureteroscopic access is much easier for lesions in the upper portion of the collecting system[38,39,40] (Fig. 12.19).

For a percutaneous procedure, the diverticulum is punctured directly. Optimally, a guidewire is then passed through the neck of the diverticulum into the collecting system and the tract is subsequently dilated. The nephroscope can then be placed through a dilated tract to treat any calculus present and to dilate or incise the neck of the diverticulum and also obliterate the mucosa lining the diverticulum in an attempt to cause it to collapse. If the wire cannot be passed into the collecting system, then it may be coiled in the diverticulum and dilated to that point. Often, under direct vision, the neck of the diverticulum can be visualized or by instilling contrast or blue dye into the collecting system, the opening of the neck may be identified.

Retrograde flexible ureteroscopy can be used to access the neck of the diverticulum from within the collecting system. It can be difficult to identify small openings and it also can be difficult to reach those in the lower pole. This technique is optimal for the mid to upper portion of the collecting system. Once identified, the neck of the diverticulum can be accessed with a guidewire. The neck can then be dilated with a balloon placed over the wire or passed directly through the ureteroscope. It can also be incised with an electrosurgical device or holmium laser. There is a risk of hemorrhage from damage to vessels coursing through the area of the neck with incision.

Both endoscopic techniques can treat stones and diverticula. Percutaneous treatment appears to offer a more successful immediate removal of stone and thorough ablation of the diverticulum. The ureteroscopic approach can fragment stones and enlarge the neck but it is more difficult to achieve complete obliteration of the diverticulum.

Endoscopic treatment of the kidney

Percutaneous nephroscopy and ureteroscopy have been used successfully for the treatment of numerous lesions of the kidney. Improvements in the working devices used through the flexible ureteroscope have expanded the applications of this technique. Often, the two procedures are complementary and can be used together. Further improvements with the downsizing of nephroscopes and ureteroscopes can be expected to minimize the risks and morbidity of these procedures further.

REFERENCES

1. Gittes RF. Operative nephroscopy. J Urol. 1976;116:148–52.
2. Gittes RF, Varady S. Nephroscopy in chronic unilateral hematuria. J Urol. 1981;126:297–300.
3. Hopkins HH. The modern urological endoscope. In: Gow JG, Hopkins HH, eds. A handbook of urological endoscopy. Edinburgh: Churchill Livingstone; 1978:20–33.
4. Honey RJ. Assessment of a new tipless nitinol stone basket and comparison with an existing flat wire basket. J Endourol. 1998;12(6) 529–31.
5. Goodwin WE, Casey WC, Woolf W. Percutaneous trocar (needle) nephrostomy in hydronephrosis. JAMA. 1955;157:891.
6. Fernstrom I, Johansson B. Percutaneous pyelolithotomy: a new extraction technique. Scand J Urol Nephrol. 1976;10:259.
7. Wickham JEA, Kellet MJ, Miller RA. Elective percutaneous nephrostolithotomy in 50 patients: an analysis of the technique, results and complications. J Urol. 1983;129:904–6.
8. Lingeman JE, Siegel YI, Steele B. Nykus SW, Woods JR. Management of lower pole nephrolithiasis: a critical analysis. J Urol. 1994;151: 663–7.
9. Lam HS, Lingeman JE, Barron M, et al. Staghorn calculi: analysis of treatment results between initial percutaneous nephrostolithotomy and extracorporeal shock-wave lithotripsy monotherapy with reference to surface area. J Urol. 1992;147:1219–25.
10. Winfield HN, Clayman RV, Chaussy CG, Weyman PJ, Fuchs GJ, Lupu AN. Monotherapy of staghorn renal calculi: a comparative study between percutaneous nephrolithotomy and extracorporeal shock-wave lithotripsy. J Urol. 1986;135:1138.
11. Bagley DH. Ureteroscopic lithotripsy. Diagn Therap Endosc. 1997;4(1):1–7.
12. Fabrizio M, Behari A, Conlin MJ, Bagley DH. Ureteroscopic management of intrarenal calculi. J Urol. 1998;1139–43.
13. Grasso M, Conlin M, Bagley DH. Retrograde ureteropyeloscopic treatment of large upper urinary tract (>2cm) and minor staghorn calculi. J Urol. 1998;160:346–51.
14. Tawfiek ER, Bagley DH. Ureteroscopic evaluation and treatment of chronic unilateral hematuria. J Urol. 1998;160:700–2.
15. Abdel-Razzak OM, Ehya H, Cubler-Goodman A, Bagley DH. Ureteroscopic biopsy in the upper urinary tract. Urology. 1994;44(3):451–7.
16. Bian Y, Ehya H, Bagley DH. Cytologic diagnosis of upper urinary tract neoplasms by ureteroscopic sampling. Acta Cytol. 1995;39(4):733–40.
17. Tawfiek ER, Bibbo M, Bagley DH. Ureteroscopic biopsy: technique and specimen preparation. Urology. 1997;50:117–9.
18. Keeley FX, Bibbo M, Bagley DH. Ureteroscopic treatment and surveillance of upper tract transitional cell carcinoma. J Urol. 1997;157: 1560–5.
19. Keeley FX, Kulp DA, Bibbo M, McCue P, Bagley DH. Diagnostic accuracy of ureteroscopic biopsy in upper tract transitional cell carcinoma. J Urol. 1997;157:33–7.
20. Kulp DA, Bagley DH. Does flexible ureteropyeloscopy promote local recurrence of transitional cell carcinoma? J Endourol. 1994;8(2):111–3.
21. Clark PE, Streem SB, Geisinger MA. 13-year experience with percutaneous management of upper tract transitional cell carcinoma. J Urol. 1999;161:772–6.
22. Bagley DH. Ureteroscopic laser treatment of upper urinary tract tumors. J Clin Laser Med Surg. 1998;16(1):55–9.
23. Jarrett TW, Sweetser PM, Weiss GH, Smith AD. Percutaneous management of transitional cell carcinoma of the renal collecting system: 9 year experience. J Urol. 1995;154:1629–35.
24. Lee BR, Jabbour ME, Marshall FF, Smith AD, Jarrett TW. 13-year survival comparison of percutaneous and open nephroureterectomy approaches for management of transitional cell carcinoma of renal collecting system: Equivalent outcomes. J Endourol. 1999;13(4): 289–94.
25. Chen GL, El-Gabry EA, Bagley DH. Surveillance of upper urinary tract transitional cell carcinoma: the role of ureteroscopy, retrograde pyelography, cytology and urinalysis. J Urol. 2000 (in press).
26. Cassis AN, Bramen GE, Bush WH. Endopyelotomy: review of results and complications. J Urol. 1991;146:1492.
27. Motola JA, Badlani GH, Smith AD. Results of 212 consecutive endopyelotomies: An 8 year follow-up. J Urol. 1993;149:453.
28. Inglis JA, Tolley DA. Ureteroscopic pyelolysis for pelvic ureteric obstruction. Br J Urol. 1986;58:250.
29. Meretyk I, Meretyk S, Clayman RV. Endopyelotomy: comparison of ureteroscopic retrograde and antegrade percutaneous techniques. J Urol. 1992;148:775.
30. Thomas R. Endopyelotomy for ureteropelvic junction obstruction and ureteral stricture disease: a comparison of antegrade and retrograde techniques. Curr Opin Urol. 1994;4:174.
31. Conlin MJ, Bagley DH. Ureteroscopic endopyelotomy in a single setting. J Urol. 1998;159:727–31.
32. Tawfiek ER, Liu J-B, Bagley DH. Ureteroscopic treatment of ureteropelvic junction obstruction. J Urol. 1998;160:1643–7.
33. Van Cangh PJ, Nesa S, Galeon M. Vessels around the ureteropelvic junction: significance and imaging by conventional radiology. J Endourol. 1996;10:147.
34. Gupta M, Smith AD. Crossing vessels at the ureteropelvic junction: do they influence endopyelotomy outcome? J Endourol. 1996;10:183.
35. Keeley FX, Moussa SA, Miller J, Tolley DA. A prospective study of endoluminal ultrasound versus computerized tomography angiography for detecting crossing vessels at the ureteropelvic junction. J Urol. 1999;162:1938–41.

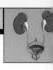

36. Siegel CL, McDougall EM, Middleton WD, et al. Preoperative assessment of ureteropelvic junction obstruction with endoluminal sonography and helical CT. AJR. 1997l168:623–6.

37. Yamada S, Ono Y, Ohshima S, Miyake K. Transurethral ureteroscopic ureterotomy assisted by a prior balloon dilation for relieving ureteral strictures. J Urol. 1995;153:1418–21.

38. Hulbert JH, Reddy PK, Hunter DW, et al. Percutaneous techniques for the management of caliceal diverticula containing calculi. J Urol. 1986;135:225.

39. Bellman GC, Silverstein JI, Blickenderfer S, et al. Techniques and follow up of percutaneous management of caliceal diverticula. Urology. 1993;42:21.

40. Grasso M, Lang GS, Loisides P, Bagley DH. Endoscopic management of the symptomatic anterior caliceal diverticular calculus. J Urol. 1995;153:1878–81.

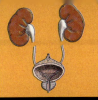

Chapter 13

Laparoscopy

Kevin R Anderson

INTRODUCTION

Since the advent of laparoscopic cholecystectomy in 1987, use of the laparoscopic approach to surgery has been applied to almost all facets of urology. Many procedures traditionally managed via an open approach are now routinely carried out through three or four small incisions. A skilled laparoscopist can remove a kidney, repair a bladder, or diagnosis cryptorchidism through incisions no larger than 1cm[1–3]. In general, laparoscopic urology can be divided into three categories – diagnostic, ablative, and reconstructive. In addition, the technical demands to perform such procedures increases in the same order. Initially, laparoscopic procedures were performed mainly in the realm of gynecology and (on a limited basis) in urology purely for diagnostic purposes in boys with cryptorchidism. Improved imaging technologies, concomitant with refinements of laparoscopic instrumentation, have allowed a rapid increase in the ability to perform meticulous surgery. After the initial popularity of laparoscopic cholecystectomy, initial attempts using laparoscopic approaches were made for most procedures that were open.

The urologist, however, faces a unique challenge in that most of the structures effected by urologic disease exist outside the peritoneal cavity, either in the retroperitoneum or extraperitoneal spaces. The one exception to this is the cryptorchid testis. For this reason, laparoscopy has not been embraced by the urologic community as it has been by our general surgical colleagues.

Unique equipment is necessary to create a laparoscopic environment. Such equipment includes imaging and insufflation technologies, trocars, and instrumentation[4].

IMAGING

Advances in video technology have been essential to enable advanced laparoscopic techniques. Now everyone in the room can view the same image simultaneously, which therefore allows first and second assistants to maintain exposure and countertraction for the surgeon. A basic imaging system includes the laparoscope, light source, camera, and monitor. Most laparoscopes do not have a working channel and have a fixed rod-lens system for image transmission. The initial laparoscopes measured 10mm in diameter, while new minilaparoscopes are only 2mm in diameter and use fiberoptics to provide excellent image transmission. The light source is external to the system and light is transmitted via a fiberoptic cable from a cold xenon light source of high intensity. The aperture setting on the light source is either manual or automatic. In an automatic system feedback through the camera automatically adjusts the light intensity to maintain the optimum image.

In the past the laparoscopist looked directly through the eyepiece, which greatly limited the ability to perform any type of manipulation and completely excluded others in the room from participating in the procedure. Currently, all laparoscopy is carried out with a camera system connected to a monitor. Newer camera systems commonly employ three chips for image resolution (Fig. 13.1), often with digital enhancement. These cameras, coupled with a high-resolution monitor, provide a crisp and accurate depiction in two dimensions of three-dimensional reality. With the loss of the third dimension some surgeons feel that they lose depth perception. Therefore advanced systems have been developed to provide true three-dimensional imaging of the anatomy. These systems, however, are very expensive and often cumbersome to use. It is unclear whether they offer any significant advantage over two-dimensional systems.

INSUFFLATION

Laparoscopy is based on the concept of creating a working environment through which the desired anatomy can be visualized and thereby manipulated. Generally, endoscopic maneuvers within the urinary tract are visualized through a liquid medium

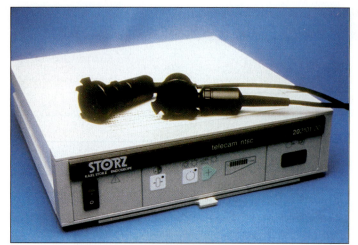

Figure 13.1 Digital 3-chip camera system.

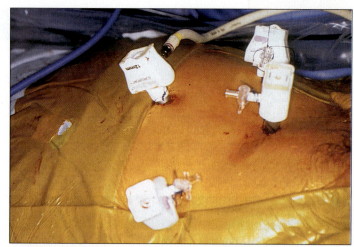

Figure 13.2 Trocars positioned for a laparoscopic dissection of a pelvic lymph node.

such as saline or sorbitol. Working inside the peritoneum the best visualizing media is gas; for laparoscopy the most commonly used gas is carbon dioxide. The advantages of carbon dioxide include that it is both nonflammable and readily absorbed into the blood stream. The disadvantage is that it reacts with the peritoneal surface to give carbonic acid and therefore can cause peritoneal irritation once the patient has recovered from anesthesia. An often-seen complication of laparoscopy is hypercarbia, which in general is benign and can be managed by hyperventilation. However, in rare circumstances a carbon dioxide embolus can occur and can have dire consequences.

The insufflator maintains the intra-abdominal pressure at or below a level specified by the surgeon. Most laparoscopic procedures are carried out at pressures between 10 and 15mmHg (1.3 and 2.0kPa). Sterile tubing is connected from the insufflator to one of the working ports. Initial insufflation can be carried out by blind puncture using a Veress needle[5], which is usually placed at or near the umbilicus as this location is most often free of vessels or adhesions. The Veress needle has a spring-loaded retractable tip so that once it enters the peritoneal cavity it tends not to cause puncture injuries to tissues that can be freely moved away from the tip. The gas is then passed through the Veress needle until the abdomen is insufflated. During insufflation routine maneuvers that help to assure good position of the Veress needle are:

- saline is infused in the needle and if it cannot be withdrawn the needle is generally not inside a hollow viscus; and
- upon insufflation intraperitoneal pressure should remain low as the flow of gas begins (i.e. the pressure should remain at 2–5mmHg (0.27–0.67kPa) – an immediate rise to 15mmHg (2.0kPa) suggests that the tip of the Veress needle is not within the peritoneal space and it should therefore be replaced).

In some cases, because of previous surgery or suspected adhesions, a Veress needle is not used and an open technique is performed whereby visual dissection is carried out with standard instruments to the level of the peritoneum. The peritoneum is opened and, under direct visualization, a blunt tip, or Hassan cannula, is introduced into the abdominal cavity and a purse string suture is placed around the trocar to maintain an airtight seal. Some surgeons feel that this technique is inherently safer than the Veress needle, but injuries can occur with both techniques.

TROCARS

Trocars (or ports) are passed through the abdominal wall to allow access from the outside into the gas-filled working environment. The ideal trocar should maintain a gas-tight seal within the abdominal cavity and allow easy passage of instruments into the abdomen and removal of tissue or other foreign bodies out of the abdomen (Fig. 13.2) Generally, trocars come with a side port for insufflation and a one-way flap valve to allow placement of the instrument without egress of gas. The initial trocar is often placed blindly once the abdomen has filled with gas, but the remaining trocars are placed under direct vision from inside using the laparoscope. Trocars come in varying sizes; it is preferable to use as small a port as possible for a given procedure, since the degree of pain and postoperative complications increases with the size of the trocar. Common trocar sizes include 5mm, 10mm, and 12mm and are utilized according to the type of instruments that that are essential for a specific case. Minilaparoscopy uses 2–3mm trocars and allows passage of a number of newly developed smaller instruments.

INSTRUMENTATION

Specialized instrumentation has been developed for laparoscopy. These instruments fall into the following categories:
- tissue dissection;
- tissue fixation;
- vascular control;
- tissue retrieval;
- hemostasis; and
- tissue apposition and closure.

Common to the design of all these instruments is the essential ability to pass them through trocars or ports that measure generally a maximum diameter of 12mm. They must be long enough to both extend through the abdominal cavity and be handled ergonomically by the surgeon. Initially, instrumentation

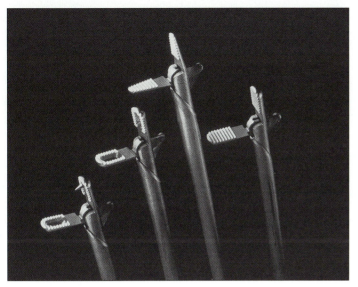

Figure 13.3 Various nondisposable 5mm laparoscopic dissectors.

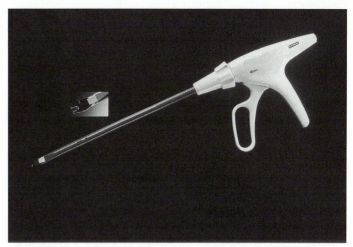

Figure 13.4 Laparoscopic clip applier.

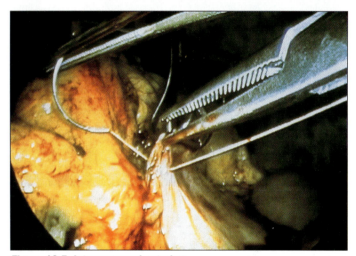

Figure 13.5 Intracorporeal suturing.

design paralleled the function of standard open instrumentation [i.e. laparoscopic scissors, forceps, graspers, clamps, etc. (Fig. 13.3)]. More recently, instruments have been uniquely designed for the laparoscopic environment.

Tissue dissection

Tissue dissection can be carried out by direct mechanical manipulation (such as with scissors or graspers). Electrocautery can be applied to a variety of instruments (scissors or angled-tip probes) to cause thermal separation of the tissues. Various types of lasers have been utilized for tissue dissection, such as a laser that combines a yttrium–aluminum–garnet with a potassium titanyl phosphate crystal. Both hydrodissection with high-pressure saline jet and pneumodissection with high-pressure carbon dioxide through a nozzle have been used to rapidly dissect through connective tissue and fat[6]. Recently, balloon dilation has been utilized, especially in the extraperitoneal space, to create a large working environment rapidly. This is achieved by inserting a balloon into a potential space and filling it with gas or fluid[7].

Tissue fixation

Certain procedures, such as bladder neck suspensions and hernia repairs, require fixation of tissue to solid structures or the application of graft material to a hernia defect. This may be carried out with either intracorporeal suturing techniques or special types of laparoscopic clips. Intracorporeal suturing can be tedious and difficult and, therefore, in most circumstances an automatic clip applier is utilized first (Fig. 13.4). In certain circumstances laparoscopic suturing is necessary and these technical skills need to be developed and practiced. Both intracorporeal and extracorporeal knots can be tied (Fig. 13.5)[8]. Automatic suturing devices have been developed that greatly facilitate the technique of intracorporeal suturing.

Hemostasis and vascular control

Electrocautery is most commonly used to manage superficial oozing and bleeding after dividing tissue, and is very effective; however, occasionally large vessels are encountered and these

should be clipped prior to their division. Generally, laparoscopic clip appliers, which utilize a V-shape clip, are used (Fig. 13.6). For small veins, generally one clip is placed on either side and the vessel is divided. For larger vessels, such as the renal artery and renal vein, generally three clips are placed on both sides of the vessel and the vessel is then divided. Currently, most clip appliers pass through a 10F port; however, newer clip appliers have been manufactured that will also go through a 5mm port and are of great use in pediatric laparoscopy. For a very large vessel, such as the renal vein, often the 9mm clip is not long enough; in such cases an automatic stapling device, which places three rows of staples on either side of the incision, is used to divide the vein (Fig. 13.7). Critical is that the device be positioned correctly prior to activation.

A right angle clip applier has also been developed to allow the laparoscopist to visualize more easily the tip of the staple prior to its closure.

Aspiration irrigation

Another essential tool for laparoscopy is an aspiration–irrigation device that can both wash away blood and aspirate fluids, such as irrigation fluid, blood, and smoke. These can be freestanding

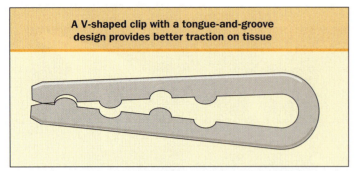

Figure 13.6 A V-shaped clip with a tongue-and-groove design provides better traction on tissue.

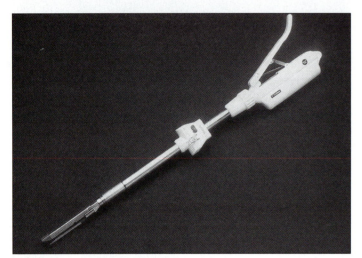

Figure 13.7 Automatic stapling device staples and divides the tissue simultaneously.

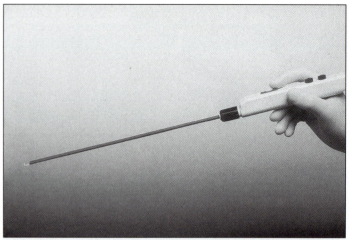

Figure 13.8 Right-angle electrode that combines electrocautery, aspiration, and irrigation into one device.

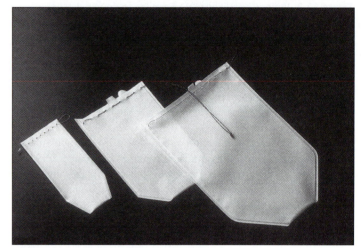

Figure 13.9 Laparoscopic entrapment sacks of tough nylon design allow for morcellation within the sack.

devices that serve only to provide aspiration and irrigation through a separate probe or they can be combined with other instrumentation, such as a combination retractile right-angle electric probe and aspiration irrigator (Fig. 13.8). Generally, the fluid irrigated contains heparin (5000U/L) as well as a broad-spectrum antibiotic, such as cefazolin.

Tissue retrieval

Ablative laparoscopic procedures often require tissue or organs to be removed from the body. Small pieces of tissue, such as lymph node biopsies or small testicles, can be removed through a 10mm port purely by grasping the tissue and pulling it through. In such situations it is important to open a flap valve manually to prevent the tissue from being trapped inside the port. Larger solid organs often have to be morcellated prior to removal. In such cases laparoscopic retrieval bags or sacks are employed to capture the organ so that it can be controlled during the removal process[9]. If a large solid organ, such as a kidney, is removed a sturdy laparoscopic bag should be used (Fig. 13.9). This is an impermeable nylon bag that does not rip with manipulation of the organ. Either a tissue morcellator can be used or the tissue can be fragmented with a Kelly clamp or ring forceps. For smaller, floppier tissue a number of commercially produced laparoscopic sacks are available that have a spring-loaded opening and allow easy 'scooping' of the tissue with subsequent retrieval.

LAPAROSCOPIC UROLOGIC PROCEDURES

Cryptorchid testis

The first laparoscopic diagnosis of a nonpalpable cryptorchid testis was performed by Cortesi in 1976[10]. Currently widely utilized, this is a simple way to make a rapid diagnosis of an intra-abdominal testis or absent testis[3,11]. Recent advances in laparoscopic equipment now allow the surgeon to use a 2mm laparoscope that combines a Veress needle and a 2mm port. A diagnosis can be made within minutes through a needle opening that requires no closure or sutures. A Veress needle is placed through a small puncture at the umbilicus. The abdominal cavity is inflated to approximately 10mmHg (1.3kPa) and the 2mm scope is introduced. In a patient with unilateral cryptorchidism, the contralateral 'normal' side is visualized and the vas and gonadal vessels are seen traversing the internal ring (Fig. 13.10). On the side that has no palpable testis, if a vas and vessels are seen coursing through the internal ring (in the absence of a hernia sac) it is highly unlikely that a normal testis will be found within the canal[3].

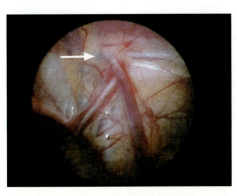

Figure 13.10 Normal vas and vessels entering the internal ring (no hernia defect).

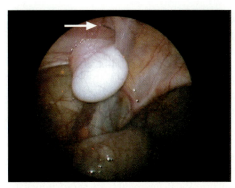

Figure 13.12 Intra-abdominal testis. Note the hernia defect at the internal ring (arrow).

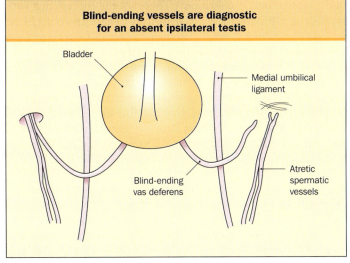

Blind-ending vessels are diagnostic for an absent ipsilateral testis

Bladder

Medial umbilical ligament

Blind-ending vas deferens

Atretic spermatic vessels

Figure 13.11 Blind-ending vessels are diagnostic for an absent ipsilateral testis.

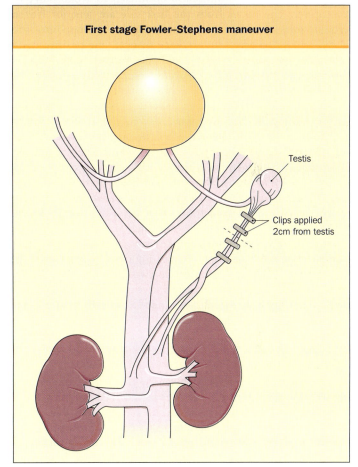

First stage Fowler–Stephens maneuver

Testis

Clips applied 2cm from testis

Figure 13.13 First stage Fowler–Stephens maneuver. The gonadal vessels are clipped (without disturbing the testis).

Most urologists still explore the inguinal canal through either an external open incision or, in some cases, a laparoscopic dissection, because gonadal tissue has been found at the tip of the vessels. If blind-ending vessels are seen above the internal ring, the diagnosis of an absent testis is made (Fig. 13.11). If an intra-abdominal testis is identified, immediate orchiopexy can be carried out with either open or laparoscopic techniques (Fig. 13.12). If it appears that the length of the gonadal vessels is insufficient to allow an immediate orchiopexy, a first stage Fowler–Stephens maneuver is carried out laparoscopically by dissecting the gonadal vessels superior to the testis (Fig. 13.13)[12,13]. Care is taken not to disturb the testis or its peritoneal attachments and thereby preserve the secondary blood supply to the testis. Once the gonadal vessels are dissected free, a clip is placed across the vessels to occlude the gonadal artery. This allows hypertrophy of the vasal and cremasteric arteries to the testis, such that an orchiopexy can be carried out at a later date (generally 4–6 months after the first stage) by dividing the clipped gonadal artery and thereby allowing for greater mobility of the testis. This maneuver can be achieved through a second 5mm port using a 5mm clip applier. Kavoussi and colleagues reported on 515 patients who underwent the laparoscopic evaluation of a nonpalpable testis, with a success rate of 98.5%. Absent testis occurred in 32% of patients, with abdominal testis found in 39% and inguinal testis in 28%. Complications occurred in only 1% of patients and usually related to insufflation of the preperitoneal space[14].

Pelvic lymphadenectomy

One of the earliest uses of laparoscopy in urology was to stage prostate cancer. The initial site for metastatic disease in prostate cancer is generally the pelvic lymph nodes. Sampling of these lymph nodes may indicate advanced disease and thereby obviate the need for radical surgery or radiation therapy. Schuessler and colleagues described the first laparoscopic dissection of a pelvic lymph node in 1989, after which this found wide acceptance among urologists throughout the world[15]. Currently, the indications for a laparoscopic dissection of the pelvic lymph nodes for prostate cancer are limited to patients with a high likelihood of metastatic disease (i.e. prostate-specific antigen >20ng/mL, Gleason score of 8–10, or evidence of pelvic lymphadenopathy on computer tomography)[16]. The procedure is carried out with the patient in the supine position, and generally four ports are used in a diamond configuration. A 10mm port is used at the umbilicus with a 10–12mm port in the midline above the pubic bone and two 5mm ports laterally (see Fig. 13.2). Dissection can be performed either transperitoneally or extraperitoneally (using a dissecting balloon). In the transperitoneal approach an incision is made in the peritoneum, the vas identified and divided. The landmarks of dissection are the medium umbilical ligament, pubic bone, external iliac vein, and obturator nerve. The entire nodal package is dissected and care is taken to stay medial to the medium umbilical ligaments, to avoid injury to the ureter. The nodes from the first side are sent for frozen section analysis. If these nodes are negative the opposite side is dissected; however, the presence of even one positive node indicates metastatic disease and no further dissection is necessary. Winfield and colleagues compared standard open lymphadenectomy with laparoscopic lymph node dissection in 30 patients[17]. All patients then underwent a radical retropubic prostatectomy. It was found that an average of 10 lymph nodes per side was retrieved doing the laparoscopic approach, with an additional three nodes per patient removed by means of an open procedure. There were no major complications in either group in this particular study. Kavoussi and colleagues performed a multi-institutional study to examine complications of laparoscopic pelvic lymphadenectomy. They reported on 329 pelvic laparoscopic node dissections, of which major complications occurred in 8% and minor complications in 6%. Intraoperative complications included six vascular injuries, ureteral injury in two patients, bladder injuries in two patients, and bowel perforation in one patient. Postoperative complications included urinary retention in two patients, and prolonged ileus, lymphedema, and lymphocele formation in 1%, each. There was no operative mortality[18].

Varicocelectomy

Laparoscopic varicocele ligation can be utilized in patients who present with symptomatic varicoceles[19]. Most commonly these varicoceles are unilateral and occur on the left, but some patients do present with bilateral varicoceles. The laparoscopic varicocele ligation is carried out generally through a transperitoneal approach using 2–3 ports; care is taken to dissect the gonadal veins away from the gonadal artery and to clip the gonadal veins independently, leaving the artery intact. The indications for varicocele repair are subfertility with testicular atrophy or scrotal pain related to a large varicocele. The laparoscopic approach is especially useful in patients who have bilateral varicoceles, with a great reduction in morbidity as two inguinal incisions are avoided.

Laparoscopic surgery on the kidneys and ureters

Laparoscopic nephrectomy has become an accepted and widely practiced procedure for both benign and malignant lesions of the kidney. Clayman and colleagues performed the first laparoscopic nephrectomy in 1990[1]. Prior to the initial laparoscopic nephrectomy animal studies had been carried out to develop the equipment necessary to remove a solid organ. Concurrently, a strong laparoscopic entrapment sack and a high-speed tissue morcellator were developed.

Indications for laparoscopic simple nephrectomy include renal vascular hypertension, chronic obstruction and infection, chronic pain associated with poorly functioning kidney, or a multicystic kidney. In addition, many surgeons have performed laparoscopic radical or total nephrectomies for patients with solid renal tumors. Generally, these are carried out in patients who have tumors that measure ≤ 5cm in diameter. Initially, many of these kidneys were morcellated, but they can also be removed intact via a lap sack through a small suprailiac or midline incision. Recently, with the development of the pnuemo-sleeve, this procedure has become more popular now that the surgeon can actually place one hand into the abdominal cavity to assist with retraction and dissection under laparoscopic visualization[20]. There is some concern that with laparoscopic nephrectomy for malignant disease there might be spillage of tumor[21–23]; but to date no evidence of fossa recurrence has been attributed solely to the laparoscopic approach.

To perform a laparoscopic simple nephrectomy, generally the patient is positioned in the lateral decubitus position (Fig. 13.14). A total of 4–5 ports are used, and lateral insufflation is performed by placing the Veress needle lateral to the rectus muscle rather than at the umbilicus. A 10mm laparoscope with a 30° lens is utilized. The peritoneum lateral to the colon is incised and the colon is reflected medially. The ureter or kidney is identified. In cases of benign renal disease associated with obstruction or reflux the ureter or kidney may often be dilated and therefore more readily visible. Once the ureter has been identified it is dissected free and grasped with forceps to allow traction on the kidney (Fig. 13.15). The kidney is dissected laterally, posteriorly, inferiorly, and, finally, medially to expose the hilum (Fig. 13.16). The hilar vessels are carefully dissected free and the renal artery is clipped with 9 mm clips using at least three clips on the aorta side and two clips on the kidney side (Fig. 13.17). The artery is then sharply divided. If the renal vein is small enough, a similar clipping maneuver is sufficient to divide the vein. However, for large renal veins a vascular automatic stapler is used to both staple and divide the vein in one move.

Once the renal vessels are divided the remainder of the dissection is performed. The adrenal is left *in situ* and the freed kidney is placed in an entrapment sack (Fig. 13.18). If there is a significant volume of solid parenchyma the stronger lap sack should be employed. If it is a hydronephrotic or small multicystic kidney, generally it can be removed using a spring-open entrapment bag that is simpler to insert and employ; however, the bags are made of weaker material and can break if not used carefully. The mouth of the bag is pulled through the abdominal wall. A Kelly clamp or ring forceps is used to tear the tissue piece by piece from inside the bag and out through the abdominal wall. The tissue is sent to pathology. The renal fossa is inspected at low pressure [5mmHg (0.67kPa)] to confirm that there is no venous bleeding, which can be compressed at the higher pressures [15mmHg (2.0kPa)] and begin to bleed later once the abdomen is deflated and closed. Each port is removed under visual inspection. If no bleeding occurs at the port sites, the larger port sites are closed either with an endo-close device or with standard suture material. It is important to close trocar sites that are 10–12mm in diameter to prevent herniation of abdominal contents.

There is a definite learning curve to performing laparoscopic nephrectomies and the initial series reported operating times that ranged from 3–6 hours. Most current studies report

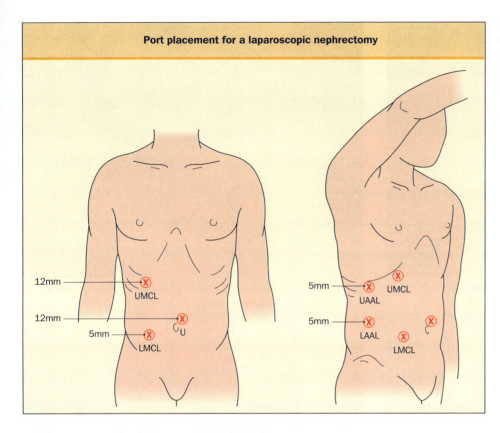

Port placement for a laparoscopic nephrectomy

12mm — UMCL
12mm
5mm — LMCL
U

5mm — UMCL / UAAL
5mm — LAAL / LMCL

Figure 13.14 Port placement for a laparoscopic nephrectomy. LAAL, lower anterior–axillary line; LMCL, lower midclavicular line; U, umbilicus; UAAL, upper anterior–axillary line; UMCL, upper midclavicular line.

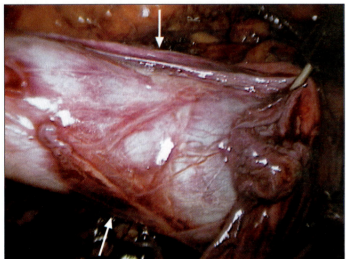

Figure 13.15 Dissection of a dilated ureter (arrows).

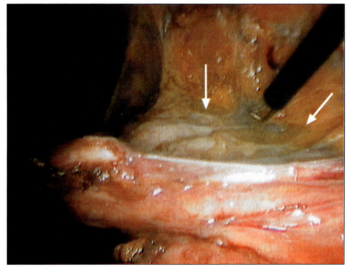

Figure 13.16 The decompressed hydronephrotic kidney is reflected medially away from the side wall (arrows).

operating times between 2 and 4 hours. Gill and associates reported that in a multi-institutional study most complications occurred early in the learning curve and that the complication rate for laparoscopic nephrectomies is 16%[24]. In patients who present with reflux nephropathy and poor renal function a laparoscopic nephroureterectomy is indicated. The initial dissection is carried out just as the laparoscopic nephrectomy, but once the kidney is freed the ureter is dissected down to the level of the bladder. In patients with no transitional cell carcinoma it is not necessary to take a bladder cuff; therefore, the ureter can be clipped just above its entrance into the bladder, divided, and removed.

In children no additional ports are necessary to carry out this maneuver; however, in adults sometimes a fifth port in the lower abdomen is necessary to finish the distal ureteral dissection.

Laparoscopic unroofing of renal cysts

The laparoscope is ideal for treating patients with symptomatic renal cysts[25,26]. The patient may have a single, simple large renal cyst that is symptomatic or can be unroofed or the patient may have multiple cysts, such as those of adult polycystic kidney disease. In the latter case a laparoscopic approach is used to unroof scores of cysts. Generally, these patients present with prolonged

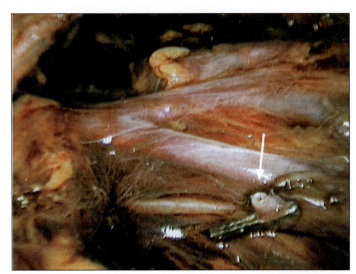

Figure 13.17 A small arterial branch has been clipped (arrow). The renal vein remains intact.

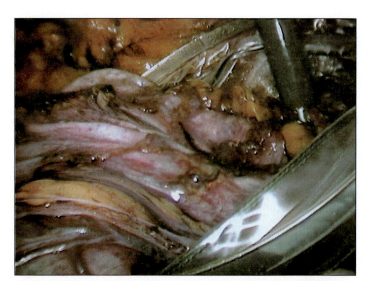

Figure 13.18 The kidney (now completely freed) is placed into a spring-opening entrapment sack.

and incapacitating pain. In the procedure the kidney is exposed in a similar fashion as for the laparoscopic nephrectomy. Gerota's fascia is opened and the cysts are dissected and exposed. Using a right-angle electrode the cysts can be punctured. The cyst wall is grasped and completely removed. The edges and base of the cyst can be fulgurated using an argon beam coagulator. In the case of adult polycystic disease, multiple cysts are encountered and the goal is to unroof as many as possible. It has been shown that unroofing of cysts does not adversely affect renal function in patients with adult polycystic kidney disease. It is very important to inspect the cyst base in patients who present with complex cysts to rule out cancer and, if indicated, to perform a biopsy. Segura and colleagues reported an initial success rate with the laparoscopic approach for unroofing polycystic kidney disease as 50%[27]. These patients had relief of their symptoms for up to 2 years in follow-up; however, as is the case with all treatments of adult polycystic disease new cysts do grow and the pain often recurs.

Laparoscopic lymphocele drainage

Pelvic lymphoceles may occur after pelvic lymph node dissections or in association with renal transplants. In both cases permanent drainage of a lymphocele can be achieved with a laparoscopic approach[28]. It is important to differentiate a true lymphocele that surrounds a transplant kidney from a urinoma. Prior to marsupialization of a lymphocele, it is prudent to needle aspirate it and send the fluid for both culture and creatinine level. The lymphocele is treated by identifying its wall (which can be facilitated by either overfilling the lymphocele cavity, if there is a tube already draining it, with a solution of saline and indigo carmine). The lymphocele is opened and the edges are marsupialized using either a laparoscopic tacking clip applier or by tacking omentum into the lymphocele cavity (Fig. 13.19). This prevents closure and reformation of the lymphocele.

Laparoscopic bladder neck suspension

In women with stress urinary incontinence a multitude of procedures have been utilized to reposition the bladder neck to

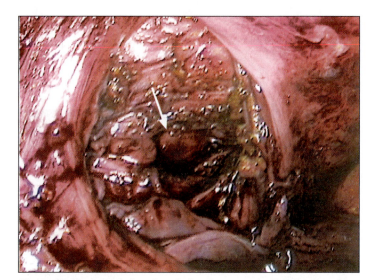

Figure 13.19 A pelvic lymphocele has been opened, drained, and marsupialized (arrow) with tacking clips.

prevent descent during micturition and thereby stop incontinence. In patients with documented Type I or Type II stress urinary incontinence a laparoscopic bladder neck suspension can be carried out[29]. A diagnosis is generally made by physical examination and video urodynamics.

The procedure can be performed through either a transperitoneal or extraperitoneal approach; however, the extraperitoneal approach provides the advantage of access to the anterior aspect of the bladder and bladder neck. This is carried out by first placing a tissue dilating balloon into the extraperitoneal space (Fig. 13.20). A 1cm incision is made midway between the symphysis pubis and the umbilicus, and carried through the rectus muscles into the supravesical space. Initially, finger dissection creates a space whereby the dilating balloon can be placed and inflated. A blunt or Hassan trocar is inserted and this extraperitoneal space is inflated to 15mmHg (2.0kPa) with carbon dioxide.

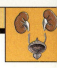

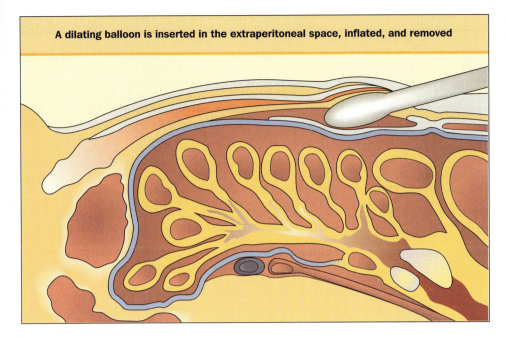

A dilating balloon is inserted in the extraperitoneal space, inflated, and removed

Figure 13.20 A dilating balloon is inserted in the extraperitoneal space, inflated, and removed.

Further dissection is carried out around the bladder neck, assisted by transvaginal palpation with the index finger to demonstrate the anterior vaginal wall on either side of the urethra. Cooper's ligament is dissected and exposed. Fixation sutures are placed in the anterior vaginal wall, and to Cooper's ligament. Intracorporeal suturing techniques are utilized to bring the tissue laterally to the ligament. It is important not to tie the sutures too tightly, but enough to provide support to prevent descensus of the bladder neck. Initial studies by McDougall revealed that the laparoscopic bladder neck suspension provided equivalent relief from incontinence as the Stamey–Raz needle suspension procedure; however, the patients were able to void sooner than those who had the needle suspension procedure[30].

Laparoscopic live donor nephrectomy

Interest in performing laparoscopic live donor nephrectomies has been increasing. Gill and colleagues pioneered the initial work in the animal model and it was found that the right kidney could be laparoscopically removed in a porcine model[31]. These kidneys were then transplanted and functioned normally. This procedure has now been performed in multiple centers throughout the country with good success. The warm ischemia time is short and the kidney is removed through a small midline incision. Recently, other investigators have employed the Pneumo-sleeve to help with dissection of the kidney and utilize the incision for the Pneumo-sleeve to remove rapidly the intact donor kidney. There is some concern, however, that the additional manipulation of the kidney and possible increased warm ischemia time may have a deleterious effect on the survival of some of these kidneys[32].

Adrenalectomy

The laparoscopic approach has become the procedure of choice with which to remove adrenal glands for benign disease[33,34]. Adrenal glands have been removed for diagnoses such as pheochromocytoma, adrenal hyperplasia, bilateral adrenal hyperplasia, and adrenal adenoma. The approach is similar to that of a laparoscopic nephrectomy. It is important to gain adequate exposure on the right by reflecting the liver anteriorly, and on the left by reflecting the colon and spleen. Special care is taken to clip all adrenal vessels adequately, especially the adrenal vein. Laparoscopic adrenalectomy has almost completely replaced the open approach for the removal of adrenal glands.

SUMMARY

Laparoscopy in urology is here to stay. Certainly, we have seen in the past decade marked benefits from this new technology (Fig. 13.21). As the technology advances and we continue to hone our skills in visualizing, dissecting, and reconstructing tissues, we will continue to see an expanding use of laparoscopy in the management of urologic disease.

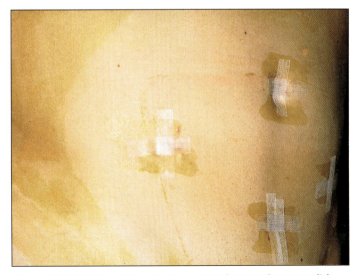

Figure 13.21 Minimally invasive laparoscopic procedures result in smaller scars.

REFERENCES

1. Clayman RV, Kavoussi LR, Soper NJ, et al. Laparoscopic nephrectomy: initial case report. J Urol. 1991:146:278–82.

2. Das S. Laparoscopic removal of bladder diverticulum. J Urol. 1992:148:1837–9.

3. Weiss RM, Seashore JH. Laparoscopy in the management of the non-palpable testis. J Urol. 1987:138:382–5.

4. Goldstein DS, Chandhoke PS, Kavoussi LR. Laparoscopic equipment. In: Clayman RV, McDougall EM, eds. Laparoscopic urology. St Louis: Quality Medical Publishing; 1993:97–101.

5. Veress J. Neues instrument zur ausfuhrung von Brust-oder bauch-punktionen und pneumothorax behandlung. Dtsche Med Wochenschr. 1938;64:1480–2.

6. Gardner SM, Clayman RV, McDougall EM, et al. Laparoscopic pneumodissection: a unique means of tissue dissection. J Urol. 1995;154:591–4.

7. Gaur DD, Agarwal DK, Purohit KC. Retroperitoneal laparoscopic nephrectomy: initial case report. J Urol. 1993;149:103–5.

8. McDougall EM. Laparoscopic knot tying. In: Clayman RV, McDougall EM, eds. Laparoscopic urology. St Louis: Quality Medical Publishing; 1993:122–54.

9. Kavoussi LR, Clayman RV, Brunt LM, Soper NJ. Organ entrapment system for removing nodal tissue during laparoscopic pelvic lymphadenectomy. J Urol. 1992;147:879–80.

10. Cortesi N, Ferrari P, Zumbarda E, Manenti A, Baldina A, Pgnatti-Morano F. Diagnosis of bilateral abdominal crytorchidism by laparoscopy. Endoscopy. 1976;8:33–4.

11. Diamond DA, Caldomone AA. The value of laparoscopy for 106 impalpable testes relative to clinical presentation. J Urol. 1992;148:632–4.

12. Bloom DA. Two-step orchiopexy with pelviscopic clip ligation of the spermatic vessels. J Urol. 1991;145:1030–3.

13. Elder JS. Laparoscopy and Fowler–Stephens orchiopexy in the management of the impalpable testis. Urol Clin North Am. 1989;16:399–411.

14. Kavoussi LR. Pediatric applications of laparoscopy. In: Clayman RV, McDougall EM, eds. Laparoscopic urology. St Louis: Quality Medical Publishing; 1993:220–2.

15. Schuessler WW, Vancaillie TG, Reich H, Griffith DP. Transperitoneal endosurgical lymphadenectomy in patients with localized prostate cancer. J Urol. 1991;145:988–91.

16. Smith JA Jr, Seaman JP, Gleidman JB, Middleton RG. Pelvic lymph node metastasis from prostatic cancer: Influence of tumor grade and stage in 452 consecutive patients. J Urol. 1983;130:290–2.

17. Winfield HN, Donovan JF, See WA, Loening SA, Williams RD. Laparoscopic pelvic lymph node dissection for genitourinary malignancies: indications, techniques, and results. J Endourol. 1992;2:103–11.

18. Kavoussi LR, Sosa E, Chandhoke PS, et al. Complications of laparoscopic pelvic lymph node dissection. J Urol. 1993;149:322–5.

19. Donovan JF, Winfield HN. Laparoscopic varix ligation. J Urol. 1992;147:77–81.

20. Wolf JS Jr, Moon TD, Nakada SY. Hand assisted laparoscopic nephrectomy: comparison to standard laparoscopic nephrectomy. J Urol. 1998;160:22–7.

21. Stockdale AD, Pocock TJ. Abdominal wall metastasis following laparoscopy: a case report. Eur J Surg Oncol. 1985;11:373–5.

22. Cava A, Roman J, Quintela AG, Martin F, Aramburo P. Subcutaneous metastasis following laparoscopy in gastric adenocarcinoma. Eur J Surg Oncol. 1990;16:63–7.

23. Dobronte Z, Wittmann T, Karacsony G. Rapid development of malignant metastases in the abdominal wall after laparoscopy. Endoscopy. 1978;10:127–30.

24. Gill IS, Kavoussi LR, Clayman RV, et al. Complications of laparoscopic nephrectomy in 185 patients: a multi-institutional review [see comments]. J Urol. 1995;154:479–83.

25. Morgan C Jr, Rader D. Laparoscopic unroofing of renal cyst. J Urol. 1992;148:1835–6.

26. Stoller ML, Irby PB III, Carrol PR, Osman M. Laparoscopic renal cyst resection. J Endourol. 1992;6:S56 (Abstract).

27. Brown JA, Torres VE, King BF, Segura JW. Laparoscopic marsupialization of symptomatic polycystic kidney disease. J Urol. 1996;156:22–7.

28. McCullough CS, Soper NJ, Clayman RV, So SSK, Jendrisak MD, Hanto DW. Laparoscopic drainage of a posttransplant lymphocele. Transplantation. 1991;51:725–7.

29. Albala DM, Schuessler WW, Vancaillie TG. Laparoscopic bladder neck suspension. J Endourol. 1992;6:137–41.

30. McDougall EM. Correction of stress urinary incontinence: retropubic approach. J Endourol. 1996;10:247–50.

31. Gill IS, Carbone JM, Clayman RV, et al. Laparoscopic live-donor nephrectomy. J Endourol. 1994;8:143–8.

32. Schulam PG, Kavoussi LR, Cheriff AD, et al. Laparoscopic live donor nephrectomy: the initial 3 cases. J Urol. 1996;155:1857–9.

33. Gagner M, Lacroix A, Bolte E. Laparoscopic adrenalectomy in Cushing's syndrome and pheochromocytoma (Letter). N Engl J Med. 1992;327:1033.

34. Schuessler WW, Pharand D. Laparoscopic adrenalectomy: case report. J Endourol. 1992;6:S158 (Abstract).

Chapter 14

Congenital Diseases of the Upper Urinary Tract

David FM Thomas

KEY POINTS

- Approximately one-third of all congenital abnormalities affect the genitourinary tract.
- Prenatal diagnosis has brought new problems to light at an early stage of development.
- Normal development of the urinary tract reflects the pivotal role of the ureteric bud.
- Multicystic dysplastic kidney is far more prevalent than was ever suspected.
- The management of prenatal hydronephrosis continues to be unclear, although a consensus is emerging.

INTRODUCTION

Approximately one-third of all congenital abnormalities affect the genitourinary tract. In contrast to anomalies of the external genitalia or lower urinary tract, congenital abnormalities of the upper urinary tract often provide few clinical clues to their existence and, in many instances, are destined to remain asymptomatic and clinically undetectable throughout the affected individual's lifetime.

Assessment of the clinical significance of a congenital upper tract anomaly was more straightforward when only those lesions that had declared their potential for morbidity by presenting with urinary infection, pain, etc. came to medical attention. Invasive investigations and possible surgical intervention could be readily justified on clinical grounds, but with the advent of prenatal diagnosis the decision-making process is more problematic since the majority of infants with prenatally detected upper tract anomalies are asymptomatic.

In the absence of overt morbidity, investigation and management must be guided by an assessment of the potential risk of morbidity and a prediction of the likely natural history of the anomaly in question.

CLINICAL EMBRYOLOGY OF THE UPPER URINARY TRACT

For a more detailed account of the embryology of the genitourinary tract see Chapter 2. The normal embryologic development of the upper tract reflects the pivotal role of the ureteric bud (Fig. 14.1). In turn the site of origin of the ureteric bud on the mesonephric duct is a crucial determinant of ureteric morphology

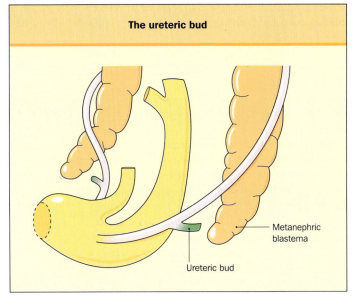

The ureteric bud

Metanephric blastema

Ureteric bud

Figure 14.1 The ureteric bud arises from the mesonephric duct early in the fifth week of gestation. It is a crucial determinant of the embryologic development of the upper tract.

and the successful induction of nephrogenesis. Faulty or failed interaction between the ascending ureteric bud and metanephric mesenchyme results in renal agenesis or different patterns of renal dysplasia. In cases of complete ureteric duplication, the ureter derived from the more cephalad of the two ureteric buds remains more closely associated with the descending mesonephric duct – thus explaining the paradoxic pattern of ureteric anatomy whereby the upper pole ureter drains in a more caudal (and sometimes ectopic) position in the definitive urinary tract – as described by the Meyer–Weigert law[1,2].

Bifurcation of the ureteric bud accounts for cases of incomplete ureteric duplication. According to the ureteric bud hypothesis proposed by Mackie and Stephens[3], a ureteric bud that arises from an abnormal site on the mesonephric duct is more likely to interact with one of the peripheral zones of metanephric tissue, with a limited potential for nephrogenesis. The 'ureteric bud hypothesis' neatly explains the observation that the upper pole renal parenchyma of a duplex kidney drained by an ectopic ureter is invariably dysplastic.

A group of renal anomalies, which includes pelvic kidney, horseshoe kidney, and crossed renal ectopia, can be clearly attributed to the period of renal ascent between the sixth and ninth weeks when the embryonic kidney acquires transient segmental blood supply at different levels until the definitive lumbar position is reached[4].

Ureteropelvic junction (UPJ) obstruction is a heterogeneous entity that exhibits a broad spectrum of severity. Most cases of congenital UPJ obstruction appear to derive from the mid-to-late stages of fetal development, rather than when the embryonic kidney makes its appearance in the first 10 weeks.

RENAL AGENESIS

One or both kidneys may be congenitally absent, either as part of a syndrome or as an isolated anomaly. In the absence of co-existing anomalies, unilateral renal agenesis generally remains undiagnosed unless it comes to light as an incidental ultrasound or autopsy finding.

Etiology

Three etiologies are an intrinsic defect of the embryonic mes-enchyme, failed induction of nephrogenesis, and involution of multicystic dysplastic kidney (MCDK).

Intrinsic defect of the embryonic mesenchyme

Renal agenesis from an intrinsic defect of the embryonic mes-enchyme explains the association in girls of unilateral renal agenesis with ipsilateral agenesis of paramesonephric duct derivatives.

Failed induction of nephrogenesis

Failure of ureteric bud development or abortive interaction with the metanephric blastema results in renal agenesis, which is typically associated with the cystoscopic appearance of deficiency of the ipsilateral hemi trigone. The high incidence (37%) of contralateral vesicoureteric reflux (VUR)[5] in children with unilateral renal agenesis provides further evidence of the involvement of the ureteric bud.

Involution of multicystic dysplastic kidney

Involution of MCDK is a common prenatally detected renal anomaly and has been shown to involute spontaneously both *in utero*[6] and in postnatal[7] life to mimic the radiologic (and possibly autopsy) findings of renal agenesis.

Incidence

Data from autopsy and radiologic studies suggest that the preva-lence of unilateral renal agenesis in the general population is approximately 0.1–0.3%[8]. Curiously, unilateral renal agenesis is rarely diagnosed prenatally despite the accuracy with which fetal kidneys can be imaged with ultrasound from the 17th week onward. This observation has been interpreted as evidence to link involution of MCDKs to adult renal agenesis. The inci-dence of bilateral renal agenesis is about 1:10,000–1:15,000 pregnancies and it accounts for approximately one-third of terminations of pregnancy for urologic malformations[9].

Genetics

The empiric recurrence risk quoted for bilateral renal agenesis is 3.5%[10]. Roodhoft et al. found asymptomatic urinary tract mal-formations in 7.4% of parents of children with bilateral renal agenesis[11].

The inheritance of 'silent' or nonsyndromic forms of unilateral renal agenesis is less amenable to study and remains poorly doc-umented. Experimental forms of renal agenesis or hypoplasia have been created in mice by ablating the WT1, RET, and PAX2 genes[12]. As yet these experimentally induced anomalies have not been mirrored by comparable findings in humans.

Prognosis

The widely held belief that unilateral renal agenesis has little if any impact on longevity must be qualified by the following reservations:

- the high incidence of contralateral VUR poses a potential threat of pyelonephritic damage to the solitary kidney; and
- case reports and long-term follow-up studies[13] that reveal proteinuria, hypertension, and reduced creatinine clearance in a percentage of individuals with solitary kidneys indicate that hyperfiltration damage leading to glomerulosclerosis cannot be dismissed as a purely theoretic risk.

MULTICYSTIC DYSPLASTIC KIDNEY

Congenital cystic malformations of the kidney and genetically determined polycystic renal disease constitute common forms of renal pathology in childhood and adult life. The advent of prenatal ultrasound has shed important new light on the natural history and prevalence of cystic renal pathology – notably MCDK. It is now known that MCDK is far more prevalent in the general population than was previously suspected. In the majority of affected individuals, however, the lesion is unilateral and clinically undetectable at birth (Fig. 14.2).

Etiology

Almost invariably MCDK is associated with complete ureteric obstruction, which usually takes the form of proximal ureteric atresia. Attempts to reproduce the anomaly by experimentally induced fetal ureteric obstruction have proved unsuccessful and defective interaction between the ureteric bud and metanephric

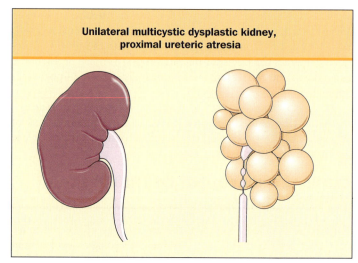

Unilateral multicystic dysplastic kidney, proximal ureteric atresia

Figure 14.2 Unilateral multicystic dysplastic kidney, proximal ureteric atresia.

mesenchyme now seems a more plausible explanation. The high incidence of coexisting ipsilateral and contralateral VUR and the association with renal agenesis (which also carries a high incidence of VUR) suggests that MCDK, renal agenesis, and VUR belong to a spectrum of ureteric bud anomalies – which in some instances may be genetically determined.

Genetics

Although MCDK is generally (and probably correctly) regarded as a sporadic anomaly its pattern of inheritance has not been systematically researched. Case reports of MCDK in siblings and other family members suggest that within affected families MCDK exhibits autosomal dominant inheritance with variable penetrance[14].

Pathology

Macroscopically, MCDK consists of an irregular aggregation of tense cysts of variable dimensions. The collecting system is absent or vestigial and the ureter at the level of the UPJ is atretic. Renal parenchyma is absent or limited on microscopy to vestigial plates of thinned dysplastic tissue interposed between the cysts. The cysts themselves are lined by cuboidal or flattened tubular epithelium.

Incidence

Data published in 1988 put the prevalence at 1:4300 live births[15]. A more recently published estimate, obtained over a 10 year period with more modern, sensitive ultrasound equipment, indicates a prevalence of MCDK in an unselected district general hospital population of 1:2400 live births[16]. The incidence of bilateral MCDK is approximately 1:15,000–1:20,000 pregnancies.

Presentation

Clinical

Rarely, MCDK presents clinically as an abdominal mass in the neonatal period. In contrast to other congenital renal masses that are smooth in contour, such as hydronephrosis or the autosomal recessive polycystic kidney, the surface of an MCDK is typically irregular and 'knobbly' on palpation.

Asymptomatic

The discovery of MCDK may occur during routine evaluation of infants with other congenital anomalies such as esophageal atresia.

Prenatal ultrasound

Although most prenatally detected MCDKs are detected on the initial fetal anomaly scan performed between 17 and 19 weeks gestation, Liebeshuetz[16] and colleagues noted that 20% of prenatally detected MCDKs were only evident on scans performed later in pregnancy. Bilateral MCDK, or MCDK associated with contralateral renal agenesis, is associated with marked oligohydramnios on the second trimester scan – at a time when parents can still opt for termination of pregnancy.

With modern ultrasound equipment in the hands of an experienced ultrasonographer, MCDK can be diagnosed with a high degree of accuracy *in utero*.

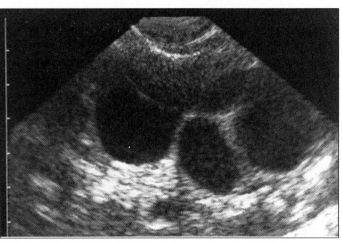

Figure 14.3 Characteristic postnatal ultrasound appearances of multicystic dysplastic kidney.

Postnatal evaluation

Ultrasound

The diagnostic features on postnatal ultrasound (Fig. 14.3) comprise:

- presence of interfaces between the cysts;
- nonmedial location of the largest cyst (in contrast with the dilated renal pelvis of gross hydronephrosis);
- absence of identifiable renal sinus;
- multiplicity of noncommunicating, round cysts; and
- absence of parenchymal tissue.

Isotope renography

Total absence of isotope uptake (i.e. 0% function) of ^{99m}Tc-dimercaptosuccinic acid (^{99m}Tc-DMSA) is a diagnostic feature of MCDK. In some centers dynamic renography with ^{99m}Tc-mercaptoacetyltriglycine (^{99m}Tc-MAG3) is preferred as this may yield additional information on drainage in the contralateral kidney.

Investigation of coexisting urologic anomalies

Vesicoureteric reflux

An incidence of contralateral or ipsilateral VUR of 18%[17] to 43%[18] has been reported at those centers in which every newborn infant with a prenatally detected MCDK is investigated by micturating cystourethrography (MCU). However, such VUR is generally low grade and destined to resolve spontaneously. The necessity for a routine MCU in the absence of ureteric or contralateral upper tract dilatation on ultrasound is therefore unclear. If an MCU is not carried out the parents and family doctor should be advised of the possible risk of urinary tract infection (UTI) and the need to proceed to an MCU in the event of an unexplained febrile illness or documented UTI.

Contralateral ureteropelvic junction obstruction

The incidence of contralateral UPJ obstruction in infants with prenatally detected MCDK is between 5% and 10%[9]. Diagnostic criteria are the same as for other forms of prenatally detected UPJ obstruction (see below).

Management

Abdominal mass

Nephrectomy is indicated in those infants whose MCDK presents with a sizeable mass in the neonatal period. Surgery is rarely a matter of urgency and can be reasonably deferred for several weeks, until a full diagnostic work-up has been completed.

Nephrectomy is also unquestionably justified in those rare instances when MCDK is genuinely associated with hypertension or some other complication.

Asymptomatic prenatally detected multicystic dysplastic kidney

The rationale for 'prophylactic' nephrectomy for asymptomatic prenatally detected MCDKs is unclear. The arguments center on the natural history of asymptomatic MCDKs and the perceived risk of complications, notably hypertension and malignant potential.

Natural history

The potential for MCDKs to disappear completely on serial ultrasound scans has been well documented by several studies. The assumption that involution represents the disappearance of cyst fluid to leave some residual tissue (collapsed cyst wall, etc.) *in situ*, while logical, remains unverified since the renal bed remains unexplored in such cases. In the series of 64 prenatally detected MCDKs reported from Great Ormond Street Hospital, 35% disappeared during the course of follow-up, mostly in the first year of life[19]. Data from the American MCDK Registry indicate that approximately 50% of MCDKs can be expected to involute spontaneously in the first 5 years of life. Further long-term follow-up data are awaited.

Hypertension

Unquestionably, MCDK is associated with a risk of hypertension, but is this risk of sufficient magnitude to justify submitting every asymptomatic child with a prenatally detected MCDK to 'prophylactic' nephrectomy?

Manzoni and Caldemone[20] have recently published a literature review spanning 30 years, during which period 13 cases of hypertension linked to MCDK were reported. In the 11 cases for which follow-up information was available blood pressure reverted to normal after nephrectomy. Closer scrutiny of the original case reports[21] reveals one in which the diagnosis of MCDK was incorrect and two in which the diagnosis of hypertension was arguable[22]. Viewed against the prevalence of MCDK (1:2000–1:4:000 live births) and the number of individuals with unrecognized MCDKs born in the USA and UK during this time the risk of hypertension revealed by the published literature does not appear to justify routine 'prophylactic' nephrectomy.

It could be argued that hypertension is an under-reported complication and the published cases represent only the tip of the iceberg. However, if unreported hypertension occurs on an appreciable scale, it should, nevertheless, be expected to figure prominently as a cause of hypertension presenting in later childhood. This is not the case. In a series of 454 children with renal hypertension managed at Great Ormond Street Hospital, London, Deal and colleagues did not encounter a single case of MCDK (personal communication cited in Thomas and Fitzpatrick[22]).

In children who underwent nephrectomy for 'surgical' forms of renal hypertension no cases of MCDK were reported in two surgical series totaling 64 children[23,24].

The true risk of hypertension is difficult to quantify but the available evidence points to a low order of risk (e.g. 0.01–0.1%). In the author's view this risk does not justify routinely submitting asymptomatic infants to 'prophylactic' nephrectomy.

Malignancy

Manzoni and Caldemone's[20] review identified five published cases of Wilms' tumor in children with MCDKs, and renal cell carcinoma linked to MCDK in five adults aged between 15 and 68 years. As with hypertension it is important that the perceived risk of malignancy is not distorted by erroneously ascribing pathology to a lesion that is not MCDK.

Estimating the lifetime risk of developing malignancy in an asymptomatic MCDK is difficult, but the available evidence suggests a figure of about 1:2000–1:3000. The risk of dying from an associated Wilms' tumor in childhood is considerably less, having been calculated by Noe et al.[25] as approximately 1:20,000.

Nonoperative management

Follow-up of MCDK comprises further ultrasound scans at 6 months and 12 months of age with annual ultrasound scans thereafter until the age of 5 years. If the MCDK has disappeared on ultrasound by this stage, no further ultrasound follow-up is required. Even when residual appearances of MCDK are evident on ultrasound at this age, it is arguable whether further follow-up serves any purpose other than for clinical research. Blood pressure is checked annually, although it must be acknowledged that this can be technically problematic in infants or fractious young children.

Surgery

When indicated, nephrectomy can be accomplished through a small incision anterior to the twelfth rib or, ideally, via a posterior lumbotomy approach. Cyst puncture and aspiration of cyst fluid prior to mobilization and delivery of the kidney facilitates the use of a small incision. The benefits claimed for laparoscopic nephrectomy are unclear in view of the limited morbidity and discomfort associated with conventional extraperitoneal nephrectomy in this age group.

POLYCYSTIC KIDNEY DISEASE

Both the autosomal dominant form of polycystic kidney disease (ADPKD) and the recessive pattern (ARPKD) are characterized by pathologic changes throughout the renal parenchyma of both kidneys. The recessive form occurs in children, whereas the impact of ADPKD is borne mainly in adult life.

Autosomal recessive polycystic kidney disease

A rare disorder, ARPKD has an estimated incidence between 1:10,000 and 1:40,000 (Fig. 14.4)[26].

Pathology

Both kidneys are enlarged and the renal parenchyma is diffusely infiltrated with small cysts, typically <2mm in diameter.

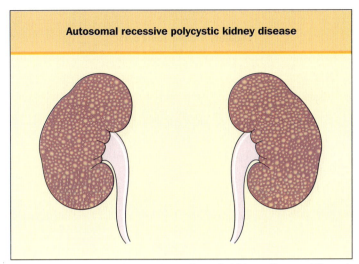

Figure 14.4 Autosomal recessive polycystic kidney disease. Bilateral renal enlargement and diffuse parenchymal infiltration with small cysts.

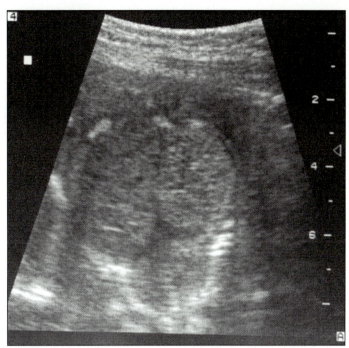

Figure 14.5 Characteristic prenatal ultrasound appearances of autosomal recessive polycystic kidney disease.

Invariably, ARPKD is accompanied by hepatic manifestations that include biliary dysgenesis and periportal fibrosis.

Presentation

On the basis of characteristic ultrasound findings, ARPKD can now be detected prenatally (Fig. 14.5). When diagnosed by ultrasound at the second trimester, termination of pregnancy can be considered; however, the condition is not always apparent on ultrasound at this stage in gestation. If not detected prenatally, ARPKD usually presents in the neonatal period with palpable renal abdominal masses, respiratory insufficiency, or clinical features of impaired renal function. Rarely, the underlying renal pathology remains undetected until later childhood when complications of liver involvement supervene.

Diagnosis

Ultrasound, intravenous urography (IVU), and computed tomography (CT) all yield characteristic findings, although in practice the combination of two imaging modalities is usually sufficient. Renal biopsy is not routinely indicated.

Management

Severely affected infants with pulmonary hypoplasia may require ventilatory support in the neonatal period. Management of ARPKD is primarily medical and aimed at actively treating hypertension and the complications of chronic renal failure, such as anemia, malnutrition, and renal bone disease. The onset of end-stage renal failure, which is variable in timing, demands conventional renal replacement therapy with dialysis and transplantation. Nephrectomy may be indicated for the treatment of hypertension or to facilitate transplantation. In addition to the management of renal failure, specific measures may be required to treat the complications of hepatic involvement.

Prognosis

The presence or absence of pulmonary hypoplasia is now the main determinant of prognosis. For infants who survive the neonatal period, survival rates of 85% at 3 months, 79% at 12 months, 51% at 10 years, and 46% at 15 years have been reported[27].

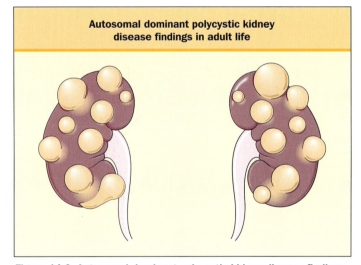

Figure 14.6 Autosomal dominant polycystic kidney disease findings in adult life.

Autosomal dominant polycystic kidney disease

In contrast to ARPKD, the autosomal dominant variant (Fig. 14.6) is a common disorder that affects 1:500–1:1000 individuals[28] and accounts for approximately 10% of adults on end-stage renal failure programs. There is considerable individual variation in the natural history, rate of progression, and severity of renal impairment.

Pathology

In adults, cysts lined by epithelium are interspersed throughout the renal cortex with compression and glomerulosclerosis of the intervening parenchyma. Multisystem involvement may include hepatic, pancreatic, or splenic cysts and cerebral aneurysms.

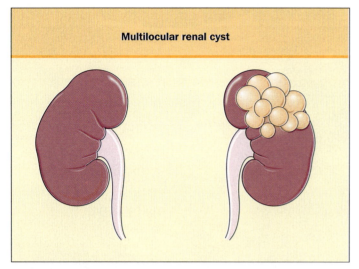

Figure 14.7 Multilocular renal cyst. Localized multilocular cystic lesion in an otherwise normal kidney.

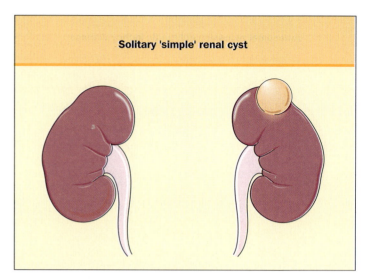

Figure 14.8 Solitary 'simple' renal cyst.

Genetics

The genetic basis for ADPKD has been established following the discovery of the *PKD1* gene located on chromosome 16[29]. A second mutation on chromosome 4 has been implicated in a minority of cases[30].

Presentation

Ultrasound screening of the offspring and young family members of affected adults may reveal the presence of renal cysts at an asymptomatic stage. Most patients still present in adult life with hypertension or symptoms that relate to the enlarged cystic kidneys. As with ARPKD a reliable diagnosis can be established on the basis of diagnostic imaging without the need for renal biopsy.

Management

Management is aimed principally at detecting and actively managing hypertension and the metabolic manifestations of chronic renal insufficiency. Surgical involvement is limited to nephrectomy in patients with severe hypertension, symptoms attributable to the cysts, or complications such as calculi or hemorrhage.

Prognosis

When evident on prenatal ultrasound, ADPKD carries a poor prognosis. However, the detection of asymptomatic cysts on ultrasound screening in later childhood does not appear to carry a poorer long-term prognosis. It has been estimated that when ADPKD is diagnosed in an asymptomatic young adult, the risk of developing end-stage renal failure by the age of 40 years is <5%[31].

MULTILOCULAR RENAL CYST

It is unclear whether multilocular renal cyst (Fig. 14.7), a rare renal lesion, represents a congenital anomaly or a benign form of acquired renal neoplasia. The age distribution is bimodal with one incidence peak in childhood and a second in mid–late adult life. Presenting symptoms in childhood include hematuria, pain,

or the discovery of an abdominal mass. The lesion is usually unilateral, but very rare bilateral cases have been reported. The diagnosis is made by ultrasound and CT and in most circumstances the most appropriate treatment consists of nephrectomy rather than nephron-sparing surgery.

SOLITARY RENAL CYST

Despite the frequency with which solitary ('simple') renal cysts (Fig. 14.8) are diagnosed in adult urologic practice, they are encountered in children only rarely. Thus it can be inferred that solitary renal cysts in adults represent acquired rather than congenital renal pathology.

When diagnosed in childhood, simple renal cysts are best managed conservatively. It is important that misguided intervention is not undertaken for unrelated symptoms such as nonspecific abdominal pain incorrectly ascribed to the ultrasound finding of an asymptomatic cyst.

OTHER MALFORMATIONS OF THE RENAL PARENCHYMA

A detailed consideration of the nonsurgical (i.e. 'nephrologic') congenital disorders of renal parenchyma is beyond the scope of this chapter. The term 'renal hypoplasia' is used to describe global reduction in renal size that is nevertheless accompanied by preservation of normal renal architecture ('a smooth small kidney'). Low-to-moderate grades of intrauterine VUR may be associated with this finding. In contrast, renal dysplasia is characterized by distinctive histologic features that denote a major insult to the process of embryogenesis (e.g. the presence of primitive tubules and metaplastic tissue such as cartilage). Intrauterine infravesical obstruction, notably by posterior urethral valves, is also a potent cause of dysplasia. In the absence of fetal VUR or obstructive uropathy the etiology of isolated renal hypoplasia or dysplasia is not usually apparent.

Medullary sponge kidney is essentially a radiologic finding of mild congenital dilatation of the collecting ducts. Although of

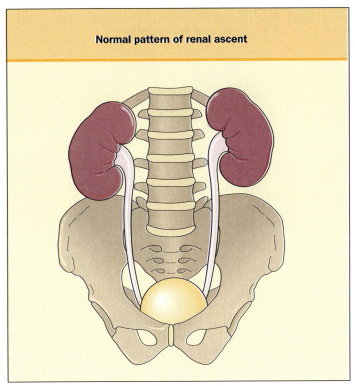

Figure 14.9 Normal pattern of renal ascent.

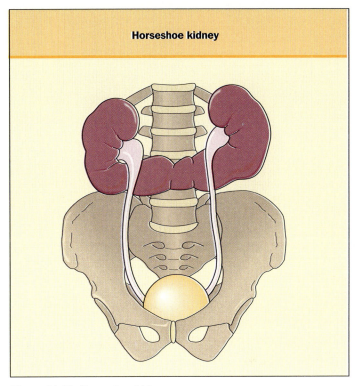

Figure 14.10 Horseshoe kidney.

little clinical significance in childhood, stasis of urine within the collecting ducts may give rise to infection or stone formation in later life.

ABNORMALITIES OF RENAL ASCENT AND FUSION

The embryologic basis of anomalies of normal renal ascent and fusion (Fig. 14.9) is considered above. Abnormally sited kidneys frequently exhibit hypoplasia and are associated with an increased incidence of obstruction and VUR.

Horseshoe kidney
One of the most common renal anomalies, horseshoe kidney (Fig. 14.10), has a reported autopsy incidence of 1:400. Fusion of the lower poles of metanephric tissue distorts the normal mechanisms of renal ascent, vascularization, and rotation. Postnatally, this is manifest as kidneys that are fused across the midline via their lower poles by an isthmus, which may vary from a fibrous strand to a substantial, well-vascularized bridge of renal parenchyma. The collecting systems are rotated with the renal pelves lying anteriorly.

Presentation
Most horseshoe kidneys do not give rise to complications and are only detected as incidental findings at autopsy or during urinary tract imaging of children with other congenital anomalies – notably Turner's syndrome, which carries a 5–10% risk of horseshoe kidney. Symptoms generally reflect the presence of coexisting VUR or UPJ obstruction, which predispose to urinary infection or calculi.

Diagnosis
Ultrasound complemented by ^{99m}Tc-DMSA provides good visualization of the horseshoe anatomic configuration of renal parenchyma. Dynamic renography with ^{99m}Tc-MAG3 and MCU may be indicated if obstruction or VUR are suspected.

Management
In the absence of complications the majority of horseshoe kidneys merit no treatment or follow-up (other than perhaps an occasional ultrasound scan in children under 5 years of age). Pyeloplasty for the correction of UPJ obstruction in a horseshoe kidney is best performed via an anterolateral incision and trans-peritoneal approach, reflecting the hepatic or splenic flexure to gain access to the kidney. Where it is evident that conventional pyeloplasty will not ensure adequate dependent drainage or after a previous failed pyeloplasty, ureterocalicostomy is preferable to an ill-judged attempt at division of the renal isthmus.

Pelvic kidney
Pelvic kidneys (Fig. 14.11) are often hypoplastic and are prone to reflux and obstruction.

Diagnosis
Poorly functioning kidneys located within the bony pelvis are easily overlooked – both on ultrasound and IVU. The most sensitive modality with which to visualize a poorly functioning pelvic kidney is ^{99m}Tc-DMSA, although CT or magnetic resonance imaging (MRI) may be required to demonstrate the presence of a nonfunctioning dysplastic ectopic kidney. Surgical exposure should be undertaken with caution in view of the risk to the adjacent vascular anatomy.

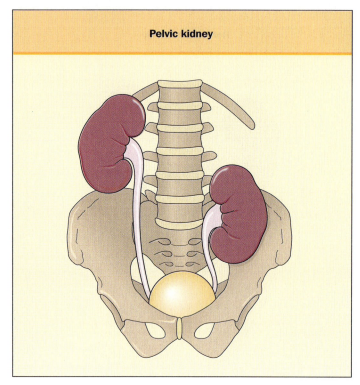

Figure 14.11 Pelvic kidney.

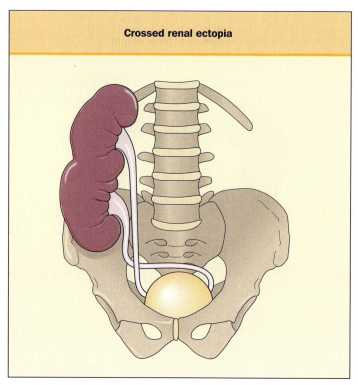

Figure 14.12 Crossed renal ectopia.

Crossed renal ectopia

Crossed renal ectopia (Fig. 14.12) is usually an incidental finding or comes to light following inadvertent abdominal palpation of the lower pole of the fused renal mass. Apart from low-grade VUR, other anomalies are rare and the condition rarely gives rise to clinical problems.

UPPER TRACT DUPLICATION

Duplication is the most common structural anomaly of the upper urinary tract, with a prevalence of approximately 1:125[32]. The varied spectrum of anatomic patterns encountered in clinical practice reflects the site of origin and morphology of the ureteric bud. Ureteric duplication is conventionally classified as either complete (Fig. 14.13) or incomplete (Fig. 14.14), depending on whether the ureters fuse above their point of entry into the lower urinary tract. In all cases of complete ureteric duplication the course of the upper pole ureter crosses the lower pole ureter to drain via the more caudal of the two ureteric orifices (the Meyer–Weigert law)[1,2].

Genetics

The occurrence of ureteric duplication within some families indicates a pattern of autosomal dominant inheritance with incomplete penetrance.

Clinical significance

Neither complete nor incomplete duplication poses a specific threat to health and the majority of uncomplicated duplications remain entirely asymptomatic and largely undetected. Symptoms arise as the result of VUR, obstruction (usually in the presence of a ureterocele) or marked ureteric ectopia. Since the majority of uncomplicated duplications are not associated with

dilatation they are not readily detected by ultrasound, either pre- or postnatally. Ureteroceles and dilated upper renal pole collecting systems can be visualized on prenatal ultrasound – duplications identified in this way account for 8.4% of significant prenatally detected uropathies[33].

Vesicoureteric reflux in duplex systems

As a result of its insertion into the bladder with a shorter submucosal tunnel, VUR occurs predominantly in the lower pole ureter. Reflux into both ureters or the common stem of an incomplete duplication accounts for 10–15% of VUR in duplex systems (see Fig. 14.13)[34]. Isolated reflux into an upper pole ureter can occur if the ureter drains ectopically into the bladder neck or when a ureterocele has been punctured iatrogenically (during MCU) or therapeutically.

Diagnosis

Ultrasound, MCU, and ^{99m}Tc-DMSA scans are used to grade the severity of VUR and to document differential renal function between the two kidneys and within the upper and lower moieties of the duplex kidney.

Management

The indications for ureteric reimplantation are comparable to those for single refluxing systems and center principally on the occurrence of breakthrough infection. To minimize the risk of damaging blood supply shared with the ipsilateral upper pole ureter it is important that both the upper and lower pole ureters are mobilized and reimplanted (*en bloc*) within their common sheath. Lower pole heminephroureterectomy is more appropriate in the presence of severe lower pole scarring or dysplasia. Considerable care is needed to avoid injury to vessels that supply the upper pole moiety and its ureter.

Anatomic variants associated with complete ureteric duplication and summary of treatment options

Uncomplicated	Lower pole vesicoureteric reflux	Ureterocele	Ectopic ureter

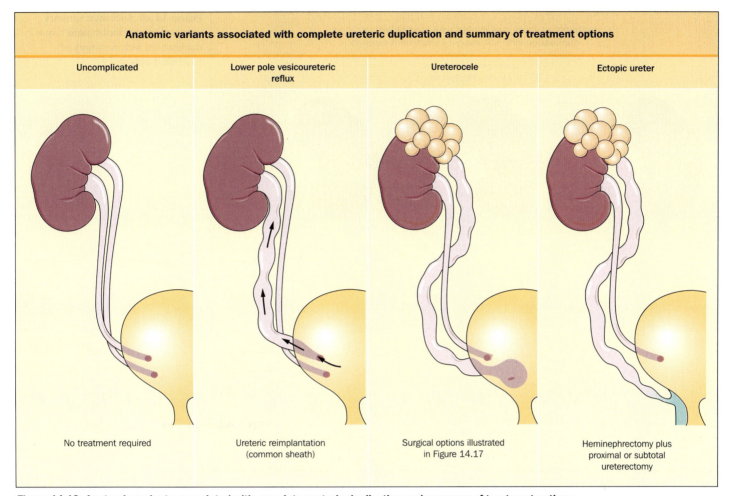

| No treatment required | Ureteric reimplantation (common sheath) | Surgical options illustrated in Figure 14.17 | Heminephrectomy plus proximal or subtotal ureterectomy |

Figure 14.13 Anatomic variants associated with complete ureteric duplication and summary of treatment options.

Ureterocele

A ureterocele (see Fig. 14.13) is defined conventionally as a cystic terminal dilatation of the intravesical ureter. The historic, descriptive classification of ureteroceles ('sphincteric', 'stenotic', 'cecoureterocele', etc.) is complex and largely unhelpful. For practical purposes, ureteroceles can be subdivided into those associated with upper pole duplex ureters (duplex ureteroceles, see Fig. 14.13) and 'simple' or single-system ureteroceles (Fig. 14.15, and considered below). Duplex ureteroceles may be confined within the bladder or may extend or prolapse beyond the bladder neck. The quoted incidence of duplex ureteroceles is 1:4000 with a female:male ratio of approximately 6:1[35].

Presentation

Prenatal

Dilatation of the obstructed upper pole moiety and its associated ureter is readily detectable on prenatal ultrasound – although this may not be apparent on the second trimester scan.

Postnatal

A prolapsed duplex ureterocele may (rarely) present as an introital swelling in the newborn female. However, the most common presentation of a previously undiagnosed duplex ureterocele is with urinary infection. Within the obstructed upper pole system, urinary infection may progress to pyonephrosis with high fever and marked systemic symptoms. On ultrasound pyonephrosis is evident by the presence of infective echogenic debris within the dilated collecting system.

Diagnosis

When dilatation is detected prenatally or when a child presents with symptoms (usually related to UTI), a full evaluation is required, including ultrasound (Fig. 14.16), conventional contrast MCU, ^{99m}Tc-DMSA imaging, and IVU. Renal function (as assessed by isotope uptake) is either absent or grossly impaired in more than 90% of upper pole moieties drained by ureters terminating in a ureterocele[36]. The discovery of unilateral duplication always prompts consideration of the presence of a contralateral and possibly occult duplex system.

Management

Prolapsed introital ureterocele

Decompression of the obstructed upper pole system can be achieved by local incision or partial excision of the prolapsed ureterocele. Definitive management, which can usually be deferred beyond the neonatal period, comprises upper pole heminephrectomy and subtotal ureterectomy.

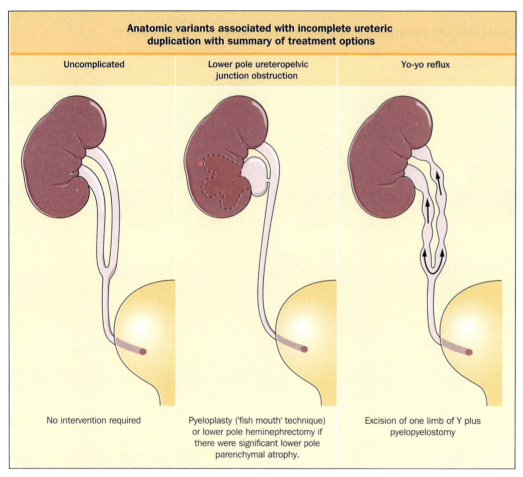

Anatomic variants associated with incomplete ureteric duplication with summary of treatment options

Uncomplicated	Lower pole ureteropelvic junction obstruction	Yo-yo reflux
No intervention required	Pyeloplasty ('fish mouth' technique) or lower pole heminephrectomy if there were significant lower pole parenchymal atrophy.	Excision of one limb of Y plus pyelopyelostomy

Figure 14.14 Anatomic variants associated with incomplete ureteric duplication, with summary of treatment options.

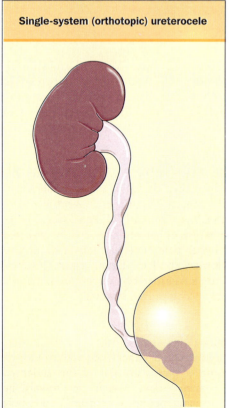

Single-system (orthotopic) ureterocele

Figure 14.15 Single-system (orthotopic) ureterocele.

Urinary infection

Once the presenting infection has been treated effectively, antibiotic prophylaxis is instituted pending a full radiologic evaluation and possible surgical intervention. Pyonephrosis or severe infection that does not respond promptly to parenteral antibiotics is best treated initially by percutaneous nephrostomy to decompress and drain the obstructed system.

Surgical considerations

In the past, definitive surgical management usually took the form of upper pole heminephrectomy, excision of the dilated upper pole ureter, and intravesical excision of the ureterocele (often combined with lower pole ureteric reimplantation) – a lengthy and sometimes challenging operation that requires two incisions. The past 15 years have seen the emergence of a more selective and less invasive approach[37] in recognition that no single operation can successfully encompass all the different variants of duplication encountered in clinical practice (Fig. 14.17). Cystoscopic incision or puncture of the ureterocele represents the least invasive way of facilitating drainage within the obstructed upper pole system. This approach is well suited to the management of prenatally detected duplex ureteroceles in asymptomatic infants[38,39]. Endoscopic treatment, however, is not appropriate for every ureterocele and the best results are obtained when treatment is individualized according to factors such as age of the child, mode of presentation, and the particular variant of duplex anatomy.

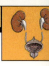

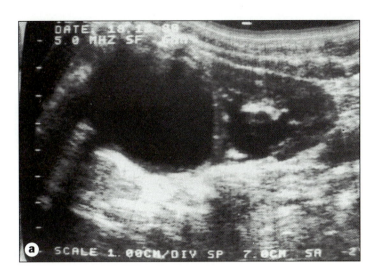

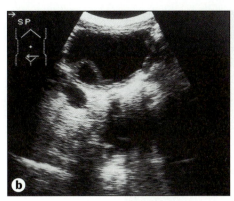

Figure 14.16 Ultrasound appearances of duplex kidney. (a) Grossly dilated upper pole, with normal lower pole renal parenchyma. (b) Transverse view of bladder demonstrating ureterocele and dilated upper pole ureter.

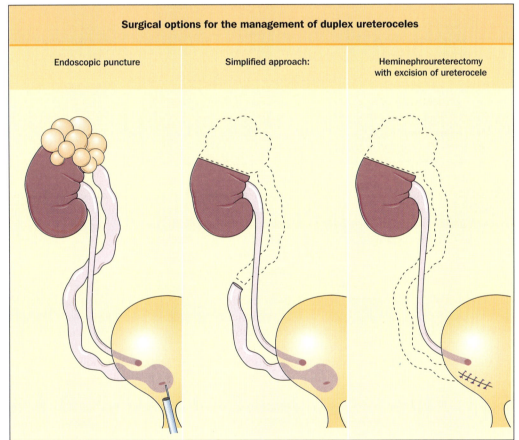

Surgical options for the management of duplex ureteroceles

Endoscopic puncture	Simplified approach:	Heminephroureterectomy with excision of ureterocele

Figure 14.17 Surgical options for the management of duplex ureteroceles. (Left) Endoscopic puncture. (Center) Simplified approach: heminephrectomy plus proximal ureterectomy, one incision. (Right) Heminephroureterectomy with excision of ureterocele (plus lower pole ureteric reimplantation).

Single-system ureteroceles

In contrast to duplex ureteroceles, single-system ureteroceles (see Fig. 14.15) occur more commonly in boys and are associated with better preservation of renal function. Presentation is usually with urinary infection, sometimes complicated by the presence of calculi. Ultrasound and isotope imaging are the principle diagnostic modalities, but also IVU is often an instructive investigation. Treatment was previously by open excision of the ureterocele and ureteric reimplantation, but this approach has been superseded by endoscopic decompression with a Bugbee electrode (Figs 14.16 & 14.18). Drainage is reliably achieved and the incidence of clinically significant reflux is low.

Ectopic ureter

The possibility of an ectopic upper pole ureter must always be considered in a girl with a lifelong history of urinary incontinence. Typically, the incontinence is dribbling in nature and superimposed on a pattern of normal voiding. Where there is evidence of dilatation in the upper pole and the ectopic ureter, the diagnosis is usually straightforward. However, to demonstrate the existence of a poorly functioning 'occult' upper pole system with a nondilated ureter can be a challenging and frustrating diagnostic exercise. The most useful modalities are ^{99m}Tc-DMSA, MRI, and delayed IVU films. Upper pole heminephrectomy with excision of the proximal and midportion of

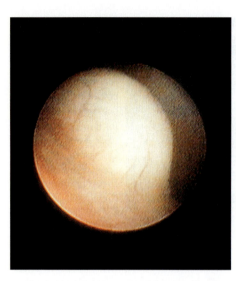

Figure 14.18
Endoscopic appearances of ureterocele prior to endoscopic puncture.

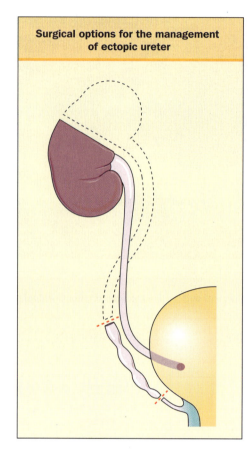

Surgical options for the management of ectopic ureter

Figure 14.19
Surgical options for the management of ectopic ureter associated with a poorly functioning upper pole. Heminephrectomy plus proximal ureterectomy (simplified approach) or subtotal ureterectomy to avoid the risk of iatrogenic damage to the continence mechanism of the bladder neck and of a striated sphincter. Reimplantation of the ectopic ureter is another option, but upper pole renal function is rarely sufficient to justify preservation.

the ureter is generally sufficient. If more extensive ureterectomy is judged necessary it is important to avoid unnecessary dissection of the terminal portion of the ectopic ureter to minimize the risk of iatrogenic damage to bladder neck and of a striated continence mechanism (Fig. 14.19).

Ectopic ureters are rare in males and tend to present with urinary infection or epididymo-orchitis rather than urinary incontinence – which reflects the close embryologic relationship with the mesonephric duct. The discovery of an abnormal kidney indicates the existence of a single-system ectopic ureter, but it may be particularly difficult to confirm the presence of a suspected ectopic duplex ureter associated with a small, dysplastic, poorly functioning upper pole. Treatment is guided by the level of function in the relevant kidney, but as function is usually grossly impaired treatment is likely to consist of nephrectomy plus subtotal ureterectomy.

Single ectopic ureter

Ureteric ectopia is not confined to duplex systems. Unilateral single ectopic ureter is associated with some deficiency of the trigone and bladder neck, but continence is preserved. In contrast, the condition of bilateral single ectopic ureters is accompanied by marked deficiency of the bladder neck and striated sphincter. The ureters drain into the urethra rather than into the bladder, which is greatly reduced in capacity. Incontinence is a common feature of bilateral single ectopic ureters. Surgical management comprises ureteric reimplantation followed, where indicated, by bladder neck surgery in later childhood.

CONGENITAL URETERIC OBSTRUCTION

Congenital ureteric obstruction may be extrinsic (e.g. retrocaval ureter) or intrinsic and may occur at any level in the ureter. Stenotic obstruction of the distal ureter accounts for the overwhelming majority of congenital nonrefluxing megaureters.

Presentation

In the past, obstructed megaureters generally presented with urinary infection, loin pain (in older children), or calculi. While some children continue to present clinically, the majority are now identified by prenatal ultrasound. Obstructed megaureter accounts for approximately 10% of infants with significant prenatally detected uropathy[33].

Diagnosis

Pre- or postnatal appearances of ureteric dilatation on ultrasound usually initiate the diagnostic process. Despite any presumption of obstruction as the cause of this dilatation, a MCU is mandatory to exclude VUR (which may coexist with obstruction). Dynamic isotope renography with ^{99m}Tc-diethylenetriamine pentaacetic acid (^{99m}Tc-DTPA) or ^{99m}Tc-MAG3 is the most sensitive indicator of obstruction, but interpretation of the drainage curve data may prove problematic. Even with frusemide (furosemide) washout it may be difficult to distinguish between genuine obstruction and stasis within a grossly dilated ureter (Fig. 14.20). In older children the relative degree of ureteric and caliceal dilatation and the caliceal morphology on IVU may give a useful clue to the severity of obstruction.

Management
Clinical presentation
Surgical intervention is usually indicated once the diagnosis of obstruction has been confirmed and differential function assessed. Preliminary percutaneous nephrostomy should be considered when infection fails to respond to parenteral antibiotic treatment.

Prenatal diagnosis
Significant impairment of differential renal function (<35%) in conjunction with evidence of obstruction justifies surgical

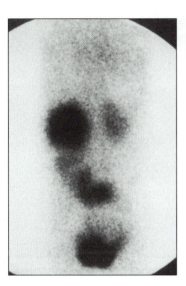

Figure 14.20 Accumulation of tracer (^{99m}Tc-DTPA) within a grossly dilated obstructed right megaureter. To distinguish between obstructive and nonobstructive dilatation may prove difficult, despite the administration of a diuretic.

intervention, although this is best deferred until at least 6 months (ideally 12) of age. When more urgent relief of obstruction is indicated (e.g. in a solitary system or to control infection) the open placement of an indwelling JJ catheter has been advocated in preference to ureteric reimplantation of a megaureter in the first year of life[40].

The majority of infants with prenatally detected obstructed megaureter can be managed conservatively since they are asymptomatic and their obstruction is associated with good preservation of renal function. The indications for intervention mirror those for UPJ obstruction (i.e. deteriorating differential function, onset of complications – pain, infection, etc.). Baskin and colleagues reported an excellent medium-term outcome in 17 children with prenatally detected megaureter managed nonoperatively for a mean of 7.5 years[41]. In a series of 67 children followed for a mean of 3.1 years, Liu and colleagues reported that only 17% required surgical intervention[42].

Surgical considerations

Surgery for the obstructed megaureter generally consists of extravesical mobilization of the ureter and excision of the terminal obstructing segment prior to ureteric reimplantation. Plication of the ureter (e.g. by the Starr technique) is desirable, particularly if the ureter is flabby and aperistaltic and its diameter exceeds 1cm (Fig. 14.21). If it is evident that an antireflux submucosal tunnel of the appropriate dimensions cannot be achieved by the transtrigonal technique, the Leadbetter–Politano method of reimplantation may be preferable – ideally in combination with a psoas hitch (Fig. 14.22).

URETEROPELVIC OBSTRUCTION (HYDRONEPHROSIS)

The most common form of congenital obstructive uropathy is UPJ obstruction. It exhibits a broad spectrum of severity and considerable variability in its natural history. Resolution of prenatally detected hydronephrosis is well documented, as are instances of unequivocal UPJ obstruction arising *de novo* in kidneys that were previously of normal appearance and nondilated on ultrasound or IVU.

Pathology

Operative findings in congenital hydronephrosis consist of narrowing and tortuosity of a segment of proximal ureter, which is often bound to the dilated pelvis by flimsy adhesions (Fig. 14.23). In infants and young children the extrinsic compression of the UPJ by aberrant renal vessels is an exceptionally rare finding – although it is implicated in the etiology of fixed or intermittent UPJ obstruction in older children. Histologic examination of the resected ureter is generally uninformative.

Genetics

Generally, UPJ obstruction behaves as a sporadic anomaly, but familial occurrence has been documented[43], as has the association

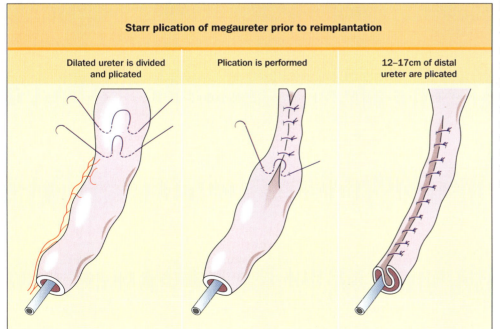

Starr plication of megaureter prior to reimplantation

Dilated ureter is divided and plicated	Plication is performed	12–17cm of distal ureter are plicated

Figure 14.21 Starr plication of megaureter prior to reimplantation. (Left) The dilated ureter is divided proximal to the stenotic segment and plicated over a 10Ch feeding tube or catheter. (Center) Plication is performed by placing a series of 4/0 absorbable sutures, taking care to preserve the vascularity of the ureter. (Right) 12–17cm of distal ureter are plicated – depending on the child's age and the technique of reimplantation. On completion of the plication the 10Ch tube is replaced by a stent of smaller caliber.

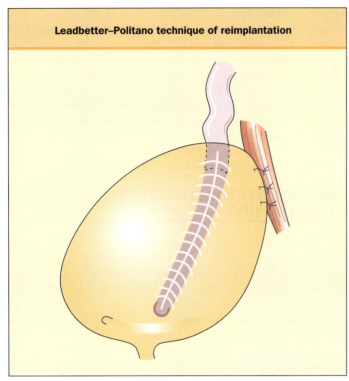

Leadbetter–Politano technique of reimplantation

Figure 14.22 Leadbetter–Politano technique of reimplantation. This combined with a psoas hitch provides a longer, more effective antireflux submucosal tunnel.

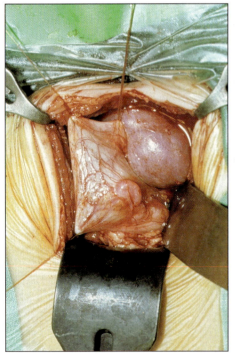

Figure 14.23 Operative findings at pyeloplasty for prenatally detected hydronephrosis. Gross dilatation of renal pelvis, good preservation of renal parenchyma, and tortuous ureteropelvic junction.

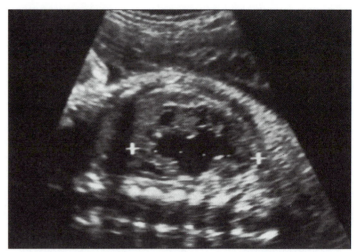

Figure 14.24 Prenatal ultrasound appearances of hydronephrosis (ureteropelvic junction obstruction).

Presentation

Prenatal ultrasound

Dilatation may become apparent on ultrasound at any stage from the second trimester onward (Fig. 14.24). Normal appearances of a nondilated fetal urinary tract on a second trimester ultrasound (e.g. 17–19 weeks) do not preclude the subsequent development of significant UPJ obstruction in later pregnancy. In a study designed to examine the correlation between postnatal renal function and the timing and severity of dilatation *in utero* it was noted that 31% of prenatally detected UPJ obstructions did not give rise to detectable dilatation at the time of routine second trimester ultrasound. The onset and severity of dilatation was only broadly linked to the prognosis for postnatal renal function, except for a renal pelvis diameter >15mm in the second trimester which was associated with significant reduction in renal function[44].

Obstruction of the UPJ accounts for 35–50% of all significant prenatally detected uropathies[33,45].

Incidental postnatal ultrasound finding

Asymptomatic, active, or 'burned out' UPJ obstruction may be detected incidentally in older children undergoing investigation for unrelated symptoms.

Clinical presentation

Clinical presentation is by:
- neonatal abdominal mass (although hydronephrosis of this severity is usually already evident prenatally);
- urinary infection represents the most common form of presentation in infants and young children with previously unsuspected UPJ obstruction (Fig. 14.25);
- pain associated with UPJ obstruction is typically localized to the loin, but may (confusingly) be referred to the epigastrium or central abdomen – the duration and severity of pain, which is often accompanied by vomiting, serves to distinguish it from the more transient nonspecific abdominal pain of childhood; and
- other modes of presentation, which include hematuria and hypertension.

with certain genetic syndromes (e.g. Johanson–Blizzard syndrome). There is a slight male predominance, and the left kidney is more commonly affected than the right.

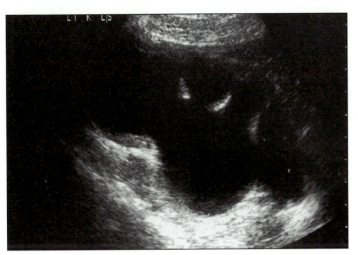

Figure 14.25 Gross hydronephrosis presenting with pain and infection. Infective debris was visible in the renal pelvis. A rapid symptomatic improvement followed percutaneous nephrostomy, with definitive pyeloplasty undertaken 2 weeks later.

Correlation between anteroposterior diameter of the renal pelvis and the requirement for pyeloplasty	
Anteroposterior diameter of renal pelvis (mm)	'Risk' of requirement for pyeloplasty (%)
<15	2
15–20	7
20–30	29
30–40	61
40–50	67
>50	100

Figure 14.26 Correlation between anteroposterior diameter of the renal pelvis and the requirement for pyeloplasty. The anteroposterior diameter is the maximum figure documented on any pre- or postnatal ultrasound scan. The requirement for pyeloplasty is determined by impaired renal function at presentation or deteriorating renal function on follow-up.

Diagnosis

In older children who present clinically, diagnostic imaging is similar to that for adults (i.e. ultrasound followed by dynamic isotope renography with ⁹⁹ᵐTc-DTPA or ⁹⁹ᵐTc-MAG3; see Chapter 23). In the presence of grossly reduced renal function ⁹⁹ᵐTc-DMSA provides the more reliable guide to prognosis and may help determine between pyeloplasty or nephrectomy. For medicolegal reasons many urologists still insist on an IVU before embarking on either procedure.

Investigation of prenatally detected ureteropelvic junction obstruction

Current thinking on the management of prenatally detected UPJ obstruction in healthy asymptomatic newborn infants revolves principally around the interpretation of information provided by ultrasound and isotope renography. The IVU is of little or no value in this context. In some centers all children with prenatally detected dilatation are routinely submitted to MCU, but this is not the author's practice if the ureters are undilated and the ultrasound configuration of the pelvis and calices is characteristic of UPJ obstruction.

Ultrasound

A well-documented correlation exists between severe dilatation [anteroposterior diameter (AP) >50mm] and reduced function in the obstructed kidney at the time of initial evaluation. Correspondingly, mild-to-moderate dilatation (AP diameter < 20mm) is generally associated with good preservation of renal function despite renographic evidence of obstruction[46]. The findings of prospective trials undertaken at Great Ormond Street Hospital, London, also demonstrated that severity of renal pelvic dilatation (as measured by the maximum AP diameter of the renal pelvis encountered at any stage on pre- or postnatal ultrasound) is a valuable predictor of the risk of functional deterioration on nonoperative management (Fig. 14.26)[46].

Dynamic isotope renography

Postnatal dynamic renography with ⁹⁹ᵐTc-MAG3 or ⁹⁹ᵐTc-DTPA is indicated when the pattern of dilatation is suggestive of UPJ obstruction (dilatation of the renal pelvis accompanied by caliceal dilatation) and where the AP diameter of the renal pelvis exceeds 15 mm. Although ultrasound confirmation of prenatally detected dilatation should be obtained within the first few days of life, practical clinical management is rarely influenced by the findings of dynamic renography at this stage. Wherever possible, isotope imaging should be deferred until 4–6 weeks of age in view of the greatly reduced glomerular and tubular function of the normal newborn kidneys. Even at 6 weeks of age, drainage curve data may be very difficult to interpret reliably.

Demonstration of a washout response on diuretic renography is evidence of nonobstructive dilatation (see chapter 10). In such cases, follow-up imaging can be limited to ultrasound unless there is evidence of increasing dilatation. However, in infants the absence of washout on a diuresis renography curve should not be automatically interpreted as evidence of significant obstruction. In the first few months of life, this may simply reflect immature tubular function in the period of so-called transitional nephrology. The pitfalls of basing a diagnosis of obstruction on drainage curve data in infants are highlighted by Ransley and Manzoni[47], who advocate that initial management protocols should be based not on drainage curve data but on the level of differential isotope uptake (differential function) in the hydronephrotic kidney.

Management

Submitting a healthy asymptomatic infant to pyeloplasty is easier to justify when the diagnosis of obstruction is accompanied by evidence of impaired renal function in the affected kidney. However, in two-thirds of prenatally detected hydronephrotic kidneys, normal levels of renal function are preserved despite evidence of obstruction as defined by isotope renography. Moreover, the potential for prenatally detected UPJ obstruction to resolve spontaneously in postnatal life is well documented[48].

While the management of prenatally detected hydronephrosis continues to divide opinion, a broad consensus has emerged in recent years. In the UK, current thinking on the indications and timing of pyeloplasty can be summarized as follows:

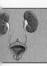

- pyeloplasty is indicated if the initial postnatal evaluation yields evidence of functional impairment (differential function <40%) and/or gross hydronephrosis (AP diameter >30mm), but the risk of further rapid functional deterioration is low and pyeloplasty is rarely justified below 3 months of age;
- conservative management is indicated if the initial figure for differential function exceeds 40% and the maximum recorded AP diameter of the renal pelvis is <30mm (in practice, an AP diameter <20mm almost, but not entirely, excludes the likelihood of pyeloplasty being required on grounds of reduced or deteriorating function in the obstructed kidney).

Moderate hydronephrosis (AP diameter 20–30mm) poses a dilemma since a substantial proportion of children with prenatally detected UPJ obstruction fall within this category. Conservative management comprises antibiotic prophylaxis during the first year of life combined with follow up protocol of ultrasound and isotope imaging.

In a prospective trial of conservative versus surgical management of prenatally detected UPJ obstruction, 48 children were managed by early pyeloplasty whereas 52 were managed conservatively[46]. Of the conservatively managed kidneys, nine (17%) came to pyeloplasty because of deteriorating function during the period of follow-up. Recovery of function was observed in the majority following pyeloplasty. Of the conservatively managed kidneys, 14 showed evidence of resolving obstruction, whereas 29 remained stable with no evidence of functional deterioration.

Indications to abandon conservative management in favor of pyeloplasty are:

- deteriorating renal function (falling to <40% on follow-up);
- increasing dilatation (which often precedes deterioration of function); and
- persisting obstruction with no evidence of improving drainage after 4–5 years of conservative management.

Management of the poorly functioning kidney (differential function <15%)

In the early days of prenatal diagnosis percutaneous drainage was employed to demonstrate any potential for functional recovery of poorly functioning kidneys before a decision to proceed to nephrectomy. Apart from the technical difficulty in maintaining reliable percutaneous nephrostomy drainage in this age group, it soon became apparent that useful recovery of function rarely occurred in kidneys that have sustained a severe obstructive insult *in utero*. Nephrectomy is considered if the contralateral kidney is normal and when a differential function <15% has been documented on ^{99m}Tc-DMSA (^{99m}Tc-DTPA is unreliable for this purpose). Ideally, functional assessment should be carried out on more than one occasion.

Bilateral ureteropelvic obstruction

Differential isotope uptake ceases to be a reliable guide to renal function in the presence of bilateral renal pathology. In practice, bilateral UPJ obstruction is not usually of equal symmetric severity and isotope renography data are therefore of some value when considered within the context of the ultrasound findings. Bilateral UPJ obstruction is not necessarily a contraindication to conservative management, but it may be more appropriate to manage the more severely hydronephrotic kidney surgically and monitor the contralateral kidney. Occasionally, bilateral simultaneous or staged pyeloplasty may be required. Each case must be judged on its merits.

Surgical considerations

The Anderson–Hynes procedure is employed almost universally in children. An anterolateral extraperitoneal exposure is favored in infants in view of their broad subcostal angle, but a supra twelfth rib loin incision is more appropriate in the older age group. The posterior lumbotomy incision undoubtedly results in less postoperative discomfort, but is less flexible if unexpected operative findings occur. Postoperative extrarenal drainage and a brief period of bladder catheter drainage generally suffice. After a difficult pyeloplasty the use of a temporary indwelling JJ stent is superseding external nephrostomy drainage.

REFERENCES

1. Meyer R. Anatomie und Entwicklungsgeschickte der Ureter verdoppelung. Virchows Arch (A). 1907;187:408–34.
2. Weigert C. Ueber einige Bildungsfehler der Ureteren. Virchows Arch (A). 1877;70:490–501.
3. Mackie GG, Stephens FD. Duplex kidneys: a correlation of renal dysplasia with the position of the ureteric orifice. J Urol. 1975;14:274–80.
4. McDonald JH, McClellan DS. Crossed renal ectopia. Am J Surg. 1957;93: 995–1002.
5. Song JT, Ritchey ML, Zerin JM, Bloom DA. Incidence of vesico-ureteral reflux in children with unilateral renal agenesis. J Urol. 1995;153:1249–51.
6. Mesrobian H-GJ, Rushton HG, Bulas D. Unilateral renal agenesis may result from in utero regression of multicystic renal dysplasia. J Urol. 1993;150:793–4.
7. Avni EF, Thoua Y, Lalmand B, et al. Multicystic dysplastic kidney: natural history from in utero diagnosis and post-natal follow up. J Urol. 1987;138:1420–4.
8. Woolf AS. The single kidney. In: Stringer MD, Oldham KT, Mouriquand PDE, Howard ER, eds. Paediatric surgery and urology: long-term outcome. London: WB Saunders; 1998:625–31.
9. Thomas DFM, Fitzpatrick MM. Cystic renal disease in childhood. In: Thomas DFM, ed. Urological disease in the fetus and infant. Oxford: Butterworth–Heinemann; 1997:237–49.

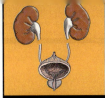

Chapter 15

Congenital Diseases of the Lower Urinary Tract

John P Gearhart and Linda A Baker

KEY POINTS

- The goals of management of the exstrophy–epispadias complex include closure of the bony pelvic ring, closure of the bladder and posterior urethra, closure of the abdominal wall defect, closure, straightening, and lengthening of the epispadiac penis in the male and reconstruction of the external genitalia in the female, bladder neck reconstruction, correction of vesicoureteral reflux, and achievement of an adequate bladder capacity.
- The goals of management of hypospadias include correction of chordee by degloving penile skin, dorsal plication sutures, division of urethral plate, or patch graft to ventral corporotomy, glanuloplasty, and construction of a neourethra.

Anomalies of closure of the ventral midline that affect the urogenital tract include classic bladder exstrophy, cloacal exstrophy, epispadias, and hypospadias. It is believed that classic bladder exstrophy, cloacal exstrophy, and epispadias share a similar mechanism of embryonic maldevelopment. These rare anomalies are grouped as the exstrophy–epispadias complex and discussed in the first part of this chapter. The second part of the chapter is devoted to the common birth defect, hypospadias.

THE EXTROPHY–EPISPADIAS COMPLEX

Classic bladder exstrophy

The most common anomaly in this complex, which occurs in 1:35,000 births[1], is classic bladder exstrophy. Easily recognized at birth and occasionally recognized on prenatal ultrasound, this anomaly is three times more common in males than females. No strong genetic inheritance pattern has been appreciated, although few males have fathered children. A detailed embryological account of the disorder is described in Chapter 2.

The anatomic composition of this anomaly includes a cup-like bladder plate of various sizes exteriorized in the suprapubic region. The size and pliability of the bladder plate are factors in the decision as to whether the bladder should be closed. The bony pelvis does not make a complete ring, for the pubic bones are spaced widely apart, externally rotated, and foreshortened. The ventral abdominal wall musculature is well formed, but widely splayed on either side of the exstrophic bladder, with the medial edges of each rectus sheath inserting on each pubic

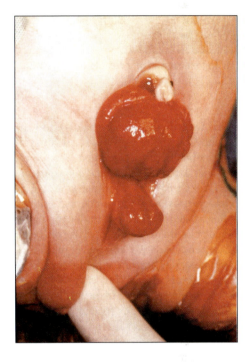

Figure 15.1 Lower ventral abdominal wall of a male neonate with classic bladder exstrophy.

tubercle. In the male (Fig. 15.1), the penis is completely epispadiac, with the posterior and anterior urethra open and superior to the corpora cavernosae. The penis is shorter and wider, with dorsal chordee and an open urethral plate. In the female (Fig. 15.2), the mons and clitoris are bifid and the entire urethra is open dorsally. Otherwise, in both sexes, the reproductive organs are normal. The pelvic floor musculature is splayed anteriorly. The anus is anterior on the perineum and may be prone to prolapse.

Care of the neonate with bladder exstrophy includes ligation of the umbilical cord with a nonabsorbable suture instead of a plastic clamp, which can tear the delicate bladder mucosa. The bladder should be covered with Saran wrap to prevent desiccation and denuding. It is extremely unusual for any other anomalies to be present and these babies are typically very healthy. The child may be fed as any other neonate. Referral to an exstrophy center is often the best course of action, for a successful first surgical attempt at bladder closure gives the highest success rate of creating a normal voiding child.

Surgical reconstruction of the urogenital anomalies of classic bladder exstrophy is clearly controversial at every stage of the reconstruction. The management scheme must be tailored to the severity of the anomalies in each child and modified if complications arise. The surgical management of classic bladder exstrophy should begin within the first week of life with an examination

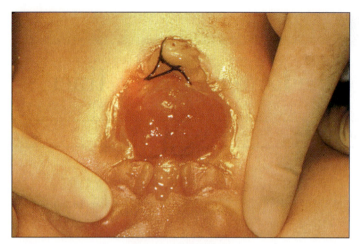

Figure 15.2 Lower ventral abdominal wall of a female neonate with classic bladder exstrophy.

under anesthesia, at which time the bladder is evaluated for its size and quality and the pubic bones are assessed for severity of diastases and mobility. If the bladder is not deemed suitable for reconstruction, it can be given 4–6 months to grow before reconstruction is attempted[1]. Other surgeons recommend a urinary diversion in this case[2]. However, if the bladder is deemed suitable for reconstruction, the first stage is carried out under the initial anesthesia. The goals include closure of the bony pelvic ring (with or without osteotomies, depending on age and pelvic mobility), closure of the bladder and posterior urethra, and closure of the abdominal wall defect without loss of renal function. The operative technique is depicted in Figure 15.3. In males, this first surgical stage converts the bladder exstrophy patient into a complete epispadias, while in females the external genitalia are reconstructed completely at this stage. Meticulous attention to surgical details and postoperative care are crucial to the success of this stage. These include complete urinary diversion and modified Bryant's traction for 3–4 weeks in the neonate without osteotomies, or external fixation for 6–8 weeks with light Buck's traction for 2–4 weeks in the child who requires osteotomies[1].

Some surgeons have performed simultaneous reconstruction of the epispadiac penis in the newborn with good preliminary results. Formerly, the staged functional reconstruction proposed by Jeffs required the epispadias repair to be carried out at 3 years of age. However, Gearhart and Jeffs[3] found an improvement in bladder capacity when the epispadias repair was performed earlier, at around 6 months to 1 year of age. Several surgical methods have been used to achieve closure, straightening, and lengthening of the epispadiac penis, but long-term outcomes best support the use of the modified Cantwell–Ransley repair[4]. This operative technique is depicted in Figure 15.4.

Annually, the bladder growth is assessed by gravity cystogram and cystoscopy, which allows measurement of bladder capacity and detection of vesicoureteral reflux. Bladder capacity is the single best predictor of eventual urinary continence and if the bladder achieves an 85cm³ capacity by 4–5 years of age, the final stage of surgical reconstruction, bladder neck reconstruction for urinary continence, can be considered[1]. It is crucial to factor the maturity of the child into the timing of this reconstruction, for the child must desire urinary continence and be cooperative with

a voiding regimen. The surgical technique is depicted in Figure 15.5 and entails bilateral cephalotrigonal ureteral reimplantation and Young–Dees–Leadbetter bladder neck reconstruction.

Reconstructive failures can occur at any point in this operative cascade and are best managed at an exstrophy center. After bladder closure, bladder dehiscence or prolapse can occur and requires reclosure after 6 months of healing. Stricturing of the neourethra can be obstructive and has disastrous sequelae (renal damage and diminished likelihood of bladder reconstructive success) if not detected and promptly managed[5]. The most common complication of epispadias repair is fistula formation, which may resolve spontaneously or require surgical excision. Urethral stricture, residual dorsal chordee, and poor cosmetic results can also complicate this surgery, but fortunately are rare with the Cantwell–Ransley repair. Despite successful bladder and epispadias closure, some bladders do not grow to adequate capacity. In such cases, attempts at constructing a continence mechanism are futile. Bladder augmentation with a bowel segment is typically performed with simultaneous transection of the bladder neck and creation of an appendicovesicostomy for catheterization. Fortunately, this is necessary in only 5% of patients[1]. If the patient has undergone all three stages of reconstruction but urinary incontinence is a persistent problem, diagnostic studies must define the etiology of the incontinence before therapy can be instituted.

The staged functional reconstruction of the classic bladder exstrophy is an amazing success story in 75–85% of patients, and yields patients who spontaneously void and are continent for 3 hours during the day and dry at night, with preservation of renal function and excellent cosmetic results[6].

Cloacal exstrophy

Cloacal exstrophy is a malformation of multiple organ systems that occurs in one of 200,000–400,000 births[1]. It is fortunate that it is very rare, for this constellation of anomalies can lead to demise. Prior to 1960, no survivors were reported. However, with advances in neonatology, nutritional support, anesthesia, antibiotic therapy, and surgical reconstruction, long-term survivors (83–100%) with excellent quality of life are now common.

The diagnosis and presentation is often by prenatal ultrasound or at birth. This malformation severely affects formation of the lower abdominal wall and pelvis, genitourinary tract, and intestinal tract[7]. The most common anatomic variety of cloacal exstrophy is delineated in Figure 15.6, but many cloacal variants have been observed. Superiorly, an omphalocele is present in 90% of cases. The ileocecum is exstrophic in the suprapubic region, with flanking hemibladders that may meet superiorly. Each hemibladder typically has its own ureteral orifice, although a kidney may be absent or ectopic in 20–50% of patients. On the ileocecal plate are openings to the terminal ileum superiorly and distal colon (hindgut) inferiorly. The terminal ileum often prolapses to yield an 'elephant-trunk' deformity. Orifices to one or two appendices are also present. The hindgut is short and may be partially or completely duplicated. Most patients have gut malrotation and short-gut syndrome is also a common source of significant morbidity and mortality (25–50% of cases). The anus is imperforate. Partial or complete duplication or absence of portions of the female reproductive tract occurs in 25–90% of cases, but the ovaries are normal. In the males (Fig. 15.7), the phallus is completely bifid and very widely spaced, since the pelvic bone

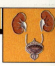
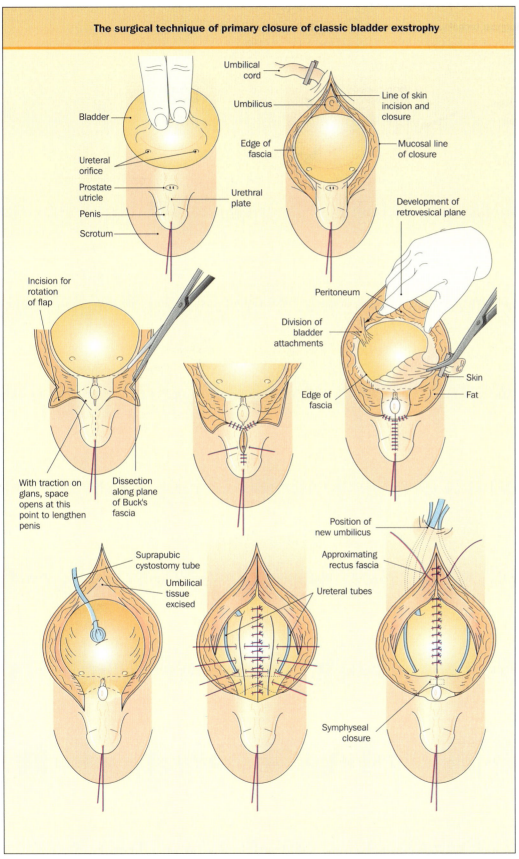

The surgical technique of primary closure of classic bladder exstrophy

Umbilical cord

Umbilicus

Line of skin incision and closure

Bladder

Edge of fascia

Mucosal line of closure

Ureteral orifice

Development of retrovesical plane

Prostate utricle

Urethral plate

Penis

Scrotum

Incision for rotation of flap

Peritoneum

Division of bladder attachments

Edge of fascia

Skin

Fat

With traction on glans, space opens at this point to lengthen penis

Dissection along plane of Buck's fascia

Position of new umbilicus

Suprapubic cystostomy tube

Approximating rectus fascia

Umbilical tissue excised

Ureteral tubes

Symphyseal closure

Figure 15.3 The surgical technique of primary closure of classic bladder exstrophy. (Adapted with permission from Gearhart and Jeffs[1].)

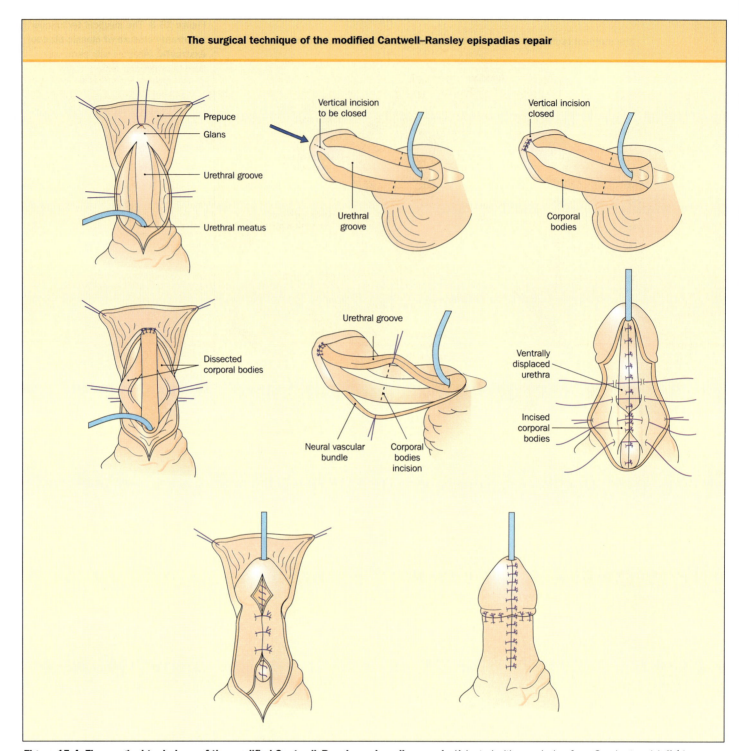

The surgical technique of the modified Cantwell–Ransley epispadias repair

Figure 15.4 The surgical technique of the modified Cantwell–Ransley epispadias repair. (Adapted with permission from Gearhart and Jeffs[1].)

is foreshortened and malformed to yield a severe pubic diastases. In 30% of males the penis is absent. The testes are often intra-abdominal if not palpable in the groin. The scrotum may be absent or split in varying degrees. In 40–60% of cases, a lumbar or sacral myelomeningocele, meningocele, or lipomeningocele is present and the lower limbs are often significantly malformed.

The embryologic theory that accounts for this malformation is based upon the cloacal membrane[8], a bilaminar structure composed of ectoderm and endoderm that covers the cloaca in the

2.5–3 week human embryo. This structure normally ruptures after the cloaca has been septated into the urogenital sinus and the anorectum. If it ruptures prematurely, it is thought that the undivided cloaca everts. Anatomic variants are produced by different locations and timing of the rupture.

Surgical management must be tailored to the anatomy and physiologic status of the neonate[1]. If a myelomeningocele is present, it must be repaired promptly. Once healed, the initial surgery upon the cloacal exstrophy must consider the need for a staged

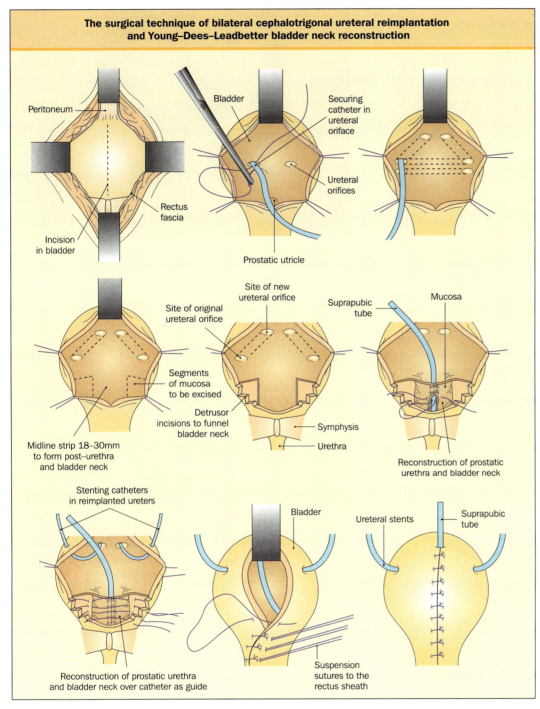

The surgical technique of bilateral cephalotrigonal ureteral reimplantation and Young–Dees–Leadbetter bladder neck reconstruction

Peritoneum

Rectus fascia

Incision in bladder

Bladder

Securing catheter in ureteral oriface

Ureteral orifices

Prostatic utricle

Site of new ureteral orifice

Site of original ureteral orifice

Suprapubic tube

Mucosa

Segments of mucosa to be excised

Detrusor incisions to funnel bladder neck

Symphysis

Urethra

Midline strip 18–30mm to form post–urethra and bladder neck

Reconstruction of prostatic urethra and bladder neck

Stenting catheters in reimplanted ureters

Bladder

Ureteral stents

Suprapubic tube

Reconstruction of prostatic urethra and bladder neck over catheter as guide

Suspension sutures to the rectus sheath

Figure 15.5 The surgical technique of bilateral cephalotrigonal ureteral reimplantation and Young–Dees–Leadbetter bladder neck reconstruction. (Adapted with permission from Gearhart and Jeffs[1].)

repair. It is paramount to retain all segments of the bowel and not discard the hindgut or appendices, which might be used in future reconstructions. In addition, the need for gender reassignment in the male child must be assessed at this time, with a multidisciplinary team involved in the decision.

Hurwitz and Manzoni describe a two-stage procedure[9]. In the first stage the omphalocele is excised, and the ileocecal plate is separated from the hemibladders and then tubularized. The blind-ending hindgut is brought out as a colostomy in the left upper quadrant. The hemibladders are approximated in the midline if they are small. In the second stage the bladder plate is closed similarly to the procedure for a classic bladder exstrophy with

osteotomies. Alternatively, both stages can be carried out simultaneously in a single-stage repair, but this is a long surgical endeavor that requires a strong child with a large bladder template. Other surgeons leave the ileocecal plate attached to the hemibladders as an augmentation, close the bladder, anastomose the hindgut to the terminal ileum, and create a colostomy. Alternatively, the hindgut remnant may be matured as a mucous fistula.

If the phallic structures in the genetic male cloacal exstrophy patient meet the criteria of micropenis and do not respond to androgen stimulation, gender conversion is recommended with early orchiectomy and phallectomy, usually at the initial surgery on the cloacal exstrophy.

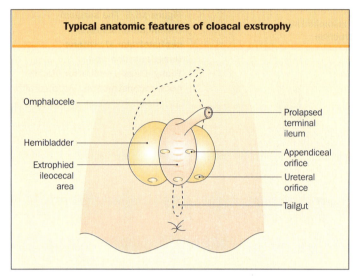

Figure 15.6 Typical anatomic features of cloacal exstrophy. (Adapted with permission from Gearhart and Jeffs[1].)

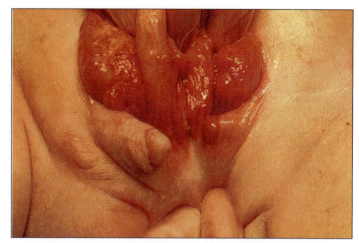

Figure 15.7 Lower ventral abdominal wall of a male neonate with cloacal exstrophy after ileostomy and first stage closure. Note the cecal plate between the hemibladders and the diminutive right hemiphallus.

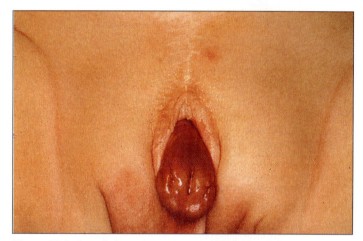

Figure 15.8 Dorsal view of a male with complete epispadias status post primary closure of classic bladder exstrophy.

Subsequent surgeries deal with cosmetic issues, creation of a neovagina, and attainment of urinary continence. If bowel segments such as the hindgut are available, they may be used for vaginal reconstruction, bladder augmentation, or creation of a colon conduit or catheterizable stoma. Stomach has also been a source of bowel for augmentation or for catheterizable stoma. Bladder neck surgeries, such as the Young–Dees-Leadbetter or Kropp, have been used with success to achieve urinary continence. The urinary continence status is known in 32 of our 37 cloacal exstrophy patients treated at Johns Hopkins Hospital[7]; 11 are continent with clean intermittent catheterization via a continent catheterizable stoma, five are continent with catheterization per urethra, and one patient is dry and spontaneously voiding. Of the others, four failed incontinence surgery, eight await continence surgery, and three have ileal conduits.

In summary, the surgical reconstruction of cloacal exstrophy requires a multidisciplinary approach with close attention to surgical details and tissue conservation; it yields a 90–100% survival rate and high functional states.

Epispadias

The term epispadias (Greek *epi*, upon; Greek *spadon*, a rent) describes the urethral malformation in which the urethral meatus opens in a proximal position on the dorsum of the penis followed by a distal dorsal urethral plate. Epispadias in the male occurs in 1 of 117,000 live births[1], is an uncommon anomaly when not associated with bladder exstrophy, and can present as complete epispadias (penopubic or subsymphyseal epispadias), penile epispadias, and glandular (balanitic) epispadias forms. Of these locations, the complete variety (Fig. 15.8) is the most common and glandular is the least common defect. It has been observed that the more distal the urethral meatus lies, the more likely it is that continence will be achieved without surgical intervention. In the female, epispadias is even more rare, occurring in 1 of 484,000 births[1].

The epispadiac penis can be reconstructed by several methods, but the modified Cantwell–Ransley epispadias repair has enjoyed widespread application with the greatest success. Closure of epispadias of the female urethra is depicted in Figure 15.9. In males or females, if urinary incontinence is also present, a Young–Dees–Leadbetter bladder neck reconstruction with suspension and ureteral reimplantation (see above) are carried out when a sufficient bladder capacity is attained and the child is psychologically mature. With carefully planned and executed surgical techniques, the reconstruction should yield a straight, dependent, potent penis with urinary continence and preservation of renal function.

HYPOSPADIAS

Male hypospadias, a congenital anomaly in which the urethral meatus is located on the ventral surface of the penis instead of at the tip of the penis, occurs in 3.2 of 1000 live male births[10] and can vary in severity from the glandular position to the perineal position. Fortunately, the more distal varieties are both the most common and the simplest to reconstruct.

The growth and embryologic differentiation of the male external genitalia from its anlagen, the genital tubercle, urethral folds,

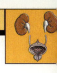
The surgical technique of female epispadias repair

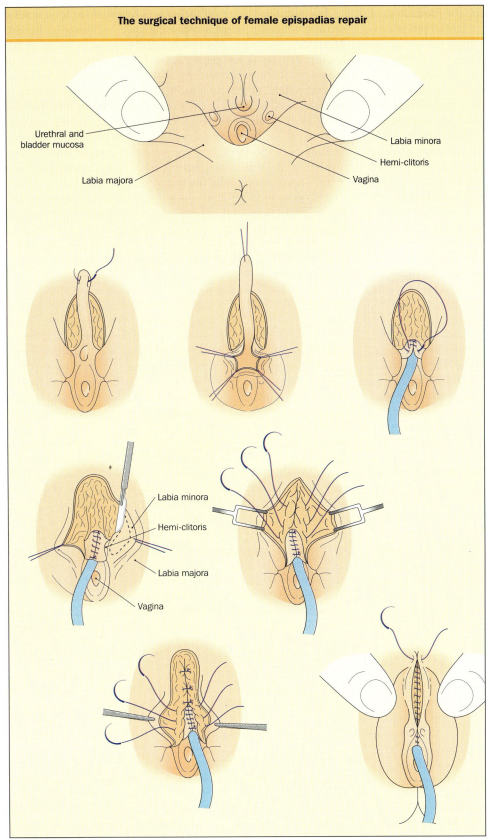

Urethral and bladder mucosa

Labia minora

Hemi-clitoris

Labia majora

Vagina

Labia minora

Hemi-clitoris

Labia majora

Vagina

Figure 15.9 The surgical technique of female epispadias repair. (Adapted with permission from Gearhart and Jeffs[1].)

genital swellings, and urogenital sinus, require the production of testosterone. Secreted by the fetal testis, testosterone is converted into dihydrotestosterone by 5α-reductase within the tissues of the male external genitalia. Dihydrotestosterone causes the genital tubercle to enlarge as the shaft and glans penis, while the urethral folds fuse in the ventral midline, to create the tubular urethra. Although several factors have been investigated and implicated in the development of hypospadias, no single defect explains the embryologic anomaly. It can run in families – 8% of patients have affected fathers and 14% have affected male siblings[10].

The anatomic findings vary in severity and are worse in cases in which the meatus is more proximally located. All hypospadic patients have an incomplete foreskin, called a dorsal hood because the foreskin is absent on the ventral surface of the penis. The ventral chordee or curvature of the erect penis may vary in severity and location. The intact urethra proximal to the meatus may have segments that are quite thin ventrally and must be unroofed. Distal to the meatus, the urethral plate may vary from shallow, thin, and narrow to deep, thick, and wide. Other anomalies, which include penile torsion or penoscrotal transposition, may be present and require surgical intervention. Cryptorchidism is present in 9% of all cases, but it is present in 32% of cases of posterior hypospadias[11]. The presence of an undescended testis must raise the concern of intersex, which is seen in as many as 27% of hypospadic patients with an undescended testis[12]. Mixed gonadal dysgenesis is the most common intersex disorder in this group. When a patient with proximal hypospadias (10% of penoscrotal hypospadias patients and 50% of perineal hypospadias patients) is catheterized an enlarged prostatic utricle can be problematic and rarely may lead to recurrent urinary tract infections or utricular stones, which warrants transtrigonal resection[13].

Surgical reconstruction is the only means of correction and offers the patient improved penile cosmesis (circumcision, normal meatal location, and a straight penis), a straight urinary stream in the standing position, and the potential for improved fertility, especially in cases of proximal hypospadias. Typically, the surgery is carried out between 6 and 18 months of life, with optical magnification, and a general anesthetic with or without penile or caudal block. Some surgeons favor testosterone injection at 2 and 5 weeks prior to the surgery to promote vascular supply to the penile skin and urethral plate. Most cases are undertaken on an outpatient basis with urethral stenting via a soft silicone catheter for 7–10 days.

Many surgical techniques have been described to correct hypospadias, reflecting the need for versatility during the reconstruction. The urologic surgeon must be equipped with a variety of options, for each case may vary in tissue quality, urethral plate and proximal urethral tube quality, degree and location of penile chordee, quantity and quality of penile or preputial skin, and location of the meatus. Surgical goals of reconstruction include correction of penile chordee (orthoplasty), creation of a hairless, straight uniform urethral tube (neourethra) to elongate the urethra to the tip of the glans (urethroplasty), creation of a conical glans with a vertical slit-like meatus (meatoplasty, glanuloplasty) and cosmetic skin coverage of the penile shaft. Functional goals include a cosmetic penis with normal urinary and sexual functions (straight erections and forceful ejaculation) and normal penile growth.

The number of surgical techniques reported for hypospadias reconstructions prevent a comprehensive presentation herein. Therefore, the most commonly used surgical procedures for hypospadias repair are presented and are grouped according to their application to the severity of the hypospadias. In the intraoperative state, not the preoperative state, the urethral meatus is anterior in 50% (glandular or coronal), middle in 30% (on the penile shaft – distal penile, midshaft, or proximal penile), and posterior in 20% of cases (penoscrotal, scrotal, or perineal)[14]. The distinction between intraoperative state and preoperative state is important since once the penile skin has been degloved and any penile chordee corrected, the meatus may be in a different position. Therefore a different surgical approach may be necessary. Figure 15.10 depicts an algorithm that helps guide the decision making in this process.

Surgical techniques to correct penile chordee (orthoplasty)

The first surgical maneuver is to create a Firlit cuff by incising the penile shaft skin just below the corona. Initially, the urethral plate is left intact. The penile skin is degloved between Buck's fascia and the subcutaneous tissue. In some cases, degloving is all that is required to release penile skin and/or Dartos fascia chordee. However, it is prudent to induce an artificial erection (Fig. 15.11) with a penile tourniquet and intracorporeal saline injection, as described by Gittes and McLaughlin, to assure a straight penis[15]. If chordee is still present, the urethral plate can be left intact and any fibrous chordee tissue about the urethral meatus, which may be abundant even in the normal proximal urethra, is resected. At this point, mild chordee can be corrected with one of several types of Nesbit plication sutures (Fig. 15.12) on the dorsal surface of the penis[16,17]. If the chordee is more severe, which is more common with proximal hypospadias, it may be more prudent to divide the urethral plate and resect any ventral fibrous tissue present about the urethral plate and meatus. Some surgeons advocate elevating the urethral meatus to excise this tissue beneath the meatus. 'Fairy cuts', a technique described by Belman wherein ventral transverse incisions are made in the tunica albuginea, may gain small amounts of ventral length. In some cases, there is intrinsic corpora cavernosal disproportion. To reconstruct severe chordee, a ventral corporotomy is patched with an elliptic free dermal graft[18] or a tunica vaginalis parietalis testis graft[19].

It is crucial to check an artificial erection repeatedly throughout the orthoplasty. A straight penis is required prior to any further stages of hypospadias reconstruction. One-stage hypospadias repair[20] is feasible with all of the above maneuvers, except when the urethral plate is divided and when the penile tunica albuginea is patch grafted.

Surgical techniques to reconstruct anterior hypospadias

Most anterior or distal (glandular or coronal) hypospadias defects, if there is adequate urethral mobility and no chordee, can be corrected by the meatal advancement and glanuloplasty technique (MAGPI)[21]. This technique is not applicable to the hypospadiac patient with a patulous 'fish-mouthed' meatus, the noncompliant fibrotic meatus, or the meatus with proximal hypoplasia of the urethra[22]. Therefore, proper patient selection is critical and can be assessed by testing urethral meatal mobility

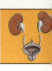

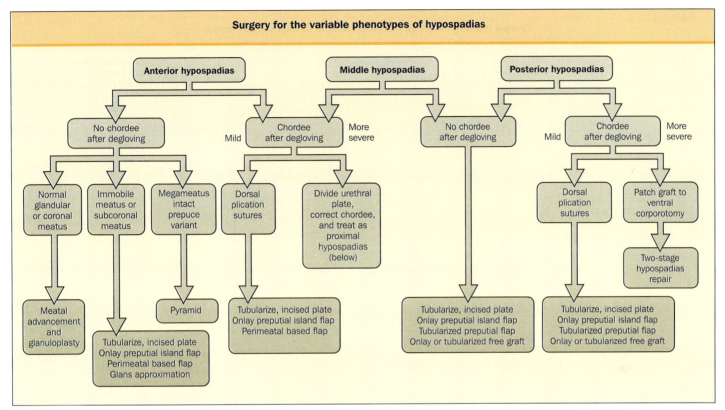

Figure 15.10 An algorithm to help guide the application of proper surgical techniques to the variable phenotypes of hypospadias.

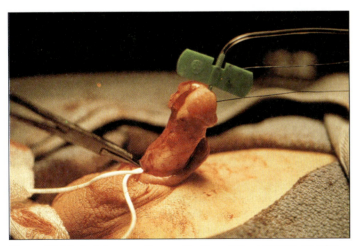

Figure 15.11 An intraoperative application of the artificial erection by Gittes and McLaughlin.

prior to incision with fine toothed forceps. To begin MAGPI (Fig. 15.13), a Firlit cuff incision is followed by penile degloving. Chordee is assessed and corrected. Meatal advancement is achieved by creating a small dorsal incision in the midline roof of the hypospadic meatus. This vertical incision is closed horizontally with 7–0 Vicryl, thereby advancing and widening the meatus and flattening the dorsal bridge of tissue present, which can deflect the urinary stream ventrally. The ventral edge of the urethral meatus is advanced simultaneously as the glanuloplasty. Three holding sutures are placed in the edge of the Firlit cuff,

two laterally on the ventrum and one in the ventral midline. This final suture is pulled distally to the tip of the penis while 5–0 Vicryl sutures are placed in the tunica of the glans. A second subepithelial layer is placed here and the glans skin is closed cosmetically. Excess dorsal hood is removed and the penile skin is closed. A 10–12F Bougie should pass through the meatus without difficulty in a 6- to 12-month-old child. Urethral catheterization is not required after this hypospadias repair.

If the distal hypospadic meatus is not conducive to repair by the MAGPI procedure, the glans approximation procedure or pyramid procedure[23] may be a useful repair. Good for the subcoronal glans with a deep urethral groove or the megameatus intact prepuce variant, these repairs (Fig. 15.14) involve de-epithelializing perimeatal skin with microscissors and closing the cut edges to the tip of the penis, thereby reconstituting the ventral floor of the urethra. To prevent fistula formation, a vascular flap of de-epithelialized prepuce can be placed over the suture line and the glans skin then closed. A urethral catheter is used in this case to divert the urine.

Surgical techniques to reconstruct midshaft hypospadias
Several techniques are useful to reconstruct the hypospadic meatus that is located more proximal than the corona. The degree of penile chordee present may limit the use of some of these techniques. A recently reported technique, the tubularized, incised plate urethroplasty, advocated by Snodgrass (Fig. 15.15)[24], involves incision of the intact urethral plate from the meatus to the tip of the glans on the lateral edges and in the dorsal midline, exposing the corporeal bodies. The two urethral plate halves are then anastomosed in the ventral midline,

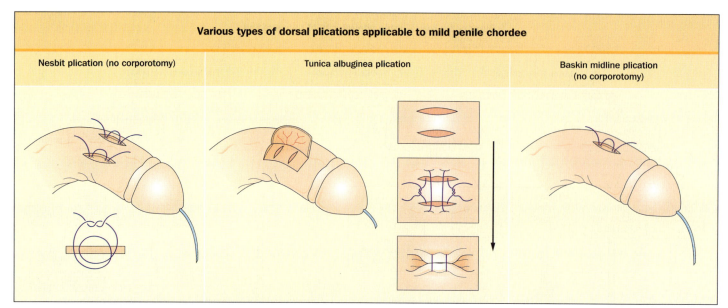

Various types of dorsal plications applicable to mild penile chordee		
Nesbit plication (no corporotomy)	Tunica albuginea plication	Baskin midline plication (no corporotomy)

Figure 15.12 Various types of dorsal plications applicable to mild penile chordee.

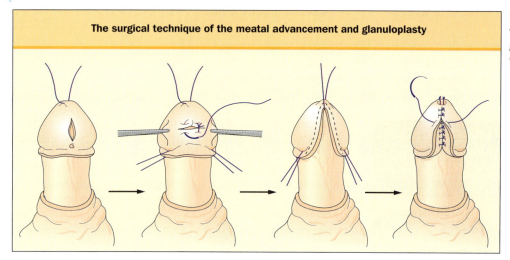

The surgical technique of the meatal advancement and glanuloplasty

Figure 15.13 The surgical technique of the meatal advancement and glanuloplasty. (Adapted with permission from Duckett[21].)

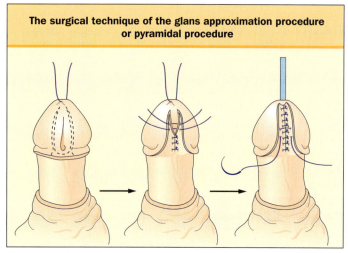

The surgical technique of the glans approximation procedure or pyramidal procedure

Figure 15.14 The surgical technique of the glans approximation procedure or pyramid procedure.

a layer of vascularized subcutaneous tissue is placed to cover the neourethra, and the glans wings are reapproximated. In this urethroplasty, the urethral plate is left intact and not divided to correct penile chordee. In some instances, this useful technique can be used even in proximal (penoscrotal or perineal) hypospadias repair. A 5.5% complication rate has been reported when applied to distal and proximal shaft hypospadias.

Other more traditional methods include perimeatal based flaps (Fig. 15.16), such as the Beck, Mathieu, Barcat, or Devine–Horton[25], and require the presence of thick, normal urethra and penile skin immediately proximal to the hypospadiac meatus. Once chordee is eliminated, the urethral plate is prepared to receive a perimeatal-based flap. A penile shaft skin flap, based just proximal to the meatus and parallel to the urethra, is created of sufficient length to reach the glans tip, flipped distal, and anastomosed. Mobilization of a thick vascular pedicle for the flip–flap is crucial and a second layer of soft-tissue coverage is obtained.

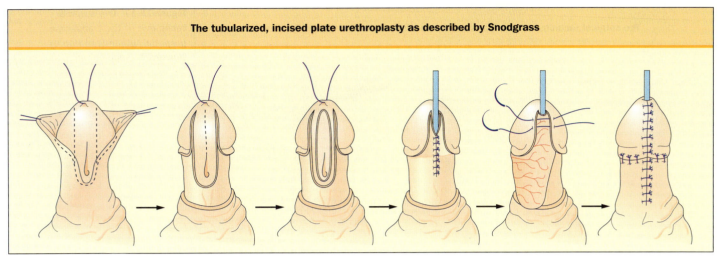

Figure 15.15 The tubularized, incised plate urethroplasty as described by Snodgrass[24]. (Adapted with permission.)

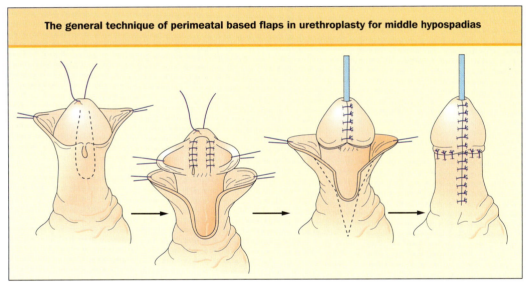

Figure 15.16 The general technique of perimeatal based flaps in urethroplasty for middle hypospadias.

Duckett advocated the transverse preputial tubularized or onlay[26] island flap technique (Figs 15.17 & 15.18) for proximal and middle hypospadias. A rectangular inner preputial skin flap, as long as 5–6cm, is created with care to maintain blood supply to this flap and the penile shaft skin. If the 4–6mm wide urethral plate is intact, this flap may be used as an onlay, but if the urethral plate has been divided to manage chordee, the skin flap may be rolled into a tube and fashioned as the distal urethra. The tubed repair was found to have more frequent complications by this group of surgeons[27].

In some cases, the hypospadiac urethra can be mobilized circumferentially in the proximal direction to such a degree that it reaches the tip of the penis without the creation of a neourethra and without inducing chordee[28,29]. Free grafts[25], derived from preputial skin, buccal mucosa, bladder mucosa, or extragenital skin that is not hair-bearing, can either be tubularized or applied as an urethral plate onlay to create a neourethra. Since the complication rate is greater (stricture or graft loss), these are used only when other more successful sources are not available.

Surgical techniques to reconstruct posterior hypospadias

Penoscrotal, scrotal, and perineal hypospadias are classified as posterior hypospadias; it is fortunate that these are the least common variety as they are the most difficult to reconstruct. Historically speaking, hypospadias surgery has proceeded from multistage repairs toward single-stage repairs. However, in cases of posterior hypospadias, the hurdles typically include a small penis, severe chordee, paucity of penile skin, and the need for a long urethroplasty. Often preoperative parenteral or topical testosterone may stimulate penile growth, improve penile skin vascularity, and increase penile skin. However, despite these measures, in many cases the chordee is so severe that the urethral plate must be sacrificed. Here the best surgical outcome may result from a staged repair.

In the first stage of a two-stage hypospadias repair (Fig. 15.19), a Firlit cuff is created, leaving the urethral plate intact. The penis is degloved and an artificial erection is created to assess chordee. Various maneuvers are employed to achieve a straight phallus [see above, Surgical techniques to correct penile chordee (orthoplasty)].

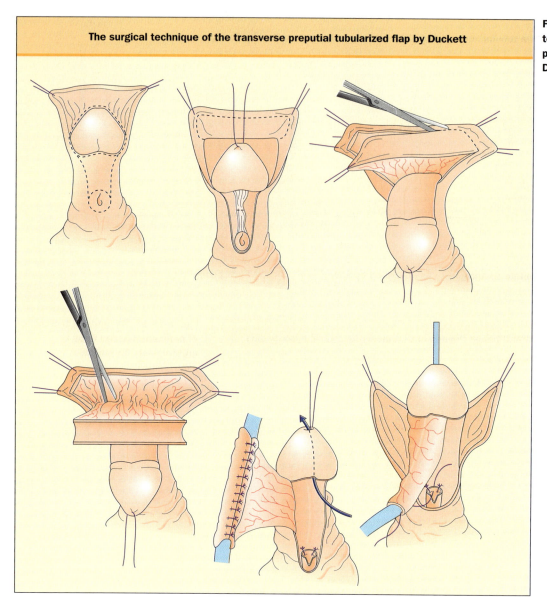

The surgical technique of the transverse preputial tubularized flap by Duckett

Figure 15.17 The surgical technique of the transverse preputial tubularized flap by Duckett[26]. (Adapted with permission.)

Often the urethral plate must be sacrificed in the orthoplasty. Once straight, the glans is incised on the ventral midline to create glans wings. Byers flaps are fashioned by splitting the dorsal hood of the prepuce, and the inner preputial skin is unfurled, which allows the dorsal skin to be rotated to the ventrum for a cosmetic skin closure. This penile skin is sutured into the glans groove. Alternatively, a glans dimple may be left intact and the Byers flaps can be fashioned, with excess skin being left distally so that the neourethra can be placed through a glans tunnel at the second stage[30,31]. Many variations upon this theme exist for the first stage of this repair. The second stage is performed 6 months or more after the first stage and involves tubularization of a 15mm urethral plate once the penis is verified as straight. Multiple layers of vascularized tissue are closed over this tube to prevent fistulae, including a tunica vaginalis vascular flap[32].

If the penis is straight without ventral corporeal patch grafting or without sacrifice of the urethral plate, an onlay flap may be used to construct the neourethra as previously described[26].

Flaps, based on a vascular supply, are always preferred over free grafts of skin, which are more likely to contract or die. Other options include free grafts of bladder mucosa, buccal mucosa, or a composite of multiple sources (see below). Buccal mucosa is the current favorite for this application and, although this source allows a single-stage surgical procedure for a highly complex surgical problem, even this technique is associated with a complication rate of 23–27%.

Postoperative care, complications, and reoperative hypospadias surgery

Postoperative care includes dressings, which act to immobilize tissue, diminish edema, and maintain sterility. Tegaderm adhesive dressing achieves these goals well. Pain is controlled by oral analgesics, such as oxycodone or acetaminophen with codeine. Oxybutynin and diazepam can control bladder spasms. The use of antibiotics immediately postoperatively is unclear, but they are necessary after catheter removal at 7–10 days.

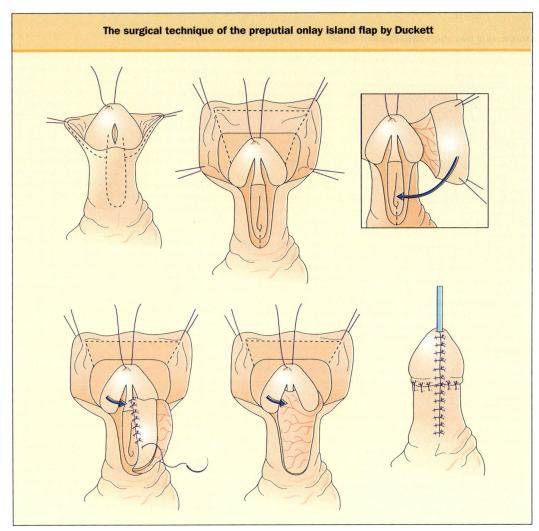

The surgical technique of the preputial onlay island flap by Duckett

Figure 15.18 The surgical technique of the preputial onlay island flap by Duckett[26]. (Adapted with permission.)

Several complications have been described, including residual penile chordee, urethral stricturing, fistula, meatal stenosis, prolapse or regression, urethral diverticular formation, loss of the flap or graft in the urethra or the penile shaft skin coverage, and morbidity associated with the donor site. The most common complication, urethrocutaneous fistulae, varies in frequency depending upon the urethroplasty carried out (Fig. 15.20). To diminish the likelihood of fistula formation, highly vascularized soft-tissue flaps[34] have been interposed between the skin and the urethroplasty. Retik and colleagues de-epithelialized the preputial flap[35] and Snow used the tunica vaginalis flap for this purpose[32]. These soft-tissue flaps must be immobilized to Buck's fascia to minimize shear effects and to maximize inosculation.

Reoperative surgery is typically performed no sooner than 6 months after the initial surgery for urethrocutaneous fistulae, urethral stricture, or urethral diverticuli, or for loss of urethral reconstruction. In the last case, the limiting factor is often tissue sources for subsequent attempts at urethral reconstruction. Many sources have been used for this purpose, including free grafts from the forearm, thigh, buccal mucosa, bladder mucosa, or scro-tal skin. Bladder mucosa has fallen out of favor because of meatal mucosal prolapse, meatal stenosis, and morbidity associated with the graft harvest. To prevent meatal prolapse, bladder mucosal grafts must be composite with local skin used at the meatus. Buccal mucosa has become favored since it is hairless, is harvested with minimal discomfort and no scar, is a thick epithelium with a rich vascular supply, and is limitlessness as a source[36]. It is best applied as an onlay, for tube grafts have a higher complication rate.

SUMMARY

The surgical reconstruction of congenital anomalies of the genitourinary tract may be achieved in a number of ways, but all require a broad knowledge of surgical techniques, as well as appropriate patient selection and options of management. The surgeon must be meticulous to minor details of tissue handling and plastic surgical techniques. With proper application, successful reconstruction with excellent functional and cosmetic results can be expected.

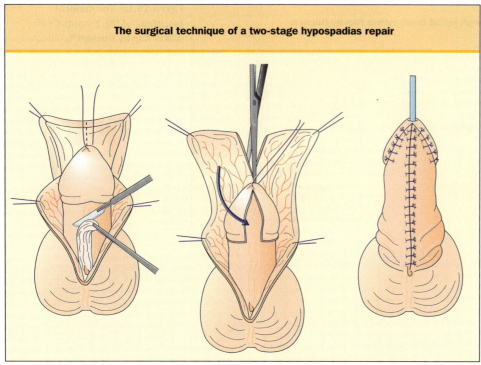

The surgical technique of a two-stage hypospadias repair

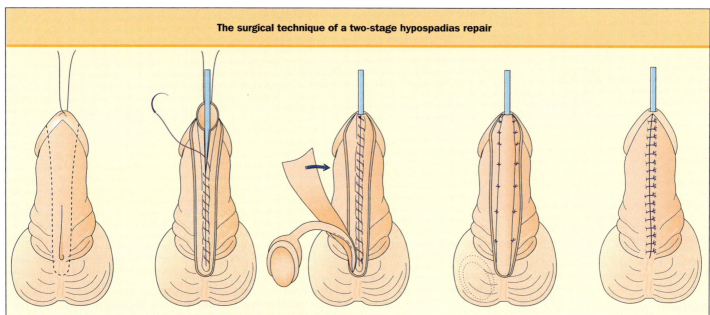

The surgical technique of a two-stage hypospadias repair

Figure 15.19 The surgical technique of a two-stage hypospadias repair.

Urethrocutaneous fistula rates in various types of urethroplasties	
Urethroplasty technique	Fistula rates reported (%)
Meatal advancement and glanuloplasty	0.5–10
Flip–flap repairs	2.2–35
Island pedicle tubed repairs	4–33
Free graft tubed repairs	15–50
Urethral advancement	1.0–16.7
Pyramid procedure	<5

Figure 15.20 Urethrocutaneous fistula rates vary depending upon the type of hypospadias repair used. (Adapted with permission from Shapiro[33].)

REFERENCES

1. Gearhart JP, Jeffs RD. Exstrophy–epispadias complex and bladder anomalies. In: Walsh PC, Retik AB, Vaughan ED Jr, Wein AJ, eds. Campbell's textbook of urology, 7th edn. Philadelphia: WB Saunders; 1998:1939–90.

2. Koo HP, Avolio L, Duckett JW Jr. Long-term results of ureterosigmoidostomy in children with bladder exstrophy. J Urol. 1996;156:2037–9.

3. Gearhart JP, Jeffs RD. Bladder exstrophy: increase in capacity following epispadias repair. J Urol. 1989;142:525–7.

4. Gearhart JP, Leonard MP, Bingers JK, Jeffs RD. The Cantwell–Ransley technique for repair of epispadias. J Urol. 1992;148:851–4.

5. Baker LA, Jeffs RD, Gearhart JP. Posterior urethral obstruction after primary bladder exstrophy closure: what is the fate of the genitourinary tract? J Urol. 1999;161:618–21.

6. Lakshmanan Y, Peppas DS, Gearhart JP, Jeffs RD. Bladder exstrophy: a twenty-one year experience with functional reconstruction in 88 consecutive patients followed from birth. J Urol. 2000 (in press).

7. Mathews R, Jeffs RD, Reiner WG, Docimo SG, Gearhart JP. Cloacal exstrophy – improving the quality of life: the Johns Hopkins experience. J Urol. 1998;160:2452–6.

8. Johnston TB. Extroversion of the bladder, complicated by the presence of intestinal openings on the surface of the extroverted area. J Anat. 1913;48:89–106.

9. Hurwitz RS, Manzoni GM. Cloacal exstrophy. In: O'Donnell B, Koff SA, eds. Pediatric urology, 3rd edn. Oxford: Butterworth–Heinemann; 1997:514–25.

10. Duckett J. Hypospadias. In: Walsh PC, Retik AB, Vaughan ED Jr, Wein AJ, eds. Campbell's textbook of urology, 7th edn. Philadelphia: WB Saunders; 1998:2093–119.

11. Khuri FJ, Hardy BE, Churchill BM. Urologic anomalies associated with hypospadias. Urol Clin North Am. 1981;8:565–9.

12. Rajfer J, Walsh PC. The incidence of intersexuality in patients with hypospadias and cryptorchidism. J Urol. 1976;116:769–72.

13. Monfort G. Transvesical approach to utricular cysts. J Pediatr Surg. 1982;17:406–9.

14. Duckett JD, Snyder HM. The MAGPI hypospadias repair after 1000 cases: avoidance of meatal stenosis and regression. J Urol. 1992;147:665–9.

15. Gittes RF, McLaughlin API. Injection technique to induce penile erection. Urology. 1974;4:473–6.

16. Nesbit RM. Congenital curvature of the phallus: report of three cases with description of corrective operation. J Urol. 1965;93:230–3.

17. Hinman FJ. Atlas of pediatric urologic surgery. Philadelphia: WB Saunders; 1994.

18. Devine CJ, Horton C. Chordee without hypospadias. J Urol. 1973;110:264–8.

19. Das S. Peyronie's disease: excision and autografting with tunica vaginalis. J Urol. 1980;124:818–21.

20. Hendren WH, Caesar RE. Chordee without hypospadias: experience with 33 cases. J Urol. 1992;147:107–11.

21. Duckett JW. MAGPI (meatoplasty and glanuloplasty). A procedure for subcoronal hypospadias. Urol Clin North Am. 1981;8:513–20.

22. Gibbons MD, Gonzales ET. The subcoronal meatus. J Urol. 1983;130:739–42.

23. Duckett JW, Keating MA. Technical challenge of the megameatus intact prepuce hypospadias variant: the pyramid procedure. J Urol. 1989;141:1407–9.

24. Snodgrass W. Tubularized, incised plate urethroplasty for distal hypospadias. J Urol. 1994;151:464–5.

25. Devine CJ, Horton CE. Hypospadias repair. J Urol. 1977;118:188–93.

26. Duckett JW. The island flap technique for hypospadias repair. Urol Clin North Am. 1981;8:503–12.

27. Baskin LS, Duckett JW, Ueoka K. Changing concepts of hypospadias curvature lead to more onlay island flap procedures. J Urol. 1994;151:191–6.

28. Koff SA. Mobilization of the urethra in the surgical treatment of hypospadias. J Urol. 1981;125:394–7.

29. Spencer JR, Perlmutter AD. Sleeve advancement distal hypospadias repair. J Urol. 1990;144:523–5.

30. Broadbent TR, Woolf RM, Toksu E. Hypospadias: one-stage repair. Plastic Reconstr Surg. 1961;27:154–9.

31. Fuqua F. Renaissance of urethroplasty: the belt technique of hypospadias repair. J Urol. 1971;106:782–5.

32. Snow BW. Use of tunica vaginalis to prevent fistulae in hypospadias surgery. J Urol. 1986;136:861.

33. Shapiro SR. Fistula repair. In: Ehrlich RM, Alter GJ, eds. Reconstructive and plastic surgery of the external genitalia: adult and pediatric, 1st edn. Philadelphia: WB Saunders; 1999:132–6.

34. Smith ED. A de-epithelialized overlap flap technique in the repair of hypospadias. Br J Plast Surg. 1973;26:106–14.

35. Retik AB, Mandell J, Bauer SB, Atala A. Meatal based hypospadias repair with the use of a dorsal subcutaneous flap to prevent urethrocutaneous fistula. J Urol. 1994;152:1229–32.

36. Duckett J, Coplen D, Ewalt D, Baskin L. Buccal mucosal urethral replacement. J Urol. 1995;153:1660–4.

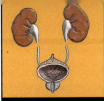

Chapter 16 Pediatric Neoplasia

Christopher S Cooper and Howard M Snyder III

KEY POINTS

- Wilms' tumor is the most common neoplasm of the urinary tract in children, and accounts for 8% of all solid tumors.
- The majority present with an asymptomatic mass that rarely crosses the midline.
- Neuroblastoma may arise from multiple sites that give a variety of presentations; a mass, commonly present, often extends across the midline.
- Rhabdomyosarcoma may arise from any part that contains embryonal mesenchyme; 20% of these tumors arise in the genitourinary tract.

WILMS' TUMOR

Incidence

The most common malignant neoplasm of the urinary tract in children is Wilms' tumor, which comprises 8% of all the solid tumors in children. Of Wilms' tumors, 75% afflict children between 1 and 5 years of age, and 90% occur in children younger than 7 years of age. The peak incidence occurs in children between 3 and 4 years of age. Boys and girls are almost equally affected by Wilms' tumor (ratio of 0.97:1.0)[1].

Etiology and pathophysiology

Wilms' tumor presumably originates from abnormal renal histogenesis in which proliferation of metanephric blastema without normal differentiation into tubules and glomeruli occurs. Nephrogenic rests or nephroblastomatosis may be precursor lesions that have the potential to undergo change and become a Wilms' tumor. A nephrogenic rest consists of a focus of abnormally persistent nephrogenic cells. Nephroblastomatosis describes the condition when multifocal or diffuse nephrogenic rests exist.

Nephrogenic rests occur in 1% of infant autopsy examinations. When the kidneys from children with Wilms' tumor are examined, up to 44% have nephrogenic rests. This incidence of nephrogenic rests approaches 100% in a child with bilateral synchronous Wilms' tumors. Genetic predisposition likely increases the incidence of nephrogenic rests and a second factor may induce the transformation of these rests into malignancies[2].

Nephrogenic rests are classified in two categories based on their position relative to the renal lobe. Intralobar nephrogenic rests (ILNRs) consist of rests anywhere within the renal lobe, sinus, or pelvicaliceal system. Perilobar nephrogenic rests (PLNRs) occur in the lobar periphery. The latter rests likely occur later in development, since the renal lobe develops in a centrifugal fashion. They occur more frequently than ILNRs and are associated with hemihypertrophy and the Beckwith–Wiedemann syndromes. The ILNRs present in a younger age group, are less common, and are often associated with the WAGR (Wilms' tumor, aniridia, genitourinary abnormality, and mental retardation) and Denys–Drash syndromes (described below).

The majority of nephrogenic rests undergo regression and become sclerotic or obsolescent. Some rests may grow and become hyperplastic, but even these hyperplastic rests may regress. Unfortunately, a dormant, hyperplastic, or regressing rest maintains neoplastic potential. Adding to the physician's dilemma, the microscopic appearance of Wilms' tumor and nephrogenic rests can be indistinguishable. This implies that the diagnosis of Wilms' tumor may depend on the shape and growth characteristics of the lesion. With hyperplasia a rest tends to maintain its original shape, unlike a neoplasm, which is often spheric. Serial imaging studies to determine the growth characteristics of a lesion offer useful clues as to the malignant potential of the lesion[2].

Various genes and gene mutations have been identified and associated with the development of Wilms' tumor. The Wilms' tumor 1 gene (WT1) is located in the 11p13 region and is critical for normal genitourinary development. Mutations in this gene have been associated with the development of Wilms' tumor as well as associated syndromes such as the Denys–Drash or WAGR syndromes. Other gene mutations distal to the WT1 gene in the 11p15 (WT2) region are associated with Wilms' tumors that occur in the Beckwith–Wiedemann syndrome[3].

Associated anomalies

Congenital abnormalities occur in about 15% of children with Wilms' tumor (Fig. 16.1)[4]. Aniridia consists of hypoplasia of the iris and the sporadic form occurs in 1 in 50,000 people. The incidence of aniridia in children with Wilms' tumors increases to 1 in 70. The familial form of aniridia is not associated with Wilms' tumor, but 33% of children with the sporadic form of aniridia develop Wilms' tumor[5]. The WAGR syndrome includes Wilms' tumor, aniridia, genitourinary anomalies, and mental retardation. Children afflicted with the WAGR syndrome generally present before 3 years of age and also have deformities of the external ear and may have facial or skull dysmorphism[6].

Hemihypertrophy, in which an asymmetry of the body exists, occurs in 1 in 14,300 people; however, it occurs in 1 in 32 (2.9%) children with Wilms' tumor. The tumor may occur on either side

Anomalies associated with Wilms' tumor
Aniridia
WAGR syndrome (Wilms' tumor, aniridia, genitourinary abnormalities, mental retardation)
Hemihypertrophy
Beckwith–Wiedemann syndrome (gigantism, macroglossia, omphalocele, genitourinary anomalies)
Musculoskeletal
Dermatologic
Genitourinary (renal anomalies, hypospadias, cryptorchidism)
Denys–Drash (ambiguous genitalia, progressive renal failure, Wilms' tumors)

Figure 16.1 Anomalies associated with Wilms' tumor.

of the patient. These children have an increased incidence of genitourinary anomalies and other cancers, including adrenal cortical carcinomas and hepatoblastomas.

Children with the Beckwith–Wiedemann syndrome develop enlargement of the adrenal cortex, kidney, liver, pancreas, and gonads. Other anomalies associated with the Beckwith–Wiedemann syndrome include omphalocele, hemihypertrophy, microcephaly, mental retardation, and macroglossia. Neoplasia occurs in one out of 10 children with this syndrome and affects the same organs as affected in those children with hemihypertrophy, including the liver, adrenal cortex, and kidney[7].

Denys–Drash syndrome occurs from a mutation in the *WT1* gene. This mutation results in testicular dysgenesis, male pseudohermaphroditism, and a nephropathy characterized by mesangial sclerosis. These children also develop Wilms' tumors. Bilateral nephrectomy and transplantation is indicated in patients with Denys–Drash because of their progressive nephropathy and high risk of Wilms' tumors in the native kidneys[8].

Almost 3% of children with Wilms' tumor have musculoskeletal anomalies. Dermatologic lesions, including hemangiomas, multiple nevi, and café-au-lait spots, occur in 7.9% of children with Wilms' tumors. Genitourinary anomalies, which include renal hypoplasia, ectopia, fusions, duplications, cystic disease, hypospadias, cryptorchidism, and pseudohermaphroditism, occur in 4.4% of children with Wilms' tumors[9].

Pathology

Wilms' tumor frequently consists of an encapsulated solitary tumor that occurs in all parts of the kidney. Necrosis within the tumor is common and may lead to hemorrhage. Occasionally the tumor contains true cysts. The tumor rarely grows into the renal pelvis, where it can cause obstruction or hematuria. Multiple lesions may occur with nephroblastomatosis. Invasion of the renal vein by the tumor occurs up to 20% of the time. The lymph nodes are frequently enlarged at the time of surgery without metastatic disease, which renders gross assessment of nodal involvement unreliable.

Microscopically, the tumor demonstrates a triphasic histology consisting of blastemal, epithelial, and stromal cells. The 'nephrogenic' cells demonstrate a tubuloglomerular pattern against a background of 'stromagenic' cells (Fig. 16.2a). The stromal component may differentiate into striated muscle, cartilage, or (rarely) fat or bone. The epithelial component varies from a well-differentiated (resembling mature tubules) to a very primitive appearance.

The histologic demonstration of anaplasia portends a worse prognosis (Fig. 16.2b). Anaplasia consists of a three-fold variation in nuclear size, with hyperchromatism and abnormal mitotic figures. Anaplasia occurs more frequently in older children. Diffuse distribution of anaplasia throughout the lesion or at any extrarenal site conveys a worse prognosis than focal anaplasia, in which sharply localized clusters of anaplastic cells are contained only in the primary tumor. The rhabdoid tumor and clear-cell sarcoma of the kidney were once considered forms of Wilms' tumor with poor prognoses, but are now considered to be separate entities[10].

Other pediatric renal neoplasms

Pediatric renal neoplasms other than Wilms' tumor are listed in Figure 16.3.

Cystic nephroma or multilocular cystic nephroma

Cystic nephroma, or multilocular cystic nephroma, is a round and smooth tumor externally with multiple cysts internally. The septae of the cysts in the pediatric tumor are composed of fibrous tissue and may contain well-differentiated tubular structures. It usually occurs in only one kidney and its incidence

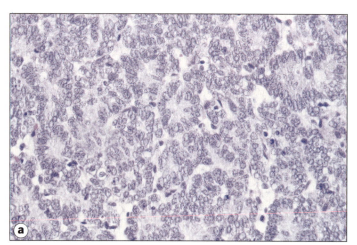

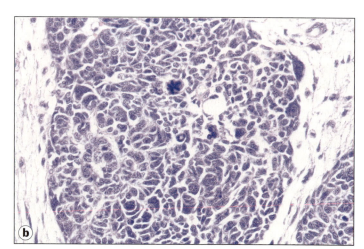

Figure 16.2 Wilms' tumor histology. (a) Well-differentiated Wilms' tumor with tubular formation. (b) Anaplastic Wilms' tumor with evident mitotic activity. (Courtesy of Dale S Huff.)

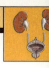

Figure 16.3 Primary pediatric renal neoplasms (excluding Wilms' tumor).

Primary pediatric renal neoplasms (excluding Wilms' tumor)	
Neoplasm	**Characteristics, treatment and prognosis**
Renal cell carcinoma	Most common primary renal neoplasm of childhood other than Wilms' tumor
	Presentation – hematuria, flank pain, mass, weight loss
	Metastasis – lymph nodes, bones, lungs, liver
	Increased incidence with von Hippel–Lindau disease and polycystic kidney disease
	Survival – 50%
	Treatment – radical nephrectomy
Rhabdoid tumor	Large cells with eosinophilic inclusions like rhabdomyoblasts but no muscle
	Metastasis – brain
	Very lethal (survival, 18%)
	Treatment – no clearly effective chemotherapy yet defined
Clear cell sarcoma	Metastasis – bone and brain
	Predominately male infants
	Treatment – chemotherapy with doxorubicin improves prognosis
Multilocular cyst	Usually unilateral
	Pediatric age peak has blastema in septa of cysts which may become Wilms' tumor
	Adult age peak usually in females; has fibrous septa and is benign
	Treatment – local excision, but frozen section essential to identify partially differentiated cystic nephroblastoma
Congenital mesoblastic nephroma	Infant tumor associated with polyhydramnios, usually boys
	Massive, firm with local infiltration of margins (nonencapsulated)
	Treatment – nephrectomy
Rare Neoplasms	
Rhabdomyosarcoma	Unlike rhabdoid tumor contains fetal striated muscle
Neuroblastoma	
Leiomyosarcoma	
Fibroma	
Hemangiopericytoma	
Cholesteatoma	
Lymphangioma	
Hamartoma (including angiomyolipoma)	
Transitional cell carcinoma	

reflects a bimodal age peak distribution. The peak incidence occurs in the pediatric age group, and it usually affects boys. This tumor has the potential to develop into a classic Wilms' tumor, although without this transformation it remains benign. Treatment of the multilocular cystic nephroma requires local excision, but the kidney may be preserved. The second peak incidence of multilocular cyst occurs in the adult and usually in women. This tumor frequently has mature fibrous tissue in the wall and also follows a benign course[11].

Cystic, partially differentiated nephroblastoma
Cystic, partially differentiated nephroblastoma mimics cystic nephroma and may be a variant of it. In this case the septae contain blastema and may or may not contain other embryonal or epithelial cell types. Frozen-section analysis is essential to plan surgical treatment, since a nephrectomy is indicated for treatment of the cystic, partially differentiated nephroblastoma[11].

Congenital mesoblastic nephroma
The most common solid renal tumor of the neonate is the congenital mesoblastic nephroma, which frequently is associated with polyhydramnios and occurs most often in boys[12]. It is a firm tumor that grossly resembles a leiomyoma (Fig. 16.4). Histologic evaluation demonstrates sheets of spindle-shaped uniform cells with a fibroblastic appearance. The margins of the tumor often demonstrate local infiltration. Treatment involves complete excision of this benign lesion with a nephrectomy (partial nephrectomy is not appropriate for this nonencapsulated tumor). On occasion a cellular variant of congenital mesoblastic nephroma occurs and proves difficult to distinguish from a clear-cell sarcoma of the kidney[13].

Rhabdomyosarcoma
The rhabdomyosarcoma tumor of the kidney is a Wilms' tumor variant. This tumor, unlike the rhabdoid tumor, has a favorable

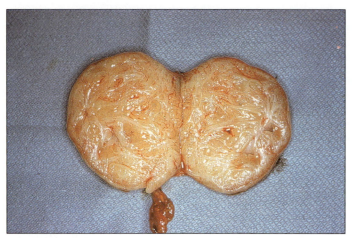

Figure 16.4 Congenital mesoblastic nephroma. Gross specimen demonstrates the dense interlacing bundles.

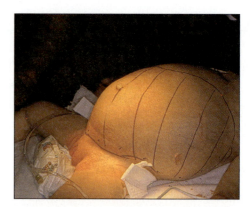

Figure 16.5 Preoperative image of a child with a large abdominal mass from a Wilms' tumor.

outcome. The rhabdomyosarcoma contains fetal striated muscle that distinguishes it from the rhabdoid tumor, which does not contain muscle[14].

Presentation

Most children with Wilms' tumor present with an abdominal mass (Fig. 16.5) or increasing abdominal girth, which underscores the need to include Wilms' tumor in the differential diagnoses of childhood abdominal masses (Fig. 16.6). About 30% of patients present with abdominal pain, but most children with Wilms' tumor appear well and are asymptomatic. Occasionally, a sudden subcapsular hemorrhage creates an acute onset of pain and fever associated with anemia and hypertension. Tumor rupture may present with an acute abdomen[15].

Physical examination of the child with Wilms' tumor reveals a firm, nontender, smooth mass that rarely crosses the midline. This contrasts with the nodular neuroblastoma that grows across the midline and presents in a child of ill appearance. Hypertension occurs in up to 63% of children afflicted with Wilms' tumor and may result from elevated renin secondary to renal ischemia caused by the pressure of the tumor. With tumor propagation into the vena cava a child may develop a varicocele or even congestive heart failure.

Radiographic evaluation

With the advent of ultrasound, computed tomography (CT), and magnetic resonance imaging (MRI), the use of intravenous pyelography (IVP) to evaluate Wilms' tumor has declined. The intrarenal mass distorts and deforms the caliceal morphology seen on the IVP. Ultrasonography permits identification of hydronephrosis and multicystic kidneys, which also may present as an abdominal mass. Wilms' tumor characteristically demonstrates a heterogeneous echo pattern on ultrasonography and can vary from predominately cystic to solid. Ultrasonography allows assessment of the renal vein and inferior vena cava for tumor thrombus.

Magnetic resonance imaging accurately evaluates the extent and size of Wilms' tumor, which frequently gives variable signal intensities (Figs 16.7 & 16.8). Areas of hemorrhage show increased signal intensity on T1- and T2-weighted pulse sequences. Regions of necrosis demonstrate a decreased signal on

Differential diagnoses for childhood abdominal masses	
Benign	**Malignant**
Hydronephrosis	Wilms' tumor
Congenital mesoblastic nephroma	Neuroblastoma
Multicystic dysplastic kidney	Renal cell carcinoma
Abscess	Clear cell carcinoma
Xanthogranulomatous pyelonephritis	Rhabdoid tumor
Multilocular cyst	Hepatoblastoma
Polycystic kidney	Lymphoma, lymphosarcoma
Glomerulocystic kidney	Rhabdomyosarcoma
Angiomyolipoma	
Teratoma	
Pseudotumor	

Figure 16.6 Differential diagnoses for childhood abdominal masses.

T1- but not on T2-weighted pulse sequences[16]. CT also provides precise anatomic delineation of the renal and retroperitoneal anatomy. Despite the accuracy with these techniques, false negative results do occur and a contralateral renal exploration by opening Gerota's fascia and inspecting all surfaces of the kidney is still required, since bilateral Wilms' tumor occurs in close to 10% of children.

Treatment

Effective treatment of Wilms' tumor relies on the appropriate use of surgery, radiation, and chemotherapy. The addition of single-agent chemotherapy to the combination of surgery and radiation increased cure rates from 40% to 89%[17]. Subsequent refinements with radiation and multiagent chemotherapy have further increased survival and minimized side effects.

Surgery

Prior to removal of the primary tumor, the extent of the tumor is evaluated, as well as the renal vessels, inferior vena cava, liver, and lymph nodes. Preoperative imaging misses over 7% of bilateral Wilms' tumors and therefore the contralateral kidney must be explored by opening Gerotas' capsule and inspecting the entire surface at the time of surgery[18]. Biopsy of any suspicious lesions is required.

If the primary tumor has invaded surrounding organs and cannot be removed safely it is prudent to wait until after treatment with chemotherapy and/or radiation. When the kidney can

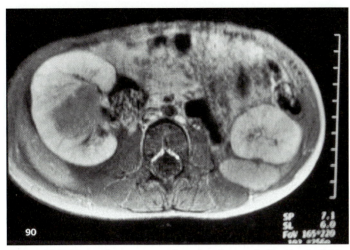

Figure 16.7 Magnetic resonance imaging demonstrating large right-sided Wilms' tumor and smaller left-sided tumor.

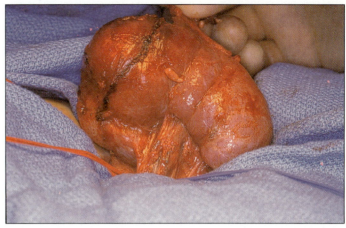

Figure 16.8 Intraoperative appearance of upper pole Wilms' tumor prior to partial nephrectomy.

be removed it is taken along with the adrenal gland if the tumor involves the upper pole. As with other renal tumors the renal artery and vein should be ligated prior to tumor mobilization to avoid hematogenous spread, if possible. Tumor rupture with diffuse spillage increases the chance of abdominal relapse. Preoperative radiation in addition to chemotherapy decreases this risk. A formal lymph node dissection does not improve survival, although biopsies of nodes should be taken since positive nodes portend a worse prognosis[3].

Chemotherapy

Preoperative chemotherapy can be used selectively and is appropriate for extensive tumors, tumors with major vena cava invasion, or bilateral tumors. International Society of Pediatric Oncology investigators routinely administer preoperative chemotherapy to all patients with the presumptive diagnosis of Wilms' tumor. This approach may shrink the tumor and produce lower morbidity, although it does not influence long-term survival and carries the risk of downstaging the tumor with the potential for undertreatment of a stage III tumor. Dactinomycin, vincristine, and doxorubicin have been effective in the treatment of Wilms' tumor. The usage of these agents as well as radiotherapy varies with the tumor stage and histology[3].

The staging system employed by the National Wilms Tumor Study (NWTS) group is outlined in Figure 16.9[19].

A summation of the current treatment for Wilms' tumor stages I–IV employed by NWTS V is outlined in Figure 16.10. The treatment of bilateral disease (stage V) employs a biopsy followed by preoperative chemotherapy and bilateral partial nephrectomies. When metastatic or recurrent disease is encountered doxorubicin is given routinely if the patient has received only dactinomycin and vincristine. For those patients who have already received three-agent chemotherapy there is no well-established regimen.

Radiation

The routine uses of radiation in the treatment of Wilms' tumor are incorporated in Figure 16.10. Radiation to the flank of children is given 1–3 days after surgery. Supplemental radiation is directed to regions with residual tumor. Pulmonary metastases

Wilms' tumor stages	
Stage	**Description**
I	Tumor within the kidney and completely excised
II	Tumor beyond the kidney and completely excised; may have invaded vessels or a local confined spill may have occurred
III	Tumor left within the abdomen and can include positive lymph nodes, positive surgical margins, peritoneal metastases, diffuse unconfined tumor spillage
IV	Metastatic disease via hematogenous route
V	Bilateral Wilms' tumor

Figure 16.9 Staging of Wilms' tumor.

result in radiation to both lungs, regardless of the number or location of metastases.

Bilateral Wilms' tumor

Synchronous bilateral Wilms' tumor occurs in about 6% of children with Wilms' tumor and metachronous bilateral Wilms' tumor affects another 1%. Nephrogenic rests occur in all cases of bilateral Wilms' tumors. These children frequently present at an earlier age and tend to have older mothers. They have more genitourinary anomalies and a higher incidence of hemihypertrophy than do children with unilateral Wilms' tumor. The incidence of unfavorable histology is 10%, which is similar to children with unilateral disease. Anaplasia is less frequent in children under the age of 2 years with bilateral Wilms' tumor and, accordingly, the younger children tend to have a better prognosis.

The overall survival of patients with synchronous bilateral Wilms' tumor is 76% at 3 years. This is in contrast to those patients who develop a metachronous bilateral Wilms' tumor, of whom only 39% are free of disease 2 years after developing the second Wilms' tumor. The stage of the most advanced lesion, histology, and presence of lymph node metastases are important prognostic indicators with bilateral Wilms' tumor.

A correct preoperative diagnosis of bilateral Wilms' tumor is made about two-thirds of the time. Hence the importance of a contralateral kidney exploration even when the disease appears

Summary of treatment for Wilms' tumor stages I–IV	
Stage	**Treatment**
I	Dactinomycin and vincristine
II	Favorable histology, as for stage I
	Unfavorable histology: cyclophosphamide, etoposide, vincristine, doxorubicin, and radiation
III, IV	Favorable histology: dactinomycin, vincristine, doxorubicin, and radiation
	Unfavorable histology: as for unfavorable histology in stage II

Figure 16.10 Summary of treatment for Wilms' tumor stages I–IV.

to be unilateral, since one-third of bilateral diagnoses are made in this manner. Previously, the approach to treatment was to carry out a nephrectomy for the larger tumor and a biopsy of the smaller one. At present, the treatment after diagnosis by radiographic imaging and/or biopsy is chemotherapy and then surgery. This frequently permits a renal-sparing approach with partial nephrectomy or excisional biopsy; at times the larger tumor responds better to chemotherapy than the smaller one. Of children treated in this manner, 80% retain normal renal function 6 years after treatment[20]. Bilateral nephrectomy and renal transplantation are rarely required with bilateral Wilms' tumor, but may be appropriate for those patients with diffuse anaplasia.

Complications

Multiple potential complications of chemotherapy and radiation therapy for Wilms' exist (Fig. 16.11). One of the most common is acute hematologic toxicity as a result of the suppressive effects of chemotherapy on the bone marrow. Chemotherapy also frequently induces an acute gastrointestinal toxicity manifest by nausea, vomiting, and diarrhea.

Radiation has the potential to affect any exposed organ adversely and can do so over a long period of time. One of the most distressing complications is the occurrence of second malignant neoplasms that occur in 1.6% of survivors 15 years after diagnosis. Abdominal irradiation increases the risk of second malignant neoplasms and doxorubicin potentiates this effect[21].

Prognosis

The 4-year postnephrectomy survival results from the National Wilms' Tumor Study III are listed in Figure 16.12[19]. The most important prognostic factor in Wilms' tumor is histology. Diffuse anaplasia is an unfavorable histology characterized by a three-fold enlargement in the nuclei, mitotic figures, and hyperchromatism. Approximately 5% of children with Wilms' tumor have anaplasia, which occurs more frequently in the older child. Children with anaplasia develop four times more relapses and are nine times more likely to die from their disease than children without anaplasia. When anaplasia is well circumscribed and focally contained within the primary tumor, it is not considered unfavorable. Focal anaplasia in a stage I Wilms' tumor does not alter the prognosis when treated with a total nephrectomy[10].

Hematogenous metastases also worsen the child's prognosis and are present at diagnosis in 10–15% of patients. Metastatic disease to the lungs occurs most often (85%), followed by metastases to the liver, bone, or brain. Metastases to the lymph nodes also predict a worse outcome with increased risk of local recurrence, and thus abdominal radiotherapy is added to chemotherapy. A tumor with renal vasculature invasion carries a higher risk of local relapse.

NEUROBLASTOMA

Etiology and pathophysiology

The most common malignant tumor of infancy and the second most common malignant solid tumor of childhood is neuroblastoma. This neoplasm arises from cells of the neural crest that normally form the sympathetic ganglia and adrenal medulla. The clinical behavior of neuroblastoma is variable and probably reflects a number of different genetic abnormalities that determine the tumor phenotype. A dominant transmittable mutation has been detected in about 20% of children with neuroblastoma and a hypothesized neuroblastoma suppressor gene is located on the short arm of chromosome 1[22].

A ganglioneuroma is thought to arise from a similar cell line as the neuroblastoma, but is a benign lesion. On occasion a neuroblastoma undergoes spontaneous maturation to give a benign ganglioneuroma. Between the ganglioneuroma and neuroblastoma is the ganglioneuroblastoma, which can behave in either a benign or malignant manner[23].

Complications of chemotherapy and radiation for Wilms' tumor	
Complication	**Cause**
Bone marrow toxicity	Chemotherapy
Gastrointestinal toxicity	Chemotherapy-induced nausea, vomiting, diarrhea, or radiation enteritis
Hepatic toxicity	Chemotherapy or radiation
Vertebral hypoplasia and scoliosis	Radiation
Renal	Chemotherapy-induced tubular necrosis or radiation-induced nephritis
Pulmonary	Acute interstitial radiation pneumonitis, reduced lung capacity
Cardiac	Doxorubicin-induced cardiomyopathy, increased when combined with irradiation
Gonads	Ovarian failure after radiation, or oligospermia after chemotherapy or radiation
Secondary neoplasms	1.6% of long-term survivors (sarcomas, adenocarcinomas, leukemias); most develop within radiation fields

Figure 16.11 Complications of chemotherapy and radiation therapy for Wilms' tumor.

Wilms' tumor 4-year survival (%) after nephrectomy and chemotherapy with or without radiotherapy		
Stage	Survival rate (%)	
	Favorable histology	Unfavorable histology
I	97	68
II	92	55
III	87	45
IV	83	4

Figure 16.12 Wilms' tumor 4-year survival rates after nephrectomy and chemotherapy ± radiotherapy.

Boys are slightly more affected than girls by a ratio of 1.1 to 1. One half of the cases of neuroblastoma occur in children under the age of 2 years and by 4 years of age more than 75% of cases of neuroblastoma have developed. Brain and skull abnormalities occur in 2% of children with neuroblastoma[24].

The tumor frequently forms a pseudocapsule and tends to infiltrate through this capsule into surrounding tissues as it grows. Multiple, small, round cells that resemble lymphocytes or neuroblasts make up the neuroblastoma. Along with Ewing's sarcoma, non-Hodgkin's lymphoma, primitive neuroectodermal tumors, and rhabdomyosarcoma, the neuroblastoma is considered one of the 'small blue round cell' tumors of childhood. With well-differentiated tumors the cells form themselves into rosettes and neurofibrils. These rosettes can be seen on bone marrow aspirate of marrow infiltrated with neuroblastoma[23].

Presentation

Neuroblastoma occurs in multiple sites along the sympathetic chain from head to pelvis (Fig. 16.13). The multiple sites create a variety of presentations, of which a mass is the most common symptom. Neuroblastoma is characteristically fixed, irregular, firm, nontender, and extends beyond the midline. This contrasts with the smooth Wilms' tumor, which does not frequently cross the midline (Fig. 16.14).

In the early stages of the disease, neuroblastomas usually do not cause symptoms, and up to 70% of patients have metastases by the time of diagnosis. Metastases in the younger child tend to occur in the liver, and in the older child they arise more often in the bone[25]. Manifestations of disseminated disease include fever, malaise, anorexia, weight loss, irritability, bone pain, and pallor secondary to anemia. These symptoms create a child of unwell appearance, in contrast to the child afflicted with Wilms' tumor. Occasionally, tumor secretion of catecholamines creates paroxysmal attacks of sweating, pallor, headaches, hypertension, palpitations, and flushing. Secretion of vasoactive intestinal peptide may lead to intractable diarrhea and hypokalemia (Kerner–Morrison syndrome)[23].

Two-thirds of abdominal neuroblastomas originate in the adrenal gland and these metastasize less frequently than do nonadrenal abdominal neuroblastomas. Neuroblastomas that arise from an abdominal paravertebral sympathetic ganglion have the potential to grow through an intervertebral foramen and compress the spinal cord[26]. Tumors in this location therefore require evaluation, usually with MRI, for possible intraspinal extension.

In the infant the liver is involved most frequently by metastatic disease. Bone pain and a limp (Hutchinson's syndrome) may

Location and various presentations of primary neuroblastoma	
Location (%)	Presentation
Head (2)	Nasal obstruction, epistaxis, periorbital ecchymosis ('Raccoon eyes') or edema, proptosis
Neck (5)	Horner's syndrome (ptosis, myosis, and anhydrosis), hoarseness
Chest (13)	Cough, dyspnea, pulmonary infection
Abdomen (55)	Adrenal 67%, nonadrenal 33%
Pelvis (4)	Urinary frequency and/or retention, constipation
Unknown and/or other location (21)	Opsomyoclonus (myoclonic jerking and random eye movement, possible cerebellar ataxia)

Figure 16.13 Location and various presentations of primary neuroblastoma.

Comparison of Wilms' tumor and neuroblastoma	
Wilms' tumor	Neuroblastoma
Frequent associated congenital anomalies	Low incidence of associated anomalies (except a 2% incidence of brain and skull defects)
Presents in well child	Presents in sick child
Usually unilateral mass	Often mass crosses midline
Peak age 3–4 years	Peak age 22 months
Arises in the kidney	Primary renal neuroblastoma very rare
Occasional calcification in egg-shell pattern	'Stippled' calcification on plain films in 50%, and in 80% by CT

Figure 16.14 Comparison of Wilms' tumor and neuroblastoma. CT, computed tomography.

signal metastatic bone lesions. Over half of children with neuroblastoma have bone marrow metastases and may not demonstrate radiographic changes in the bone[27]. Bone marrow replacement may lead to thrombocytopenia or anemia. Metastases to the periorbital region may cause periorbital ecchymoses, edema, and proptosis. Disseminated metastatic disease occurs much more frequently in children over 1 year of age.

Subcutaneous metastatic nodules frequently present in infants. The nodules often have a bluish 'blueberry muffin' appearance. When these nodules occur in combination with hepatomegaly and tumor cells in the bone marrow without bone lesions, the child is classified as having 4S disease. Children with stage 4S disease have a strong likelihood of spontaneous regression and are considered to have 'favorable disease' with a survival rate of 80% (Fig. 16.15) [23].

Evaluation

The history and physical examination provide clues as to whether the child may have a localized favorable tumor or a metastatic unfavorable tumor. An infant of healthy appearance with an asymptomatic mass is likely to have favorable disease. An older child who presents with constitutional symptoms probably suffers from disseminated metastases.

A bone marrow aspiration from each of the posterior iliac crests is a required part of the evaluation of neuroblastoma. Up to 70% of bone marrow aspirates are positive with neuroblastoma, many of which do not show skeletal metastases by radiographic evaluation[27]. The aspirate can be carried out at the time of primary surgery for a child who probably has favorable disease. In the child with unfavorable disease a preoperative bone marrow aspiration may prevent the need for an open-tissue biopsy. Histologic demonstration of the characteristic rosettes confirms the diagnosis, but in cases with very undifferentiated cells the pathologist relies on positive staining for neuron-specific enolase or neuroblastoma-specific monoclonal antibodies.

The two major metabolites of catecholamine production by neuroblastoma are vanillylmandelic acid and homovanillic acid. These metabolites are elevated in the urine in 95% of patients with neuroblastoma and have been used for mass screening studies in Japan, Europe, and North America. Imaging studies have proved useful and those recommended in the evaluation of neuroblastoma include a CT scan and/or MRI, chest radiography, skeletal survey, and 1-meta-iodobenzylguanidine (MIBG) radionuclide scanning. Secretory vesicles of catecholaminergic cells within most primary and metastatic neuroblastomas take up MIBG[23].

Staging

The international neuroblastoma staging system (INSS) of neuroblastoma is outlined in Figure 16.15[23].

Treatment and prognosis

As with Wilms' tumor the appropriate use of surgery, chemotherapy, and radiotherapy depends on the patient's prognostic factors. Patients' prognoses may be grouped into 'favorable' or 'unfavorable' according to age, stage, tumor markers, and biologic factors, which include histology. Stage is the most important prognostic factor and age at diagnosis is the only other independent clinical prognostic factor. Stages 3 or 4 and over 1 year of age are both considered unfavorable prognostic factors. Elevated ferritin, lactic dehydrogenase, or neuron-specific enolase levels portend a worse prognosis. Histologic characteristics considered unfavorable include poorly differentiated neuroblasts, a nodular stroma, and increased mitotic activity. The *MYCN* oncogene is frequently amplified with tumors that contain unfavorable histology. A diploid DNA content also confers a worse prognosis[22].

The role of the initial surgery is to establish the diagnosis and stage the tumor, provide tumor tissue for evaluation, and excise the tumor if possible without undue morbidity. A staging lymph node sample is taken as there is no evidence that a radical node dissection improves survival. A second surgery may be used to remove residual disease. Chemotherapeutic agents used for neuroblastoma include cyclophosphamide, doxorubicin, etoposide, and platinum-based agents. Radiation may be used as an ablative method prior to bone marrow transplant, as well as to control local and metastatic disease[23].

Most patients with favorable disease (stages 1 and 2) can be cured with complete surgical excision alone. The 5-year survival rates approach 95% in this group of patients. Subsequent surgery is performed only in the event of local recurrence. Chemotherapy in these patients does not appear to improve survival, nor does the addition of radiotherapy. Patients with 4S disease have a high rate of spontaneous regression and require no treatment if they are asymptomatic. On occasion these patients may develop respiratory distress caused by hepatomegaly and can receive limited chemotherapy and/or local irradiation.

A group of patients considered to be at intermediate risk include those infants with INSS stages 3 and 4 who lack *MYCN* amplification, as well as children with INSS stage 3 tumors that contain favorable biologic features. These children should be treated with multiagent chemotherapy and surgery; survival ranges from 55% to 90%.

Figure 16.15 International neuroblastoma staging system.

International neuroblastoma staging system	
Stage	**Description**
1	Tumor within area of origin completely excised, with or without microscopic residual disease
2A	Tumor does not cross midline and there is incomplete gross resection
2B	Tumor does not cross midline, with ipsilateral positive lymph nodes
3	Tumor crosses midline, and may involve regional lymph nodes bilaterally
4	Distant metastases, except as defined in stage 4S
4S	Localized stage 1 or 2 and spread to liver, skin, or bone marrow (<10% of nucleated marrow cells are malignant and no bony lesions on skeletal survey)

Children at high-risk include those over 1 year of age with stage 3 tumors and unfavorable biology, as well as all children with stage 4 disease. Also included in the high-risk group are infants with stages 3, 4, or 4S and *MYCN* amplification as well as older children with stage 2 and unfavorable histology. Survival in this group ranges from <10% to 30%, despite aggressive multimodal therapy.

Therapeutic approaches aimed at improving the outcome of high-risk patients include bone marrow transplant after a combination of chemotherapy and total body irradiation. Targeted radiation with labeled MIBG or monoclonal antibodies to treat neuroblastoma is also being evaluated. Gene therapy remains as a possible future therapeutic option[22].

RHABDOMYOSARCOMA

Incidence

Rhabdomyosarcoma is the most common soft-tissue sarcoma and accounts for about 50% of all soft-tissue sarcomas in children. Sarcomas are the fifth most common solid tumor in children after central nervous system tumors, lymphomas, neuroblastomas, and Wilms' tumor. Rhabdomyosarcoma affects boys more often than girls in a ratio of 3:1[28]. Most cases occur between 2 and 6 years of age, although a second age peak occurs between 15 and 19 years of age. As many as 20% of these tumors arise from the genitourinary tract and 10% from pelvic or retroperitoneal sites[29].

Etiology and pathophysiology

Familial aggregations of rhabdomyosarcoma have been reported and give evidence of a genetic component. Patients with neurofibromatosis have an increased incidence of rhabdomyosarcoma. The alveolar subtype occurs in association with a translocation between chromosomes 2 and 13[29].

Rhabdomyosarcomas arise from any part of the body that contains embryonal mesenchyme. This normally differentiates into skeletal muscle. The most common sites of rhabdomyosarcoma within the genitourinary tract involve the prostate, bladder (usually in area of trigone), and anterior vaginal wall. Other sites that present to the urologist include paratesticular and pelvic locations.

Rhabdomyosarcoma grows rapidly and invades adjacent tissue, which renders complete surgical excision difficult despite a deceptively well-circumscribed appearance. It is an unencapsulated and locally infiltrating tumor that spreads both by the lymphatic and vascular system. When patients develop metastases, 80% are evident within 1 year of diagnosis[30].

Several histologic types of rhabdomyosarcoma have been described and include embryonal, alveolar, and pleiomorphic. Embryonal rhabdomyosarcoma accounts for 60% of cases and is usually seen in younger children. Sarcoma botryoides is a polypoid type of embryonal rhabdomyosarcoma that tends to arise in hollow organs, such as the bladder or vagina, and looks like a cluster of grapes. Histologically, embryonal rhabdomyosarcoma resembles developing skeletal muscle from a 7–10 week fetus.

The alveolar form occurs most often in adolescents and young adults and accounts for 20% of rhabdomyosarcomas. This tumor most commonly arises in the extremities and trunk rather than the genitourinary tract. Histologically, it resembles skeletal muscle in the 10–21 week fetus. Pleiomorphic rhabdomyosarcoma accounts for only 1% of rhabdomyosarcomas in children, but it is

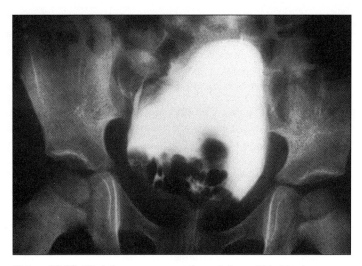

Figure 16.16 Rhabdomyosarcoma of prostate and bladder base.
Contrast agent in the bladder demonstrates characteristic polypoid configuration.

the most common form in adults. It also occurs predominately in the extremities and trunk. Other histologic types include mixed rhabdomyosarcoma, as well as up to 20% that are so undifferentiated they cannot be placed in a standard classification[31].

Presentation

As with neuroblastoma, the multiple possible sites of rhabdomyosarcoma create a variety of presentations. A large palpable mass is the single most common presentation for rhabdomyosarcoma. With involvement of the bladder or prostate, the child may have symptoms of lower urinary tract obstruction or hematuria (Fig. 16.16). With sarcoma botryoides the tumor may prolapse through the urethra or vagina. A pelvic tumor may grow large before it produces symptoms by impinging on the rectum or genitourinary tract. Other rare pelvic and bladder tumors to be considered in the differential diagnosis are listed in Figure 16.17.

Evaluation

Radiographic evaluation should employ chest radiographs, CT or MRI of the primary tumor, bone marrow examination, and routine blood tests. Cystoscopy and vaginoscopy may help delineate the site of tumor. A histologic diagnosis is established by biopsy. Since 20% of genitourinary rhabdomyosarcomas have spread to the retroperitoneal lymph nodes by the time of diagnosis, an inspection and sampling of these nodes is required to accurately stage the tumor[31].

Staging

The staging groups for rhabdomyosarcoma previously utilized by the Intergroup Rhabdomyosarcoma Study (IRS) is outlined in Figure 16.18. This staging system suffered criticism as it varied with operative techniques and excluded prognostic factors such as the size and site of the tumor. Hence, the IRS Committee currently employs a modification of the TNM (tumor, nodes, and metastasis) staging system (Fig. 16.18). Most studies now use both the clinical grouping system and the TNM staging system[31].

Rare pelvic and bladder tumors of childhood

Tumor	Description and treatment
Transitional cell carcinoma of bladder	Usually low grade and/or stage; endoscopic resection usually curative, recurrence infrequent
Leiomyosarcoma of bladder	Less aggressive than rhabdomyosarcoma; local excision
Adenocarcinoma of bladder	Originates from urachus or exstrophy of the bladder
Neurofibroma of bladder	Occurs in patients with neurofibromatosis; local excision
Lymphohemangioma	May arise in pelvis and invade bladder and/or ureters; local excision
Adenocarcinoma of infant vagina	Very rare and highly malignant

Figure 16.17 Rare pelvic and bladder tumors of childhood.

Intergroup Rhabdomyosarcoma Study staging system and TNM staging

System	Stage	Description
Rhabdomyosarcoma Study	Group I	Localized disease completely excised
	Group IA	Confined to area of origin
	Group IB	Infiltration outside area of origin
	Group IIA	Tumor resected with 'microscopic' residual disease
	Group IIB	Complete resection of regional disease and positive regional nodes
	Group IIC	Regional disease with involved nodes removed, but 'microscopic' residual disease
	Group III	Gross residual disease
	Group IV	Distant metastatic disease at diagnosis
TNM staging	T1	Tumor confined to organ tissue of origin
	T1a	Tumor ≤ 5cm in greatest diameter
	T1b	Tumor >5cm
	T2	Tumor outside organ tissue of origin
	T2a	Tumor ≤ 5cm in greatest diameter
	T2b	Tumor >5cm
	N0	Regional nodes not clinically involved
	N1	Regional nodes clinically involved
	M0	No distant metastases
	M1	Metastases present

Figure 16.18 Intergroup Rhabdomyosarcoma Study staging system and TNM (tumor, nodes and metastasis) staging.

Treatment

Historically, treatment with surgical excision alone resulted in a 40% survival rate for patients with vaginal tumors and 73% for patients with bladder or prostate rhabdomyosarcoma[32]. Survival rates have improved with the use of multimodal therapy. The survival results with genitourinary tumors are better than those for rhabdomyosarcoma in other parts of the body, but this may be related to earlier symptoms and detection. Radiation and chemotherapy are effective treatment modalities. Chemotherapy alone was not effective in the IRS-II study, in which 75% of patients with bladder or prostate tumors also required radiotherapy[33].

Current treatment usually begins after tumor biopsy and consists of vincristine, dactinomycin, and cyclophosphamide (VDC) or other active antisarcoma drugs for 8 weeks. Even patients in group I, who appear to have the tumor completely excised, receive vincristine and dactinomycin. If no response occurs after treatment with VDC, either surgical excision or radiotherapy is carried out. The authors' current approach utilizes surgical excision of gross residual disease after chemotherapy. In some of these patients the disease removed harbors no viable tumor cells and the patient is spared treatment with radiotherapy. When evidence of positive surgical margins or metastatic disease is found, the patient receives further treatment with radiotherapy or chemotherapy. An alternative approach for patients with residual disease after treatment with primary chemotherapy is radiotherapy followed by surgical excision of any remaining tumor[29]. The pathologic analysis of tissue removed after radiotherapy is difficult to interpret, and this reason along with the impaired wound healing imparted by radiation, support the authors' preference to eliminate all bulk disease before radiotherapy.

Using a combination of primary chemotherapy and radiation in the IRS-III study improved both survival and bladder salvage. The 5-year survival rates in patients with local disease in IRS group I equaled 93%. The survival rates for those in groups II and III equaled 81% and 74%, respectively[29]. At present about one half of the patients with bladder–prostate tumors retain their bladders. Conservative surgery after chemotherapy and radiation has also produced excellent disease-free survival for patients with vaginal and vulvar tumors.

Prepubertal testis tumor types and relative frequencies	
Type	**Relative frequency (%)**
Yolk sac	62
Teratoma	15
Gonadal stromal (Leydig, Sertoli, juvenile granulosa cell, undifferentiated)	9
Epidermoid cyst	2
Gonadoblastoma	1
Others: sarcomas benign tumors of supporting tissue secondary tumors (lymphoma, leukemia)	11

Figure 16.19 Prepubertal testis tumor types and distribution.

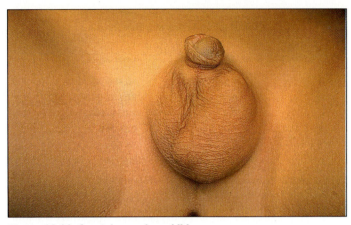

Figure 16.20 Scrotal mass in a child.

Unfortunately, the outlook for patients with metastatic disease remains dismal. The evolution of treatment for these patients involves intensified chemotherapy regimens and also radiation to the sites of metastatic lesions. Despite these efforts the long-term survival rates are only 20%. The side effects from chemotherapy and radiation are similar to those with Wilms' tumor (see Fig. 16.11)[31].

PREPUBERTAL TESTICULAR TUMORS

Incidence
Testicular tumors account for 2% of all pediatric solid tumors. The peak incidence of pediatric testicular tumors is in 2 year olds and effects up to two out of 100,000 children. Germ cell tumors account for 60–77% of testicular tumors in children[34], as against the 95% of adult testicular tumors that are germ cell tumors. This implies that up to one-third of pediatric testicular tumors are benign; however, any testicular mass is considered malignant until proved otherwise[35].

Classification
Figure 16.19 illustrates various types and relative frequencies of prepubertal testis tumors[34].

Presentation and evaluation
Most testicular tumors in children present as a painless scrotal swelling (Fig. 16.20). The differential diagnosis includes epididymitis, testicular torsion, inguinal hernia, and hydrocele. Importantly, 10–25% of malignant testicular tumors present with a hydrocele[36]. On physical examination a hard mass may be palpable; however, a normal physical examination is not sufficient to exclude a tumor. Ultrasonography permits a rapid, non-invasive method of examining the testicle and it helps to distinguish an extratesticular mass from an intratesticular mass (Fig. 16.21). A serum α-fetoprotein (AFP) level should also be obtained prior to treatment of a testicular mass.

The diagnosis of the type of testicular tumor is made following an inguinal orchiectomy. When suspicion of a benign lesion is high, the testis and cord can be delivered through an inguinal incision and the tumor excised from the testis. With intraoperative histologic confirmation of a benign lesion a testicular-sparing surgery may be performed. The type of tumor determines the need for further evaluation and follow-up[37].

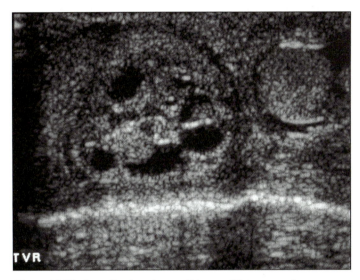

Figure 16.21 Juvenile granulosa cell tumor. Ultrasonography demonstrates heterogeneous intratesticular echogenicity.

Germ cell tumors
Prepubertal germ cell tumors include yolk-sac tumors, teratoma, teratocarcinoma, and seminoma. The seminoma is extremely rare before puberty and is managed as in the adult. The most common germ cell tumor, as well as the most common prepubertal testicular tumor, is the yolk-sac tumor[34]. Histologic evaluation of the yolk-sac tumor demonstrates eosinophilic inclusions positive to periodic acid–Schiff in the cytoplasm of clear cells that consist of AFP. Schiller–Duval bodies may be seen histologically in the perivascular region of a yolk-sac tumor and resemble a yolk sac[38].

Levels of AFP are elevated in about 80% of boys with yolk-sac carcinomas and may be used as a tumor marker. The half-life of AFP is about 5 days and should return to normal (<20ng/mL) within 1 month of complete removal of the tumor. Normally, AFP levels are elevated in the neonate and age-specific values should be utilized (Fig. 16.22). Persistent elevations of AFP postoperatively may indicate tumor metastases or recurrence. Liver dysfunction may lead to false-positive elevations of AFP[39].

Most yolk-sac tumors occur in infants younger than 2 years of age. Spread of the tumor occurs predominantly to the lungs

Normal infant levels of α-fetoprotein	
Time after birth (weeks)	Level (ng/mL)
0	48,406–34,718
2	33,113–32,503
4	2,654–3,080
8	323–278
16	74–56
32	8.5–5.5

Figure 16.22 Normal infant levels of α-fetoprotein.

Prepubertal testicular staging		
Stage	Description	
I	Tumor confined to testis and completely resected, tumor markers normalize	
II	Trans-scrotal orchiectomy; microscopic disease in scrotum or high in spermatic cord, retroperitoneal node involvement (≤ 2cm diameter), persistently abnormal tumor markers	
III	Retroperitoneal lymph nodes involved (≥ 2cm)	
IV	Distant metastases	

Figure 16.23 Prepubertal testicular staging system.

(20%) and, unlike the adult testicular tumor, spread via the lymphatics to the retroperitoneal nodes occurs infrequently (4–5%)[40]. About 9% of patients diagnosed with yolk-sac tumor die from their disease[34].

Teratoma and teratocarcinoma contain elements derived from more than one of the three germ tissues – endoderm, mesoderm, and ectoderm. These tumors are often cystic and on cut section various tissues, such as the skin, hair, bone, and even teeth, may be present. Despite containing areas of dedifferentiation with a malignant appearance, teratomas are consistently benign in children younger than 2 years of age. In the older patient with a testicular teratocarcinoma, multimodal chemotherapy results in a cure rate of 80% in those with metastatic disease[41].

Gonadal stromal tumors

Gonadal stromal tumors include Leydig cell tumors, Sertoli cell tumors, and intermediate forms such as the juvenile granulosa cell tumor. Leydig cell tumors are the most common gonadal stromal tumor in children and adults. They occur most frequently in boys 4–5 years old and synthesis of testosterone may produce precocious puberty and gynecomastia. Unlike true precocious puberty, the levels of luteinizing hormone and follicle-stimulating hormone are at low prepubertal level. Leydig cell tumors must also be differentiated from hyperplastic nodules that develop in boys with poorly controlled congenital adrenal hyperplasia. Most of these nodules regress with the administration of corticosteroids[42].

Sertoli cell tumors are the second most common gonadal stromal tumors. These tumors tend to appear as a painless mass in a boy younger than 6 months of age. Sertoli cell tumors usually produce no endocrinologic effects. Both Leydig cell and Sertoli cell tumors are usually benign and can be treated with local excision with testis preservation[40].

Although the juvenile granulosa cell tumor accounts for only 15% of all gonadal stromal tumors and 1% of all prepubertal testis tumors, it accounts for 27% of neonatal testicular tumors. These tumors tend to be nodular with thin walled cysts of variable size. Although there have been no reports of metastatic disease in neonates with this tumor, 10% of all granulosa cell tumors develop metastases to the nodes, liver, or lungs, usually within 5 months[34].

Gonadoblastoma

Gonadoblastoma occurs in children with intersex disorders; 80% are phenotypic females with intra-abdominal testes or streak gonads. The putative gonadoblastoma gene is on the Y chromosome and the tumor almost always develops in a child whose karyotype contains a Y chromosome. The streak gonads in patients with mixed gonadal dysgenesis often develop gonadoblastomas. The peak incidence occurs at puberty, which accounts for the current recommendations for early gonadectomy in patients at risk for gonadoblastoma. Metastatic spread of a gonadoblastoma is uncommon[34].

Staging

The staging for testicular tumors is given in Figure 16.23.

Treatment

The treatment for yolk-sac tumor is inguinal orchiectomy and close surveillance. Follow-up should include monthly serum AFP levels and chest radiography every 3 months for the first year, followed by serum AFP levels every 2 months for a second year. Routine imaging of the retroperitoneum by CT or MRI has also been recommended. Since spread to the retroperitoneal lymph nodes occurs infrequently, a routine prophylactic node dissection is not undertaken. Chemotherapy is given for patients with radiographic evidence of metastatic disease or persistently elevated serum AFP. The use of combination chemotherapy with VDC, with or without doxorubicin, has proved effective for patients with metastatic disease, with salvage rates approaching 60%. Survival for all patients with yolk-sac tumor is about 90%[43].

Chemotherapy is recommended for all patients with yolk-sac tumors and stage II disease. Boys with persistent elevation of tumor markers after chemotherapy may require a retroperitoneal lymph node dissection. Boys with stage III or IV germ cell tumors are treated with chemotherapy. If elevated markers or retroperitoneal disease persists, a biopsy or resection of residual tumor is undertaken[43].

Prepubertal testicular teratoma, epidermoid cyst, Leydig cell, and Sertoli cell tumors are benign and an orchiectomy or testicular-sparing surgery with complete excision is curative. Stage II or higher teratocarcinomas require treatment with cisplatin, bleomycin, and vinblastine. The recommended treatment for juvenile granulosa cell tumor includes inguinal orchiectomy with periodic postoperative chest radiography and retroperitoneal imaging for 1 year[34].

Treatment of gonadoblastoma involves removal of the gonad. These tumors may be hormonally active and may produce elevated serum levels of β-human chorionic gonadotrophin. The use of β-human chorionic gonadotrophin as a tumor marker with gonadoblastoma has yet to be defined[44].

TUMORS IN THE UNDESCENDED TESTIS

Of germinal tumors of the testis, 10% develop in an undescended testis[45]. The risk of malignancy in an undescended testis is 35 times greater than normal. An intra-abdominal testis has a 5% risk of developing a tumor, compared to a 1% risk for a tumor within the inguinal canal. With bilateral cryptorchidism the incidence of bilateral tumors is 25%[46]. An increased risk of tumor development also occurs in the contralateral normally descended testis. The most common tumor that arises in an undescended testis is a seminoma; in the testis brought down into the scrotum the most common is an embryonal carcinoma[47].

Prepubertal orchiopexy may reduce the risk of testis cancer. The relative risk of testis cancer in a series of 1075 boys who underwent orchiopexy in Great Britain is reported as 7.5 times greater than normal[48]. In this series, the age at which orchiopexy occurred did not appear to affect this risk, although few patients underwent orchiopexy prior to 5 years of age. Postpubertal orchiopexy does not diminish the risk of malignancy[29].

Orchiopexies are now routinely performed at 6 months of age. Given the increased chance of testicular malignancy, boys should be instructed in testicular self-examination beginning after puberty. The average age of tumor development in a formerly undescended testis is 40 years, so continued awareness of the tumor risk must be emphasized. The treatment of adult testicular tumors is discussed in Chapter 29.

PARATESTICULAR RHABDOMYOSARCOMA

Presentation and evaluation

Of rhabdomyosarcomas, 7–10% arise from the distal spermatic cord and present as a scrotal mass. The tumor may invade the testis, epididymis, or surrounding envelopes and it may be associated with a hydrocele. As with other scrotal masses, the initial investigation should be an ultrasound to further evaluate the mass. Benign scrotal tumors must be included in the differential diagnosis and are listed in Figure 16.24. Most (97%) of the paratesticular rhabdomyosarcomas are embryonal and up to 70% of patients have involvement of the retroperitoneal lymph nodes at the time of diagnosis. Distant metastases to the lungs, cortical bone, or bone marrow occur in 20% of cases at diagnosis. Further evaluation of patients with a paratesticular rhabdomyosarcoma includes a CT scan to evaluate the retroperitoneal nodes, as well as a chest radiograph, bone marrow

Benign scrotal tumors
Adenomatoid tumors
Lipoma
Leiomyoma
Epidermoid cyst
Teratoma
Fibroma
Hemangioma
Neurofibroma

Figure 16.24 Benign scrotal tumors.

aspiration, and bone scan to further assess metastases. These studies may be performed before or after histologic confirmation of the diagnosis[28].

Staging

The tumor staging for paratesticular rhabdomyosarcoma conforms to the TNM system previously discussed with other rhabdomyosarcomas (see Fig. 16.18).

Treatment

For histologic confirmation of the suspected diagnosis the testical should be removed using a radical inguinal orchiectomy. Trans-scrotal biopsies are absolutely contraindicated because of the likelihood of seeding the tract with this tumor. If the scrotum has been violated, or appears involved by tumor, a hemi-scrotectomy should be carried out.

With the advent of effective chemotherapy it became apparent that routine retroperitoneal lymph node dissection did not improve survival. The exception to this is for boys with bulky disease after chemotherapy.

At present, for children under 10 years of age, the recommended treatment is a radical orchiectomy followed by retroperitoneal imaging. If this is negative, chemotherapy alone is given and long-term survival is close to 95% in these patients. For children with a T2 stage tumor or metastatic disease, treatment frequently consists of chemotherapy and radiation to the involved region. Some investigators advocate surgery first, and radiotherapy only after a failed surgery and a second course of chemotherapy. Children over the age of 10 years have a worse prognosis and no well-established treatment protocol exists[28].

REFERENCES

1. Young JLJ, Heise HW, Silverberg E, et al. Cancer incidence, survival and mortality for children under 15 years of age. Professional Education Publication. Atlanta: American Cancer Society; 1978.
2. Beckwith JB. Precursor lesions of Wilms' tumor: clinical and biological implications. Med Pediatr Oncol. 1993;21:158–68.
3. Petruzzi MJ, Green DM. Wilms' tumor. Pediatr Clin North Am. 1997;44:939–52.
4. Pendergrass TW. Congenital anomalies in children with Wilms' tumor. Cancer. 1976;37:403–8.
5. Haicken BN, Miller DR. Simultaneous occurrence of congenital aniridia, hamartoma and Wilms' tumor. J Pediatr. 1971;78:497–502.

6. Narahara K, Kikkawa K, Kimira S, et al. Regional mapping of catalase and Wilms' tumor: aniridia, genitourinary abnormalities, and mental retardation triad loci to the chromosome segment 11p1305 p1306. Hum Genet. 1984;66:181–5.
7. Sotelo-Avila C, Gonzalez-Crussi F, Fowler JW. Complete and incomplete forms of Beckwith–Wiedemann syndrome: their oncogenic potential. J Pediatr. 1980;96:47–50.
8. Rudin C, Pritchard J, Fernando ON, et al. Renal transplantation in the management of bilateral Wilms' tumor (BWT) and of Denys Drash syndrome (DDS). Nephrol Dial Transplant. 1998;13:1506–10.

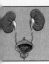
9. Stay EJ, Vawter G. The relationship between nephroblastoma and neurofibromatosis (von Recklinghausen's disease). Cancer. 1977;39:2550–5.

10. Faria P, Beckwith JB, Mishra K, et al. Focal versus diffuse anaplasia in Wilms tumor – new definitions with prognostic significance. Am J Surg Pathol. 1996;20:909–20.

11. Joshi VV, Beckwith JB. Multilocular cyst of the kidney (cystic nephroma) and cystic, partially differentiated nephroblastoma: terminology and criteria for diagnosis. Cancer. 1989;66:466–79.

12. Blank E, Neerhout RC, Burry KA. Congenital mesoblastic nephroma and polyhydramnios. JAMA. 1978;240:1504–5.

13. Hartman DS, Lesar MSL, Madewell JE, et al. Mesoblastic nephroma: radiologic–pathologic correlation of 20 cases. Am J Roentgenol. 1981;136:69–74.

14. Harms D, Gutjahr P, Hohenfellner R, et al. Fetal rhabdomyomatous nephroblastoma: pathologic histology and special clinical and biological features. Eur J Pediatr. 1980;133:167–72.

15. Ramsay NK, Dehner LP, Coccia PF, et al. Acute hemorrhage into Wilms' tumor: a cause of rapidly developing abdominal mass with hypertension, anemia and fever. J Pediatr. 1977;91:763–5.

16. Hricak H, Thoeni RF, Carroll PR, et al. Detection and staging of renal neoplasms: a reassessment of MR imaging. Radiology. 1988;166:643–9.

17. Farber S. Chemotherapy in the treatment of leukemia and Wilms' tumor. JAMA. 1966;198:826–36.

18. Ritchey ML, Green DM, Breslow NB, et al. Accuracy of current imaging modalities in the diagnosis of synchronous bilateral Wilms' tumor. A report from the National Wilms' Tumor Study Group. Cancer. 1995;75:600–4.

19. D'Angio GJ, Breslow N, Beckwith JB, et al. Treatment of Wilms' tumor: Results of the Third National Wilms' Tumor Study. Cancer. 1989;64:349–60.

20. Kumar R, Fitzgerald R, Breatnach F. Conservative surgical management of bilateral Wilms tumor: results of the United Kingdom Children's Cancer Study Group. J Urol. 1998;160:1450–3.

21. Breslow NE, Takashima JR, Whitton JA, et al. Second malignant neoplasms following treatment for Wilm's tumor: a report from the National Wilms' Tumor Study Group. J Clin Oncol. 1995;13:1851–9.

22. Katzenstein HM, Cohn SL. Advances in the diagnosis and treatment of neuroblastoma. Curr Opinion Oncol. 1998;10:43–51.

23. Castleberry RP. Biology and treatment of neuroblastoma. Pediatr Clin North Am. 1997;44:919–37.

24. Miller RW, Fraumeni JF, Hill JA. Neuroblastoma: epidemiologic approach to its origin. Am J Dis Child. 1968;115:253–61.

25. Bond JV. Neuroblastoma metastatic to the liver in infants. Arch Dis Child. 1976;51:879–82.

26. Akwari OE, Payne WS, Onofrio BM, et al. Dumbbell neurogenic tumors of the mediastinum: diagnosis and management. Mayo Clin Proc. 1978;54:353–8.

27. Finklestein JZ, Eckert H, Issacs H, et al. Bone marrow metastases in children with solid tumors. Am J Dis Child. 1970;119:49–52.

28. de Vries JD. Paratesticular rhabdomyosarcoma. World J Urol. 1995;13:219–25.

29. Prowse OA, Reddy PP, Barrieras D, et al. Pediatric genitourinary tumors. Curr Opinion Oncol. 1998;10:253–60.

30. Heyn RM, Holland R, Newton WA Jr, et al. The role of combined chemotherapy in the treatment of rhabdomyosarcoma in children. Cancer. 1974;34:2128–42.

31. Pappo AS, Shapiro DN, Crist WM. Rhabdomyosarcoma: biology and treatment. Pediatr Clin North Am. 1997;44:953–72.

32. Green DM, Jaffe N. Progress and controversy in the treatment of childhood rhabdomyosarcoma. Cancer Treatment Rev. 1978;5:7–27.

33. Crist W, Gehan EA, Ragab AH, et al. The Third Intergroup Rhabdomyosarcoma Study. J Clin Oncol. 1995;13:610–30.

34. Levy DA, Kay R, Elder JS. Neonatal testis tumors: a review of the Prepubertal Testis Tumor Registry. J Urol. 1994;151:715–17.

35. Visfeldt J, Jorgensen N, Muller J. Testicular germ cell tumors of childhood in Denmark, 1943–1989: incidence and evaluation of histology using immunohistochemical techniques. J Pathol. 1994;174:39–47.

36. Karamehmedovic O, Woodtli W, Pluss HJ. Testicular tumors in childhood. J Pediatr Surg. 1975;10:109–14.

37. Skoog SJ. Benign and malignant pediatric scrotal masses. Pediatr Clin North Am. 1997;44:1229–50.

38. Kurman RJ, Scardino PT, McIntire KR, et al. Cellular localization of α-fetoprotein and human chorionic gonadotrophin in germ cell tumors of the testis using an indirect immunoperoxidase technique: a new approach to classification utilizing tumor markers. Cancer. 1977;40:2136–51.

39. Wu JT, Book L, Sudar K. Serum α-fetoprotein (AFP) levels in normal infants. Pediatr Res. 1981;15:50–2.

40. Brosman SA. Testicular tumors in prepubertal children. Urology. 1979;18:581–8.

41. Einhorn LH, Donohue JP. Combination chemotherapy in disseminated testicular cancer: The Indiana University experience. Semin Oncol. 1979;6:87–93.

42. Urban MD, Lee PA, Plotnick LP, et al. The diagnosis of Leydig cell tumors in childhood. Am J Dis Child. 1978;132:494–7.

43. Connolly JA, Gearhart JP. Management of yolk sac tumors in children. Urol Clin North Am. 1993;20:7–14.

44. Schanne FJ, Cooper CS, Canning DA. False-positive pregnancy test associated with gonadoblastoma. Urology (Online). 1999;54:162

45. Gallager HS. Pathology of testicular and paratesticular neoplasms. In: Johnson DE, ed. Testicular tumors, 2nd edn. Flushing: Medical Examination Publishing; 1976.

46. Campbell HE. The incidence of malignant growth of the undescended testicle: a reply and reevaluation. J Urol. 1959;81:663–668.

47. Batata MA, Whitmore WF Jr, Chu FC, et al. Cryptorchidism and testicular cancer. J Urol. 1980;124:382–7.

48. Swerdlow AJ, Higgins MC. Risk of testicular cancer in cohort of boys with cryptorchidism. Br Med J. 1997;314:1507–11.

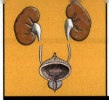

Section 3 Pediatric Urology

Chapter 17

Intersex

David CS Gough

KEY POINTS

- The normal female phenotype is the 'default' state for development and will occur in the absence of the *SRY* gene, testis and male hormones.
- Congenital adrenal hyperplasia is the commonest abnormality of the newborn with ambiguous genitalia.
- Associated salt-losing disorder may constitute a medical emergency.
- Surgical correction of intersex-related disorders depends on both the severity and time of diagnosis of the underlying condition.

Well then take a good heart and counterfeit to be a man, so I do: but i' faith, I should have been a woman by right.

William Shakespeare, *As you Like It*, Act IV scene 3.

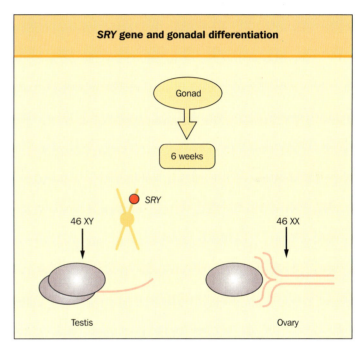

Figure 17.1 *SRY* gene and gonadal differentiation.

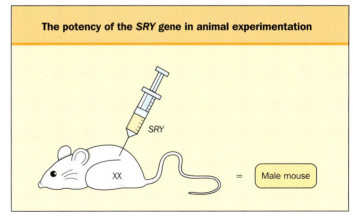

Figure 17.2 The potency of the *SRY* gene in animal experimentation.

INTRODUCTION

Abnormalities of sexual differentiation are uncommon and have complex etiologies. The most dramatic forms of intersex present as newborns with genital ambiguity and of necessity this chapter will essentially concentrate on the surgical aspects of intersex. As is usual in surgical texts, the complex psychosocial aspects of intersexuality and gender identity will be given scant coverage and this chapter will therefore seem to minimize the enormous psychological burdens born by families and patients with these conditions.[1] Additional detail is covered in Chapter 2.

GENETICS

Sexual differentiation is a widely used but poorly defined term to describe the process by which an embryo develops into a fetus with male or female characteristics. In general, genotype determines phenotype but this chapter is about exceptions to that rule.

In the human there are 46 paired chromosomes and the sex chromosomes are known as XX in the female and XY in the male. The piece of genetic material that induces the gonad to develop into a testis and therefore determines male sexual development is known as the *SRY* gene (Fig. 17.1).[2]

It is generally accepted that this piece of genetic material is responsible for normal male development. Yet other factors may influence this gene and suppress its activity, such as an extra X chromosome as seen in Klinefelter's syndrome[3].

This piece of chromatin, the *SRY* gene, is, however, very powerful and can induce male development when inserted experimentally into the genetic make-up of a female mouse embryo (Fig. 17.2).

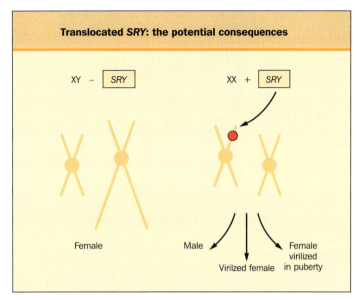

Figure 17.3 Translocated SRY: the potential consequences.

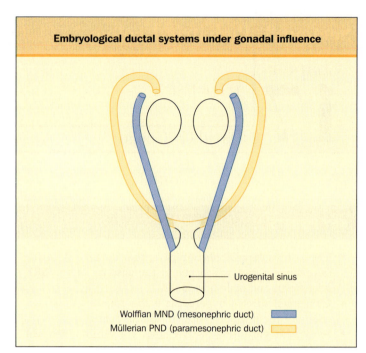

Figure 17.4 Embryological ductal systems under gonadal influence.

The genetics of intersex are complicated by the fact that the SRY gene can be translocated to the X chromosome in meiosis, giving rise to an XX male, or it may be mutated and therefore less than fully active.

The consequences of this are that the phenotype does not seem to match the genotype. While it is easy to describe some of these events, such as translocation of SRY, it is less easy to determine the phenotype from this event, which can range from apparently normal male through to ambiguous genitalia in the newborn period or even a 'normal female' who may virilize in puberty with an androgen surge (Fig. 17.3).

THE FEMALE PHENOTYPE

Normal female development occurs when the genetic makeup is 46XX and has been termed 'the default' state of development that occurs in the absence of the SRY gene, testis, and male hormones – even in the absence of ovarian tissue.

The female phenotype develops independently of the fetal gonad, and estrogen is not needed for normal prenatal sex differentiation along female lines. This can be best illustrated in mice who have 46XX with aromatase deficiency and in whom there are no estradiol receptors. These mice develop normal female phenotype. Therefore, provided that there are two X chromosomes and no translocation of the SRY, there will be normal female development. Even if the ovary fails to develop or becomes a streak gonad, there should be normal female internal and external development.

Abnormal development in the female
Congenital adrenal hyperplasia
The female fetus can be masculinized by exogenous testosterone from a maternal adrenal or ovarian tumor. Adrenal adenomas or ovarian androblastomas, luteoma, or a Krookenberg tumor may all occasionally do this.

The female fetus can also be masculinized by endogenous male hormone when enzyme defects in the adrenal gland lead to an overproduction of male hormonal precursors. This condition, a virilized female child, is called congenital adrenal hyperplasia.

Normal ovarian development
Both the long and the short arm of the X chromosome are needed for normal ovarian development and a situation in which there is deletion of the short arm of the X chromosome will lead to a Turner-like syndrome.

THE MALE PHENOTYPE

The mechanisms of sexual differentiation depend on normal development of the gonad, which under the power of the SRY gene on the Y chromosome and with no adverse effects from additional or abnormal genetic material, form a testis.

Physiology
Normal testicular development
The fetal testis at 7 weeks is secreting müllerian inhibiting substance (MIS) from the Sertoli cell following which placental human chorionic gonadotrophin (hCG) stimulates the Leydig cells to produce testosterone at 8 weeks. In later pregnancy, luteinizing hormone from the fetal pituitary takes over the role of placental hCG and continues to stimulate Leydig cells to produce testosterone.

These hormones act locally and may do so by diffusing down the ductal system that they influence. MIS causes regression of the female (müllerian) ductal system and testosterone causes the wolffian duct to develop into epididymis, vas, and seminal vesicles (Fig. 17.4).

When MIS is not present there can be persistence of müllerian structures, and where testosterone is absent, the epididymis, vas, and seminal vesicles do not develop (Fig. 17.5).

The effect of the gonad on the embryological ductal systems

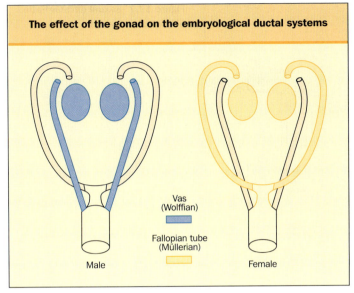

Vas
(Wolffian)

Fallopian tube
(Müllerian)

Male   Female

Figure 17.5 The effect of the gonad on the embryological ductal systems. Involution of the müllerian system in the male and involution of the wolffian system in the female.

The persistent müllerian duct syndrome secondary to müllerian inhibiting substance failure in a dysgenetic gonad

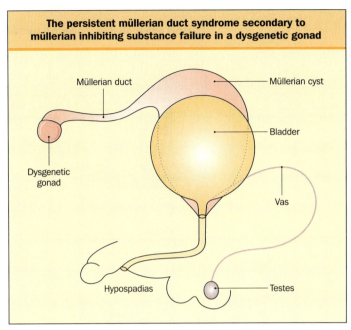

Müllerian duct   Müllerian cyst

Bladder

Dysgenetic
gonad

Vas

Hypospadias   Testes

Figure 17.6 The persistent müllerian duct syndrome secondary to müllerian inhibiting system failure in a dysgenetic gonad (usually associated with hypospadias).

This part of the development process is *local* and *lateral* and is responsible for unilateral abnormal development in patients with mixed gonadal dysgenesis when the genotype is 45XO or 46XY. One gonad is usually very abnormal, often 'streak' in nature, and there is persistence of müllerian duct structures on this side. On the side with a normal testis there is regression of müllerian structures and normal development of epididymis, vas, and seminal vesicles (Fig. 17.6).

The combination of genetic and consequent hormonal abnormalities in this syndrome causes failure of normal sexual differentiation and a degree of genital ambiguity at birth[4].

Abnormal development in the male
Failure of normal male sexual differentiation may occur where there is an obvious defect in the Y chromosome leading to a gonadal abnormality, or where the *SRY* gene is translocated or mutated, and therefore the chromosome may be morphologically normal.

Once the testis fails to develop or develops abnormally, a number of abnormalities in sexual development may occur, which will depend on the degree of abnormality induced in the testis by the genetic accident.

Abnormal pathways
The most profound of these (Fig. 17.7) occurs in XY gonadal agenesis. There is a female phenotype and the situation only becomes apparent at puberty. There is complete failure of puberty in the female and the condition comes to light on investigation.

Where there is XY gonadal dysgenesis there may be a female phenotype until puberty, and then with the testosterone surge at puberty masculinization occurs. Children with this form of dysgenesis may have severe abnormalities of the gonads, which may be streak in nature, despite a normal *SRY* gene, and there is a very high risk of gonadoblastoma in this condition, which is known as Swyer's syndrome.

In pediatric urology practice, XY gonadal dysgenesis frequently presents with a degree of sexual ambiguity at birth. There is testicular asymmetry and internally one frequently finds persistent müllerian structures and a streak gonad (Fig. 17.8).

Severe forms of gonadal dysgenesis can lead to sexual reassignment because of the inability surgically to reconstruct the patient as a male.

Syndromal association and gonadal dysgenesis
A number of other syndromes have been associated with ambiguous genitalia (Fig. 17.8), such as the Denys–Drash syndrome, in which there is a global testicular deficiency both of MIS and testosterone thought to be due to a mutation in the 11p13 'Wilms tumor' gene. This leads to a high incidence of Wilms tumor, severe glomerulonephritis, and associated ambiguous genitalia.

Another syndrome in which there is likely to be abnormality of renal development leading to Wilms tumor is the WAGR (Wilms' tumor, aniridia, genitourinary abnormality, and mental retardation) syndrome in which there is a dysgenetic gonad, again thought to be related to 11p13 genetic mutation or the Pax 6 aniridia gene malformation.

EXTERNAL SEXUAL DIFFERENTIATION

Without androgens the fetus will assume the external appearance of a female. Androgen stimulation virilizes the external genitalia. Even with androgen present there can be a failure to virilize because of local enzyme deficiency in the end-organ target cells.

If there is failure of testosterone production, this can be caused by biosynthetic defects; these are usually recessively inherited and are uncommon[5].

Testosterone is metabolized to dihydrotestosterone (DHT) intracellularly which increases its potency by a factor of 4. Its action depends on intracellular binding sites being present.

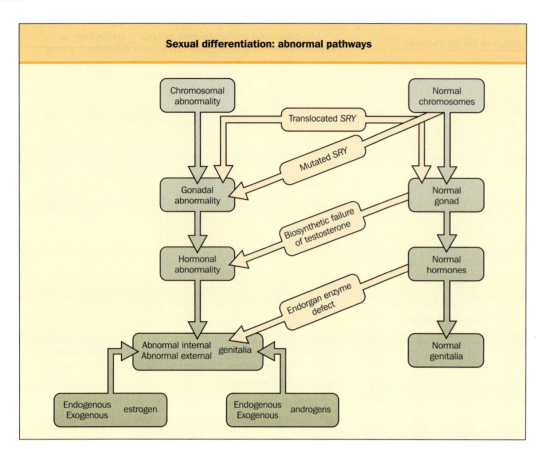

Figure 17.7 Sexual differentiation: abnormal pathways.

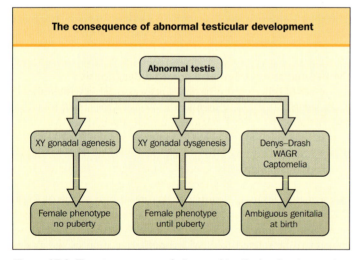

Figure 17.8 The consequence of abnormal testicular development.
WAGR, Wilms' tumor, aniridia, genitourinary abnormality, and mental retardation.

Complete absence of binding sites for DHT leads to the testicular feminization syndrome.

Here there is a genetically normal male who forms testes that do not descend but produce both MIS and testosterone. This causes complete internal virilization but the complete intracellular block of DHT action stops any external male development; and the child is born an apparently normal female at birth. The clitoris and lower third of the vagina are quite normal. All internal development above this level is entirely male as the müllerian duct, which produces the tube, uterus, cervix, and upper vagina, has been suppressed by MIS.

The children present with primary amenorrhea or with testicles present in the sac of an inguinal hernia that come to light when the hernia is repaired. The condition can be familial.

Intersexuality at birth

The commonest abnormality that affects newborn with ambiguous genitalia is congenital adrenal hyperplasia (CAH). In this condition there is an enzyme block for steroid production by the adrenal gland, and the biofeedback mechanism that suppresses the stimulation of the adrenal is therefore bypassed and there is gross overproduction of androgenic precursors by the adrenal cortex. This affects external genital development, which in the female consists of enlargement of the clitoris and suppression of development of the lower vagina. This results in a varying degree of masculinization of the external genitalia, with genital ambiguity. The clue to the diagnosis rests in the fact that gonads are impalpable and the chromosomal sex can rapidly be identified as 46XX; measurement of the plasma shows both to be grossly elevated and confirms the diagnosis. In both these common forms of CAH plasma testosterone concentrations are elevated to normal adult ranges and are responsible for virilization of the female external genitalia[5] (Fig. 17.9).

Approaches on examining the newborn with ambiguous genitalia

A patient with ambiguous genitalia is an undervirilized male or an overvirilized female (Fig. 17.10). In practice, 70% of the patients will be overvirilized females with a congenital adrenal

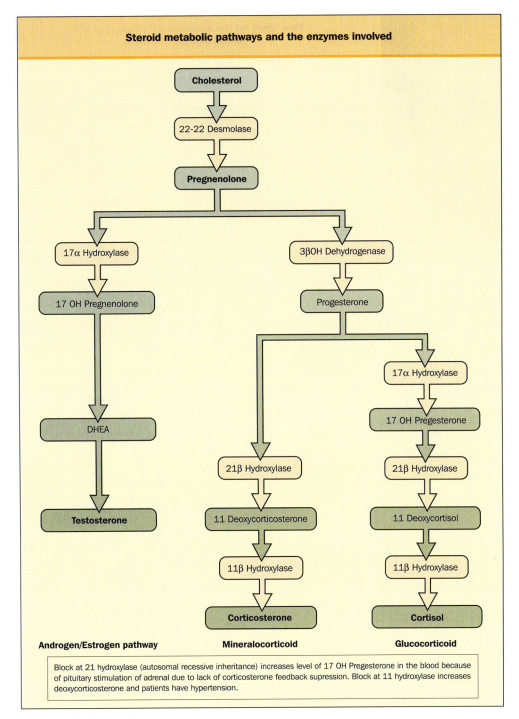

Figure 17.9 Steroid metabolic pathways and the enzymes involved. DHEA, dihydroepiandrosterone

hyperplasia. These patients need an urgent strategy for diagnosis in the newborn period because of the high risk of salt-losing crisis and mortality. This is a medical and surgical emergency.

If the patient does not have an obvious diagnosis then the surgeon is going to be involved with interpretation of the radiology in the form of a genitogram, and possibly cystourethroscopy of the genitourinary sinus and laparoscopy and gonadal biopsy in order to make a diagnosis.

Approaching a family where the sex of a child has yet to be determined is one of the most daunting responsibilities that a pediatric urologist can face. Clinical examination of the infant is most helpful and if a gonad is palpable it is almost always a testis; this has led Aaronson to develop a scheme that is

recommended as a flow chart to follow when examining the infant to determine what investigations subsequently take place (Fig. 17.11).

Nearly 70% of all children with genital ambiguity at birth will have absent gonads and are almost always suffering from CAH. This is a medical rather than a surgical emergency in order to determine whether the child has a salt-losing state and requires urgent medical treatment[5].

If CAH is present and the child is genetically 46XX then the sexual assignment is to the female gender. Medical treatment is used to prevent further masculinization by exogenous steroid administration. Surgical reconstruction of the genitalia is along female lines – a feminizing genitoplasty.

17

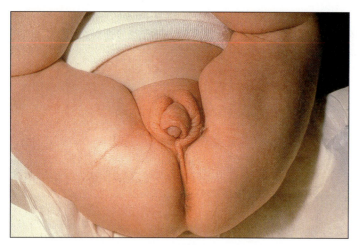

Figure 17.10 Genital ambiguity at birth. No gonads palpable; high incidence of probability that the diagnosis is congenital adrenal hyperplasia.

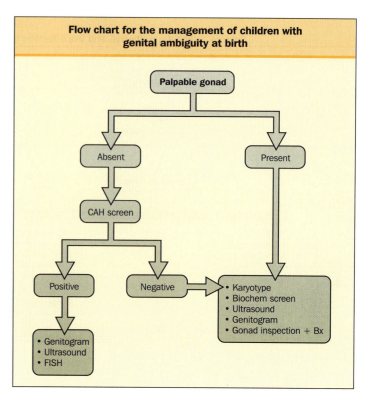

Figure 17.11 Flow chart for the management of children with genital ambiguity at birth. CAH, congenital adrenal hyperplasia. (Courtesy of I Aaronson.)

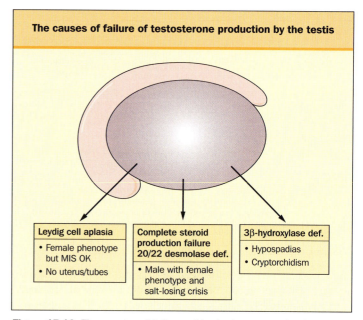

Figure 17.12 The causes of failure of testosterone production by the testis. def, deficiency; MIS, müllerian inhibiting substance.

This approach has been challenged, however, and patients who have severe salt-wasting and are extensively masculinized at birth can suffer serious crises of sexual identity through childhood, adolescence, and early life[7]. Some give consideration to formal gender reassignment in these patients.

If male sex is assigned by accident and the diagnosis comes to light after the age of 6 months, it is generally believed that the patient should remain in the sex assigned at birth and that surgical reconstruction should be undertaken, with excision of the vagina and ovaries and testicular prostheses placed at the appropriate moment.

This remains a very controversial area and those who defend the current mainstream approach of raising all CAH patients with 46XX as females state that the historical medical and surgical treatment has been less than effective, as has counseling and psychological support. We are looking therefore at the end results of less than perfect medical, surgical, and psychological treatment and there is no reason to suppose that current medical, surgical, and psychological treatment will lead to the same outcome as these historical 'controls.'

Very careful medical supervision and adequate steroid replacement is vital if further masculinization is not to occur from undertreatment, which would allow testosterone levels to rise.

In another enzyme abnormality of the adrenal gland, the 20/22 desmolase deficiency syndrome (Fig. 17.9) there is complete steroid production failure by the adrenal gland. The gland gets swollen with lipid and the patient will also suffer a salt-losing crisis shortly after birth. These are males with a female phenotype, who become very ill with salt-losing in the first few days of life as a result of an addisonian crisis.

A milder form of failure of steroid production caused by 3β-hydroxylase deficiency leads to patients with hypospadias and cryptorchidism (Fig. 17.12).

If the patient does not have congenital adrenal hyperplasia then the flow chart recommended by Aaronson can be followed. A decision will need to be taken about the sex of rearing. Some believe that chromosomal sex plays very little part in the decision-making process at this time, which will depend more on the state of virilization of the external genitalia and presence or absence of internal female structures. The other view is that, as a general rule, the genetic sex of the individual does play a crucial role in the decision-making process and should be respected. The psychological risk of gender reassignment can be very difficult to predict[8].

Surgery may be undertaken to inspect the internal genitalia and perform gonadal biopsy in order to assist diagnosis and to determine the sex of rearing.

Where androgen insensitivity is suspected, a short course of hCG in order to determine phallic responsiveness and the possibility of male reconstruction would be appropriate[9].

Raising the child as male will normally depend on the reconstructability or the size, length, and diameter of the stretched penis in comparison with normal males. The range of normality has previously been documented in children[10].

Failure of testosterone production from an apparently normal gonad

Leydig cell aplasia can lead to a female phenotype but normal internal male genitalia, as MIS is secreted normally. Therefore there is no uterus or tube formation but an apparently normal female who fails to develop secondary sex change at puberty because of lack of any hormone production at that time (Fig. 17.12).

Androgen insensitivity syndrome

Complete androgen insensitivity syndrome (AIS; Fig. 17.13) is a rare X-linked disorder in which the patient presents with primary amenorrhea or inguinal hernia in infancy. At puberty there is characteristically primary amenorrhea and a complete lack of pubic hair. It has been thought that this condition is prevalent in 1–2% of all females with inguinal hernias[11].

Characteristically, patients with partial AIS are either raised female or have an ambiguous phenotype and are found to have 46XY male chromosomes with normal testosterone production and metabolism. Occasionally, testosterone levels are found to be relatively low but an hCG test of 1,500U daily × 3 will indicate normal responsiveness of testicular tissue and a rise in testosterone production. There should be a five- to ten-fold rise in testosterone levels with a normal hCG test and a normal testis.

There can sometimes be significant debate as to the appropriate sex of rearing in partial AIS patients who have a micropenis with chordee, perineal hypospadias, and a bifid scrotum. A gonad may or may not be palpable. Some general principles are that if there is fusion of the labial scrotal folds with a palpable gonad, then the patient is probably best reared male, but where there is nonfusion, then female sexual assignment is perhaps appropriate[12]. A novel approach to determining sex of rearing has been the use of the sex hormone binding globulin response to androgens and this has been advocated as an investigation that can help determine sex of rearing[13]. Unfortunately, this opinion is yet to be validated in long-term studies.

The diagnosis of AIS is suspected by the phenotype and confirmed when normal hormonal response is induced from the gonad by an hCG test. It can be further confirmed by an absence of abnormal structures on ultrasound and a gonadal biopsy. Genital skin biopsy taken at the time of genitoplasty can be used for fibroblast culture and assessing the 5α-reductase assay.

Patients with AIS who are raised female should have the gonads removed as early as possible and estrogen therapy commenced early in puberty or in late childhood in order to improve skeletal maturation.

With 5α-reductase deficiency the patient is normally born with ambiguous genitalia and may well be recognized and raised as a male but, where mistakes have been made, there will of course be severe masculinization in puberty as the testosterone surge occurs.

Less prominent end-organ enzyme defects of this type result in a patient with Reifenstein's syndrome, in which there is a small penis and cryptorchidism.

THE SURGERY OF INTERSEX

Feminizing genitoplasty

Almost 70% of patients presenting with ambiguous genitalia are females who have been born with congenital adrenal hyperplasia. They will be relatively severely masculinized and will come to light during investigation of ambiguous genitalia.

Once the patient is stable, surgical treatment to reduce the clitoris and open the vagina on to the surface will be necessary.

The most commonly practiced form of clitoroplasty is one in which the clitoris is mobilized and the neurovascular bundles are identified separate from the corpora cavernosa. The neurovascular bundles are then lifted from the corpora, which are resected down to their bifurcation, and the vascularized, innervated glans of the clitoris is replaced on to this area (Fig. 17.14).

In the majority of patients the excess of skin around the clitoral hood can be opened up and reconstructed as labia minora and the vagina can be opened into the vulva. The main controversy in this condition exists when the vagina is very high and very short, and there have been some innovative approaches to dealing with vaginal reconstruction or pull through in this situation[14–16].

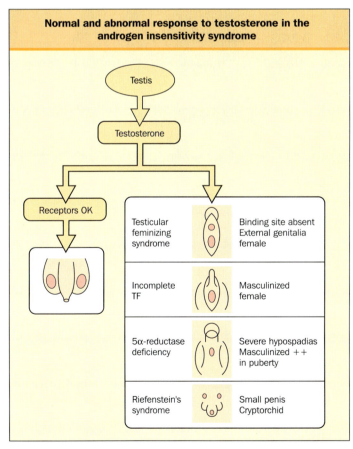

Figure 17.13 Normal and abnormal response to testosterone in the androgen insensitivity syndrome. The clinical consequences. TF, testicular feminization.

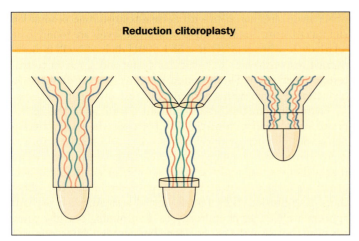

Figure 17.14 Reduction clitoroplasty

Most attempts at surgical reconstruction to the high genito-urinary sinus are likely to lead to a stenosis in the mid portion of the vagina, with hair-bearing skin being taken into the lower vaginal reconstruction[17].

Simply waiting until puberty can induce enormous changes in vaginal capacity (Fig. 17.15). At puberty, with the onset of menstruation, there is usually 'tissue expansion' of the vagina, which leads to relatively straightforward perineal procedure to open the vagina into the vulva (Fig. 17.16).

This approach in patients with CAH of early clitoroplasty and then late vaginoplasty has also been recommended by others[18].

Menstruation normally commences quite young in patients with congenital adrenal hyperplasia and is signaled by episodic lower abdominal pain and increasing size of the vaginal tissues on ultrasound. This indicates the 'correct' timing for surgical reconstruction.

Controversies in congenital adrenal hyperplasia
Sex reassignment

Some patients are born with such severe masculinization that either hypospadias reconstruction is attempted or the patient has a urethral opening at the tip of the phallus and is raised male without thought of the diagnosis. Where there is no evidence of salt-losing in this situation, the patient may then go on to develop normally until puberty, when some form of complication occurs with the genitourinary sinus. If it is discovered, it is normally recommended that the sexual assignment is not changed and the internal genitalia are removed at this point.

Because of the psychological problems associated with CAH and severe salt-losing states, there are those that recommend such patients are raised as male, even when the diagnosis has been identified at birth. This is a controversial area and many people believe that adequate and complete medical therapy does not leave girls with severe CAH in a bad psychological state at puberty, but historically this has happened and has led many to consider reassigning the gender at birth.

Vaginal replacement
A number of different approaches to the type and the timing of vaginal replacement have been suggested. The most commonly used organ for substitution is the large bowel, either the cecum or the sigmoid colon[19–22].

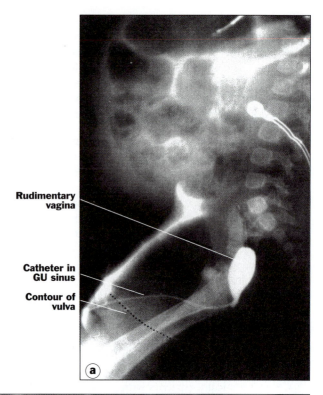

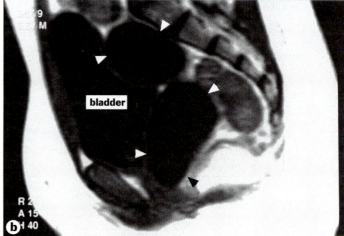

Figure 17.15 Patient with severe congenital adrenal hyperplasia.
(a) The size of the vagina and length of the genitourinary sinus (no surgery in the newborn period apart from clitoroplasty). (b) The same patient as in (a) beginning to experience the menarche aged 10. The increasing size of the vagina is outlined with arrows.

Controversy still exists on the timing of this therapy, many people believing that it should be deferred until puberty, when there will be co-operation and understanding of the type of surgery involved and the probability of dilatations of the vaginal introitus being necessary. There are those, however, who suggest that treatment can and should take place in the newborn period. At present there is no professional agreement on these issues.

Genitoplasty in non-congenital adrenal hyperplasia patients
In patients where there is vaginal atresia the uterine structures are usually cord-like and there is not normally a cervix. It is generally considered that these uterine structures have significant

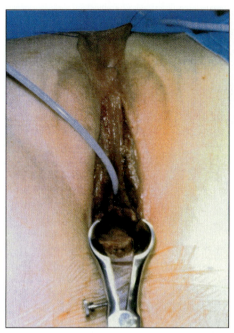

Figure 17.16 Patient with severe congenital adrenal hyperplasia. The same patient as in Figure 17.15 before construction of the labia minora. The vagina has been opened into the vulva without any special flap procedures.

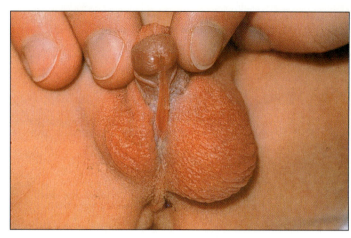

Figure 17.17 Patient with mixed gonadal dysgenesis. Severe hypospadias and marked testicular asymmetry with impalpable right gonad. Chromosomes 45 XO–XY with 20% of the cell lines XO. Reconstructed male with hypospadias surgery and excision of the right gonad.

malignant potential and that, as there is no normal cervix to retain a pregnancy and no normal uterus, they should be excised rather than reconstructed. The artificial vagina is inserted at the time that these structures are removed. Early forms of vaginal replacement were generally performed in patients who had a congenitally absent vagina, such as those with Meyer–Rokitansky–Kuster–Hauser syndrome, in which there is absence of the vagina, renal disorders, skeletal dysplasia, and an absence of puberty in the female.

Tissues used for reconstruction/replacement of the vagina

Split skin was used on a former by McIndoe in 1950 and the problems with this particular form of reconstruction were that the vagina was often short, needed continued dilatation and required lubrication[23].

The use of intestine, sigmoid colon or cecum was described by Baldwin in 1904 but it was not until relatively recently that the long-term results of this type of vaginal replacement have been studied. Reconstruction with colocecum has been quite successful, with 50% of patients becoming sexually active. There were, however, a significant number of revisional procedures with this type of reconstruction[19]. The use of sigmoid colon has been reported, with 70% of the patients being sexually active and one in five of the group being married, but then divorced. Some 5% of patients experienced painful intercourse, but most were not dilating[20].

Long-term outlook

In patients with congenital adrenal hyperplasia, normal sexual activity and fertility can be anticipated with modern treatment. Yet historical studies show that less than half of female patients with CAH have evidence of fertility and those with the salt-losing form were less likely to marry or have children[24].

Another rare problem for long-term consideration in these patients where pull through of the vagina has been undertaken is that there is a risk of malignant change[25].

In the majority of other instances where a feminizing genitoplasty or vaginal replacement has been done, there is either failure of development of normal ovarian or follicular tissue, or failure of normal development of the uterus and cervix, which will lead to sterility.

Surgery to the vagina – removal

There will be a number of instances where a genitourinary sinus or a müllerian remnant will need to be removed as the patient is being raised as a male. This occurs most commonly in müllerian duct syndrome, usually associated with mixed gonadal dysgenesis XO–XY. These patients are normally born with severe hypospadias or ambiguous genitalia and a decision may be taken to raise them as male or female. This will depend on the severity of the condition and the ease of reconstruction along male lines. Although the majority of the literature suggests raising such children as female, my own experience has been that in each instance when I have found XO–XY mixed gonadal dysgenesis, with unilateral cryptorchidism and severe hypospadias, the patient has been assigned the male sex before referral and it has been quite appropriate to reconstruct them along those lines (Fig. 17.17).

General principles in this condition are as follows.

- The severe hypospadias may often require novel methods of reconstruction, such as the use of buccal or bladder mucosa, because of local tissue deficiency[26].
- The cryptorchid testis is usually severely abnormal, may be crossed to the other side and ectopic, and will need to be removed because of the risk of later malignancy.
- The müllerian remnant may or may not be obvious at birth but it may become so after hypospadic reconstruction.
- There is controversy in this condition whether both gonads should be removed. Many would leave the normally descended testis in this situation (Fig. 17.18).
- Patients with XO–XY mixed gonadal dysgenesis are normally sterile.

A number of different approaches to the müllerian remnant have been suggested, both perineal and trans- or pararectal (Pena approach). The transtrigonal approach can be accomplished

17

241

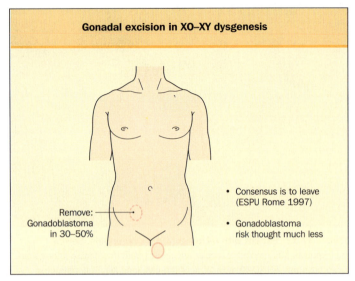

Gonadal excision in XO–XY dysgenesis

Remove:
Gonadoblastoma
in 30–50%

• Consensus is to leave
  (ESPU Rome 1997)

• Gonadoblastoma
  risk thought much less

Figure 17.18 Gonadal excision in XO–XY dysgenesis. The consensus from the European Society of Paediatric Urology (ESPU) meeting 1997 was to leave the normally descended gonad.

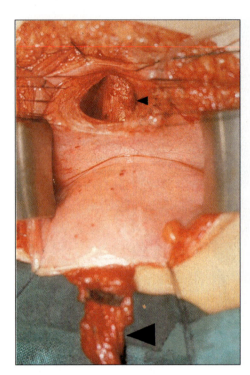

**Figure 17.19
Excision of
müllerian remnant
by the transtrigonal
procedure.** The
müllerian remnant
has been arrowed
where it has been
mobilized behind the
bladder and then it
disappears behind
the open bladder and
reappears in the
transtrigonal opening
that has been
surgically created
(arrow shows the
excision about to be
completed). -

without moving the patient during anesthesia, as the whole of the müllerian duct system will require removal both by laparotomy and transtrigonal excision (Fig. 17.19) The main anxiety with transrectal excision is that, should some form of sepsis occur, then there will almost invariably be a rectourethral fistula.

Gonadal excision

The gonads should always be excised as soon as possible in patients in whom the sex of rearing is different to the chromosomal/gonadal sex (Fig. 17.20). This will include such patients as XY females with the testicular feminizing syndrome, and as a general principle all intra-abdominal gonads that contain an element of testis with Y chromatin should be excised as there is a high risk of malignant transformation and gonado-blastoma development. This occurs in 30% of patients with these abnormalities.

TRUE HERMAPHRODITISM

This occurs in 10% of cases of intersex and there may be a testis and a separate ovary, or more usually ovotestes. The uterus is usually present but may be bicornuate or hypoplastic and the ductal structures that remain depend entirely on the gonad: its influence and the phenotypic effects may be quite variable. When biopsying the gonad a longitudinal biopsy is usually undertaken rather than a transverse one in order to pick up abnormalities of gonadal origin; again all intra-abdominal material inconsistent with sex of rearing should be removed. This applies to all intra-abdominal gonads with testicular histology.

Masculinizing genitoplasty

This type of surgery essentially consists of hypospadias repair, which in the majority of incidences in patients with intersex will involve extensive reconstruction of the phallus (Fig. 17.21).

Controversies exist as to the timing of surgical repair – either early, within the first few months of life, or after the age of

Gonadal incision in intersex

• Testicular feminization syndrome
• Turner type with Y chromation
• Sex of rearing changes
  – XO/XY or XXX, or XO with streaks
  – XY micropenis

Figure 17.20 Gonadal excision in intersex.

3 years, when double drainage of the bladder via suprapubic and urethral catheters can be accomplished more easily. The patient is less likely to have problems with urinary leakage through the repair.

At whatever time the reconstruction is undertaken, it is quite possible that extra tissue will need to be mobilized in order to complete the repair. This can be done by either staging the procedure and transferring skin into the area as free or pedicled skin grafts, as in the repairs advocated by Durham Smith and Bracka, or using a one-stage repair and, where tissue is at a premium, reconstructing the urethra out of buccal mucosa.

The risks of this type of surgery are not inconsiderable, and reoperation rates in the region of 10–20% are commonplace for complications such as stricture or fistula. Where buccal mucosa is used as a tube replacement of the urethra then a 30% reoperation rate will be encountered.

The phallus will almost always have severe chordee and Horton's test is used during the procedure with Nesbitt-type corrections of the tunica albuginea to obtain a straight erection.

Where there is a 'shawl' scrotum, then a scrotal transposition will be an important part of the cosmetic procedure and this is normally accomplished after hypospadias repair has been undertaken and successfully completed.

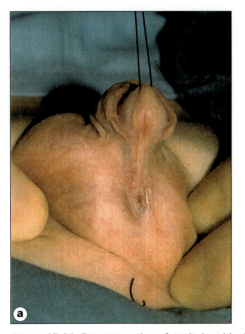

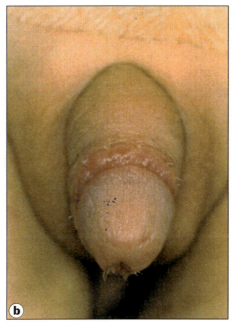

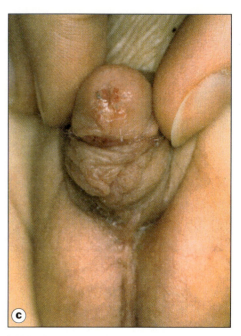

Figure 17.21 Reconstruction of genital ambiguity along male lines. (a) Before operation. (b, c) Following surgery with buccal mucosa graft.
A patient with 46XY syndromal association with severe hypospadias.

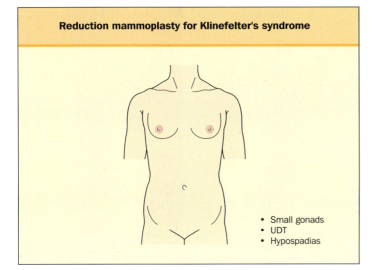

Reduction mammoplasty for Klinefelter's syndrome

- Small gonads
- UDT
- Hypospadias

Figure 17.22 Reduction mammoplasty for Klinefelter's syndrome.
UDT, undescended testis.

Hernia uteri inguinale

- Contents of male hernia found to be
  – Uterus
  – Fallopian tube
- Müllerian inhibiting substance failure
- Excise: usually with gonadal excision also

Figure 17.23 Hernia uteri inguinale.

CONDITIONS CONFUSED WITH INTERSEX

Adhesions of the labia minora
This is a relatively common finding in young girls under the age of 7–8 years. It is thought to be hormonally based, because it responds to the local application of estrogen cream, but seldom causes any symptoms, is often recurrent, and never requires any surgical treatment.

The characteristic thin gray line of adhesion can be seen when the labia majora are gently separated (Fig. 17.24). The condition is never present at birth because of the hormonal influence that occurs during the pregnancy and affects the fetus.

Buried penis
This condition generally affects slightly overweight or obese young boys. Its surgical treatment is far from satisfactory and circumcision of the standard variety should be avoided as this can sometimes denude the entire shaft of the penis, leading to significant deformities and difficulties as adolescence advances. It may be difficult, but it is always advisable to delay or defer surgical intervention. At puberty, a fair degree of self-correction of the abnormality will occur (Fig. 17.25).

Masculinizing surgery
Other forms of surgical treatment in patients with intersexual chromosomal abnormality are rare in the male, but occasionally reduction mammoplasty in patients with XXY Klinefelter's syndrome is needed at puberty (Fig. 17.22).

One also occasionally encounters abnormal content in a hernial sac during herniotomy in the male and this occurs when there is a degree of MIS failure and abnormal contents, in the form of a uterus or perhaps fallopian tube, are found in the sac. The advice in this situation is to excise the abnormal tissue with gonadal excision and hernia repair (Fig. 17.23).

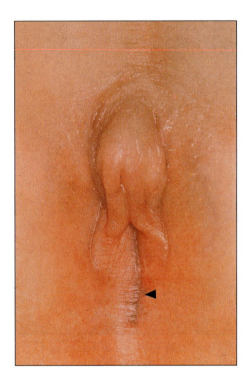

Figure 17.24 Labial adhesions in the female. The gray line indicating fusion is arrowed.

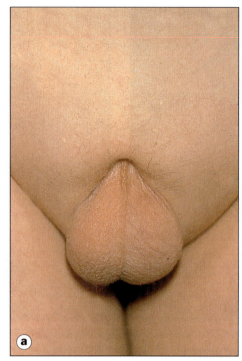

Figure 17.25 Buried penis.
(a) Appearance before puberty. (b) Situation at puberty without treatment.

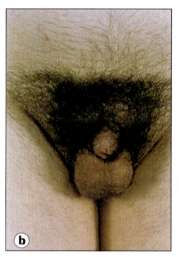
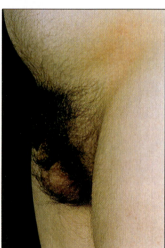

A number of procedures have been described to disinter the penis, but most of these are relatively unsatisfactory and, although the surgeon may be pleased with the result, the patients and the family seldom are.

Diagnosis based on the evidence of chromosomes, physiology, radiology, and surgery can give us a clear path to tread in treating patients with intersex states, yet in the final analysis the feeling of maleness or femaleness is an unmeasurable but concrete quality.

Doctors can get it wrong and in this condition it can take nearly 20 years to realize it.

Oh time, thou must untangle this, not I: it is too hard a knot for me to untie.
William Shakespeare, *Twelfth Night*, Act II scene 2.

REFERENCES

1. Mayer-Bahlberg HFL. Intersexuality and the diagnosis of gender identity disorder. Arch Sexual Behav. 1994;23:21–40.
2. Sinclair AH, Berta P, Palmer MS, et al. A gene from the human sex determining region encodes a protein with homology to a concerned DNA binding motif. Nature. 1990;346:240–4.
3. Mittowoch U. Sex determination and sex reversal: genotype, phenotype, dogma and semantics. Hum Genet. 1992;89:467–79.
4. Robboy SJ, Muller T, Donahoe PK, et al. Dysgenesis of testicular and streak gonads in the syndrome of mixed gonadal dysgenesis. Hum Pathol. 1982;13:700–16.
5. Hughes IA, Mouriquand PDE. Ambiguous genitalia in the newborn. Surgery. 1995;13:265–271
6. Wilson JD. Syndromes of androgen resistance. Biol Reprod. 1992; 46:168–73.
7. Mulaikal RM, Migeon CJ, Rock JA. Fertility rates in female patients with congenital adrenal hyperplasia due to 21-hydroxylase deficiency: New Engl J Med. 1987;316:178–82.
8. Money J. Hormones, hormonal anomalies, and psychologic health care. In: Kappy MS, Blizzard RM, Migeon CJ, eds. The diagnosis and treatment of endocrine disorders in childhood and adolescence. Springfield, IL: Charles C. Thomas; 1994:1141–78.
9. Almaguer MC, Saenger P, Linder BL. Phallic growth after hCG: a clinical index of androgen responsiveness. Clin Pediatr. 1993; 32:329–33.
10. Beheshti M, Churchill BM, Hardy BE, Daneman D. Gender assignment in male pseudo hermaphrodite children. Urology. 1983; 22:604–7.
11. Jagiello G, Atwell J. Prevalence of testicular feminisation. Lancet 1962;1:329–31.

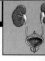
12. Viner RM, Teoh Y, Williams DM, et al. Androgen insensitivity syndrome: a survey of diagnostic procedures and management in the UK. Arch Dis Child. 1997;77:305–9.

13. Sinnecker GH, Hiort O, Nitsche EM, et al. Functional assessment and clinical classification of androgen insensitivity in patients with mutations of the androgen receptor gene. Eur J Paediatr. 1997;156:7–14.

14. Passerini-Glazel G. A new one stage procedure for clitero-vaginoplasty in severely masculinised female pseudo hermophrodites. J Urol. 1989;142:565–9.

15. Benedetto B, Giovale M, Bagnara V, et al. The anterior sagittal trans ano-rectal approach: a modified approach to one stage clitero-vaginoplasty in severely masculinised female pseudo hermaphrodites – preliminary results. J Urol. 1997;157:330–2.

16. Pena A, Filma B, Bonila E, et al. Trans ano-rectal approach for the treatment of uro-genital sinus: preliminary report. J Pediatr Surg. 1992;27:681–3.

17. Newman K, Randolph J, Anderson K. The surgical management of infants and children with ambiguous genitalia: lessons learned from twenty five years. Ann Surg. 1992;215:644–53.

18. Hensle TW, Kennedy WA II. The surgical management of intersexuality. In: Walsh PC, et al, eds. Campbell's urology. Philadelphia, PA: WB Saunders; 1998:2155–71.

19. Turner-Warwick R, Kirby R. The construction and reconstruction of the vagina with the colo-caecum. Surg Gynecol Obstet. 1990;170:132–6.

20. Dean GE, Hensle TW. Intestinal vaginoplasty. Curr Surg Tech Urol. 1994;7:1–8.

21. Wesley JR, Coran AG. Intestinal vaginoplasty for congenital absence of the vagina. J Pediatr Surg. 1992;27:885–9.

22. Hitchcock RJI, Malone PS. Colovaginoplasty in infants and children. Br J Urol. 1994;73:196–9.

23. McIndoe A. Discussion of treatment of congenital absence of vagina with emphasis on long term results. Proc R Soc Med. 1959;52:952–4.

24. Kuhnle U, Bullinger M, Schwartz HP. The quality of life in adult female patients with congenital adrenal hyperplasia: a comprehensive study of the impact of genital malformations and chronic disease on female patients' life. Eur J Pediatr.1995;154:708–16.

25. Schober JM. Feminising genitoplasty for intersex. In: Stringer MD, Mouriquand PDE, Oldham KT, Howard ER, eds. Pediatric surgery and urology: long term outcomes. London: WB Saunders; 1998:549–58.

26. Ahmed S, Gough DCS. Buccal mucosa graft for secondary hypospadias repair and urethral replacement. Br J Urol. 1997;80:328–30.

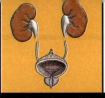

Chapter 18

Vesicoureteric Reflux

Duncan T Wilcox, Margaret L Godley, and Pierre DE Mouriquand

KEY POINTS

- Vesicoureteric reflux (VUR) descibes the retrograde flow of urine from bladder to kidneys.
- It is a complex condition with a wide diversity of urinary pathology.
- VUR exposes the upper tract to lower tract pressure changes and infection.
- The consequences of VUR, known as reflux nephropathy, can lead to renal insufficiency and hypertension.
- In the majority of cases VUR resolves spontaneously; medical management to avoid infection and treat bladder dysfunction is the rule, with surgery reserved for selected severe cases.

INTRODUCTION

Vesicoureteric reflux (VUR) is the retrograde flow of urine from the bladder into the upper urinary tract (Fig. 18.1). It is a dynamic event, which exposes the upper urinary tract to pressure changes and to urine usually confined to the bladder, and it facilitates ascending urinary infection. The term is used to describe a common childhood problem associated with urinary infection and renal scarring, otherwise called 'reflux nephropathy', which can lead to renal insufficiency and hypertension.

The VUR disorder has a wide diversity of features. Reflux can be unilateral or bilateral. The upper tracts may appear normal or severely dilated and individual ureters can be affected differently. The kidneys may be abnormal from acquired disease or from maldevelopment; alternatively they may be normal. The disorder can present differently in boys and girls. The reflux resolves spontaneously in most children, but in some it does not. Such variations imply that compound factors are likely to operate in the genesis of VUR and in the pathogenesis of the associated upper tract anomalies. Not all of these factors are well understood. The aim here is to provide a simple understanding of this complex problem and its clinical management.

THE URETEROVESICAL JUNCTION

The normal ureterovesical junction (UVJ) functions like a valve to separate the upper and lower urinary tracts while allowing the passage of urine into the bladder. The upper tracts have small capacity and low pressure. The bladder is a high-capacity,

Figure 18.1 Vesicoureteric reflux. Appearance during micturating cystourethrography. Contrast medium infused into the bladder extends to both the renal pelvis (distended) and the calyces, which are outlined. The ureters are dilated.

low-pressure storage system, which generates high pressures at intervals to void urine. Prevention of VUR at the UVJ requires integration of structural (passive) and functional (active) components.[1] The structural requirements are that the ureter enters the bladder with an oblique intramural course through the detrusor muscle and that it extends in a submucosal tunnel to open on to the trigone in a correct location (Fig. 18.2, left). Longitudinal muscle fibers that extend from the terminal ureter to the trigone and proximal urethra contribute an active component. Reflux is prevented by occlusion of the submucosal ureter, which requires compression of the ureteral orifice between bladder mucosa and detrusor muscle. During micturition contraction of the ureterotrigonal muscles assists with closure of the ureteral meatus and prevents lateral displacement of the ureteric orifice, which in itself can predispose to VUR.

THE ABNORMAL URETEROVESICAL JUNCTION

The UVJ may be abnormal from primary or secondary causes. Primary reflux results from immaturity, or from maldevelopment of the ureterovesical junction. In general this is caused by a short submucosal tunnel, attributable to delayed maturity (Fig. 18.2, right). Secondary reflux occurs when the UVJ is

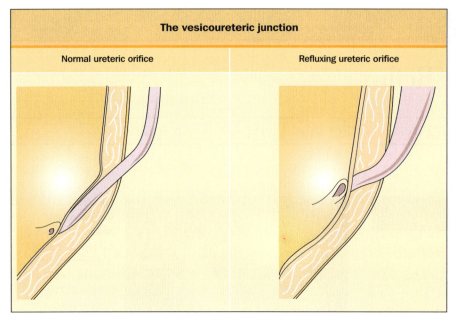

The vesicoureteric junction

Normal ureteric orifice	Refluxing ureteric orifice

Figure 18.2 The vesicoureteric junction. (Left) The normal junction with a long submucosal tunnel compared with a refluxing ureteric orifice with a short submucosal tunnel (right). (Adapted from Hutch JA. Vesicoureteral reflux and pyelonephritis. New York: Appleton-Century-Crofts;1972.)

distorted by changes in the bladder wall secondary to other pathology (Fig. 18.3).

The distinction between primary and secondary reflux is crude and is not always clear; for example, some primary reflux may be secondary to abnormal lower tract function or, more controversially, due to inflammation at the UVJ. As the complexities of the VUR disorder are better understood further stratification of primary reflux may be required. The importance of the 'primary' or 'secondary' distinction lies in recognizing that for any child presenting with VUR the possible presence of attributing pathology needs to be identified or excluded, since secondary reflux often resolves after the underlying condition is treated. While any pathophysiologic effects of the reflux are the same for primary and secondary VUR, this chapter only concerns primary VUR.

DETECTING AND GRADING VESICOURETERIC REFLUX

Micturating cystourethrography is the standard investigation for diagnosing the presence of VUR. Radiographic contrast media instilled into the bladder may be observed to pass into the ureter only or extend into the renal pelvis (Fig. 18.1). The ureter may appear radiographically normal or dilated and tortuous. These appearances have formed the basis of a number of three-, four- or five-point classification systems. The five-point International Classification used widely since 1981 has now become the convention (Fig. 18.4)[2].

The nature of the VUR disorder, which can be transient, variable or depend on underlying conditions in the lower tract, inevitably confers inconsistencies in the detection and grade of VUR observed. Methodologic variables contribute further to poor reproducibility. The bladder filling volume and changes in intravesical pressure induced by the filling procedure are likely to affect the radiographic grading appearances of upper tract distention and the extent of retrograde flow. A simpler classification system that is more tolerant of the methodologic variables may have merit: the distinction between mild, nondilating (grade I, II) and severe, dilating (grade IV, V) reflux may be more robust.

Causes of secondary vesicoureteric reflux
Posterior urethral valves
Duplex systems
Detrusor instability
Neurogenic bladder
Non-neurogenic neurogenic bladder

Figure 18.3 Causes of secondary vesicoureteric reflux.

EPIDEMIOLOGY

Vesicoureteric reflux itself is generally asymptomatic and is identified during infancy and childhood only by investigations for other urinary tract problems. The two most common problems are 1) urinary infection and 2) fetal urinary tract dilatation detected during routine prenatal ultrasound screening. In children without urinary infection or any urologic anomalies the prevalence of VUR is difficult to ascertain but possibly lies between 0.4% and 1.8% of the pediatric population[3]. In children with symptomatic infection and those identified with covert bacteriuria during screening programs, the prevalence of VUR is typically about 30% for children aged 2–18 years[4, 5] and approximately 50% for neonates[6]. In affected children the prevalence and features of VUR vary with age, gender and ethnic origin; up to 10 times more North American white children have VUR than their Afro-American compatriots[7].

Males with VUR are likely to be identified in infancy (less than 1 year of age), most of them after prenatal detection, otherwise with signs of infection. By contrast, females are more likely to be identified between 2 and 8 years of age following urinary infection (Fig. 18.5). Whereas the older group are predominately female[4,8], in the infant group identified after prenatal detection males exceed females by approximately 4:1[9,10]. Twice as many of these males as females feature upper tract dilatation. Furthermore, 'reflux nephropathy' of the type likely to be a maldevelopment is

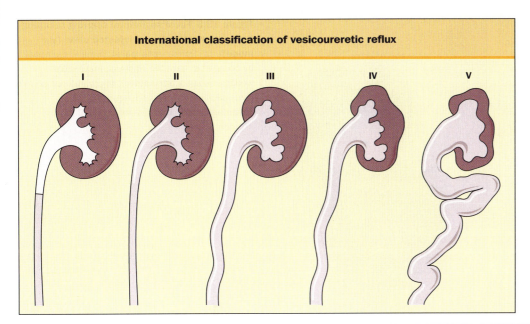

Figure 18.4 International classification of vesicoureteric reflux. Appearances at micturating cystourethrography. Grades: I, reflux into the ureter; II, reflux extending to the renal pelvis; III, extended reflux as in grade II but with mild dilatation of the ureters and renal pelvis; IV, extended reflux with upper tract dilatation; V, includes blunting of the calyces and ureters grossly dilatated and tortuous.

associated with the severe (dilating) reflux most often found in males[10–12]. Most of the female infants (and a proportion of males) have normal kidneys. By contrast, the older group, which is mostly female, is more likely to feature acquired 'reflux nephropathy' of the type associated with urinary infection. These data suggest that the reflux disorder exists in at least two distinct forms.

Familial vesicoureteric reflux

Siblings of patients with reflux have a 45% chance of reflux compared with approximately 1% in the general pediatric population[13], females being more commonly affected. The children of parents with reflux also have a higher than average risk, with 69% of them having reflux[14], and there have been reports of VUR in twins. It is apparent that in some patients the VUR disorder is inherited. Despite active research the mode or modes of inheritance remains uncertain[15].

Spontaneous resolution

Vesicoureteric reflux disappears during childhood in a high proportion of cases. This accounts for its rarity in adults and its higher prevalence in neonates compared with older children. Resolution occurs with maturation at the UVJ when the intravesical ureter lengthens to improve competence in preventing reflux[16]. Other factors may also be involved, such as maturation of neuromuscular components and voiding dynamics.

Whether or not there is spontaneous resolution depends on factors that include the patient's age, the reflux grade, and whether the reflux was unilateral or bilateral. The grade of reflux influences resolution but it does not determine whether or not resolution occurs[4,17,18]. At age 10 years, mild reflux can have a resolution rate of 90% in girls and 81% in boys compared with a resolution rate for severe reflux of 50% in boys and 65% in girls[18]. There is no difference in resolution rate between boys and girls when the grade of reflux is considered[18].

It appears that the younger the child is at presentation the more likely the reflux is to resolve. In an infant series with VUR identified after prenatal detection, reflux resolved at 15 months of age in 70% (78 of 112) of ureters with the mild forms of reflux (without significant dilatation) and 43% (35 of 81) of

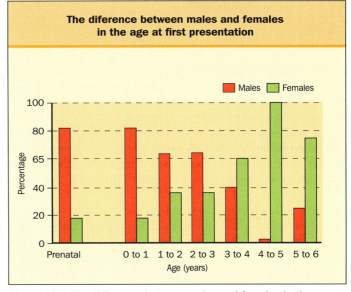

Figure 18.5 The difference between males and females in the age at first presentation. The percentage of males and females (Y axis) after prenatal diagnosis (see text) and with age (X axis; postnatal data derived from Lenaghan et al.[8]). Males present earlier in life than females.

those with severe reflux. By comparison, the International Reflux Study Committee reported a 28% rate of resolution in their older population of school-age children[2]. This last report also noted that 54% of unilateral but only 12% of bilateral cases resolved. Others, however, have noted no difference in resolution rate between bilateral and unilateral reflux patients[18].

The high spontaneous resolution rate for reflux has influenced the nonoperative approach to management of VUR, which instead aims to prevent urinary tract infections.

Vesicoureteric reflux and urinary tract infection

The association between vesicoureteric reflux and urinary infection is well established but uncertainties about the causal relationships between infection and the reflux event are less widely considered.

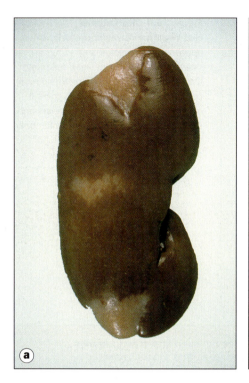

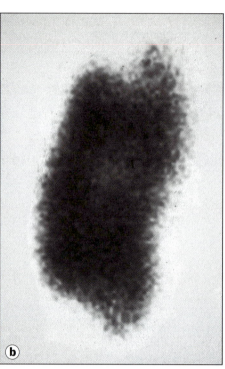

Figure 18.6 Focal segmental scarring resulting from intrarenal reflux of infected urine (pig model). (a) Normal renal parenchyma is replaced by collagen to form the classical, irreversible, wedge-shaped scars that typically overlie compound renal papillae. (b) The corresponding ^{99m}Tc-dimercaptosuccinic acid renal image of focal segmental scars.

Vesicoureteric reflux is thought to predispose children to infection, because after micturition refluxed urine returns from the ureter to the bladder so that complete bladder emptying is never achieved. Bacteria that have ascended into the bladder are never completely expelled during each void but instead are able to colonize the bladder and the upper tract. However, the incidence of urinary infection does not seem to be altered when the reflux is successfully stopped by surgical repair[19]. Kunin and colleagues examined a group of children with recurrent urinary infection with and without reflux and found that those patients with reflux had a lower incidence of infection[5]. These data cast doubt over the traditional concept that reflux causes urinary infection.

An alternative theory is that urinary infection causes reflux. It has been proposed, and there is supporting evidence, that infection causes inflammatory changes at the UVJ so that the valve mechanism is unable to close effectively, resulting in vesicoureteric reflux. The concept has been reviewed recently; it remains controversial, with an increasing body of evidence suggesting that infection does not cause reflux but that infection and reflux often coexist as independent variables[20,21].

REFLUX-ASSOCIATED NEPHROPATHY

The term 'reflux nephropathy' was introduced to emphasize the well established association between vesicoureteric reflux and renal damage[22]. The term suggests that the nephropathy is causally linked to reflux. Instead, there are likely to be several mechanisms explaining why a kidney associated with a refluxing ureter is abnormal.

Between 30% and 60% of infants and children with VUR have abnormal kidneys, most of them identified at first presentation. In general, the renal abnormality features focal or segmental areas of fibrous scarring replacing the normal renal parenchyma (hence the term renal scarring; Figs 18.6 & 18.7). The poles of the kidney are the areas most often affected. The normally smooth renal

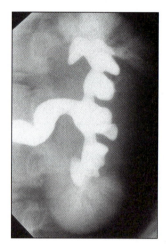

Figure 18.7 Intrarenal reflux. Contrast medium extends into the renal parenchyma at the renal poles. (Courtesy of PG Ransley.)

outline may instead appear contracted and lobulated. However, 'reflux nephropathy' can also feature diffuse or generalized damage with or without a segmental component. The renal abnormalities associated with the reflux event can be acquired, usually from the reflux of infected urine, or they may result from maldevelopment.

Acquired renal damage

A series of experimental and morphologic studies has led to the present understanding of the pathogenesis of acquired renal damage. The important factors are intrarenal reflux, urinary infection and less commonly extreme urodynamic abnormalities.

Intrarenal reflux

Intrarenal reflux is the retrograde passage of urine into the collecting ducts (Fig. 18.7). It allows the egress of urine and urinary pathogens into the renal parenchyma, where it may cause renal scarring. Intrarenal reflux occurs more commonly at the polar regions of the kidney than in the hilar region. This segmental

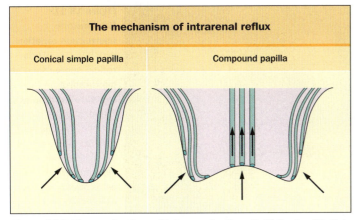

The mechanism of intrarenal reflux

| Conical simple papilla | Compound papilla |

Figure 18.8 The mechanism of intrarenal reflux. (Left) Ducts of Bellini on convex surfaces of the conical simple papilla do not allow intrarenal reflux. (Right) The wide ductal openings on flat or concave surfaces of compound papillae allow intrarenal reflux. (Adapted with permission from Ransley PG. Intrarenal reflux: anatomical, dynamic and radiological studies. Urol Res. 1977;5:61–69 © Springer-Verlag.)

distribution is due to variation in papillary morphology. Not all renal papillae allow intrarenal reflux (Fig. 18.8). During embryologic development, fusion between individual lobes results in compound papillae with a flattened area cribrosa, which allows intrarenal reflux (Fig. 18.9a). Simple papillae with the more typical conical shape do not allow intrarenal reflux (Fig. 18.9b). Compound papillae are usually located at the poles of the kidney, which correlates well with the polar siting of segmental renal scarring. However, only two thirds of human kidneys have compound papillae, which may explain why some patients appear to be protected from scar formation[23–25].

Infected vesicoureteric reflux

Ransley and colleagues clearly demonstrated from experimental work that the retrograde passage of infected urine can result in the formation of new renal scars (see Fig. 18.6)[25]. They further showed that when the infection was treated within a week, or during the acute inflammatory phase, renal scar

formation could be avoided or minimized. Treatment instituted after this early phase did not prevent or reverse the formation of renal scars[26,27].

Sterile vesicoureteric reflux

In the absence of urinary infection reflux itself does not damage the kidney. Experimental studies by Ransley et al.[28] using the growing pig have shown that VUR does not affect renal growth or renal function. The subject was contentious for many years following Hodson's earlier experimental work showing that sterile reflux did cause renal scarring[22]. It is now recognized that sterile reflux can only induce scarring in the presence of non-physiologic bladder pressures such as occur with bladder outflow obstruction, when residual urine volumes and upper tract dilatation are also features[29]. In general clinical practice sterile 'primary' VUR does not cause renal damage. Sterile scars may occur only when reflux is secondary to infravesical obstruction of structural, functional or neurogenic origin.

New renal scars

These experimental data show that new scarring requires the intrarenal reflux of infected urine. If a urinary infection is left untreated for more than a week then renal scars are likely to form; this has been referred to as the 'big bang' theory.

Renal maldevelopment

It is now clear that the extent of reflux-associated nephropathy acquired from the intrarenal reflux of infected urine has been overemphasized while the contribution of developmental abnormalities has been underestimated. Recent studies of infants with VUR identified after prenatal diagnosis have shown that many have renal abnormalities[9–12]. In one large series of 155 infants, 40% had abnormal kidneys, most without any exposure to urine infection. Most (91%) of the abnormal kidneys were associated with severe reflux, which predominantly affected males, as has been noted by others. The abnormal kidneys featured imaging appearances indicating the generalized rather than the purely focal type of renal damage[10] (Fig. 18.10). These results suggest that many kidneys associated with a refluxing

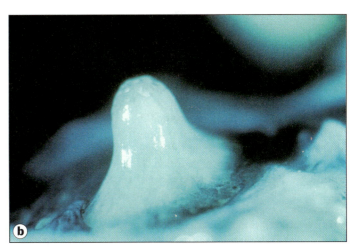

Figure 18.9 Renal papillae stained with methylene blue. (a) A complex 'compound' papilla formed during fusion of the embryonic renculi. The central ductal openings are on flat or concave surfaces and are wide and gaping. (b) A 'simple' conical renal papilla. The ducts of Bellini open on the convex tip of the papilla, formed from a single embryonic renculi. (Courtesy of PG Ransley and RA Risdon.)

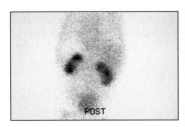

Figure 18.10 ^{99m}Tc-DMSA renal image in an infant with prenatal dilatation and no urinary infection. Shows poor DMSA uptake (with high background activity). The images appear patchy with uneven uptake typical of generalized, rather than segmental, renal damage. These kidneys often display increased echogenicity with ultrasound imaging.

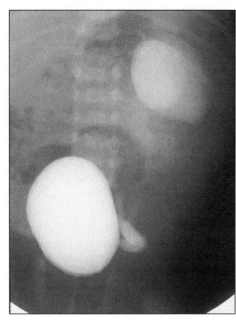

Figure 18.11 Pelviureteric obstruction together with vesicoureteric reflux: appearance at micturating cystourethrography. The renal pelvis opacified by reflux of contrast medium from the bladder. Contrast medium remains in the pelvis after it has been expelled from all but the most distal portion of the ureter.

ureter are damaged in utero, or that they develop abnormally. Indeed, the concept that abnormal development leads to both reflux and renal damage concurs with Mackie and Stephens's earlier report that abnormal development of the ureteric bud would lead to anomalous renal development and renal dysplasia as well as reflux[30]. That renal dysplasia does account for a proportion of reflux-associated nephropathy is further supported by clinicopathologic studies[31].

Associated anomalies

Pelviureteric junction obstruction can be associated with vesicoureteric reflux[32]. This may be an association, or reflux may cause kinking at the pelviureteric junction resulting in obstruction. Pelviureteric junction obstruction should be considered if the renal pelvis is dilated out of proportion to the degree of reflux seen (Fig. 18.11).

Hutch diverticulae are associated with reflux. These diverticulae usually occur lateral to the ureteric orifice, but occasionally they involve the ureteric orifice. Bladder diverticulae do not affect the natural resolution of reflux and so they do not alter management.

DIAGNOSIS

Presentation after prenatal detection

Following the introduction of prenatal ultrasound an increasing number of neonates are being identified with fetal uropathies. Fetal urinary tract dilatation occurs in between 1/150 and 1/1200 live births; 25% of these neonates have primary vesicoureteric reflux detected postnatally[33]. To identify the cause of a fetal dilatation, the following sequence of investigations is recommended (Fig. 18.12).

Presentation after symptoms

Postnatal diagnosis of vesicoureteric reflux

The most common presentation of a child with vesicoureteric reflux is a urinary infection. Up to 50% of children who present with a urinary infection have proven reflux[2]. Occasionally, children will present with vague flank pain not associated with an infection but related to micturition. Children can also present with hypertension and/or symptoms of renal insufficiency. The high prevalence of reflux in children with urinary infection emphasizes the importance of adequately investigating all urinary infections in the pediatric age range.

Physical examination is usually normal. It is important, however, to look for pathology that would predispose to secondary reflux. In particular the spine and external genitalia should be carefully examined and any abnormality further investigated.

The most important investigation, for children presenting with a suspicion of urinary infection, is a midstream urine culture. It is essential that the urinary infection is confirmed before the child is subjected to numerous invasive tests. It is necessary to identify how the urine was collected for culture and to confirm that there was a pure growth of more than 100,000 colony forming units per milliliter of urine. It is surprising how often children are referred with a urinary tract infection based only on symptoms. Once the infection is proved then imaging is undertaken to diagnose the underlying cause. The imaging of a child with a urinary infection will not be elaborated on here. However, it is important to remember that ultrasound scanning is particularly inaccurate at diagnosing reflux[34].

INVESTIGATION

Micturating cystourethrogram

The micturating cystourethrogram is still the 'gold standard' investigation for the diagnosis of vesicoureteric reflux (Fig. 18.1). A small catheter is placed into the bladder under aseptic conditions. It is normal practice to cover the procedure with prophylactic antibiotics. Radio-opaque contrast media at body temperature, to prevent irritation of the trigone, is instilled into the bladder. This is done under gravity control to avoid overfilling the bladder. Once the bladder is filled reflux is looked for, the child is then asked to void and close attention is paid to the bladder neck, urethra and vesicoureteric junction. Once voiding is completed, then reflux is again considered and the bladder residual volume is estimated. The accuracy for detecting reflux can be increased by up to 15% if the investigation is immediately repeated. The advantage of the micturating cystogram over other diagnostic modalities is that it provides good anatomic detail of the lower urinary tract. This method is therefore used in all boys with suspected reflux so that bladder outlet obstruction, especially posterior urethral valves, can be excluded.

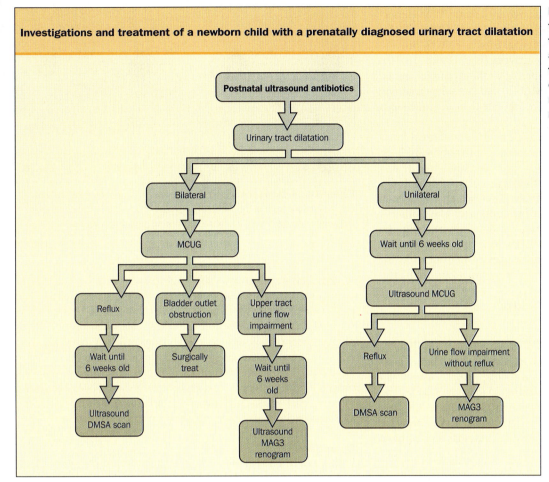

Investigations and treatment of a newborn child with a prenatally diagnosed urinary tract dilatation

Postnatal ultrasound antibiotics

Urinary tract dilatation

Bilateral

MCUG

Reflux

Bladder outlet obstruction

Upper tract urine flow impairment

Wait until 6 weeks old

Surgically treat

Wait until 6 weeks old

Ultrasound DMSA scan

Ultrasound MAG3 renogram

Unilateral

Wait until 6 weeks old

Ultrasound MCUG

Reflux

Urine flow impairment without reflux

DMSA scan

MAG3 renogram

Figure 18.12 Algorithm outlining the basic investigations and treatment of a newborn child with a prenatally diagnosed urinary tract dilatation. DMSA, dimercaptosuccinic acid; MAG3, mercaptoacetyltriglycline; MCUG, micturating cystourethrogram.

Direct isotope cystography

This investigation is similar in technique to a micturating cystourethrogram except that radionuclide isotopes, usually technetium-99m pertechnetate, are instilled into the bladder instead of radio-opaque contrast. The advantage of this method is that there is a significant reduction in the radiation dose when compared to a standard cystogram[35]. The main disadvantage is that anatomic details are poorly represented. This makes the technique suitable for following patients with vesicoureteric reflux and for identifying girls with reflux where bladder outlet problems are not suspected (Fig. 18.13).

Indirect radionuclide cystography

In this technique radioisotope is injected intravenously and the isotope is cleared by the kidney and excreted into the urine. Approximately 20 minutes after injection the isotope has entered the bladder; reflux can then be identified during both the filling and voiding phases (Fig. 18.14)[36]. This method has the advantage that the bladder does not have to be catheterized and that the bladder fills under physiologic conditions. The disadvantages are that only patients who have normal urinary control can undertake the investigation; that patients need good renal function to excrete the isotope; and that there is a significant false-negative rate when compared with the micturating cystogram. This modality is therefore reserved for children over 3 years of age who do not require any further anatomic imaging. It is most commonly used for following patients known to have reflux.

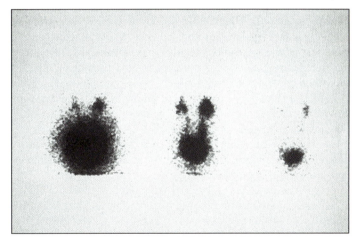

Figure 18.13 Direct isotope cystogram. Final sequence of images (5s acquisitions) with pertechnetate instilled into the bladder. Bilateral reflux observed at the end of bladder filling (first frame) and during micturition (second frame). After micturition (third frame) drainage from the upper tracts contributes a residue in the bladder.

Static renography

Once reflux has been detected it is important to identify the presence and extent of the associated nephropathy, which affects between 33% and 60% of kidneys at the time of diagnosis[4,10].

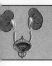
Reflux nephropathy is best evaluated by a static ^{99m}Tc-dimercaptosuccinic acid (^{99m}Tc-DMSA) nuclear isotope scan. ^{99m}Tc-DMSA is taken up by the proximal renal tubular cells to provide an image of functioning renal parenchyma (Figs 18.6 & 18.10). For identifying renal scars it is superior to the dynamic agents, such as mercaptoacetyltriglycine (MAG3) and diethylenetriamine pentaacetic acid (DTPA), and is more accurate than an intravenous urogram[37].

Static renal imaging does not provide a measure of renal function, although the ratio of the functional contribution by individual kidneys can be obtained (differential function). If any renal damage has been identified, then a test of renal function is recommended; first a plasma creatinine level, which if abnormal should be followed by a glomerular filtration rate. The glomerular filtration rate together with the radionuclide imaging can provide a baseline for future investigations and management decisions. Even in unilateral disease it can be helpful to know about overall renal function, especially in situations when the affected kidney appears from imaging to have deteriorated, or renal damage is later found to be bilateral.

MANAGEMENT

Studies comparing surgical and medical treatments have influenced current management protocols, which historically favored surgical correction of the reflux. We know that in the majority of patients the reflux will resolve. As sterile reflux does not cause new scar formation, this has led to a nonoperative approach to the management for these patients, with an emphasis on maintaining sterile urine.

Medical

The rationale of medical management is to keep patients infection-free, allowing them to grow out of their reflux problem without further damaging the kidneys. Medical management involves teaching patients a regular voiding habit that minimizes residual urine collection. Constipation is actively treated as it may increase the risk of infection[38].

The use of low-dose prophylactic antibiotics to keep the urine sterile is widely accepted as the mainstay of medical treatment[39]. Recently, however, this approach has been questioned[20]. Since Edwards's original study proposing this treatment modality there have been no controlled studies comparing low-dose antibiotics with a placebo.

Until the issue is resolved by controlled studies the use of low-dose prophylactic antibiotics is recommended, but when this should stop is another contentious question. As the majority of new scars occur during the first 2 years following diagnosis many believe that antibiotics should be continued for this period. Other, more conservative units, recommend continuing until the reflux has been shown to have resolved.

If breakthrough infections continue despite medical management then further therapy is required. Before embarking on surgical correction of reflux some centers now recommend circumcision for the boys as this has been shown to significantly reduce urinary tract infections[40].

Surgical

The indications for the surgical repair of vesicoureteric reflux are controversial. These include breakthrough infections, new renal

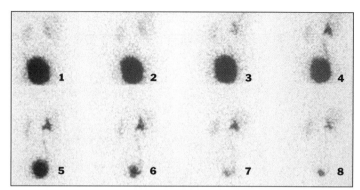

Figure 18.14 Indirect isotope cystogram. After renal clearance and upper tract drainage of intravenously injected ^{99m}Tc-MAG3. Vesicoureteric reflux into the right kidney is observed during micturition (frames 4–6).

scarring, presence of associated diverticulae and high grades of reflux. Increasingly these indications are being questioned. The rate of breakthrough infections does not appear to be altered by successful surgical correction of reflux[19], although the incidence of pyelonephritis is reduced. Infections without new scar formation are no longer an indication for surgery. As has been already discussed, high-grade reflux can resolve and should also be observed. The current indication for repair should be the presence of new renal scars, assuming that underlying bladder pathology has been excluded by appropriate urodynamic evaluation.

Operations

Reflux can be corrected endoscopically or by open surgery. Open techniques involve both transhiatal and suprahiatal procedures.

The sting procedure

The endoscopic injection of a nonbiodegradable material to treat reflux was first reported in 1981 but it was Puri and O'Donnell who popularized the technique[41]. The patient is placed in the lithotomy position. A cystoscopic examination is performed and the two ureteric orifices are observed. A 20G needle is placed through the scope and the needle tip is placed so that it enters the urothelium 5mm distal to the ureteric orifice. The nonbiodegradable material is slowly injected while the needle is advanced towards the ureteric orifice. The aim of the procedure is to obliterate the ureteric orifice; this usually takes 1–2ml (Fig. 18.15). Once the orifice is obliterated the needle is left in place for a few minutes to minimize extravasation of material. Using this technique, success rates of between 65% and 95% have been reported[42,43], although these may have required more than one procedure. Many published reports, however, have been criticized for treating patients with grade I and II reflux, which could have resolved spontaneously.

The advantage of the sting procedure is that it can be performed as an outpatient procedure with minimal morbidity to the patient. If the procedure initially fails the operation can easily be repeated. The short-term complication is that although the early success is high the injected material often settles with time and this can reduce the effectiveness. The major theoretic disadvantage is migration of the material. Migration of polytetrafluoroethylene (PTFE), an early material used, has been demonstrated in animals[44], although no adverse reaction has been

The Sting procedure

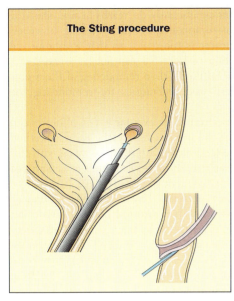

Figure 18.15 The sting procedure. The bulking agent is inserted into the submucosal layer just proximal to the ureteric orifice; agent is inserted until a volcanic bulge is seen. (Adapted from Spitz L, Coran AG, eds. Rob and Smith's operative surgery: pediatric surgery, 5th edn. London: Chapman & Hall; 1995.)

Cohen reimplantation technique

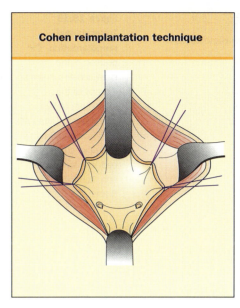

Figure 18.16 Cohen reimplantation technique: exposing the trigone. The diagram shows the bladder open with the Denis Browne ring inserted retracting the muscle but not the bladder. By retracting the dome of the bladder caudally the trigone is well exposed. (Adapted from Spitz L, Coran AG, eds. Rob and Smith's operative surgery: pediatric surgery, 5th edn. London: Chapman & Hall; 1995.)

Cohen reimplantation technique

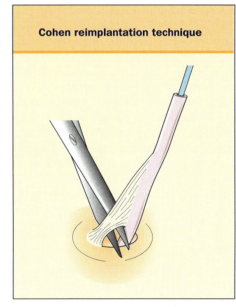

Figure 18.17 Cohen reimplantation technique: mobilizing the ureter. The ureter is mobilized from within the bladder, using Reynolds scissors. The dissection is commenced below the ureteric orifice and continues circumferentially. By removing the attached detrusor fibers the ureter can be completely freed. (Adapted from Spitz L, Coran AG, eds. Rob and Smith's operative surgery: pediatric surgery, 5th edn. London: Chapman & Hall; 1995.)

reported in human studies. This concern has led to a search for biologic material, which includes collagen, muscle and fat. To date none have been as successful as PTFE but there is still considerable research being carried out in this field.

Transhiatal reimplantation of the ureter

This method was first described by Cohen and has become the most widely used surgical procedure to reimplant the ureter and prevent vesicoureteric reflux[45].

An extraperitoneal approach to the bladder is used. The bladder is opened in the midline, extending to within 2cm of the bladder neck. A ring retractor is then placed with the blades placed outside the bladder. The blades should not be placed in the bladder as excessive retraction may cause damage to the bladder; the blades may impair access to the lateral walls of the bladder and thirdly if the bladder is stretched too much the submucosal dissection is more difficult. Moist swabs are placed in the dome of the bladder to help expose the trigone (Fig. 18.16).

A ureteric catheter is placed into the ureter and a stay suture is then inserted and secured to the catheter. This allows traction on the ureter, simplifying the dissection of the ureter from the detrusor, it also minimizes handling of the urothelium, which bleeds easily. The ureteric orifice is circumcised and the distal 2cm of the ureter is mobilized with diathermy. A plane is created between the ureter and the detrusor until the ureter is mobilized free of the bladder. It is essential to enter the correct plane between the bladder and the transparietal ureter, starting below the ureteric orifice. Reynolds scissors are used to elevate the muscle fibers that attach the ureter to the detrusor. These fibers are coagulated and then divided. The dissection continues until the ureter is free and an adequate length has been mobilized to perform the transhiatal reimplantation. In boys it must be remembered that the vas deferens loops over the distal ureter and can be damaged (Fig. 18.17).

A submucosal tunnel is then created from the old ureteric hiatus to a position superior and lateral to the contralateral orifice. If both ureters are to be reimplanted then two separate tunnels are created. It is important to create a submucosal tunnel that is five times the diameter of the ureter in length[46]. If the

ureter is too dilated to allow this then refashioning the ureter either by plication or tapering is necessary. When the tunnel is completed the ureter is placed into the tunnel, the distal portion of the ureter is excised back to fresh tissue and the end is spatulated to prevent stenosis. The bladder is then closed (Fig. 18.18).

A ureteric stent is left in place by some surgeons, usually for 2 days. The bladder is drained by either a transurethral or a suprapubic catheter for 5 days.

Suprahiatal reimplantation of the ureter

The main indication for the suprahiatal reimplantation is a megaureter. This is a difficult procedure, which should be performed by experienced pediatric urologists.

The bladder is approached by an extraperitoneal incision. The peritoneum covering the dome and the lateral walls of the bladder is pushed superiorly. The obliterated umbilical arteries are ligated, which allows mobilization of the peritoneum so that the

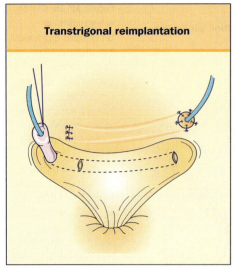

Transtrigonal reimplantation

Figure 18.18 Transtrigonal reimplantation. The position of the submucosal tunnels at the end of the procedure. (Adapted from Spitz L, Coran AG, eds. Rob and Smith's operative surgery: pediatric surgery, 5th edn. London: Chapman & Hall; 1995.)

iliac vessels can be identified. The ureter can be located as it passes over the iliac vessels close to the origin of the hypogastric arteries. The ureter is mobilized down to the bladder, preserving the blood supply. The ureter is divided at its entrance into the bladder; it is then redirected over the vas deferens to help straighten it out. Once the ureter is fully mobilized it is remodeled as necessary and the bladder is opened as described above.

The ureter should enter the bladder medially and high up on the posterior surface of the bladder. This enables a straight submucosal tunnel to the trigone to be developed. The ureter should be passed through the new hiatus in the bladder and via the submucosal tunnel to the trigone. It is essential that this is done without twisting or kinking the ureter (Fig. 18.19).

Most surgeons place a ureteric stent, especially if ureteric remodeling has occurred; this is left for 2–10 days. The bladder is closed and drained using a urethral or suprapubic catheter.

Remodeling the ureter

If after mobilizing the ureter it appears too dilated to reimplant then the first step is to excise the narrow distal portion of the ureter. Often the ureter significantly decreases in size, allowing reimplantation without remodeling of the ureter. If, however, the diameter of the ureter is too great, so that a submucosal tunnel to ureter diameter ratio of 5:1 can not be created (i.e. Paquin's law cannot be fulfilled), then remodeling of the ureter is required[46]. There are two techniques for remodeling the ureter.

- *Ureteric tapering* is performed by excising a strip of ureter and then re-anastomosing the ureter over a catheter; this method was popularized by Hendren[47]. Care must be taken with this method as excising the strip of ureter can result in ischemia of the distal ureter and subsequent stenosis (Fig. 18.20).
- *Plication of the ureter* is performed by marking the redundant portion of the ureter, which is sutured creating two distal lumens to the ureter. The excess lumen is then plicated over the true lumen of the ureter (Fig. 18.21)[48]. The advantage of plication over excision is that the vascular supply to the ureter is unaffected; however, infolding can result in obstruction of the ureter[49].

Whichever technique is performed it is only necessary to remodel the portion of the ureter that lies in the submucosal tunnel. Both these techniques to remodel a dilated ureter and the subsequent reimplantation are technically challenging procedures that even in experienced hands have significant morbidity[50].

Complications

Reimplantation of a refluxing ureter is subject to all the general complications of surgery including infection, hematoma, hemorrhage and urinary leakage from the bladder. There are however two problems that are specific to reimplantation: these are reflux and obstruction.

Vesicoureteric reflux

Reflux can occur in the ipsilateral ureter following surgery; this is probably due either to edema, which prevents coaptation of the ureter, or to postoperative bladder dysfunction, which is usually transient. In some patients the previously normal contralateral ureter begins refluxing; this may be a result of damage to the valve mechanism during bladder dissection or of transient

Suprahiatal reimplantation

Figure 18.19 Suprahiatal reimplantation. The ureter must enter the bladder medially and high on the posterior wall of the bladder, in order to prevent kinking of the ureter. The submucosal tunnel, as shown in the diagram, is straight towards the trigone. (Adapted from Spitz L, Coran AG, eds. Rob and Smith's operative surgery: pediatric surgery, 5th edn. London: Chapman & Hall; 1995.)

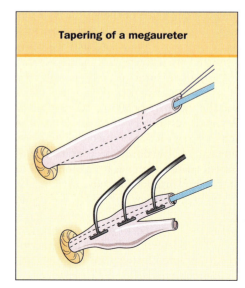

Tapering of a megaureter

Figure 18.20 Tapering of a megaureter. This is performed by resecting the distal portion of the ureter. Clamps are placed over a ureteric catheter (usually 10F), the redundant ureter is excised, and the ureter is closed in two layers. (Adapted from Spitz L, Coran AG, eds. Rob and Smith's operative surgery: pediatric surgery, 5th edn. London: Chapman & Hall; 1995.)

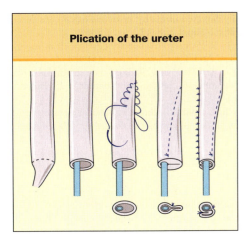

Plication of the ureter

**Figure 18.21
Plication of the
ureter.** This is
performed by excising
the distal ureter. The
redundant portion of
the ureter is then
plicated as shown in
the diagram. (Adapted
from Spitz L, Coran AG,
eds. Rob and Smith's
operative surgery:
pediatric surgery, 5th
edn. London: Chapman
& Hall; 1995.)

time but in some a temporary nephrostomy or a ureteric stent is required. If a transtrigonal reimplantation has been performed then cystoscopic placement of a ureteric stent can be technically challenging and a nephrostomy tube is preferable. Once the edema has settled the drainage tube can be removed.

Late obstruction may be continuous or intermittent. Continuous obstruction is normally due to fibrosis secondary to ischemia at the time of the original operation; only meticulous care during the original procedure can prevent this. Fibrotic obstruction requires reoperation. Intermittent obstruction occurs when the ureter kinks as the bladder fills. If the new insertion of the ureter is high on the posterior or lateral wall the ureter is subject to kinking. If this is suspected by intermittent symptoms it is important in making the diagnosis to perform a dynamic radioisotope scan with the bladder full and empty. Usually this requires a second reimplantation; occasionally the bladder can be fixed posteriorly, i.e. by a psoas hitch that prevents kinking on bladder filling.

postoperative bladder dysfunction. In the vast majority of patients early postoperative reflux settles and can be treated expectantly.

If reflux persists following reimplantation it is usually either due to an inadequate length of submucosal tunnel or because a secondary cause to the reflux was not diagnosed. It is necessary to exclude a secondary cause before embarking on further surgery[51]. If no secondary cause is found then further surgery is indicated only if the patient has persistent symptoms or progressive renal nephropathy.

Obstruction

Early obstruction can occur as a result of postoperative edema; it may present with a transient rise in serum creatinine. Some surgeons place a ureteric stent at the time of surgery to avoid this complication. In more severe cases the child presents with pain, nausea and vomiting 1–2 weeks following the operation. Impairment to urine flow can be diagnosed by increasing hydronephrosis on ultrasound and delayed excretion on dynamic radioisotope scanning. The majority of patients improve with

SUMMARY

Primary vesicoureteric reflux represents a wide diversity of urinary pathology. In infants two distinct forms of the disorder can be distinguished: boys with high-grade reflux and abnormal kidneys and boys and girls with low-grade reflux and normal kidneys. In older children with urinary infection the disorder is predominately found in girls. Reflux-associated nephropathy can be a fetal maldevelopment or acquired from intrarenal reflux of infected urine.

The days of surgical reimplantation as the panacea of all primary vesicoureteric reflux have gone. Increasingly we are aware that maintaining an infection-free urinary tract and treating any underlying bladder dysfunction are the goals of treatment. Ureteric reimplantation has only a small part in an overall treatment armamentarium that requires continuous updating and careful patient monitoring.

REFERENCES

1. Tanagho EA, Hutch JA, Meyers FH, Rambo ONJ. Primary vesicoureteral reflux: Experimental studies of its etiology. J Urol. 1965;93:165–76.
2. Committee IRS. Medical versus surgical treatment of vesicoureteric reflux. Pediatrics. 1981;67:392–400.
3. Bailey R. Vesicoureteric reflux in healthy infants and children. In: Hodson JA, Kincaid-Smith P (eds). Reflux nephropathy. New York: Masson. 1979:59–61.
4. Smellie J, Edwards D, Hunter N, Normand IC, Prescod N. Vesicoureteric reflux and renal scarring. Kidney Int Suppl. 1975;Suppl 4: S65–72.
5. Kunin C, Deutscher R, Paquin AJ. Urinary tract infection in school children: an epidemiological, clinical and laboratory study. Medicine (Baltimore). 1964;43:91–130.
6. Winberg J, Anderson H, Bergstrom T, et al. Epidemiology of symptomatic urinary tract infection in childhood. Acta Paediatr Scand. 1974;252:1–20.
7. Askari A, Belman A. Vesicoureteric reflux in black girls. J Urol. 1982;127:747.
8. Lenaghan D, Whitaker J, Jensen F, Stephens F. The natural history of reflux and long-term effects of reflux on the kidney. J Urol. 1976;115:728–30.
9. Elder JS. Commentary: Importance of prenatal diagnosis of vesicoureteric reflux. J Urol. 1992;148:1750–4.
10. Yeung CK, Godley ML, Dhillon HK, et al. The characteristics of primary vesico-ureteric reflux in male and female infants with pre-natal hydronephrosis. Br J Urol. 1997;80(2):319–27.
11. Gordon AC, Thomas DF, Arthur RJ, Irving HC, Smith SE. Prenatally diagnosed reflux: a follow-up study. Br J Urol. 1990;65(4):407–12.
12. Crabbe D, Thomas D, Gordon A, et al. Use of ^{99m}technetium-dimercaptosuccinic acid patterns of renal damage associated with prenatally detected vesicoureteric reflux. J Urol. 1992;148:1229–31.
13. Noe H. The long-term result of prospective sibling reflux screening. J Urol. 1992;148:1739.
14. Noe H, Wyatt R, Peeden JJ, et al. The transmission of vesicoureteral reflux from parent to child. J Urol. 1992;148:1869.

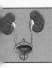

15. Eccles MR, Bailey RR, Abbott GD, Sullivan MJ. Unraveling the genetics of vesicoureteric reflux: a common familial disorder. Hum Mol Genet. 1996;5 Spec No:1425–9.

16. Hutch JA. Theory of maturation of the intravesical ureter. J Urol. 1961;86:534–8.

17. Tamminen-Mobius T, Brunier E, Ebel KD, et al. Cessition of vesicoureteral reflux for 5 years in infants and children allocated to medical treatment. The international reflux study in children. J Urol. 1992;148 (5 pt 2):1662–6.

18. Goldraich N, Goldraich I. Follow up of conservatively treated children with high and low grade vesicoureteral reflux: a prospective study. J Urol. 1992;148:1688–92.

19. Elo J, Tallgreen L, Sarna S, Alfthan O, Stenstrom R. The role of vesicoureteral reflux in pediatric urinary tract infection. Scand J Urol Nephrol. 1981;15:243–8.

20. Garin E, Campos A, Homsy Y. Primary vesicoureteral reflux: review of current concepts. Pediatr Nephrol. 1998;12:249–56.

21. Gross GW, Lebowitz RL. Infection does not cause reflux. AJR. 1981;137(5):929–32.

22. Hodson CJ, Maling TM, McManamon PJ, Lewis MG. The pathogenesis of reflux nephropathy (chronic atrophic pyelonephritis). Br J Radiol. 1975;Suppl 13:1–26.

23. Ransley PG, Risdon RA. Renal papillary morphology and intrarenal reflux in the young pig. Urol Res. 1975;3(3):105–9.

24. Ransley PG, Risdon RA. Renal papillary morphology in infants and young children. Urol Res. 1975;3(3):111–3.

25. Ransley PG, Risdon RA. Reflux and renal scarring. Br J Radiol. 1978;Suppl 14:1–35.

26. Ransley PG, Risdon RA. Reflux nephropathy: effects of antimicrobial therapy on the evolution of the early pyelonephritic scar. Kidney Int. 1981;20(6):733–42.

27. Risdon RA, Godley ML, Gordon I, Ransley PG. Renal pathology and the ^{99m}Tc-DMSA image before and after treatment of the evolving pyelonephritic scar: an experimental study. J Urol. 1994;152(4):1260–6.

28. Ransley PG, Risdon RA, Godley ML. Effects of vesicoureteric reflux on renal growth and function as measured by GFR, plasma creatinine and urinary concentrating ability. An experimental study in the minipig. Br J Urol. 1987;60(3):193–204.

29. Ransley PG, Risdon RA, Godley ML. High pressure sterile vesicoureteral reflux and renal scarring: an experimental study in the pig and minipig. Contrib Nephrol. 1984;39:320–43.

30. Mackie G, Stephens F. Duplex kidneys: A correlation of renal dysplasia with position of the ureteral orifice. J Urol. 1975;114:274–80.

31. Risdon RA, Yeung CK, Ransley PG. Reflux nephropathy in children submitted to unilateral nephrectomy: a clinicopathological study. Clin Nephrol. 1993;40(6):308–14.

32. Hollowell J, Altman H, Snyder H et al. Coexisting ureteropelvic junction obstruction and vesicoureteral reflux: diagnostic and therapeutic implications. J Urol. 1989;142:490.

33. Thomas D. Prenatally detected uropathy: epidemiological considerations. Br J Urol. 1998;81(Suppl 2):8–12.

34. Tibballs JM, De Bruyn R. Primary vesicoureteric reflux – how useful is postnatal ultrasound? Arch Dis Child. 1996;75(5):444–7.

35. Blaufox M, Gruskin A, Sandler P et al. Radionuclide scintigraphy for detection of vesicoureteral reflux in children. J Pediatr. 1971;79:239–46.

36. Peters AM, Morony S, Gordon I. Indirect radionuclide cystography demonstrates reflux under physiological conditions. Clin Radiol. 1990;41(1):44–7.

37. Wallin L, Bajc M. The significance of vesicoureteric reflux on kidney development assessed by dimercaptosuccinate renal scintigraphy. Br J Urol. 1994;73(6):607–11.

38. O'Regan S, Yerbeck S, Schick E. Constipation, bladder instability, urinary tract infection syndrome. Clin Nephrol. 1985;23:152.

39. Edwards D, Normand IC, Prescod N, Smellie JM. Disappearance of vesicoureteric reflux during long-term prophylaxis of urinary tract infection in children. Br Med J. 1977;2(6082):285–8.

40. Wiswell T, Roscelli J. Corroborative evidence for the decreased incidence of urinary tract infections in circumcised male infants. Pediatrics. 1986;79:338.

41. Puri P, O'Donnell B. Correction of experimentally produced vesicoureteric reflux in the piglet by intravesical injection of Teflon. Br Med J Clin Res Educ. 1984;289(6436):5–7.

42. Puri P. Endoscopic correction of primary vesicoureteric reflux by subureteric injection of polytetrafluoroethylene. Lancet. 1990;335(8701):1320–2.

43. Frey P, Whitaker RH. Prevention of vesicoureteric reflux by endoscopic injection. Br J Urol. 1992;69(1):1–6 [published erratum appears in Br J Urol. 1992;70(4):459].

44. Aaronson I, Rames R, Greene W, et al. Endoscopic treatment of reflux: migration of Teflon to the lungs and brains. Eur Urol. 1993;23:394–9.

45. Cohen J. Ureterozystoneostomie. Eine neue Antirefluxtechnik. Aktuel Urol. 1975;6:1.

46. Paquin A. Ureterovesical anastomosis. The description and evaluation of a technique. J Urol. 1959;82:573.

47. Hendren W. Operative repair of megaureter in children. J Urol. 1969;101:491–507.

48. Kalicinski Z, Kanzy K, Kotarvinska B, Joszt W. Surgery of megaureters – modification of Hendren's technique. J Pediatr Surg. 1977;12:183–8.

49. Perdzynski W, Kalicinski Z. Long-term results after megaureter folding in children. J Pediatr Surg. 1996;31:1211–7.

50. Mollard P, Valla V, Sarkissan J. Les echecs du traitement chirurgical des mega-uretères primitifs de l'enfant. J Urol (Paris). 1979;85:625–38.

51. Noe H. The role of dysfunctional voiding in the failure or complication of ureteral reimplantation for primary reflux. J Urol. 1985;134:1172.

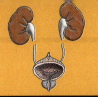

Chapter 19

Urologic Nephrology

Donald Fraser and Mike Venning

KEY POINTS

- Reliance on plasma creatinine alone when measuring renal function may be misleading.
- National guidelines emphasize the importance of early referral to a nephrologist for chronic renal failure patients.
- Typical clinical syndromes may indicate likely underlying renal pathology.
- Accurate assessment of fluid balance is of critical importance to the renal patient.
- Resuscitation skills for patients with acute renal failure should be second nature to the urologic surgeon.
- The nephrotoxicity of common therapeutic agents should be appreciated.

INTRODUCTION: THE FUNCTIONS OF THE KIDNEY

Excretory functions of the kidney

The kidneys are responsible for the excretion of nitrogenous waste products and for maintaining the balance of water, electrolytes, and hydrogen ions in the body. There are approximately 1,000,000 nephrons in each human kidney, each essentially functioning independently to achieve these aims.

Renal blood flow in health accounts for about 20% of cardiac output, or 1200mL/min. Filtration occurs in the glomeruli, producing a total of approximately 125mL of ultrafiltrate per minute in a healthy adult human. This is equivalent to 180L/24 hours, and is referred to as the glomerular filtration rate (GFR). The filtrate passes through the nephron, where resorption of water and electrolytes occurs, leaving the filtered waste products in a concentrated solution to be excreted. Waste products are typically neither reabsorbed nor secreted in great amounts further down the nephron. Therefore, whatever the final volume of urine produced (usually about 1mL/min), the volume of plasma cleared of most waste products corresponds to the original GFR of 125mL/min.

The handling of some endogenous compounds, electrolytes, and drugs, is more complex. Many of these are metabolized, reabsorbed, and excreted at different points along the nephron. Particularly with respect to electrolytes, this allows the kidneys tightly to control homeostasis of these compounds and makes their excretion less dependent on the glomerular filtration rate.

Nonexcretory functions of the kidney

The kidney has important synthetic activity. It produces erythropoietin, which stimulates red blood cell production in the bone marrow, and renin. It is responsible for the 1α-hydroxylation of vitamin D, and so plays a part in bone turnover and the regulation of calcium and phosphate in blood and bone. It filters and metabolizes insulin and low-molecular-weight proteins (such as β_2-microglobulin).

THE SPECTRUM OF RENAL DISEASE

Renal disease can be considered according to clinical presentation, histopathologic appearance, and etiology. The problem lies in the lack of concordance between the three classifications. However there are a number of classic clinical syndromes, which in their pure form indicate the likely pathology (Figs 19.1 & 19.2). Although this is a simplified approach and there is considerable overlap between them, these syndromes provide a useful basis for the practical evaluation of the patient[1]. A further classification according to a combination of pathology and etiology is given in Figures 19.3–19.7.

THE SYNDROMES OF RENAL DISEASE

Nephritis

This syndrome is the clinical manifestation of an inflammatory response within the kidney. It can be further divided into glomerulonephritis and interstitial nephritis.

Glomerulonephritis is recognized by the presence of hematuria (phase contrast microscopy may reveal red cell casts or 'glomerular' dysmorphic red cells); evidence of acutely disordered renal function (oliguria, decreased GFR); edema and hypertension. Proteinuria is also common in glomerular disease, which may alternatively present with the nephrotic syndrome.

Interstitial nephritis presents in a similar fashion, usually without hematuria. Hypertension and edema tend to be less evident, and proteinuria above 3g/24 hours is very rare. Elevated serum IgE, eosinophilia and eosinophiluria are relatively common in acute allergic interstitial nephritis, and may be of diagnostic value.

The nephrotic syndrome

Proteinuria in excess of 3g/day is referred to as within the nephrotic range. When it is associated with edema and hypoalbuminemia (less than 30g/L), the nephrotic syndrome[2] is said to be present. Hyperlipidemia and a hypercoagulable state typically accompany this state. The nephrotic syndrome is pathognomonic of glomerular damage, and a renal biopsy is usually

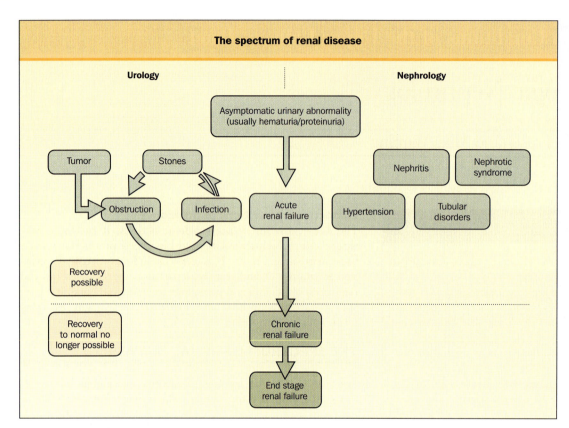

The spectrum of renal disease

Urology | Nephrology

Asymptomatic urinary abnormality (usually hematuria/proteinuria)

Tumor · Stones · Nephritis · Nephrotic syndrome

Obstruction · Infection · Acute renal failure · Hypertension · Tubular disorders

Recovery possible

Recovery to normal no longer possible

Chronic renal failure

End stage renal failure

Figure 19.1 The spectrum of renal disease.

necessary. A notable exception to the need for renal biopsy is the nephrotic syndrome in children, in whom 90% have minimal change disease. This is characterized by highly selective proteinuria and remission with steroid therapy.

Asymptomatic urinary abnormality

Moderate proteinuria and hematuria are usually caused by nephritis, renal failure, urinary tract infection, obstruction, hypertension, or renal stones. In the older patient, malignancy must be excluded. There may be other evidence of these conditions in the history, examination, and initial investigations of the patient. Other causes of each of these urinary abnormalities are shown in Figure 19.2.

Acute and chronic renal failure

Acute renal failure (ARF) must be distinguished from chronic (CRF), as many causes of ARF are potentially reversible, and delay in therapy may cause irreversible loss of renal function. If renal failure is of long duration (6 months or longer) recovery is unlikely, and it may be possible to avoid invasive and potentially hazardous investigations such as renal biopsy or arteriography. In the absence of previously documented renal function, it is often difficult to distinguish ARF from CRF.

Anuria or oliguria indicates that GFR is insufficient for survival, and at least some of the renal impairment must be acute. Renal failure without anemia is indicative of ARF, provided that there is no other reason why the hemoglobin might be normal (for example renal cysts, polycythemia, or erythropoietin-producing tumors).

The presence of symptoms of uremia for months before presentation, physical or biochemical evidence of renal osteodystrophy

Other causes of asymptomatic urinary abnormality	
Hematuria	Alport's syndrome (hereditary nephritis and deafness)
	Thin basement membrane nephropathy
	Hemoglobinuria (includes 'march hematuria', prosthetic heart valves, paroxysmal nocturnal hemoglobinuria)
Proteinuria **(usually less than 1g/day)**	Pyrexia
	Cardiac failure
	Uncontrolled diabetes mellitus
	Exercise
	Upright posture in some individuals (orthostatic proteinuria)

Figure 19.2 Other causes of asymptomatic urinary abnormality.

(corneal calcification, pseudoclubbing, elevated alkaline phosphatase, and parathyroid hormone levels) and small kidneys (e.g. on ultrasound) all indicate CRF. Anemia and abnormal serum calcium and phosphate levels may develop rapidly in the presence of ARF and are not reliable indicators of CRF.

Once CRF is established it is usually difficult to determine the original disease process as the differences between the various syndromes become increasingly blurred.

Urinary tract infection, obstruction, and nephrolithiasis

These entities are described in detail in chapters 21, 22, 23, and 30.

Disorders of the renal tubules

Renal disease of any type is likely to lead to some abnormality of tubular function, but sometimes the tubular disorder is the major or sole cause of the clinical disease. Most of the clinical manifestations of renal tubular disorders result from failure to adequately reabsorb solutes that have been filtered through the glomerulus or, in the case of renal tubular acidosis, failure to adequately acidify urine. Many inherited and acquired disorders of tubular function have been described. The commonest clinical features of tubular disorders are listed elsewhere in this book.

Hypertension

Hypertension may coexist with any of the causes of renal failure. Occasionally hypertension may be the sole cause of renal failure.

CLASSIFICATION OF RENAL DISEASE ACCORDING TO PATHOLOGY AND ETIOLOGY

Diseases in the kidney can be classified according to whether the histopathologic changes seen are acute or chronic, whether they predominantly affect the blood vessels, the glomeruli, or the tubulointerstitium, and whether the disease is a primary renal one or secondary to disease elsewhere.

Renal vascular disease

Renal disease resulting from vascular pathology is listed in Figure 19.3.

Renal artery occlusion leads to complete loss of function of the kidney in the absence of collateral blood supply. As a primary event this is rare, but it is much commoner in those with pre-existing renal artery stenosis.

Renal artery stenosis may be due to atheromatous deposits or to fibromuscular dysplasia. The risk of sudden occlusion is lessened by correcting the stenosis. Blood pressure and existing renal impairment may also be improved, particularly in arterial fibrodysplasia. Angioplasty with or without stent insertion is gaining favor, although surgical techniques are still important. Angiotensin-converting enzyme (ACE) inhibitors may reduce GFR in the affected kidney(s) and should be avoided, although some use them after radiologic or surgical correction of the stenosis. Smaller-vessel arterial disease within the kidney may be under-recognized in the elderly and represents a hazard of ACE inhibitor therapy.

Atheromatous renovascular disease typically presents with hypertension. Modest proteinuria, slowly progressive renal impairment, and flash pulmonary edema (or pulmonary edema disproportionate to left ventricular function) may occur if bilateral disease is present. It is more prevalent in those with known disease in other vascular territories, including cerebrovascular disease, ischemic heart disease, aortic aneurysm, and peripheral vascular disease. Some 25–50% of patients undergoing angiography for disease in other areas will have coexistent atheromatous renovascular disease[3].

Renal artery fibrodysplasia usually presents with severe hypertension before the age of forty. It is commoner in females[4].

Atheromatous embolization down the renal arteries may cause acute renal failure, sometimes with fever and an elevated ESR. Peripheral blood eosinophilia and low complement levels are characteristic associations. A livedo reticularis rash and

Diseases of the renal vasculature	
Primary	Renal artery stenosis (fibromuscular dysplasia)
	Renal artery occlusion
	Renal vein thrombosis
Secondary	Renal artery stenosis (caused by atheroma)
	Cholesterol embolization
	Medium vessel vasculitis (e.g. PAN)
	Hypertensive nephrosclerosis
	Thrombotic microangiopathy (HUS/TTP, scleroderma renal crisis, postpartum ARF, malignant hypertension)

Figure 19.3 Diseases of the renal vasculature. ARF, acute renal failure; HUS/TTP, hemolytic uremic syndrome and thrombotic thrombocytopenic purpura; PAN, polyarteritis nodosa.

gangrenous toes from embolization of the lower limb arteries are suggestive findings. There is a characteristic renal biopsy appearance. There is a strong association with aortic atheroma, both in those with known aortic disease and from postmortem studies. Risk factors include atheromatous renal artery stenosis, recent aortic surgery or angiography, and anticoagulation. Treatment is supportive[5].

Renal vein thrombosis presents with acute renal failure, hematuria and heavy proteinuria. It is commoner in those with a procoagulant tendency, and is an important cause of ARF in those with the nephrotic syndrome.

Medium vessel vasculitis affecting the kidneys typically involves branch or more distal vessels. Polyarteritis nodosa is the commonest example; this can cause renal infarction associated with partial or complete renal artery occlusion.

Glomerular disease[6,7]

Diseases affecting the renal glomeruli (Fig. 19.4), excluding diabetic nephropathy, account for about 15% of those reaching end-stage renal failure[8]. Patients with primary glomerular disease usually present with asymptomatic hematuria, nephritis, the nephrotic syndrome, or chronic renal failure. Renal biopsy is almost always necessary to establish the diagnosis: the severity and rate of deterioration of associated renal impairment determine the urgency of investigation. As well as distinguishing between primary and secondary glomerular disease, glomerulonephritis can be classified as proliferative or nonproliferative according to the degree of cellular proliferation within the glomeruli. A complete description of glomerular disease is beyond the scope of this chapter, but key features of the more important conditions are included below.

Primary glomerular disease

Glomeruli are the sole or predominant tissue involved. Extrarenal abnormalities are secondary to the glomerular damage. Their pathogenesis is currently incompletely understood.

Immunoglobulin A nephropathy is the commonest form of proliferative glomerulonephritis worldwide. Patients commonly present with isolated asymptomatic microscopic hematuria or with episodes of macroscopic hematuria, commonly following

Common glomerular diseases		
Primary	Rapidly progressive glomerulonephritis	Typically necrotizing and crescentic
	Proliferative	IgA nephropathy Mesangiocapillary glomerulonephritis Diffuse proliferative glomerulonephritis
	Nonproliferative:	Minimal change disease Focal segmental glomerulosclerosis Membranous nephropathy
Secondary	Rapidly progressive glomerulonephritis	Small vessel vasculitis Anti-glomerular basement membrane disease
	Proliferative	Myeloma Lupus erythematosus Henoch–Schönlein purpura Related to liver cirrhosis Shunt nephritis Post infectious glomerulonephritis Infective endocarditis Cryoglobulinemia
	Nonproliferative	Diabetic nephropathy Amyloid HIV-associated nephropathy

Figure 19.4 Common glomerular diseases.

respiratory tract infections. The disease progresses to end-stage renal failure (ESRF) in approximately one third of patients. No specific therapies have been proved to be effective, although some trials suggest that immunosuppressive therapy can be of benefit.

Mesangiocapillary glomerulonephritis may be a primary glomerular disease but may also be secondary to a variety of systemic inflammatory conditions and infections. Its association with infections such as bacterial endocarditis, viral hepatitis, malaria, and schistosomiasis make it a relatively common condition in some parts of the world.

Membranous nephropathy is associated with malignancy in one third of cases. The malignancy may present some time after the glomerular disease.

Secondary glomerular disease

Glomerular damage occurs in conjunction with damage to other organs in a variety of diseases. The clinical presentation is similar to the primary glomerular diseases, with evidence of the underlying condition also.

Diabetic nephropathy warrants specific mention as the commonest glomerular disease leading to ESRF: it is responsible for 38% of those reaching ESRF in the USA[8]. It tends to develop 10–20 years after diagnosis of type 1 diabetes but may be present at diagnosis in type 2 (where there is likely to have been subclinical hyperglycemia for some years before diagnosis). Steadily increasing proteinuria precedes renal impairment and treatment with ACE inhibitors improves prognosis.

Small vessel vasculitis commonly presents with ARF associated with hematuria, moderate proteinuria, and hypertension, but little edema. This may occur in isolation, or with evidence of involvement of other organs. Lung and brain involvement may be life threatening. Antineutrophil cytoplasmic antibodies (ANCA) are often positive. Urgent referral to a specialist center for renal biopsy and immunosuppressive treatment is required.

Prerenal causes of acute renal failure
Salt and water depletion
Hemorrhagic shock
Burns
Hypercalcemia
Low-output heart failure
Hepatorenal syndrome

Figure 19.5 Prerenal causes of acute renal failure.

Tubulointerstitial disease

As well as diseases of the tubular compartment of the kidneys, tubulointerstitial damage is often seen in conjunction with damage to the vascular or glomerular compartments[9] (Fig. 19.6). The extent and severity of tubulointerstitial damage are often a better predictor of long-term outcome than the changes in the other compartments, even in diseases considered to be primarily glomerular or vascular.

Primary tubular disorders

Nephrogenic diabetes insipidus. Failure of the kidneys to respond to vasopressin can be inherited as an X-linked condition. This leaves the kidneys unable to concentrate the urine, resulting in polyuria. Minor abnormalities of urinary concentration may also be responsible for familial enuresis, with an underlying genetic basis[10].

Fanconi syndrome. The proximal tubule is responsible for reabsorbing amino acids, glucose, phosphate, and bicarbonate. Proximal tubular damage leads to the presence of these in the urine. The phosphaturia leads to rickets (osteomalacia in adults) and the bicarbonate loss to acidosis. The whole clinical picture is referred to as the Fanconi syndrome.

Cystinuria. An isolated defect in dibasic amino acid reabsorption in the proximal tubule leads to the presence of cystine, ornithine, arginine, and lysine in abnormal quantities in the urine. This occurs in approximately 1 in 7,000 live births. The elevation in urinary cystine concentration leads to precipitation and stone formation. Renal failure does not usually occur.

Renal tubular acidosis. Failure of proximal tubular bicarbonate reabsorption or of distal tubular hydrogen ion secretion will result in metabolic acidosis with a normal anion gap and high serum chloride level. In the case of proximal renal tubular acidosis, defects in reabsorption of other electrolytes are likely, and the full Fanconi syndrome may be present.

Secondary tubular disorders

Acute tubular necrosis[11] is the term that has come to be used for acute renal failure (often oliguric) following circulatory or nephrotoxic insult, where complete recovery is expected if the patient survives the original condition. Common predisposing factors include sepsis, hypoxia, hypotension, tissue damage (e.g. pancreatitis), anesthesia, and pre-existing renal impairment. Recovery is often preceded by a period of polyuria during which careful attention to fluid and electrolyte balance is required. It is the commonest cause of ARF in patients following surgery and on the intensive care unit; the most important differential diagnosis is usually prerenal uremia.

Acute interstitial nephritis usually presents with oliguric acute renal failure of variable severity. It may be associated with eosinophilia or eosinophiluria: the latter is highly suggestive. It is often caused by drugs: especially nonsteroidal anti-inflammatory drugs (NSAIDs) and antibiotics (penicillins and cephalosporins). Virtually any drug may be implicated, however. Interstitial nephritis due to NSAIDs is often distinguished by nephrotic-range proteinuria[12]. Acute interstitial nephritis can also follow infections, particularly streptococcal infections in children. There is anecdotal evidence for benefit from steroid therapy. Many cases recover completely with or without treatment, although temporary dialysis may be required.

Chronic interstitial nephritis is seen following a wide variety of insults to the kidney. Many toxic nephropathies show a chronic interstitial nephritis on renal biopsy. In most cases chronic interstitial nephritis causes slowly progressive renal impairment.

Acute renal failure caused by toxins. Tumor lysis syndrome, rhabdomyolysis, and massive hemolysis cause ARF with deposition of pigment casts in tubules. Alkalinization of urine with intravenous sodium bicarbonate probably helps, by reducing pigment precipitation. In the case of massive hemolysis exchange transfusion may also be required. Nephrotoxic drugs are often given to sick patients in whom many other potential causes of ARF may coexist, and it is important to remember that they may be contributory in their own right.

Papillary necrosis begins as patchy medullary ischemia. This spreads to the papillary tip, leading to papillary sloughing and cortical scarring. Common associations are obstructive uropathy, analgesic nephropathy, sickle-cell disease, and diabetes mellitus.

Miscellaneous

In many cases the etiology of renal disease does not fit neatly into one of the above categories and is linked to specific pre- and postrenal causes (Fig. 19.5 and Chapter 30), drugs and other toxic agents (Fig. 19.7), and specific conditions such as multiple myeloma and chronic pyelonephritis.

ASSESSMENT OF THE PATIENT WITH RENAL IMPAIRMENT

History and examination

A comprehensive and directed history is the most important step in establishing a diagnosis in a patient with renal impairment. A complete record of all recent medication, including nonprescription items, is essential, as idiosyncratic drug reactions are a common cause of renal impairment. Coexisting disease should be sought, such as evidence of autoimmunity, vascular disease, malignancy, or infection.

The single most important part of the examination in the renal patient is the assessment of fluid balance. No single clinical parameter will be reliable in isolation, and information from several sources has to be considered (Fig. 19.8).

The examination may provide evidence of chronic renal failure. There may be evidence of the cause of the renal impairment, such as a distended urinary bladder, vasculitic rash, absent pulses, or vascular bruits.

Tubulointerstitial diseases	
Primary	Inherited tubular disorders
Secondary	Acute tubular necrosis
	Cast nephropathy (myeloma kidney, rhabdomyolysis, acute hemolysis, tumor lysis syndrome)
	Acute interstitial nephritis
	Chronic interstitial nephritis
	Obstruction
	Papillary necrosis

Figure 19.6 Tubulointerstitial diseases.

Causes of toxic nephropathies	
Acute	**Chronic**
Aminoglycosides	Analgesic nephropathy
Amphotericin	Antirejection agents (e.g. cyclosporin)
X-ray contrast medium (see Fig. 19.20)	Chemotherapeutic agents
Myoglobin (rhabdomyolysis)	NSAIDs
Hemoglobin (massive hemolysis)	Lithium
Urate, phosphate, xanthine (Tumor lysis)	Heavy metals
Dextran (lipoid nephrosis)	Hydrocarbons

Figure 19.7 Causes of toxic nephropathies. NSAIDs, nonsteroidal anti-inflammatory drugs.

Laboratory investigation of urine
Blood and protein

Urinalysis is an invaluable aid in the investigation of the kidney. The two principal substances tested for are hemoglobin (usually in intact red blood cells) and protein. Dipsticks may be falsely positive for blood with hemoglobinuria, myoglobinuria, or the presence of many bacteria in the urine. False-negative tests for blood can occur in those taking high doses of vitamin C.

Other substances (tubular function)

If the amount of a substance in the ultrafiltrate exceeds the rest of the nephron's ability to reabsorb (maximal tubular absorptive capacity) or metabolize it then it will be present in the urine, and for each substance in excess a number of mechanisms can be identified (Fig. 19.9).

Renal tubular damage is complex both in the number of possible underlying causes and in the variety of clinical syndromes produced. Figure 19.10 lists abnormalities that suggest an underlying tubular syndrome. Early signs include hypophosphatemia (from renal phosphate wasting), proteinuria (predominantly of low-molecular-weight proteins, usually less than 2g/day), and in some cases acidosis – typically with a normal anion gap. Hypercalciuria can cause nephrolithiasis, which may be the presenting feature of a tubular syndrome.

Urine microscopy

The microscopic examination of a fresh sample of urine can be helpful in several ways. Hemoglobin detected on dipstick

Assessment of fluid balance	
Blood pressure	A low blood pressure suggests dehydration but a normal blood pressure does not exclude it. Postural tachycardia and hypotension is strongly suggestive, and so daily lying and standing (or sitting) pulse and blood pressure can be very informative.
Weight	Daily weighing gives a guide as to changes in hydration state but the accuracy of the scales and changes in amount of clothes worn often render this relatively unhelpful. If changes in weight are to be used to guide fluid replacement, it is vital that the same set of scales is used each day.
Edema	The presence of sacral or lower limb edema is suggestive of overhydration. However it is possible to be edematous and yet intravascularly volume depleted, usually because of a low plasma oncotic pressure (low albumin, e.g. from burns, chronic illness, sepsis, nephrotic syndrome, liver disease) but also in the presence of right-sided heart failure.
Other signs	Other clinical indicators of dehydration are a reduction of skin turgor and dry mucous membranes. Overhydration is evidenced by coarse crackles at the lung bases and pulmonary edema on chest X-ray, a third heart sound, and possibly raised blood pressure.
Right heart filling pressure	Reduction or elevation of the jugular venous pressure is a valuable guide to right heart filling pressure, which reflects intravascular volume if the heart is normal. An alternative is to measure right atrial pressure via a central line.
Left heart filling pressure	If there is significant cardiac or pulmonary disease then right heart pressure may not be an accurate guide to ideal intravascular volume. The information gained by insertion of a pulmonary artery flotation catheter (Swan–Ganz catheter) to measure left heart filling pressure has to be weighed against the risks of this procedure. Clinical assessment and chest X-ray may be sufficient.

Figure 19.8 Assessment of fluid balance.

Reasons that maximal tubular absorptive capacity may be exceeded	
Substance in excess: glucose	
Mechanism	**Example**
Increased blood concentration	Diabetes mellitus
Increased single-nephron GFR	Pregnancy or chronic renal failure
Reduced tubular absorptive capacity	Proximal tubular damage

Figure 19.9 Reasons that maximal tubular absorptive capacity may be exceeded. GFR, glomerular filtration rate.

Clinical and laboratory evidence of disorders of tubular function	
Primary defect in	**Clinical manifestation**
Urinary concentration	Polyuria
Glucose reabsorption	Glycosuria
Phosphate reabsorption	Phosphaturia, rickets
Amino acid reabsorption	Amino aciduria, nephrolithiasis
Hydrogen ion excretion	Renal tubular acidosis
Potassium handling	Hypokalemia or hyperkalemia
Calcium handling	Hypo- or hypercalciuria, nephrolithiasis
Tubular protein secretion	Modest proteinuria

Figure 19.10 Clinical and laboratory evidence of disorders of tubular function.

Measurement of renal function

The assumption that the ability of the kidneys to perform their excretory functions is directly proportional to remaining GFR underpins current laboratory assessment of renal function. GFR can be determined by using a substance that is secreted into the plasma at a constant rate, freely filtered at the glomerulus, and neither secreted nor reabsorbed further down the nephron. Under these conditions, clearance can be calculated using the formula:

Clearance = UV/P,

where U = urine concentration, V = urine flow rate (mL/min), and P = plasma concentration.

No endogenous compound fits this ideal exactly. Measurement of the clearance of infused inulin is the current gold standard test of GFR, but is too time-consuming and expensive for routine clinical use. Radioisotope measurement of GFR is an alternative technique for use when accuracy is critical, e.g. when calculating doses of drugs for cancer chemotherapy. Urea and creatinine are the two endogenous compounds routinely used to assess GFR.

Urea is a product of protein breakdown and so high dietary protein intake and catabolic states increase urea generation and thus its concentration in the blood. It is freely filtered by the glomerulus. It is reabsorbed to a variable degree in the distal nephron, so that urea clearance underestimates GFR by up to 40%. Urea reabsorption is dependent on water reabsorption and so is greatest when the kidneys are avidly conserving salt and water. This causes the disproportionate rise in urea seen in dehydration.

urinalysis can be confirmed to be due to intact *red blood cells*, and these can be examined for dysmorphic features ('glomerular' red cells, suggestive of glomerular disease). *Casts* (cylindrical bodies formed within the renal tubules) are more likely to be detected if a fresh urine sample is centrifuged and the precipitant resuspended. Hyaline (clear) and occasionally granular casts can be seen in normal individuals, but casts consisting of red blood cells are strongly suggestive of glomerular disease. White blood cell casts and abundant urinary eosinophils are usually seen in interstitial nephritis. White cell casts can be difficult to distinguish from the tubular cell casts commonly seen in acute tubular necrosis.

Crystals of urate, calcium oxalate, or triple phosphate may be seen in those under evaluation for renal stone disease. *Microorganisms* may be seen in those with suspected urinary tract infection.

Creatinine is produced by muscle, and so the amount produced daily is dependent on the total muscle mass in the body. It is also freely filtered by the glomerulus, but is secreted into the distal tubule: creatinine clearance overestimates GFR by about 10% in health. As GFR declines, the relative importance of this tubular secretion to the total amount of creatinine excreted rises, and so does the degree of overestimation of GFR. Cimetidine blocks tubular secretion of creatinine and so can be used to produce a more accurate result. Alternatively, some centers average urea clearance and creatinine clearance.

If muscle mass remains constant then the equation above predicts that serum creatinine is inversely proportional to GFR; thus serial measurements of plasma creatinine may be sufficiently informative once GFR has been established. It is important to appreciate that the relationship between serum creatinine and GFR is not linear: a halving of creatinine clearance leads to a doubling in plasma creatinine. With mild renal impairment large losses of GFR lead to small increments in serum creatinine while with advanced renal impairment the converse holds true. See also Chapter 10.

The hazard of reliance on plasma creatinine: example

A large muscular man has a serum creatinine of 1.24mg/dL. A 24 hour urine collection contains 2,000mL of urine and has a creatinine concentration of 101.7mg/dL. His creatinine clearance is 114mL/min. An elderly lady has a serum creatinine of 110μmol/L also. She passes 1,000mL of urine with a creatinine concentration of 56.5mg/dL. Her creatinine clearance is 32mL/min. In both cases a doubling of serum creatinine approximates to a halving of GFR. The man would have a GFR of approximately 57mL/min and relatively mild renal impairment. In contrast, the woman would be near to dialysis, with a GFR of 16mL/min. If his creatinine clearance were to fall to this value his serum creatinine would be expected to rise to above 800μmol/L.

Cockcroft and Gault formula for creatinine clearance[13]:

Formulas have been devised that predict creatinine clearance from serum creatinine, age, sex, and weight. The best known is reproduced below.

$$\text{Creatinine clearance} = \frac{(140 - \text{age}) \times \text{body weight in kg}}{72 \times \text{serum creatinine in mg/dL}}$$

In women, multiply the result by 0.85.

It is often difficult to be certain that a timed urine collection is complete (patient error is common), and so calculation from the above formula may be more accurate than that derived from a 24 hour urine sample in many patients.

Imaging the kidneys

Imaging and functional assessment of the upper urinary tract is important and is discussed in detail in section 2.

Renal biopsy

Renal biopsy is undertaken to establish the diagnosis, suggest prognosis, and direct therapy (Fig. 19.11). Its ability to achieve these aims is often controversial. Accurate diagnosis of intrinsic renal disease usually requires a renal biopsy. Sometimes the clinical features of a patient allow the diagnosis to be secure

Common indications for renal biopsy
Diagnosis of nephrotic syndrome
Diagnosis of acute nephritis
Diagnosis and prognosis post renal transplantation
Diagnosis of asymptomatic urinary abnormality
Prognosis and diagnosis in systemic lupus erythematosus and other multisystem diseases
Evaluation of response to therapy

Figure 19.11 Common indications for renal biopsy.

Resuscitation – life-threatening features of renal failure
Hyperkalemia
Fluid overload
Acidosis
Uremic syndrome

Figure 19.12 Resuscitation – life-threatening features of renal failure.

without this being necessary. This is most often true for acute tubular necrosis, minimal change nephropathy, and Alport's syndrome.

Renal biopsy is relatively safe, with an observed mortality rate of 0.2%. Pain at the biopsy site occurs in 15% and macroscopic hematuria in 3–10%; both are usually self-limiting. Surgical exploration is required in 0.4%[14]. The likelihood of the result of the biopsy altering the patient's management must be weighed against these risks. Renal biopsy is more hazardous in those with a bleeding diathesis or a single functioning kidney. It is also seldom indicated in those with small kidneys, which may be at greater risk of hemorrhage and usually indicate untreatable chronic renal disease.

ACUTE RENAL FAILURE

Acute renal failure can occur in patients with previously normal kidneys or in those with pre-existing renal impairment (acute on chronic renal failure). In either case, management can be divided into immediate resuscitation, subsequent supportive care, establishing the diagnosis, and giving specific treatment.

Oliguric and nonoliguric renal impairment

If the kidneys remain capable of maximally concentrating urine, a normal adult requires a minimum urine output of about 400mL/day for obligate solute excretion. Lower rates of urine flow almost certainly indicate at least a degree of acute renal failure. Nonoliguric acute renal failure is a sudden decline in GFR (usually detected as a rise in urea and creatinine) with a urine flow rate of more than 400mL/day[15].

Resuscitation

Urgent action may be required with respect to the life-threatening features of ARF (Fig. 19.12).

Benign Conditions of the Upper Urinary Tract

Hyperkalemia[16]

Hyperkalemia is the complication of acute renal failure most often encountered in routine clinical practice. It occurs because the kidney is responsible for excreting 95% of ingested potassium (5% is lost in the feces). Acidosis exacerbates hyperkalemia in acute renal failure by reducing renal potassium excretion and by reducing the active transport of potassium into cells.

Hyperkalemia causes profound reduction in resting cell membrane potential. This has effects on all electrically active cells: those on the myocardium are life threatening (Fig. 19.13). The serum potassium concentration at which electrocardiogram (ECG) abnormalities will begin to develop depends on patient sensitivity and the rapidity of development of hyperkalemia: a serum potassium of 6mmol/L or more should lead to ECG monitoring. ECG changes indicate a need for urgent control of hyperkalemia. This can be achieved by:

- Rapid protection of the heart from the effects of a high serum potassium (immediate intravenous injection of 10mL of 10% calcium gluconate). ECG improves within 5min and protection lasts 30–60min.
- Lowering serum potassium by increasing cellular potassium uptake (10 units soluble insulin in 50mL 50% dextrose intravenously over 5min). Begins to lower potassium within 20min, effect lasts up to 6 hours. β_2 agonists are also effective.
- Lowering serum potassium by increasing urinary excretion (250mg furosemide intravenously over 30min). May help prevent hyperkalemia by maintaining urinary potassium loss in the ARF patient.
- Lowering serum potassium by increasing excretion via the gut (kayexalate 60g orally or per rectum three times daily). Onset within 2 hours, effect of each dose lasts about 6 hours.
- Removing potassium from the circulation by dialysis.
- Correction of acidosis increases cellular potassium uptake and increases urinary potassium excretion. It is relatively inefficient at both compared with the above methods, but may be used over several days.

Fluid overload

This may be iatrogenic in the acute renal failure patient. Scrupulous assessment of fluid balance is an important part of day to day management (Fig. 19.8). Fluid overload is avoided (or treated) by establishing a diuresis with loop diuretics, which will have an immediate venodilatory effect as well as their delayed diuretic action. Loop diuretics are organic acids that need to be secreted into the renal tubules in order to work; the accumulation of other organic acids in renal failure means that large doses will be required[17]. A dose of 250–1,000mg of furosemide (frusemide) by infusion over 1h is acceptable for those with severe renal insufficiency. Patients with the nephrotic syndrome are especially resistant to diuretics; this can sometimes be overcome by infusing diuretics together with albumin. Fluid overload unresponsive to loop diuretics is an indication for dialysis. If dialysis is not immediately available the use of other venodilators (such as glyceryl trinitrate) or venesection (initially 400mL) may provide sufficient reduction in preload for a short period in those with life-threatening fluid overload.

Acidosis

In acute renal failure, acidosis occurs because the kidney fails to excrete the nonmetabolizable acids produced by the body. The

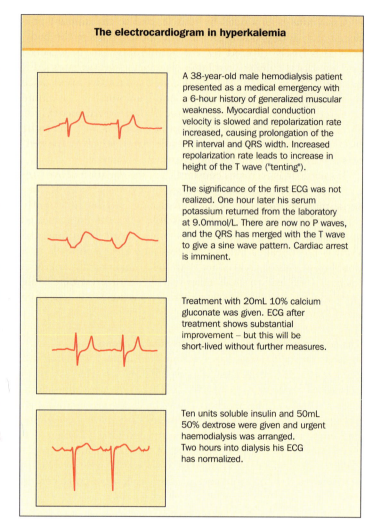

The electrocardiogram in hyperkalemia

A 38-year-old male hemodialysis patient presented as a medical emergency with a 6-hour history of generalized muscular weakness. Myocardial conduction velocity is slowed and repolarization rate increased, causing prolongation of the PR interval and QRS width. Increased repolarization rate leads to increase in height of the T wave ("tenting").

The significance of the first ECG was not realized. One hour later his serum potassium returned from the laboratory at 9.0mmol/L. There are now no P waves, and the QRS has merged with the T wave to give a sine wave pattern. Cardiac arrest is imminent.

Treatment with 20mL 10% calcium gluconate was given. ECG after treatment shows substantial improvement – but this will be short-lived without further measures.

Ten units soluble insulin and 50mL 50% dextrose were given and urgent haemodialysis was arranged. Two hours into dialysis his ECG has normalized.

Figure 19.13 The electrocardiogram (ECG) in hyperkalemia. Each ECG recorded from limb lead II.

most serious consequences include hyperkalemia, impaired cardiac performance, reduced resistance to infection, and malnutrition caused by hypercatabolism. Severe acidosis can be fatal. Mild to moderate acidosis can be treated with bicarbonate infusion, but this may be limited by the risk of sodium or water overload or associated hypocalcemia, and more severe acidosis commonly necessitates dialysis. If bicarbonate is used it should be noted that an 8.4% solution contains 1mmol/mL. An appropriate initial dose is 500mL of a 1.4% solution (contains 83mmol) or 50mL of an 8.4% solution (50mmol).

Uremic syndrome

The life-threatening components of the uremic syndrome are *pericarditis* and *encephalopathy*. Both are absolute indications for urgent dialysis. The clinical features suggestive of each of these conditions are summarized in Figure 19.14. *Pericarditis*: hypotension, Kussmaul's sign, or pulsus paradoxus suggest that cardiac tamponade is developing. An echocardiogram will demonstrate excess fluid in the pericardial sac and may show evidence of cardiac tamponade. Pericardial aspiration may be required in advance of dialysis. *Encephalopathy* often begins as mild disorientation and confusion. The patient becomes progressively obtunded over days. Convulsions may occur.

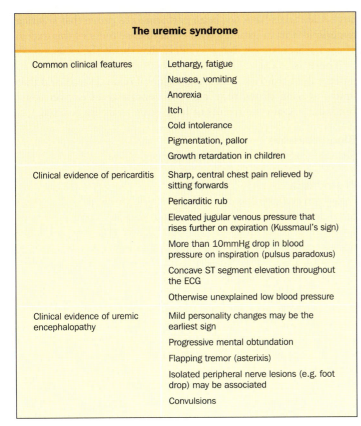

The uremic syndrome	
Common clinical features	Lethargy, fatigue
	Nausea, vomiting
	Anorexia
	Itch
	Cold intolerance
	Pigmentation, pallor
	Growth retardation in children
Clinical evidence of pericarditis	Sharp, central chest pain relieved by sitting forwards
	Pericarditic rub
	Elevated jugular venous pressure that rises further on expiration (Kussmaul's sign)
	More than 10mmHg drop in blood pressure on inspiration (pulsus paradoxus)
	Concave ST segment elevation throughout the ECG
	Otherwise unexplained low blood pressure
Clinical evidence of uremic encephalopathy	Mild personality changes may be the earliest sign
	Progressive mental obtundation
	Flapping tremor (asterixis)
	Isolated peripheral nerve lesions (e.g. foot drop) may be associated
	Convulsions

Figure 19.14 The uremic syndrome. ECG, electrocardiogram.

None of these signs of advanced uremia are due solely to urea. Rather there is a large array of other toxins cleared by the kidney that accumulate in renal failure. There is no blood level of urea that can be used as a guide for their development, but they are very unlikely to occur below a concentration of 30mmol/L. This is often used as the cutoff for initiation of dialysis in intensive care patients.

Hypocalcemia

This is a common accompaniment to acute renal failure, although it is rarely severe enough to cause tetany or convulsions. However it is important to remember that acidosis protects against the effects of a low serum calcium by reducing its binding to plasma proteins and hence increasing the fraction of serum calcium that is ionized. Therefore, correction of acidosis can rapidly lower plasma ionized calcium and cause convulsions in a hypocalcemic patient.

If urgent correction is necessary, this is easily achieved with intravenous calcium carbonate (typically 10mL of a 10% solution). It is important not to give this via a drip that has been used for sodium bicarbonate infusion, as insoluble calcium carbonate (chalk) will be formed. The resulting tissue damage can lead to severe skin necrosis with the need for skin grafting. Similar damage can be caused by hypertonic calcium solution alone if extravasation occurs. When possible, concentrated calcium solution should be administered via a central line.

Supportive care

Patients with established renal failure need attention to many facets of their care. These are detailed in the section on chronic

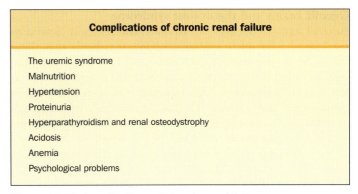

Complications of chronic renal failure
The uremic syndrome
Malnutrition
Hypertension
Proteinuria
Hyperparathyroidism and renal osteodystrophy
Acidosis
Anemia
Psychological problems

Figure 19.15 Complications of chronic renal failure.

renal failure. In the acute renal failure patient it is also important to be wary of the complications of immobility, such as deep venous thrombosis, pulmonary embolism, osteoporosis, hypercalcemia, muscle wasting, and pressure sores. There is also an increased risk of peptic ulceration.

There have been many attempts to improve renal recovery and patient survival in acute renal failure by the administration of drugs, mostly vasoactive substances (especially dopamine) and diuretics. No compound has been shown to be of unequivocal benefit, although the use of diuretics can make oliguric renal failure easier to manage by increasing the urine output and so 'making room' in the circulation for drugs and nutrition. Until adequate evidence of effectiveness is forthcoming, use of other agents such as dopamine is controversial[18,19].

Establishing the cause and giving specific treatment

It is important to remember that acute renal failure is not in itself a diagnosis. The underlying cause must be rapidly determined to allow specific treatment and the best chance of renal recovery. Dehydration and obstruction are common and should be excluded by assessment of fluid balance and by renal ultrasound. Intrinsic renal disease other than acute tubular necrosis should be looked for with urine dipstick and microscopy.

CHRONIC RENAL FAILURE

Inevitably, and despite the best care, most patients with CRF slowly lose residual renal function, possibly through the increased burden placed upon the remaining nephrons[20].

As nephron loss progresses the homeostatic and synthetic functions of the kidney fail, causing a variety of clinical problems (Fig. 19.15). These problems are often relatively easy to deal with when they first occur, but if not managed appropriately they can become irretrievable. Most of these complications present insidiously and must be carefully looked for during the follow-up of the CRF patient. Early assessment by a nephrologist is advisable in those at risk of progressive CRF. National guidelines recommend referral at or before serum creatinine of 2mg/dL (1.5mg/dL in women)[21] or 150mmol[22].

Although a gradual loss of function is often inevitable, it is important that this occurs as slowly as possible. Care must be taken to limit exposure of the patient to nephrotoxic agents and to control parameters known to influence rate of nephron loss, particularly blood pressure and proteinuria.

Uremic toxins and the uremic syndrome

As renal function declines the various toxins normally cleared by the kidney accumulate within the body. It is likely that these toxins are responsible for the collection of symptoms and the increase in incidence of certain diseases that are referred to as the uremic syndrome[23]. The importance of urea as a toxin is controversial and it is now felt that the accumulation of a range of other chemicals is of equal or greater importance[24]. At present these remain unmeasured and the assessment of the severity of the uremic syndrome has to take place on clinical grounds.

Diet and nutrition[25]

Malnutrition is multifactorial in CRF patients (Fig. 19.16). Indicators of malnutrition have been shown to be predictive of increased mortality in patients with chronic renal failure, especially those on dialysis[26]. It is hard to reverse malnourishment once it is present. It is easily overlooked among the other factors requiring attention in the CRF patient. Various dietary restrictions are likely to become necessary as GFR falls (Fig. 19.17). The attention of a dietitian skilled in dealing with renal failure patients is valuable in preventing malnutrition and for advice on dietary restriction.

Low protein diets

There is evidence from animal and patient studies that a low protein diet retards the progression of chronic renal failure. However, a large prospective randomized trial of low protein diets in patients with CRF has failed to show a beneficial effect[27]. Patients on low protein diets require careful monitoring to ensure that they do not become malnourished, and so they are not in widespread use.

Lipids and renal disease

Patients with renal disease have higher blood lipid levels and an increased incidence of cardiovascular disease. Sufficiently large-scale trials have not been performed to prove that treating hyperlipidemia in patients with renal disease reduces this excess of cardiovascular risk, but it is likely that this is the case.

There is some evidence that hyperlipidemia may be an independent risk factor for progression of renal disease, and that lipid-lowering drugs may exert a beneficial effect on renal function[28]. Again the results of large-scale trials are awaited.

Blood pressure

See under Hypertension and the kidney, below.

Proteinuria

Heavy proteinuria has been shown to be predictive of a more rapid decline in renal function[29]. Blood pressure control reduces proteinuria. ACE inhibitors are particularly effective, probably because of their renal hemodynamic effects[30,31].

In some disorders, particularly diabetic nephropathy, reduction of proteinuria by the prescription of an ACE inhibitor has been shown to retard the progression of renal impairment. An ACE inhibitor may thus be the initial drug of choice in managing hypertension in patients with CRF, except where renal artery stenosis is a possibility. They may also have a role in reducing proteinuria in normotensive patients, particularly those with diabetic nephropathy.

Angiotensin receptor antagonists are a relatively new class of drugs that may share the benefits of ACE inhibitors, although there is less evidence to support their use[32]. At present they should be reserved for those patients who are intolerant of ACE inhibitors, particularly as a result of a cough. Nondihydropyridine calcium channel blockers may have a similar effect on proteinuria, but the evidence for their use is also not secure[33].

Smoking

Smoking compounds the high cardiovascular risk of the CRF patient. It also reduces bone density, increasing the risk of

Factors contributing to the risk of malnutrition in renal failure patients	
Reduced energy intake	Nausea and anorexia from uremic toxins and from chronic illness
	Dietary restrictions and fluid restriction
	Large number of tablets, some of which are bulky (phosphate binders, iron, bicarbonate)
	Increase in gastrointestinal symptoms and disease
	Missing meals because of hemodialysis sessions and investigations
	Feeling of fullness from intraperitoneal dialysis fluid (in the CAPD patient)
Increased energy expenditure	Increased protein catabolism as a result of acidosis and dialysis
	Possible increase in resting energy expenditure
	Catabolism during periods of acute illness (e.g. sepsis)

Figure 19.16 Factors contributing to the risk of malnutrition in renal failure patients. CAPD, continuous ambulatory peritoneal dialysis.

Dietary restrictions likely to be necessary in the chronic renal failure patient		
Item	Accumulation causes	Foods to avoid or restrict
Potassium	Risk of arrhythmias and cardiac arrest	Coffee, chocolate, bananas, orange juice, potatoes, salt substitutes
Phosphate	Secondary hyperparathyroidism and ectopic calcification	Cheese, milk, yogurt
Protein	Increased acidosis and rate of nephron loss	Meat (animal protein is especially problematic)
Sodium	Edema, hypertension, cardiac failure	Table salt, most tinned foods, soups
Water	Edema, hypertension, cardiac failure	Necessary to limit total fluid intake to less than 500ml/day in some dialysis patients
Cholesterol	High risk of cardiovascular disease	Saturated fats

Figure 19.17 Dietary restrictions likely to be necessary in the chronic renal failure patient.

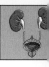
osteoporosis, which will already be high in those on long-term corticosteroids (many patents with glomerulonephritis or a renal transplant). There is evidence for an increased rate of progression of CRF in smokers compared to nonsmokers, particularly in those with diabetes mellitus[34].

The skeleton and parathyroid dysfunction
The kidney is responsible for the 1α-hydroxylation of vitamin D and the excretion of phosphate in health. The failure of these two functions causes the hyperparathyroidism and renal osteodystrophy often seen in CRF patients. The end result is hypocalcemia and hyperphosphatemia with grossly elevated parathyroid hormone (PTH) and bone turnover. Lytic lesions cause bone pain and predispose to fractures. Elevation of the calcium phosphate product risks calcification in the tissues and the vessel walls, causing accelerated ischemic heart disease and peripheral vascular disease. These risks can be minimized by the judicious use of alfa-calcidol (in low dose to increase calcium absorption from the gut or in high dose to suppress PTH) and phosphate binders (commonly calcium salts). Left untreated, the parathyroid glands enlarge to the point where the only option is parathyroidectomy.

Anemia
The kidney produces erythropoietin, the hormone responsible for stimulating red cell production and maturation in the bone marrow. Recombinant erythropoietin is now available and has transformed the management of the anemia of chronic renal failure. These patients are often functionally iron-deficient and fail to respond to oral iron, and so may also require intravenous iron therapy.

As with the other signs of advancing uremia, there is no level of glomerular filtration rate below which anemia will occur. It is likely to be the cause in those with a GFR below 25mL/min who present with a normochromic normocytic anemia and no evidence of iron deficiency. Symptoms suggestive of another cause for the anemia, or a failure to respond as expected to erythropoietin, should lead to a search for other causes, usually by imaging the upper and lower gastrointestinal tract given the increased incidence of gastritis/peptic ulcer disease.

Acidosis
Chronic acidosis causes catabolism of proteins, increases leaching of calcium and phosphate from the bones, reduces resistance to infection, and reduces response to insulin and erythropoietin. Acidosis is associated with increased mortality in dialysis patients[26], and correction of acidosis probably improves nutritional status in CRF patients[35]. Correction with oral sodium bicarbonate may be possible, but the sodium load that this represents may worsen hypertension and edema.

Psychologic care
Renal failure brings an increasing burden to people's lives, both in terms of medical intervention (time in hospital, invasive investigations and therapies, medication) and in reduction of wellbeing (from advancing uremia, anemia, side effects of therapy, admissions with complications such as infection). Fear of the need for interventions such as dialysis and transplantation, fear of loss of employment and independence, and fear of death

also take their toll. There is a high incidence of breakdown of marriage and long-term relationships in those on dialysis.

It is important that all of the members of the multidisciplinary team caring for the patient are aware of these issues so that appropriate counseling can be given.

Patient education
Information about a patient's prognosis and the probable time before dialysis is required will reduce anxiety and, by allowing patients to make informed decisions on their care, will ensure the minimum possible impact on their normal life.

Compliance with drugs and with restrictions on diet and fluids will be improved by explaining why these are necessary. Anxiety concerning what dialysis will mean for an individual can be reduced by arranging a visit to the dialysis unit and providing special educational materials such as books and videos.

Long periods of ill health, frequent admissions to hospital, and the time required for dialysis make continuing in full-time employment very difficult for many CRF patients. Financial advice from a social worker knowledgable in the special needs of these patients can be of great help to them.

Preparation for renal replacement therapy
This is covered in the section on the patient needing renal replacement therapy.

Care of the family members
The cause of renal impairment may have implications for the health of family members. Genetic counseling may be required,

The family of the patient (including the patient's partner) may wish to be considered as kidney donors. The partner will have anxieties about the patient's life expectancy and likely morbidity.

Pregnancy and renal disease[36]
The prognosis for pregnancy in the presence of renal disease is now more optimistic than in the recent past, particularly with respect to fetal outcome. The underlying diagnosis appears less important than the degree of renal impairment present. Levels of risk are relatively well defined (Fig. 19.18) although greater caution is required in those with systemic inflammatory diseases such as systemic lupus erythematosus or vasculitis. All pregnancies in the presence of renal disease should be regarded as high-risk and require careful multidisciplinary management.

HYPERTENSION AND THE KIDNEY

Secondary hypertension
Renal disease is the commonest cause of secondary hypertension: CRF of any cause commonly leads to hypertension and in atheromatous renal artery stenosis and glomerulonephritis hypertension may precede reduction in GFR.

Hypertension and chronic renal impairment
Lowering blood pressure is known to retard the rate of progression of renal impairment. Hypertension is often hard to control in the setting of renal impairment: four or more drugs may be required[37]. Blood pressure targets are lower than in the general population and so effective treatment of the blood pressure of a patient with CRF is often a challenge.

Pregnancy in renal disease: fetal and maternal prognosis	
Serum creatinine at booking (μmol per L/mg per dL)	**Risks to mother and fetus**
Abnormal but less than 180/2.03 (130–150/1.5–1.7 for diabetic nephropathy)	Fetal loss rate 7–16%, little risk of deterioration in maternal renal function
180/2.03 to 250/2.8	Increasing risk of fetal loss, preterm delivery, and intrauterine growth retardation; concomitant increase in permanent deterioration in maternal renal function
Greater than 250/2.8	High risk of fetal loss or severe complications; high risk of maternal renal function deteriorating to dialysis dependency
The presence of uncontrolled hypertension or heavy proteinuria greatly increases the level of risk.	

Figure 19.18 Pregnancy in renal disease: fetal and maternal prognosis.

Blood pressure targets

Targets for instituting antihypertensive therapy remain controversial. The aim of treatment is reduction of cardiovascular risk and prevention of progression of end-organ damage. The absolute benefit that individuals stand to gain from treatment depends on their level of risk for these diseases. In other words, the target blood pressure for an individual should take account of the comorbid conditions present. This is reflected in recent guidelines[38,39]. Renal impairment of any cause should lead to lower blood pressure targets than those employed for the general population. A blood pressure target of less than 140/80 is widely accepted in diabetics[39], and may be appropriate in patients with nondiabetic renal disease who do not yet require dialysis.

Treatment of hypertension

Weight loss, regular aerobic exercise, and moderation of alcohol and sodium intake have all been shown to reduce blood pressure effectively and should be considered in all hypertensive patients[40]. Where possible, known pressor agents such as the oral contraceptive pill, licorice, and tobacco should be avoided. Relaxation therapies may be useful in selected individuals.

A number of additional considerations affect choice of agent in the CRF patient (Fig. 19.19).

Accelerated hypertension

This is a clinical syndrome characterized by marked elevation in blood pressure and widespread arteriolar injury. Diastolic blood pressure (DBP) is usually at least 110mmHg, but in children may be as low as 100mmHg. Before effective antihypertensive therapy was available this condition had a 90% 1-year mortality.

Retinal hemorrhages and exudates may be diagnostic, although acute rises in blood pressure can lead to convulsions without these fundal changes. The term *malignant hypertension* is generally reserved for those cases where papilledema is also present

Choice of antihypertensives for the patient with renal impairment	
Drug class	**Comment**
ACE inhibitors	Drug of choice in those with diabetes mellitus or proteinuria; avoid if renal artery stenosis is suspected
Angiotensin II receptor antagonists	As ACE inhibitors but beneficial effects less well established
Calcium channel blockers	Rate limiting calcium channel blockers e.g. verapamil, may be renoprotective, but trials are not conclusive
Beta blockers	Effective
Alpha blockers	Effective
Thiazide diuretics	Ineffective: avoid (except metolazone)
Loop diuretics	Drug of choice in those with edema or fluid overload; risk of dehydration
Methyldopa (centrally acting; predominantly alpha agonist)	Effective; causes depression in higher doses; safe in pregnancy
Moxonidine (centrally acting; predominantly imidazoline-1 antagonist)	Effective
Arteriolar vasodilators (hydralazine, minoxidil)	Risk of tachycardia; also of fluid retention with Minoxidil – requires coprescription of beta blocker and diuretic

Figure 19.19 Choice of antihypertensives for the patient with renal impairment. ACE, angiotensin-converting enzyme.

(grade IV retinopathy); there is often encephalopathy also. Fibrinoid necrosis in the renal arterioles and glomeruli commonly cause acute renal failure.

The aim in management (in the absence of convulsions or hypertensive heart failure) should be to lower the DBP to a value approximately halfway between the initial DBP and 90mmHg in the first 24 hours, and to reduce it below 100mmHg over the next several days. Over-rapid blood pressure reduction carries a high risk of cerebral infarction, as autoregulation of cerebral perfusion is impaired. The initial drug chosen should reflect this aim: sublingual nifedipine is not a good choice as its effects are unpredictable and can be profound[41]. A longer-acting preparation of a calcium channel blocker or a beta-blocker is a safer alternative[42]. Methyldopa, hydralazine, and ACE inhibitors are acceptable alternatives. Some authorities still favor continuous infusions of hydralazine, labetolol, or sodium nitroprusside. The latter has the shortest duration of action, allowing very precise blood pressure control. Intra-arterial blood pressure monitoring is required with this agent. Whatever agent is used, very close supervision of the patient is required.

Atheromatous renovascular disease

This is an underdiagnosed cause of hypertension and renal impairment. It is especially worth considering in those with atheroma in other vascular areas and in those with severe hypertension that develops below the age of 40.

DRUGS AND THE PATIENT WITH RENAL IMPAIRMENT

Drug pharmacology in the presence of renal impairment

Renal impairment has profound effects on the pharmacokinetics and pharmacodynamics of many drugs. The gastrointestinal absorption of many drugs is reduced by a range of factors, including the phosphate binders prescribed in renal failure. Plasma protein binding of drugs in the circulation is often reduced, which may enhance the activity of the drug for a given dose or plasma level and may also enhance clearance of the drug. Apparent volume of distribution of drugs varies enormously. The rate of metabolism and excretion of drugs is also variable in the presence of renal impairment but excretion is often reduced. Drugs may be cleared by dialysis sessions, requiring extra doses to maintain therapeutic levels.

Drug prescribing in the patient with renal impairment

The net effect is often a requirement for a normal loading dose of the drug, with substantial reduction in subsequent doses or prolongation of dose interval, or both. Unfortunately, the variety in these effects with respect to individual drugs means that few other generalizations can be made. When prescribing for the patient with renal impairment it is advisable to check the necessary dosage adjustment and safety of all drugs before using them. General pharmaceutical literature may be sufficient. Alternatively, an excellent short reference book has been published by the American College of Physicians[43]. Some of the common pitfalls with specific drugs are outlined below.

No drug should be prescribed to the patient with renal impairment without first carefully considering the alternatives. In other words, is a drug necessary in this situation and, of the possible effective agents, is this the one least likely to cause problems? All drugs should be considered to be potentially nephrotoxic and the patient should be monitored accordingly even if the answer to both questions is yes. Figure 19.20 indicates the drugs and other compounds most likely to cause additional problems in those with renal impairment. Particular issues with other drugs are listed in Figure 19.21.

THE PATIENT REQUIRING RENAL REPLACEMENT THERAPY

The goal of renal replacement therapy is to provide a substitute for all the functions of the kidneys with the minimum of risks and inconvenience to the patient. At present only renal transplantation can hope fully to replace the activity of the native kidneys, but brings with it a significant morbidity in terms of operative risk and immunosuppressive burden. Dialysis and transplantation are relatively new treatments; there have been large improvements in their efficacy, tolerability, and durability since they were introduced. It can be expected that this trend will continue.

Modalities of renal replacement therapy

Dialysis attempts to replace the excretory functions of the kidney. Blood is exposed to dialysis solution across a selectively permeable membrane, which allows low-molecular-weight compounds to move freely between the two solutions but restricts

Drugs to be used with particular caution in those with renal impairment	
ACE inhibitors	Avoid in those with renal artery stenosis. Renal blood flow is dependent on efferent arteriolar tone, and reduction of this by ACE inhibition may seriously damage renal function, sometimes irreversibly. Risk of profound hypotension in patients with heart failure or volume depletion. These hazards are shared by angiotensin-receptor antagonists.
Aminoglycosides	Very narrow therapeutic range and, with prolonged treatment, toxic within it. Predominantly renal excretion. High risk of ototoxicity and nephrotoxicity in those with renal impairment. Toxicity mainly relates to trough plasma concentration, so once-daily (or less frequent) dosing may be safer if their use is essential. Netilmicin is probably the least nephrotoxic.
NSAIDs	Risk of nephrotoxicity, partly from effect on prostaglandin-mediated renal vasoregulation. Damage caused by other insults to the kidney (e.g. hypoxia, hypotension, or sepsis) is likely to be enhanced. Increased risk of peptic ulceration in the uremic patient.
Tetracyclines	These have an antianabolic effect, increasing blood urea, and should be avoided in those with renal impairment.
X-ray contrast medium	Toxicity enhanced by renal failure, particularly with diabetes mellitus, myeloma, dehydration, and low cardiac output states. Even nonionized contrast can cause ARF. IVU relies on the excretion of the contrast by the kidney and so will not be helpful in the presence of advanced renal failure. See also Chapter 7.

Figure 19.20 Drugs to be used with particular caution in those with renal impairment. ACE, angiotensin-converting enzyme; ARF, acute renal failure; IVU, intravenous urogram.

the passage of larger molecules. In hemodialysis the membrane is contained in a disposable dialyser cartridge; in peritoneal dialysis it is the patient's own peritoneum[44].

Chronic dialysis: hemodialysis

Intermittent hemodialysis is used in CRF. The aim is to provide the optimal dose of dialysis in the shortest possible time, but there is no consensus on the ideal duration; three 3–4 hour sessions per week is usual. This is usually provided in-center, although home hemodialysis can be successful in motivated and capable individuals. The best survival outcomes have been achieved in centers undertaking long-hours dialysis, with up to 45% of patients surviving 20 years[45].

Chronic dialysis: peritoneal dialysis

Continuous ambulatory peritoneal dialysis (CAPD) is the usual method. The patient performs exchanges of dialysate fluid (usually) four times per day via a tunneled peritoneal catheter (Tenckhoff catheter). There is always dialysate in the peritoneal cavity, allowing low-efficiency continuous removal of fluid and solutes. Peritoneal dialysis tends to have limited durability compared to hemodialysis as a result of patient burnout and technique failure.

Important considerations with the prescription of other drugs

Antimicrobial agents

Many are renally excreted, with lower doses and extended dose intervals required

Aciclovir	Risk of accumulation and encephalopathy: reduce dose
Amphotericin	Nephrotoxic: liposomal and colloid dispersed formulation probably less so
Vancomycin	Nephrotoxic and greatly reduced clearance

Cardiovascular agents

Digoxin	Cleared by the kidney: reduce dose Increased risk of toxicity in hemodialysis caused by transient hypokalemia on dialysis
Diuretics (potassium-sparing)	Risk of hyperkalemia: caution (avoid in severe renal impairment)
Diuretics (other)	Organic acids that rely on secretion into tubular lumen: efficacy reduced in renal impairment so (much) larger doses required (loop diuretics) or are ineffective and should be avoided (thiazides except metolazone)
Procainamide	Clearance of drug and active metabolite reduced leading to unpredictable efficacy and toxicity: avoid if possible

Drugs active on the CNS

Benzodiazepines, barbiturates, tricyclic antidepressants and phenothiazines	Drugs and active metabolites accumulate with prolonged use in CRF: risk of drowsiness
Opioids and opiates	Accumulation of drugs and metabolites: caution required, particularly in those with ESRF (Fig. 19.22); meperidine (pethidine) is probably the safest. Newer agents may prove to have important advantages
Phenytoin	Reduced protein binding means that lower total plasma levels are therapeutic (and toxic); there is also reduced clearance of drug

Diabetic medication

Insulin	Reduced metabolism of insulin by the kidney: dose reduction usually required
Metformin	Lactic acidosis: avoid in severe renal impairment
Sulfonylureas	Prolonged half-life: risk of hypoglycemia, gliclazide, tolbutamide, and glipizide are preferred as they are the shortest-acting drugs of this class

Other drugs

Allopurinol	Toxic metabolite accumulates. Reduce dose. Avoid in those prescribed azathioprine (risk of fatal bone marrow suppression)
Antacids	May contain enough sodium to exacerbate thirst and edema. Avoid those containing aluminum (risk of bone disease and dementia)
H_2 receptor antagonists, particularly cimetidine	Accumulate and cause drowsiness or confusion: reduce dose
Immunosuppressants and cytotoxic agents	Risks of toxicity and drug accumulation are enhanced

Figure 19.21 Important considerations with the prescription of other drugs. CNS, central nervous system; CRF, chronic renal failure; ESRF, end-stage renal failure.

Acute dialysis

Continuous filtration techniques are often used in ARF, allowing precise fluid and electrolyte control and gentle correction of uremia.

Transplantation

Patients under consideration for transplantation need assessment to ensure that they are fit for the operation and that they are likely to survive sufficiently long for it to be worthwhile pursuing. They should be known to be free of conditions that would make immunosuppression particularly hazardous: those with chronic infections such as hepatitis B or C and human immunodeficiency virus infection need very careful assessment. Further information on renal transplantation is provided in Chapter 20.

Ideally, patients with ESRF are prepared for transplantation before requiring dialysis, but this is often not possible. Wherever possible the decision on modality of dialysis is taken by the patient, after they have been educated sufficiently to make an informed choice. Peritoneal dialysis has potential advantages early in the course of renal replacement therapy and should be offered to all suitable new patients[46].

Initiation of renal replacement therapy

Acute renal failure. Conventional indications for urgent dialysis are life-threatening hyperkalemia, fluid overload, acidosis, or uremia unresponsive to other treatments. In those with ARF, dialysis may be instituted prophylactically when serum urea is greater than 30mmol/L[47].

Chronic renal failure. Timing of renal replacement therapy in CRF requires judgment. Creatinine clearance of less than 10mL/min is a common guide, but the clinical condition of the patient is of primary importance. Old, frail, diabetic, or malnourished patients may benefit from earlier dialysis. When the need for dialysis is predictable, suitable access to the peritoneal cavity or bloodstream should be planned (see below).

Special considerations in the care of the dialysis patient

Provided the patient has been carefully managed in the predialysis phase, management of the complications of renal failure can continue much as before. Unfortunately, many have acquired complications before starting dialysis and it may be difficult to reverse problems such as severe hyperparathyroidism or malnutrition once they are established. Such problems are often avoidable with good predialysis care in those whose renal impairment is detected early.

Particular areas of a patient's care require special attention in the dialysis patient.

Drugs

Patients on dialysis usually have a glomerular filtration rate of 15mL/min or less. This has profound implications for their clearance of drugs and metabolites. These may also be cleared by their dialysis treatments, so the timing of drug doses with respect to dialysis can be important. Examples of drugs that are used differently in the patient on dialysis are provided in Figure 19.22.

Drugs that require very different prescription in the dialysis patient	
Drug	**Notes**
Vancomycin	A large molecule poorly cleared by all forms of dialysis (but may be cleared to a greater degree by continuous hemofiltration techniques). Dose of 1g once weekly usually results in consistently therapeutic drug levels (usual dose 1g twice daily).
Aminoglycosides, e.g. netilmicin	Cleared to a variable degree by both hemodialysis and peritoneal dialysis. Dose likely to be greatly reduced (e.g. one third of usual daily dose every 2 days) and monitoring of plasma levels required. Note that even if nephrotoxicity is no longer an issue, ototoxicity is still a serious complication of therapy
Morphine	Smaller doses are likely to be effective. Accumulation of metabolites normally cleared by the kidney such as morphine-6 glucuronide can cause profound narcosis and respiratory depression. Morphine-6 glucuronide is not cleared by dialysis, and clearance will take days to weeks in the anephric patient
Meperidine	Accumulation of normeperidine (a metabolite) can cause seizures: great care needed with use for longer than 24 hours
Digoxin	Reduced clearance. Transient profound hypokalemia is common on hemodialysis, increasing the risk of arrhythmia with digoxin.

Figure 19.22 Drugs that require very different prescription in the dialysis patient.

Access

Access to the circulation is required for hemodialysis, and to the peritoneal cavity for peritoneal dialysis (Fig. 19.23). The more durable types of access are desirable for those who will require long-term dialysis, but these are more invasive to place and usually require a period of maturation before they can be used. Note that in any patient likely to require long-term dialysis the forearm veins should not be used for venepuncture or cannulation to avoid loss of a potential fistula site.

The importance of residual renal function

There is a trend to start people on dialysis increasingly early in the course of their chronic renal failure. At one time most patients would not start dialysis until their GFR was below 5mL/min. In an effort to prevent complications taking hold before dialysis is initiated, this has gradually shifted to the extent that some patients now begin dialysis with a GFR above 15mL/min.

Dialysis patients with some residual renal function survive longer than those without[48]. They will need less severe dietary restriction and a lower dose of dialysis, meaning a shorter time on hemodialysis or less fluid exchanges per day with peritoneal dialysis. It is very important to safeguard residual renal function in the dialysis patient by avoiding nephrotoxic agents and by scrupulous attention to fluid balance at times of intercurrent illness or surgical procedures.

Figure 19.23 Dialysis access.

Dialysis access		
Type	**Usable**	**Comments**
Hemodialysis		
Central venous catheter (femoral/jugular/subclavian) Avoid subclavian where possible	Immediately	Usual maximum life of 2 weeks. Complications include venous stenosis, which may prevent subsequent fistula or graft from being successful (particularly with subclavian catheters)
Tunneled central venous catheter	Immediately	May last 1 year or more. Main complications are sepsis and catheter blockage.
Arteriovenous fistula	2–6 weeks	May last indefinitely. Requires adequate artery and vein: Doppler studies can be helpful in assessing patients with diabetes mellitus and peripheral vascular disease. Avoid cannulation of the veins of the forearm and wrist in those likely to require fistula formation.
Arteriovenous graft	1–2 weeks	More prone to thrombosis and infection than a fistula. Alternative for those whose vessels are inadequate for fistula formation.
Peritoneal dialysis access		
Hard cannula	Immediately	Usable for 1 week
Tenckhoff catheter	2 weeks	Can be placed by minilaparotomy, laparoscopy, or percutaneous technique. Risk of fluid leaks increased by using the catheter sooner than 2 weeks.

REFERENCES

1. Coe FL. Clinical and laboratory assessment of the patient with renal disease. In: Brenner BM, Rector FC, eds. The kidney, 2nd edn. Philadelphia: WB Saunders, 1981:1135–80.
2. Orth SR, Ritz MD. The nephrotic syndrome. N Engl J Med. 1998;338:1202–11.
3. Scoble JE. The epidemiology and clinical manifestations of atherosclerotic renal disease. In: Novick A, Scoble J, Hamilton J, eds. Renal vascular disease. London: WB Saunders; 1996:303–14.
4. Stanley JC. Renal artery fibrodysplasia. In: Novick A, Scoble J, Hamilton J, eds. Renal vascular disease. London: WB Saunders; 1996:21–33.
5. Phinney MS, Smith MC. Atheroembolic renal disease. In: Novick A, Scoble J, Hamilton J, eds. Renal vascular disease. London: WB Saunders; 1996:63–74.
6. Couser WG. Glomerulonephritis. Lancet. 1999;353:1509–15.
7. Hricik DE, Chung-Park M, Sedor JR. Glomerulonephritis. N Engl J Med. 1998;339:888–99.
8. Incidence and prevalence of ESRD. Am J Kidney Dis. 1997;30(Suppl 1):S40–53.
9. Rastegar A, Kashgarian M. The clinical spectrum of tubulointerstitial nephritis. Kidney Int. 1998;54:313–27.
10. Super M, Postlethwaite RJ. Genes, familial eneuresis and clinical management. Lancet. 1997; 350:159–60.
11. Firth JD. Medical treatment of acute tubular necrosis. Q J Med. 1998;91, 5:321–3.
12. Clive DM, Stoff JS. Renal syndromes associated with nonsteroidal anti-inflammatory drugs. N Engl J Med. 1984:310;563.
13. Cockcroft DW, Gault MH. Prediction of creatinine clearance from serum creatinine. Nephron. 1976;16:31–41.
14. Parrish AE. Complications of percutaneous renal biopsy: a review of 37 years experience. Clin Nephrol. 38:135, 1992.
15. Nissenson AR. Definition and pathogenesis of ARF. Kidney Int. 1998;53(Suppl 66):S7–10.
16. Weiner ID, Wingo CS. Hyperkalaemia: a potential silent killer. J Am Soc Nephrol. 1998;9:1535–43.
17. Brater DC. Diuretic therapy. N Engl J Med. 1998;339:387–95.
18. Conger J. Prophylaxis and treatment of acute renal failure by vasoactive agents: the fact and the myths. Kidney Int. 1998;53(Suppl 64):S23–6.
19. Star RA. Treatment of acute renal failure. Kidney Int. 1998; 54:1817–31.
20. Meyer TW, Baboolal K, Brenner BM. Nephron adaptation to renal injury. In: Brenner BM, Rector FC, eds. The kidney, 2nd edn. Philadelphia: WB Saunders, 1981:2011–48.
21. National Institutes of Health. Consensus conference statement. Morbidity and mortality of renal dialysis. Ann Intern Med. 1994; 121:62–70.
22. UK Renal Association. Treatment of adult patients with renal failure: recommended standards and audit measures, 2nd edn. London: Royal College of Physicians; 1997;10:62.
23. Vanholder RC, Ringoir S. The uraemic syndrome. In: Cameron S, Davison AM, Grunfeld JP, et al, (eds). Oxford textbook of clinical nephrology. Oxford: Oxford Medical Publications; 1992:1236–50.
24. Ringoir S. An update on uraemic toxins. Kidney Int. 1997;52 (Suppl 62):S2–4.
25. Ikizler TA, Hakim RM. Nutrition in end-stage renal disease. Kidney Int. 1996;50:343–57.
26. Lowrie EG, Lew NL. Death risk in hemodialysis patients: the predictive value of commonly measured variables and an evaluation of death rate differences between facilities. Am J Kidney Dis. 1990;15:458–82.
27. Klahr S, Levey A, Beck A, et al. The effects of dietary protein restriction and blood pressure control on the progression of chronic renal failure. N Engl J Med. 1994;330:877–84.
28. Oda H, Keane W F. Lipids in progression of renal disease. Kidney Int. 1997;52(Suppl 62):S36–8.
29. Garella S. Pathophysiology and clinical implications of proteinuria. Nephrol Dial Transplant. 1990;Suppl 1:10–5.
30. Gansevoort RT, Sluiter WJ, Hemmelder MH, de Zeeuw D, de Jong PE. Antiproteinuric effect of blood-pressure-lowering agents: a meta-analysis of comparative trials. Nephrol Dial Transplant. 1995;10:1963–74.
31. Remuzzi G and Bertani T. Pathophysiology of progressive nephropathies. New Engl J Med. 1998;339, 20:1448–56.
32. Geiger H. Are angiotensin II receptor blockers superior to angiotensin converting enzyme inhibitors with regard to their renoprotective effect? Nephrol Dial Transplant. 1997;12:640–2.
33. Mene P. Calcium channel blockers: what they can and what they can't do. Nephrol Dial Transplant. 1997;12:25–8.
34. Orth SR, Ritz E, Schrier RW. Renal risks of smoking. Kidney Int. 1997;51:1669–7.
35. Walls J. Effect of correction of acidosis on nutritional status in dialysis patients. Miner Electrolyte Metab. 1997;23:234–6.
36. Jungers P, Chauveau D. Pregnancy in renal disease. Kidney Int. 1997;52:871–85.
37. UK Prospective Diabetes Study Group. Efficacy of atenolol and captopril in reducing risk of macrovascular and microvascular complications. Br Med J. 1998;317:713–20.
38. International Society of Hypertension. Guidelines for the management of hypertension. J Hypertens. 1999;17:151–83.
39. Ramsay L, Williams B, Russel G, et al. Guidelines for management of hypertension: report of the third working party of the British Hypertension Society. Journal of Human Hypertension. 1999; 13:569–92.
40. Treatment of Mild Hypertension Research Group. The treatment of mild hypertension study: a randomised placebo-controlled trial of nutritional-hygiene regimen alone with various drug monotherapies. Arch Intern Med. 1991;151:1413–23.
41. Grossman E, Messerl FH, Grodzicki T, et al. Should a moratorium be placed on sublingual nifedipine capsules given for hypertensive emergencies and pseudoemergencies? JAMA. 1996;276:1328–31.
42. Kaplan NM. Management of hypertensive emergencies. Lancet. 1994;344:1335–8.
43. Bennett WM, Aronoff GR, Golper TA, et al. Drug prescribing in renal failure, 3rd edn. American College of Physicians; 1994.
44. Fraser D, Venning M. Principles of haemodialysis. Medicine. 1999; 27, 6:44–6.
45. Covic A, Goldsmith DJ, Venning MC, Ackrill P. Long-hours home haemodialysis – the best renal replacement therapy method? Q J Med. 1999;92:251–60.
46. Coles GA, Williams JD. What is the place of peritoneal dialysis in the integrated treatment of renal failure? Kidney Int. 1998; 54:2234–40.
47. Bellomo R, Ronco C. Indications and criteria for initiating renal replacement therapy in the intensive care unit. Kidney Int. 1998; 53(Suppl 66):S106–9.
48. Gotch FA. The CANUSA study. PD International 1997;17(Suppl 2):5111–14.

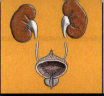

Chapter 20

Renal Transplantation

Charles S Modlin and Andrew C Novick

KEY POINTS

- Renal transplantation is the preferred method of treatment for end-stage renal disease.
- Improvements in surgical technique and immunosuppressive therapy have led to increases in successful graft survival.
- 1-, 5-, and 10-year survival rates are currently >85%, 60–70%, and 40–50% respectively.

INTRODUCTION

With recent improvements in surgical technique and immunosuppressive therapy renal transplantation has emerged as the preferred method for treatment of end-stage renal disease (ESRD) in the appropriately selected candidate. Transplantation offers an improved quality of life via superior physical and psychosocial rehabilitation and reduced cost over chronic dialysis[1]. Overall, 1-, 5-, and 10-year graft survival rates are currently >85%, 60–70%, and 40–50%, respectively. Despite improved quality of life, renal transplantation in matched studies does not prolong patient longevity over dialysis[2,3]. In this chapter an overview is given of the pretransplantation evaluation and selection of candidates for renal transplantation, the process of histocompatibility testing, organ procurement, immunosuppression protocols, kidney transplant, and donor nephrectomy operations; also, commonly encountered postoperative management issues and complications are reviewed.

PRETRANSPLANT EVALUATION

Evaluation and selection of candidates for renal transplantation

To be a candidate for renal transplantation, renal failure must be of a permanent (nonreversible) nature. In most cases, renal transplantation is not carried out until the patient has started chronic maintenance dialysis. However, with respect to living-donor transplantation, the transplant may be timed to occur just before the initiation of dialysis. Results of renal transplantation for the management of kidney failure are superior to those of chronic dialysis in the appropriately selected patient. The purpose of pretransplant medical evaluation is to identify during the pretransplant period any correctable conditions or medical contraindications to transplantation. The pretransplant evaluation consists of a general medical evaluation and assessment of multisystem disease risk factors commonly seen in the renal failure population. Thorough cardiovascular, peripheral vascular, urologic, and gastrointestinal evaluations are carried out, as well as a general survey for infection. In addition, as several etiologies of renal disease have different impacts upon the outcome of renal transplantation, the etiology of ESRD must be considered when patients for renal transplantation are evaluated.

The reported causes of ESRD (Fig. 20.1) include insulin-dependent diabetes mellitus (IDDM; 31% of transplantations), chronic glomerulonephritis (28%), polycystic kidney disease (12%), nephrosclerosis (9%), systemic lupus erythematosus (3%), interstitial nephritis (3%), immunoglobulin A (IgA) nephropathy (2%), and Alport's syndrome (1%). The most common causes are insulin-dependent diabetes mellitus in whites, hypertensive nephrosclerosis in blacks, and chronic glomerulonephritis in Hispanics and Asians[4,5].

Contraindications and adverse risk factors for renal transplantation

The absolute contraindications to renal transplantation are listed in Figure 20.2. Primary oxalosis is a contraindication to primary renal transplantation because of the inevitable recurrence and allograft loss, although combined liver–kidney transplantation is a possibility. Active infection and recently treated or uncontrolled malignancy are contraindications to immunosuppressive therapy. Obviously, patients with severe extrarenal disease that precludes surgery are eliminated from consideration for transplantation. Patients with active drug or alcohol abuse and those with a history of repeated noncompliance (prior failed transplant from noncompliance, noncompliance with medications and/or dialysis) are excluded based upon their likely unreliability post-transplant.

Patients with active systemic disease that could lead to renal failure are not candidates for renal transplantation because of the heightened risk that the systemic disease will destroy the allograft; the patient can be considered for transplantation once the systemic disease is quiescent. Patients with systemic lupus erythematosus (manifesting as cerebritis), pericarditis, myocarditis, vasculitis, or recent (<6 months) nephritis are not accepted for transplantation[6]. The exact role for serologic testing in lupus to determine transplant candidacy is unclear; however, severely depressed serum complement levels or high anti-DNA antibody titers may be a relative contraindication[7]. Lupus patients who require more than 10mg of maintenance prednisone therapy daily should await transplantation[8]. Patients with antiglomerular basement membrane (anti-GBM) disease should have a negative

Causes of renal failure that indicate renal transplantation		
Glomerulonephritis	**Reflux nephropathy, chronic pyelonephritis Hereditary renal failure**	**Metabolic disorders**
Idiopathic and postinfectious crescentic Membranous Mesangiocapillary (Type I) Mesangiocapillary (Type II dense-deposit disease) Immunoglobulin A nephropathy Antiglomerular basement membrane Focal glomerulosclerosis Henoch–Schönlein	Polycystic kidneys Nephronophthisis (medullary cystic disease) Nephritis (including Alport's syndrome) Tuberous sclerosis	Diabetes mellitus Hyperoxaluria Cystinosis Fabry's disease Amyloid Gout Porphyria Hemolytic uremic syndrome
Obstructive uropathy Toxic	**Multisystem diseases**	**Tumors**
Analgesic nephropathy Opiate abuse	Systemic lupus erythematosus Vasculitis Progressive systemic sclerosis	Wilm's tumor Renal cell carcinoma Incidental carcinoma Myeloma
Congenital disorders	**Irreversible acute renal failure**	**Trauma**
Hypoplasia Horseshoe kidney	Cortical necrosis Acute tubular necrosis	

Figure 20.1 Causes of renal failure that indicate renal transplantation[4,5].

Contraindications to renal transplantation and immunosuppression
Active systemic renal disease (e.g. active lupus; active antiglomerular basement membrane disease; active antinuclear cytoplasmic antibody-positive glomerulonephritis)
Oxalosis (combined liver–kidney transplant recommended)
Active infection
Uncontrolled local or disseminated malignancy
Recently treated malignancy within recommended cancer-free survival waiting period
Prohibitive surgical risk from severe extrarenal disease (e.g. cardiac, peripheral vascular disease, pulmonary, etc.)
Active substance abuse or alcohol abuse
Patient noncompliance
Uncontrolled psychiatric disorders

Figure 20.2 Contraindications to renal transplantation and immunosuppression.

Adverse risk factors for renal transplantation
Elderly recipient (upper age limit not rigid)[11]
Very young recipient (<1 year old)
Prior failed transplants each in early post-transplant period (early recurrent disease; hypercoagulability)
Obesity (body mass index >30kg/m²)[10]
Diabetes
Renal disease prone to recurrence (see Fig. 20.5)
Hypercoagulability

Figure 20.3 Adverse factors for renal transplantation.

anti-GBM antibody for at least 6 months prior to transplantation and those with Wegener's granulomatosis and other forms of antinuclear cytoplasmic antibody-positive glomerulonephritis need to have low antinuclear cytoplasmic antibody levels before transplantation[8].

A number of factors, although not absolute contraindications to transplantation, represent relative contraindications, especially in combination with one another, because of their potential adverse impact upon patient and graft survival (Fig. 20.3). These relative contraindications include advanced age, age <1 year[9], obesity with a body mass index[10] (BMI) >30kg/m², and transplantation in the setting of prior graft losses that all occurred shortly after transplantation. Diabetics as well as obese patients are at heightened risk for pre- and post-transplant morbidity and mortality related to silent cardiovascular disease[10]. Those patients with a BMI >30kg/m² must be carefully screened for existing pretransplant cardiac disease[10]. There is no upper age limit to transplantation, but patients over the age of 65 years comprise approximately 35% of patients who undergo dialysis. Mortality inevitably increases as age increases, but a marked variation in risk occurs between individual patients of the same age, depending in particular on the degree of cardiovascular disease[11]. At the Cleveland Clinic Foundation, provided that a patient is cleared to undergo transplantation from a medical standpoint (i.e. cardiovascular, pulmonary, gastrointestinal, urologic, etc.) and has a life expectancy of at least 5 years, then age alone is not used as an exclusionary criterion. Elderly prospective recipients waiting for a cadaver kidney are reevaluated more frequently than younger counterparts, to monitor for any change in their health status while awaiting transplantation.

For patients who have had a prior kidney transplant, particular issues need to be considered in the pretransplant evaluation. The reason for the failed allograft must be defined clearly to determine the risk of retransplantation. It must be determined whether graft loss occurred as a result of noncompliance, hypercoagulability, or recurrence of native kidney disease in the allograft, or as a result of early and aggressive immunologic rejection. Regardless of the reason for the failed first allograft, graft survival rates of subsequent kidney transplants are inferior to those of the first[12–15].

Risk factors in living-related renal transplantation are to transplant patients with IgA nephropathy, hemolytic–uremic syndrome, or diabetes with kidneys from relatives, because of the high risk of recurrence of renal disease in the allograft as well as the possibility that the kidney donor might develop the disease in the future.

TISSUE TYPING, CROSSMATCHING, AND IMMUNOLOGIC MONITORING

The purpose of tissue typing and crossmatching prior to transplantation is to select the most appropriate donor–recipient pair. The first requirement of crossmatching is that the recipient's and donor's ABO blood types must be compatible. Prior to transplantation the donor and recipient must also have a negative crossmatch. The principal of the crossmatch is to detect preformed recipient antibodies against the prospective donor. The crossmatch is performed by mixing recipient sera with donor lymphocytes and complement. A positive crossmatch is indicated when preformed recipient antidonor antibodies lyse the donor cells, which contraindicates transplantation. A transplant performed in this setting results in hyperacute rejection, in which the allograft is immediately destroyed following revascularization. Figure 20.4 outlines the crossmatching algorithm used at the Cleveland Clinic.

RENAL DISEASE PRONE FOR RECURRENCE POST-TRANSPLANT

Recurrent renal disease may affect approximately 25% of renal allografts, but is responsible for allograft failure in fewer than 5% of cases. Glomerulopathies that demonstrate a rapid pretransplant course in the native kidneys recur in the allograft more commonly than others. Patients and families must be informed of the risk of recurrent disease, especially when living-donor renal transplantation is considered. Primary hyperoxaluria is a contraindication to transplantation because of the very high incidence of early recurrence, which results in a 3-year graft survival of only around 20%[16]. In primary hyperoxaluria, good results can be achieved with combined liver–kidney transplantation[17].

Serologic evidence of disease quiescence must be documented prior to transplants in patients who have renal disease prone to recurrence in the allograft. Membranoproliferative glomerulonephritis (MPGN) type I, MPGN type II, IgA nephropathy, focal segmental glomerulosclerosis, anti-GBM disease, fibrillary glomerulonephritis, diabetic nephropathy, Henoch–Schönlein purpura and hemolytic uremic syndrome are prone to recurrence, but cause graft loss with a variable rate.

True recurrent disease must be differentiated from rejection, as must be histologic lesions previously present in the donor kidney or that occurred secondary to the harvesting process. Recurrent disease may be categorized into systemic versus primary renal disease[18]. Figure 20.5 list those causes of ESRD that recur in the allograft[18,19].

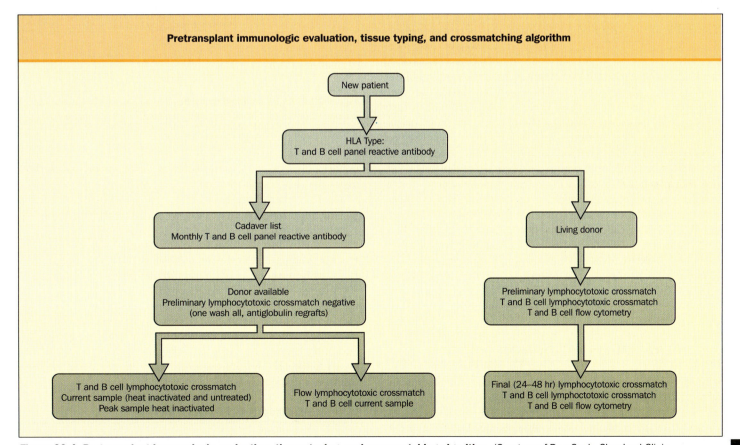

Figure 20.4 Pretransplant immunologic evaluation, tissue typing, and crossmatching algorithm. (Courtesy of Dan Cook, Cleveland Clinic Foundation Allogen Histocompatibility Laboratory.)

Recurrent diseases in renal allografts	
Systemic diseases	**Primary renal diseases**
Systemic lupus erythematosus	Focal and segmental glomerulosclerosis
Hemolytic uremic syndrome	Immunoglobulin A nephropathy
Henoch–Schönlein purpura	Membranoproliferative glomerulonephritis type I
Diabetes mellitus	Membranoproliferative glomerulonephritis type II
Monoclonal gammopathies and mixed cryoglobulinemia: essential mixed cryoglobulinemia multiple myeloma Waldenström's macroglobulinemia light chain deposition disease fibrillary glomerulonephritis	Membranous glomerulonephritis Antiglomerular basement membrane
Amyloidosis	
Wegener's granulomatosis	
Primary hyperoxaluria Type I	
Cystinosis	
Fabry's disease	
Sickle cell disease	
Systemic sclerosis (scleroderma)	
Alport's syndrome	

Figure 20.5 Recurrent disease in the renal allograft[18].

CADAVERIC KIDNEY PROCUREMENT

The information required to evaluate the potential cadaver donor includes blood type, donor age, donor weight, past medical history (systemic infection, local infection, malignancy, etc.), current medical history (trauma, hypertension, renal disease, pressor requirements, other organ disease), vital signs (hypotension, oxygen tension, urine output), laboratory tests [electrolytes, blood urea nitrogen (BUN) and creatinine, urinalysis, serologies, electrocardiogram, chest radiography]. The goal of the evaluation is to provide the best possible organs for kidney transplantation. As the number of patients who await kidney transplantation grossly outnumbers the availability of ideal cadaver organs, many transplant centers have expanded inclusion criteria to allow kidneys from 'marginal donors' or high-risk donors. These so called 'marginal donor kidneys' include those from pediatric donors transplanted as single pediatric kidneys[20] or *en bloc*[21], elderly donor kidneys as single or as dual allografts, kidneys from donors with a history of hepatitis transplanted into hepatitis-positive recipients, and kidneys from nonheartbeat donors. Figure 20.6 shows the surgical technique for cadaveric kidney removal.

PREOPERATIVE LIVING-DONOR WORK-UP

The first reported successful renal transplant was between living identical twins in 1956[22]. Living-related (genetically) and living-unrelated transplantations provide superior short and long-term results than do cadaveric donor transplantations. Living-unrelated donation (i.e. spouse, nonblood relative, friend) has been controversial, but is gaining widespread acceptance. Living-unrelated donors must satisfy the same criteria as living-related

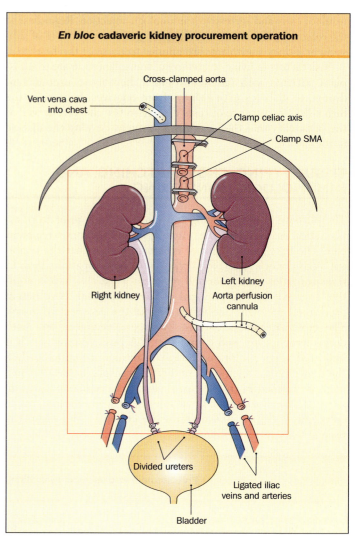

Figure 20.6 *En bloc* cadaveric kidney procurement operation. The structures within the box are removed *en bloc* during the procurement process.

donors. Living-donor transplantation offers many advantages over cadaveric transplantation:
- elective scheduling;
- closer human leukocyte antigens (HLA) matching (in living-related cases);
- shorter cold ischemia preservation times
- improved patient and graft survival; and
- lower immunosuppression requirements.

A thorough evaluation of the potential kidney donor must occur to detect any medical or social condition that would exclude kidney donation and to minimize the risk of postoperative complications[23]. The living donor should have perfect health with minimum anesthetic risks (American Society of Anesthesia class I or II risk), no transmissible infection or tumor, and two well-functioning kidneys[24].

LIVING-DONOR NEPHRECTOMY

Donor preoperative preparation

The donor is admitted to the hospital either the night prior to surgery or on the morning of surgery. Careful attention to

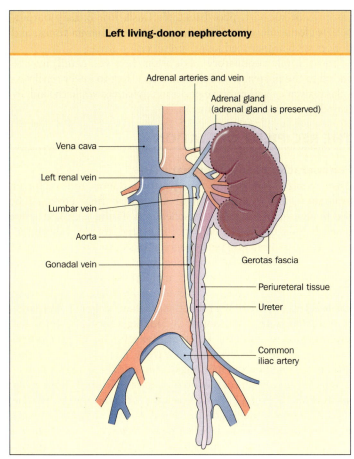

Figure 20.7 Left living-donor nephrectomy operation. Periureteral tissue is preserved (flank approach preferred).

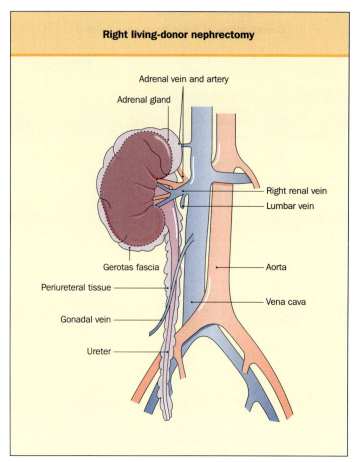

Figure 20.8 Right living-donor nephrectomy (flank approach preferred).

vigorous preoperative, intraoperative, and postoperative hydration in the donor is essential to maintain excellent renal function in the allograft as well as in the remaining kidney of the donor. Some centers administer oral verapamil (240mg) to the donor the day before surgery to lessen the risk of arterial vasospasm induced in the kidney by operative manipulation and cyclosporine[23]. Informed consent is obtained. The patient is instructed in incentive spirometry.

Donor nephrectomy

The aim of operative strategies for living-donor nephrectomy is to obtain excellent exposure to the kidney and reduce trauma to the renal vasculature. Techniques have been described to utilize kidneys from live donors previously considered inappropriate because of anatomic concern (e.g. kidneys with multiple arteries, ureteropelvic junction (UPJ) obstruction, renal cysts, kidneys with arterial dysplasia[25,26]), as well as kidneys from older donors. Proper positioning of the donor is crucial to obtain the intended exposure of the renal vasculature. Our preferred method is the extraperitoneal flank approach, with or without excision of the 11th or 12th rib (Figs 20.7 & 20.8). Alternative approaches to living donor nephrectomy include transabdominal transperitoneal (chevron or midline) incisions as well as laparoscopic donor nephrectomy.

Long-term follow-up of all living donors is mandatory to reassess postnephrectomy risk continually. Several large series of

living-donor nephrectomies identify a major postoperative complication rate of 1.8–7%. This rate includes complications such as myocardial infarction, pulmonary embolism, pneumonia, major infection, hepatitis, pancreatitis, splenic injury, and renal failure (Fig. 20.9)[23,27–31]. The renal donor is not at increased risk over age-matched controls for the development of renal failure or hypertension. Long-term studies suggest that donors have a higher incidence of proteinuria, but this is not clinically significant.

ORGAN PRESERVATION

Figure 20.10 lists the commonly utilized hypothermic preservation solutions in renal transplantation. Kidneys can be stored (cold preservation) for 48 hours at 4°C (39.2°F), but cold ischemia times >24 hours result in a higher incidence of delayed graft function. An alternative to simple cold storage is pulsatile pump perfusion, whereby the cadaver donor kidney is placed on a pump apparatus and mechanically perfused with organ preservation solution (Fig. 20.11). Compared to simple cold storage, longer total ischemia times can be achieved with pulsatile pump perfusion. In addition, donor perfusion parameters, such as donor kidney renal vascular resistance, can be measured in an effort to ascertain the possibility of post-transplant delayed graft function (Fig. 20.12). Pulsatile pump preservation is often used in cases that involve kidneys from elderly donors (>50 years old), donors with a history of hypertension,

Complications of living-donor nephrectomy		
Procedures	Complications	Incidence, >1500 cases (%)
Aortogram	Prolonged discomfort	0.5
	Femoral thrombosis or aneurysm	0.4
Intraoperative	Splenic laceration	0.3
	Pancreatic injury, pseudocyst	0.2
Nephrectomy wound	Prolonged discomfort	2.1
	Infection	2.0
	Hernia	0.5
	Hematoma	0.5
Pulmonary	Atelectasis	13.5
	Pneumothorax or pneumomediastinum	9.1
	Pneumonitis or pleural effusion	4.3
Urinary tract	Infection	8.6
	Late proteinuria	3.0
	Retention	1.6
	Tyrosine-negative oculocutaneous albinism	0.9
Other	Hypertension	15.0
	Prolonged ileus	2.6
	Thromboembolism with or without pulmonary embolus	1.9
	Peripheral nerve palsy	1.1
	Hepatic dysfunction (late)	0.9
	Acute depression	0.6

Figure 20.9 Complications of living-donor nephrectomy[31].

vasopressor support, poor backtable flush, low urinary output, >10% glomerulosclerosis on biopsy, warm ischemia times, and donors with anticipated longer preservation times.

In addition, vasodilatory medications (e.g. verapamil) may be added to the preservation solution in an effort to lower renal vascular resistance and improve perfusion dynamics while the kidney is undergoing pulsatile perfusion.

THE RECIPIENT OPERATION

Perioperative recipient preparation

After completion of the preoperative donor and recipient evaluation, and confirmation of a negative final crossmatch, the living-donor transplant is scheduled. If the recipient is on hemodialysis, this is carried out, if indicated, the day before surgery. Those patients on peritoneal dialysis drain their peritoneal cavities on call to the operating room. Preoperative broad spectrum intravenous antibiotics are administered (Vancomycin 1g, Gentamicin 1mg/kg). Patients are instructed in incentive spirometry. For the living-related transplant recipient, immunosuppression with cyclosporine 3–5mg/kg every 12 hours and mycophenolate mofetil 1g q12h (except in HLA-identical cases) is started 2 days preoperatively. A cyclosporine blood level is obtained on the morning of surgery. The patient receives 250mg methylprednisolone intravenously on call to surgery and an additional 750mg in three divided doses post-transplant (the total dose of solumedrol on the day of surgery is 1g). Recipients of living-unrelated or cadaver kidneys receive the same regimen of solumedrol and mycophenolate mofetil, but receive induction polyclonal antithymocyte therapy with antithymocyte globulin (ATG) or murine monoclonal low-dose orthoclone muromonab-CD3 (OKT3; 2.5mg) or baxiliximab with delayed introduction of cyclosporine.

Commonly utilized hypothermic preservation solutions				
Hypothermic renal preservation solutions				
University of Wisconsin solution			Collins	EuroCollins
Substance	Concentration	Substance	Concentration	Concentration
Potassium lactobionate	100mmol/L	KH_2PO_4	15mmol/L	15mmol/L
KH_2PO_4	25mmol/L	$MgSO_4$	5mmol/L	0
$MgSO_4$	5mmol/L	KCl	15mmol/L	15mmol/L
Raffinose	30mmol/L	K_2HPO_4	42.5mmol/L	42.5mmol/L
Adenosine	5mmol/L	$NaHCO_3$	10mmol/L	10mmol/L
Glutathione	3mmol/L	Glucose	25g/L	35g/L
Allopurinol	1mmol/L			
Hydroxyethyl starch	50g/L			
Insulin	40U/L			
Dexamethasone	16mg/L			
Penicillin	200,000U/L			
Osmolarity (mOsmol/L)	320		360	375

Figure 20.10 Commonly utilized hypothermic preservation solutions.

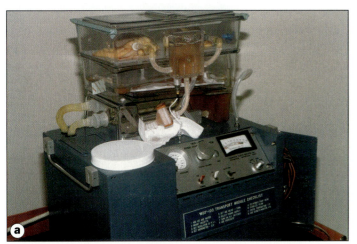

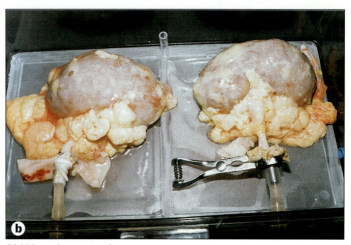

Figure 20.11 Organ preservation. (a) Kidney pump apparatus; (b) kidneys in preservation.

Pulsatile pump organ preservation – optimal pump parameters	
Parameter	Optimum value
Perfusion pressure	<45/25mmHg (6.0/3.3kPa) systolic/diastolic
Perfusion flow rate	>100mL/minute
Flow resistance	<0.3

Figure 20.12 Pulsatile pump organ preservation: optimal pump parameters.

Operative procedure

The transplant operative procedure has been described in detail in surgical texts (Fig. 20.13). The right pelvic fossa is generally chosen for implantation because the right external iliac vein is more superficial on the right compared to the left. Following anesthesia, a curvilinear incision is made from the pubic symphysis to a point four finger breadths superior to the anterior superior iliac spine. In males the spermatic cord is preserved and in females the round ligament is divided. The inferior epigastric vessels are ligated and divided and the peritoneal cavity retracted medially. The venous anastomosis is carried out first. Thereafter, an end-to-end renal artery to hypogastric anastomosis, or renal artery to external or common iliac anastomosis, is carried out, followed by an extravesical ureteral reimplantation. The decision to use a ureteral stent is at the discretion of the surgeon, although it is desirable in most cases and its benefits outweigh its risks [stent breakage, migration, encrustation, and urinary tract infection (UTI)].

Bench table vascular reconstruction

For a right donor kidney, it is necessary to ensure adequate renal venous length for transplantation, especially if it is anticipated that the recipient iliac vein is deep in the pelvis or the renal vein is short. For living-donor transplants, a cuff of donor vena cava is usually harvested in continuity with the renal vein. In cadaveric transplantation, to lengthen the renal vein the edges of the vena cava may be sewn together to effect renal vein extension. Several techniques have been described to refashion the attached donor vena cava to provide for renal venous extension (Fig. 20.14). Accessory renal veins are ligated, with the dominant renal vein preserved for implantation.

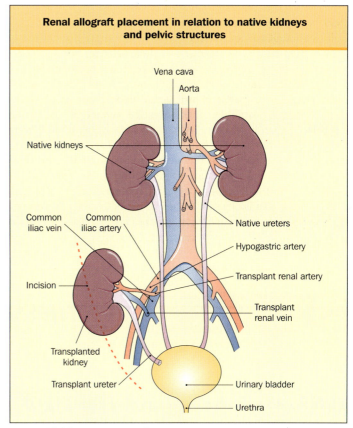

Renal allograft placement in relation to native kidneys and pelvic structures

Figure 20.13 Renal allograft placement in relation to native kidneys and pelvic structures.

For cases in which the donor kidney has multiple renal arteries, several techniques exist for bench arterial reconstruction prior to implantation (Figs 20.15 & 20.16). Effort must be made to preserve all the arteries; the only exception is the tenuous small upper polar artery, which is not attached to an aortic cuff, is widely separated from the main renal artery, and is estimated to supply <10% of the renal parenchyma. Lower polar arteries usually supply the transplant ureter and are preserved whenever possible. For situations in which lower polar arteries are traumatized or ligated, it is routine to use ureteral stents post-transplant as the risk of urinary fistulization is heightened.

Orthotopic renal transplantation

Orthotopic renal transplantation is a technique used to implant the transplant kidney in the physiologic native kidney retroperitoneal space; it is indicated in situations that contraindicate graft placement in the pelvis. Such indications are determined on an individual basis, but include vena caval resection, agenesis, or thrombosis, severe iliac artery atheromatosis disease, aortoiliac bypass, or in recipients of multiple transplantations[32]. This technique is based upon anastomosis of the transplant renal artery end-to-end to the splenic artery (or end-to-side to the aorta), the transplant renal vein to the native renal vein (or, rarely, the splenic vein), and the allograft renal pelvis anastomosed to the native renal pelvis (pyelo–pyelo) over a stent. Demonstration of a patent and adequately sized splenic artery (intravenous digital subtraction angiography with sequential planes), a normal native renal vein, and a normal native ureter (retrograde ureteropyelography) is mandatory.

Peri- and postoperative care

Full perioperative care for the renal transplantation recipient is provided, with special attention to fluid balance, urine output, insensible losses, and daily weight. There is a positive association between delayed graft function and delayed onset of urine output with poor graft survival. Renal blood flow can often be improved using albumen, intraoperative verapamil and other calcium channel blockers, and occasionally, although more controversially, renal doses of dopamine. On postoperative day one, a radionuclide renal scan is carried out to assess renal blood flow and excretion, and to exclude urine extravasation. The bladder catheter is left in for 5–7 days and removed when a repeat radionuclide scan is negative for urinary leakage. An appropriate diet is instituted and patients continue to receive antifungal prophylaxis for 3 months and antibacterial prophylaxis for 12 months. In addition, all patients receive antiplatelet inhibitors (aspirin or dipyridamole 50mg daily).

IMMUNOSUPPRESSION

Figures 20.17 & 20.18 outline the current immunosuppression protocols used at the Cleveland Clinic Foundation for living and cadaver donor transplants.

Experimental and future trends in immunosuppression
Human monoclonal antibody induction therapy
The ultimate goal of monoclonal antibody therapy is to suppress only selected T cell subsets or functions[33,34]. The first monoclonal agent to demonstrate remarkable immunosuppressive effects was OKT3. Extensive clinical trials are underway with other monoclonal antibodies directed against selected accessory molecules essential to the interaction between T cells and histocompatibility antigens[35]. One of the more promising additions to the monoclonal antibody field is the recombinant DNA technology used to humanize murine or rat preparations. Such humanized preparations will hopefully be less immunogenic than OKT3 (ameliorating dangerous side effects and the development of antimurine antibodies that limit the effectiveness of the monoclonal antibody) and more effectively directed to specific cellular targets that contribute to the rejection process[35].

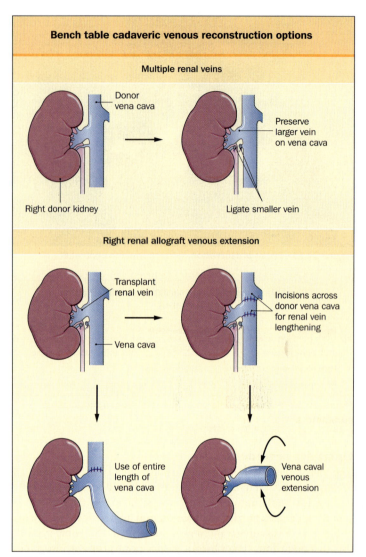

Figure 20.14 Bench table cadaveric venous reconstruction options. (Top) Multiple renal veins and (bottom) right renal allograft venous extension.

ASSESSMENT OF ALLOGRAFT DYSFUNCTION

Causes of renal transplant dysfunction within the first 6 months can be divided into medical and surgical complications. The main differential diagnoses of early renal transplant dysfunction (Fig. 20.19) include acute tubular necrosis (ATN), ischemic damage that results from organ procurement, prolonged ischemia times and reperfusion injury, cyclosporine toxicity, and rejection[36], with rarer causes related to hemorrhage, ureteral obstruction, urine leak, venous thrombosis, renal transplant arterial stenosis, or occlusion and infection. Rejection is a common cause of graft dysfunction in the early post-transplant period, as is cyclosporine toxicity or other drug toxicity. Delayed graft function (DGF) is usually defined as the requirement for dialysis in the first week after transplantation and occurs in approximately 20% of cadaver transplant recipients. It is associated with reduced short- and long-term graft survival. Once the above potential causes of early transplant dysfunction are ruled out, ATN is usually the cause of early graft dysfunction. Aggressive peri- and postoperative fluid management, in

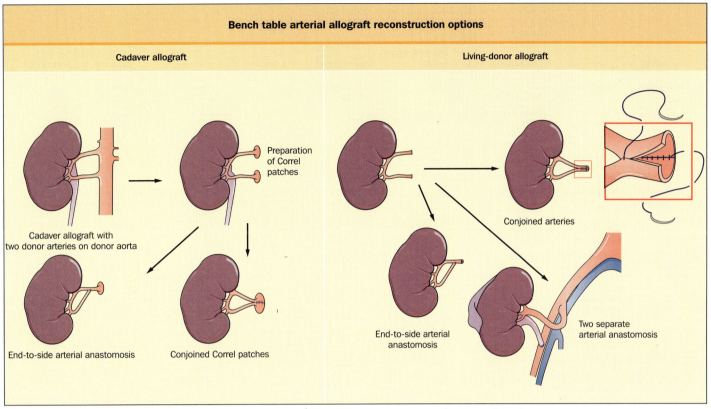

Figure 20.15 Bench table arterial allograft reconstruction options. Cadaver allograft and living-donor allograft.

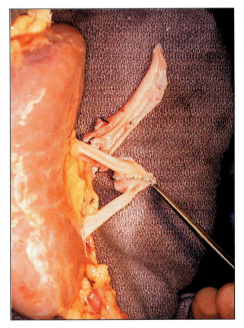

Figure 20.16 Conjoined arterial anastomosis of two donor renal arteries.

particular maintenance of a central venous pressure of 10–20cmH$_2$O (1.0–2.0kPa), promotes renal perfusion and thereby reduces the incidence of DGF. Reports are unclear on the utility of renal dose dopamine to promote renal vasodilation and to improve allograft hemodynamics.

Late allograft dysfunction most often results from chronic rejection, chronic cyclosporine or drug toxicity, ureteral obstruction, infection, renal artery stenosis, fluid status, or (infrequently)

recurrent or de-novo renal disease in the allograft (Fig. 20.19). Acute rejection can occur in the late period also, often secondary to noncompliance, which is increasingly the cause of late graft loss. Cyclosporine-induced nephrotoxicity in the short term is dose dependent and responds to dose reduction. However, late allograft dysfunction can occur as a result of cyclosporine glomerulopathy.

Chronic cyclosporine nephrotoxicity is a histologic diagnosis that can be difficult to differentiate from chronic rejection. Cyclosporine causes vasoconstriction of the glomerular afferent arterioles, which leads to diminished glomerular filtration rate and renal blood flow. Routine monitoring of cyclosporine level is necessary to maintain it in the therapeutic but nontoxic range. Cyclosporine is metabolized in the liver cytochrome P-450 system; several medications can affect cyclosporine blood concentrations by either inhibition or stimulation of the P-450 enzyme system. The majority of antibiotics (excluding the antituberculous antibiotics) compete with cyclosporine in metabolism by the P-450 system and thus act to raise cyclosporine blood levels. Cyclosporine concentrations are also increased by calcium channel blockers (diltiazem) and decreased by antiepileptic drugs. Early and late graft dysfunction may occur as a result of use of medication nephrotoxic to the allograft and medication that alters allograft perfusion such as nonsteroidal anti-inflammatory drugs (NSAIDs) and angiotensin-converting enzyme (ACE) inhibitors.

RENAL ALLOGRAFT REJECTION

The features of renal allograft rejection have both a clinical basis and a histopathologic basis. The essential finding is renal

20

283

Cleveland Clinic adult immunosuppression protocols

Time period	Cyclosporine*	FK506 (tacrolimus)	Mycophenolate mofetil†	Azathioprine‡	Prednisone	Antithymocyte globulin‡	OKT3 (orthoclone muromonoclonal antibody)
Pretransplant	Cadaver: none LUR: begin 2 days preoperatively 3–5mg/kg q12h; obtain cyclosporine level	LUR: Same time as cyclosporine Begin 2mg orally q12h; 2 days preoperatively; obtain tacrolimus level	1.0g	1.5–2.0mg/kg per day	250mg solumedrol bolus	None	None
Recovery room postoperatively	Cadaver: none LUR: dose per level	Cadaver: none LUR: dose per level	1g orally		250mg i.v. (three doses) solumedrol	10–15mg/kg with premedications	2.5mg i.v. with premedications
Post-transplant, year one	Begin cyclosporine when kidney diuresis serum creatinine <4.0mg/dL	Same as cyclosporine	1g 12qh	1.0–1.5mg/kg per day	Prednisone taper (see text)	Antithymocyte globulin daily for 10–14 days, discontinue when therapeutic cyclosporine level	Continue 7–10 days postoperatively
	Target TDx cyclosporine levels 200–250 ng/mL year one, target levels 150–200 thereafter	Target tacrolimus levels 5–15	Monitor white blood cell count	Monitor white blood cell count	Goal is 0.1mg/kg per day by end of first year	If delayed graft function continue every other day postoperatively for days 14–28 (total doses = 21)	Discontinue with therapeutic level cyclosporine
		Tacrolimus used in selected situations (see text)				Monitor CD2 subsets	Monitor CD3 subsets

LUR, living unrelated.
*Begin cyclosporine low dose in recipients of pediatric kidneys and in patients with delayed graft function >14 days. Use either cyclosporine or tacrolimus.
†Use either mycophenolate mofetil or azathioprine.
‡Use either antithymocyte globulin or OKT3 induction.

Figure 20.17 Cleveland Clinic adult immunosuppression protocols: cadaver and living-unrelated donors. i.v., intravenous.

Cleveland Clinic adult immunosuppression protocols

Time period	Cyclosporine*	FK506 (tacrolimus)	Mycophenolate mofetil†	Azathioprine‡	Prednisone	Antithymocyte globulin‡	OKT3 (orthoclone muromonoclonal antibody)
Begin 2 days pretransplant	3–5mg/kg orally q12h	2.0mg orally q12h (use in selective situations)	1.0g orally q12h	1–2mg/kg orally q12h	None	None	None
On-call to transplant	3–5mg/kg orally Obtain morning trough level	2.0mg orally Obtain morning trough level	1.0mg orally	1–2mg/kg orally	250mg solumedrol	None	None
Post-transplant	Titrate to TDx level 200–250 year one; levels 150–200 after year one	Titrate to target levels 5–15	1.0g orally q12h	1–1.5mg/kg orally q12h	250mg solumedrol times 3		
					Day of transplant, then prednisone taper (see text)	None	None

*Use cyclosporine or tacrolimus
†Use mycophenolate mofetil or azathioprine; withhold if HLA identical.
‡Use either antithymocyte globulin or OKT3 induction.

Figure 20.18 Cleveland Clinic adult immunosuppression protocols: living-related donors. HLA, human leukocyte antigens.

Assessment of allograft dysfunction	
Early dysfunction	**Late dysfunction**
Delayed graft function	Chronic rejection
Acute rejection	Acute rejection
Arterial thrombosis	Urinary obstruction
Arterial stenosis	Cyclosporine/tacrolimus toxicity
Venous thrombosis	Drug toxicity
Cyclosporine/tacrolimus toxicity	Infection
Drug toxicity	Hydration status: prerenal/postrenal
Urine leak or obstruction	Renal artery stenosis
Hemorrhage	Recurrent or de-novo kidney disease
Metabolic/endocrine disturbances	Renal calculi
	Metabolic/endocrine disturbances
Prerenal states	
Cirrhosis with ascites	
Congestive heart failure	
Severe salt depletion	
Diuresis-induced volume contraction	
Metabolic/endocrine disturbances	

Figure 20.19 Assessment of allograft dysfunction.

dysfunction – manifested as an elevated serum creatinine and BUN from baseline values. High molecular weight proteinuria may also occur. Patients may be completely asymptomatic or have significant symptoms. The symptoms may be:
- systemic – fever, chills, rigors, lassitude, headache;
- local – graft swelling, tenderness, overlying tissue edema; or
- result from decreased kidney function – oliguria, hypertension, weight gain, hyperkalemia, pulmonary or peripheral edema.

It is important to rule out other causes of post transplant renal dysfunction that can mimic rejection. The most common are infection, drug-induced nephrotoxicity, lymphocele, technical problems (urine leak, obstruction), hyperglycemia, congestive heart failure, and de-novo and/or recurrent renal diseases. Many causes can be ruled out after a careful history and physical examination, blood chemistries, urine analysis, chest radiography, blood and urine cultures, serologies, ultrasound examination, and isotopic scanning of the transplant kidney.

In most cases percutaneous transplant renal biopsy is used to confirm the clinical suspicion of rejection and remains the gold standard for diagnosis. The diagnosis of rejection cannot be made on radiographic grounds. Immunologic assessment via T and B cell flow cytometry may accurately suggest the diagnosis of antibody-mediated rejection. Most acute rejections are cellular mediated, although antibody-mediated (vascular) rejections occur.

Solez and a consortium of the transplant community have developed an international standardized grading system to characterize the diagnosis and reports of rejections[37], termed the 'Banff' system for acute and chronic rejection. The goal of this standardized histologic grading system is to correlate histologic findings on biopsy with a prognosis for therapeutic response to antirejection therapy and long-term function[38]. The biopsies are graded according to the

Banff criteria (I, II, III). The morbidity of rejection not only arises from damage to the allograft, but also from complications in antirejection therapy – infection, malignancy, gastrointestinal bleeding, etc. It is considered prudent to limit antirejection therapy to two or three episodes as overimmunosuppression can lead to significant morbidity. While each case must be carefully considered, the outline given is appropriate for most patients.

Hyperacute rejection
Hyperacute rejection is caused by preformed cytotoxic antibodies to allograft major histocompatibility complex (MHC) antigens. It results in sudden graft malfunction and thrombosis, usually intraoperatively, but always within 24–48 hours of transplant. Isotopic renal scans demonstrate no blood flow. There is no effective treatment and a nephrectomy is required. Hyperacute rejection can usually be prevented by careful pretransplant donor specific crossmatching.

Accelerated rejection
Accelerated rejection can occur during the first week post-transplant and implies some form of cellular presensitization (it occurs prior to the 7–10 days required for a primary immune response). It can be very aggressive clinically, with a resultant large swollen graft that may rupture or thrombose.

Accelerated rejection is less common when induction therapy with an antilymphocyte agent is employed. When it occurs, intense antirejection therapy is required to salvage the graft. These rejection episodes may be rapid in onset, and necessitate the use of temporary dialysis until they have been reversed.

Acute cellular rejection
Acute cellular rejection is the most commonly observed form of rejection and can occur at anytime after the transplant. As the name implies, the predominant histologic feature is an acute cellular infiltrate. It occurs with diminishing frequency as time elapses after the transplant and is most frequently encountered during the first 3 months. Acute rejection occurs in approximately 50% of transplant recipients and is an important cause of early graft loss. Late acute rejections may be triggered by a coexistent infection or it may suggest patient noncompliance with medications. These rejections are usually reversed with high-dose corticosteroid therapy, but some rejections may require the addition of antilymphocyte preparations.

Acute cellular rejections may be mild and result in only a slight increase in the serum creatinine over several days, or they may have an abrupt onset and result in severe oliguria and a rapid daily rise in serum creatinine. Temporary dialysis may be necessary to stabilize patients until rejection reversal occurs.

Chronic rejection
Chronic rejection is usually encountered beyond 6 months post-transplant. Chronic rejection is the most common cause of late graft loss and is manifested as a gradual, progressive decline in renal function that eventually results in allograft failure. Chronic rejection is often accompanied by hypertension and proteinuria. The diagnosis of chronic rejection is usually made late after irreversible changes in the allograft have occurred. The etiology of chronic rejection is believed to be multifactorial and related to repeated immunologic insults of acute rejection (caused by

antidonor directed antibody that is unresponsive to immuno-suppression), persistently low concentrations of cyclosporine or nonimmunologic in etiology.

The histologic diagnosis of chronic rejection is characterized by intimal proliferation of graft arteries and arterioles, interstitial cellular infiltration and fibrosis, tubular atrophy, and glomerular sclerosis[38]. Vessels are often occluded and demonstrate intimal and medial proliferation.

Treatment of chronic rejection is limited and directed at the control of other factors that can cause a decline in graft function, such as hypertension, hyperlipidemia, diabetes, drug toxicities, and a low protein diet. There are experimental case reports of the administration of dietary fish oils, prostacycline analogs, and NSAIDs to aid in the treatment of chronic rejection[39].

Currently, no immunosuppressive medications can prevent rejection completely. Methods to reduce the incidence of acute and chronic rejection currently center on adequate induction and maintenance immunosuppressive therapy as well as attempts to match the donor and recipient HLA closely.

Treatment of rejection

The most frequently employed agents to treat biopsy-confirmed acute rejection include corticosteroids, either as a pulse dose or as a tapered or 'recycled' daily reducing dose over a period of days to weeks. If after 48–72 hours renal function does not begin to improve or a significant component of vascular rejection is present, antilymphocyte agents may be instituted. These may include anti-CD3 antibody or antithymocyte globulin. Also, OKT3 monoclonal antibody may be used for acute rejection. A number of recipients who undergo rejection develop low titers of antidonor MHC antibody and in such cases plasmapheresis may be a useful adjunct. When post-transplant flow cytometry indicates rising T and B cell antibody titers, pheresis three times per week for 2 weeks may provide additional rejection therapy for those grafts injured by antibody-mediated mechanisms.

UROLOGIC COMPLICATIONS POSTTRANSPLANTATION

Early post-transplant urologic complications most commonly represent technical failures of the ureterovesical anastomosis that result in urinary fistulization and ureteral obstruction (Fig. 20.20). The reported incidence of urologic complications is 3–14%. Streem[40] and Pardalidis et al.[41] have provided comprehensive reviews of the endourologic management of urologic complications following renal transplantation. When considering endourologic intervention, prophylactic antibiotics should be started before the nephrostomy puncture and continued for as long as a drainage tube is indwelling.

Ureteral obstruction

Urinary obstruction can manifest any time post-transplant, but in current series occurs in <5% of renal allograft recipients. Ureteral obstruction accounts for up to one-third of all significant urologic complications. Early obstruction may be a consequence of mechanical obstruction caused by a peritransplant fluid collection (urinoma, hematoma, lymphocele), improper anastomotic technique, ureteral blood clot after renal biopsy, or a redundant kinked ureter. Late ureteral obstructions most

Post-transplant surgical management issues
Assessment of allograft dysfunction
Early dysfunction
Late dysfunction
Evaluation and treatment of transplant surgical complications
Vascular complications
Renal artery stenosis
Renal artery thrombosis
Renal vein thrombosis
Allograft rupture
Arteriovenous fistulization
Urologic complications
Urine leak
Urinary obstruction
Urinary tract infections
Urinary calculi
Impotence and infertility post-transplant

Figure 20.20 Post-transplant surgical management issues.

often result from distal ureteral ischemia, fibrosis, or necrosis secondary to damage to the ureteral blood supply during graft procurement, preservation, or implantation.

The diagnosis is usually established during the evaluation of progressive azotemia. Routine radiographic screening with ultra-sonography results in early diagnosis of this complication. In cases of normal renal function, intravenous urography (IVU) may assist the diagnosis of obstruction location, but usually renal insufficiency limits the use of IVU. The preferred diagnostic modalities include ultrasonography, antegrade pyelography, and on occasion diuretic nuclear renography. Management is usually initiated by placement of a percutaneous nephrostomy tube, which assists in resolution of infection and azotemia. After infection has resolved and renal function stabilized, antegrade pyelography is performed to localize the site of obstruction (Fig. 20.21).

Ureteral obstruction is usually managed by conventional percutaneous techniques with nephrostomy drainage and stenting[40,42–45], but open surgical procedures may be required.

Endourologic techniques include percutaneous ureteral balloon dilation, percutaneous endoscopic incisional ureterotomy, and (rarely) retrograde endourologic management. Following either open or endourologic repair, stents are usually removed 6 weeks postoperatively. Following stent removal, continued life-long surveillance by monitoring renal function, cultures, and imaging studies is mandatory.

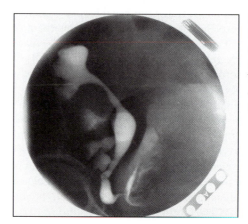

Figure 20.21 Percutaneous antegrade pyelography. Transplant ureteral obstruction with hydroureteronephrosis.

Ureteropelvic junction obstruction of the transplants may occur as a result of angulation of the ureter at the time of transplant or of an unrecognized intrinsic problem. Percutaneous endopyelotomy is now widely accepted as the initial treatment of UPJ obstruction. Standard open pyeloplasty is contraindicated because of the risk that the transplant ureteral blood supply may be interrupted. Therefore, in endoscopic UPJ treatment failures or in cases for which endoscopic treatment is contraindicated, open ureteropyelostomy using the native ureter is indicated for the repair of UPJ obstruction.

Urinary fistula

Early urine leaks are a result of improper surgical technique and most often occur in the distal third of the ureter or at the ureterovesical anastomosis. After the immediate postoperative period, the majority of urine leaks result from distal ureteral ischemia and necrosis. Ischemia and necrosis occur as a result of damage to the blood supply to the transplant ureter, which is derived solely from the renal artery. Injury to the renal artery (especially a lower pole accessory vessel) during retrieval, bench repair, or implantation makes the ureter vulnerable to ischemia.

Urinary extravasation is usually suspected clinically by the findings of fever, allograft pain and tenderness (often associated with peritoneal signs of rebound tenderness and rigidity), nausea, vomiting, urinary incisional drainage (with aspirated BUN and creatinine fluid concentrations markedly elevated over that of serum BUN and creatinine levels), and a drop in urine output with consequent deterioration of allograft function. Diagnosis of urine extravasation is most often made by nuclear isotope scanning with demonstration of extraurinary isotope (Fig. 20.22). Ultrasonography often reveals the presence of a peritransplant fluid collection. In addition, cystography with oblique views and postwash exposure often reveals the location of the extravasation to be at the site of the ureteroneocystostomy. A percutaneous antegrade nephrostogram often helps to delineate anatomically the site of urinary extravasation or obstruction.

Treatment of a urine leak depends on the location and severity of the urinary fistula. Small leaks from the ureteroneocystostomy can often be managed conservatively with urinoma aspiration, prolonged bladder catheterization (with or without percutaneous nephrostomy tube drainage and antegrade ureteral stenting), and antibiotic prophylaxis. More complicated situations that involve necrosis of a portion of the ureter or the entire transplant ureter, or larger and persistent leaks at the ureteroneocystostomy require individualized treatments that involve urinary reconstructions generally well known to the urologist. Options include repeat ureteroneocystostomy, open surgical exploration with transplant to native ureteroureterostomy, transplant pelvis to native ureter (pyeloureterostomy), transplant pelvis to bladder (pyelocystostomy), transplant calix to native ureter (calicoureterostomy), transplant calix to bladder (calicocystostomy), Boari flap with or without psoas hitch, and (rarely ureteral) replacement with an ileal ureter. The surgeon should consider native nephrectomy when ligating the native ureter proximal to the repair to avoid potential cases of symptomatic hydronephrosis of the native kidney. Caliceal fistulization is more often seen after cadaver transplantation with multiple renal arteries and inadvertent interruption of small polar vessels during retrieval; percutaneous nephrostomy drainage often permits closure of a caliceal fistula[46].

Stone disease

Renal calculi develop in <2% of transplant recipients, and occur usually as a result of hyperparathyroidism and recurrent UTIs. Other predisposing factors for stones in the transplanted kidney include renal tubular acidosis, hypercalciuria, hyperoxaluria, papillary necrosis, nonabsorbable suture material, and obstruction[41]. As the renal allograft is denervated, patients are often

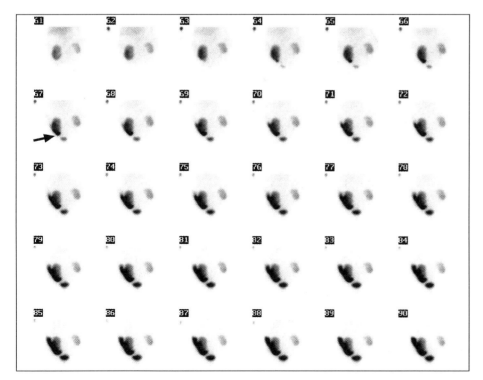

Figure 20.22 Post-transplant ^{99m}Tc-MAG3 renal scan of a 'dual transplant' with extraurinary extravasation of isotope lateral to transplanted kidney in right pelvic fossa. Note the delayed uptake of isotope in the contralateral left pelvic fossa allograft (consistent with acute tubular necrosis). Arrow indicates extraurinary isotope extravasation. (Courtesy Richard Brunken, Department of Nuclear Medicine, Cleveland Clinic Foundation.)

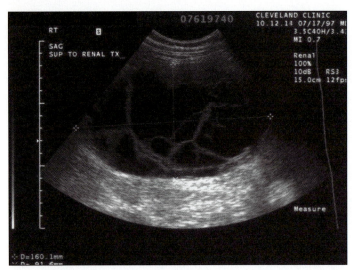

Figure 20.23 Peritransplant lymphocele. The sonogram demonstrates multiloculated peritransplant lymphocele.

asymptomatic without renal colic, but present with either a UTI or a rise in serum creatinine. Almost all calculi that occur in renal allografts can be treated successfully with percutaneous techniques or extracorporeal shock-wave lithotripsy[47].

Perinephric fluid collections
Lymphoceles
All transplant recipients develop perinephric fluid collections, but most are clinically insignificant. Perinephric fluid collections include lymphoceles, hematomas, urinomas, and abscesses. Lymphoceles originate from severed donor and/or recipient lymphatic channels, with an incidence that ranges from 0.5 to 20%. Lymphoceles present clinically, usually within the first 6 months post-transplant, with:

- graft dysfunction that results from ureteral obstruction or allograft compression, ipsilateral lower extremity edema, or deep venous thrombosis from external iliac vein compression;
- voiding dysfunction as a result of bladder compression, pelvic discomfort, swelling, or lymphatic leakage from the wound.

Diagnosis of the lymphocele is confirmed via pelvic sonography (Fig. 20.23) or computed tomography (CT)-guided aspiration (without placement of an indwelling drain) of the symptomatic fluid collection; the fluid is analyzed for BUN and creatinine content as well as culture and sensitivity. Lymphoceles usually recur rapidly postaspiration and must be repaired. Options for repair for the noninfected lymphocele include:

- open surgical transabdominal marsupialization (creation of a large peritoneal window to drain the lymphocele fluid into the peritoneal cavity, in which the fluid is reabsorbed; Fig. 20.24);
- laparoscopic marsupialization or percutaneous aspiration; and
- lymphocele cavity sclerosis.

Proponents of laparoscopic approaches report shorter hospitalization and recovery postlymphocele repair. Infected lymphoceles are best treated with either percutaneous aspiration and external catheter drainage or (rarely) open surgical drainage with external marsupialization.

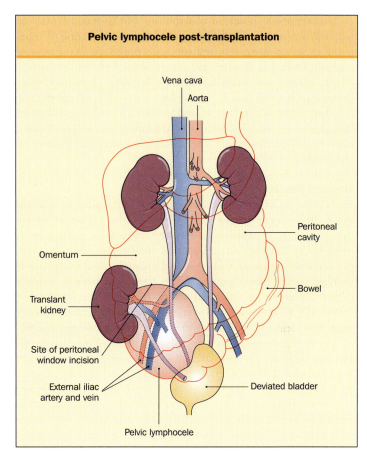

Pelvic lymphocele post-transplantation

Vena cava
Aorta
Peritoneal cavity
Omentum
Bowel
Translant kidney
Site of peritoneal window incision
External iliac artery and vein
Deviated bladder
Pelvic lymphocele

Figure 20.24 Pelvic lymphocele post-transplantation. Note anatomic proximity of lymphocele to allograft ureter, pelvic vessels, and urinary bladder. With a transperitoneal incision, the lymphocele wall (posterior peritoneum) is identified and incised to create the 'peritoneal window'.

Hematomas
Large symptomatic hematomas (pain, graft dysfunction, falling hematocrit, infection) require exploration and evacuation. Usually, no obvious site of bleeding is found upon exploration. The bleeding is often attributed to platelet dysfunction secondary to uremia.

Urinomas
Diagnosis and treatment of urinomas are discussed above under Urinary fistula.

VASCULAR COMPLICATIONS POST-TRANSPLANT

Renal artery stenosis
Transplant renal artery stenosis (TRAS) is the most frequent vascular complication of renal transplantation, with a reported incidence between 1 and 15%, depending on the method of diagnosis and definition of TRAS. Renal artery stenosis represents a potentially reversible cause of hypertension and allograft loss.

Hemodynamically, significant stenosis is generally defined as >70% stenosis with a pressure gradient >15mmHg (2.0kPa). Usually, TRAS occurs weeks or months after transplantation and is considered a late vascular complication. A variety of causes include arterial injury during allograft procurement or preservation, narrowing of the arterial anastomosis at the time of grafting, arteriosclerosis of the donor or recipient artery, idiopathic fibrosis, or vascular rejection. Renal artery stenosis occurs at the site of the anastomosis or in the postanastomotic artery, as in the case of vascular rejection.

Clinically, TRAS commonly presents as recent onset, refractory, or poorly controlled renin-mediated hypertension, with or without a bruit over the allograft, and with or without insidious onset of allograft dysfunction. Often, TRAS is suspected clinically with development of acute renal insufficiency after the addition of an ACE inhibitor for the treatment of hypertension. Consequently, before an ACE inhibitor is introduced to treat hypertension in renal transplant recipients, duplex sonography is needed to rule out hemodynamically significant renal artery stenosis. The presence or absence of an arterial bruit over the allograft is not a reliable predictor of TRAS[48].

With this clinical scenario, often the diagnosis is suggested initially by findings of significant arterial stenosis (>60–70%) on noninvasive duplex Doppler sonography or provocative testing with captopril renography[49]. Duplex sonography for the diagnosis of significant renal artery stenosis is reported to have a high sensitivity, but a specificity of only 75% and a positive predictive value of only 56%, which suggests that although this test may be a valuable screening tool, angiographic confirmation is still required[49]. Isotopic renography carried out before and after administration of a dose of captopril is reported to be highly predictive of physiologically significant renal artery stenosis, with a sensitivity of 75% and specificity of 67% (Fig. 20.25)[49,50].

The gold standard for confirmation of the diagnosis of renal transplant arterial stenosis and anatomic detail is angiography (Fig. 20.26a). Selective renal vein renin analysis may help when uncontrollable hypertension that results from native kidney hypersecretion of renin is a possibility. The specificity of peripheral plasma renin concentrations in patients with TRAS before and after captopril administration is low[51]. Research is in progress with magnetic resonance angiography[52] and spiral CT scanning to diagnosis renal artery stenosis. Spiral CT can provide three-dimensional reconstruction of the renal arteries, avoids arterial puncture, and requires less intravenous contrast than does conventional angiography[53]. In addition, carbon dioxide angiography has been utilized to visualize renal arterial stenosis as it avoids the use of nephrotoxic agents and hypersensitivity reactions[54].

Treatment of TRAS historically was by open surgical reanastomosis, either via direct arterial reimplantation, saphenous interposition bypass grafting, patch grafting, or localized endarterectomy; however, as a result of the intense inflammatory reaction around the renal artery the incidence of graft loss from attempted revascularization is high (15–20%)[55], and also variable rates of success (63–92%) with surgical intervention have been reported[56]. Transluminal angiographic balloon angioplasty (Fig. 20.26b) with or without the insertion of an intra-arterial stent has shown success in the treatment of TRAS[57] and is now usually the preferred initial mode of therapy for TRASs that are short, linear, and relatively distal from the anastomosis[56]. Stenosis at the anastomosis has a lower success rate after percutaneous angioplasty with a high complication rate[58,59]. Percutaneous angioplasty also has a low success rate in TRAS that results from arterial kinking[59,60].

After correction, TRAS is considered cured if antihypertensive medication is eliminated. It is considered improved post-treatment if the dosage of antihypertensive medications decreases or diastolic blood pressure is reduced by >10%[61]. Surgical back-up should always be available prior to attempted renal artery angioplasty as complications can occur in as many as 10% of cases[56].

Renal artery thrombosis

Renal artery thrombosis usually occurs within 24 hours of transplantation and is manifest by the initial nonfunction of the graft or a sudden decline in urine output. Diagnosis is confirmed on nuclear renal isotope scanning (photopenic effect in region of allograft). Early renal artery thrombosis usually occurs at the site of the arterial anastomosis as a result of anastomotic stenosis or formation of an intimal flap. Arterial kinking is also a known rare etiology of renal arterial occlusion. Other causes include dehydration and hypotension. The incidence of renal artery thrombosis is <5% of transplants. The treatment necessary is usually transplant nephrectomy. The risk of vascular thrombosis can be reduced by appropriate surgical technique during retrieval, bench preparation and transplantation, correct positioning of the kidney to avoid vascular kinking, and attention to proper fluid management intraoperatively and in the immediate postoperative period.

Renal vein thrombosis

Thrombosis of the renal vein is a rare complication of renal transplantation with a reported overall incidence of 0.3–4.2%[62]. It occurs in the early postoperative period, is usually diagnosed after allograft infarction, and almost universally results in allograft nephrectomy. Renal vein thrombosis usually results from venous anastomotic technical complications (i.e. venous kinking or stenosis), extrinsic venous compression from peritransplant hematoma, or a hypercoagulable state, such as in patients with membranous glomerulonephritis and severe nephrotic syndrome and loss of antithrombin III. Also implicated in the etiology of renal vein thrombosis are OKT3 induction immunosuppression and cyclosporine. In addition, renal venous occlusion by progression of lower extremity or caval venous thromboses have been reported.

Renal vein thrombosis is suggested clinically by the abrupt onset of oliguria or anuria, hematuria, acute allograft tenderness, and swelling. An acute increase in allograft venous pressure often causes acute graft rupture and hemorrhage. Radiographically, acute renal vein thrombosis is suspected with the absence of perfusion on renal nuclear scintigraphy [^{99m}Tc-diethylenetriaminepentaacetic acid or ^{99m}Tc-mercaptoacetyltriglycine (^{99m}Tc-MAG3)] in the setting of detection of an arterial signal with reversal of diastolic flow on duplex Doppler sonography[62]. Differential diagnosis includes allograft rejection and ATN; however, neither of these conditions is associated with the absence of perfusion on nuclear scan[62]. Arterial occlusion is associated with a photopenic region in the area of the allograft, whereas in venous thrombosis radiotracer uptake by the allograft resembles that of background activity[62].

Treatment options include prompt exploration and thrombectomy and/or clot lysis using infusion of either systemic[63] or selective intravenous and/or intra-arterial streptokinase. There is limited documented experience with the use of fibrinolytic agents in transplant renal vein thrombosis. However, it appears that selective intra-arterial infusion with high-dose streptokinase may lead to early resolution of thrombus in small venules, which may be critical to graft reperfusion.

Allograft rupture
Graft rupture results from venous thrombosis or hyperacute or accelerated severe rejection; it usually results in loss of the allograft.

Anastomotic hemorrhage and pseudoaneurysms
Significant hemorrhage requires prompt surgical exploration with attempted repair of the bleeding site, as well as transfusion and

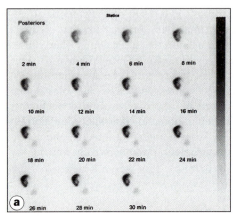

correction of coagulopathy. Anastomotic hemorrhage is suspected clinically with an abrupt drop in blood pressure, widened pulse pressure, tachycardia, acute abdominal and allograft pain, and a drop in hematocrit. Sonography and/or CT scanning aid in radiographic diagnosis. Angiography is carried out in selected cases of suspected pseudoaneurysm. Early causes of anastomotic hemorrhage include technical error and coagulopathy. Late anastomotic hemorrhage, although rare, occurs secondary to pseudoaneurysm formation and vascular anastomotic infection, which results in mycotic aneurysm formation and rupture.

Arteriovenous fistulae
Arteriovenous fistulae (AVFs) occur frequently after allograft percutaneous biopsy, but they are seldom of clinical consequence. Diagnosis is confirmed by color flow Doppler (CFD) sonography, which demonstrates foci of turbulent flow. Most AVFs close spontaneously and require no intervention. Asymptomatic AVFs that are radiographically <1.8cm may be observed with CFD every 3 months with minimal risks of hemorrhage. Those that are asymptomatic but larger than 1.8cm may enlarge and bleed and therefore must be followed with CFD monthly. Those that persist and are symptomatic (hematuria, high-output cardiac failure, renal dysfunction, hypertension) require intervention most commonly with percutaneous transcatheter embolization or (rarely) open surgical closure or nephrectomy.

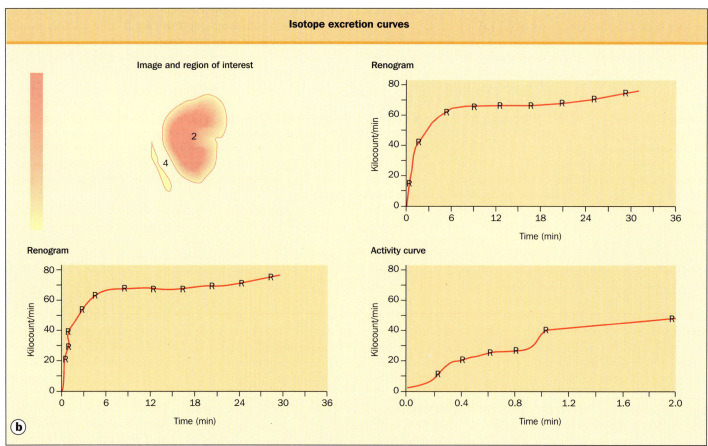

Figure 20.25 Provocative captopril renography in diagnosis of transplant renal artery stenosis. (a) ^{99m}Tc-MAG3 nuclear renal scan after oral captopril 25mg; (b) isotope excretion curves.

LONG-TERM COMPLICATIONS AFTER TRANSPLANTATION

Despite better short-term patient and graft survival results of renal transplantation as a result of improvements in immuno-suppression, long-term patient and graft survival has not increased in recent years. The annual mortality in the second decade after transplantation is 3–4% and an additional 2–3% of patients suffer graft loss each year[64]. The major causes of death are atherosclerotic vascular occlusive disease, sepsis, hepatic failure, and malignancy. In recent years the proportion of infection-related deaths has decreased with an associated increase in the proportion of cardiovascular-related deaths. Chronic rejection is known to be the major cause of late graft loss. Other factors that contribute to late graft loss include recurrent or de-novo renal disease and nonimmunologic factors such as chronic cyclosporine toxicity, nephrotoxicity, hypertension, diabetes, hyperfiltration, and hyperlipidemia[65].

Post-transplant diabetes

Post-transplant diabetes is generally attributed to the use of corticosteroids. Cyclosporine as well tacrolimus (FK506) have been implicated in the occurrence of post-transplant diabetes[66]. The prevalence of post-transplant corticosteroid-induced diabetes has ranged from 3.4 to 46%, depending on the criteria for diagnosis and the duration of follow-up. Post-transplant diabetes may be either insulin or noninsulin dependent and has been reported to occur as early as 3 weeks post-transplant and as late as 19 years post-transplant[66]. For patients with pretransplant diabetes and for those at high-risk of the development of post-transplant diabetes, corticosteroid-free immunosuppressive protocols have been developed[67]. Patients with post-transplant diabetes have poorer patient and graft survival, with increased mortality because of infectious complications[68].

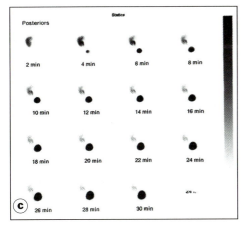

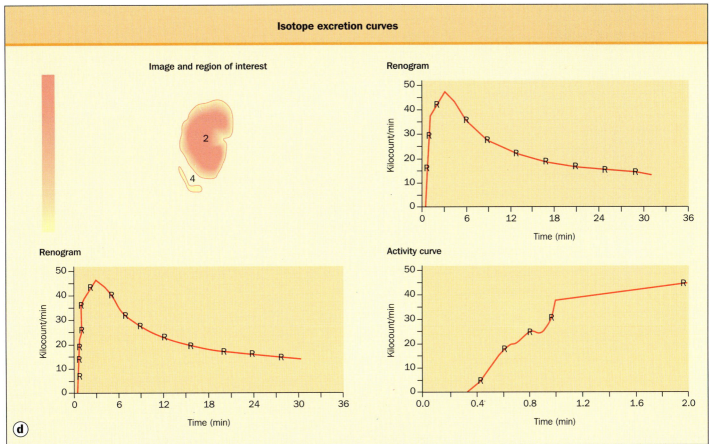

Figure 20.25 Provocative captopril renography in diagnosis of transplant renal artery stenosis (cont'd). (c) ^{99m}Tc-MAG3 nuclear renal scan in same patient as in (a) 1 day later without captopril; (d) isotope excretion curves – note the superior function and excretion compared with those in (b), which indicates a positive captopril renogram consistent with transplant renal artery stenosis.

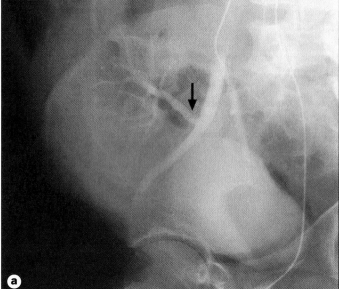

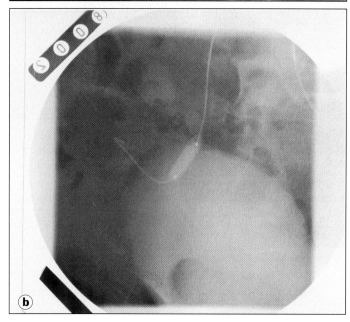

Figure 20.26 Diagnosis of renal transplant arterial stenosis.
(a) Transplant renal arterial stenosis (arrow) arteriography and (b) balloon angioplasty.

Post-transplant malignancies

The incidence of cancer after renal transplantation is significantly higher than that in the nontransplant population. Higher incidences of both specific cancers and cancer in general are well-documented in transplant recipients[69]. Over recent years the pattern of malignancies has changed.

The tumor types that occur with greatest frequency include squamous and basal cell carcinomas of the skin, non-Hodgkin's lymphoma, Kaposi's sarcoma, cervical and vulvar carcinoma, renal cell carcinoma, and hepatobiliary carcinoma. There are observed differences in the types of cancer that occur in recipients of nonrenal organs – lymphomas predominate over skin cancer, and carcinoma of the cervix, vulva, and anus predominate in the renal transplant recipients[69].

The natural history of tumors associated with immunosuppression may be more aggressive than that expected in non-immunosuppressed patients. Post-transplant malignancies occur in a young population (mean age 41 years), with an average time of appearance of malignancies after transplant of 61 months. Certain tumors appear at fairly distinct time intervals post-transplant – Kaposi's sarcoma appears at an average time of 33 months, lymphomas at 33 months, and cancers of the vulva and perineum at 107 months[69]. Malignancies commonly seen in the general population, such as lung, breast, prostate, colon, and invasive uterine carcinoma, show no increase in frequency in the transplant population. The only other common malignancy in the general population seen also in transplant patients is in-situ uterine cervical carcinoma (3% of tumors). The development of these tumors most likely arises from overimmunosuppression with quadruple therapy (antilymphocytic agents such as ATG, antilymphocyte globulin or OKT3, cyclosporine, azathioprine, and prednisone).

Post-transplant lymphoproliferative disorder

The estimated rate of post-transplant lymphoproliferative disorder (PTLD) is 1.0% for renal transplant recipients[70]. The majority of post-transplant lymphomas are non-Hodgkin's lymphomas (93% of all lymphomas versus 65% in the non-transplant general population). Post-transplant non-Hodgkin's lymphomas differ from their counterparts in many respects[71]. In the transplant population there is a greater incidence of extra-nodal involvement – 28% involve the central nervous system multicentrically (as compared to 1% in the general population). The allograft is involved either microscopically or macroscopically in 18% of cases. The incidence of post-transplant lymphomas in the cyclosporine era is greater than that noted in the azathioprine era. Of patients with PTLD, 60% eventually die of the disease.

Pregnancy post-transplant

Successful pregnancy is possible in the female renal transplant recipient. Penn et al.[71] reported 67 pregnancies caused by 50 male renal transplant recipients and 56 pregnancies in 37 female renal transplant recipients. Major risks to the female recipients included a 27% incidence of pre-eclampsia and a 7% risk of permanent renal allograft impairment, with those mothers who had preexisting hypertension or impaired renal function at greatest risk. The pelvic position of the allograft caused no mechanical dystocia during labor. In this series, the incidence of premature labor and delivery was 49%, of which 30% had one or more complications of the neonatal period. Additional observations included chromosomal aberrations in the lymphocytes of offspring of female recipients, but to date no evidence indicates that the offspring of renal transplant recipients have an increased incidence of hematopoetic malignancies. Recommendations for the renal transplant recipient include birth control for 18 months post-transplant to optimize graft function. In addition, patients with impaired allograft function are advised of the high likelihood that pregnancy could lead to further allograft functional deterioration as the pregnancy continues[72].

Male infertility and impotence post-transplant

The effects of uremia and hemodialysis on fertility are known to cause subnormal levels of serum testosterone, perhaps secondary to toxic effects on Leydig cell function[73]. Typically, ESRD patients have an intact hypothalamic–pituitary axis with an appropriate rise in serum luteinizing hormone (LH) and follicle-stimulating hormone (FSH) levels after stimulation by gonadotropin-releasing hormone, but do not have a corresponding rise in serum testosterone[74]. Studies with testicular biopsy show that these men generally have significantly decreased numbers of mature spermatocytes, spermatids, spermatozoa, and total germinative cells, with evidence of spermatogenic arrest[75,76]. Semen analysis is abnormal in patients with renal failure, with decreased sperm density, motility, and number of normal forms[73,75–77]. The spermatogenic insult caused by uremia is not reversed by the institution of hemodialysis, yet it shows significant improvement after successful renal transplantation. Of uremic patients on hemodialysis, 85% are infertile, whereas approximately 50% show improvement in sperm density and sperm motility within 6 months of transplantation[77], with restoration of an appropriate serum testosterone level and subsequent fall in LH and FSH into the normal range[75,78]. Impregnation rates in male renal transplant recipients range from 0 to 42%[73,78]; the suboptimal impregnation rates are believed to occur because of residual, nonreversible gonadotoxicity from long-standing uremia.

Holdsworth et al. reported that persistently elevated serum FSH levels after successful renal transplantation may serve as a marker of irreversible spermatogenic damage[75]. Killion and Rajfer provided an excellent review of the evaluation and management of male infertility following solid-organ transplantation[72].

REFERENCES

1. Christensen AJ, Holman JM, Turner CW, Slaughter JR. Quality of life in end-stage renal disease. Influence of renal transplantation. Clin Transplant. 1989;3:46–53.
2. Hutchinson TA, Thomas DC, Lemieux JC, Harvey CE. Prognostically controlled comparison of dialysis and renal transplantation. Kidney Int. 1984;26:44–51.
3. Burton PR, Walls J. Selection-adjusted comparison of life-expectancy of patients on continuous ambulatory peritoneal dialysis, haemodialysis, and renal transplantation. Lancet 1987;i:1115–9.
4. Suthanthiran M, Strom TB. Renal transplantation. N Engl J Med. 1994;331:365–76.
5. Mitsuishi Y, Cecka JM. Disease effects and associations. In: Terasaki PI, Cecka JM, eds. Clinical transplants 1992. Los Angeles: UCLA Tissue Typing Laboratory; 1993:371–81.
6. McKay DB, Milford EL, Sayegh MH. Clinical aspects of renal transplantation. In: Brenner BM. The kidney. London: WB Saunders; 1996:2602–52.
7. Nossent HC, Swaak TJ, Berden JH. Systemic lupus erythematosus after renal transplantation: patient and graft survival and disease activity. Ann Intern Med. 1991;114:183–8.
8. Hunt J. Pretransplant evaluation and outcome. Semin Nephrol. 1992;12:227–33.
9. Loirst C, Ehrich JHH, Geerlings W, Jones EHP, et al. Report on management of renal failure in children in Europe, XXIII, 1992. Nephrol Dial Transplant. 1994;9(Suppl 1):26–40.
10. Modlin CS, Flechner SF, Goormastic M, et al. Should obese patients lose weight before receiving a kidney transplant? Transplantation 1997:64:599–604.
11. Briggs JD. Patient selection for renal transplantation. Nephrol Dial Transplant. 1995;10(Suppl. 1):10–13.
12. Opelz G, Mickey MR, Terasaki PI. Calculations on long term graft and patient survival in human kidney transplantation. Transplant Proc. 1977;9:27–30.
13. Tilney NL, Milford EL, Aranjo JL, et al. Experience with cyclosporine and steroids in clinical renal transplantation. Ann Surg. 1984;200:605–13.
14. Stratta RJ, Oh CS, Sollinger HW, et al. Kidney transplantation in the cyclosporine era. Transplantation 1988;45:40–5.
15. Goldfarb D, Kapoor, Modliin CS, et al. The Cleveland Clinic experience with third transplant kidney grafts. Submitted for publication.
16. Broyer M, Brunner FP, Brynger H, et al. Kidney transplantation in primary oxalosis: data from the EDTA Registry. Nephrol Dial Transplant. 1990;5:332–6.
17. Watts RWE, Danpure CJ, DePauw L, et al. Combined liver-kidney and isolated liver transplantations for primary hyperoxaluria type 1: the European experience. Nephrol Dial Transplant. 1990;6: 502–11.
18. Ramos EL, Tisher CC. Recurrent diseases in the kidney transplant. Am J Kidney Dis. 1994;24:142–54.
19. Mathew TH. Recurrent disease in renal allografts. Am J Kidney Dis 12: 85–96, 1988.
20. Modlin C, Novick AC, Goormastic M, Mastrioanni B, Myles J. Long-term results with single pediatric donor kidney transplants in adult recipients. J Urol. 1996;156:890–5.
21. Hobart M, Modlin CS, Kapoor A, Flechner SM, Goldfarb DA, Novick AC. Long-term results of transplanting pediatric en bloc cadaveric kidneys into adult recipients. Transplantation 1998;66:1689–94.
22. Merrill JP, Murray JE, Harrison JH, et al. Successful homotransplantation of the human kidney between identical twins. JAMA. 1956;160:277–82.
23. Lowell JA, Taylor RJ. The evaluation of the living renal donor, surgical techniques and results. Semin Urol. 1994;12:102–7.
24. Benedetti E, Hakim NS, Perez EM, Matas AJ. Renal transplantation. Acad Radiol. 1995;2:159–66.
25. Serrano D, Flechner SP, Modlin CS, Streem SB, Goldfarb DA, Novick AC. The use of kidneys from living donors with renal vascular abnormalities: expanding the donor pool. J Urol. 1997;157:1587–91.
26. Jones J, Payne WD, Matas AJ. The living donor: risks, benefits, and related concerns. Transplant Rev. 1993;7:115–28.
27. Bay WH, Hefert LA. The living donor in kidney transplantation. Ann Int Med. 1987;106:719–27.
28. Dunn JR, Richie RE, MacDonell RC, et al. Living related kidney donors: a 14-year experience. Am Surg. 1986;203:637–43.
29. Ringden O, Friman L, Lundgren G, et al. Living related kidney donors: complications and long-term renal function. Transplantation 1978;25:221–3.
30. Spanos PK, Simmons RL, Lampe E. Complications of related kidney donation. Surgery 1974;76:741–7.
31. Cosimi AB. The donor and donor nephrectomy. In: Morris PJ, ed. Kidney transplantation: principles and practice, 4th edn. London: WB Saunders; 1994:56–70.

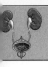

32. Gil-Vernet JM, Gil-Vernet A, Caralps A, et al. Orthotopic renal transplant and results in 139 consecutive cases. J Urol. 1989;142:248–52.

33. Cosimi AB, Burton RC, Colvin RB, et al. Treatment of acute renal allograft rejection with OKT3 monoclonal antibody. Transplantation 1981;32:535–9.

34. Cosimi AB, Colvin RB, Burton RC, et al. Use of monoclonal antibodies to T-cell subsets for immunologic monitoring and treatment in recipients of renal allografts. N Engl J Med. 1981;305: 308–14.

35. Cosimi AB. The future of monoclonal antibody immunosuppression in solid organ transplantation. Transplant Sci. 1992;2:28–31.

36. Frauchiger B, Bock A, Spoendlin M, et al. Early renal transplant dysfunction due to arterial kinking stenosis. Nephrol Dial Transplant. 1994;9:76–9.

37. Solez K, Axelsen RA, Benediktsson H, et al. International standardization criteria for the histologic diagnosis of renal allograft rejection. Kidney Int. 1993;44:411–2.

38. Rigg KM. Renal transplantation: current status, complications and prevention. J Antimicrob Chemother. 1995;36(Suppl B):51–7.

39. Paul LC, Fellstrom B. Chronic vascular rejection of the heart and the kidney. Transplantation 1992;53:1169–79.

40. Streem SB. Endourological management of urological complications following renal transplantation. Semin Urol. 1994;12:123–33.

41. Pardalidis NP, Waltzer WC, Tellis VA, Jarrett TW, Smith AD. Endourologic management of complications in renal allografts. J Endourol. 1994;8:321–7.

42. Lieberman RP, Glass NR, Crummy AB, et al. Nonoperative percutaneous management of urinary fistulae and strictures in renal transplantation. Surg Gynecol Obstet. 1992;155:667–72.

43. Streem SB, Novick AC, Steinmuller DR, et al. Percutaneous techniques for the management of urological renal transplant complications. J Urol. 1986;135:456–9.

44. Bennett LN, Voegeli DR, Crummy AB, et al. Urologic complications following renal transplantation. Role of interventional radiologic procedures. Radiology 1986;160:531–4.

45. Swierzewski SJ III, Konnak JW, Ellis JH. Treatment of renal transplant ureteral complications by percutaneous techniques. J Urol. 1993;149:986–7.

46. Schiff M Jr, McGuire EJ, Weiss RM, Lytton B. Management of urinary fistulae after renal transplantation. J Urol. 1976;115:251–5.

47. Caldwell TC, Burns JR. Current operative management of urinary calculi after renal transplantation. J Urol. 1988;140:1360–3.

48. Gray DWR. Graft renal artery stenosis in the transplanted kidney. Transplantation Rev. 1994;8:15–21.

49. Erley CM, Duda SH, Wakat J-P, et al. Noninvasive procedures for diagnosis of renovascular hypertension in renal transplant recipients: a prospective analysis. Transplantation 1992;54:863–7.

50. Shamlou KK, Drane WE, Hawkins IF, Fennell RS. Captopril renogram and the hypertensive renal transplantation patient: a predictive test of therapeutic outcome. Radiology 1994;190:153–9.

51. Idrissi A, Fournier H, Renaud B, et al. The captopril challenge test as a screening test for renovascular hypertension. Kidney Int. 1988;34(Suppl 25):138–41.

52. Lewin JS, Laub G, Hausmann R. Three-dimensional time-of-flight MR angiography: applications in the abdomen and thorax. Radiology 1991;179:261–4.

53. Rubin GD, Dake MD, Napel SA, McDonnell CH, Jeffrey RB Jr. Three-dimensional spiral CT angiography of the abdomen: initial clinical experience. Radiology 1993;186:147–52.

54. Kuo PC, Peterson J, Semba C, Alfrey EJ, Dafoe DC. CO_2 angiography: a technique for vascular imaging in renal allograft dysfunction. Transplantation 1996;61:652–4.

55. Merkus JWS, Huymans FTM, Hoitsma AJ, Buskens FGM, Skotnicki SH, Koene RAP. Renal allograft artery stenosis: results of medical treatment and intervention: a retrospective analysis. Transplant Int. 1993;6:111–5.

56. Benoit G, Moukarzel M, Hiesse C, Verdelli G, Charpentier B, Fries D. Transplant renal artery stenosis: experience and comparative results between surgery and angioplasty. Transplant Int. 1990;3:137–40.

57. Newman-Sander APG, Gedroyc WG, Al-Kutouby MA, Koo C, Taube D. The use of expandable metal stents in transplant renal artery stenosis. Clin Radiol. 1995;50:245–50.

58. Chandrasoma P, Aberle AM. Anastomotic line renal artery stenosis after transplantation. J Urol. 1986;135:1159–62.

59. Sutherland RS, Spees EK, Jones JW, Fink DW. Renal artery stenosis after renal transplantation: the impact of the hypogastric artery anastomosis. J Urol. 1993;149:980–5.

60. Fauchald P, Vatne K, Paulsen D, et al. Long term clinical results of percutaneous transluminal angioplasty in transplant renal artery stenosis. Nephrol Dial Transplant. 1992;7:256–9.

61. Greenstein S, Verstanding A, McLean G, et al. Percutaneous transluminal angioplasty. Transplantation 1987;43:29–32.

62. Duckett T, Bretan PN, Cochran ST, Rajfer J, Rosenthal JT. Noninvasive radiological diagnosis of renal vein thrombosis in renal transplantation. J Urol. 1991;146:403–6.

63. Chiu AS, Landsberg DN. Successful treatment of acute transplant renal vein thrombosis with selective streptokinase infusion. Transplant Proc. 1991;23:2297–300.

64. Rao TKS, Gupta SK, Butt KHM, Kountz SL, Friedman EA. Relationship of renal transplantation to hypertension in end-stage renal failure. Arch Intern Med. 1978;138:1236–41.

65. Modlin CS, Hafez K. Clinical significance of positive CMV urine culture in renal transplant patients with cytomegaloviral septicemia (Abstract). American Society Transplant Physicians 1997.

66. Freidman EA, Shyh Tai-ping, Beyer MM, Manis T, Butt KMH. Posttransplant diabetes in kidney transplant recipients. Am J Nephrol. 1985;5:196–202.

67. Hariharan S, Schroder TJ, Weiskittel P, et al. Prednisone withdrawal in HLA identical and one haplotype-matched live related donor and cadaver renal transplants. Kidney Int. 1993;44:S30–5.

68. Sumrani NB, Delaney V, Ding Z, et al. Posttransplant diabetes. Transplantation 1991;51:343–7.

69. Penn I. Cancers complicating organ transplantation. N Engl J Med. 1990;323:1767–9.

70. Nalesnik M, Makowka L, Starzl T. The diagnosis and treatment of posttransplant lymphoproliferative disorders. Curr Prob Surg. 1988;25:371–472.

71. Penn I, Makowski E, Harris P. Parenthood following renal and hepatic transplantation. Transplantation 1980;30:397–400.

72. Killion D, Rajfer J. The evaluation and management of male infertility following solid-organ transplantation. Semin Urol. 1994;12:140–6.

73. Rodrigues Netto N, Pecoraro G, Sabbaga E, et al. Spermatogenesis before and after renal transplant. Int J Fertil. 1980;25:131–3.

74. Baumgarten SR, Lindsay GK, Wise GJ. Fertility problems in the renal transplant patient. J Urol. 1977;118:991–3.

75. Holdsworth SR, Atkins RC, DeKrester DM. The pituitary–testicular axis in men with chronic renal failure. N Engl J Med. 1977;296:1245–9.

76. Phadke AG, MacKinnon KJ, Dossetor JB. Male fertility in uremia: restoration by renal allografts. Can Med Assoc J. 1970;102:607–8.

77. Reinberg Y, Bumgardner GL, Aliabadi H. Urological aspects of renal transplantation. J Urol. 1990;143:1087–92.

78. Penn I, Makowski E, Droegemueller W, et al. Parenthood in renal homograft recipients. JAMA 1971;216:1755–61.

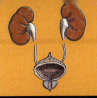

Chapter 21

Urinary Tract Infections

Kent T Perry Jr and Anthony J Schaeffer

KEY POINTS

- 'Simple' urinary tract infections may become life-threatening in the presence of complicating factors.
- The presence of pili may explain the predilection of certain bacteria for different anatomic sites.
- Deficient host defense mechanisms may be critically important in some recurrent infections.
- Treatment of patients with complicated infections requires careful consideration of all risk factors.
- Patients with 'prostatitis' may have a spectrum of disorders requiring accurate diagnosis for successful treatment.

INTRODUCTION

Fundamentally important to the clinical and scientific practice of urology is an understanding of the pathogenesis, diagnosis, and treatment of urinary tract infections. Many urologic referrals will be for the evaluation and treatment of recurrent or severe urinary tract infections (UTIs) and prostatitis syndromes. It is important to evaluate correctly, diagnose, and treat patients who are at higher risk for severe sequelae because of an underlying functional or anatomic disorder. Conversely, it is desirable to minimize evaluation and treatment for patients with uncomplicated UTIs when not necessary, in order to reduce morbidity and risk of serious sequelae. We physicians are fortunate to be practicing medicine at a time where we have seen the development of excellent diagnostic capabilities, particularly in the field of imaging techniques. Additionally, we have seen the development of new broad-spectrum oral antimicrobials that attain excellent urinary tract penetration, and we have began to understand in more detail the pathogenesis of urinary tract infections, which should aid in our ability to better diagnose and treat patients with UTIs.

DEFINITIONS

Urinary tract infection

Urinary tract infection is bacterial invasion of the urothelium resulting in an inflammatory response[1], which usually presents as frequency, urgency, and dysuria with associated pyuria and bacteriuria. Fever and flank pain suggest infection of the kidney.

Complicated or potentially complicated infection

This is a urinary tract infection that is at moderate to high risk of resulting in sepsis, tissue destruction, or other significant morbidity and mortality. Additionally, a severe infection may uncover an anatomic, functional, or metabolic abnormality of the urinary tract, previously unknown to the patient and clinician, that will require more extensive evaluation and a change in treatment strategy. The majority of urinary tract infections, particularly in sexually active women, are not severe infections that require extensive imaging or prolonged antimicrobial therapy. However, some infections are associated with either an anatomic or a functional abnormality of the urinary tract that decreases the ability of the host to mount an effective response to and subsequently eliminate the pathogen. Figures 21.1–21.3 list some factors that should alert the urologist to an increased likelihood of severe or complicated infection.

Isolated infection

This is a first infection or an infection temporally isolated from previous infection by more than 6 months[1]. Approximately 50% of all women report that they have had a UTI by their late 20s[2]. An isolated infection may occur in men, but these are much less common.

Unresolved infection

This is an infection that fails to respond to an appropriate course of antimicrobial therapy, with persistent symptoms and without

Factors increasing the likelihood of complicated urinary tract infection
Male sex
Elderly
Febrile UTI
Symptoms for more than 7 days
Signs or symptoms of obstruction
Hematuria
History of nephrolithiasis
Recently hospitalized
Urinary tract instrumentation
Concurrent pregnancy, diabetes or immunosuppression
Infection with drug-resistant organism
Functional or structural abnormality (see Fig. 21.2)

Figure 21.1 Factors increasing the likelihood of complicated urinary tract infection (UTI).

Common functional and anatomic abnormalities

Indwelling catheter

Postvoid residual urine greater than about 100mL

Functional or neurogenic disturbances of micturition

Vesicoureteral reflux

Poorly functioning renal unit with resulting urinary stasis

Surgically created urinary diversion

Figure 21.2 Common functional and anatomic abnormalities.

Common complicating medical situations

Diabetes mellitus

Decreased renal function

Immunosuppressive illness

Figure 21.3 Common complicating medical situations.

Causes of unresolved bacteriuria in descending order of importance

Bacterial resistance to chosen antimicrobial agent

Acquired resistance from initially susceptible bacteria

Bacteriuria caused by two different species with mutually exclusive susceptibilities

Rapid reinfection with a new, resistant species during treatment for the original organism

Azotemia

Papillary necrosis

Giant staghorn calculi in which the critical mass of sensitive bacteria is too great for antimicrobial inhibition

Patient failing to take antimicrobial medication

Figure 21.4 Causes of unresolved bacteriuria in descending order of importance.

Common community and nosocomial urinary tract infection pathogens

Escherichia coli

Staphylococcus saprophyticus

Proteus spp. (most common in men)

Providencia spp. (more common in men)

Klebsiella spp.

Pseudomonas spp.

Citrobacter spp.

Serratia spp.

Enterococcus faecalis

Figure 21.5 Common community and nosocomial urinary tract infection pathogens.

---

resolution by culture at any time during therapy. The physician can miss this type of infection if cultures are not obtained during therapy or if cultures with less than 10^5 bacteria are misinterpreted as negative. Figure 21.4 lists the most common causes of unresolved bacteriuria.

The most important factor is bacterial resistance to the chosen empiric antimicrobial regimen. This is not completely unavoidable but can be minimized by knowledge of the bacterial antimicrobial profile of the uropathogens most frequently encountered in the local environment. Occasionally, an originally sensitive organism may acquire resistance to an antimicrobial during treatment or a resistant phenotype present in low numbers may persist. This occurs in approximately 5% of patients on antimicrobial therapy[3] and can be minimized by using adequate dosing regimens and emphasizing patient compliance. Additionally, two or more phenotypes or species of bacteria may be involved with differing, nonoverlapping sensitivities. During initial treatment, as the susceptible pathogen is eliminated, a selection bias favors growth of the resistant species. Azotemia and papillary necrosis increase the likelihood of an unresolved UTI because decreased renal concentrating ability may prevent antimicrobial concentrations from reaching bacteriostatic or bacteriocidal levels. Staghorn calculi can produce a 'critical mass' of bacteria that are too numerous to clear and become a focus of continued bacterial infection. Finally, a common reason for unresolved infection, which may frequently be erroneously attributed to any of the above scenarios, is failing to take the prescribed treatment.

Recurrent infection

Recurrent infection is characterized by UTI following resolution of initial infection as defined by negative culture during therapy. Recurrence may occur as a result of either reinfection from a source outside the urinary tract or bacterial persistence within the urinary tract. Reinfection is responsible for over 95% of recurrent UTIs in women[1] and 25% of all women with a first UTI will have a reinfection[4]. Bacterial persistence is more common in males and may imply an anatomic anomaly or obstruction

where surgical intervention may be required. Additionally, bacterial persistence usually gives rise to a shorter interval between infections and occurs with the same bacteria.

PATHOGENESIS

There are several factors that influence the probability of developing a UTI. Additionally, there are factors that help to predict the potential severity of an infection. Much work has been done recently to advance our knowledge of UTIs regarding the route of infection and, in particular, the bacterial virulence factors that augment attachment of bacteria to epithelial cell surfaces. Additionally, we continue to increase our knowledge of the bacteria most likely to be involved in a given setting and the evolving sensitivity spectra of these organisms.

Organisms

The majority of urinary tract pathogens are Gram-negative facultative anaerobes (Fig. 21.5), which are generally present in the bowel flora. Gram-positive organisms, including *Staphylococcus saprophyticus* and *Enterococcus faecalis*, may also cause urinary tract infections. Anaerobes are much less common as solitary infecting organisms. However, they must be suspected in a symptomatic patient with a negative urine culture who has a urine Gram stain-positive for Gram-positive rods or Gram-negative cocci. Anaerobes are very commonly found as one of many pathogens in an abscess and are frequently responsible for gas production within an abscess cavity. It has been observed that 88% of scrotal, prostatic, and perinephric abscesses are positive for anaerobic organisms[5].

In the community-acquired setting, *Escherichia coli* causes approximately 85% of UTIs in women. Other Gram-negative Enterobacteriaceae that are found less frequently and cause between 5–10% of UTIs in women include *Proteus* spp. and *Klebsiella* spp. *Staphylococcus saprophyticus*, a Gram-positive organism, is seen in 10–30% of UTIs in young adult females, depending on the season[6]. Additionally, one may find *E. faecalis* in the community setting.

The nosocomial UTI has similar pathogens to those found in the community, with differing prevalences. Additionally, one sees organisms not generally found in the community setting. Importantly, these organisms, as with other nosocomial infections, tend to be resistant to many of the antimicrobials that one would consider as a first-line treatment for a noncomplicated urinary tract infection. For example, at our institution, 26% of *E. coli* specimens are resistant to trimethoprim–sulfamethoxazole (TMP-SMX)[7]. In terms of prevalence, *E. coli* is again the most frequent species, but at 50% is less than found in the community. In contrast to the community setting, *E. faecalis* is a frequently encountered pathogen[8], but exhibits near-100% susceptibility to penicillins and aminopenicillins[7]. Other common Gram-negative bacteria include *Pseudomonas* spp., *Citrobacter* spp., and *Serratia* spp.

Although the majority of UTIs occur in women, and the majority of research efforts focus on UTIs in the female, males are also susceptible. In fact, 12% of men between the ages of 14 and 61 report a history of kidney, bladder, or urine infection. The organisms responsible for UTI in men differ from those seen in the female population. As in females, nearly three quarters of UTIs in men are caused by Gram-negative bacilli. However, only approximately 25% are caused by *E. coli*[9]. With the majority consisting of other Gram-negative species, particularly *Proteus* spp. and less frequently *Providencia* spp., Gram-positive organisms, in particular enterococci and coagulase-negative staphylococci, account for about 20% of UTIs in men[10]. In contrast to females, *S. saprophyticus* is rarely a uropathogen in men[11].

Genitourinary fungal infections are much less common than bacterial infections but they are of increasing prevalence in a broad population and are not an uncommon occurrence in the intensive care units at any institution. *Candida albicans* is the most common genitourinary fungal pathogen, followed by other *Candida* spp. and *Turulopsis glabrata*[12]. *Candida* is quite common in humans. It is frequently found as a component of the vaginal flora and is present in the feces of 10–20% of normal subjects[13]. Originally, it was believed that candiduria could be found in 0–4% of healthy subjects. Subsequently, it was determined that a properly collected urine specimen that grows any number of *Candida* colonies should be considered as pathologic and treated appropriately. This is especially important when one considers that the kidney is the most frequently involved organ in systemic candidiasis and that systemic candidiasis is universally fatal if not treated.

Mycobacterium tuberculosis has declined in prevalence and mortality but it is frequently not appreciated that tuberculosis is still one of the most lethal of the infectious diseases. Genitourinary (GU) tuberculosis frequently presents as sterile pyuria. It has been identified in all regions of the genitourinary system from the kidneys to the genitals. It is found most commonly in the epididymis and prostate in terms of GU extrapulmonary tubercular disease. It may present in a myriad of signs and symptoms. Systemic symptoms typically include cachexia and febrile spikes, which generally occur in the evening. Pathologies specific to the GU tract include: sterile pyuria; ureteral involvement, which may appear radiographically as a ureteral stricture; and renal involvement, varying from miliary tuberculosis to caseous decay of renal parenchyma. In a recent epidemiologic study it was demonstrated that renal tuberculosis was present in 0.6% of the population at autopsy. Additionally, renal involvement was found in 52–68% of the population with pulmonary miliary tuberculosis[14].

Bacterial virulence factors

It has been well established that most bacteria reach the urinary tract in an ascending manner. Bacteria are normal flora in the bowel, ascend from the rectum to the vagina where they adhere and colonize, and then migrate through the urethra and bladder. The bacteria must overcome host defense factors such as the flow of urine and mucus secretion. Bacteria have developed specific virulence factors that greatly increase their probability of success in terms of establishing infection. These virulence factors include bacterial adhesins, which mediate attachment to glycoprotein on the urothelium. Most of these interactions take place between rod-shaped pili (or fimbriae) and glycolipids found on the epithelial cell surface. In addition to pili, bacteria may also secrete substances such as toxins that damage the urothelium, or protease to enhance their survivability in an acidic environment. Figure 21.6 lists bacterial virulence factors.

Bacterial adherence

Before a bacterium is able to colonize and invade the urinary tract, it must first be able to adhere to the surface of the urothelium. Bacteria express structures known as pili (or fimbriae), which are rod-like structures that extend from the outer bacterial membrane and express adhesins that attach to various glycolipids of the host cell (Fig. 21.7). They are historically defined by their ability to agglutinate erythrocytes in either the presence or absence of mannose.

Bacterial virulence factors	
Factor	**Action**
Type I pili	Most commonly expressed adherence factor
P pili	Pili most strongly associated with pyelonephritis
Hemolysin	*Escherichia coli* secreted toxin that lyses erythrocytes
Urease	Produced by *Pseudomonas*, *Klebsiella*, *Proteus*, and *S. saprophyticus*, generates nitrogen/struvite stones
Swarming motility	Phenotypic change in *P. mirabilis* that enhances many virulence factors
CNF1	Toxin produced by *E. coli* ?cytotoxic effect on the kidney

Figure 21.6 Bacterial virulence factors.

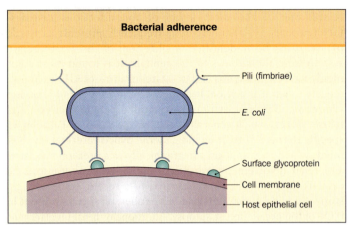

Figure 21.7 Bacterial adherence. Bacterial adhesins attach to surface glycolipids of the host epithelial cell. Each bacterium expresses 100–400 pili.

Type I pili, a mannose-sensitive hemagglutinin, bind to uroplakins Ia and Ib[15], which are membrane proteins found in the urothelium. This is the most common type of pilus expressed in *E. coli*[16] and is found in the majority of isolates that produce cystitis and about half of those that produce pyelonephritis[17]. The majority of *E. coli* possess fim genes coding for type I pili but the expression of pili is subject to phase variation between states of expression and nonexpression of pili. Nonfimbriated phenotypes are more likely to be seen as bacteria suspended in the urine, whereas the piliated phenotypes are found on the urothelium. In one study, O1:K1:H7 pathogenic *E. coli* expressing type I pili caused more pyuria and higher colony counts than the same serogroup that was a null construct for the type I pili. Additionally, when the type I pili gene was reintroduced to the bacteria, the virulence again increased[18].

P pili, a mannose-insensitive hemagglutinin, are so named for both their frequent association with pyelonephritis, and their binding site to P blood group antigens. The P pili bind poorly to the bladder epithelium and preferably to the urothelium lining the collecting system of the kidney. The location and severity of infection correlates with the expression of P pili. P pilus expression is found in 80% of isolates causing pyelonephritis, compared to 30% of isolates causing cystitis[19]. Additionally, P pilus adherence to the urothelium may play a role in inducing *E. coli* expression of other virulence determinants, such as hemolysin, in response to the environment[20].

There are several other piliated and nonpiliated adhesins that have more recently been discovered and their roles in the pathogenesis of UTIs is not as well defined. *Proteus mirabilis* is known to express several types of fimbria, some of which have been implicated in pyelonephritis. *Klebsiella* spp. produce a mannose-resistant hemagglutinin. This is a pilus that mediates attachment to epithelial cells of the kidney and lung. Additionally, there are bacterial surface proteins, such as the Dr adhesins of *E. coli*, that bind to a glycoprotein that protects epithelial cells from complement-mediated damage. While the roles of many of these other adhesins are not yet well studied, they offer additional targets for future UTI therapies and infection prevention.

Toxin production

The *E. coli* that cause UTI are a select subset of the organisms that comprise the *E. coli* of the colonic flora. In 1953, it was recognized that *E. coli* that produced hemolysin, a toxin that causes lysis of erythrocytes, led to infections that were more lethal than those *E. coli* isolates that did not produce the toxin[21]. Soon after this, serologic typing of *E. coli* showed that specific O:K:H groups were more likely to cause infection. In 1966, it was demonstrated that serogroups O1, O4, O6, O18, and O75 accounted for 72% of the hemolytic strains isolated[22]. Further epidemiologic studies have demonstrated that hemolytic *E. coli* are isolated twice as often from the upper urinary tract as from the lower tract. Additionally, in a mouse model, hemolysin-positive strains that colonized the kidney produced death in 66% of the animals. When the same bacteria was mutated to a hemolysin-negative strain and allowed to colonize the kidney, none of the mice died[23]. Cytotoxic necrotizing factor type 1 (CNF1) is a second toxin produced by some pathogenic strains of *E. coli* that is similar in structure to a dermonecrotic toxin[17]. Evidence suggests that CNF1 probably does not act alone to produce its cytotoxic effect in the kidney. However, one study found that 37% of *E. coli* strains producing pyelonephritis were positive for CNF1 compared to only 3% of isolates of colonic *E. coli*[24].

Urease is produced commonly by various strains of *Pseudomonas*, *Klebsiella*, and *Proteus*, and *S. saprophyticus*. There are some rare strains of *E. coli* that produce a plasmid-encoded urease[25]. Urease is used to generate a useful nitrogen source for the bacteria by the breakdown of urea to produce ammonia and carbamate. Additionally, the ammonia elevates the pH of the urine, producing a more favorable environment for these organisms. The ammonia also promotes the formation of magnesium ammonium phosphate (struvite) calculi. These calculi further promote bacterial pathogenesis by causing obstruction and acting as a nidus for bacterial persistence.

Swarming motility is a phenotypic change that can be observed in *P. mirabilis*. When *P. mirabilis* is grown in liquid media the bacteria appear as short, fimbriated rods with fewer than 10 flagella. However, when grown on solid media these bacteria differentiate into cells that are not fimbriated but express thousands of flagella[26]. This differentiation occurs in response to a change in the viscosity of the environment in which the bacteria are established. Several observations about the swarming characteristic lead to the conclusion that this is a significant virulence factor in *P. mirabilis*. First, the increased expression of flagellar genes greatly increases the motility of each bacterium. Second, there is an associated 30–80 times overexpression of other virulence factors such as urease, hemolysin, and proteases in the swarmer cells compared to the nonswarming phenotype[27]. Finally, mutant *P. mirabilis* that had lost the ability to express the swarmer phenotype failed to establish kidney infections in mice, whereas the wild type effectively colonized the mouse renal epithelium[28].

Host factors

There are several host factors that play a role in the defense against and the development of UTI. These factors include urine, voiding, and the receptivity of the vaginal epithelium. Species of *E. coli* that cause UTI grow well in urine through their own adaptive measures. However, urine is bactericidal to most species of bacteria and to most fecal isolates of *E. coli*[29]. There are several factors in urine that are inhibitory to bacterial growth. These factors include urine acidity, urine osmolality, urea, organic acids, and secreted inhibitory factors. Bacterial growth is inhibited by very dilute urine, supporting the widely held belief that increased fluid intake decreases the occurrence of UTIs. Additionally, a high osmolality when associated with a low pH is highly inhibitory[30].

The physical act of micturition and the flow of urine in an antegrade fashion flush bacteria from the urinary tract and are important host defense mechanisms[31]. Defects in micturition and urine flow such as benign prostatic hypertrophy, vesico-ureteral reflux, and stricture disease greatly predispose to the development of urinary tract infections. Bacteria frequently reach the bladder via the urethra and only infrequently does a UTI ensue. One of the major defenses against the establishment of adherent bacteria in adequate numbers is the constant flow of urine washing away nonadherent bacteria and maintaining the sterility of urine. It has been experimentally demonstrated that the ability of bacteria to divide and colonize the bladder is frequently exceeded by the dilution and displacement of bacteria in urine through micturition[31].

Secreted factors in urine also play an important role as inhibitors of bacterial growth. The most important of these factors is the Tamm–Horsfall glycoprotein (THP) or uromodulin. THP is produced by the tubular epithelial cells of the ascending loop of Henle and the distal convoluted tubule and is secreted into the urine[32]. THP is the most abundant protein in human urine and can be seen in clumps, alone or associated with exfoliated epithelial cells, under light microscopy. THP acts as a receptor matrix for type I and type S fimbriated bacteria, thereby inhibiting the adherence of bacteria to the uroepithelium[33]. Additionally, THP binds to neutrophils and enhances phagocytosis[34]. However, THP does not bind to the P pili of *E. coli*, possibly partially explaining the increased virulence of P-piliated strains. THP is also produced in decreased quantity in the elderly population, possibly contributing to the increased incidence of bacteriuria in the elderly population.

Vaginal epithelial cell receptivity is an important host factor for UTI. Vaginal epithelial cells from women with a history of recurrent UTIs were significantly more receptive for virulent *E. coli* strains than were cells from healthy women[35]. Additional studies have suggested that a genetic susceptibility may play a role in UTI development. For example, possessing the HLA A3 antigen more than quadruples the risk of developing recurrent UTIs in women[36]. Furthermore, the expression of specific blood group antigens plays a role in UTI susceptibility. The Lewis blood group antigens control fucosylation of membrane proteins. The phenotype that expresses this antigen is known as a secretor, whereas nonsecretors do not exhibit these antigens on cell surfaces. The nonsecretor phenotypes, Le (a– b–) and Le (a+ b–), are overexpressed in women with recurrent urinary tract infections[37]. This suggests that fucosylation at the cell surface decreases the ability of bacteria to attach to cell surface antigens of the uroepithelium.

DIAGNOSIS

Diagnosis of urinary tract infection involves the appropriate collection of urine to minimize possible contamination, microscopic examination of the urine, appropriate interpretation of data received from the urine culture, and knowledge of localization procedures.

Urine collection

There are three ways to collect urine for diagnostic purposes. They are, in order of increasing risk of contamination, suprapubic aspiration, urethral catheterization, and midstream or two-glass voided specimens. Suprapubic bladder aspiration is safe but relatively unpleasant (Fig. 21.8). It is seldom required but may be useful in newborn infants and paraplegics[1]. Bladder aspiration should be performed when the bladder is palpably full. The appropriate site for needle puncture is in the midline, two fingerwidths above the pubic symphysis. The area should be shaved and cleaned with an antiseptic. Cutaneous anesthesia should be established by the raising of a wheal with 1% lidocaine with a 25G needle. A 22G 3.5" (90mm) spinal needle should then be inserted through the wheal into the bladder and 20mL of urine is aspirated into the syringe. A small amount is sent for culture and the remainder is spun and examined under light microscopy. The needle should be gently withdrawn and a small sterile bandage placed over the aspiration site.

Urethral catheterization

Urethral catheterization for urine culture should be performed only in the female patient. The labia minora and urethral meatus are cleaned with soap and water. While the labia minora are spread, a small 10–14F red rubber catheter is inserted through the urethra into the bladder. At least 20mL of mid-stream urine should be collected into a sterile container. Obviously, introducing infection by catheterizing to obtain a specimen is an undesirable but potential risk. The risk of urinary tract infection from catheterizing a female patient varies from 0.5% to 1% in the outpatient setting and from 10% to 20% in the hospital setting[38]. In order to decrease the risk of urinary tract infection, a single dose of an antimicrobial may be given at the time of catheterization.

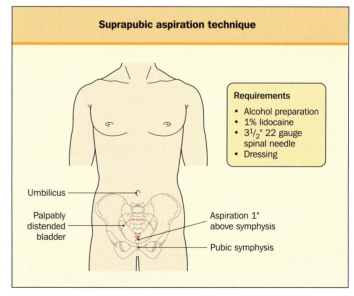

Suprapubic aspiration technique

Requirements
• Alcohol preparation
• 1% lidocaine
• 3½" 22 gauge spinal needle
• Dressing

Umbilicus

Palpably distended bladder

Aspiration 1" above symphysis

Pubic symphysis

Figure 21.8 Suprapubic aspiration technique. Aspiration as described in text should only be performed if the bladder can be detected (palpation or ultrasound) above the pubic symphysis with confidence.

Midstream urine collection

Midstream urine collection in the female, or two-glass urine collection in the male is the easiest and most frequently used method for urine collection. The midstream collection in the female involves instructing the patient to spread the labia and wipe the periurethral area with a clean, tap-water-moistened gauze in a cephalad to caudal nature. The middle portion of the void is collected in the sterile container provided to the patient. In men a two-glass specimen comprising the first 10mL of urine can be collected as the urethral sample, also known as the VB_1. The bladder portion, the VB_2, is collected after an additional 100–150mL of urine has been voided. No preparation is required for circumcised men. If uncircumcised, the patient should retract the foreskin and wipe the glans with a wet gauze, followed by a dry gauze.

Localization cultures

Localization cultures are essential in the male patient who is being evaluated for chronic bacterial prostatitis. After collection of the VB_1 and VB_2 specimens, the physician performs prostatic massage and collects the expressed prostatic secretion (EPS) from the urethra on to a glass slide for microscopic examination. The patient is then asked to void the initial 10mL into a sterile container labeled VB_3[39]. To confirm the diagnosis of bacterial prostatitis, the VB_3 culture should have 10 times the bacterial count of the VB_1 and VB_2 specimens[39]. Upper tract localization procedures are performed by ureteral catheterization and collection of urine from the kidney.

Urinalysis

After collecting a urine specimen a dipstick test and microscopic urinalysis should be performed on the specimen. In addition to pH, protein, and glucose, the dipstick can provide indirect evidence of bacteria (nitrite) and leukocytes (leukocyte esterase), which is helpful as a screening examination for asymptomatic patients. Next, the centrifuged sediment should be examined for white blood cells (WBCs), WBC casts, red blood cells, and bacteria. White and red blood cells in urine are one of the hallmarks of UTI. Pyuria with a negative routine culture may be indicative of nephrolithiasis, tuberculosis, or tumor. The excretion of 400,000WBCs per hour into the urine has been demonstrated to be the upper limit of normal[40]. This is approximately 10WBCs per high-power field (hpf) of urine and is indicative of significant inflammation. The volume of urine represented by one high-power field is $1/30,000mL^1$. Thus, if a specimen being examined has only 1 bacterium/hpf, that equals approximately 30,000 bacteria/mm³. Since a urinary tract infection may be present with bacterial counts of less than 30,000, the absence of bacteriuria does not exclude a urinary tract infection. Conversely, lactobacilli from the vaginal mucosa may contaminate the voided urine and give a false-positive urinalysis. The presence of vaginal epithelial cells should be noted, as they suggest contamination.

Urine culture

Regardless of how carefully a urine specimen is collected there are almost always a few contaminant bacteria present. To prevent bacterial growth prior to culture, urine should be stored in a refrigerator immediately upon collection and cultured within 24 hours of collection.

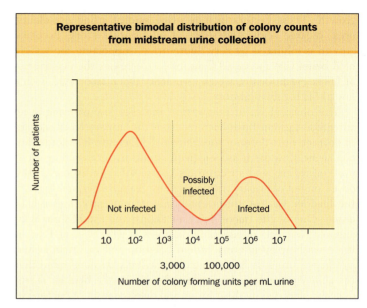

Figure 21.9 **Representative bimodal distribution of colony counts from midstream urine collection.**

The number 10^5cfu (colony forming units)/mL of urine was not derived arbitrarily. When midstream urine cultures are examined in a large number of patients, a bimodal distribution of colony counts is found (Fig. 21.9). The first, largest distribution with lower colony counts represented specimens that were either badly contaminated or were delayed in their transport to the lab. The second, smaller distribution represented patients with a probable infection. Virtually all patients with colony counts above 10^5 had a urinary tract infection. On the other hand, nearly all patients with counts below 3,000 did not have a UTI[40]. Approximately 70% of patients with UTI will have 10^5cfu/mL and 30% will have 10^2–10^4cfu/mL. Therefore, there is a moderate sized area beneath these curves that represent the intermediate probability of infection being present, those with counts between ~3000–100,000.

The interpretation of results in the intermediate probability patients can be aided by an understanding of factors that might decrease the number of organisms cultured in a patient that does indeed have a UTI. These factors include high urine flow rates, current antimicrobial treatment, and frequent voiding. Other factors that favor infection include pyuria, a specimen that was collected carefully, a single pathogenic organism, and the same organism found on repeat culture. Additionally, the technique of urine collection influences the reliability of the urine culture results (Fig. 21.10).

TREATMENT OF LOWER TRACT INFECTION

Uncomplicated acute cystitis

The selection of the appropriate antimicrobial agent is simple but requires minor forethought. Factors that influence the choice of agent include probable pathogen, recent antimicrobial exposure or institutionalization (high risk of resistant organism), patient allergy, potential side effects, and cost.

Most uncomplicated acute cystitis can be treated with urine culture and 3 days of antimicrobial therapy. Single-dose therapy

Factors that favor the presence of urinary tract infection
>10cfu/mL from suprapubic aspiration
>100cfu/mL from catheter specimen
>1000cfu/mL from midstream specimen
Symptoms present
Pyuria present
Single organism present
Same organism present on repeat culture
Intermediate cfu/mL culture results in the presence of   1) use of antimicrobials, 2) high fluid intake, 3) frequent voiding

Figure 21.10 Factors that favor the presence of urinary tract infection.

Groups at increased risk for severe sequelae resulting from urinary tract infection
Elderly people
Males
Pregnant women
Diabetics
Immunosuppressed people
Those with a functional or anatomic urinary tract anomaly

Figure 21.11 Groups at increased risk of severe sequelae resulting from urinary tract infection.

has been advocated by some in uncomplicated acute cystitis, but has higher recurrence rates[41,42]. A 3-day course with either TMP-SMX or a quinolone will cure 85% and 95% of women respectively[43]. Cystitis complicated by pregnancy, diabetes, elderly, recurrent UTI, or the presence of symptoms for more than a week prior to the initiation of treatment should be treated with culture and antimicrobials for 7–10 days. The presence of fever and/or flank pain suggests pyelonephritis and should be treated as such (see Pyelonephritis). More severe complicating factors, including oliguria, renal insufficiency, anatomic or functional abnormalities of the urinary tract, immunocompromised states, and other host-compromising illnesses, require culture and 14 days of therapy.

Complicating factors
The diagnosis of UTI requires special consideration in several groups. They may be at increased risk for treatment failure, have increased morbidity from UTI, or require a different treatment from conventional patients with a urinary tract infection (Fig. 21.11).

Infection in the elderly
The prevalence of urinary tract infection increases significantly with increasing age. The prevalence of bacteriuria increases from 5–10% in those aged 70 years to 20% in those aged 80 years or more[44]. The rate of bacteriuria increases with degree of functional impairment.

Urinary tract infections are the most common source of bacteremia in the elderly population[45]. Additionally, elderly women with nonobstructed pyelonephritis are more likely to become bacteremic than their younger counterparts[46]. On the other hand, because of the high prevalence of bacteriuria in the elderly population, it is unlikely that fever in an asymptomatic elderly individual with bacteriuria is secondary to a urinary source[47].

The elderly population requires a modified approach to treatment of urinary tract infections. There is no definitive proof that the treatment of asymptomatic bacteriuria significantly decreases the incidence of symptomatic urinary tract infection. Additionally, this approach would be costly and probably increase the incidence of multi-drug-resistant organisms in this population. For those with symptomatic UTI, the best approach is to treat with the goal of eliminating symptoms, as sterilizing the urine may be nearly impossible[47]. Elderly women with cystitis should receive 7 days of

an appropriate oral antimicrobial. Women with pyelonephritis will require at least 14 days of antimicrobial therapy; those with more severe infections will require these antimicrobials intravenously. Elderly men with UTI frequently have associated prostatitis and may receive an initial 14-day antimicrobial trial, but may require 6 weeks for a higher likelihood of cure.

Infection in males
Urinary tract infections are much more prevalent in women than in men. However, there are approximately 76 office visits per 1,000 men annually for UTI[48]. Additionally, the rate of urinary tract infection is higher in male infants and children. This is caused by an increased incidence of urinary tract abnormalities. This rate is higher yet in uncircumcised male infants as a result of bacterial colonization of the prepuce.

The pathophysiology of UTI in the male is less well understood than that of the female. However, urinary tract infections in the male should be considered complicated until proved otherwise. This is because over a quarter of young men with a first time UTI will be found to have an abnormality on intravenous pyelogram (IVP)[49] and elderly men have even higher rates of anatomic anomalies. Possible anomalies include prostatic hypertrophy, calculi, bladder tumor, urethral stricture, vesicoureteral reflux, ureteropelvic junction obstruction, and others. Chronic bacterial prostatitis occurs in 9% of men diagnosed with recurrent UTI[50]. Additionally, the male urinary tract is interconnected with the epididymis, which may develop an infection secondarily to an urinary tract infection or vice versa.

The organisms that cause UTI in men are somewhat different from those most common in women. For instance, the proportion of UTIs in men caused by *E. coli* is only around 25%[51]. Other Gram-negative pathogens, including Proteus spp. and *Providencia* spp., compromise the majority of UTI pathogens in men. *Staphlycoccus saprophyticus* is rarely a pathogen in men[52].

Treatment of UTI in men should be started immediately and continued for 7–10 days if the prostate is not infected. If the prostate is involved, 6 weeks of therapy is necessary. Men are more likely then women to have a resistant pathogen. Fluoroquinolones may be preferred in men because of their broad spectrum and excellent prostatic penetration. The necessity for radiographic studies in men after a single UTI is controversial. However, there is no doubt that men who have pyelonephritis or a recurrent infection, or who respond poorly to treatment, should be studied[53]. The appropriate studies in middle-aged men and older include IVP and cystoscopy. Male children should have a renal ultrasound and voiding cystourethrogram, as one needs to

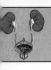

rule out vesicoureteral reflux, duplicated collecting system, UPJ obstruction, and, in very young children, posterior urethral valves. An uncircumcised male infant with recurrent UTI and no identified anatomic anomaly should be considered for circumcision.

Infection in pregnancy

The rate of asymptomatic bacteriuria in pregnant females is 4–7%, which is twice as high as the comparable nonpregnant population. The incidence of pyelonephritis is 2% in pregnancy[54], which is behind only anemia and hypertension in terms of medical problems complicating pregnancy[55]. There have been a number of studies that have examined pregnancy outcomes in women with asymptomatic bacteriuria in terms of birthweight and prematurity. No definitive conclusion can be drawn from these studies. However, it is known that pyelonephritis is a risk factor for preterm labor, and prompt diagnosis and aggressive treatment are warranted.

Treatment of UTI in pregnancy is complicated by the fact that tetracyclines, quinolones, trimethoprim, chloramphenicol, and sulfonamides are contraindicated during pregnancy[55]. Pregnant patients with pyelonephritis should be treated with intravenous gentamicin or cephalosporins. There is evidence that nonbacteremic patients can be treated with oral antimicrobials (cephalosporins) as outpatients with equal success[56]. For cystitis, treatment with a cephalosporin or aminopenicillin for 3 days is a good choice. Screening and treatment of asymptomatic bacteriuria is probably not cost-effective because of the small proportion of bacteriuric patients who develop infection[57].

Infection in diabetes

Urinary tract infections in diabetics are more common than in the general population. Furthermore, the risk of complication as a result of infection, including the development of emphysematous infections, is much higher. This is because of the increased likelihood of functional abnormalities within the diabetic urinary tract and the abnormal leukocyte function in diabetics.

Diabetic women are two to three times as likely to develop urinary tract infection as the general population[58,59]. Diabetics are also more likely to develop nosocomial urinary tract infections[60]. Additionally, the diabetic patient has four times the risk of developing pyelonephritis and is at increased risk of abscess development[61]. Emphysematous complications of urinary tract usually occur in diabetic patients. The increased risk in diabetics is related to three conditions: the presence of gas-forming organisms, decreased tissue perfusion, and high levels of glucose[62].

The urinary functional abnormalities in the diabetic that result in an increased frequency of UTIs most probably result from diabetic cystopathy[63]. This is a condition of weakened detrusor function and decreased filling sensation that culminates in increasing bladder distention and increased postvoid residual volumes. Most studies have failed to demonstrate an increase in the incidence of actual structural abnormalities in diabetics.

Treatment of UTI in the diabetic requires a thoughtful approach. First, most diabetic patients with pyelonephritis should have a screening ultrasound to look for obstructive or emphysematous complications. Although cystitis may be treated the same way as the general population, some would advocate treating asymptomatic bacteriuria in the diabetic population[64]. Pyelonephritis in the diabetic should always be treated with intravenous antibiotics until fever and symptoms have resolved for 24 hours, at which time oral antibiotics should be given for a total of 14 days of therapy. The oral agent should be chosen on the basis of culture sensitivity data. Although TMP-SMX is an excellent first-line therapy for most UTIs, diabetics taking oral antihyperglycemics may see potentiation of the effects of these medications[65].

Antimicrobial prophylaxis

Instrumentation of the urinary tract, as with other invasive procedures, produces some risk of inducing infection. The presence of infection prior to an invasive urologic procedure carries a high incidence of sepsis. This situation requires pretreatment with antibiotics until resolution of infection unless an emergency situation dictates otherwise. In the noninfected patient, the risk of inducing infection is dependent on the procedure being performed and the area in which the procedure is taking place. The simple introduction of a Foley catheter in the outpatient setting carries a 0.5–1% risk of infection. In the nosocomial setting, the risk increases to 5% for men and 10–20% for women[38]. Foley catheters that remain in place carry an infection risk of 4–7.5% per day; limiting length of catheterization is therefore an important preventative measure. Endoscopy of the urinary tract carries a slightly higher risk than catheterization because of the increased trauma of the cystoscope, possible contamination from the eyepiece, and the increased length of the procedure. Although the topic is controversial, patients undergoing simple catheterization or simple cystoscopy who have a negative urine culture probably do not benefit from antimicrobial prophylaxis.

Many studies have examined the role of antimicrobial prophylaxis in transurethral resection of the prostate (TURP). Again, urine culture should be performed and if it is found to be positive, the patient should be treated prior to undergoing any procedure. In patients with a urine culture that shows no growth prior to the procedure, the rate of bacteriuria following procedure without prophylaxis ranges from 6% to 43%[66]. Complicating the situation is the fact that most patients require an indwelling Foley catheter for 2–3 days following TURP, further increasing the risk of urinary tract infection. Therefore, the question of whether prophylaxis that continues until the catheter is removed is treating the risk of infection from the procedure or from the catheter has not been established. On the basis of known data, it is recommended that most patients undergoing TURP be treated prophylactically with a first-generation cephalosporin, a fluoroquinolone, or gentamicin. The agent must be given at least 1 hour before surgery and continued for 24 hours. Additionally, broad-spectrum antimicrobials (TMP-SMX or a fluoroquinolone) should be restarted the evening prior to catheter removal and continued for 3 days after its removal.

Transurethral resection of bladder tumor (TURBT) is also associated with possible UTI. There is up to a 38.7% risk of UTI following TURBT without prophylaxis[67]. Additionally, some authors have found evidence that the tumors themselves harbor bacteria[68]. Therefore, the same guidelines should be followed as those above for TURP.

Transrectal prostate needle biopsy also carries a high risk of infectious complications. The urinary infections include prostatitis, epididymitis, and pyelonephritis. Additionally, the risk of sepsis is a concern as 76% of patients are transiently bacteremic following biopsy[69]. A fluoroquinolone started the evening before biopsy and continued for 24 hours is effective.

Open urologic procedures follow the same prophylaxis guidelines as all other procedures, depending on whether they are classified as clean, clean-contaminated, or contaminated.

TREATMENT OF UPPER TRACT INFECTION

Upper tract infections involve mainly the nephric and perinephric regions, although collecting system and ureteral involvement is possible.

Acute pyelonephritis
Acute pyelonephritis is defined as inflammation of the renal parenchyma and the renal pelvis.

Diagnosis
Diagnosis of pyelonephritis versus cystitis is typically made clinically on the basis of the presence of fever, chills, and costo-vertebral angle tenderness. Bacteremia and sepsis are common, particularly in high-risk patient groups. Other symptoms of pyelonephritis include abdominal pain, nausea, vomiting, diarrhea, urinary frequency, dysuria, and urgency. Laboratory findings include pyuria, WBC casts, bacteriuria, and positive urine culture. Additional hematologic findings include an elevated white count, elevation of acute phase reactants such as C-reactive protein, and an elevated erythrocyte sedimentation rate (ESR). Rarely, acute pyelonephritis may be associated with renal failure and an increased serum creatinine. Blood cultures should be obtained as a diagnostic and treatment aid in very ill and high-risk patients.

Bacteriology
The majority of pyelonephritis pathogens are the enteric Gram-negative bacteria that are responsible for cystitis, with *E. coli* being the most prevalent. The subgroup of *E. coli* that is responsible for 80% of pyelonephritis episodes expresses P pili on its surface[19]. Gram-positive organisms, particularly *E. faecalis*, can be responsible in some cases.

Imaging studies
Routine imaging in low-risk patients with pyelonephritis is not indicated. However, diabetics, children, men, and patients with suspected obstruction should be imaged, as well as patients not responding to antimicrobial therapy within 72 hours and those who deteriorate during appropriate therapy. Ultrasound is an effective, safe means of demonstrating obstruction in all patients, although it is not able to demonstrate lobar nephronia or scarring as well as other methods. IVP demonstrates focal or general renal enlargement in 20% of cases of pyelonephritis[70], and will demonstrate anatomic anomalies and stone disease. Computed tomography (CT), however, is better at demonstrating focal inflammatory abnormalities and previous renal scarring as wedge-shaped or linear zones of decreased attenuation (Fig. 21.12) and is able to give information on anatomy, stone disease, and the presence of abscess or gas formation within the nephric or perinephric space. Additionally, many nonspecific IVP or ultrasound abnormalities will require a CT scan for additional information in order to arrive at a diagnosis.

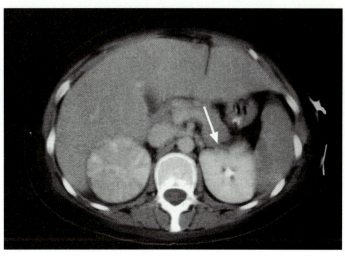

Figure 21.12 Acute pyelonephritis. Computed tomography scan showing acute pyelonephritis on the right side, demonstrating linear zones of decreased attenuation.

Treatment of acute noncomplicated pyelonephritis in women			
Circumstances	**Route**	**Drug**	**Duration**
Outpatient – moderately ill, no vomiting	Oral	TMP-SMX Fluoroquinolone	10–14 days
Inpatient – severely ill, possible sepsis	Parenteral	TMP-SMX Ampicillin and gentamicin Fluoroquinolone Ceftriaxone *until afebrile, then*	14 days
	Oral	TMP-SMX or fluoroquinolone	
Pregnant	Parenteral	Ceftriaxone Ampicillin and gentamicin Aztreonam *until afebrile, then*	14 days
	Oral	Cephalexin	

Figure 21.13 Treatment of acute noncomplicated pyelonephritis in women. TMX-SMX, trimethoprim-sulfamethoxazole.

Treatment
The appropriate treatment of acute pyelonephritis involves subdividing patients into relative risk groups: 1) complicated versus uncomplicated, and 2) the degree of illness that the patient exhibits. Figures 21.13 & 21.14 demonstrate appropriate antimicrobial therapy regimens based on the risk evaluation of the patient. Urine cultures should be repeated 4 days after initiation of treatment and 10 days after completion of therapy, because there is a 10–30% relapse rate.

Chronic pyelonephritis
Chronic pyelonephritis is a disease of recurring pyelonephritis diagnosed by the pathologic finding of chronic tubulointerstitial nephritis with scarring and/or the radiographic finding of atrophic, shrunken kidneys. Chronic pyelonephritis is causative of end-stage renal disease and renal insufficiency in 25% of the

Treatment of complicated urinary tract infections			
Circumstances	Route	Drug	Duration
Outpatient – moderately ill, no nausea or vomiting	Oral	Fluoroquinolone	10–14 days
Inpatient – severely ill, possible sepsis	Parenteral	Fluoroquinolone Ampicillin and gentamicin Ceftriaxone Ticarcillin–clavanulate Imipenem–cilastatin Aztreonam *Until afebrile, then*	14–21 days
	Oral	Fluoroquinolone	

Figure 21.14 Treatment of complicated urinary tract infections.

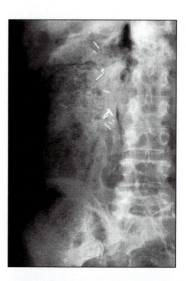

Figure 21.15 Severe right-sided emphysematous pyelonephritis. Note the gas overlying the right kidney. The surgical clips are from a prior, unrelated, procedure.

population[71]. Several animal model studies have demonstrated the adverse affect of even a single episode of untreated pyelonephritis on the renal parenchyma, resulting in vessel kinking and atrophy, complement activation, and increased thromboxane A_2 levels[72,73]. The end result is renal vasoconstriction, inflammation, ischemia, and finally atrophy. The association of chronic pyelonephritis with vesicoureteral reflux is controversial and difficult to prove clinically as not all patients with VUR develop renal scarring. However, animal studies using the pig demonstrated that only infected urine that refluxed caused scarring in specific regions of the kidney. Noninfected urine did not induce scarring[74].

Emphysematous pyelonephritis
Emphysematous pyelonephritis is a severe, necrotizing form of acute bacterial pyelonephritis in which gas is present either in the kidney or perirenally. The mortality rate is between 20% and 43%[75,76].

Diagnosis
The diagnosis of emphysematous pyelonephritis requires a high index of suspicion. Some 70–90% of reported cases have occurred in diabetics[77]. The three most common predisposing clinical factors are: diabetes mellitus, recent or remote pyelonephritis, and obstruction. Common presenting signs are similar to those of acute pyelonephritis. Additionally, 50% of patients will have a palpable flank mass and, rarely, crepitation over the flank or thigh will be present. Typical laboratory findings are similar to those of pyelonephritis with the addition of hyperglycemia and glycosuria.

Etiology
The majority of cases are caused by *E. coli*; other Gram-negative organisms make up the majority of the remainder of cases. The etiology of the gas formation is not exactly defined. The fermentation of sugar, which exists in high concentrations in the urine and tissues of diabetics, to produce carbon dioxide is one hypothesis[78]. Another possible mechanism is the breakdown of products from necrotic tissue. Regardless of the exact mechanism, three conditions seem to be necessary: the presence of gas forming organisms, high glucose levels, and impaired perfusion.

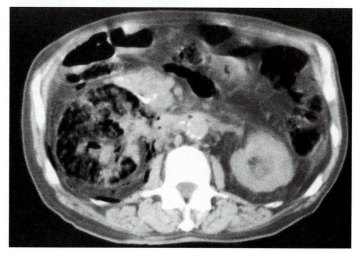

Figure 21.16 Severe right-sided emphysematous pyelonephritis. Computed tomography scan demonstrating parenchymal and retroperitoneal gas. This is the same patient as in Figure 21.15.

Imaging
Plain abdominal films will demonstrate gas over the involved kidney in 85% of cases[77] (Fig. 21.15). This is frequently mistaken for bowel gas. IVP plays no role. Ultrasound will demonstrate the presence of gas and obstruction, if present. However, if emphysematous pyelonephritis is suspected, CT is the study of choice. A CT scan allows for accurate assessment of the severity of disease for planning treatment. Initially, there are diffuse hypodensities in the renal parenchyma with gas along the renal pyramids. As the disease progresses, more severe necrosis is observed and gas is found in Gerota's fascia, and may even extend into the retroperitoneum (Fig. 21.16). Additionally, a renal scan is helpful in determining differential function in a risk–benefit analysis when considering nephrectomy.

Treatment
Antimicrobial agents, correction of hyperglycemia, and fluid resuscitation should begin immediately. With medical therapy alone, there is a 60–80% mortality rate, depending on the severity of disease. This is not improved by surgical drainage of

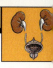

Causes of obstruction in xanthogranulomatous pyelonephritis	
Cause	Frequency
Nephrolithiasis	Common
Ureteropelvic junction obstruction	Unusual
Severe vesicoureteral reflux disease	Rare
Renal cell carcinoma	Rare
Transitional cell carcinoma	Rare

Figure 21.17 Causes of obstruction in xanthogranulomatous pyelonephritis.

affected area[76,79]. Surgical removal of the kidney lowers mortality rates to 20% or less[80]. Therefore, except for very select cases in which disease is minimal and dialysis would most probably result from nephrectomy, nephrectomy is the treatment of choice.

Xanthogranulomatous pyelonephritis

Xanthogranulomatous pyelonephritis (XPN) is characterized by diffuse renal parenchyma destruction with granulomatous infiltrates containing lipid-laden macrophages. The disease is rare, and can affect children[81], although it is most common in women in the fifth to seventh decades. Obstructive uropathy secondary to nephrolithiasis is usually involved. It is, however, frequently misdiagnosed as a renal tumor and has been described as 'the great imitator'[82,83].

Diagnosis

Most patients present with nonspecific signs including fever, flank pain, weight loss, and malaise. Additionally, 62% present with a palpable flank mass and 35% have a history of nephrolithiasis[84]. Rarely, the patient may present with a cutaneous draining fistula. The onset of symptoms is usually subacute to chronic with 80% of patients having symptoms for more than a month at presentation[84]. Laboratory findings are similar to those of pyelonephritis; an elevated creatinine is more common in XPN because of the massive tissue destruction that is usually present. Definitive diagnosis can be made only upon pathologic examination of the nephrectomy specimen.

Etiology

The exact pathogenesis of XPN remains unresolved. However, two factors necessary for its development are obstruction and urinary tract infection. Obstruction due to calculi is present in between 38–83% of reported cases[84–87]. Other causes of obstruction reported in XPN include ureteropelvic junction (UPJ) obstruction, severe vesicoureteral reflux, and renal or transition cell carcinomas (Fig. 21.17).

Positive urine cultures are found in 50–75%[88] of XPN patients; however, kidney tissue cultures are positive in over 90% of cases[84]. This may be explained by the obstruction that frequently occurs in XPN. The most common organisms isolated are *Proteus* spp., *E. coli* is also commonly cultured[86]. There are several other factors that have a weaker association with XPN than obstruction and infection. These factors are listed in Figure 21.18 and should increase clinical suspicion of XPN.

Host factors in xanthogranulomatous pyelonephritis
Obstruction – very common
Urinary tract infection – very common
Prior genitourinary surgery/instrumentation
Diabetes mellitus
Immunosuppression
Altered leukocyte function
Abnormal lipid metabolism
Lymphatic obstruction
Arterial insufficiency
Alcoholism
Malnutrition
Hyperparathyroidism
Renal transplantation

Figure 21.18 Host factors in xanthogranulomatous pyelonephritis.

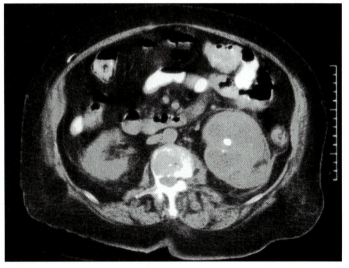

Figure 21.19 Left-sided xanthogranulomatous pyelonephritis. Computed tomography scan demonstrating central calcification and reniform mass.

Imaging

Computed tomography scan is the most helpful imaging technique to clinically diagnose XPN and to evaluate the extent of involvement. A CT scan typically demonstrates a large, reniform mass tightly surrounding a central calcification but without pelvic dilation[89,90] (Fig. 21.19). The renal parenchyma is replaced by water-density parenchymal lesions. The walls of these lesions typically enhance, while the lesions remain unenhanced, thus differing significantly from the typical CT appearance of renal cell carcinoma. IVP does not provide as much information as a CT scan. It usually demonstrates an enlarged, ill-defined renal outline. Renal calculi are also demonstrated in the majority of these patients and various degrees of delayed contrast uptake and excretion can be observed. Renal scan will demonstrate various degrees of nonfunction depending on whether diffuse or focal XPN is present. Ultrasound will reveal an enlarged kidney with hypoechoic parenchyma and a large central echogenic region[91].

21

Treatment

Nephrectomy is curative and is the treatment of choice for XPN. Antimicrobial therapy should be initiated once the diagnosis is made or if there is a high level of suspicion. Partial nephrectomy may be considered if focal XPN is demonstrated by a CT scan and confirmed intraoperatively. Some authors have made reasonable arguments for a limited role of conservative management in young patients with focal XPN[88]. This may be appropriate in select patients in whom malignancy can be excluded with a reasonable degree of probability. However, this is difficult to do even with intraoperative frozen sections, as the lipid-laden macrophages closely resemble clear cell adenocarcinoma.

Malacoplakia

Malacoplakia is a rare chronic inflammatory process that most commonly affects the urinary tract. It is usually caused by *E. coli*. The lesions consist of foamy macrophages containing the pathognomic Michaelis–Gutmann bodies.

Diagnosis

Malacoplakia involves the urinary tract in 58% of cases[92], although it has been described involving multiple organ systems. In the urinary tract, the bladder, renal parenchyma, and ureter are most frequently involved[92]. Urinary tract involvement presents with hematuria and recurrent UTIs. Symptoms of obstruction may develop from larger masses. When renal lesions are present the patient may present with fever, flank pain, and a palpable mass[92,93]. Urine culture will usually be positive. Hematologic findings include elevated ESR, anemia, and leukocytosis[94]. More extensive lesions may also present with anemia, weight loss, fever, and night sweats[94]. Nearly 50% of patients with malacoplakia are immunosuppressed or have a serious systemic disease[92].

Etiology

Escherichia coli is a consistent finding in malacoplakia lesions and suggests a causative role. The second important factor appears to be the diminished capacity for macrophages to completely lyse bacteria that are phagocytosed. One study found decreased levels of cyclic guanosine monophosphate (cGMP) in macrophages from a patient with malacoplakia[95]. This decrease could inhibit the fusion of lysosomes with bacteria contained in phagosomes. However, some other studies have failed to reproduce these results[96,97]. Increased α_1-antitrypsin levels in macrophages have been suggested by others to play a role[98].

Imaging

Computed tomography scanning and gallium scintigraphy are both useful modalities in assessing malacoplakia. A CT scan reveals heterogeneous masses that enhance poorly with contrast, and allows for evaluation of the local extent of disease[93]. Gallium scintigraphy will also detect lesions that may not be clinically evident[94].

Treatment

The primary management involves antibiotic treatment in combination with surgery. From a large retrospective analysis of malacoplakia patients and treatment modalities[94], the following were derived:

- Stop immunosuppressive agents if possible.
- Perform surgical excision in combination with ciprofloxacin administration.

- If surgery is not possible use ciprofloxacin 500mg twice-daily.
- The addition of bethanechol and ascorbic acid may be of some benefit. The latter is thought to increase macrophage cGMP levels.

The overall mortality rate from this disease is 15%. This mortality varies by extent and location of disease, with renal lesions carrying the highest risk (22%)[94].

Perinephric abscess

Perinephric abscess is an abscess that forms within Gerota's fascia, either from a hematogenous seeding or by direct extension secondary to pyelonephritis. The abscess may extend beyond Gerota's fascia to the pararenal space; it is then called a pararenal abscess. Pararenal abscesses tend to migrate inferiorly because of nonfusion of the renal fascial layers (Fig. 21.20)[99]. The mortality from this disease is reported to be as high as 20–50%[100] as a result of frequent delay in diagnosis.

Diagnosis

A high level of clinical suspicion is required to diagnose a perinephric abscess and not just to assume that pyelonephritis is the culprit. The typical history is of a patient with an infection involving the ipsilateral kidney, urinary tract, dentition, or skin approximately 2 weeks before the onset of fever and flank pain. In an older, but very large review of the presenting symptoms of perinephric abscess it was noted that fever and flank pain were very common. Rigors, dysuria, nausea, and vomiting were less common. Additionally, nearly half of patients present with a palpable flank mass as well as flank tenderness[101]. Laboratory findings are nonspecific and may resemble pyelonephritis; they include pyuria, leukocytosis, and anemia.

Etiology

Most perinephric abscesses are caused by retrograde ascent from the urinary tract. Thus, the organisms most commonly

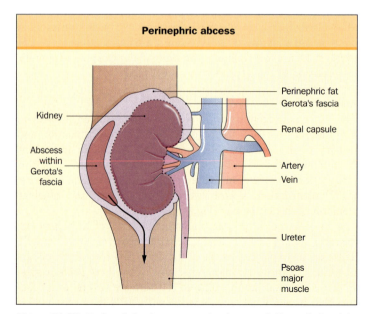

Figure 21.20 Perinephric abscess: anatomic associations. Perinephric abscess contained within Gerota's fascia usually tracks inferiorly down the surface of the psoas muscle and, if undetected, may present in the groin.

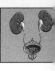
involved include *E. coli*, *Proteus* spp., *Klebsiella* spp., and *Pseudomonas* spp. Before the advent of antibiotics, these lesions were referred to as renal carbuncles and were usually the result of the hematogenous spread of *Staphylococcus aureus*. Hematogenous spread is still seen often in intravenous drug users and in patients with cutaneous disorders. Occasionally, paranephric abscesses may be secondary to a gastrointestinal source, in which case anaerobes are commonly associated[102].

Imaging
Renal ultrasound and CT scanning have greatly aided in the diagnosis of the perinephric abscess. A CT scan is the radiographic study of choice for diagnosing and evaluating perinephric abscesses. The findings on CT are typically those of nonspecific renal inflammation with the presence of perirenal fluid or gas; psoas muscle enlargement may also be noted[103,104] (Fig. 21.21). Plain films of the abdomen may reveal nonspecific findings such as loss of psoas shadow, loss of renal contour, and retroperitoneal gas, and are abnormal in 60% of cases[105]. IVP is frequently nonspecifically abnormal. Frequent findings include calyectasis, distortion of the collecting system, or displacement of the kidney. The most frequent finding is delayed uptake or absence of uptake[105]. Ultrasound has a high false-negative rate but frequently demonstrates an irregular cystic lesion outside the kidney, with echogenic debris frequently visible.

Treatment
Drainage of the abscess is of primary importance. It has been demonstrated repeatedly that mortality rates remain between 75% and 100% for those receiving antibiotics alone and that mortality drops dramatically in those who are drained[105,106]. The best initial approach is through ultrasound- or CT-guided percutaneous drainage in combination with intravenous antimicrobials. This minimizes morbidity rates and preserves the renal parenchyma. It is not unusual for the patient not to be adequately drained by percutaneous drainage alone; in that case the patient will require immediate surgical exploration and abscess evacuation. If there is involvement of the kidney, nephrectomy is usually required. Several drains should be placed into the evacuated abscess pocket and the skin should be left open to close by secondary or tertiary intention. Intravenous antimicrobial selection should be based on Gram stain and culture results, but initial therapy should be broad-spectrum and cover anaerobes and Gram-negative organisms. An ampicillin, gentamicin, nitroimidazole combination is a good initial choice.

PROSTATITIS

Prostatitis is a multifaceted syndrome with many etiologies. It is so common that 50% of men will experience symptoms of prostatitis during their lifetime[107]. The term prostatitis is misleading in that it implies inflammation when not all patients with a prostatitis syndrome have prostatic inflammation. Drach classified patients with symptoms of prostatitis into four major groupings: acute bacterial prostatitis, chronic bacterial prostatitis, nonbacterial or abacterial prostatitis, and prostadynia[108]. Another pathologic entity known as granulomatous prostatitis frequently presents as a suspicious prostatic nodule. This usually occurs following a prostatic needle biopsy, resolving urinary tract infection, or prostatitis. Occasionally, it may represent a local manifestation of a systemic disease such as tuberculosis or Wegener's disease[109]. Most cases resolve spontaneously and require no treatment. However, the presence of a systemic granulomatous disease should be sought.

Acute bacterial prostatitis
Acute bacterial prostatitis (ABP) is a serious, sometimes life-threatening bacterial infection of the prostate associated with intense inflammation and frequent septicemia. It is relatively unusual in that it accounts for less than 5% of prostatitis cases, but its presentation is dramatic. The most common presenting signs and symptoms include: fever, chills, malaise, pelvic and low back pain, frequency, urgency, and, sometimes, urinary retention. Digital rectal examination (DRE) will reveal an exquisitely tender, warm, and swollen prostate. DRE must be done very gently and urinary tract instrumentation is contraindicated. The most common organism causing ABP is *E. coli*, which causes 80% of cases. Species of *Pseudomonas*, *Klebsiella*, *Proteus*, and *Serratia* are also common. Enterococci are found in 5–10% of cases[110]. Other occasional causes of ABP include *Neisseria gonorrhoeae*, *Mycobacterium tuberculosis*, *Salmonella* spp., and mycotic organisms[111]. Fluoroquinolones have better prostatic penetration than TMP-SMX[112]. Patients who present with septicemia or urinary retention, or who have an underlying systemic illness, should be hospitalized and given broad-spectrum intravenous antimicrobials such as ampicillin and an aminoglycoside until cultures are back to normal. Urinary retention should be addressed by the placement of a suprapubic catheter. Treatment should be continued as an outpatient with oral antimicrobials for a total of 3–4 weeks. Prostatic abscess can occasionally occur as a result of ABP, particularly in immuno-compromised patients or those with urethral catheters[111]. These abscesses may feel fluctuant, can be identified by ultrasound, and are treated by an unroofing TURP.

Chronic bacterial prostatitis
Chronic bacterial prostatitis (CBP) usually presents as recurrent urinary tract infection associated with genitourinary pain,

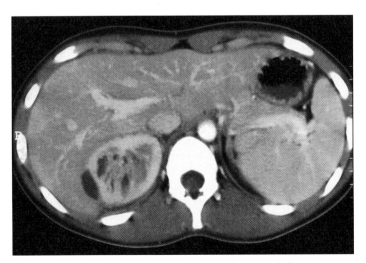

Figure 21.21 Right perinephric abscess and intrarenal abscess (computed tomography scan). Note the parenchymal and perinephric gas and fluid.

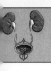

frequency, and urgency. Digital rectal examination occasionally reveals a tender, boggy, swollen, or firm prostate but the prostatic examination is usually normal. The diagnosis is made by expressed prostatic secretion (EPS) examination and localization culture techniques (see Localization Cultures, above). EPS usually reveals more than 10 WBC/hpf and the VB_3 culture should grow colony counts one log higher than the VB_1. CBP is caused by the same organisms as ABP; again, *E. coli* is the most common pathogen. The stasis of prostatic secretions in the peripheral zone of the prostate, with ductal fibrosis and stone formation, are thought to contribute to the development of CBP[111]. There are several reports in the literature suggesting an association of CBP with infertility and that treatment has resulted in improvement in sperm analysis parameters and in spouses becoming pregnant.

Treatment of CBP focuses on elimination of bacteria from the prostate. This can be difficult to achieve and is frustrating to both the urologist and to the patient. Additionally, in patients in whom bacteriologic cure is achieved it is not unusual for relapse to occur. The best treatment is TMP-SMX or fluoroquinolones. Both of these antimicrobials achieve adequate prostatic concentrations because of their lipid solubility, pKa, and weak alkalinity[39]. Treatment should be for 6 weeks. If cure is not achieved, treatment should be continued to 12 weeks. Long-term suppression doses are also a possibility in patients who are prone to frequent recurrences or who fail treatment. For patients who are refractory to antimicrobial agents, TURP may be considered as a last resort but is not always effective. The majority of infections lie in the peripheral regions of the gland; hence there is a chance that infected gland might be left behind. The cure rate after TURP has been reported to be anywhere from 30% to 100%[111].

Nonbacterial prostatitis

Nonbacterial prostatitis (NBP) is the most common of all the prostatitis groupings. Patients with NBP outnumber those with CBP eightfold[113]. Patients with NBP present with similar symptoms to those with CBP, including genitourinary pain, pain on ejaculation, frequency, urgency, and dysuria. The distinguishing characteristic is that patients with NBP have cultures that are repeatedly negative. Inflammation is present, more than 10 WBC/hpf as well as lipid-laden macrophages are seen in the expressed prostatic secretion. Two major schools of thought exist as to the etiology of NBP. The first implicates the reflux of urine into the prostatic ducts as the cause of inflammation in the prostate[114]. The second has focused on an infectious cause, such as *Chlamydia* or *Ureaplasma* spp. However, most authors have not found a causative role for these pathogens[115,116]. One recent study found evidence by biopsy that some patients diagnosed with NBP actually had micro-organisms present in their prostatic tissue[117]. Treatment initially should consist of an antimicrobial trial as if one were treating CBP. If *Chlamydia* or *Ureaplasma* are suspected pathogens, then a 2-week trial of tetracycline, erythromycin, minocycline, or doxycycline should be tried. Alpha-blockers have been demonstrated to increase urine flow rates and to decrease symptom scores in patients with NBP and prostadynia[39]. Other treatments that have shown some success include transurethral incision of the prostate, pollen extracts, nickel, and allopurinol. Symptomatic treatment

composed of sitz baths and nonsteroidal anti-inflammatory drugs (NSAIDs) are of benefit to some patients. Recently, transurethral microwave thermotherapy was shown to improve AUA symptom scores and quality of life in a randomized, double-blind study[118].

Prostadynia

Prostadynia or prostatodynia is a chronic syndrome with pain or discomfort referred to the prostate but with negative cultures and without evidence of prostatic inflammation. The presenting symptoms are similar to those of NBP and include urgency, frequency, dysuria, and genitourinary pain in the perineal, scrotal, penile, or suprapubic locations. Painful ejaculation may also be reported. The etiology is attributed to increased tone or spasm of the bladder neck and to spasm or contraction of the pelvic floor musculature that may lead to urinary reflux into the prostatic ducts[114,119]. Treatment options include alpha-blockers with or without the addition of diazepam to relax the pelvic floor musculature. Biofeedback has been demonstrated to be of benefit to many patients. Symptomatic relief may also be obtained with sitz baths and NSAIDs. Patients who have irritative voiding symptoms may benefit from oxybutynin, but they should be evaluated for transitional cell carcinoma before initiating therapy. These patients are typically more refractory to therapy. Many options might need to be pursued before an effective regimen is discovered. Furthermore, some patients who fail therapy should be offered psychologic counseling, if required, as 50% of such patients meet the diagnostic criteria for major depression[39].

EPIDIDYMO-ORCHITIS

Epididymo-orchitis (EO) is an inflammation, usually infectious, involving the epididymis and the testicle. EO occurs in all age groups and, particularly in children, must be differentiated from testicular torsion. The typical presentation includes the gradual onset of testicular pain and swelling, sometimes accompanied by scrotal erythema. In children, color duplex sonography or radionuclide imaging should be obtained if the diagnosis of EO is not certain, to rule out testicular torsion. Urinalysis and urine culture should be obtained in all cases. Gonococcal and chlamydial cultures should be obtained in most sexually active patients. Some cases of EO, particularly in children, are noninfective. The etiology of EO is variable and depends upon the age of the patient, though there is considerable overlap in these groups. In men under 35 years old, the predominant organism is *Chlamydia trachomatis*, followed by *E. coli* and *N. gonorrhoeae*[120,121]. In men over the age of 35 years, Gram-negative bacteria, particularly *E. coli*, are responsible in the majority of cases[120]. The etiology in children is usually abacterial, and is usually idiopathic or occurs as a result of trauma. Treatment of EO depends upon the age group. In children with negative urinalysis and culture, NSAIDs and rest are usually helpful and antimicrobials are not required[122]. In men under 35 years of age, doxycycline for 7 days or ofloxacin for 10 days is recommended for the treatment of *Chlamydia trachomatis*. If gonorrhea is suspected, a one-time intramuscular dose of ceftriaxone should be added to doxycycline. Sexual partners will also require culture and treatment. In men over the age of 35, TMP-SMX or

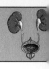
a fluoroquinolone should be prescribed for 10–14 days. If treatment failure occurs, prostatic involvement or abscess should be considered.

FOURNIER'S GANGRENE

Fournier's gangrene is a true urologic emergency that must be recognized and dealt with immediately and appropriately. It is a necrotizing infection involving the perineum and external genitalia. Patients typically present with fever and toxemia late in the course. Local findings include perineal and external genitalia that are swollen, warm, and erythematous. Crepitation may be present, indicating the presence of gas-forming *Clostridium* spp. Late local findings might also include necrosis and eschar formation. Frequently, the patient may describe colorectal complaints or surgery preceding infection. This indicates that a colorectal source is likely, which indicates that more widespread disease may be present[123]. A history of some sort of immunosuppression, such as HIV, diabetes, or systemic disease, is common.

The etiology is a synergistic infection comprising enteric Gram-negative organisms, Gram-positive staphylococci or streptococci, and anaerobes. The infection results in an obliterative endarteritis[124]. Usually the source is colorectal or genitourinary in nature. Treatment includes intravenous antimicrobials and surgical debridement of all necrotic tissue. Penicillin, clindamycin, and an aminoglycoside is the traditional treatment and all are needed to cover the entire spectrum of pathogens that may be present until specific culture information is available. Surgical debridement is best accomplished from the dorsal lithotomy position. Careful evaluation of the urethra and rectum can be accomplished with cystoscopy and proctoscopy. Those patients with significant penile or urethral involvement will require suprapubic cystotomy and patients with significant rectal involvement will require a diverting colostomy. Debridement of all necrotic tissue should be performed and left open with placement of copious drains. The patient should return to the operating room after 24 hours to reassess all wounds and to do further debridement as necessary.

REFERENCES

1. Schaeffer A. Infections of the urinary tract. In: Walsh PC, Retik AB, Vaughan ED, Wein AJ, eds. Campbell's urology, 7th edn. Philadelphia: WB Saunders; 1997:533–614.

2. Zielske J, Lohr K, Brook R, et al. Conceptualization and measurement of physiologic health for adults: urinary tract infection. Rand Corporation 1981:Report R2262/16-HHS.

3. Pewitt E, Schaeffer A. Urinary tract infection in urology, including acute and chronic prostatitis. Infect Dis Clin North Am. 1997; 11:623–45.

4. Foxman B. Recurring lower urinary tract infections: occurence and determinants. Am J Publ Health. 1990;80:331–3.

5. Bartlett J, Gorbach SL. Anaerobic bacteria in suppurative infections of the male genitourinary system. J Urol. 1981;125:376.

6. Svanborg C, Godaly G. Bacterial virulence in urinary tract infection. Infect Dis Clin North Am. 1997;11:513–29.

7. Hospital PaTDCoNM. Optimizing drug use at NMH. Chicago: Northwestern Memorial Hospital; 1998:168.

8. Hall L, Duke B, Urwin G, et al. Epidemiology of *Enterococcus faecalis* urinary tract infection in a teaching hospital in London, United Kingdom. J Clin Microbiol. 1992;30:1953–7.

9. Maskell R, Pead L, Hallett R. Urinary pathogens in the male. Br J Urol. 1975:691–4.

10. Lipsky B. Urinary tract infection in men. Ann Intern Med. 1989;110:138–50.

11. Kauffman C, Hertz C, Sheagren J. *Staphylococcus saprophyticus*: role in urinary tract infections in men. J Urol. 1989:493–4.

12. Michigan S. Genitourinary fungal infections. J Urol. 1976; 110:390–7.

13. Schonebeck J, Winblad B, Ansehn S. Renal candidosis complicating caeco-cystoplasty. Case report with scanning EM studies. Scand J Urol. 1972;6:129.

14. Schubert G, Haltaufderheide T, Golz R. Frequency of urogenital tuberculosis in an unselected autopsy series from 1928 to 1949 and 1976 to 1989. Eur Urol. 1992;21:216–23.

15. Wu X, Sun T, Medina J. In vitro binding of type1-fimbriated *Escherichia coli* to uroplakins Ia and Ib: relation to urinary tract infections. Proc Natl Acad Sci USA. 1996;93:9630–5.

16. Lichodziejewska M, Steadman R, Kate V, et al. Variable expression of P fimbriae in *Escherichia coli* urinary tract infection. Lancet. 1989:1414–7.

17. D'Orazio S, Collins C. Molecular pathogenesis of urinary tract infections. Curr Topics Microbiol Immunol. 1998;225:137–64.

18. Connell H, Agace W, Klemm P, et al. Type I fimbrial expression enhances *Escherichia coli* virulence for the urinary tract. Proc Natl Acad Sci USA. 1996;93:9827–32.

19. Donnenberg M, Welch R. Virulence determinants in uropathogenic *E. coli*. In: Mobley H, Warren J, eds. Urinary tract infection: molecular pathogenesis and clinical management. Washington, DC: American Society for Microbiology. 1996:135–74.

20. Zhang J, Normark S. Induction of gene expression in *Escherichia coli* after pilus mediated adherence. Science. 1996;273:1234–6.

21. Kallenius G, Mollby R, Winberg J, et al. The Pk antigen as a receptor for the hemagluttination of pyelonephritogenic *E. coli*. FEMS Microbiol Lett. 1980;7:297–302.

22. McGeachie J. Hemolysis by urinary *E. coli*. Am J Clin Pathol. 1966;45:222–4.

23. O'Hanley P, Lalonde G, Ji G. Alpha-hemolysin contributes to the pathogenicity of piliated digalactoside-binding *E. coli* in the kidney: efficacy of an alpha-hemolysin vaccine in preventing renal injury in the BALB/c mouse model of pyelonephritis. Infect Immun. 1991;59:1153–61.

24. Caprioli A, Falbo V, Ruggeri F, et al. Cytotoxic necrotizing factor production by hemolytic strains of *E. coli* causing extraintestinal infections. J Clin Microbiol. 1987;25:146–9.

25. Collins C, Falkow S. Genetic analysis of *E. coli* urease genes: evidence for two distinct loci. Mol Microbiol. 1990;9:907–13.

26. Belas D, Erskine D, Flaherty D. *Proteus mirabilis* mutants defective in swarmer cell differentiation and multicellular behavior. J Bacteriol. 1991;173:6279–88.

27. Allison C, Lai H, Hughes C. Co-ordinate expression of virulence genes during swarm-cell differentiation and population migration of *Proteus mirabilis*. Mol Microbiol. 1992;6:1583–91.

28. Allison C, Emody L, Coleman N, et al. The role of swarm cell differentation and multicellular migration in the uropathogenicity of *Proteus mirabilis*. J Infect Dis. 1994;169:1155–8.

29. Kaye D. Antibacterial activity of human urine. J Clin Invest. 1968;47:2374–90.

30. Sobel J. Pathogenesis of urinary tract infection. Infect Dis Clin North Am. 1997;11:531–47.

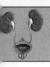

31. Cox C, Hinman F. Experiments with induced bacteriuria, vesicle emptying and bacterial growth on the mechanism of bladder defense to infection. J Urol. 1961;86:739–51.

32. Sikri K, Foster C, Bloomfield F, et al. Localization by immunofluorescence and by light and electron microscopic techniques of Tamm–Horsfall glycoprotein in adult hamster kidney. Biochem J. 1979;181:525–32.

33. Orskov I, Ferencz A, Orskov F. Tamm–Horsfall protein or uromucoid is the normal urinary slime that traps type I fimbriated *Escherichia coli*. Lancet. 1980;1:887.

34. Toma G, Bates J, Kumar S. Uromodulin (Tamm–Horsfall protein) is a leukocyte adhesion molecule. Biochem Biophys Res Commun. 1994;200:275–82.

35. Fowler JJ, Stamey T. Studies of introital colonization in women with recurrent urinary tract infections. VII. The role of bacterial adherence. J Urol. 1977;117:472–6.

36. Schaeffer A, Radvany R, Chmiel J. Human leukocyte antigens in women with recurrent urinary tract infections. J Infect Dis. 1983; 148:604.

37. Kinane D, Blackwell C, Brettle R, et al. ABO blood group, secretor status and susceptibility to recurrent urinary tract infection in women. Br Med J. 1982;285:7–9.

38. Amin M. Antibacterial prophylaxis in urology. Am J Med. 1992; 92:114S–7S.

39. Britton JJ. Prostatitis. AUA Update Ser. 1998;17:154–60.

40. Brumfitt W. Urinary cell counts and their value. J Clin Pathol. 1965;18:550–5.

41. Finn S, Johnson C, Roberts P, et al. Trimethoprim/sulfamethoxazole for acute dysuria in women: a single dose or 10 day course. Ann Intern Med. 1988;108:350–7.

42. Stamm W, Hooton T, Johnson J, et al. Urinary tract infections: from pathogenesis to treatment. J Infect Dis. 1989;159:400–6.

43. Andriole V. Urinary tract infections in the 90's: pathogenesis and management. Infection. 1992;20:S251–4.

44. Boscia J, Kobasa W, Knight R, et al. Epidemiology of bacteriuria in an elderly ambulatory population. Am J Med. 1986;81:979–82.

45. Muder R, Brennen C, Wegener M, et al. Bacteriuria in a long-term care facility: a five year prospective study of 163 consecutive episodes. Clin Infect Dis. 1992;14:647–54.

46. Gleckman R, Bradley P, Roth R, et al. Bacteric urosepsis: a phenomenon unique to elderly women. J Urol. 1985;133:174–5.

47. Nicolle L. Urinary tract infection in the elderly. J Antimicrob Chemother. 1994;33:99–109.

48. Lipsky B. Urinary tract infections in men. Ann Intern Med. 1989; 110:138–50.

49. Booth C, Whiteside C, Milroy E, et al. Unheralded urinary tract infection in the male: a clinical and urodynamic assessment. Br J Urol. 1981;53:270–3.

50. Krieger J, Egan K. Comprehensive evaluation and treatment of 75 men referred to chronic prostatitis clinic. Urology. 1991;38:11–9.

51. Maskell R, Pead L, Hallett R. Urinary pathogens in the male. J Urol. 1975;47:691–4.

52. Kauffman C, Hertz C, Sheagren J. *Staphylococcus saprophyticus* role in urinary tract infections in men. J Urol. 1983;130:493–4.

53. Schaeffer A. Urinary tract infections in urology: a urologist's view of chronic bacteriuria. Infect Dis Clin North Am. 1987;1:875–92.

54. Gilstrap L, Cunningham F, Whalley P. Acute pyelonephritis in pregnancy: an anterospective study. Obstet Gynecol. 1981;57:409–13.

55. Maclean A. Urinary tract infection in pregnancy. Br J Urol. 1997;80:10–3.

56. Angel J, O'Brien W, Finan M, et al. Acute pyelonephritis: a prospective study of oral versus intravenous antibiotic therapy. Obstet Gynecol. 1990;76:28–32.

57. Campbell-Brown M, McFadyen I, Seal D. Is screening for bacteriuria in pregnancy worthwhile? Br Med J. 1987;294:1579–82.

58. Ooi B, Chen B, Yu M. Prevalence and site of bacteriuria in diabetes mellitus. Postgrad Med J. 1974;50:497–99.

59. Vejlsgaard R. Studies in urinary infections in diabetics: bacteriuria in relation to long-term diabetic manifestations. Acta Med Scand. 1966;179:173–89.

60. Platt R, Polk B, Murdock B, et al. Risk factors for nosocomial urinary tract infection. Am J Epidemiol. 1986;124:977–85.

61. Patterson J, Andriole V. Bacterial urinary tract infections in diabetics. Infect Dis Clin North Am. 1995;9:25–33.

62. Huang J, Chen K, Ruann M. Mixed acid fermentation of glucose as a mechanism of emphysematous urinary tract infection. J Urol. 1991;146:148–51.

63. Ellenbarg M. Diabetic neuropathy: clinical aspects. Metabolism. 1976;25:1627–55.

64. Zhanel G, Harding G, Guay D. Asymptomatic bacteriuria: which patients should be treated? Arch Intern Med. 1990;150:1389–96.

65. Baciewicz A, Swafford WJ. Hypoglycemia induced by the interaction of chlorpropamide and co-trimoxazole. Drug Intell Clin Pharmacol. 1984;18:309–10.

66. Christensen M, Madsen P. Antimicrobial prophylaxis in transurethral surgery. Urology. 1990;35:11–4.

67. Appell R, Flynn J, Paris A, et al. Occult bacterial colonization of bladder tumors. J Urol. 1980;124:345–6.

68. Badenoch D, Murdoch D, Tipsaft R. Microbiological study of bladder tumors, their history and infective complications. J Urol. 1990;35:5–8.

69. Ashby E, Reese M, Dowding C. Prophylaxis against systemic infections after transrectal biopsy for suspected prostatic carcinoma. Br Med J. 1978;2:1263–4.

70. Silver T, Kass E, Thornbury J, et al. The radiological spectrum of acute pyelonephritis in adults and adolescents. Radiology. 1976; 118:65–71.

71. Mayrer A, Miniter P, Andriole V. Immunopathogenesis of chronic pyelonephritis. Am J Med. 1983;Infect Dis Symp:59–70.

72. Hill G. Renal infection. In: Hill G, ed. Uropathology, vol. 1. New York: Churchill Livingstone, 1989:333–6.

73. Roberts J. Pathogenesis of pyelonephritis. J Urol. 1983;129:1102–6.

74. Ransley P, Risdon R. The pathogenesis of reflux nephropathy. Contrib Nephrol. 1979;16:90–7.

75. Freiha F, Messing E, Gross D. Emphysematous pyelonepthritis. J Contin Urol Educ. 1979;18:9–13.

76. Lautin E, Gordon P, Friedman A, et al. Emphysematous pyelonephritis: optimal diagnosis and treatment. Urol Radiol. 1979; 1:93–6.

77. Evanoff G, Thompson C, Foley R, et al. Spectrum of gas with in the kidney: emphysematous pyelonephritis and emphysematous pyelitis. Am J Med. 1987;83:149–54.

78. Schainuck L, Fouty R, Cutler R. Emphysematous pyelonephritis, a new case and review of previous observations. Am J Med. 1968;44:134–9.

79. Schultz E, Klorfein E. Emphysematous pyelonephritis. J Urol. 1962; 87:762–6.

80. Micheli J, Mogle P, Perlberg S, et al. Emphysematous pyelonephritis. J Urol. 1984;131:203–7.

81. Hammedah M, Nicholls G, Calder C, et al. Xanthogranulomatous pyelonephritis in childhood: pre-operative diagnosis is possible. Br J Urol. 1994;73:83–6.

82. Malek R. Xanthogranulomatous pyelonephritis: a great imitator. J Contin Educ Urol. 1978;17–28.

83. Tolia B, Iloreta A, Freed S, et al. Xanthogranulomatous pyelonephritis: detailed analysis of 29 cases and a brief description of atypical presentations. J Urol. 1981;126:437–42.

84. Malek R, Elder J. Xanthogranulomatous pyelonephritis: a critical analysis of 26 cases and the literature. J Urol. 1978:589–93.

85. D'Costa G, Nagle S, Wagholikar U, et al. Xanthogranulomatous pyelonephritis in children and adults – an 8 year study. Indian J Pathol Microbiol. 1990;33:224–9.

86. Chuang C, Lai M, Chang P. Xanthogranulomatous pyelonephritis: experience in 36 cases. J Urol. 1992;147:333–6.

87. Levy M, Baumal R, Eddy A. Xanthogranulomatous pyelonephritis in children. Etiology, pathogenesis, clinical and radiologic features, and management. Clin Pediatr. 1994;33:360–6.

88. Brown PJ, Dodson M, Weintrub P. Xanthogranulomatous pyelonephritis: report of nonsurgical management of a case and review of the literature. Clin Infect Dis. 1995;22:308–14.

89. Goldman S, Hartman D, Fishman E, et al. CT of xanthogranulomatous pyelonephritis: radiologic–pathologic correlation. AJR. 1984; 142:963–99.

90. Solomon A, Braz F, Papo J. Computerized tomography in xanthogranulomatous pyelonephritis. J Urol. 1983;130:323–5.

91. VanKirk O, Go R, Wedel V. Sonographic features of xanthogranulomatous pyelonephritis. AJR. 1980;134:1035–9.

92. Stanton M, Maxted W. Malacoplakia: a study of the literature and current concepts of pathogenesis, diagnosis and treatment. J Urol. 1981;125:139–46.

93. Hartman D. Radiologic pathologic correlation of infectious granulomatous diseases of the kidney. Monogr Urol. 1985;6:3–43.

94. Van der Voort P, Ten Velden J, Wassenaar R, et al. Malacoplakia: two case reports and a comparison of treatment modalities based on a literature review. Arch Intern Med. 1996;156:577–83.

95. Abdou N, Pombejara C, Sagawa A. Malacoplakia: evidence for monocyte lysosomal abnormality correctable by cholinergic agonist in vitro and in vivo. N Engl J Med. 1977;297:1413–9.

96. Biggar W, Crawford L, Cardella C, et al. Malacoplakia and immunosuppressive therapy. Am J Pathol. 1985;119:5–11.

97. Webb M, Pincott J, Marshall W, et al. Hypogammaglobulinaemia and malacoplakia: response to bethanechol. Eur J Paediatr. 1986; 145:297–302.

98. Callea F, Van Damme B, Desmet V. Alpha-1-antitrypsin in malakoplakia. Virchows Arch A. 1982;395:1–9.

99. Mitchell G. The renal fascia. Br J Surg. 1950;37:257–66.

100. Hutchison F, Kaysen G. Perinephric abscess: the missed diagnosis. Med Clin North Am. 1988;72:993–1010.

101. Atcheson D. Perinephric abscess with a review of 117 cases. J Urol. 1941;46:201–8.

102. Clemens J, Schaeffer A. Renal and retroperitoneal abscesses. In: Graham S, ed. Glenn's urologic surgery. Philadelphia: Lippincott-Raven; 1998.

103. Bova J, Potter J, Arevalos E, et al. Renal and perirenal infection. J Urol. 1985;133:375–8.

104. Gerzof S, Gale M. Computed tomography and ultrasonography for diagnosis and treatment of renal and retroperitoneal abscesses. Urol Clin North Am. 1982;9:185–93.

105. Thorley J, Jones S, Sanford J. Perinephric abscess. Medicine. 1974;53:441–51.

106. Malgieri J, Krush E, Persky L. The changing clinicopathological pattern abscesses in or adjacent to the kidney. J Urol. 1977;118:230–32.

107. Stamey T. Pathogenesis and treatment of urinary tract infections. Baltimore: Williams & Wilkins; 1980.

108. Drach G, Fair W, Meares E, et al. Classification of benign diseases associated with prostatic pain: prostatits or prostadynia? J Urol. 1978;120:266.

109. Stillwell T, Engen D, Farrow G. The clinical spectrum of granulomatous prostatitis: a report of 200 cases. J Urol. 1987;138:320–3.

110. Lopez-Plaza I, Bostwick D. Prostatitis. In: Bostwick D, ed. Pathology of the prostate. New York: Churchill Livingstone; 1990:15–30.

111. Roberts R, Lieber M, Bostwick D, et al. A review of clinical and pathological prostatitis syndromes. Urology. 1997;49:809–21.

112. Bergeron M, Thabet M, Roy M, et al. Norfloxacin penetration into human renal and prostatic tissues. Antimicrob Agents Chemother. 1985;28:349.

113. Schaeffer A, Wendel E, Dunn J. Prevalence and significance of prostatic inflammation. J Urol. 1981;125:215.

114. Kirby R, Lowe D, Bultitude M, et al. Intraprostatic urinary reflux: an etiologic factor in abacterial prostatitis. Br J Urol. 1982;54:729.

115. Weidner W, Schiefer H, Krauss H, et al. Chronic prostatitis: a thorough search for etiologically involved microorganisms in 1461 patients. Infection. 1991;19:S119–25.

116. Berger R, Krieger J, Kessler D, et al. Case-control study of men with suspected chronic idiopathic prostatitis. J Urol. 1989; 141:328–31.

117. Shortliffe L, Sellers R, Schachter J. The characterization of nonbacterial prostatitis: the search for an etiology. J Urol. 1992; 148:1461–6.

118. Nickel J, Sorensen R. Transurethral microwave thermotherapy for nonbacterial prostatitis: a randomized double-blinded sham controlled study using new prostatitis specific assessment questionnaires. J Urol. 1996;155:1950–5.

119. Meares E. Prostatitis. Med Clin North Am. 1991;75:405–24.

120. De Jong Z, Pontonnier F, Plante P, et al. The frequency of *Chlamydia trachomatis* in acute epididymitis. Br J Urol. 1988;62:76–8.

121. Doble A, Taylor-Robinson D, Thomas B, et al. Acute epididymitis: a microbiological and ultrasonographic study. Br J Urol. 1989;32:90–4.

122. Lau P, Anderson P, Giacomantonio J, et al. Acute epididymitis in boys: are antibiotics indicated? Br J Urol. 1998;81:179–80.

123. Weiner D, Lowe F. Gangrene of the male genitalia. AUA Update Ser. 1998;17:42–7.

124. Jones R, Hirschmann J, Brown G, et al. Fournier's syndrome: necrotizing subcutaneous infection of the male genitalia. J Urol. 1979; 122:279–82.

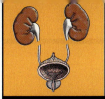

Chapter 22 Urinary Tract Stones

Ravi Munver and Glenn M Preminger

KEY POINTS

- Stone disease affects 1–5% of the population, with a lifetime risk of 10–20%.
- Attention to pathophysiology identifies etiology in over 90% of cases.
- Metabolic screening should be tailored to individual cases.
- Medical management can reduce recurrence rates.
- 10–20% of cases will require surgical intervention.

INTRODUCTION AND EPIDEMIOLOGY

Incidence

Urolithiasis is a disorder characterized by the presence of urinary calculi at any point along the collecting system. These abnormal concretions consist of crystalline components incorporated into an organic matrix and are among the most common afflictions of the urinary tract. Calculous disease affects approximately 1–5% of the population in industrialized countries, the annual incidence rate of this disorder being as high as 1% in middle-aged Caucasian men.

The most common type of calculus contains calcium and oxalate, occurring alone or in combination with hydroxyapatite. Calcareous calculi account for approximately 80% of all types of urinary calculi, the remaining 20% being noncalcareous in nature (Fig. 22.1).

The lifetime risk for stone formation in adult Caucasian men approaches 20%, while it is only approximately 5–10% for women. In addition, the recurrence rate of urolithiasis is reported to be as high as 50% within 5 years of the initial stone occurrence[1]. In general, stone disease in adult Caucasian men is one fourth to one third more common than in black men. However, black patients demonstrate a higher incidence of calculi associated with urinary tract infection by urea-splitting organisms[2].

Age and gender

Although the highest incidence of urinary calculi occurs in the 20–50 age group, a substantial number of patients report onset of the disease before the age of 20[3,4]. While some investigators have reported on equal tendencies toward stone formation in men and women during childhood, adult men are affected three times as often as women[5].

Heredity

The incidence of stone disease appears to be greatest in areas of the world populated by Caucasians and Asians. Alternatively, urinary calculi are seen with less frequency in blacks and native Americans. Nephrolithiasis has been shown to be associated with a polygenic defect and partial penetrance; however, heredity may be only one of several responsible factors[6,7]. Hereditary disorders that promote the development of calculi include familial renal tubular acidosis (RTA), cystinuria, dehydroxyadeninuria, and xanthinuria. Metabolic, environmental, and dietary factors, along with the amount of fluid intake, are the other major contributors to stone formation.

PATHOPHYSIOLOGY OF NEPHROLITHIASIS

Advances in pathophysiologic elucidation and analytic methodology have allowed the identification of causes for urinary calculi formation in more than 97% of patients. Low urinary volume is by far the most common combined abnormality and the single most important factor that may be corrected in order to avoid recurrent stone disease (Fig. 22.2)[8].

Calcium nephrolithiasis

Hypercalciuria

Hypercalciuria is defined as the excretion of urinary calcium exceeding 200mg/24 hours collection (or an excess calcium of 4mg/kg/24 hours). The association of hypercalciuria with recurrent calcium nephrolithiasis has long been recognized, although the exact nature of this relationship continues to be debated. Nephrolithiasis resulting from hypercalciuria is heterogeneous in origin and is comprised of several entities.

Kidney stone composition	
Crystal composition	Percentage of stones analyzed
Calcium oxalate	60
Calcium phosphate	20
Uric acid	10
Cystine	3
Struvite	7
Total	100

Figure 22.1 Kidney stone composition.

22

Classification of nephrolithiasis		
	% sole occurrence	% combined occurrence
Absorptive hypercalciuria	20	40
Type I		
Type II		
Renal hypercalciuria	5	8
Resorptive hypercalciuria (primary hyperparathyroidism)	3	8
Unclassified hypercalciuria	15	25
Hyperoxaluric calcium nephrolithiasis	2	15
Dietary hyperoxaluria		
Enteric hyperoxaluria		
Primary hyperoxaluria		
Hyperuricosuric calcium nephrolithiasis	10	40
Hypocitraturic calcium nephrolithiasis	10	50
Distal renal tubular acidosis		
Chronic diarrheal syndrome		
Thiazide-induced hypocitraturia		
Idiopathic hypocitraturia		
Hypomagnesuric calcium nephrolithiasis	5	10
Gouty diathesis	15	30
Cystinuria	<1	
Struvite (infection) lithiasis	1	5
Low urine volume	10	50
No pathologic disturbance and miscellaneous	<3	
Total	100	

Figure 22.2 Classification of nephrolithiasis.

Absorptive hypercalciuria

The primary abnormality in absorptive hypercalciuria is increased intestinal absorption of calcium[9]. The precise cause for the hyperabsorption of calcium is not fully understood. This increased serum calcium concentration enhances the renal filtered load and suppresses parathyroid function. The combination of an increase in the filtered load and a decrease in renal tubular reabsorption of calcium, caused by parathyroid suppression, results in development of hypercalciuria and stone formation (Fig. 22.3). The excessive renal loss of calcium compensates for the intestinal hyperabsorption, thereby maintaining serum calcium in the normal range.

Absorptive hypercalciuria type I (AH-I) is a more severe form of hypercalciuria characterized by a urine calcium level above 200mg/day, with high or low dietary calcium intake. In AH-I, patients have normal serum levels of calcium and phosphorus and a normal or low serum level of parathyroid hormone (PTH). Fasting urinary calcium is normal, while an oral calcium load results in exacerbated hypercalciuria.

Absorptive hypercalciuria type II (AH-II) is a mild to moderate form of this disorder in which hypercalciuria only occurs with high calcium intake. AH-II is similar to AH-I and is considered to be a less severe form of this disorder. These patients have normal urinary calcium excretion either while fasting or on a restricted calcium diet.

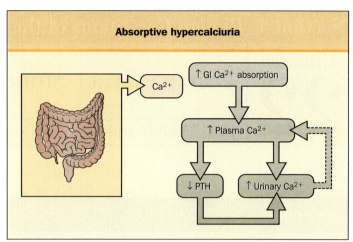

Figure 22.3 Absorptive hypercalciuria. Increased gastrointestinal (GI) absorption of calcium (Ca) leads to an elevated serum calcium concentration, which suppresses parathyroid hormone (PTH) secretion and enhances the renal filtered load. The combination of a decrease in renal tubular reabsorption of calcium, caused by parathyroid suppression, and an increase in the renal filtered load results in an elevated urinary calcium concentration. Solid arrow, positive stimulation; dashed arrow, negative feedback.

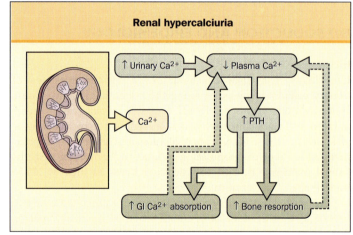

Figure 22.4 Renal hypercalciuria. An impairment in renal tubular reabsorption of calcium leads to an elevated urinary calcium (Ca) concentration. The consequent reduction in serum calcium concentration stimulates parathyroid hormone (PTH) secretion, which results in enhanced gastrointestinal (GI) absorption of calcium and mobilization of calcium from bone. Solid arrow, positive stimulation; dashed arrow, negative feedback.

Renal hypercalciuria

The underlying abnormality in renal hypercalciuria (or 'renal leak' hypercalciuria) is thought to be an impairment in renal tubular reabsorption of calcium[9]. The consequent reduction in serum calcium concentration stimulates parathyroid function. PTH excess results in mobilization of calcium from bone and enhanced intestinal absorption of calcium, with ensuing stimulation of renal synthesis of $1,25\text{-}(OH)_2D$ (Fig. 22.4). These events lead to an increase in the circulating concentration and renal filtered load of calcium, often causing significant hypercalciuria,

Resorptive hypercalciuria

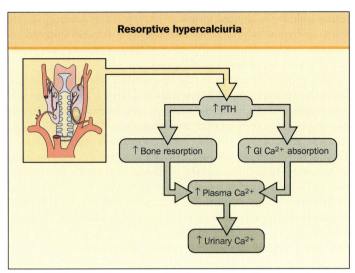

↑ PTH

↑ Bone resorption   ↑ GI Ca²⁺ absorption

↑ Plasma Ca²⁺

↑ Urinary Ca²⁺

Figure 22.5 Resorptive hypercalciuria. Hypersecretion of parathyroid hormone (PTH) results in excessive bone resorption and an increase in serum calcium levels. Gastrointestinal (GI) absorption of calcium is secondarily elevated because of the PTH-dependent stimulation of renal synthesis of 1,25-(OH)$_2$D. These effects lead to elevated serum and urinary calcium concentrations.

Differential diagnosis of hypercalciuria

	Serum calcium	Parathyroid function	Fasting urinary calcium	Intestinal calcium absorption
Absorptive	Normal	Decreased	Normal	Increased (primarily)
Renal	Normal	Increased (secondarily)	Increased	Increased (secondarily)
Resorptive	Increased	Increased (primarily)	Increased	Increased (secondarily)
Unclassified	Normal	Normal	Increased	Increased

Figure 22.6 Differential diagnosis of hypercalciuria.

Causes of secondary hypercalciuria

With hypercalcemia
  Granulomatous diseases
  Immobilization (prolonged)
  Lymphoma
  Metastatic bone disease
  Multiple myeloma
  Paget's disease of bone
  Primary hyperparathyroidism
  Sarcoidosis
Endocrine disorders
  Cushing's syndrome
  Hyperthyroidism
Medications
  Acetazolamide
  Calcium ingestion (excessive)
  Furosemide (frusemide)
  Milk–alkali syndrome
  Vitamin D intoxication
Renal tubular acidosis

Figure 22.7 Causes of secondary hypercalciuria.

even in the fasting state. Unlike in primary hyperparathyroidism, patients have a normal serum calcium level. As the elevated level of PTH (secondary hyperparathyroidism) is a subsequent event in response to the renal leakage of calcium, an oral calcium load may suppress the hyperparathyroidism.

Resorptive hypercalciuria

Primary hyperparathyroidism is the etiology behind resorptive hypercalciuria. The initial event is hypersecretion of PTH that results in excessive bone resorption and an increase in serum calcium levels. Intestinal absorption of calcium is often secondarily elevated because of the PTH-dependent stimulation of renal synthesis of 1,25-(OH)$_2$D. These effects lead to significant hypercalciuria through an increase in the circulating concentration and renal filtered load of calcium (Fig. 22.5). The elevated level of serum PTH enhances renal reabsorption of calcium and excretion of phosphate. Fasting urinary calcium levels remain elevated, as they do in renal hypercalciuria.

Unclassified hypercalciuria

In some patients with hypercalciuria, the cause of their increased urinary calcium excretion cannot be determined with certainty. This unclassified, or idiopathic, hypercalciuria is represented by patients having normal serum calcium and PTH levels, and an elevated fasting urinary calcium level without parathyroid stimulation[10]. This disorder exhibits features of both absorptive and renal hypercalciuria; however, it lacks the characteristics required for differentiation. Fasting hypercalciuria suggests a renal calcium leak, although hyperparathyroidism is not evident. A lack of PTH elevation resembles absorptive hypercalciuria, but fasting urinary calcium is elevated. The differences among the various types of hypercalciuria are presented in Figure 22.6. Secondary hypercalciuria can also be seen in several conditions (Figure 22.7).

A trial of sodium cellulose phosphate (SCP) may assist in elucidating the nature of this condition[11]. SCP binds to intestinal calcium and prevents its absorption, thereby eliminating the potential confusion surrounding patients with inadequate dietary preparation prior to the standard fast and calcium load. In these patients, there may be an incomplete renal clearance of intestinally absorbed calcium. Under these circumstances, patients with absorptive hypercalciuria may have the appearance of fasting hypercalciuria, while those with renal hypercalciuria may not exhibit parathyroid stimulation, which occurs from the suppressive effect of the absorbed calcium. SCP is therefore helpful in allowing for discrimination between absorptive and renal hypercalciuria.

Impact of dietary calcium

Early recommendations suggested that a low calcium diet would decrease urinary calcium excretion, thereby reducing the risk of recurrent calcium stone formation. However, recent studies have suggested that a low calcium diet may place some stone-formers at risk for either recurrent stone formation or other problems such as reduced bone density. Recent investigations assessing the bone mineral content of the radius in patients with idiopathic calcium stone disease have demonstrated low bone density. Therefore, a calcium-restricted diet may place these patients at further risk for bone problems such as osteopenia or osteoporosis[12].

More recently, large epidemiologic studies have demonstrated that a low calcium diet may place patients at increased risk of recurrent stone formation. In a study of 45,000 men with no history of stones, 4-year follow-up demonstrated that calcium intake was inversely associated with stone formation. Similarly, the Nurses Health Study, which followed 97,000 women for an average of 12 years of follow-up, also found that calcium intake might be inversely associated with stone formation. Both of these studies suggest that a low calcium diet may raise urinary oxalate, thereby placing these patients at increased risk for stone formation[13,14]. However, these epidemiologic studies could not control for confounding variables such as an apparent increase in urinary potassium, phosphorus, magnesium, and water, all factors that would decrease the risk of recurrent stone formation. Moreover, these large epidemiologic studies did not look specifically at patients whose underlying pathophysiology was absorptive hypercalciuria. One would assume that placing patients with absorptive hypercalciuria on a high calcium diet would have exacerbated their stone formation.

Physiologic studies have demonstrated that patients with normal intestinal tracts will develop intestinal adaptation to high calcium intake. Therefore, after a prolonged period of high calcium diet, vitamin D production will be downregulated, thereby reducing intestinal calcium absorption. However, patients with absorptive hypercalciuria appear to have lost their ability for intestinal adaptation, which is no longer regulated by vitamin D. Therefore, these patients continue to hyperabsorb calcium, even in the face of a high calcium intake.

Therefore, our current approach is not to place patients routinely on a severe calcium restriction. We recommend a moderate calcium restriction in patients with absorptive hypercalciuria. In addition, all patients are advised to limit excessive intake of dairy products, high oxalate foods (spinach, tea, chocolate, nuts), and dietary sodium. These moderate dietary limitations should avoid exacerbation of hypercalciuria and/or hyperoxaluria.

Hyperoxaluria

Hyperoxaluria is defined by urinary oxalate excretion in excess of 45mg/day. A mild to moderate elevation (45–80mg/day) may be caused by dietary hyperoxaluria. At levels above 80mg/day, the diagnosis of nephrolithiasis is likely due to either enteric or primary hyperoxaluria.

Dietary hyperoxaluria

Between 80% and 90% of urinary oxalate is synthesized in the liver, while the remainder is from dietary oxalate or ascorbic acid (vitamin C). Therefore, dietary overindulgence in oxalate-rich foods, or excessive ascorbic acid ingestion, can contribute to hyperoxaluria through intestinal absorption of oxalate.

Enteric hyperoxaluria

The cause of calcium stone formation in the majority of hyperoxaluric patients is enteric hyperoxaluria[15,16]. Ileal disease is responsible for increased intestinal absorption of oxalate, which leads to hyperoxaluria. This disorder may be encountered in patients with inflammatory bowel disease, gastric or small bowel resection, or jejunoileal bypass[17].

Two processes are probably responsible for the intestinal hyperabsorption of oxalate. Bile salts and fatty acids increase the permeability of the intestinal mucosa, which results in a primary increase in the intestinal transport of oxalate. Fat malabsorption, characteristic of ileal disease, leads to calcium soap formation. This factor limits the amount of free calcium that can complex with oxalate, thereby raising the oxalate pool available for absorption and promoting the development of stones.

In enteric hyperoxaluria, stone formation may also be the result of additional factors such as low urinary output from intestinal fluid loss, low urinary citrate caused by hypokalemia and metabolic acidosis, and low urinary magnesium caused by impaired intestinal magnesium absorption.

Primary hyperoxaluria

Primary hyperoxaluria type I is an autosomal recessive disorder resulting from a defect of the hepatic enzyme alanine–glyoxylate aminotransferase (AGT). In the normal liver, AGT functions by catalyzing the transamination of glyoxylate to glycine in hepatic peroxisomes. The deficiency or altered migration of this enzyme in primary hyperoxaluria type I results in the conversion of glyoxylate to oxalate, leading to increased urinary excretion of oxalic, glycolic, and glyoxylic acids[18,19]. This condition is characterized by nephrocalcinosis, oxalate deposition in tissues (oxalosis), and renal failure, resulting in death before the age of 20 when untreated[20]. The diagnosis can definitively be made by assaying the amount and distribution of AGT in liver specimens obtained by percutaneous biopsy.

Primary hyperoxaluria type II is very rare and results in deficiency of the hepatic enzymes D-glycerate dehydrogenase and glyoxylate reductase, leading to increased urinary oxalate and glycerate excretion. Both types of primary hyperoxaluria cause stone formation beginning in childhood, with subsequent development of nephrocalcinosis, tubulointerstitial nephropathy, and chronic renal failure. In addition to high levels of urinary oxalate, serum oxalate levels are also elevated.

Hyperuricosuria

The only recognizable physiologic abnormality occurring in about 10% of patients with calcium oxalate nephrolithiasis is hyperuricosuria[21]. While excessive uric acid excretion can be found in primary gout, it may also be seen in secondary conditions of purine overproduction, which include myeloproliferative states, glycogen storage disease, and malignancy. Dietary indulgence in purine-rich foods is another potential cause for this condition. Possible etiologies for hyperuricosuric calcium oxalate nephrolithiasis can be found in Figure 22.8. It is believed that monosodium urate is formed in a supersaturated environment in hyperuricosuric patients. Monosodium urate (colloidal or crystalline) may then initiate calcium stone formation through direct induction of heterogeneous nucleation of calcium oxalate or by adsorption of certain macromolecular inhibitors of stone formation[22]. The features of hyperuricosuric calcium oxalate nephrolithiasis include elevated urinary uric acid (>600mg/day), a normal serum calcium level, normal urinary calcium and

Causes of increased urinary uric acid
Abnormal production
Genetic overproduction
Enzymatic mutation (i.e. HGPRT deficiency)
Acquired overproduction
Myeloproliferative disorders
Obesity
Alcohol ingestion
Abnormal excretion
Diet high in purines
Uricosuric drugs

Figure 22.8 Causes of increased urinary uric acid. HGPRT, hypoxanthine–gnanine phosphoribosyl–transferase.

oxalate levels, normal fasting and calcium load response, and urinary pH typically above 5.5.

Hypocitraturia

Hypocitraturic calcium nephrolithiasis may exist as an isolated abnormality (10%) or in combination with other metabolic disorders (50%)[3,4,23]. Acid–base status, acidosis in particular, is the most important factor affecting the renal handling of citrate, with increased acid levels resulting in diminished endogenous citrate production.

Citrate lowers urinary saturation of calcium salts by forming soluble complexes with calcium, as well as directly inhibiting the crystallization of calcium salts[24,25]. In the setting of low urinary citrate, the urinary environment is more supersaturated with respect to calcium salts, thus promoting nucleation, growth, and aggregation, resulting in stone formation. Mean normal urinary citrate excretion is 640mg/day, while the lower limit of normal is 320mg/day[3,4,26].

Distal renal tubular acidosis

One of the more common causes of hypocitraturia is distal RTA. Acidosis impairs urinary citrate excretion by enhancing renal tubular reabsorption of citrate as well as by reducing its synthesis[24]. Distal RTA may occur in a complete or incomplete form. The complete form is characterized by hyperchloremic metabolic acidosis, hypokalemia, and elevated urinary pH, while the incomplete form is characterized by normal serum electrolyte levels and an inability to acidify urine following an ammonium chloride load. In both of these forms, hypercalciuria and profound hypocitraturia may be associated. In combination with alkaline urine, the patient is at risk for developing calcium oxalate or calcium phosphate stones[27].

Chronic diarrheal syndrome

Patients with this condition lose alkali in the form of bicarbonate via their gastrointestinal tract[28]. This results in metabolic acidosis with a subsequent impairment in citrate synthesis. Decreased citrate production is responsible for the lower urinary concentration of citrate. Besides hypocitraturia, patients with chronic diarrheal syndrome may have additional risk factors for stone formation such as low urine volumes and hyperoxaluria (see Enteric hyperoxaluria).

Thiazide-induced hypocitraturia

Thiazide diuretics can produce hypokalemia that leads to intracellular acidosis. The acidotic state inhibits the synthesis of citrate, resulting in hypocitraturia. The essential mechanism is the inhibition of citrate production, which is a consequence of chronic acidosis[29,30].

Idiopathic hypocitraturia

This entity includes hypocitraturia occurring alone as well as in conjunction with other abnormalities (i.e. hypercalciuria or hyperuricosuria). Mechanisms that account for hypocitraturia in this condition include a high animal protein diet (with an elevated acid-ash content), strenuous physical exercise (causing lactic acidosis), high sodium intake, and intestinal malabsorption of citrate.

Hypomagnesuria

Magnesium is known to be an inhibitor of calcium nephrolithiasis by apparently increasing the solubility product of calcium oxalate and calcium phosphate. Hypomagnesuria is defined as urinary magnesium excretion below 50mg/day. This condition may coexist with hypocitraturia in approximately 65% of patients, and low urine volume (<1L/day) in approximately 40% of patients[31]. Many patients with nephrolithiasis will report a limited intake of magnesium-rich foods such as nuts and chocolate, suggesting the dietary basis of this condition.

Gouty diathesis

Gouty diathesis may appear in a latent or an early phase of classic gout, or it may manifest fully with gouty arthritis and hyperuricemia. In this disorder, patients develop renal stones composed purely of uric acid, uric acid in combination with calcium oxalate or calcium phosphate, or stones that contain only calcium oxalate or calcium phosphate. Certain patients may alternately form uric acid and calcium stones[32].

The invariant feature of this condition is persistently acidic urine (pH<5.5), in which uric acid is sparingly soluble in the absence of intestinal alkali loss or dietary acid load. No specific cause has been detected for the unusually low urinary pH. The undue acidity of urine causes high levels of undissociated uric acid, which favors crystallization. These uric acid crystals can induce formation of calcium stones by urate-induced heterogeneous nucleation of calcium salts.

Noncalcareous nephrolithiasis
Uric acid stones

The essential factors responsible for pure uric acid lithiasis are urinary pH less than the dissociation constant for uric acid (5.47) and profound hyperuricosuria, with urinary uric acid levels above 1,500mg/day. Uric acid stones may form in the presence of gouty diathesis or as a result of secondary causes of purine overproduction, such as myeloproliferative states, glycogen storage disease, and malignancy. Chronic diarrheal states, such as Crohn's disease and ulcerative colitis, or jejunoileal bypass surgery may cause uric acid lithiasis, through a loss of bicarbonate (net alkali deficit) thereby lowering urinary pH, or through a reduction in urine volume (augmentation of urinary concentration of uric acid).

Cystine stones

Cystinuria is an autosomal recessive familial disorder involving an inborn error of metabolism characterized by a disturbance in renal and intestinal transport of dicarboxylic acids, including cystine. Stone formation occurs in a minority of patients (of the homozygous genotype) and is the result of the low solubility of cystine in urine and its excessive renal excretion. Cystine solubility is pH-dependent, with its lowest solubility being at the low range of urinary pH. A gradual increase in solubility is noted with a rise in pH to 7.5, and a rapid increase in solubility as the pH rises above 7.5.

The main determinant of cystine crystallization is urinary supersaturation. Urine that is supersaturated with respect to cystine will invariably result in the precipitation of cystine. As the urinary saturation of cystine exceeds 250mg/L, cystine will precipitate out of solution. If the cystine concentration can be maintained below 200mg/L, cystine stones typically should not form. Recent studies have demonstrated that 18–44% of patients with cystinuria have associated metabolic defects (hyperuricosuria, hypocitraturia, etc.) which may further complicate their cystine stone disease[33].

The diagnosis of cystinuria should be suspected in patients with an early onset of nephrolithiasis, a significant family history, or recurrent stone disease. A positive sodium nitroprusside urine test or the presence of flat, hexagonal crystals in urinary sediment provides a presumptive diagnosis of cystine stone disease. Quantitative urine amino acid measurements or identification of cystine calculi on stone analysis provides the definitive diagnosis. Urinary cystine excretion of more than 250mg/day is usually diagnostic of homozygous cystinuria.

Struvite (infection) stones

Infection lithiasis comprises 10–15% of all cases of nephrolithiasis and is three times more common in women than in men. This disorder is rather ambiguous as it has been described as several different entities. Depending on the investigator, 'infection stones' may designate staghorn stones (with various compositions), struvite stones [magnesium ammonium phosphate (MAP) or calcium carbonate apatite] produced by urea-splitting bacteria, calcium oxalate stones (with secondary infection), or mixed struvite stones (a combination of two or more of these).

A recent study was performed to clarify the etiology, composition, and nomenclature of these stones[34]. The results suggest that stones composed purely of struvite were produced solely by ureolysis. The primary pathophysiologic event in patients with struvite stones is infection of the urinary tract with urea-splitting organisms. Figure 22.9 lists the more common urea-splitting organisms, which include not only Gram-negative and Gram-positive bacteria but also mycoplasma and yeasts. The critical mechanism of stone formation involves the formation of ammonia in urine through the enzymatic degradation of urea by the bacterial enzyme urease[35]. The ammonia undergoes hydrolysis to form ammonium and hydroxyl ions. The resulting urine alkalinity enhances the dissociation of phosphate to form triphosphate ions, which reduce the solubility of struvite. Hence, the urinary environment becomes supersaturated with respect to struvite. In patients with struvite calculi, urinary pH is generally high (pH>7.5), as is the ammonium content in urine.

Struvite stones are most commonly found in patients with chronic infections as well as in those with anatomic or functional abnormalities of their urinary tracts that favor stasis of urine and chronic bacteriuria, including urinary diversions, neurogenic bladder, diverticuli, strictures, etc[34]. In patients with pure struvite stones, metabolic abnormalities are not responsible for ureolysis or stone formation. Stones composed of struvite along with calcium oxalate, or other mixed struvite variations, suggest an underlying metabolic abnormality (i.e. hypercalciuria, hypocitraturia, etc.), which may contribute to stone formation. In these patients there is a need for a complete metabolic evaluation to identify the underlying etiology of their stone disease. The classic radiographic finding is a radiopaque staghorn calculus.

Common urea-splitting organisms in struvite calculus formation			
Gram-negative bacteria	**Gram-positive bacteria**	**Mycoplasma**	**Yeasts**
Proteus mirabilis*	**Corynebacterium hofmannii**	**Mycoplasma (T-strain)**	**Candida humicola**
Proteus morganii	**Corynebacterium ovis**	**Ureaplasma urealyticum**	**Cryptococcus spp.**
Proteus rettgeri	**Corynebacterium renale**		**Rhodotorula spp.**
Proteus vulgaris	**Corynebacterium ulcerans**		**Sporobolmyces spp.**
Providencia stuartii	**Micrococcus varions**		**Trichosporon cutaneum**
Haemophilus influenzae	**Staphylococcus aureus**		
Yersinia enterocolitica	Corynebacterium equi		
Bacteroides corrodens	Corynebacterium murium		
Bordetella pertussis	Clostridium tetani		
Brucella spp.	Peptococcus asaccharolyticus		
Flavobacterium spp.	Staphylococcus epidermidis		
Citrobacter spp.			
Haemophilus parainfluenzae			
Klebsiella pneumonia			
Klebsiella oxytoca			
Pasteurella spp.			
Pseudomonas aeruginosa			
Serratia marcescens			

Figure 22.9 Common urea-splitting organisms in struvite calculus formation. Bold type, more common isolates; *, most common isolate.

Other causes of nephrolithiasis
Low urine volume
Low urine volume is defined by urine output of less than 1L/day. For patients who are prone to developing stones, less than 2L of urine output per day is inadequate to prevent recurrent stone disease. The typical etiology behind this condition is low fluid intake, however low urine volume can also be associated with chronic diarrheal syndromes that result in large fluid losses from the gastrointestinal tract. Low urine output contributes to the development of all types of urinary stones by providing a concentrated environment for substances that initiate stone formation, such as calcium, oxalate, uric acid, and cystine.

No pathologic disturbance
In approximately 3–5% of the stone-forming population, no identifiable risk factor for stone formation can be found[36]. This group includes individuals with normal serum calcium and PTH, normal fast and calcium load response, normal values for urinary volume, and normal pH, calcium, oxalate, uric acid, citrate, and magnesium levels, in the presence of calcium nephrolithiasis. In the future, new promoters and inhibitors of urinary stones may be discovered that will assist in clarifying the basis behind nephrolithiasis in these patients.

Drug-induced nephrolithiasis
Ephedrine calculi
Ephedrine and its metabolites (norephedrine, pseudoephedrine, and norpseudoephedrine) are sympathomimetic agents that have been used for the treatment of enuresis, myasthenia gravis, narcolepsy, and rhinorrhea[37]. In addition to numerous side effects, ephedrine and its derivatives have been associated with the production of urinary stones[38]. The estimated incidence of these stones is 1/1,500 renal calculi[37]. Consequently, it is important to consider ephedrine use in the differential diagnosis of patients with radiolucent calculi on radiographic films.

The urine solubility characteristics of ephedrine nephrolithiasis are incompletely characterized. It has been observed that a number of patients reported to form these calculi consume 1,000–3,000mg/day of ephedrine, of which 70–80% is excreted unchanged in urine[38]. The diagnosis of these calculi is similar to that of other radiolucent calculi. Twenty-four-hour urine metabolic analyses can aid in identifying ephedrine or its respective metabolites.

Guaifenesin calculi
Guaifenesin is a widely used expectorant that has also recently been associated with nephrolithiasis. These calculi are radiolucent and present in patients who ingest an excess of this medication, which may often be found in over-the-counter stimulants. The true incidence and prevalence of these calculi is difficult to accurately assess because of the limited data and reports regarding their occurrence.

A total intake of slightly more than 10g of guaifenesin is sufficient for enough production of the guaifenesin metabolite, β_2-methoxyphenoxy-lactic acid, to form a calculus composed predominately of this metabolite [39,40]. Twenty-four hour urine metabolic analyses can aid in the identification of guaifenesin or β_2-methoxyphenoxy-lactic acid.

Indinavir calculi
A number of pharmacologic agents have been directed at managing the progressive immune system failure in patients with acquired immune deficiency syndrome (AIDS). Indinavir sulfate is currently one of the protease inhibitors most frequently used against HIV, the virus that causes AIDS[41]. Despite its efficacy with respect to the treatment of AIDS, indinavir is not without adverse reactions. With respect to the urinary tract, crystalluria, nephrolithiasis, and renal insufficiency have been reported[42]. The management of indinavir nephrolithiasis is challenging as a result of patient comorbidities and the rapid rise in serum viral counts with discontinuation of this medication. The incidence of calculi in patients taking indinavir has been reported as ranging from 3% to 20%[43].

The precise mechanism of indinavir nephrolithiasis has not been elucidated but it has been speculated that stone formation results from both the poor solubility of indinavir in an aqueous environment and its high urinary excretion. In cases where stone analysis has been performed, indinavir has been identified as a sole constituent of the stone, or it has been found in combination with calcium oxalate and calcium phosphate[41]. Thus, indinavir calculi are radiolucent when they are pure and are radiopaque when they contain calcium.

Xanthine calculi
Xanthine calculi are exceedingly rare, with an estimated incidence of 1/2,500 stones[44]. Typically, these calculi occur in patients with hereditary xanthinuria, a recessive disorder characterized by a deficiency in the enzyme xanthine oxidase. As xanthine oxidase is responsible for the conversion of hypoxanthine to xanthine, and xanthine to uric acid, a deficiency in this enzyme results in decreased levels of serum and urinary uric acid. In turn, hereditary xanthinuria is typically discovered during the workup of incidental hypouricemia. These stones are also seen in patients treated with iatrogenic inhibition of xanthine oxidase with xanthine oxidase inhibitors for hyperuricosuria (i.e. allopurinol). Xanthine calculi present similarly to other urinary calculi and are radiolucent.

PRINCIPLES OF MANAGEMENT

Metabolic evaluation
There is much controversy regarding the selection of patients for diagnostic evaluation of nephrolithiasis. Although studies suggest that 'single-stone-formers' have a similar incidence and severity of metabolic disorders to those patients with recurrent stone disease, some patients will not develop additional stones despite the absence of further treatment[45]. In addition, many single-stone-formers who are treated conservatively with avoidance of dietary excess and increased fluid intake have demonstrated a low incidence of recurrent stone disease[46].

One approach to evaluating patients is to gauge the extent of the evaluation according to the estimation of potential risk for new stone formation (Fig. 22.10). First-time stone-formers without increased risk for recurrence can undergo an abbreviated diagnostic evaluation, whereas patients with recurrent stone disease or those first-time stone-formers who are at risk for recurrence should generally undergo extensive diagnostic evaluation. Patients

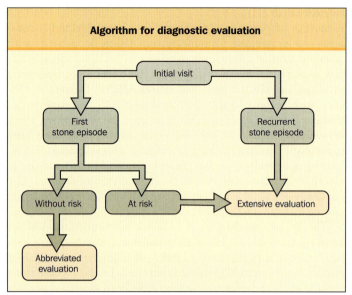

Figure 22.10 Algorithm for diagnostic evaluation.

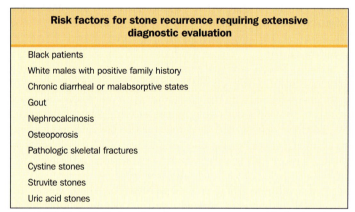

Figure 22.11 Risk factors for stone recurrence requiring extensive diagnostic evaluation.

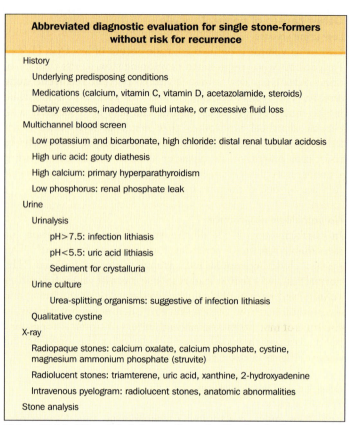

Figure 22.12 Abbreviated diagnostic evaluation for single stone-formers without risk for recurrence.

at risk include children, middle-aged Caucasian males with a family history of stones, and patients with intestinal disease (chronic diarrheal or malabsorptive states), gout, nephrocalcinosis, osteoporosis, pathologic skeletal fractures, or urinary tract infection (Figure 22.11). Any patients with stones composed of cystine, struvite, or uric acid should also undergo a complete metabolic work-up. As stone disease is relatively uncommon in black patients, a search for underlying derangements in these individuals is recommended.

The primary objective of a diagnostic evaluation of nephrolithiasis should be to efficiently and economically identify the particular physiologic defect present in a given patient in order to enable the selection of specific and rational therapy. The evaluation should be able to identify the metabolic disorders responsible for recurrent stone disease, including cystinuria, distal renal tubular acidosis, enteric hyperoxaluria, gouty diathesis, and primary hyperparathyroidism. Although many of these are relatively uncommon conditions, it is generally agreed that selective medical therapy is indicated to prevent further stone formation and to also correct underlying physiologic disturbances that may result in nonrenal complications. The relatively low cost

of a comprehensive medical evaluation might justify its wider use, especially if it averts the expense associated with additional surgery or the treatment of complications associated with stone disease[47].

Evaluating the patient with first-time stone – abbreviated diagnostic evaluation

In single-stone-formers without increased risk, the following abbreviated protocol may be applied (Fig. 22.12). A thorough history should be obtained on such patients, including dietary habits, fluid consumption, and medications. A multichannel blood screen can be helpful in identifying underlying systemic problems, such as distal renal tubular acidosis (hypokalemic, hyperchloremic metabolic acidosis), gouty diathesis (hyperuricemia), primary hyperparathyroidism (high serum calcium, low serum phosphorous), and renal phosphate leak (hypophosphatemia).

Voided urinary specimens should be obtained for comprehensive urinalysis and culture. The urinalysis should include pH determination (by electrode), since a pH greater than 7.5 is suggestive of infection lithiasis, whereas a pH less than 5.5 may be indicative of gouty diathesis. The urine sediment must be examined for crystals, since particular crystal types may provide a clue to the composition of certain stones. Urine cultures that are positive for urea-splitting organisms are consistent with struvite stones. In addition, urine should be examined for the presence of cystinuria using a qualitative examination (nitroprusside test). Abdominal plain films should also be obtained to document any residual urinary tract calculi.

Finally, all available stones should be analyzed to determine their crystalline composition. The presence of cystine crystals is diagnostic of cystinuria, whereas uric acid crystals suggest the presence of gouty diathesis. The finding of carbonate apatite or magnesium ammonium phosphate suggests infection lithiasis. A predominance of hydroxyapatite (calcium phosphate) suggests the presence of distal renal tubular acidosis or primary hyperparathyroidism. Stones composed purely or predominantly of calcium oxalate are less useful diagnostically, since they may occur in several conditions, including absorptive and renal hypercalciuria, enteric hyperoxaluria, hypocitraturic calcium nephrolithiasis, hyperuricosuric calcium nephrolithiasis, and low urine volume.

Evaluating the patient with recurrent stones – extensive diagnostic evaluation

A more extensive evaluation, directed at the identification of underlying physiologic derangements, should be performed in patients with recurrent nephrolithiasis, as well as in stone-formers at increased risk for further stone formation or with evidence of multisystem involvement.

Prior to and throughout the entire period of evaluation, the patient must be instructed to discontinue any medication that is known to interfere with the metabolism of calcium, oxalate, or uric acid. These medications include acetazolamide, antacids, calcium supplements, vitamin C, and vitamin D. Current medication for stone treatment (allopurinol, magnesium, phosphate, or thiazide) should be discontinued as well.

Three 24 hour urine samples are collected, two of which are obtained with the patient on a random diet reflective of the usual dietary intake. The third 24 hour sample is collected after 1 week on a diet restricted in calcium (less than 400mg/day), oxalate (less than 50mg/day), and sodium (less than 100mEq/day). This dietary restriction is imposed to standardize the diagnostic tests, to better assess the etiology of hypercalciuria, and to prepare for the 'fast and calcium load' test, which is performed on the second visit. Fasting urinary calcium is expressed as milligrams per deciliter of glomerular filtrate as it is reflective of renal function. To calculate this unit of measurement, the urinary calcium in milligrams per milligram of creatinine is multiplied by the serum creatinine (mg/dL). Normal fasting urinary calcium is less than 0.11mg/dL glomerular filtrate. The postload urinary calcium is best expressed as milligrams per milligram of creatinine, as it is a function of a fixed oral calcium load. The normal value for this measurement is less than 0.2mg calcium/mg creatinine.

Blood samples are collected at both visits and the two outpatient visits can be completed in less than 3 weeks. Most of the required laboratory analyses can be performed in a routine clinical laboratory with only a few of the specialized techniques being performed in a more sophisticated laboratory. The schedule of laboratory tests is outlined in Figure 22.13.

Simplified metabolic evaluation

The extensive diagnostic evaluation offers the physician a high diagnostic yield and is quite reliable. Unfortunately, some physicians find this protocol time-consuming and difficult to perform because of the inaccessibility of certain laboratory tests. A simplified diagnostic evaluation may be performed that uses the same principles and procedures as a standard outpatient evaluation and yet incorporates commercially available diagnostic assays[48]. This simplified evaluation allows all physicians the ability to evaluate patients with recurrent stones or those with single stones at increased risk.

In the simplified protocol, a full stone-risk analysis is performed on a urine sample collected from a patient on a random diet. The protocol differs in that it consists of a urine preservation method that allows the collection of urine without refrigeration and submission of an aliquot to a central laboratory for the automated analysis of various stone-forming substances[49]. The urinary constituents assayed include calcium, oxalate, and citrate (which may result from underlying metabolic problems) as well as total volume, sodium, and sulfate (which are influenced by environmental or dietary factors) (Fig. 22.14). From these determinations, the urinary saturation with respect to stone-forming salts can be calculated. A graphic display of this information may then be generated, highlighting the increased or decreased risk for each environmental, metabolic, or physicochemical factor.

After the values of all urinary constituents and saturations have been determined, a computerized printout is obtained that provides both a graphic and numeric display of the test results. These results will aid the physician in formulating a metabolic/physiologic diagnosis; however, a definitive diagnosis of a particular metabolic derangement usually requires further testing. For example, it is desirable to confirm the presence of hypocitraturia or hyperuricosuria by repeat measurements[50]. In addition, while this graphic analysis will demonstrate hypercalciuria, it is not able to differentiate between the different forms of hypercalciuria. Finally, it is important to note that the 'normal limits' cited on commercially available urine analysis packages are not the

Outline of extensive diagnostic evaluation												
	Blood					**Urine**						
	Complete blood count	Chemistry	PTH	Calcium	Uric acid	Creatinine	Sodium	pH	Total volume	Oxalate	Citrate	Qualitative cystine
Visit 1	X	X		X	X	X	X	X	X	X	X	X
Visit 2		X	X	X	X	X	X	X	X	X	X	
Fast				X		X			X			
Load				X		X			X			

Figure 22.13 Outline of extensive diagnostic evaluation. Visit 1: History and physical examination, diet history, radiologic evaluation, two 24 hour urine specimens on random diet, and dietary instruction for restricted diet. Visit 2: 24 hour urine specimen on restricted diet (400mg calcium/day and 100mEq sodium/day), fast and calcium load test. PTH, parathyroid hormone.

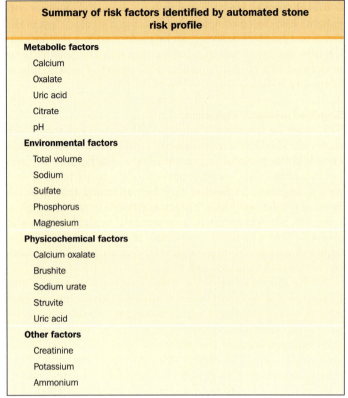

Summary of risk factors identified by automated stone risk profile
Metabolic factors
Calcium
Oxalate
Uric acid
Citrate
pH
Environmental factors
Total volume
Sodium
Sulfate
Phosphorus
Magnesium
Physicochemical factors
Calcium oxalate
Brushite
Sodium urate
Struvite
Uric acid
Other factors
Creatinine
Potassium
Ammonium

Figure 22.14 Summary of risk factors identified by automated stone risk profile.

same as those normal values that have been quoted previously, where 24 hour urinary calcium of more than 200mg/day is considered abnormal. Therefore, one should pay close attention to those patients who may fall in the 'gray zone' when using a commercially available urine analysis package.

Based on the results, a short-term dietary and/or fluid intake modification of approximately 1 week's duration should be imposed. A 24 hour urine collection should then be obtained while the patient is still on the modified diet. A limited urine analysis could be performed and the differences in values between the full and abbreviated analyses (random and modified diet) would represent changes imposed by dietary influences[51]. Additional tests, including serum PTH levels, systematic multichannel serum analysis, and urine culture, can be performed if necessary.

Asymptomatic kidney stones

Many more patients have urinary stones than those individuals who receive medical attention. Most of these stones are small and nonobstructing, and the majority of patients are not even aware of their presence. In a study of asymptomatic nephrolithiasis, patients remained asymptomatic for an average of 6 months after their stones were identified by radiologic examination[52]. In nearly 3 years of follow-up, two thirds of the patients continued to be asymptomatic. In the remaining third, who developed symptoms, approximately one half passed their stones spontaneously while the rest required urologic intervention.

Acute stone episode

The classic symptoms associated with an acutely obstructing urinary stone include colicky flank pain, with radiation to the groin, ipsilateral testicle, or labia, and hematuria (microscopic or gross). Stones in the distal ureter may also present with frequency, urgency, and dysuria. Nausea and vomiting are not uncommon and, with superimposed infection, high-grade fevers or sepsis may ensue.

If a patient demonstrates these classic findings and has a previous history of recurrent radiopaque nephrolithiasis, a plain abdominal X-ray including kidneys, ureter and bladder (KUB) is warranted to address the size and location of the stone in order to decide on the best course of treatment. Stones measuring 4mm in greatest diameter or less have more than a 95% rate of spontaneous passage with conservative measures alone; however, stones 6mm in diameter or larger have only a 10% rate of spontaneous passage[53,54].

In patients who are experiencing their first stone episode but do not present with the classic findings, or those who are known to form radiolucent stones, either a nonenhanced helical computed tomography (CT) or an intravenous pyelogram (IVP) should be performed. Ultrasonography may be used to assess hydronephrosis and intrarenal calculi but is not very accurate for the diagnosis of ureteral stones.

If the patient is clinically stable and there is no evidence of systemic infection, complete obstruction leading to renal deterioration, or obstruction of a solitary kidney, conservative management may be offered with hydration and pain medication (usually nonsteroidal anti-inflammatory or narcotic medications). However, in the presence of any of the above impending problems, urinary drainage should be performed on an emergency basis, either by ureteral stent placement or by percutaneous nephrostomy. In the case of infection, antibiotics should be administered promptly. The size and location of the stone on imaging studies will determine the need for intervention. If there is no evidence of movement or passage of a ureteral stone that has been treated conservatively after 3–4 weeks, or if pain is intractable, surgical intervention is warranted.

MEDICAL MANAGEMENT

Conservative management

Certain conservative recommendations should be made for all patients regardless of the underlying etiology of their stone disease. Patients should be instructed to increase their fluid intake to at least 3L/day, in order to maintain a urine output of at least 2,000mL/day[8,55]. In addition, all patients should be instructed on limiting their dietary oxalate and sodium intake, which should help decrease the urinary excretion of oxalate and calcium. In patients with suspected absorptive hypercalciuria without evidence of bone loss, a dietary limitation of dairy products may also be enforced. A restriction of animal proteins in those with 'purine gluttony' and hyperuricosuria should be encouraged.

With these conservative measures, a significant number of patients may be able to reduce their risk factors for urinary stone formation. In several patients, these measures alone may be necessary to keep their stone disease under control[56]. After 3–4 months on conservative management, patients should be re-evaluated. If the patient's metabolic or environmental abnormalities have been corrected by the dietary and fluid manipulations, the conservative therapy should be continued and the patient followed with repeat 24 hour urine testing every 6 months. It is believed that follow-up is essential not only to monitor the efficiency of treatment but also to encourage patient compliance. However, if a metabolic or environmental defect persists while the patient is on conservative therapy, then selective medical therapy should be considered.

Selective medical therapy

Improved elucidation of the etiology and pathophysiology of nephrolithiasis has made the adoption of selective treatment programs quite feasible[56–58]. Treatment programs should:

- reverse the underlying physicochemical and physiologic derangements;
- inhibit further stone formation;
- overcome nonrenal complications of the disease process; and
- be without serious side-effects.

The rationale for the selection of certain treatment programs is the assumption that the particular aberrations identified with given disorders are etiologically important in the formation of stones, and that the correction of these disturbances would prevent stone formation. Moreover, such a selected treatment program should be more effective and safe than 'random' treatment. For many pharmacologic agents recommended for the management of nephrolithiasis, sufficient information is now available to characterize their physicochemical and physiologic actions (Fig. 22.15).

Hypercalciuria

Absorptive hypercalciuria type I

There is currently no treatment program that is capable of correcting the fundamental abnormality of absorptive hypercalciuria type I. When SCP is administered orally, this nonabsorbable ion exchange resin binds to calcium and inhibits calcium absorption[59]. However, this inhibition is caused by limiting the amount of intraluminal calcium that is available for absorption rather than by correcting the basic disturbance in calcium transport.

The aforementioned mode of action accounts for the three potential complications of SCP therapy[60]. First, this medication may cause a negative calcium balance and parathyroid stimulation when used in patients with normal intestinal calcium absorption or with renal or resorptive hypercalciuria. Second, the treatment may cause magnesium depletion by binding magnesium. Third,

SCP may produce secondary hyperoxaluria by binding divalent cations in the intestinal tract, reducing divalent cation–oxalate complexation, and allowing for more oxalate to be available for absorption. These complications may be overcome by selecting this medication exclusively for documented cases of absorptive hypercalciuria type I, providing oral magnesium supplementation (administered independently of SCP), and imposing a moderate dietary restriction of oxalate.

When these precautions are followed, SCP (10–15g/day, taken with meals), has been shown to be clinically effective in reducing urinary calcium and the saturation of calcium salts (calcium oxalate and calcium phosphate), thereby maintaining stable bone density[61].

Thiazide is not considered a selective therapy for absorptive hypercalciuria, since it does not decrease intestinal calcium absorption in this condition[9]. However, this drug has been widely used to treat absorptive hypercalciuria because of its hypocalciuric action, as well as the high cost and inconvenience of alternative therapy (sodium cellulose phosphate).

Previous studies indicate that thiazide may have a limited long-term effectiveness in absorptive hypercalciuria type I[62,63]. Despite an initial reduction in urinary calcium excretion, the intestinal calcium absorption remains persistently elevated. These studies suggest that the retained calcium may be accreted in bone, at least during the first few years of therapy. Bone density may increase significantly during thiazide therapy for absorptive hypercalciuria. With continued treatment, however, the rise in bone density stabilizes and the hypocalciuric effect of thiazide becomes attenuated. These results suggest that thiazide treatment causes a low turnover state of bone that interferes with continued calcium accretion in the skeleton. The nonaccreted calcium would then be excreted in urine. In contrast, bone density is not significantly altered in renal hypercalciuria, where thiazide causes a decline in intestinal calcium absorption commensurate with a reduction in urinary calcium.

Recently, a new medication has been developed that might provide more selective management with absorptive hypercalciuria. UroPhos-K is a new formulation of a slow-release, neutral potassium phosphate that appears to normalize intestinal calcium absorption while reducing the risk of recurrent stone formation[64]. In a randomized, prospective, double-blind trial comparing UroPhos-K and a placebo, a significant decrease in urinary calcium

Physicochemical and physiologic effects of pharmacologic therapy				
	Sodium cellulose phosphate	Thiazide	Allopurinol	Potassium citrate
Urinary calcium	Marked decrease	Moderate decrease	No change	Mild decrease/ No change
Urinary phosphorus	Mild increase	Mild increase/ No change	No change	No change
Urinary uric acid	No change	Mild increase/ No change	Marked decrease	No change
Urinary oxalate	Mild increase	Mild increase/ Mild decrease	No change	No change
Urinary citrate	No change	Mild decrease	No change	Marked increase
Calcium oxalate saturation	Mild decrease/ No change	Mild decrease	No change	Moderate decrease
Brushite saturation	Moderate decrease	Mild decrease	No change	No change

Figure 22.15 Physicochemical and physiologic effects of pharmacologic therapy.

and desaturation of calcium oxalate was noted after 6 months of therapy[65]. In addition, urinary citrate and inhibitor activity was increased with UroPhos-K administration. In following these patients for 4 years on UroPhos-K, urinary calcium excretion continued in the normal range with a significant decrease in intestinal calcium absorption[66]. It appears that UroPhos-K reduces the intestinal calcium absorption while also reducing skeletal calcium mobilization and augmenting renal calcium absorption. All these factors result in normalization of urinary calcium while providing a significant improvement in calcium balance. It appears that, once approved, UroPhos-K may become the medication of choice for those individuals with absorptive hypercalciuria.

Absorptive hypercalciuria type II
In absorptive hypercalciuria type II, specific drug therapy may not be necessary, since the physiologic defect is not as severe as in absorptive hypercalciuria type I. In addition, many patients show disdain for drinking fluids and excreting concentrated urine. A low intake of calcium (400–600mg/day) and a high intake of fluids (sufficient to achieve a minimum urine output of more than 2L/day), would be ideal. Normal urine calcium excretion would be restored by dietary calcium restriction alone, and the increase in urine volume would help reduce urinary saturation of calcium oxalate[30].

Renal hypercalciuria
Thiazide is ideally indicated for the treatment of renal hypercalciuria. This diuretic has been shown to correct the renal leak of calcium by augmenting calcium reabsorption in the distal tubule and by causing extracellular volume depletion and stimulating proximal tubular reabsorption of calcium[67]. The ensuing correction of secondary hyperparathyroidism restores normal serum 1,25-$(OH)_2$D and intestinal calcium absorption. Thiazide may provide a sustained correction of hypercalciuria commensurate with a restoration of normal serum 1,25-$(OH)_2$D and intestinal calcium absorption up to 10 years with this therapy[63].

Resorptive hypercalciuria
There is no established medical treatment for the nephrolithiasis of resorptive hypercalciuria (primary hyperparathyroidism). Although orthophosphates have been recommended for disease of mild to moderate severity, their safety or efficacy has not been proven. This medication should be used only when surgical management cannot be undertaken. Estrogen has been reported to be useful in reducing serum and urinary calcium in postmenopausal women with primary hyperparathyroidism.

Parathyroidectomy is the optimum treatment for primary hyperparathyroidism[68]. Following removal of abnormal parathyroid tissue, urinary calcium is restored to normal levels, along with a decline in serum concentration of calcium and intestinal absorption. The urinary environment becomes less saturated with respect to calcium oxalate and brushite and the limit of metastability for these calcium salts increases.

Hyperoxaluria
Oral administration of large amounts of calcium (0.25–1.0g four times/day) or magnesium has been recommended for the control of enteric hyperoxaluria[69]. Although urinary oxalate may decrease (probably from the binding of oxalate by divalent

cations), the concurrent rise in urinary calcium may obviate the beneficial effect of this therapy, at least in certain patients[16]. A high fluid intake is recommended to assure adequate urine volume in patients with enteric hyperoxaluria. As excessive fluid loss may occur, an antidiarrheal agent may be necessary before sufficient urine output can be achieved.

Calcium citrate may theoretically have a role in the management of enteric hyperoxaluria. This treatment may lower urinary oxalate by binding oxalate in the intestinal tract. Calcium citrate may also raise the urinary citrate level and pH by providing an alkali load[70]. Finally, calcium citrate may correct the malabsorption of calcium and the adverse effects on the skeleton by providing efficiently absorbed calcium. If hypercalciuria develops during calcium citrate treatment, a thiazide agent (e.g. trichloromethiazide 4mg/day or chlorthalidone 25mg/day) may be added.

Hyperuricosuria
Allopurinol (300mg/day) is the physiologically meaningful drug of choice in patients with hyperuricosuric calcium oxalate nephrolithiasis (with or without hyperuricemia) because of its ability to reduce uric acid synthesis and lower urinary uric acid by inhibition of the enzyme xanthine oxidase[71]. Allopurinol is preferred in patients with marked hyperuricosuria (>1,000mg/day), especially if hyperuricemia coexists. The usual dose is 300mg/day but the dosage should be reduced in patients with renal insufficiency.

Potassium citrate represents an alternative to allopurinol in the treatment of this condition[72]. Use of potassium citrate in hyperuricosuric calcium oxalate nephrolithiasis is warranted since citrate has an inhibitory activity with respect to calcium oxalate (and calcium phosphate) crystallization, aggregation, and agglomeration. Administration of potassium citrate (30–60mEq/day in divided doses), may reduce the urinary saturation of calcium oxalate (by complexing calcium) and inhibit urate-induced crystallization of calcium oxalate.

Potassium citrate may be particularly useful in patients with mild to moderate hyperuricosuria (<800mg/day) in whom hypocitraturia is also present. However, allopurinol is probably preferred in patients with more marked hyperuricosuria, especially if hyperuricemia coexists.

Hypocitraturia
In patients with hypocitraturic calcium oxalate nephrolithiasis, treatment of potassium citrate is capable of restoring normal urinary citrate, lowering urinary saturation, and inhibiting crystallization of calcium salts.

Distal renal tubular acidosis
Potassium citrate therapy is able to correct metabolic acidosis and hypokalemia found in patients with distal renal tubular acidosis[27]. In addition, it will restore normal urinary citrate levels, although large doses (up to 120mEq/day) may be required for severe acidosis. Upon correction of the acidosis, urinary calcium should fall within the normal range. Since urinary pH is generally elevated in patients with renal tubular acidosis, the overall rise in urinary pH is small.

Potassium citrate therapy typically produces a sustained decline in the urinary saturation of calcium oxalate, through citrate complexation of calcium. The urinary saturation of calcium phosphate does not increase, since the rise in phosphate dissociation is relatively small and is adequately compensated by a decline in ionic calcium concentration[73]. In addition, the inhibitory activity against the crystallization of calcium oxalate and calcium phosphate is augmented by the direct action of citrate.

Chronic diarrheal states

Patients with chronic diarrheal states frequently have hypocitraturia caused by bicarbonate loss from the intestinal tract. Potassium citrate therapy has been shown to significantly reduce the stone formation rate in these patients[74]. The dose of potassium citrate is dependent on the severity of hypocitraturia in these patients. The dosage ranges from 60–120mEq/day in three to four divided doses.

It is recommended that a liquid preparation of potassium citrate be used rather than the slow-release tablet since the tablet formulation may be poorly absorbed because of rapid intestinal transit time in these patients[75]. In addition, frequent dosing schedules (3–4 times/day) are necessary for the liquid preparation, since this form of the medication has a relatively short duration of action. A less frequent dosing schedule (2–3 times/day) for the tablet is acceptable because of its slow-release property.

Thiazide-induced hypocitraturia

Thiazide therapy may induce hypocitraturia due to hypokalemia with resultant intracellular acidosis[29,30]. It should be common practice to administer potassium supplementation, preferably potassium citrate, to patients receiving thiazide for treatment of hypercalciuria. Potassium citrate has been shown to be equally as effective as potassium chloride in correcting thiazide-induced hypokalemia[29]. Moreover, the addition of potassium citrate not only prevents a fall in urinary citrate during thiazide therapy but may raise citrate excretion.

Idiopathic hypocitraturia

Stones formed in this condition are predominantly composed of calcium oxalate. Potassium citrate therapy may produce a sustained increase in urinary citrate and a decline in the urinary saturation of calcium oxalate. Thus, it is apparent that potassium citrate can be used in a variety of conditions. Combined data from a long-term clinical trial using potassium citrate showed no significant change in serum potassium, hematocrit, bone density, or endogenous creatinine clearance during treatment[74]. A solid preparation of potassium citrate given on a twice-daily schedule is generally well tolerated.

Hypomagnesuria

Hypomagnesuric calcium nephrolithiasis is characterized by low urinary magnesium, usually accompanied by hypocitraturia and low urine volume. Therefore, management might include restoration of urinary magnesium levels with oral magnesium supplementation (magnesium oxide or magnesium hydroxide), as well as correction of hypocitraturia with an oral form of citrate (potassium citrate)[31]. Currently this is accomplished with a magnesium salt preparation combined with potassium citrate. A single oral agent that provides potassium, magnesium, and citrate would be ideal in the treatment of this condition. A potentially useful medication, potassium–magnesium citrate, is currently undergoing clinical trials[76,77].

Gouty diathesis

The major objective in the management of gouty diathesis is to increase the urinary pH above 5.5, preferably to a level between pH 6.0 and 6.5[78]. In the past, urine alkalization had been accomplished with either sodium bicarbonate or various combinations of sodium and potassium alkali therapy. While sodium alkali may enhance dissociation of uric acid and inhibit uric stone acid formation by raising urinary pH, this medication may be complicated by the development of calcium-containing stones (calcium oxalate and/or calcium phosphate)[73].

Potassium citrate is the drug of choice in the management of patients with gouty diathesis[32]. Potassium citrate has been found to be an adequate alkalinizing agent, capable of maintaining urinary pH at approximately 6.5 at a dose of 30–60mEq/day in two divided doses[88]. Attempts at alkalinizing the urine to a pH of more than 7.0 should be avoided. At a higher pH, there is a possibility of precipitating calcium phosphate (hydroxyapatite) and therefore increasing the risk of calcium stone formation. If the urinary uric acid excretion is elevated or hyperuricemia exists, allopurinol (300mg/day) is recommended.

Cystinuria

The object of treatment for cystinuria is to reduce the urinary concentration of cystine to a level below its solubility limit (200–250mg/L). The initial treatment program includes a high fluid intake and oral administration of soluble alkali (potassium citrate), at a dose sufficient to maintain the urinary pH at 6.5–7.0. When this conservative program is ineffective, D-penicillamine or α-mercaptopropionylglycine (1,000–2,000mg/day in divided doses) has been used[80]. This treatment has been shown to increase cystine solubility in urine via formation of a more soluble mixed disulfide. Penicillamine has been associated with frequent side-effects including nephrotic syndrome, dermatitis, and pancytopenia. This side-effect profile appears to be less marked with α-mercaptopropionylglycine[81].

Recent studies have suggested that captopril may work in the same manner as penicillamine and α-mercaptopropionylglycine, forming a captopril–cysteine disulfide, which is 200 times more soluble in urine than cystine[82]. However, further investigations are needed to confirm the long-term effectiveness of captopril for the management of cystinuria[83].

Struvite (infection) lithiasis

If long-standing effective control of infection with urea-splitting organisms can be achieved, then new stone formation may be averted. Unfortunately, such control is difficult to obtain with antibiotic therapy. In the presence of an existing struvite stone, it is often difficult to completely eradicate the infection because the stone often harbors the organism within its interstices[84]. For this reason, the gold standard of treatment of infection stones is complete surgical removal and treatment of infection with adequate antibiotics. When the former therapies are contraindicated or unsuccessful, acetohydroxamic acid (AHA) may be used.

Acetohydroxamic acid is a urease inhibitor that retards stone formation by reducing the urinary saturation of struvite. When administered at a dose of 250mg three times per day, AHA may prevent recurrence of new stones and inhibit the growth of stones in patients with chronic urea-splitting infections[85]. In addition, in a limited number of patients, AHA has caused dissolution of

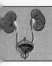

existing struvite calculi. However, some patients on chronic AHA therapy have experienced minor side-effects, and a few patients have developed deep venous thrombosis. Additional long-term studies must be done to determine the benefit-to-risk ratio of this medication.

Drug-induced nephrolithiasis

Ephedrine calculi

There are no studies that systematically address the management of these calculi. As with other calculi, a urine output of at least 2L/day is recommended. Currently, no literature exists concerning pharmacologic interventions or agents useful in the dissolution of these calculi. It is reasonable to recommend discontinuation of this agent but this is merely a preventive measure against new stone formation[38].

Guaifenesin calculi

As with ephedrine calculi, there are no reported studies regarding pharmacologic management of these calculi. Nonselective measures are likely to reduce the risk for new stone formation, as is the discontinuation of this agent.

Indinavir calculi

Initial measures in the management of these calculi should focus on hydration and analgesia as well as drug discontinuation and substitution with another protease inhibitor. In the vast majority of cases, conservative measures have led to the amelioration of symptoms[86]. Because of the relative insolubility of indinavir in physiologic urine it is recommended patients consume at least 2L of fluids per day in order to keep their urine output in the same range[96].

Xanthine calculi

The medical management of xanthine calculi is limited because the solubility of these calculi is essentially invariable within physiologic pH ranges. Currently the recommendation includes a fluid intake of at least 3L/day[88,89]. If significant quantities of other purines are present in the urine, then urinary alkalization with potassium citrate in the range of 6.0–6.5 is indicated to prevent hypoxanthine or uric acid calculi.

Chemolysis

Dissolution of existing calculi or retained stone fragments is primarily useful for stones composed of uric acid or cystine. A combination of allopurinol (300mg/day) and potassium citrate (20mEq 3 times/day) reduces uric acid stone formation and may dissolve existing stones. α-mercaptopropionylglycine or D-penicillamine (up to 2g/day) and potassium citrate may successfully dissolve cystine stones.

Acetohydroxamic acid has shown only partial success in dissolving struvite calculi. It appears that the current role for this medication is in preventing growth or recurrence of stones in patients with chronic infections. It is also useful when used prophylactically to prevent encrustation of chronic indwelling catheters[90].

SURGICAL MANAGEMENT

Approximately 10–20% of all kidney stones may cause the patient enough problems to require surgical removal. The

indications for surgical management of urinary stones include symptomatic calculi, urinary tract obstruction, staghorn calculi (symptomatic or asymptomatic), stones in high-risk patients who cannot afford an episode of renal colic (i.e. airplane pilots) or infection (transplanted patients and patients receiving a prosthesis). Surgical therapy for urinary tract calculi has changed significantly over the last 10 years. Recent improvements in fiberoptic endoscopy, fluoroscopic technology, and interventional radiologic techniques have provided the patient and the urologist with many options when choosing the means of stone removal. When open renal and ureteral surgery are the means by which all new procedures are judged, it appears that percutaneous nephrostolithotomy, ureterorenoscopy, and shock wave lithotripsy offer the patient comparable success for the stone removal with significantly diminished patient morbidity and lowered patient cost.

The advent of shock-wave lithotripsy and advances in fiberoptics, with the subsequent development of flexible instruments as well as small-caliber rigid endoscopes, allow minimally invasive treatment of all urinary calculi. As a consequence of the dramatic increase in the technologies available to the practicing urologist, some have found a dilemma with regards to the application of these new modalities in the treatment of stone disease. There are several controversies in stone management that often create difficulties in formulating absolute treatment guidelines. Yet most will agree that the composition and location of the stone(s), stone burden, anatomy, and renal function are among the most important factors in planning the appropriate approach for stone removal.

Shock wave lithotripsy

The advent of shock wave lithotripsy (SWL) revolutionized the field of endourology by offering a noninvasive technique for the management of upper urinary tract calculi. Since the first patient was successfully treated for a renal calculus with shock wave lithotripsy in 1980, its rapid acceptance and widespread use have promoted this form of stone therapy as the treatment of choice for the majority of renal and ureteral calculi. Worldwide clinical series have documented the efficacy and safety of shock wave lithotripsy[91–96] (see Chapter 42).

In properly selected patients, SWL should be the first procedure of choice for low volume stone disease of the upper urinary tract due to its reduced patient morbidity, noninvasiveness, and cost-efficiency. Yet, it is important to acknowledge that SWL has limitations and is not considered appropriate therapy for all stone patients[97–110]. SWL is associated with occasional adverse effects, including new-onset renally mediated hypertension, intrarenal hemorrhage, perinephric hematoma formation, and cortical fibrosis[101–105]. As a result, one must continue to closely monitor the total amount of energy delivered to a particular kidney in order to limit the incidence of significant renal injury.

Percutaneous nephrostolithotomy

Within a single decade, this technique has gained worldwide popularity and is now a routinely performed procedure for the management of urinary stones. Percutaneous nephrostolithotomy (PNL) is ideally suited for all patients with renal stones who are not candidates for SWL. PNL is currently indicated for the treatment of hard calculi, stones larger than 2cm, stones within the lower pole calyx or within a calyceal diverticulum, staghorn calculi, and as a salvage procedure after failed SWL[106].

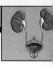

The technique relies on access to the intrarenal collecting system through a percutaneous nephrostomy tract (see Chapter 11). The nephrostomy tract is formed by dilating the skin, fascia, muscles, and renal tissues, using graduated dilators or a balloon catheter. After the nephrostomy tract has been dilated up to a 30Fr (10mm diameter) size, a hollow sheath is placed into the renal pelvis. A rigid fiberoptic endoscope may then be passed directly into the renal collecting system for visualization of the stone(s). Once the renal pelvis and accessible calyces have been visualized, flexible nephroscopy can then be performed to inspect individual calyces that may not be within the reach of the rigid instrument. With the added benefit of tip deflection and rotation, flexible instruments allow adequate visualization of the entire collecting system[107].

As the diameter of the working sheath is usually 30Fr (10mm), stones smaller than this can be extracted intact. For stones within the renal collecting system or ureter that are too large to be extracted (>1cm), four fragmentation modalities of 'power lithotripsy' are available: ultrasonic lithotripsy (UL), electrohydraulic lithotripsy (EHL), laser lithotripsy, and pneumatic lithotripsy.

Ultrasonic lithotripsy

Ultrasonic energy used to fragment kidney stones was first described in 1979[108]. Commercially available units consist of a power generator as well as an ultrasound transducer and rigid probe, which form the 'sonotrode'. A piezoceramic element in the handle of the sonotrode is stimulated to resonate and this converts electrical energy into ultrasound waves (with a frequency of 23,000–27,000Hz), which then are transmitted along the hollow metal probe, creating a vibrating action at its tip. The vibrating tip causes disintegration of the stone upon contact. The probe (10Fr or 12Fr) is passed through the straight working channel of a rigid nephroscope (24Fr or 26Fr diameter) with a 30° or 90° offset lens. Normal saline at body temperature is used as irrigant, and suction tubing can be connected to the end of the sonotrode probe, thus creating a vacuum to collect stone fragments.

Ultrasonic lithotripsy should be the procedure of choice for fragmentation of large renal stones. However, some uric acid, calcium oxalate monohydrate, or cystine stones are not amenable to UL, and may necessitate EHL or pneumatic lithotripsy for complete fragmentation. Depending on the location of the stones, retained fragments are seen in 3–35% of all cases treated with ultrasonic lithotripsy. This is not always considered a failure, because UL is often performed for the debulking of large stones, to be followed by SWL as a planned two-stage procedure.

Electrohydraulic lithotripsy

The principles of EHL were described and developed in 1950. This technology has been used extensively for the destruction of bladder stones, and in 1975, reports were published on its use for the fragmentation of kidney stones[109]. The EHL unit consists of a probe, a power generator, and a foot pedal. The probe consists of a central metal core and two layers of insulation with another metal layer between them. Probes are flexible and available in 1.9Fr, 3Fr, 5Fr, 7Fr, and 9Fr sizes for use through rigid and flexible nephroscopes.

An electrical discharge is transmitted to the probe where it generates a spark at the tip. The intense heat production in the immediate area surrounding the tip results in a cavitation bubble, which produces a shock wave that radiates spherically in all directions. Collapse of the bubble gives rise to a second shock wave, and these shock waves are repeated at a frequency of 50–100/s, which results in destruction of the stone.

Electrohydraulic lithotripsy will effectively fragment all types of urinary calculi, including the very hard cystine, uric acid, and calcium oxalate monohydrate stones. Since the probes are small and flexible, they can be used through flexible nephroscopes and ureteroscopes to fragment stones in calyces inaccessible to UL through a rigid instrument.

Overall, EHL in the kidney should be used as a secondary technique choice for routine stone fragmentation, if a flexible probe is needed and one does not have access to a holmium laser.

Laser lithotripsy

Laser lithotripsy has continuously evolved over the past three decades. Holmium laser lithotripsy is the newest laser modality, which fragments stones by plasma production resulting in the creation of mechanical shock waves. The 200μm or 365μm quartz fibers of the holmium laser are easily passed through the smallest flexible nephroscope for treatment of renal calculi[110,111]. Although the indications for use of holmium laser lithotripsy on renal calculi are similar to those of EHL, the majority of the applications for holmium laser lithotripsy are for fragmentation of ureteral or renal calculi during ureteroscopy.

Pneumatic lithotripsy

Pneumatic lithotripsy was introduced to the field of urology in 1991. In this air-powered device, a pneumatically driven solid, rigid probe is used to fragment stones via direct impact[112]. Compressed air propels a metal projectile within the handpiece against the head of the probe at 12–16Hz. After each pulse, the projectile returns to its original position and is ready for the next pulsation. Probes are available in 0.8–3.0mm diameter sizes and can be employed through rigid or semirigid endoscopes[113].

Various clinical trials have demonstrated that pneumatic lithotripsy fragments stones of all compositions and is ideal for the fragmentation of vesical, renal, or ureteral calculi. In a comparison of pneumatic, ultrasonic, electrohydraulic, and holmium laser lithotripsy, pneumatic lithotripsy produced the least amount of macroscopic and histologic urothelial injury[114]. The major advantages of pneumatic lithotripsy are its improved efficacy over the aforementioned intracorporeal lithotripsy modalities as well as its multiple applications and lack of thermal injury. In fact, laboratory studies have demonstrated that pneumatic lithotripsy is the most efficient form of intracorporeal stone fragmentation[115].

Ureterorenoscopy

The advent of ureterorenoscopy has dramatically altered the management of symptomatic ureteral calculi. Rigid ureteroscopy has been used in conjunction with pneumatic, holmium laser, and electrohydraulic lithotripsy probes to successfully fragment ureteral calculi[116,117]. However, it has been the introduction of the flexible, deflectable ureterorenoscopes that has made access to the upper ureter and intrarenal collecting system a safer and less tedious procedure[116–118]. These instruments

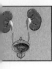

can be advanced under direct vision or fluoroscopic guidance directly to the level of the stone, which may be fragmented or extracted intact. The technique is described in detail in Chapter 12.

Open nephrolithotomy

As shock wave lithotripsy, percutaneous nephrolithotomy, and ureterorenoscopy have become widely embraced as the treatments of choice for the majority of renal and ureteral calculi, the indications for open nephrolithotomy have decreased dramatically. Currently, fewer than 1% of stones will require an open surgical procedure for removal, most commonly anatrophic lithotomy for the management of extremely large and/or complex renal calculi[119].

The more common indications for open stone removal include failure of SWL or PNL, morbid obesity, patients with multiple medical problems that may benefit from a shorter open procedure, stones in a collecting system with distal obstruction, obstructed or stenotic calyceal infundibula, and extremely large or complex branched renal calculi.

Selection of surgical therapy

Shock wave lithotripsy, percutaneous nephrostolithotomy, ureterorenoscopy, and open nephrolithotomy can effectively remove renal calculi in appropriate clinical situations. Issues important in the treatment of renal calculi are the size of the stone being treated, location of the stone within the kidney, stone composition, renal anatomy, and renal function.

Small calculi

Although various treatment options exist for small renal calculi, shock wave lithotripsy has repeatedly been shown to be extremely effective for smaller stones. As a result, percutaneous nephrostolithotomy has a less significant role in the management of small renal calculi. Although SWL is the gold-standard for treatment of renal calculi smaller than 2cm, some stones are recalcitrant to this mode of treatment.

In these cases, PNL would be the next reasonable line of therapy, as stone-free rates of more than 90–95% can be expected for renal calculi less than 2cm in size[120]. Morbidly obese patients also often require percutaneous stone removal as stone imaging and SWL are impaired by the excess tissue. Hard stones composed of cystine or calcium oxalate monohydrate are relative indications for performing percutaneous nephrostolithotomy. The failure of either of SWL and/or PNL to completely remove the renal stone burden may necessitate flexible ureterorenoscopy. Only rarely will open lithotomy be necessary for the management of small renal calculi.

Large calculi

Most large renal calculi may be managed similarly to small renal calculi; however, the physician will find a larger number of patients who require a modality other than SWL. Because the fragmentation efficiency of SWL decreases with increasing stone size, PNL may become the treatment of choice in cases of larger calculi. Previous studies have shown that the critical stone burden in considering SWL monotherapy is a stone diameter of 2cm[120]. The majority of all stones larger than 3cm treated with SWL require additional treatment. Therefore, for complete and

incomplete staghorn calculi, as well as for stones larger than 3cm in diameter, PNL should be the initial procedure, since it will occasionally be the only one required[121]. The use of PNL for stones between 2cm and 3cm depends on the preference of the physician.

Percutaneous nephrostolithotomy is indicated if there is obstruction of the urinary tract between the stone location and the ureterovesical junction (i.e. infundibular stenosis, primary or secondary ureteropelvic junction obstruction, ureteral stricture, ureterovesical junction obstruction). As with smaller stones, open surgery will be required only for stones that are resistant to previous treatment attempts. Open nephrolithotomy would not be the principal choice for large renal calculi but must always be considered in patients with existing renal anomalies or previous failures with either shock wave lithotripsy or percutaneous nephrostolithotomy.

Staghorn calculi

Treatment philosophies for staghorn calculi vary from single modality treatment of all staghorn calculi with SWL, through combined treatment with PNL and SWL, to open nephrolithotomy. The differences in opinion are based in the inferior results obtained with the treatment of renal calculi by SWL and the increased patient morbidity caused by the other modalities[121].

Initially, staghorn calculi were treated solely with open nephrolithotomy, with reasonable success rates. The advent of PNL opened new avenues for the treatment of this troublesome stone. While anatrophic nephrolithotomy renders a patient free of stones approximately 65–90% of the time, it is associated with a high complication rate (up to 50%) and a significant time is needed for convalescence[122]. Complete removal of staghorn calculi by PNL varies from 62–95% with a 20–57% complication rate[123–125]. Most physicians employ a single treatment session but sometimes require multiple nephrostomy tracts to thoroughly access a branched calculus. Often, physicians prefer to stage the percutaneous procedure with patients returning for a secondary PNL[126]. Initial attempts to treat staghorn calculi with SWL were dismal, because most patients underwent only a single treatment and follow-up was quite short. With multiple treatments, prolonged follow-up, and ureteral stenting, stone-free rates at 3–6 months have been reported from 36–72%, with a 12–64% complication rate, resembling those of PNL[127–130].

Many medical centers have recommended the combined use of PNL and SWL for the treatment of staghorn calculi. The initial treatment session is for stone debulking through a percutaneous tract with ultrasonic and/or electrohydraulic lithotripsy, and treatment of retained fragments with SWL or flexible nephroscopy, if necessary. Success rates of 80–95% have been reported with this combined approach[131].

Open pyelolithotomy or anatrophic nephrolithotomy may be considered for patients with extremely dilated collecting systems. Also, staghorn calculi with multiple calyceal extensions may best be managed with anatrophic nephrolithotomy, as multiple secondary percutaneous procedures may be required to clear all affected calices.

Lower pole calculi

As the results of the initial clinical series using shock wave lithotripsy were reported, it was clear that treatment of lower

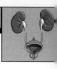

pole renal calculi by SWL was associated with a lower stone-free rate than calculi located in other parts of the kidney. In one study, PNL was provided an 85% stone-free rate compared to 59% for SWL in the treatment of solitary lower pole calculi. However, the hospital stay and recovery time were increased in the PNL group, as were the complication and retreatment/auxiliary procedure rates. SWL was therefore recommended as the treatment of choice for lower pole calculi[132]. In an attempt to overcome this apparent anatomic challenge, some physicians employ positional techniques to improve the clearance of lower pole calyceal stone debris following shock wave lithotripsy.

A recent randomized prospective clinical trial has compared SWL to PNL for the management of lower pole renal calculi[133]. This multi-institutional trial found that shock wave lithotripsy, while less invasive, is significantly less effective than percutaneous stone removal for the removal of lower pole renal calculi greater than 1cm in diameter. It appears that SWL stone-free rates are highly dependent on the stone size and renal anatomy, while stone-free rates are independent of stone burden and renal anatomy in those individuals undergoing percutaneous stone removal. The overall recommendations from the study offer that the lower pole renal calculus greater than 1cm should be considered for initial percutaneous stone removal if the goal of management is to render the patient stone-free. However, in patients with favorable lower pole renal anatomy or small volume calculi, shock wave lithotripsy offers a reasonable first choice[134]. The development of flexible ureteroscopy and lasertripsy will help further to deal with the problem of lower pole renal calculi.

SUMMARY

The management of urinary calculus disease has changed dramatically in the past two decades. The development of percutaneous techniques has allowed new access to upper tract stones. Percutaneous removal of large calculi was made possible by the development of ultrasonic and electrohydraulic lithotripsy. All upper tract calculi can now be successfully removed in 70–100% of cases, with minimal complications. Percutaneous techniques have reduced transfusion rates and hospital costs, and have markedly shortened convalescence periods when compared to open surgery.

Ureteroscopic stone procedures evolved as advanced fiber-optic technology allowed the development of the small-caliber instruments required for this procedure. Stone retrieval is successful in more than 90% of cases, with minimal complications. As percutaneous nephrostolithotomy and ureteroscopy have become available, the subspecialty of endourology has emerged and has significantly changed the management of urinary tract calculi.

The most significant advance in surgical stone management has been the design and implementation of shock wave lithotripsy. With this noninvasive technique, most renal and ureteral calculi can be effectively treated with minimal morbidity and convalescence.

Aside from surgical management of urinary tract stones, one should realize the importance of medical therapy for recurrent nephrolithiasis. Selective medical therapy of nephrolithiasis is highly effective in preventing new stone formation. With appropriate diagnosis and treatment of specific disorders resulting in nephrolithiasis, a remission rate greater than 80% can be obtained. In patients with mild to moderately severe stone disease, virtually total control of stone disease can be achieved with a remission rate greater than 95%[135]. The need for surgical stone removal may be dramatically reduced or eliminated with an effective prophylactic program. Selective pharmacologic therapy also has the advantage of overcoming nonrenal complications and averting certain side-effects that may occur with nonselective medical therapy. It is clear that selective medical therapy alone cannot provide total control of stone disease. A satisfactory response requires continued, dedicated compliance by patients with the recommended program and a commitment of the physician to provide long-term follow-up and care with the intention of improving quality of life by eliminating the symptoms caused by urinary tract stones.

REFERENCES

1. Ljunghall S. Incidence of upper urinary tract stones. Mineral Electrolyte Metab. 1987;13:220–7.
2. Sarmina I, Spirnak JP, Resnick MI. Urinary lithiasis in the black population: an epidemiological study and review of the literature. J Urol. 1987;138:14–17.
3. Pak CY. Citrate and renal calculi. Mineral Electrolyte Metab. 1987;13:257–66.
4. Pak CY. Citrate and renal calculi: an update. Mineral Electrolyte Metab. 1994;20:371–7.
5. Malek RS, Kelalis PP. Pediatric nephrolithiasis. J Urol. 1975;113:545–51.
6. McGeown MG. Heredity in renal disease. Clin Sci. 1960;19:465.
7. Resnick MI, Pridgen DB, Goodman HO. Genetic predisposition to formation of calcium oxalate renal calculi. N Engl J Med. 1968;278:1313–8.
8. Pak CY, Sakhaee K, Crowther C, Brinkley L. Evidence justifying a high fluid intake in treatment of nephrolithiasis. Arch Intern Med. 1980;93:36–9.
9. Pak CY. Physiological basis for absorptive and renal hypercalciurias. Am J Physiol. 1979;237:F415–23.
10. Pak CY, Britton F, Peterson R, et al. Ambulatory evaluation of nephrolithiasis. Classification, clinical presentation and diagnostic criteria. Am J Med. 1980;69:19–30.
11. Preminger GM, Peterson R, Pak CYC. Differentiation of unclassified hypercalciuria utilizing a sodium cellulose phosphate trial. In: Walker VR, Sutton AL, Cameron ECB, Pak CYC, Robertson WG, eds. Nephrolithiasis. New York:Plenum Press; 1989:325–40.
12. Fuss M, Pepersack T, Bergman P, Hurard T, Simon J, Corvilain J. Low calcium diet in idiopathic urolithiasis: a risk factor for osteopenia as great as in primary hyperparathyroidism. Br J Urol. 1990;65:560–563.
13. Curhan GC, Willett WC, Rimm EB, Stampfer MJ. A prospective study of dietary calcium and other nutrients and the risk of symptomatic kidney stones. N Engl J Med. 1993;328:833–8.
14. Curhan GC. Dietary calcium, dietary protein, and kidney stone formation. Mineral Electrolyte Metab. 1997;23:261–4.

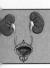
15. Smith LH, Fromm H, Hofmann AF. Acquired hyperoxaluria, nephrolithiasis, and intestinal disease. Description of a syndrome. N Engl J Med. 1972;286:1371–5.

16. Barilla DE, Notz C, Kennedy D, Pak CY. Renal oxalate excretion following oral oxalate loads in patients with ileal disease and with renal and absorptive hypercalciurias. Effect of calcium and magnesium. Am J Med. 1978;64:579–85.

17. Clayman RV, Buchwald H, Varco RL, DeWolf WC, Williams RD. Urolithiasis in patients with a jejunoileal bypass. Surg Gynecol Obstet. 1978;147:225–30.

18. Menon M, Mahle CJ. Oxalate metabolism and renal calculi. J Urol. 1982;127:148–51.

19. Danpure CJ. Molecular and cell biology of primary hyperoxaluria type I. Clin Invest Med. 1994;72:725–7.

20. Williams HE, Smith LHJ. L-glyceric aciduria: a new genetic variant of primary hyperoxaluria. N Engl J Med. 1978;278:233–8.

21. Coe FL, Kavalach AG. Hypercalciuria and hyperuricosuria in patients with calcium nephrolithiasis. N Engl J Med. 1974;291:1344–50.

22. Zerwekh JE, Holt K, Pak CY. Natural urinary macromolecular inhibitors: attenuation of inhibitory activity by urate salts. Kidney Int. 1983;23:838–41.

23. Menon M, Mahle CJ. Prevalence of hyperoxaluria in 'idiopathic' calcium oxalate urolithiasis: relationship to other metabolic abnormalities. Abstract. 1983.

24. Pak CY, Nicar M, Northcutt C. The definition of the mechanism of hypercalciuria is necessary for the treatment of recurrent stone formers. Contrib Nephrol. 1982;33:136–51.

25. Kok DJ, Papapoulos SE, Bijvoet OL. Excessive crystal agglomeration with low citrate excretion in recurrent stone-formers. Lancet 1986;1:1056–8.

26. Pak CY, Sakhaee K, Fuller C. Successful management of uric acid nephrolithiasis with potassium citrate. Kidney Int. 1986;30:422–8.

27. Preminger GM, Sakhaee K, Skurla C, Pak CY. Prevention of recurrent calcium stone formation with potassium citrate therapy in patients with distal renal tubular acidosis. J Urol. 1985;134:20–3.

28. Rudman D, Dedonis JL, Fountain MT, et al. Hypocitraturia in patients with gastrointestinal malabsorption. N Engl J Med. 1980;303:657–61.

29. Nicar MJ, Peterson R, Pak CY. Use of potassium citrate as potassium supplement during thiazide therapy of calcium nephrolithiasis. J Urol. 1984;131:430–3.

30. Pak CY, Peterson R, Sakhaee K, Fuller C, Preminger GM, Reisch J. Correction of hypocitraturia and prevention of stone formation by combined thiazide and potassium citrate therapy in thiazide-unresponsive hypercalciuric nephrolithiasis. Am J Med. 1985;79:284–8.

31. Preminger GM, Baker S, Peterson R, Poindexter J, Pak CYC. Hypomagnesiuric hypocitraturia: an apparent new entity for calcium nephrolithiasis. J Litho Stone Disease 1989;1:22–5.

32. Khatchadourian J, Preminger GM, Whitson PA, Adams-Huet B, Pak CY. Clinical and biochemical presentation of gouty diathesis: comparison of uric acid versus pure calcium stone formation. J Urol. 1995;154:1665–9.

33. Sakhaee K, Poindexter JR, Pak CY. The spectrum of metabolic abnormalities in patients with cystine nephrolithiasis. J Urol. 1989;141:819–21.

34. Lingeman JE, Siegel YI, Steele B. Metabolic evaluation of infected renal lithiasis: clinical relevance. J Endourol. 1995;9:51–4.

35. Griffith DP, Musher DM. Prevention of infected urinary stones by urease inhibition. Invest Urol. 1973;11:223–8.

36. Levy FL, Adams-Huet B, Pak CY. Ambulatory evaluation of nephrolithiasis: an update of a 1980 protocol. Am J Med. 1995;98:50–9.

37. Powell T, Hsu FF, Turk J, Hruska K. Ma-huang strikes again: ephedrine nephrolithiasis. Am J Kidney Dis. 1998;32:153–9.

38. Blau JJ. Ephedrine nephrolithiasis associated with chronic ephedrine abuse. J Urol. 1998;160:825.

39. Assimos DE. Guafenesin calculi. Personal communication, 1999.

40. Pickens CL, Milliron AR, Fussner AL, et al. Abuse of guaifenesin-containing medications generated an excess of a carboxylate salt of beta-(2-methoxyphenoxy)-lactic acid, a guaifenesin metabolite, and results in urolithiasis. Urology. 1999;54:23–7.

41. Blake SP, McNicholas MM, Raptopoulos V. Nonopaque crystal deposition causing ureteric obstruction in patients with HIV undergoing indinavir therapy. AJR. 1998;171:717–20.

42. John H, Muller NJ, Opravil M, Hauri D. Indinavir urinary stones as origin of upper urinary tract obstruction. Urol Int. 1997;59:257–9.

43. Schwartz BF, Schenkman N, Armenakas NA, Stoller ML. Imaging characteristics of indinavir calculi. J Urol. 1999;161:1085–7.

44. Brock WA, Golden J, Kaplan GW. Xanthine calculi in the Lesch–Nyhan Syndrome. J Urol. 1983;130:157–9.

45. Pak CY. Should patients with single renal stone occurrence undergo diagnostic evaluation? J Urol. 1982;127:855–8.

46. Hosking DH, Erickson SB, Van den Berg CJ, Wilson DM, Smith LH. The stone clinic effect in patients with idiopathic calcium urolithiasis. J Urol. 1983;130:1115–8.

47. Preminger GM, Peterson R, Peters PC, Pak CY. The current role of medical treatment of nephrolithiasis: the impact of improved techniques of stone removal. J Urol. 1985;134:6–10.

48. Pak CY, Griffith DP, Menon M, Preminger GM, Resnick MI. Urolithiasis. Current Practice of Medicine Series. Philadelphia, PA: Current Medicine; 1996:133–4.

49. Pak CY, Skurla C, Harvey J. Graphic display of urinary risk factors for renal stone formation. J Urol. 1985;134:867–70.

50. Brown RD, Adams BV, Pak CYC, Preminger GM. Reliability of a single 24-hour urine testing for the detection of abnormal stone-forming risk factors. In: Sutton RAL, Cameron EC, Walker V, Robertson B, Pak CYC, eds. Urolithiasis. New York: Plenum; 1989:553–6.

51. Pak CY. Southwestern Internal Medicine Conference: medical management of nephrolithiasis – a new, simplified approach for general practice. Am J Med Sci. 1997;313:215–9.

52. Glowacki LS, Beecroft ML, Cook RJ, Pahl D, Churchill DN. The natural history of asymptomatic urolithiasis. J Urol. 1992;147:319–21.

53. Morse RM, Resnick MI. Ureteral calculi: natural history and treatment in an era of advanced technology. J Urol. 1991;145:263–5.

54. Miller OF, Kane CJ. Time interval to stone passage for observed ureteral calculi: a guide for patient education. J Urol. 1999;162:688–90.

55. Borghi L, Meschi T, Amato F, Briganti A, Novarini A, Giannini A. Urinary volume, water and recurrences in idiopathic calcium nephrolithiasis: a 5-year randomized prospective study. J Urol. 1996;155:839–43.

56. Pak CY, Peters P, Hurt G, et al. Is selective therapy of recurrent nephrolithiasis possible? Am J Med. 1981;71:615–22.

57. Pak CY. Medical management of nephrolithiasis. J Urol. 1982;128:1157–64.

58. Preminger GM, Pak CY. The practical evaluation and selective medical management of nephrolithiasis. Semin Urol. 1985;3:170–84.

59. Pak CY, Delea CS, Bartter FC. Successful treatment of recurrent nephrolithiasis (calcium stones) with cellulose phosphate. N Engl J Med. 1974;290:175–80.

60. Pak CY. A cautious use of sodium cellulose phosphate in the management of calcium nephrolithiasis. Invest Urol. 1981;19:187–90.

61. Hayashi Y, Kaplan RA, Pak CY. Effect of sodium cellulose phosphate therapy on crystallization of calcium oxalate in urine. Metab Clin Exper. 1975;24:1273–8.

62. Zerwekh JE, Pak CY. Selective effects of thiazide therapy on serum 1 alpha,25-dihydroxyvitamin D and intestinal calcium absorption in renal and absorptive hypercalciurias. Metab Clin Exper. 1980;29:13–7.

63. Preminger GM, Pak CY. Eventual attenuation of hypocalciuric response to hydrochlorothiazide in absorptive hypercalciuria. J Urol. 1987;137:1104–9.

64. Breslau NA, Padalino P, Kok DJ, Kim YG, Pak CY. Physicochemical effects of a new slow-release potassium phosphate preparation

(UroPhos-K) in absorptive hypercalciuria. J Bone Mineral Res. 1995;10:394–400.

65. Breslau NA, Heller HJ, Reza-Albarran AA, Pak CY. Physiological effects of slow release potassium phosphate for absorptive hypercalciuria: a randomized double-blind trial. J Urol. 1998;160:664–8.

66. Heller HJ, Reza-Albarran AA, Breslau NA, Pak CY. Sustained reduction in urinary calcium during long-term treatment with slow release neutral potassium phosphate in absorptive hypercalciuria. J Urol. 1998;159:1451–6.

67. Barilla DE, Tolentino R, Kaplan RA, Pak CY. Selective effects of thiazide on intestinal absorption of calcium and adsorptive and renal hypercalciurias. Metab Clin Exper. 1978;27:125–31.

68. Siminovitch JM, Esselstyn CB Jr, Straffon RA. Renal lithiasis and hyperparathyroidism: diagnosis, management and prognosis. J Urol. 1981;126:720–2.

69. Sutton RA, Walker VR. Enteric and mild hyperoxaluria. Mineral Electrolyte Metab. 1994;20:352–60.

70. Harvey JA, Zobitz MM, Pak CY. Calcium citrate: reduced propensity for the crystallization of calcium oxalate in urine resulting from induced hypercalciuria of calcium supplementation. J Clin Endocrinol Metab. 1985;61:1223–5.

71. Coe FL. Hyperuricosuric calcium oxalate nephrolithiasis. Kidney Int. 1978;13:418–26.

72. Pak CY, Peterson R. Successful treatment of hyperuricosuric calcium oxalate nephrolithiasis with potassium citrate. Arch Intern Med. 1986;146:863–7.

73. Preminger GM, Sakhaee K, Pak CY. Alkali action on the urinary crystallization of calcium salts: contrasting responses to sodium citrate and potassium citrate. J Urol. 139:1988;240–2.

74. Pak CY, Fuller C, Sakhaee K, Preminger GM, Britton F. Long-term treatment of calcium nephrolithiasis with potassium citrate. J Urol. 1985;134:11–9.

75. Fegan J, Khan R, Poindexter J, Pak CY. Gastrointestinal citrate absorption in nephrolithiasis. J Urol. 1992;147:1212–4.

76. Pak CY, Koenig K, Khan R, Haynes S, Padalino P. Physicochemical action of potassium-magnesium citrate in nephrolithiasis. J Bone Mineral Res. 1992;7:281–5.

77. Ettinger B, Pak CY, Citron JT, Thomas C, Adams-Huet B, Vangessel A. Potassium-magnesium citrate is an effective prophylaxis against recurrent calcium oxalate nephrolithiasis. J Urol. 1997;158:2069–73.

78. Harvey JA, Pak CY. Gouty diathesis and sarcoidosis in patient with recurrent calcium nephrolithiasis. J Urol. 1988;139:1287–9.

79. Sakhaee K, Nicar M, Hill K, Pak CY. Contrasting effects of potassium citrate and sodium citrate therapies on urinary chemistries and crystallization of stone-forming salts. Kidney Int. 1983;24:348–52.

80. Chow GK, Streem SB. Medical treatment of cystinuria: results of contemporary clinical practice. J Urol. 1996;156:1576–8.

81. Pak CY, Fuller C, Sakhaee K, Zerwekh JE, Adams BV. Management of cystine nephrolithiasis with α-mercaptopropionylglycine. J Urol. 1986;136:1003–8.

82. Streem SB, Hall P. Effect of captopril on urinary cystine excretion in homozygous cystinuria. J Urol. 1989;142:1522–4.

83. Chow GK, Streem SB. Contemporary urological intervention for cystinuric patients: immediate and long-term impact and implications. J Urol. 1998;160:341–5.

84. Griffith DP. Struvite stones. Kidney Int. 1978;13:372–82.

85. Williams JJ, Rodman JS, Peterson CM. A randomized double-blind study of acetohydroxamic acid in struvite nephrolithiasis. N Engl J Med. 1984;311:760–4.

86. Rich JD, Ramratnam B, Chiang M, Tashima KT. Management of indinavir associated nephrolithiasis. J Urol. 1997;158:2228.

87. Reiter WJ, Schon-Pernerstorfer H, Dorfinger K, Hofbauer J, Marberger M. Frequency of urolithiasis in individuals seropositive for human immunodeficiency virus treated with indinavir is higher than previously assumed. J Urol. 1999;161:1082–4.

88. Seegmiller JE. Xanthine stone formation. Am J Med. 1968;45:780–3.

89. Greene ML, Fukimoto W, Seegmiller J. Urinary xanthine stones – a rare complication of Allopurinol therapy. N Engl J Med. 1969;280):426–7.

90. Burns JR, Gauthier JF. Prevention of urinary catheter incrustations by acetohydroxamic acid. J Urol. 1984;132:455–6.

91. Chaussy C, Schmiedt E. Shock wave treatment for stones in the upper urinary tract. Urol Clin North Am. 1982;10:743–50.

92. Chaussy C, Schmiedt E, Jocham D, Brendel W, Forssmann B, Walther V. First clinical experience with extracorporeally induced destruction of kidney stones by shock waves. J Urol. 1982;127:417–20.

93. Lingeman JE, Newman D, Mertz JH, et al. Extracorporeal shock wave lithotripsy: the Methodist Hospital of Indiana experience. J Urol. 1986;135:1134–7.

94. Riehle RA Jr, Naslund EB, Fair W, Vaughan ED Jr. Impact of shockwave lithotripsy on upper urinary tract calculi. Urology 1986;28:261–9.

95. Drach GW, Dretler SP, Fair W, et al. Report of the United States cooperative study of extracorporeal shock wave lithotripsy. J Urol. 1986;135:1127–33.

96. Brown RD, Preminger GM. Changing surgical aspects of urinary stone disease. Surg Clin North Am. 1988;68:1085–104.

97. Gilbert BR, Riehle RA, Vaughan ED Jr. Extracorporeal shock wave lithotripsy and its effect on renal function. J Urol. 1988;139:482–5.

98. Knapp PM, Kulb TB, Lingeman JE, et al. Extracorporeal shock wave lithotripsy-induced perirenal hematomas. J Urol. 1988;139:700–3.

99. Puppo P, Germinale F, Ricciotti G, et al. Hypertension after extracorporeal shock wave lithotripsy: a false alarm. J Endourol. 1989;3:401–4.

100. Smith LH, Drach G, Hall P, et al. National High Blood Pressure Education Program (NHBPEP) review paper on complications of shock wave lithotripsy for urinary calculi. Am J Med. 1991;91:635–41.

101. Williams CM, Kaude JV, Newman RC, Peterson JC, Thomas WC. Extracorporeal shock-wave lithotripsy: long-term complications. AJR. 1988;150:311–5.

102. Montgomery BS, Cole RS, Palfrey EL, Shuttleworth KE. Does extracorporeal shockwave lithotripsy cause hypertension? Br J Urol. 1989;64:567–71.

103. Lingeman JE, Woods JR, Toth PD. Blood pressure changes following extracorporeal shock wave lithotripsy and other forms of treatment for nephrolithiasis. JAMA. 1990;263:1789–94.

104. Fegan JE, Husmann DA, Alexander ME, Feagins B, Preminger GM. Preservation of renal architecture during extracorporeal shock wave lithotripsy. J Endourol. 1991;5:273–6.

105. Morris JS, Husmann DA, Wilson WT, Preminger GM. Temporal effects of shock wave lithotripsy. J Urol. 1991;145:881–3.

106. Segura JW, Patterson DE, LeRoy AJ, et al. Percutaneous removal of kidney stones: review of 1,000 cases. J Urol. 1985;134:1077–81.

107. Clayman RV, Miller RP, Reinke DB, Lange PH. Nephroscopy: advances and adjuncts. Urol Clin North Am. 1982;9:51–60.

108. Alken P. Percutaneous ultrasonic destruction of renal calculi. Urol Clin North Am. 1982;9:145–51.

109. Raney AM, Handler J. Electrohydraulic nephrolithotripsy. Urology. 1975;6:439–42.

110. Denstedt JD, Razvi HA, Sales JL, Eberwein PM. Preliminary experience with holmium: YAG laser lithotripsy. J Endourol. 1995;9:255–8.

111. Teichman JM, Rao RD, Glickman RD, Harris JM. Holmium:YAG percutaneous nephrolithotomy: the laser incident angle matters. J Urol. 1998;159:690–4.

112. Denstedt JD, Eberwein PM, Singh RR. The Swiss Lithoclast: a new device for intracorporeal lithotripsy. J Urol. 1992;148:1088–90.

113. Schulze H, Haupt G, Piergiovanni M, Wisard M, von Niederhausern W, Senge T. The Swiss Lithoclast: a new device for endoscopic stone disintegration. J Urol. 1993;149:15–8.

114. Denstedt JD, Razvi HA, Rowe E, Grignon DJ, Eberwein PM. Investigation of the tissue effects of a new device for intracorporeal lithotripsy – the Swiss Lithoclast. J Urol. 1995;153:535–7.

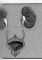
115. Teh CL, Aslan P, Preminger GM. What's new in shock wave lithotripsy? Contemp Urol. 1997;9:26–36.

116. Beck EM, Vaughan ED Jr, Sosa RE. The pulsed dye laser in the treatment of ureteral calculi. Semin Urol. 1989;7:25–9.

117. Preminger GM, Roehrborn CG. Special applications of flexible deflectable ureterorenoscopy. Semin Urol. 1989;7:16–24.

118. Huffman JL. Experience with the 8.5 French compact rigid ureteroscope. Semin Urol. 1989;7:3–6.

119. Assimos DG. Should one perform open surgery in 1994? Semin Urol. 1994;12:26–31.

120. Preminger GM, Clayman RV, Hardeman SW, Franklin J, Curry T, Peters PC. Percutaneous nephrostolithotomy vs open surgery for renal calculi. A comparative study. JAMA.1985; 254:1054–8.

121. Segura JW, Preminger GM, Assimos DG, et al. Nephrolithiasis Clinical Guidelines Panel summary report on the management of staghorn calculi. American Urological Association Nephrolithiasis Clinical Guidelines Panel. J Urol. 1994;151:1648–51.

122. Assimos DG, Wrenn JJ, Harrison LH, et al. A comparison of anatrophic nephrolithotomy and percutaneous nephrolithotomy with and without extracorporeal shock wave lithotripsy for management of patients with staghorn calculi. J Urol. 1991;145:710–14.

123. Lee WJ, Snyder JA, Smith AD. Staghorn calculi: endourologic management in 120 patients. Radiology. 1987;165:85–8.

124. Mays N, Challah S, Patel S, et al. Clinical comparison of extracorporeal shock wave lithotripsy and percutaneous nephrolithotomy in treating renal calculi. Br Med J. 1988;297:253–8.

125. Vanden Bossche M, Simon J, Schulman CC. Shock wave monotherapy of staghorn calculi. Eur Urol. 1990;17:1–6.

126. Winfield HN, Clayman RV, Chaussy CG, Weyman PJ, Fuchs GJ, Lupu AN. Monotherapy of staghorn renal calculi: a comparative study between percutaneous nephrolithotomy and extracorporeal shock wave lithotripsy. J Urol. 1988;139:895–9.

127. Constantinides C, Recker F, Jaeger P, Hauri D. Extracorporeal shock wave lithotripsy as monotherapy of staghorn renal calculi: 3 years of experience. J Urol. 1989;142:1415–8.

128. Gleeson MJ, Griffith DP. Extracorporeal shockwave lithotripsy monotherapy for large renal calculi. Br J Urol. 1989;64:329–32.

129. Karlsen S, Gjolberg T. Branched renal calculi treated by percutaneous nephrolithotomy and extracorporeal shock waves. Scand J Urol Nephrol. 1989;23:201–5.

130. Schulze H, Hertle L, Kutta A, Graff J, Senge T. Critical evaluation of treatment of staghorn calculi by percutaneous nephrolithotomy and extracorporeal shock wave lithotripsy. J Urol. 1989;141:822–5.

131. Streem SB, Yost A, Dolmatch B. Combination 'sandwich' therapy for extensive renal calculi in 100 consecutive patients: immediate, long-term and stratified results from a 10-year experience. J Urol. 1997;158:342–5.

132. Brownlee N, Foster M, Griffith DP, Carlton CE Jr. Controlled inversion therapy: an adjunct to the elimination of gravity-dependent fragments following extracorporeal shock wave lithotripsy. J Urol. 1990;143:1096–8.

133. Lingeman JE, Lower Pole Study Group. Prospective randomized trial of extracorporeal shock wave lithotripsy and percutaneous nephrostolithotomy for lower pole nephrolithiasis: initial long-term follow-up. J Endourol. 1997;11:S95.

134. Elbahnasy AM, Shalhav AL, Hoenig DM, et al. Lower caliceal stone clearance after shock wave lithotripsy or ureteroscopy: the impact of lower pole radiographic anatomy. J Urol. 1998;159:676–82.

135. Preminger GM, Harvey JA, Pak CY. Comparative efficacy of 'specific' potassium citrate therapy versus conservative management in nephrolithiasis of mild to moderate severity. J Urol. 1985;134:658–61.

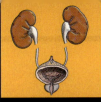

Section 4 Benign Disorders of the Upper Urinary Tract

Chapter 23 Upper Tract Obstruction

Patrick H O'Reilly

KEY POINTS

- Obstructive uropathy may be acute or chronic, unilateral or bilateral, unequivocal, or equivocal. Knowledge of its pathophysiology guides clinical management.
- Unequivocal obstruction is diagnosed predominantly by imaging techniques, but functional studies may be required to decide between renal conservation or nephrectomy.
- Equivocal obstruction requires functional and urodynamic assessment; ^{99m}Tc-mercaptoacetyltriglycine diuresis renography is the investigation of choice.
- Posture and a full or filling bladder can have a profound effect on upper tract urodynamics; this may lead to misinterpretation of investigations.
- Recovery of obstruction after its relief is biphasic, with an initial tubular phase, followed by a much slower glomerular recovery.

INTRODUCTION

Obstruction to urine flow can have its origin in the upper or the lower urinary tract, and it can be acute or chronic, complete or incomplete, and unilateral or bilateral. It has many diverse causes, each with its own specific features and yet each producing similar effects on renal function and drainage.

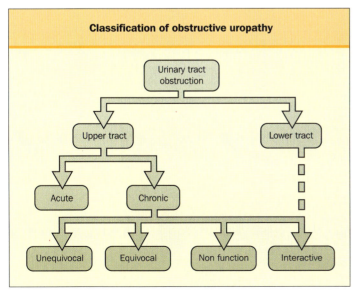

Fig. 23.1 Classification of obstructive uropathy.

It is useful to subdivide urinary tract obstruction into the categories shown in Figure 23.1. This chapter deals with obstructive conditions of the upper urinary tract.

ACUTE OBSTRUCTION

Etiology

The most common cause of acute obstruction is urinary stone disease. Sloughed renal papillae, blood clot, acute retroperitoneal pathology, and accidental ureteric ligation are less common causes.

Pathophysiology

Intrarenal pressures

Normal resting pressures within the renal pelvis and ureter are about 0–10cmH$_2$O (0–1kPa). Peristaltic pressures for urine transport vary between 20cmH$_2$O (2.0kPa) and 60cmH$_2$O (5.9kPa). In acute obstruction, there is an abrupt rise in ureteric and intrarenal pressure (see Fig. 23.2), which is proportional to the existing state of diuresis. The rise is transmitted back to the tubular lumen. The rise in pressure is short-lived, and the pressure falls gradually. This subsequent fall in pressure results from several factors:

- increasing dilatation of the renal pelvis in proportion to the compliance of the system (obeying the Law of Laplace, whereby the pressure in compliant systems falls as the radius increases);
- reduced renal blood flow (RBF) and glomerular filtration rate (GFR); and
- pyelolymphatic and pyelovenous backflow[1].

Once obstruction has become chronic, the intrapelvic pressures may be normal or even subnormal.

Renal blood flow

In the early stages of acute obstruction, RBF rises transiently (see Fig. 23.2), particularly in the inner cortex and corticomedullary regions. This is probably caused by vasodilatation induced by prostaglandin E$_2$ (pre-treatment with indomethacin reduces the effect). If the obstruction persists for more than 2 hours, vasoconstriction (mediated by thromboxane A$_2$ and other factors such as input from the renin–angiotensin system, increased renal nerve activity, and local adrenergic agonists) produces a significant decrease in RBF, which reaches 40–70% of normal by 24 hours[2–6].

Glomerular filtration rate

In acute obstruction, the GFR is initially unchanged but, before long, the increase in blood flow reduces filtration fraction and

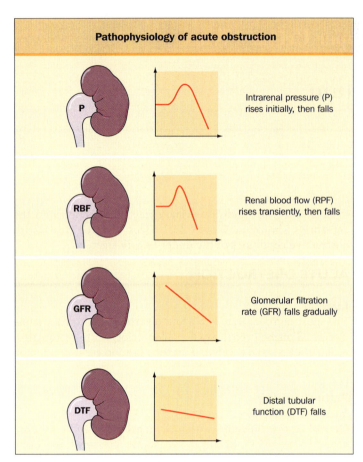

Pathophysiology of acute obstruction

Intrarenal pressure (P) rises initially, then falls

Renal blood flow (RPF) rises transiently, then falls

Glomerular filtration rate (GFR) falls gradually

Distal tubular function (DTF) falls

Fig. 23.2 Pathophysiology of acute obstruction.

thus filtration pressure. The RBF then falls and the filtration fraction increases slightly, but compensation is incomplete, so overall filtration falls steadily. Thus, within a few hours, GFR is reduced. After 1 week of unilateral acute obstruction, GFR is down to 20% of preobstruction levels (with the contralateral side increasing to 165% of preobstruction levels)[7].

Tubular function
In acute obstruction, the transit of fluid is slowed so that the column of fluid delivered to the distal nephron is reduced. Free water formation falls, salt reabsorption is increased, and the tubules become unresponsive to circulating antidiuretic hormone and cannot produce concentrated urine. Once GFR falls, nitrogen retention occurs and the solute load delivered to the nephron further impairs concentration by its osmotic effect, which results in dilute urine with a high sodium content.

Obstructive atrophy
Long periods of total obstruction cause progressive nephron loss that culminates in medullary and cortical atrophy. This series of events is called obstructive atrophy. Histologically there is dilatation and atrophy of tubules, cast formation, interstitial fibrosis, and eventual loss of glomeruli. The glomeruli are relatively better preserved than the tubules, and so more derangement of medullary than cortical function occurs after obstruction is relieved. The brunt of medullary damage is borne by the collecting and distal tubules.

The fall in GFR and RBF with short-term, acute total obstruction is temporarily reversible, but not for long. Canine kidneys tolerate only 4–7 days of total obstruction before nephron loss sets in. Relief of a total obstruction before this deadline fully restores renal function as long as there has been no infection or preexisting renal disease. Relief of total obstruction after more than 1 week is followed by only partial return of function. After 4–6 weeks of complete obstruction in animals, little glomerular function returns after reversal of the obstruction. Infection and ischemia hasten obstructive renal damage and limit the recovery of the obstructed kidney.

There are occasional reports of a return of significant GFR after periods of total obstruction ranging from 28 days to 1.5 years. Despite these exceptions, most patients with complete obstruction for long periods mimic the animal models and recover little function after obstruction is relieved[8].

Investigation and diagnosis
Intravenous urogram
Notwithstanding newer techniques, the intravenous urogram (IVU) remains the cornerstone for the investigation of acute obstruction, demonstrating as it does the pathology of the affected kidney and the integrity or otherwise of the contralateral kidney. Under normal circumstances, the density of the urographic nephrogram is greatest at 1 minute after injection. After this, the normal urogram becomes less dense as excretion produces a 50% decrease in plasma contrast levels every 50 minutes. In the early stages of acute obstruction RBF is preserved and GFR is unaffected, so intravenous contrast is delivered to the kidney. Slow intratubular transit causes increasing accumulation of contrast in the kidney, and produces the dense nephrogram (Fig. 23.3).

Other causes of a dense nephrogram, for example renal artery stenosis or thrombosis, renal vein thrombosis, intratubular

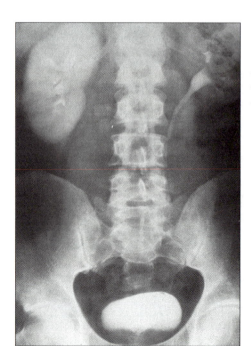

Fig. 23.3 The dense nephrogram.
Intravenous urographic appearance of the dense nephrogram in acute obstruction.

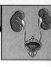
obstruction, and systemic hypotension, must be excluded; none of these other causes gives the combination of dense nephrogram, large kidney, and dilated renal pelvis and ureter. Delayed films, occasionally for as long as 24 hours, are necessary after the initial nephrogram phase to fill the collecting system and demonstrate the level of obstruction. Prone films help to empty the calices and fill the pelvis and ureter[9].

Ultrasound

Ultrasound can demonstrate hydronephrosis, and it can be useful as a quick screening test or in patients with an allergy to contrast medium.

Radionuclide studies

Radionuclide studies are of limited value, except to establish split renal function or in combination with a plain film (kidneys, ureters, bladder) and ultrasound in patients with an allergy to contrast medium.

Computed tomography

Computed tomography (CT) is occasionally used for the investigation of acute obstruction, and the findings tend to follow the urographic appearances. The increasingly dense nephrogram of acute obstruction has two phases on CT: an early cortical nephrogram develops first, followed by gradual opacification of the medulla, eventually leading to a homogeneously dense nephrogram.

Management

In patients with high-grade obstruction, for those with evidence of sepsis, those with unremitting pain, or those who are pregnant, emergency percutaneous nephrostomy (PCN) or ureteric stenting is indicated to relieve obstruction, preserve renal function, and permit subsequent appropriately controlled management of the obstructing agent (Figs 23.4 & 23.5).

UNEQUIVOCAL CHRONIC OBSTRUCTION

Unequivocal chronic obstruction refers to the finding of a dilated urinary tract in which the presence of obstruction is beyond doubt and its cause is apparent. Any lesion that arises within the lumen of the outflow tract or that compresses it from an extrinsic source can be responsible (Fig. 23.6).

Pathophysiology

As obstruction becomes established, the initially high intrarenal pressures fall to within the normal pre-obstructed range (Fig. 23.7).

The RBF declines, falling to preobstruction levels after 3–4 hours and declining further after that before stabilizing at a new, reduced level. This new level depends on the degree and duration of the obstruction[10,11].

The GFR falls progressively with time. In canine experiments in which the ureter is ligated, GFR has been shown to fall to 50% of preobstruction levels after 24 hours, and reaches 20% of preobstruction levels at 1 week. Final GFR depends on the extent and duration of obstruction[12], as does the degree of recovery after release of the obstruction.

Tubular function is affected such that the urine in chronic obstruction is persistently hypotonic and does not respond to

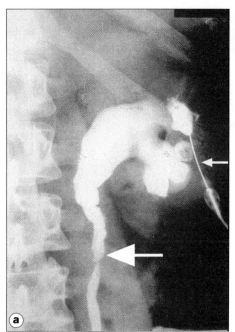

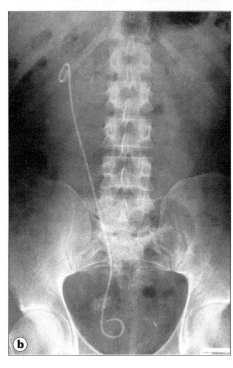

Fig. 23.4 Emergency treatment for the relief of upper urinary tract obstruction. (a) Partially obstructed left kidney caused by a ureteric calculus (large arrow). Note the percutaneous nephrostomy line (small arrow). (b) JJ stent *in situ*.

concentrating stimuli. Urinary acidification is impaired. Urinary osmolality and sodium content are increased.

There is now considerable evidence that the decline in GFR and RBF is mainly the result of preglomerular vasoconstriction. It is not known which vasoconstrictor – angiotensin II, thromboxane A_2, noradrenaline, or another agent – is responsible[13,14]. Nonetheless, the data indicating that ischemic damage accounts for so-called obstructive atrophy are compelling.

Investigation and diagnosis

The modalities available for the investigation of unequivocal chronic obstruction include intravenous urography, antegrade and retrograde ureteropyelography, ultrasound, CT scanning, magnetic resonance scanning, and other contrast studies if

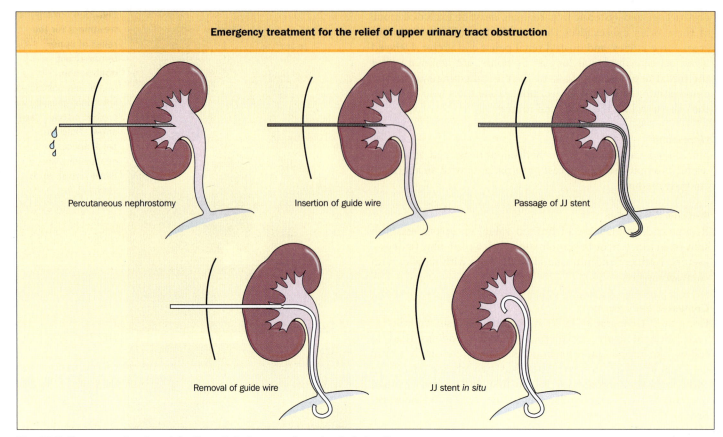

Emergency treatment for the relief of upper urinary tract obstruction

Percutaneous nephrostomy

Insertion of guide wire

Passage of JJ stent

Removal of guide wire

JJ stent *in situ*

Fig. 23.5 Emergency treatment for the relief of upper urinary tract obstruction.

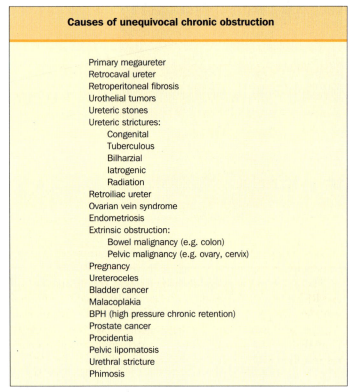

Causes of unequivocal chronic obstruction

Primary megaureter
Retrocaval ureter
Retroperitoneal fibrosis
Urothelial tumors
Ureteric stones
Ureteric strictures:
  Congenital
  Tuberculous
  Bilharzial
  Iatrogenic
  Radiation
Retroiliac ureter
Ovarian vein syndrome
Endometriosis
Extrinsic obstruction:
  Bowel malignancy (e.g. colon)
  Pelvic malignancy (e.g. ovary, cervix)
Pregnancy
Ureteroceles
Bladder cancer
Malacoplakia
BPH (high pressure chronic retention)
Prostate cancer
Procidentia
Pelvic lipomatosis
Urethral stricture
Phimosis

Fig. 23.6 Causes of unequivocal chronic obstruction.

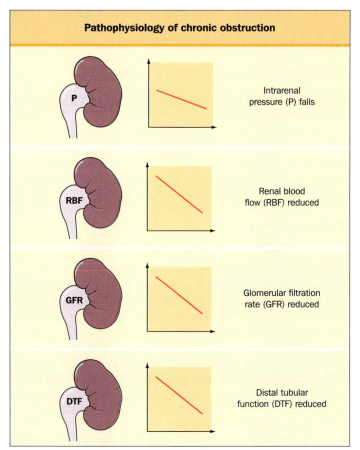

Pathophysiology of chronic obstruction

Intrarenal pressure (P) falls

Renal blood flow (RBF) reduced

Glomerular filtration rate (GFR) reduced

Distal tubular function (DTF) reduced

Fig. 23.7 Pathophysiology of chronic obstruction.

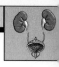

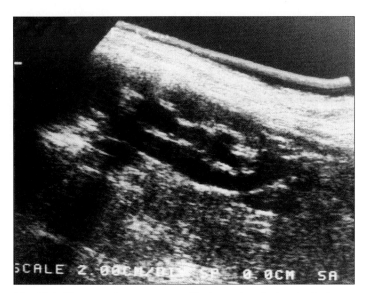

Fig. 23.8 Ultrasound appearance of hydronephrosis. Longitudinal section of the left kidney.

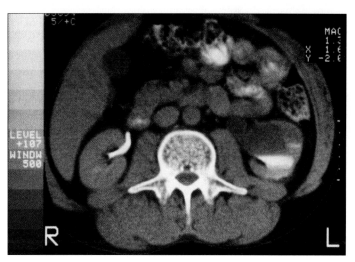

Fig. 23.9 Computed tomography appearance of hydronephrosis: postcontrast study. Note the layering of contrast in the dilated left pelvicaliceal system. The dilated proximal ureter can also be seen. The right kidney is normal.

indicated (for example, barium enema). However, their indiscriminate use is expensive and counterproductive. Conversely, wise use of these various modalities, based on appreciation of the etiologic and pathophysiologic factors responsible for the clinical picture, usually leads to correct and appropriate management decisions. Thus, clinical history, physical examination, laboratory tests, and radiology usually confirm obstruction and reveal the cause.

Intravenous urography

The presence of chronic obstruction is often detected first by intravenous urography. This remains the most comprehensive screening test of urinary tract structure, although its role as the initial investigation of suspected obstruction has largely been superseded by ultrasound.

Ultrasound

This technique is described in Chapter 8. The characteristic sonographic appearance of dilatation is separation of the renal sinus echo complex by an echo-free region. This appearance results from the fluid-filled collecting system (Fig. 23.8).

Such separation may be minimal, moderate, or severe. Minimal dilatation may be dependent on the state of hydration, and diuresis or radiographic contrast media may cause physiologic dilatation. Conversely, false-negative scans of patients in whom obstruction is in fact present may be found in dehydration or when there is coexisting sepsis. Thus, ultrasound alone does not always exclude obstruction in some uremic or septic patients with normal-sized kidneys.

In addition to dilatation of the collecting system, ultrasound also demonstrates parenchymal thickness, and thus gives a qualitative morphologic clue to underlying functional status[15,16].

Computed tomography

Computed tomography plays an important role in determining the etiology of ureteric obstruction when ultrasound, urography, and retrograde pyelography are not diagnostic[17]. It can also be used to screen for obstruction in selected cases.

Noncontrast computed tomography

Hydronephrosis is easily appreciated on noncontrast computed tomography (NCT) scans and is useful in patients who have an indeterminate ultrasound and who have contrast allergy or uremia. Dilated ureters can usually be traced to the point of obstruction on contiguous scans. Obstructive atrophy is diagnosed when hydronephrosis is accompanied by parenchymal thinning. In uremic patients screened for obstruction, CT can be as sensitive as ultrasound in detecting dilatation but, as with ultrasound, NCT has difficulty distinguishing mild, nonobstructive dilatation from obstructive hydronephrosis. False-positive scans on NCT can be caused by clubbed calices, a distensible collecting system, peripelvic cysts, megacalices, widespread papillary necrosis, and subcapsular hematoma. An upper pole cyst may resemble an obstructed upper moiety of a duplex kidney. Post-contrast scans clarify most problem cases.

Contrast-enhanced computed tomography

As with urography, the delay in opacification of the pelvicaliceal system and the degree of dilatation are determined by the severity and duration of obstruction. With moderate or severe hydronephrosis, urine-contrast layers in the dependent portion of the collecting system (which are demonstrated only occasionally by urography) are common on CT (Fig. 23.9). Also, CT is useful for evaluating parenchymal thickness.

Computed tomography to define the cause of obstruction

Urate and matrix calculi, which are often invisible on plain radiographs, have high attenuation values and can be clearly seen on CT. The principal difficulty arises with tiny stones, which must be carefully localized to ensure that they do not fall between adjacent CT slices. Contiguous scans should follow the dilated, urine-filled ureter to the point of obstruction.

It is of value in ureteropelvic junction (UPJ) obstruction in one or both limbs of a horseshoe kidney, and in the evaluation of duplex kidneys with obstruction of the upper moiety[18]. It is also useful in determining the etiology of ureteric obstruction, and CT can indicate subsequent management even when it does not provide the exact diagnosis. For example, a retroperitoneal mass at the point of extrinsic ureteric obstruction in a patient with known malignancy strongly suggests metastatic tumor (e.g. from breast, lung, ovary, or prostate), and the diagnosis can be confirmed by fine-needle aspiration biopsy under CT guidance.

Radionuclide studies

If information on underlying function is required, gamma camera renography is necessary (see Chapter 10). None of the previously mentioned imaging modalities measures renal function[19]. This simple test gives quantitative information on split renal function and urodynamics by a relatively noninvasive 30-minute procedure, and its value in obstructive uropathy cannot be overstated (Fig. 23.10).

Management

General principles

The management of unequivocal chronic obstruction is twofold:

- treatment of the causative lesion; and
- conservation or removal of the affected kidney, depending on the degree and reversibility of its function.

Where there is doubt about the recoverability of an obstructed kidney, PCN or ureteric stenting should be carried out with repeated renography after 2 weeks and, if practicable, again at 6 weeks.

Percutaneous drainage, followed by reassessment later to judge if the drainage has produced some recovery of function, is the most reliable prognostic test of renal recoverability. Radionuclides have been used to try to provide a noninvasive measure of renal function. In general, these techniques establish the renal function at the time of examination rather than the potential for recovery. However, in some patients with complete unilateral obstruction, dimercaptosuccinic acid (DMSA) split function for the obstructed kidney is found to exceed the corresponding hippuran value. Such a finding is often associated with considerable improvement in hippuran values after relief of obstruction, which

suggests that the higher DMSA level represents potential for recovery[20,21]. This is the only noninvasive prognostic guide to potential recoverability and, in practice, most urologists favor nephrostomy or stenting.

Recovery after relief of obstruction

Renal recovery after relief of obstruction, whether by PCN or surgery, has been shown to occur in two phases, a tubular phase and a glomerular phase[22].

Tubular phase

The initial or tubular phase consists of changes in fractional water and electrolyte excretion accompanied by reversal in clinical signs of salt and water retention, which frequently accompany obstructive renal failure. The major part of these changes occurs within the first few days after relief of obstruction, and in virtually all cases it is complete within 2 weeks.

Glomerular phase

Plasma creatinine and creatinine clearance also improve during this phase; however, GFR measured by the more accurate techniques of ^{99m}Tc–diethylenetriamine pentaacetic acid (^{99m}Tc–DTPA) and iohexol clearance does not change during these 2 weeks, although it does slowly improve between 3 weeks and 3 months (Fig. 23.11).

This later or glomerular phase is accompanied by further increases in creatinine clearance and plasma creatinine. The improvement in creatinine excretion during the tubular phase may be explained by the tubular secretion of creatinine that accompanies the other marked changes in tubular electrolyte handling.

Specific examples of unequivocal obstruction

Space does not permit discussion of all the causes of obstruction listed in Figure 23.6. Many causes are covered elsewhere in this book; the following section deals with some of the more common ones.

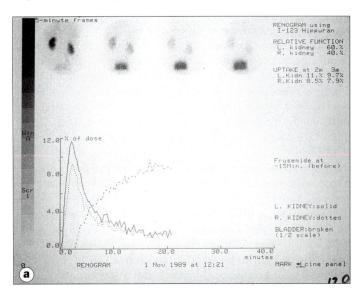

Fig. 23.10 Gamma camera renography. Normal gamma camera renogram.

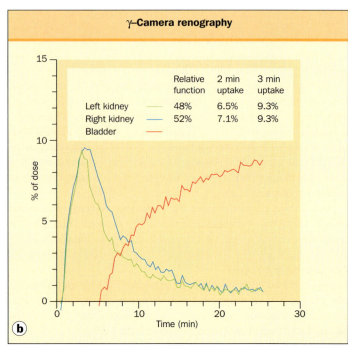

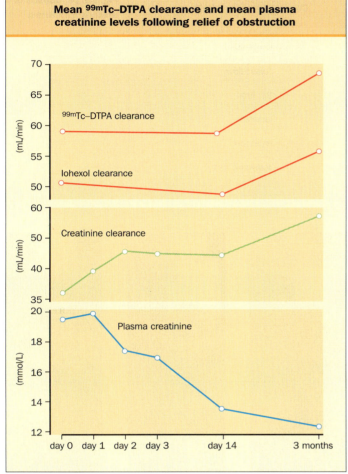

Mean ⁹⁹ᵐTc–DTPA clearance and mean plasma creatinine levels following relief of obstruction

Fig. 23.11 Mean ⁹⁹ᵐTc-DTPA, iohexol, creatinine clearance, and mean plasma creatinine levels during obstruction. Measurements are recorded on day 0, 24 hours after relief of obstruction (day 1), and on subsequent days up to 3 months. Note the biphasic nature of the recovery. (The 95% confidence limits have been omitted for clarity.)

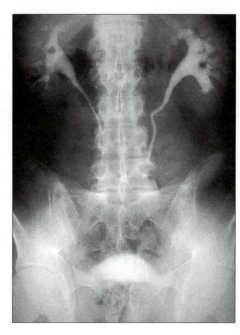

Fig. 23.12 Urographic appearance of retroperitoneal fibrosis. Note the dilated urinary tracts and medial deviation of the ureters around the level of the third to fifth lumbar vertebrae.

Retrocaval ureter

Normally the dorsal supracardinal vein forms the inferior vena cava (IVC). If the ventral subcardinal vein persists to form the infrarenal segment of the IVC, the ureter finds itself behind the IVC, describing a medial curve around it until the ureter spirals to the front of the iliac vessels. It is liable to obstruction from compression between the IVC and the vertebral column, acute bends around the vein, or kinking at the UPJ.

The condition is more common in males (by a ratio of 3:1). It typically presents as flank pain in the third or fourth decades.

Diagnosis is by urography or CT scanning, with renography to establish the extent of obstruction and functional impairment. If surgery is required, a variant of the dismembered pyeloplasty is performed, dividing the ureter at the UPJ and bringing the ureter to the front of the IVC for anastomosis to the renal pelvis.

Retroperitoneal fibrosis

Retroperitoneal fibrosis is characterized by the deposition of plaques or sheets of collagenous fibrous tissue on the posterior abdominal wall. This fibrosis pulls the ureters medially and compresses them, usually between the L2 and L5 vertebrae. The

obstruction is caused not by a blockage but by the fibrosis, which prevents bolus transmission because it limits the ability of the ureteric wall to stretch to accept the wedge-shaped bolus. Thus, chronic proximal dilatation leads to slow, insidious renal failure.

The condition occurs usually in middle age and is associated with a normocytic normochromic anemia, a high erythrocyte sedimentation rate, and raised urea and creatinine levels. Most cases are idiopathic, although some 15% are associated with inflammatory aortic aneurysms, intraperitoneal sepsis, or certain drugs (for example, ergot and beta-blockers).

Ultrasound shows hydronephrosis. Intravenous urography or retrograde ureterography demonstrates dilated urinary tracts with medial deviation of the ureters around the level of the third to fifth lumbar vertebrae (Fig. 23.12). Computed tomography may demonstrate the perianeurysmal fibrosis.

Treatment is usually surgical, unless there is evidence that an inflammatory aneurysm is the cause, in which case corticosteroids may be indicated. The principles of surgery are three-fold:
- ureterolysis;
- lateralization; and
- omental wrapping.

The ureters are released from the fibrosis, lateralized away from the predominantly medial, para-aortic fibrotic process, and wrapped in a sleeve of protective omentum. Patients with retroperitoneal fibrosis have a tendency to thromboembolism, and surgery should therefore be covered with heparin.

Urothelial tumors

Approximately 5% of all urothelial tumors arise in the ureter, and most of these cause obstruction (Fig. 23.13). The etiology of these tumors is the same as that for bladder cancer (see Chapter 25). Urothelial tumors cause obstruction by occupying the lumen of the UPJ, ureter, or ureteric orifice, or by infiltrating the ureteric wall and interfering with peristalsis. Once suspected, they can usually be detected on imaging. Ureteroscopy has assisted considerably in the early diagnosis or confirmation of urographic lesions. Three-quarters of these tumors occur in the lower one-third of the ureter, and

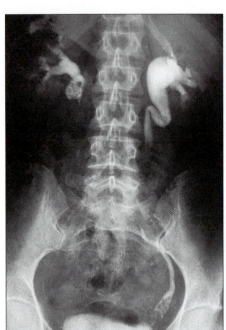

Fig. 23.13 Imaging of urothelial tumors. Urogram showing lower left ureteric tumor.

Cause of ureteric strictures
Congenital
Tuberculous
Bilharzial
Iatrogenic
Radiation
Malignant

Fig. 23.14 Causes of ureteric strictures.

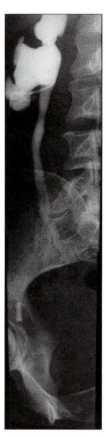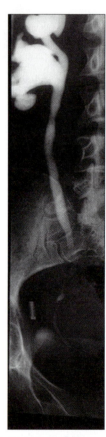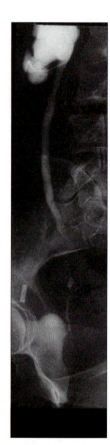

Fig. 23.15 Lower left tuberculous ureteric stricture on antegrade pyelogram.

obstruction tends to be slow and insidious since the proximal tract is compliant and can absorb the slowly progressive effects until the condition is at an advanced stage. Metastatic disease occurs early in high-grade tumors. Treatment depends on various factors (see Chapter 25).

Ureteric strictures
Ureteric strictures are uncommon causes of obstructive uropathy. Other than those caused by accidental surgical ligation, they tend to develop slowly, producing chronic obstructive uropathy. Their causes are listed in Fig. 23.14.

Congenital strictures
Congenital strictures are rare, and their contribution to the overall causes of obstructive uropathy is extremely small.

Genitourinary tuberculosis
Genitourinary tuberculosis is always blood borne and secondary to an established focus of infection elsewhere. Ureteric involvement results from spread of infection from the parenchyma via the calices and renal pelvis. Mucosal tubercles, caseation, ulceration, fibrosis, and ureteric scarring result. The lower third of the ureter is usually affected, most strictures being 2.5–5cm long (Fig. 23.15).

In the early stage, narrowing results from inflammation and edema, and it may respond to chemotherapy. Once fibrosis has occurred, progressive obstruction and renal damage is likely. Management is initially by medical treatment, with weekly single-shot full-length IVUs. If there is no improvement after 4 weeks, prednisolone is added to the regimen. If there is still no improvement after a further 4 weeks, surgery is indicated.

Bilharziasis
Ureteric strictures are the most common sequelae of urinary bilharziasis, and they are found in 25% of cases. They lead to obstruction, infection, stones, and progressive renal impairment.

The causative organism, *Schistosoma haematobium*, is endemic in many parts of the world including Egypt, central and southern Africa, Iraq, Saudi Arabia, and India. It is the most common helminthic infestation of humans, affecting 8% of the world's population, and it is predominantly a disease of young people.

Any part of the ureter can be affected, but over 80% of strictures are in the lower one-third. Calcification of the ureter is not unusual. Internally, the ureteric lumen becomes irregular, or develops papules, granulations, or 'sandy' patches (calcified helminthic ova in a fibrous stroma). Ureteritis cystica, mucosal ulceration, and papillomas may also be found. In contrast to vesical bilharziasis, the development of a carcinoma in an affected ureter is rare.

Diagnosis is by IVU or retrograde ureterography. Cystoscopy is essential to exclude vesical involvement and bladder cancer, and also to obtain histology if possible. Etiology is confirmed by isolation of ova from the urine.

Management is by specific attention to the ureteric problem, medical treatment for the underlying condition, and measures to prevent reinfestation. Surgical management is influenced by the facts that the condition is frequently bilateral and the patients are predominantly young, so conservation takes precedence over nephrectomy.

Iatrogenic strictures

Iatrogenic strictures can occur after gynecologic, general surgical, and orthopedic procedures, and even after urologic surgery (e.g. dormia basket, ureteroscopy, transurethral resection of the prostate, transurethral resection of bladder tumor). They occur most commonly after gynecologic procedures, with an overall incidence of ureteric damage of 0.8–2.5%, rising to 10% in Wertheim's hysterectomy. If the diagnosis is not revealed by early acute symptoms, late presentation occurs, with the symptoms depending on the extent and effect of the stenosis.

Radiation strictures

The overwhelming majority of radiation strictures occur as late sequelae of the management of carcinoma of the cervix.

Malignant strictures

These are usually the result of extrinsic compression, for example by colonic or metastatic tumor (Fig. 23.16).

Obstruction in pregnancy

The ureter, particularly the right ureter, often dilates in pregnancy. The causes are both hormonal and mechanical. Occasionally, genuine obstruction from stones, or compression of the ureter at the pelvic brim, can occur. Intractable pain, renal damage, or sepsis demands urgent diagnosis and treatment, either by nephrostomy drainage or ureteric stenting until parturition (Fig. 23.17).

EQUIVOCAL CHRONIC OBSTRUCTION

Urinary tract dilatation with no demonstrable organic lesion to account for it is a common urologic problem. The dilatation may be obstructive or nonobstructive. Equivocal chronic obstruction is seen in idiopathic hydronephrosis, primary megaureter, ureteric strictures, vesicoureteric reflux, or after pyeloplasty, pyelolithotomy, ureterolithotomy, ureteric reimplantation, and urinary diversions (Fig. 23.18).

The overwhelming message in managing these problems is that dilatation does not necessarily mean obstruction. It is indefensible to operate on a dilated urinary tract without definite proof that obstruction is present, and it is equally indefensible not to treat an obstructed dilated tract.

Urography, ultrasound, and the other available imaging modalities (e.g. CT, magnetic resonance imaging) cannot distinguish between obstructive and nonobstructive dilatation; neither can unmodified renography.

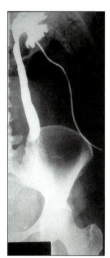

Fig. 23.17 Urinary obstruction in pregnancy. Antegrade pyelogram demonstrating high-grade obstruction at the pelvic brim.

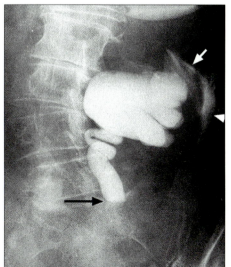

Fig. 23.16 Malignant obstruction of the left ureter demonstrated on antegrade pyelogram. Note the extravasation of contrast (white arrows) and the malignant obstruction of the colon (black arrow).

Causes of equivocal upper tract obstruction
Pelviureteric junction obstruction
Primary megaureter
Vesicoureteric junction obstruction
Urinary diversions
Previous surgery:
ureterolithotomy
reimplantation
pyeloplasty
Previous endourology:
ureteroscopy
dormia basketry
retrograde lithotripsy
Apparent ureteric strictures
Pregnancy
Infective dilatation
Duplications

Fig. 23.18 Causes of equivocal upper tract obstruction.

Investigation and diagnosis

Several techniques are available to investigate equivocal obstruction and make the distinction between obstructive and nonobstructive dilatation:

- diuresis renography;
- perfusion pressure flow studies;
- diuresis urography; and
- parenchymal transit time studies.

The first two of these modalities are those most commonly used.

Diuresis renography

Diuresis renography is now widely accepted for the evaluation of upper tract dilatation and is described in Chapter 10[23–27]. Two techniques are currently recommended, the traditional F+20 procedure (Fig. 23.19), in which the renogram is carried out and furosemide (frusemide) given 20 minutes after the radionuclide injection; and the F-15 technique, in which the furosemide is given 15 minutes before the radionuclide to ensure maximal diuresis. The radiopharmaceutical agents of choice are ^{123}I-hippuran and ^{99m}Tc-mercaptoacetyltriglycine (^{99m}Tc-MAG3), as these agents give fewer technical problems and equivocal responses than ^{99m}Tc-DTPA.

Attention to underlying renal function is necessary to ensure accurate interpretation of washout curves and to distinguish between good diuresis with impaired washout along an obstructed outflow tract, and poor diuresis with slow washout along a normal outflow tract. For a flow rate of 10mL/min to be achieved from furosemide, the single-kidney GFR must be greater than 16mL/min. Diuresis renography is widely used to assess the dilated upper urinary tract, and attention to the choice of radiopharmaceutical agent, the use of the F-15 technique, and appreciation of the roles of posture and bladder status have

resulted in reliable results with a very low rate of equivocal responses.

Perfusion pressure flow studies

Perfusion pressure flow studies are useful in some cases. The technique measures pressure changes proximal to the site of suspected obstruction during perfusion through a nephrostomy catheter at 10mL/min (Fig. 23.20). If the pressure rise is < 15cmH$_2$O (1.5kPa), obstruction is said to be excluded. A pressure rise of 15–22cmH$_2$O (1.5–2.2kPa) is equivocal, and a pressure rise > 22cmH$_2$O (2.2kPa) is consistent with obstruction. The invasive nature of this technique favors initial diuresis renography assessment, but it is useful in cases in which doubts about the presence of obstruction are not resolved by simpler techniques.

Parenchymal transit time studies

This radionuclide technique, using ^{99m}Tc-DTPA or ^{123}I-labelled orthoiodohippurate (^{123}I-OIH), relies on its ability to separate the renal parenchyma from the collecting system while replaying images from data acquired during gamma camera renography.

The influence of posture and bladder effects in dilated upper tracts

Posture

The effect of posture on the dilated upper tract must be appreciated. Stasis in a dilated upper tract can mimic obstruction on investigation, especially on renography (see Fig. 23.21). If the erect sitting position is not chosen for examination, moving the supine patient to the erect position during examination or repeating the examination erect after an initially supine study may be necessary to clarify postural effects[26]. The same can be said for urography and ultrasound studies.

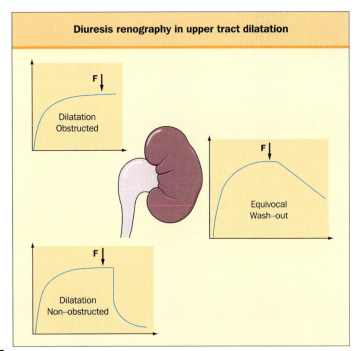

Fig. 23.19 Diuresis renography in upper tract dilatation. Three types of results are shown: obstructive dilatation, non-obstructive dilatation, and an equivocal result. (F, furosemide.)

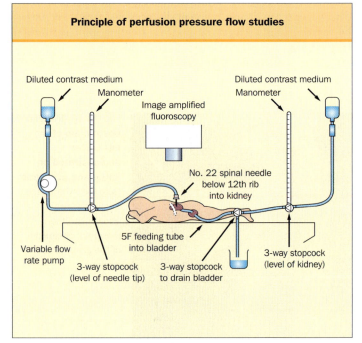

Fig. 23.20 Principle of perfusion pressure flow studies.

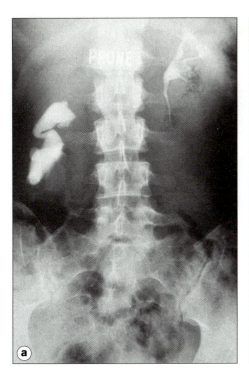

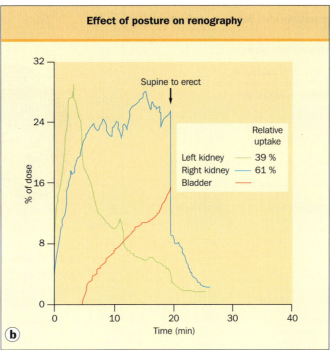

Effect of posture on renography

Fig. 23.21 Effect of posture on renography.
(a) Intravenous urogram demonstrating slightly dilated, malrotated kidney. (b) Renogram in the same patient. Note the apparently obstructive curve in the supine position and the dramatic spontaneous drainage from the kidney with the patient erect.

Interactive bladder effects

A full or rapidly filling bladder, or a bladder with poor compliance, may affect upper tract emptying, giving false-positive results for upper tract obstruction. Such results may be avoided by an indwelling open catheter, although this is not always necessary. During renography, interactive effects of the bladder on renal emptying can be investigated by asking the patient to pass urine 20 minutes into the test. Assuming that there is no voiding dysfunction, the effect of bladder emptying on the upper tracts is reflected in the curves. Certain groups of patients, however, are unable to respond to this request and require an open indwelling catheter. These patients include those with:

- lower tract obstruction;
- demonstrable postvoiding residual urine;
- known voiding dysfunction;
- neuropathic bladder; and
- vesicoureteric reflux.

Ureteropelvic junction obstruction

Ureteropelvic junction obstruction (idiopathic hydronephrosis) is a congenital condition of unknown etiology. It results in variable degrees of loin pain and obstructive uropathy. It can present at any age and afflict either sex, and it may be unilateral or bilateral (Fig. 23.22).

None of the suggested etiologies (Fig. 23.23) is proved. The presenting clinical features are listed in Figure 23.24.

Pathogenesis

In the normal kidney, pacemakers in the minor calices initiate contraction waves, which pass distally down the renal pelvis toward the ureter. Their transmission depends on urine flow rates. At low rates, proximal contractions may falter and fade away without reaching the distal pelvis. With increasing diuresis, contractions are transmitted to the distal renal pelvis, and coupling, or direct transmission of contraction from the renal pelvis to the upper ureter, occurs. At moderate flow rates, 1:1 coupling

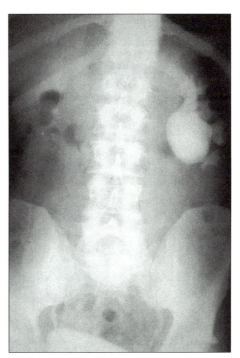

Fig. 23.22 Intravenous urogram appearance of ureteropelvic junction obstruction.

is achieved, and the renal pelvis can be regarded as pacing ureteric peristalsis (Fig. 23.25). At high flow rates, in the absence of any obstructive lesion, open tube flow occurs.

Crucial to understanding of UPJ obstruction is the appreciation that, under normal circumstances, the renal pelvis delivers urine to a proximal ureter that is open, receptive, and able to accept delivery, so that the ureter is stretched as it accepts the urine, stimulating distal bolus transmission by peristalsis.

In idiopathic hydronephrosis, the ureter is not receptive to the delivery of a renal pelvic bolus; the pressure required to open the UPJ for bolus delivery may be higher than normal, and passive ureteric filling is not seen on screening. The distal pelvis is

Suggested causes of ureteropelvic junction obstruction

Types	Suggested causes
Embryological	Physiologic constriction Adherence of ureter to renal pelvis Delayed canalization
Pediatric	Fetal folds Ureteric papillomata Vesicoureteric reflux
Predisposing features	High insertion of ureter into renal pelvis Square-shaped renal pelvis Aberrant vessels across UPJ
Congenital	Regional excess of longitudinal muscle at UPJ Absence of muscle at UPJ Cuff of collagen around UPJ Unknown etiology with non-specific secondary collagen deposition throughout renal pelvis
Associated features	Ureteric kinks Ureteric angulation Ureteric adhesions
Acquired PUJ obstruction	Ureteric tumor Ureteric stone Post-inflammatory scarring Ischemic stricture

Fig. 23.23 Suggested causes of ureteropelvic junction obstruction.

Presenting symptoms in ureteropelvic junction obstruction

Flank pain

Urinary tract infection with flank pain

Pain after drinking

Hematuria

Exercise-induced hematuria

Renal colic

Chance finding

Fig. 23.24 Presenting symptoms of ureteropelvic junction obstruction.

Physiology of urine transport

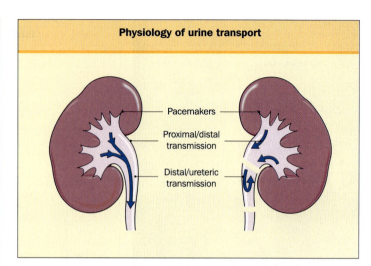

Fig. 23.25 Physiology of urine transport and pathophysiology of ureteropelvic junction obstruction. Physiology of urine transport in the normal kidney (left); pathophysiology of ureteropelvic junction obstruction (right).

Past and present operations for ureteropelvic junction obstruction

Previously used procedures

Nephroplasty
Fixation of aberrant vessels
Transposition of aberrant vessels
Renal denervation
Intubated ureterostomy
Flap (straight)
Dismembered pyeloplasty

Currently used procedures

Anderson–Hynes dismembered pyeloplasty
Foley Y–V plasty
Culp–De Weerd spiral flap

Recently introduced procedures

Percutaneous antegrade endopyelotomy
Retrograde endopyelotomy
Balloon dilatation ('endoburst')
Laparoscopic pyeloplasty

Fig. 23.26 Past and present operations for ureteropelvic junction obstruction.

dissociated from the proximal ureter and, with increasing dilatation, the proximal pelvis becomes dissociated from the distal pelvis, making transmission of pacemaker-induced contractions ineffective (Fig. 23.25).

Thus, peristaltic transmission and bolus volume are both reduced, which grossly interferes with the efficiency of urine transport. These abnormalities predispose to the further accumulation of urine in the renal pelvis and further dilatation of the pelvicaliceal system.

Investigation and diagnosis

The diagnosis of idiopathic hydronephrosis depends initially on the radiographic or ultrasound detection of a dilated renal pelvis. Once dilatation is detected, it becomes necessary to determine the significance of the finding and whether it is evidence of a genuine obstruction or of a static, nonobstructive dilatation reflecting some prior renal event that is no longer a threat to renal function. (The same applies to any of the other causes of equivocal obstruction.) Diuresis renography remains the first-choice investigation for this purpose.

Treatment of ureteropelvic junction obstruction

Various operations have been used for the correction of UPJ obstruction (Fig. 23.26). The ones discussed here are those that are in current use.

Anderson–Hynes pyeloplasty				
Line of incision	Pelviureteric junction removed (dismembered)	Pyeloplasty anastomosis begun	Posterior layer completed	Final appearance

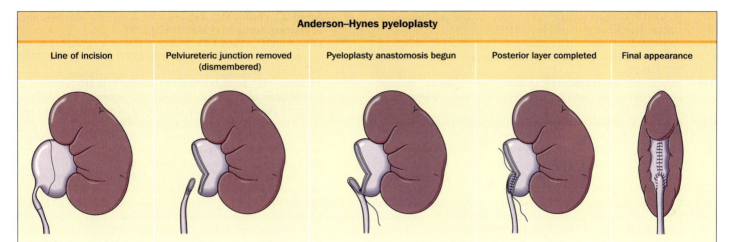

Fig. 23.27 Anderson–Hynes pyeloplasty.

Anderson–Hynes pyeloplasty

Dismembered pyeloplasty, usually by the Anderson–Hynes technique, is the most commonly performed operation for UPJ obstruction. It involves excision of the site of obstruction, the UPJ, and at the same time excision of redundant pelvis and reduction in the renal pelvic volume. The spatulated ureter is anastomosed to the inferior flap of the pelvis, to produce a wide open UPJ. The technique is appropriate to virtually all cases except those with a small tight intrarenal pelvis or long segments of ureteric stricturing. It also allows transposition of the UPJ when there are associated aberrant vessels (Fig. 23.27).

Foley Y–V plasty

The Foley Y–V plasty is most useful in small renal pelvises and ureters with high insertion. It does not allow transposition of lower pole vessels.

Culp–De Weerd spiral flap

Several procedures have been developed to produce a flap of renal pelvis that can be turned down to anastomose to the adjacent ureter to bridge long segments of narrow or strictured ureter associated with UPJ obstruction. The Culp–De Weerd spiral flap procedure is the one most commonly used.

Nonsurgical management

Some recent nonsurgical techniques for the management of UPJ obstruction include antegrade endopyelotomy, retrograde (Acusize) endopyelotomy, balloon dilatation (endoburst), and laparoscopic pyeloplasty. None has yet been shown to be superior in the long term to pyeloplasty.

Other causes

Other causes of urinary tract dilatation in which obstruction must be confirmed or excluded include primary megaureter (see Chapter 14), urinary diversions (see Chapter 31), ureteric strictures (see above), vesicoureteric reflux (see Chapter 18), and cases that occur after pyeloplasty, ureteric reimplantation, or endourologic ureteric manipulations.

REFERENCES

1. Hinman F, Lee-Brown RK. Pyelovenous backflow. Its relation to pelvic reabsorption, to hydronephrosis and to accidents of pyelography. JAMA. 1924;82:607.

2. Wilson DR. Pathophysiology of obstructive nephropathy. Kidney Int. 1980;18:281.

3. Gillenwater JY. The pathophysiology of urinary obstruction. In: Walsh PC, Gittes RF, Perlmutter AD, Stamey TA, eds. Campbell's urology, 5th edn. Philadelphia: WB Saunders; 1986: 542–75.

4. Hinman F. Experimental hydronephrosis – repair following ureterocystoneostomy in white rats with complete ureteral obstruction. J Urol. 1919;3:147.

5. Klahr S. Pathophysiology of obstructive nephropathy. Kidney Int. 1983;23:414–20.

6. Moody TE, Vaughan ED Jr, Gillenwater JY. Relationship between renal blood flow and ureteral pressure during 18 hours of total unilateral ureteral occlusion. Implications for changing sites of increased renal resistance. Invest Urol. 1975;13:246–51.

7. Vaughan ED Jr, Sorenson EJ, Gillenwater JY. The renal hemodynamic response to chronic unilateral complete ureteral occlusion. Invest Urol. 1970;8:78–90.

8. Talner L, O'Reilly PH. Urinary tract obstruction. In: HM Pollack, BL McLennan, eds. Clinical urography. Philadelphia: WB Saunders; in press.

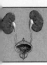

9. Bretland PM. Acute ureteric obstruction – clinical and radiological aspects. Proc R Soc Med. 1974;67:1215.

10. Yarger WE, Griffith LD. Intrarenal hemodynamics following chronic unilateral obstruction in the dog. Am J Physiol. 1974; 227:816–26.

11. Huland H, Leichtweiss H-P, Augustin HJ. Changes in renal hemodynamics in experimental hydronephrosis. Invest Urol. 1980;18:274.

12. Kerr WS Jr. Effects of complete ureteral obstruction in dogs on kidney function. Am J Physiol. 1956;184:521.

13. Huland H, Gonnermann D, Leichtweiss HP, Dietrich-Hennings R. Reversibility of preglomerular vasoconstriction in the first weeks after complete unilateral ureteral obstruction by inhibition of prostaglandin synthesis. J Urol. 1983;130:820–4.

14. Chevalier RL, Jones CE. Contribution of endogenous vasoactive compounds to renal vascular resistance in neonatal chronic partial ureteral obstruction. J Urol. 1986;136:532–6.

15. Taylor KJW, Kraus V. Grey-scale ultrasound imaging: assessment of acute hydronephrosis. Br J Urol. 1975;47:593.

16. Ellenbogen PH, Scheible FW, Talner LB, Leopold GR. Sensitivity of gray scale ultrasound in detecting urinary tract obstruction. AJR. 1978;130:731.

17. Bosniak MA, Megibow AJ, Ambos MA, et al. Computed tomography of ureteral obstruction. AJR. 1982;138:1107.

18. Cronan JJ, Amis ES, Zeman RK, Dorfman GS. Obstruction of the upper-pole moiety in renal duplication in adults: CT evaluation. Radiology. 1986:161:17.

19. Scharf SC, Blaufox MD. Radionuclides in the evaluation of urinary obstruction. Semin Nucl Med. 1982;12:254.

20. Chisholm GD, Chibber PJ, Wallace DMA, et al. DMSA scan and the prediction of recovery in obstructive uropathy. Eur Urol. 1982;8:227–30.

21. Thomsen HS, Hvid-Jacobsen K, Meyhoff H-H, Nielsen SL. Combination of DMSA-scintigraphy and hippuran renography in unilateral obstructive nephropathy. Improved prediction of recovery after intervention. Acta Radiol. 1987;28:653.

22. Jones DA, George NJR, O'Reilly PH, Barnard RJ. The biphasic nature of renal functional recovery following relief of chronic obstructive uropathy. Br J Urol. 1988;61:192.

23. O'Reilly PH, Testa HJ, Lawson RS, et al. Diuresis renography in equivocal urinary tract obstruction. Br J Urol. 1978;50:76.

24. O'Reilly PH, Aurell M, Britton K, Kletter K, Rosenthal L, Testa T. Consensus on diuresis renography for investigation of the dilated upper urinary tract. J Nucl Med. 1996;37:1872.

25. English PJ, Testa HJ, Lawson RS, et al. Modified method of diuresis renography for the assessment of equivocal ureteropelvic junction obstruction. Br J Urol. 1987;59:10.

26. Upsdell SM, Leeson SM, Brooman JC, O'Reilly PH. Diuretic-induced urinary flow rates at varying clearances and their relevance to the performance and interpretation of diuresis renography. Br J Urol. 1988;61:14.

27. Gordon I, Mialdea-Fernandez RM, Peters AM. Ureteropelvic junction obstruction: the value of a post-micturition view in ^{99m}Tc DTPA diuretic renography. Br J Urol. 1988;61:409.

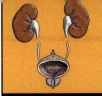

Chapter 24

Renal and Ureteric Tumors

Robert C Flanigan and Fernando J Kim

KEY POINTS

- The apparent incidence of renal cell carcinoma (RCC) is increasing.
- Renal tumors may be associated with a number of paraneoplastic syndromes.
- Studies of hereditary forms of RCC are unlocking the genetic basis of the disease.
- Nephron-sparing surgery is becoming increasingly accepted for patients in specific clinical groups.
- The prognosis for patients with metastatic RCC disease remains guarded.
- Standard treatment for transitional cell carcinoma of the upper urinary tract remains nephroureterectomy.

RENAL TUMORS

The introduction of surgical interventions for renal diseases more than 100 years ago provided the clinical and histopathologic information that formed today's current concepts of renal tumors[1].

History[2]

- 1826 – Konig first described the anatomy of kidney tumors.
- 1855 – Robin concluded that renal carcinoma arose from renal tubular epithelium.
- 1861 – Wolcott reported the first documented nephrectomy. He mistakenly operated a tumor mass he presumed was a hepatoma.
- 1869 – Simon performed the first planned nephrectomy for persistent ureteral fistula.
- 1870 – Gilmore performed the first planned nephrectomy in the USA (AL). The patient was treated for persistent urinary infection in a renal atrophic pyelonephritis.
- 1903 – Albarran and Imbert elucidated and corrected the misconception and unfortunate semantic of the term 'hypernephroma', which predominated in the literature describing parenchymal tumors of primary renal origin. Prior to that study it was conjectured that the renal clear cell tumors originated from adrenal rests.

Classification

Historically, different renal tumor classifications were created using radiographic or histologic characteristics. In 1980, Glenn simplified the comprehensive classification of renal tumors previously described by Deming and Harvard[3] (Fig. 24.1).

Pathological classification of renal tumors	
Benign	**Malignant**
Simple cyst	Renal carcinoma
Angiomyolipoma	Upper tract urothelial cancers
Oncocytoma	Lymphoma
Pseudotumor	Leiomyosarcoma
Reninoma	Hemangiopericytoma
Pheochromocytoma	Liposarcoma
Leiomyoma	Rhabdomyosarcoma
Hemangioma	Schwannoma
Cystic nephroma	Osteosarcoma
Fibroma	Fibrous histiocytoma
Arteriovenous malformation	Neurofibrosarcoma
Hemangiopericytoma	Metastatic disease
Renal artery aneurysm	Invasion by adjacent neoplasm
Inflammatory	Carcinoid
Abscess	Adult Wilms' tumor
Pyelonephritis	Wilms tumor
Xanthogranulomatous pyelonephritis	Mesoblastic nephroma
Infected renal cyst	Leukemia
Tuberculosis	
Rheumatic granuloma	

Figure 24.1 Pathological classification of renal tumors.

BENIGN RENAL TUMORS

Benign renal tumors may arise from any cell type within and around the kidney.

SIMPLE CYSTS

Renal cysts are the most common benign renal mass lesions (70% of asymptomatic renal masses). Cysts may be single or multiple and unilateral or bilateral. Usually, they are asymptomatic and have no clinical significance[4]. When lesions are not exclusively simple cysts but there are questionable malignant features, or when they present with clinical symptoms caused by growth, further evaluation must be undertaken. As a result of modern uroradiographic techniques renal cell carcinoma (RCC) can be distinguished from simple cysts with great accuracy.

Cortical adenoma

Most renal adenomas are discovered incidentally. Renal adenomas are characterized microscopically by uniform basophilic or acidophilic cells with monotonous nuclear and cellular composition[5]. Although symptoms are unusual, hematuria may occur when the tumor involves the collecting system or adjacent vessels. Small lesions (<1cm) without any malignant features (e.g. calcification, arteriovenous fistulae, or venous pooling) are indistinguishable from small renal adenocarcinoma by computed tomography (CT) or arteriography. Histologically, presence of clear cells, mitotic activity, nuclear polymorphism, cell stratification, or necrosis should suggest a small renal cell carcinoma[6]. For renal parenchymal lesions (<3cm) segmental resection or wedge resection may be appropriate but the uncertainty of malignancy may lead surgeons to treat the lesion more aggressively, as if it was RCC.

Renal oncocytoma

Renal oncocytomas are almost invariably benign tumors. The exact incidence of this pathology compared with other renal tumors is unknown; however, current studies suggest that 3–7% of solid renocortical tumors previously classified as RCCs were typical renal oncocytomas[7]. Renal oncocytomas are more common in males than in females and occur with the same age incidence as RCCs. These tumors are typically unifocal but may be bilateral (synchronous or asynchronous) in approximately 6% of cases. Renal oncocytomas are characterized histologically by highly differentiated, large, eosinophilic cells with granular cytoplasm and a typical polygonal form. Mitoses are rare, and the cells typically have a profusion of mitochondria rich in cristae with uniform and low-grade nuclei. The typical cellular appearance suggests an origin from the distal renal tubules – in particular, from the cells of the collecting tubules[8,9].

Usually the surgical specimen has the appearance of a well-circumscribed, round and encapsulated, tan or light brown lesion. The central dense fibrous band with trabeculae extending out in a stellate pattern is probably responsible for the radiographic appearance (central scar) often observed preoperatively by CT, magnetic resonance imaging (MRI), or ultrasound (US) and suggesting the diagnosis of oncocytoma preoperatively.

The arterial phase of an angiogram may reveal a characteristic spoke-wheel or stellate pattern, which is seldom associated with venous pooling or arteriovenous fistulae[10]. Oncocytomas, however, are generally felt to be radiologically indistinguishable from a hypovascular RCC[11].

The loss of chromosomes 1 and Y[12,13] and loss of human leukocyte antigen class I antigen expression have been associated with this tumor[14].

The majority of tumors are asymptomatic and are discovered incidentally on imaging studies performed for unrelated conditions. However, patients may have gross or microscopic hematuria, abdominal pain, or flank mass. Renal oncocytomas are generally managed with partial nephrectomy (including frozen section control of surgical margin) or radical nephrectomy. While high-risk or elderly patients may be considered for observation, most patients deserve renal exploration and total or partial nephrectomy with a safe excisional margin[15].

Renal angiomyolipoma

Renal angiomyolipoma (hamartoma) is a benign tumor that may occur alone or as part of the syndrome associated with tuberous sclerosis. Tuberous sclerosis is a hereditary syndrome characterized by mental retardation, epilepsy, and adenoma sebaceum. In these patients, angiomyolipomas may also be found in the brain, eye, heart, lung, and bone[16]. Patients with tuberous sclerosis require careful screening for the presence of renal tumors[17]. Younger patients often have large, symptomatic, multifocal or bilateral tumors that require surgery[18]. It is believed that extrarenal and lymph node involvement reflects multicentricity rather than metastasis[19].

The tumors are often yellow and gray in color and may clinically cause profuse hemorrhage. The microscopic features define the tumor's name: unusual blood vessels, clusters of adipocytes, and sheets of smooth muscle. Pleomorphism is common and mitotic figures are seen rarely[20].

The presence of a mass composed nearly entirely of fat on radiologic imaging is characteristic of angiomyolipoma[21]. When seen on sonography, the tumor appears highly echogenic.

Often, these tumors are detected incidentally in patients who undergo CT scans for unrelated abdominal problems or in patients with tuberous sclerosis.

When large in size, angiomyolipomas may cause local discomfort and gastrointestinal symptoms by compression of the gastrointestinal tract. Finally, massive hemorrhage within the lesion may cause sudden pain and/or severe hypotension.

The management of angiomyolipoma is controversial. Presently, the recommendation for asymptomatic simple lesions less than 4cm in diameter is observation with annual CT or ultrasound studies. Generally, these tumors do not increase in size even after many years of followup. Asymptomatic or mildly symptomatic patients, or patients with tumors more than 4cm require semiannual followup or treatment including excision or arterial embolization[22]. Selective arterial embolization or kidney-sparing surgery may be considered for patients with large angiomyolipomas or patients with symptoms. Although angio-infarction does not always decrease the size of tumors, bleeding may be prevented. Embolization should be attempted as primary treatment in patients with hemorrhage due to angiomyolipoma.

Fibroma

Fibromas may arise from renal parenchyma, the perinephric tissues, and the renal capsule[23]. These benign tumors are rare and often resemble uterine fibroids. Occasionally they are difficult to distinguish from fibrosarcomas of the retroperitoneum.

When symptoms occur, they are usually related to tumor growth with either distortion of the collecting system or invasion of adjacent structures.

Microscopically, fibromas have sheets of fibroblasts or a loose myxomatous stroma. There are no specific radiographic characteristics to distinguish these tumors from hypovascular malignant tumors. A radical nephrectomy is usually performed because of the uncertainty of the diagnosis, but awareness of their benign nature warrants partial nephrectomy or laparoscopic management in selected cases.

Other benign tumors

Other benign renal lesions include lipomas, myomas, lymphangiomas, and hemangiomas. One of the rarest is the functional renin-secreting juxtaglomerular tumor. These arise from the juxtaglomerular cells, typically in young patients[24]. They present with hypertension, elevated serum renin levels (extremely high differential renal-vein:plasma renin ratio), and hyperaldosteronism. They are usually small (2–3cm in diameter). Grossly, the tumors are gray-yellow with hemorrhagic areas; microscopically, they are typical hemangiopericytomas. Electron microscopic studies reveal the characteristics of the juxtaglomerular cells and tumor extracts may be shown to contain high concentrations of renin. This tumor is always benign and should be distinguished from the generally larger, nonfunctional, and sometimes malignant renal hemangiopericytoma.

MALIGNANT RENAL TUMORS – RENAL CELL CARCINOMA

Epidemiology
Renal cell carcinoma accounts for approximately 3% of adult malignancies. It appears that the incidence of renal cell carcinoma is increasing, probably as a result of more frequent diagnostic imaging studies (CT and US). Approximately 28,000 new cases of renal carcinoma are diagnosed annually in the USA, associated with 11,000 deaths[25].

Renal cell carcinoma is more common among males (2:1 male:female ratio) and urban residents (Fig. 24.2). Although RCC is a tumor of adults (fourth to sixth decades of life), it may occasionally occur in younger age groups. Two distinct cohorts of familial renal carcinoma have been defined: those with hereditary von Hippel–Lindau syndrome (VHL)[26] and those with hereditary papillary RCC.

Etiology
Renal cell carcinomas most commonly arise from the proximal convoluted tubule but distinct tumor types arising from the distal tubules or collecting duct cells have been identified[27] (Fig. 24.3).

Risk factors
In animal models, a number of etiologic factors have been identified for the development of RCC but no specific agent has been defined in humans. Smoking (cigarettes, pipes, or cigars) is a risk factor and the risk of RCC has been directly related to duration of smoking and inversely to the starting age[28]. No definitive relationship between occupational and industrial carcinogens and RCC has been documented. RCCs are found more commonly in patients with end-stage disease and in patients with polycystic kidney disease than in the normal population. Growth factors, such as TGF-α and TGF-β have been implicated as modulators and potentiators of RCC.

Cytogenetics
In the early 1980s, investigators observed that chromosomal deletions and translocations involving the short arm of chromosome 3 (3p) were associated with many RCCs and that the loss of a segment of chromosome 3 could be an early event in RCC development[29] (Fig. 24.4). The majority of patients with RCC also have overexpression of c-*myc*, c-Ha-*ras*, c-*fos*, c-*fms*, and f-*raf-1*, and epidermal growth factor receptor (c-*erb* B-1) mRNA and underexpression of HER-2 (*erb* B-2) mRNA[30]. Also, there is evidence that the activation of mitogen-activated protein (MAP) kinase pathway may play a pivotal role in the carcinogenesis and malignant potentiation of RCC[31].

Recent molecular studies have been very helpful in the categorization of the various types of RCC and their different prognostic characteristics[30,31] (Fig. 24.5).

Renal cell carcinoma: epidemiology
Sporadic
5th–7th decade
Male:female ratio 2:1
Cigarette smoking
Asbestos exposure
Long-term kidney dialysis
Familial
Autosomal-dominant inheritance
Von Hippel–Lindau disease (3p)
Hereditary papillary renal cell carcinoma (non 3p)
Familial clear cell renal cell carcinoma without other manifestations of von Hippel–Lindau disease (3p)

Figure 24.2 Renal cell carcinoma: epidemiology.

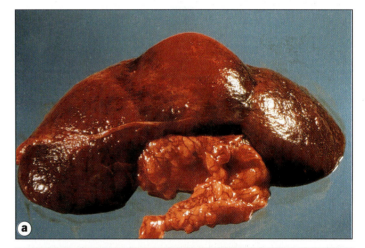

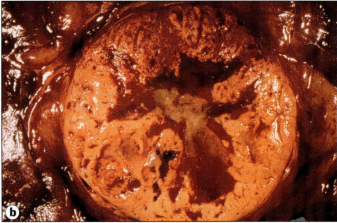

Figure 24.3 Classic renal cell carcinoma. (a) After radical nephrectomy – all fat and Gerota's fascia stripped to show central lesion. (B) Typical cross-sectional appearance of golden yellow tumour.

Chromosomal deletions and translocations of the short arm of chromosome 3 (3p) are associated with many renal cell carcinomas

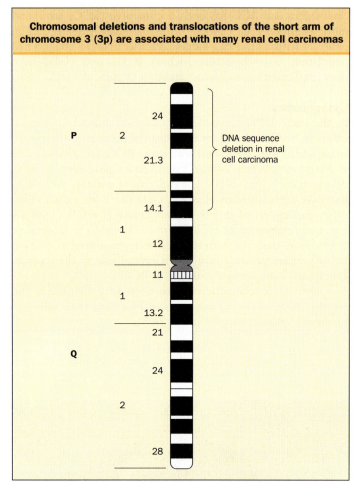

DNA sequence deletion in renal cell carcinoma

Figure 24.4 Chromosomal deletions and translocations of the short arm of chromosome 3 (3p) are associated with many renal cell carcinomas. The loss of a segment of chromosome 3 could be an early event in renal cell carcinoma development.

Hereditary papillary renal cell carcinoma may be caused by genetic mutation in the *MET* proto-oncogene

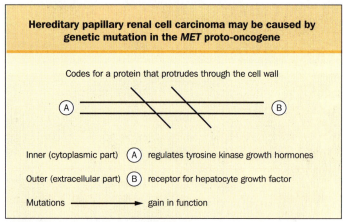

Codes for a protein that protrudes through the cell wall

Ⓐ ————————————— Ⓑ

Inner (cytoplasmic part)	Ⓐ	regulates tyrosine kinase growth hormones
Outer (extracellular part)	Ⓑ	receptor for hepatocyte growth factor
Mutations	⟶	gain in function

Figure 24.5 Hereditary papillary renal cell carcinoma may be caused by genetic mutation in the *MET* proto-oncogene.

Hereditary forms of renal cell carcinoma
Renal cell carcinoma and von Hippel–Lindau disease
Von Hippel–Lindau disease is a rare familial cancer syndrome (1 in 36,000 births) in which affected individuals tend to develop bilateral, multifocal renal tumors and cysts, hemangioblastomas

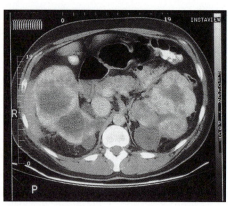

Figure 24.6 Computed tomography in patients with von Hippel–Lindau disease. Bilateral cysts and tumors present.

of the cerebellum and spine, retinal hemangiomas, pheo-chromocytomas, pancreatic islet cell tumors, and epididymal cystadenomas (Fig. 24.6). In these cases, RCC is consistently clear-cell type and when not detected and treated is the principal cause of mortality in up to 45% of patients. Studies on familial RCC not only revealed that the same gene might be involved in the origin of RCC and VHL, but also that the VHL gene had characteristics of a tumor suppressor gene. Mutant genes give rise to upregulation of endothelial growth factor. Von Hippel–Lindau syndrome occurs in equal inheritance in men and women. Furthermore, at least three exons (coding regions) of the gene have been identified that are mutated differently in different families. This gives rise to specific expression of the disease in families, e.g. (1) involvement of kidney/brain/eyes, (2) kidney/ brain/adrenal pheochromocytoma, or (3) adrenal pheochromocytoma only[32].

Hereditary papillary renal cell carcinoma
Hereditary papillary renal cell carcinoma, like VHL disease, gives rise to bilateral multiple tumors. It appears to have an autosomal dominant inheritance. The genetic change seems to be a mutation in the *MET* proto-oncogene. This proto-oncogene regulates tyrosine kinase growth hormones (Fig. 24.5).

Multidrug resistance
Renal cell carcinoma remains resistant to currently available chemotherapeutic agents. The basis for this multidrug resist-ance appears to be related to a transmembrane glycoprotein (P170) and a mechanism associated with the glutathione redox cycle, which is involved in the intracellular binding and detoxification of chemotherapeutic agents[33].

Pathology – macroscopic
Renal cell carcinomas are typically round, varying in size (Figs 24.3 & 24.7). They generally have a pseudocapsule composed of compressed parenchyma and fibrous tissue. Areas of yellowish or brownish soft tumor are usually interposed between patches of hemorrhage and necrosis. Cysts are frequent, probably resulting from segmental necrosis and resorption, and calcification can also occur. Generally, the collecting system is displaced and often invaded. The Gerota's fascia seems to provide a barrier against local spread but it may be compressed and invaded. RCC is typically unilateral but synchronous or asynchronous bilateral lesions occur in approximately 2% of cases.

Renal cancers: tumor types			
Tumor type	% of cancers	Chromosomal abnormality	Prognostic factors
Clear/granular cell (5% spindle cell)	80	Loss of 3p13	Stage, grade, and cell type
Papillary	14	Loss of 4; trisomy 7 and 17	Tendency to low grade and stage
Oncocytic	2	Loss of 4 (?1,22)	Benign unless atypical
Chromophobe	4	Loss of heterozy 3p, 5p, 17p	Better prognosis than typical renal cell carcinoma
Collecting duct carcinoma (Bellini duct)	<1	Not identified	Aggressive

Figure 24.7 Renal cancers: tumor types.

Pathology – microscopic

Clear cell variant
- Present in more than 80% of RCC.
- Microscopic features – polygonal or round cells with abundant cytoplasm. Granular cells have eosinophilic cytoplasm and abundant mitochondria.
- Immunohistochemical features – approximately 50% are vimentin-positive and almost all renal adenocarcinomas express cytokeratin 8 and 18.

Papillary variant
- Present in 14% of RCC
- Macroscopic features – small, nearly completely encapsulated, and confined to the cortex.
- Microscopic features – nuclear anaplasia is uncommon and tumors are indistinguishable from renal adenocarcinomas.
- Cytogenetic features – loss of the Y chromosome along with a trisomy of chromosomes 7 and 17.

Sarcomatoid variant
- Aggressive behavior and poor prognosis.
- Microscopic features – spindle cell pattern, may resemble pleomorphic mesenchymal cells.

Chromophobe variant
- Present in 4% of RCC
- Microscopic features – light and transparent cytoplasm, finely reticular, with moderately intense eosinophilia.
- Electron microscopic features – cytoplasm displays abundant reticular structures (microvesicles) poor in glycogen.

Oncocytic variant
- Present in 2% of RCC.
- Tends to be benign unless atypical.

Collecting duct variant
- Comprises <1% of RCC.
- Aggressive clinical behavior.

Grading
Nuclear grade probably has prognostic significance and is a predictor of survival that is independent of pathologic stage[34].

Definition of TNM staging system	
Primary tumor	Description
TX	Primary tumor cannot be assessed
T0	No evidence of primary tumor
T1	Tumor ≤ 7cm in greatest dimension limited to the kidney
T2	Tumor >7cm in greatest dimension limited to the kidney
T3	Tumor extends into major veins or invades the ipsilateral adrenal gland or perinephric tissues, but confined to Gerota's fascia
T3a	Tumor invades the ipsilateral adrenal gland or perinephric tissues, but confined to Gerota's fascia
T3b	Tumor grossly extends into the renal vein(s) involvement or vena cava below the diaphragm
T3c	Tumor grossly extends into the renal vein(s) involvement or vena cava above the diaphragm
T4	Tumor invades beyond Gerota's fascia
N1	Single ipsilateral node involved
N2	Multiple regional, contralateral, or bilateral nodes involved
N3	Fixed regional nodes
N4	Juxtaregional nodes involved
M1	Distant metastases

Figure 24.8 Definition of TNM (tumor, nodes and metastasis) staging system.

Tumors composed mainly of spindle cells seem to have a worse prognosis[34]. Although measurements of DNA ploidy may reflect the tumor heterogeneity and indicate malignant potential, the clinical value of this technique remains to be determined for RCC.

Staging
There has been a recent change in the TNM (tumor, node, and metastasis) staging system, which is the most commonly used for RCC. This change primarily involves the inclusion of tumors confined to the kidney of up to 7cm in size (Fig. 24.8).

The most common sites of metastases in RCC are the lung, liver, subcutaneous tissue, and central nervous system. Staging requires a careful history and physical examination, chest X-ray, complete medical profile [including blood urea nitrogen (BUN), creatinine level, liver function tests, and serum calcium measurement], as well as the above-mentioned radiographic studies.

Signs and symptoms
- The classic triad of pain, hematuria, and flank mass is found in few patients and generally indicates advanced disease. Pain occurs because of tumor invasion into other organs and blood vessels, or urinary outflow obstruction.
- Weight loss, fever, night sweats, and the sudden development of a varicocele in the male patient.
- Hypertension may occur as a result of segmental renal artery occlusion or renin or renin-like substances produced by the tumor.
- Paraneoplastic syndromes causing a myriad of presenting symptoms may be associated with RCC because of increased levels of prostaglandins, glucagon, erythropoietin, 1,25-dihydroxy-cholecalciferol, parathyroid hormone-like factors, human chorionic gonadotrophin, renin, and insulin[35].

Paraneoplastic syndromes related to renal cell carcinoma

Staufer's syndrome

This syndrome is associated with non-metastatic hepatic dysfunction[35]. It is characterized by:

- abnormal liver function tests;
- white blood cell loss;
- fever; and
- areas of hepatic necrosis without hepatic metastases.

Usually, these patients will have clinical improvement, returning to normal function after nephrectomy. The 1-year survival rate is 88%. Persistence or recurrence of this syndrome is almost invariably associated with recurrence of the tumor.

Hypercalcemia

Hypercalcemia may occur in up to 10% of patients with RCC. Although the cause remains unknown, a peptide produced by the tumor, analogous to regions of a parathyroid-hormone-related protein, may be related[35]. A fall in the serum calcium level may be observed after surgical removal of primary tumor. Recurrent hypercalcemia may be associated with skeletal metastases.

Hypertension and increased renin level

Hypertension and elevated serum renin level have been associated with high-stage RCC. The level often normalizes after nephrectomy[35].

Polycythemia and pyrexia of unknown origin

Tumor production of erythropoietin may identify patients with RCC responsive to immunotherapy with interleukin-2 and interferon-α[35]. Pyrexia may be related to production of necrosis factors by the tumor.

Imaging studies

Renal tumors are detected earlier and in lower stages due to increasing use of US, computed axial tomography (CAT), and MRI. Nearly, two thirds of all locally confined renal tumors are currently found serendipitously[36,37].

Intravenous pyelography

Intravenous pyelography (IVP) remains a common technique for the evaluation of patients with hematuria. When a renal mass lesion is identified with IVP, further diagnostic tests are generally required. The cost-effectiveness and accuracy of CT scan and US to evaluate renal lesions may replace the traditional IVP with contrast nephrotomography[36].

Ultrasound

Ultrasound offers an advantage in distinguishing between solid, cystic, and complex masses.

The US criteria for a simple benign cyst include:

- absence of internal echoes;
- round or oval shape;
- smooth and well-defined wall;
- acoustic shadow arising from the edges of the cyst; and
- good US transmission.

Solid masses may show a brighter or lesser echogenicity, little or no through-transmission, poorly demarcated walls, and irregular shape. Clinically insignificant pseudotumors may cause

Bosniak classification	
I (Benign)	Simple cyst
II (Probably benign)	Septated; minimally calcified; nonenhancing high-density; or obviously infected cyst
III (Suspicious)	Multiloculated hemorrhagic; coarse or pleomorphic calcifications; or nonenhancing solid components
IV (Probably malignant)	Marginal irregularity and enhancing solid component – renal cell carcinoma

Figure 24.9 Bosniak classification.

concerns, such as a prominent renal column of Bertin or fetal lobation. When the lesion is equivocal by ultrasound, it is mandatory to perform additional studies, such as radionuclide scan or CT scan, to help differentiate the cyst from a malignant tumor[36]. Highly echogenic malignant renal masses are usually benign angiomyolipomas or hemangiomas.

Magnetic resonance imaging, inferior venous cavography (IVC), and duplex Doppler US may contribute to RCC staging and are particularly useful to evaluate tumor thrombus and its extension.

Computed tomography scanning

Improvements in contrast material and technology have allowed CT to become the method of choice for detecting and staging renal carcinoma. Moreover, cystic lesion density can accurately be measured noninvasively in an outpatient setting. These lesions have been classified by Bosniak (Fig. 24.9). When correlated with angiographic and pathologic findings, CT scans diagnosed correctly cases of renal vein involvement, vena caval extension, perirenal extension, lymph node metastases, and RCC with extension to adjacent organs in up to 91%, 97%, 79%, 87%, and 96% of cases respectively[38,39]. CT is the most cost-effective method of evaluating a suspected renal mass lesion and it should be the first-line technique for that purpose[40]. The downside of CT is the false-positive readings in detecting lymph node involvement or misdiagnosing outer extension of tumor through the capsule. Therefore, one must be careful not to deny patients the potential for surgical cure on the basis of these false-positive readings. Nonetheless, the new-generation CT scanners provide a single test for diagnosis and staging of renal tumors that is minimally invasive and cost-effective.

Magnetic resonance imaging

Magnetic resonance imaging may help in evaluating neoplastic invasion of the renal vein or inferior vena cava without the need for contrast material. It may also be useful to assess bulky tumors multidimensionally, revealing the tumor extent. MRI is less sensitive than CT for solid lesions less than 3cm in diameter[40].

Selective renal arteriography

Presently, indications for selective renal angiography are:

- To evaluate a lesion in solitary kidney prior to a parenchyma-sparing procedure.
- In association with angioinfarction of large RCC or cancers with significant IV thrombus.
- Planning therapy when a metastatic lesion to the kidney is suspected. Metastatic lesions are typically hypovascular.

Prognostic factors (local regional disease)

Stage – Extension beyond capsule, positive lymph nodes – very important

Nuclear grading – Significant

Cell type – Spindle cell worse prognosis

Vena caval involvement – Decreased prognosis if vena cava invasion present; if resectable, prognosis is better (45–65% 5-year survival)

Renal pelvic invasion – ? Significant – often associated with other factors of worse prognosis

Tumor size? – Failure of most studies to control for grade or stage

Renal vein invasion – Probably not important if tumor is otherwise organ confined

Symptomatic versus incidental?

Figure 24.10 Prognostic factors (local regional disease).

Prognostic factors (metastatic disease)

Solitary resectable metastasis

Pulmonary metastasis only

Good performance status

Interval of more than 1 year between nephrectomy and metastasis

Figure 24.11 Prognostic factors (metastatic disease). (Reproduced with permission from Levy et al.[54])

The classic angiographic hallmarks of RCC include neovascularity, arteriovenous fistulae, pooling of contrast media, and accentuation of capsular vessels. Sometimes, the addition of epinephrine (adrenaline) infusion to constrict normal vessels, without constricting tumor vessels, may help with the diagnosis.

Prognosis

Prognostic factors of importance in RCC are different when one examines local/regional versus advanced disease. These factors are listed in Figures 24.10 & 24.11.

Although nuclear grade is the most important microscopic feature that independently correlates with RCC survival (all stages)[41], it seems that the single most important predictor of prognosis is pathologic stage[41]. According to Guinan et al. the 5-year survival rates for Robson's stage 1, 2, 3 and 4 were 75%, 63%, 38%, and 11% respectively[42].

Patients with tumors smaller than 5cm have better survival than those with moderate size RCC (5–10cm), while tumors larger than 10cm usually have a poor prognosis. Nuclear ploidy has been proposed as a possible prognostic marker because of reports demonstrating that the 10-year survival rates in patients with stage I disease were 92% when diploid and 63% for nondiploid tumor patterns. Additionally, patients with metastases showed a significantly better survival in diploid than aneuploid tumors[43]. The routine use of ploidy determination, however, is not yet established. Although controversy exists as to whether renal vein extension may predict poor prognosis, extension to regional lymph nodes, extension through Gerota's fascia, involvement of contiguous organs and distant metastases portend a worse prognosis[43]. In organ-confined tumors, renal vein invasion alone or inferior vena cava involvement (except invasion of the caval wall) has minimal impact on survival. Thus, for locally advanced RCC with tumor thrombus, the 5-year survival rates after complete resection of IVC tumor thrombus have ranged from 47% to 69% while those in metastatic RCC ranged from 0% to 20%. Significant impact on survival was noticed with lymph node or perinephric fat involvement. Patients with tumor extension through Gerota's fascia after incomplete tumor excision had a worse prognosis than those who developed distant metastases without local tumor recurrence[43].

Treatment

Radical nephrectomy

Radical nephrectomy remains an effective method of treatment of primary RCC (Fig. 24.3a). By definition, this procedure encompasses excision of Gerota's fascia and its contents, including the kidney, and perirenal fat. The objective is to excise all tumor with an adequate surgical margin with limited manipulation of the organ to avoid dissemination of neoplastic cells. Although the increase in survival by performing radical nephrectomy versus simple nephrectomy is unknown, radical nephrectomy has become the standard method of surgical therapy.

Adrenalectomy is often added to radical nephrectomy but recent studies have suggested that it may only be necessary in upper pole or large RCCs if the adrenal gland appears normal on radiological appearance[44]. Regional lymphadenectomy is also at times added to radical nephrectomy, and increased survival has been attributed by some authors to the removal of involved lymph nodes. Although significant controversy remains regarding lymphadenectomy in RCC, current data do suggest that patients with micrometastatic lymph node involvement in particular may benefit from regional lymphadenectomy[45].

Some factors that argue against a therapeutic role for lymphadenectomy are:

- Hematogenous and lymphatic spread have the same frequency and most patients with positive lymph nodes eventually have hematogenous metastases. Moreover, many patients without regional lymph nodes spread develop disseminated metastases.
- The lymphatic drainage of RCC is variable and may occur anywhere in the retroperitoneum.

In summary, although the practical therapeutic value of lymphadenectomy remains questionable, it can be accomplished safely and may in selected patients (usually those with high-stage disease) contribute staging information and potentially improve prognosis. The surgical approach to nephrectomy (thoracoabdominal, flank, or extraperitoneal) depends on the surgeons' preference, rather than necessity; however, early ligation of the artery and vein must be achieved to avoid neoplastic cell spread. As noted above, for small lower or mid pole tumors, removal of the ipsilateral adrenal gland is probably not routinely necessary, given the actual rarity of adrenal metastases. The thoracoabdominal incision is particularly suitable for large tumors in the upper pole of the kidney[46]. This technique may include an extraperitoneal or intraperitoneal incision. Extraperitoneal radical nephrectomy can be safely performed with excellent exposure through a flank incision (10th or 11th intercostal space).

Preoperative angiographic renal artery occlusion may reduce hemorrhage, especially in large tumors. However, this procedure does not affect survival. Complications including pain, ileus, sepsis, and dislocation of the infarcting coil may occasionally compromise the ability of the patient to tolerate surgery. The propensity of RCC to invade the renal veins and extend into the cava system is well recognized. It is therefore pivotal that a pre-operative evaluation and delineation of the extent and degree of venous involvement of the carcinoma be undertaken, using non-invasive spiral CT and MRI.

Currently, surgical excision of renal tumor and caval thrombus extension with intraoperative frozen sections of surgical margins remains the treatment of choice and can be safely performed, even with extension into the right atrium. A limited infracaval extension may be managed by local vascular control but supra-diaphragmatic and right atrial extension requires that cardio-pulmonary bypass be performed. Survival rates are reported to be about 64% for 5-year survival and 57% for 10-year survival, even when the tumor extends into the right atrium[38].

In conclusion, the long-term outcome following surgical therapy for renal carcinoma depends on many factors, including the tumor stage, grade, and histologic type.

Several investigators showed a 5-year survival rates after radical nephrectomy for RCC:[47–49].

- Stage 1 – 60–82%
- Stage 2 – 47–80%
- Stage 3 – 35–51%, depending on renal vein involvement without lymph node extension or extracapsular extension
- Stage 4 – virtually 0%.

Nephron-sparing surgery

Renal cell carcinoma may occur in a solitary kidney or bilaterally (synchronously or asynchronously). Recently, the indication for nephron-sparing surgery (NSS) has been expanded to include patients with contralateral normal kidneys (Figs 24.12 & 24.13). An understanding of renal anatomy allows this procedure to be done safely and allows for the preservation of adequate renal parenchyma to maintain life without dialysis. Nephron-sparing surgery techniques include wedge resection, enucleation, and polar amputation.

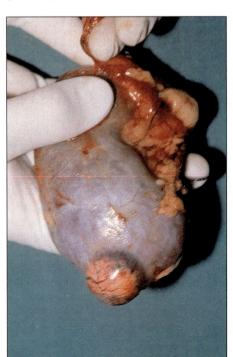

Figure 24.12 Small exophytic renal cell carcinoma. Normal contralateral kidney. This tumor would now almost certainly be removed by nephron sparing surgery.

Indications for partial nephrectomy for renal cell carcinoma
Cancer in solitary kidney
Bilateral renal cell carcinoma
Poorly functioning contralateral kidney
Small peripheral lesion
Incidentally detected tumor
Malignancy uncertain preoperatively
Renal cell carcinoma in von Hippel–Lindau disease
Normal contralateral kidney?

Figure 24.13 Indications for partial nephrectomy for renal cell carcinoma.

Very rarely, autotransplantation following ex vivo excision is needed.

Excision of tumor in a solitary kidney is associated with excellent long-term cancer-free survival and current data allow several conclusions about nephron-sparing surgery:[50,51]

- Survival is significantly better in patients with tumor in a solitary kidney (70–85%) versus bilateral (synchronous or asynchronous) tumors (50–75%).
- Complete removal of the tumor in a solitary kidney, or of bilateral renal tumors, is associated with 72% tumor-free survival at 3 years.
- Survival depends on the stage of the local tumor. Stage I tumors revealed a 3-year survival rate of 80% versus 50% for stage II.
- Bilateral nephrectomy with dialysis is seldom necessary but should be an option for selected patients in this modern era of hemodialysis and transplantation.
- Conservative surgery with enucleation or partial nephrectomy as a treatment for RCC remains controversial despite good results in terms of local control and disease-free survival.

The major disadvantage of nephron-sparing surgery for RCC is the risk of local tumor recurrence, ranging from 2% to 10%. Some of these local tumor recurrences may represent undetected pre-existent multifocal renal tumors[52]. Some surgeons feel that intraoperative sonography, using a 7.5 MHz transducer with Doppler probe, can be valuable to evaluate tumor multifocality, detect associated cysts, and determine the extent of RCC[53].

Postnephrectomy follow-up studies

Recent information suggests that clinical followup of RCCs after nephrectomy can be individualized using tumor stage as the predominant factor that indicates the frequency of testing. One such guideline described by Levy et al.[54] is shown in Figure 24.14.

Lymphadenectomy

The role of lymphadenectomy in the management of RCC remains controversial. Lymphatic involvement in RCC varies by stage of the primary tumor from less than 10% in T1 tumors to nearly 50% in T3b tumors[55]. Some authors have suggested (in nonrandomized studies) an advantage for lymphadenectomy in more advanced focal stages T2 and T3[56]. Golimbu et al. revealed a 10–15% increased 5-year survival in T3 patients after lymphadenectomy but found no advantage in T1 or T2

Stage-specific guidelines for follow-up renal cell carcinoma				
Stage	**Chest X-ray**	**LFT s/alkaline phosphatase**	**Abdominal CT scan**	**Duration**
pT1	Annual	Annual	None*	Lifetime
pT2	6 months (begin month 6)	6 months (begin month 6)	24 months	3 years
	Annual	Annual	60 months	Lifetime
pT3	6 months (begin month 3)	6 months (begin month 3)	24 months	3 years
	Annual	Annual	60 months	Lifetime

Figure 24.14 Stage-specific guidelines for follow-up renal cell carcinoma. *Unless routine laboratory tests are abnormal or patient develops symptoms. CT, computed tomography; LFT, liver function tests.

tumors[57]. To date, no clearcut consensus has been achieved regarding lymphadenectomy.

Radiation therapy

Radiation therapy has been employed as a preoperative or postoperative surgical adjunct. Besides palliative treatment of skeletal metastases, thus far no definitive studies have demonstrated effectiveness of preoperative or postoperative radiotherapy for RCC or for regional lymph node extension[58]. Although radiotherapy seems to delay local renal fossa recurrence, no significant improvement in 5-year survival rate has been demonstrated[59,60]. The role of preoperative adjunctive radiation therapy in the treatment of locally extensive carcinoma remains unclear.

Metastatic renal cell carcinoma
Chemotherapy

A number of single and combination chemotherapeutic agents have been investigated for treatment of RCC without success. However, preliminary studies using the combination of 5-fluorouracil with interleukin-2 (IL-2) and interferon-α revealed an impressive response rate of 46% with 15% complete response and only moderate toxicity among treated patients[61,62]. The reason for chemoresistance seems to be the frequency of multidrug resistance in RCC (Fig. 24.12).

Hormonal therapy

Although hormonal therapy demonstrated some efficacy in animal studies, thus far there is little evidence to support the use of hormonal agents in RCC.

Immunotherapy

The basis of immunotherapy for metastatic RCC is the unusual natural history of RCC, including spontaneous regression, delayed growth of metastatic lesions, and varying tumor-doubling times. Therefore, it suggests that host immune factors may be important in tumor control.

Historically, nonspecific immune stimulators, such as bacillus Calmette–Guérin (BCG), *Corynebacterium parvum*, and levamisole, demonstrated minimal benefit[63,64].

α-Interferon

Interferons (IFN) (particularly α-IFN) have shown efficacy (approximately 15% partial response rates) against RCCs but

Toxicity of α-interferon
Flu-like symptoms (worse at higher doses)
Anorexia, weight loss, malaise, and fatigue
Immunosuppression
Central nervous system (confusion and depression)
Increased liver enzyme levels
Nausea and vomiting
Cardiovascular

Figure 24.15 Toxicity of α-interferon.

complete responses are rare (1% of cases). Most patients who responded to α-IFN had limited metastases, especially lung metastases. Because of a low level of clinical response, the need for further trials with combination interferons and other agents have been undertaken. The range of immunologic effects with α-IFN include activation of natural killer cells, increased expression of tumor associated antigens, and modulation of HLA class I and II antigens[61,62]. Side effects employing α-IFN in metastatic RCC are reviewed in Figure 24.15.

Interleukin-2

In clinical studies with the T-cell growth factor IL-2, complete response have been achieved in 5% of patients treated while 10–15% responded partially. Some of these completely responding patients have now been disease-free for more than 7 years, suggesting very sustained responses in a minority of patients. The Food and Drug Administration (FDA) therefore approved high-dose IL-2 for the therapy of good performance status patients with metastatic RCC.

Side effects of IL-2 therapy include fever, chills, malaise, nausea, vomiting, and diarrhea. Some patients may develop prerenal azotemia with hypotension, fluid retention, respiratory distress syndrome, oliguria, and low fractional sodium excretion but cessation of drug results in a total reversal and recovery from side effects. Treatment-related mortality is less than 2%[62]. The current trend in investigations has been to test combinations of biologic response modifying agents, e.g. IL-2, and α-interferon, together or in association with other agents in outpatient regimens. Toxicities of α-interferon are listed in Figure 24.15.

Lymphocyte-activated killer cell and T1L cell approaches

Two more intensive regimens for the management of metastatic RCC are lymphocyte-activated killer (LAK) cell and T1L cell studies. Both make use of *ex vivo* stimulation of lymphocytes (peripheral in LAK cell therapy, tumor-contained in T1L therapy). Stimulation occurs *ex vivo* using IL-2 and the activated cells are returned to the patient. Results of LAK cell therapy have been summarized by Fisher et al., who found a 38% response rate in pulmonary and soft tissue metastasis, a 20% response rate on abdominal disease, and that patients with bulky disease did worse while patients with previous nephrectomy did better[65]. The side effects of LAK cell therapy are substantial, with a hypoperfusion-like injury occurring to many organ systems[66]. T1L therapy (with or without IL-2 therapy association) has been renewed by Beldgrund et al. who found

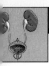

a 61% 1-year survival, which diminished to 31% at 3 years (median survival 12.2 months) in 203 patients who received IL-2+ T1L therapy.

Palliative nephrectomy

Approximately 30% of patients have metastases when the diagnosis of RCC is first made. Palliative nephrectomy may be performed for the control of severe symptoms such as severe hemorrhage or pain, paraneoplastic syndromes, and compression of adjacent viscera. These patients have an average survival of approximately 4 months, and only 10% can be expected to survive 1 year. Currently, angioinfarction provides a safer and less invasive method than surgery of managing severe hemorrhage and other severe symptoms.[67]

Adjunctive nephrectomy

To date, adjunctive nephrectomy has not been documented to increase survival significantly.

The role of adjunctive nephrectomy has recently been addressed in a clinical trial (Southwest Oncology Group trial 8949) where patients with metastatic RCC were randomized to radical nephrectomy and α-interferon versus α-interferon alone. The results of this trial are still pending.

UNUSUAL RENAL CANCERS

Sarcomas of the kidney

Sarcomas constitute only about 1–3% of malignant tumors of the kidney but increase in incidence with advancing age, and differentiation from the sarcomatoid variant of RCC is usually difficult or impossible[68]. The presenting signs and symptoms are essentially the same as RCC (e.g. pain, a flank mass, and hematuria). CT findings highly suggestive of a renal sarcoma include tumor originating from renal sinus or capsule, presence of a mass with fat or bone, and large renal tumor without retroperitoneal lymphadenopathy[69,70]. Angiographically, renal sarcomas are hypovascular without arteriovenous fistulae. About 60% of sarcomas are leiomyosarcomas that originate from smooth muscle cells. They are more frequent in females in their 3rd to 5th decades of life and are more likely to compress and displace the kidney than invade it. Leiomyosarcomas are generally large, well-encapsulated, firm, and multinodular, and may metastasize early. Although sarcomas tend to recur locally after resection, radical nephrectomy is the treatment of choice[69,70]. Complete radical excision of tumor may significantly prolong patient survival. Moreover, the evaluation of the surgical specimen may help to differentiate these tumors from renal adenocarcinoma. Prognosis in high-grade or advanced disease is generally poor despite the use of aggressive surgery, chemotherapy, or radiotherapy[70].

Rhabdomyosarcoma

Rhabdomyosarcoma in the adult is one of the rarest and most malignant renal neoplasms. It arises from striated muscle and is usually large and multinodular with a well-defined capsule. Common sites of metastases are the liver, lymph nodes, and lung.

Surgery is the only potentially curative method for these rare tumors; however, survival following surgery alone is extremely poor.

Malignant fibrous histiocytoma

Malignant fibrous histiocytoma is the most common soft tissue sarcoma of late adult life. It often grows to large size in the retroperitoneal space. Its histology is similar to that of histiocytomas arising in other areas. The therapy is radical nephrectomy, but local recurrence is frequent and radiotherapy may be effective.

Other malignancies – lymphoma

Reticulum cell sarcoma, lymphosarcoma, and leukemia uncommonly involve only the kidney without other manifestations of the systemic disease. Initially the tumor grows between the nephrons and subsequently expands and produces the typical lymphomatous tumor. Surgical treatment is seldom indicated except in the case of a solitary lesion or in the patient with severe symptoms, such as uncontrollable hemorrhage. The treatment generally involves systemic treatment of the primary disease. There are no typical radiographic features but there are suggestive patterns of involvement (often documented with CT) including multiple intraparenchymal nodules, direct contiguous lymph node masses, and diffuse infiltration of the kidney[71]. At the present time, CT appears to be the most reliable way to diagnose renal involvement by lymphoma and to monitor the progress of therapy. Aspiration biopsy under CT guidance may confirm the diagnosis without the need for open biopsy or exploration.

Metastatic tumors

The kidney is a frequent site of metastatic malignancy. Metastatic lesions are usually asymptomatic and most often discovered at autopsy. Rarely, flank pain, hematuria, and massive hemorrhage may occur. Renal metastasis may originate from breast, lung, ovarian, or gastrointestinal primary neoplasms. Commonly, imaging studies do not clearly distinguish metastatic tumors from primary renal neoplasms: CT-guided aspiration biopsy may helpful in this situation. Typically, the postcontrast CT scan may show only slight enhancement of the lesion and arteriography a round and hypovascular lesion, without the discrete neovascularity and other angiographic characteristics associated with primary renal cell carcinoma.[72,73]

TUMORS OF THE URETER AND RENAL PELVIS

Benign ureteral tumors (fibroepithelial polyps)

Primary urothelial tumors are rare, representing only 1% of all upper tract neoplasms. The most common benign ureteral tumor is the fibroepithelial polyp. Usually these tumors arise from the renal pelvis or upper third of the ureter and may resemble a smooth nodule or be pedunculated with a long stalk. Histologically they are composed of a central fibrous core surrounded by normal or hyperplastic benign urothelium. Flank pain and hematuria are the usual presenting symptoms. Radiographically, varying degrees of hydroureteronephrosis may be detected. Polyps appear as smooth filling defects that may change position if the tumor is pedunculated. Ureteroscopy (flexible/rigid) has become a pivotal diagnostic tool to confirm malignant lesions prior to treatment. Management of these benign ureteral lesions includes ureteroscopic resection, open ureterotomy with polypectomy, or partial ureterectomy. In

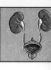

incidence of contralateral renal involvement after radical nephroureterectomy. Although no randomized studies have been performed comparing radical nephroureterectomy with more conservative therapies, an aggressive approach is justifiable in the majority of patients.

Laparoscopic ureterectomy or nephroureterectomy has also been performed in carefully selected patients. Early results are encouraging, but further followup is necessary to assess the benefits and potential complications of this form of therapy.

Selected patients (functionally or anatomically abnormal kidneys, solitary kidney, or bilateral disease) with noninvasive tumors of the ureter may be best served by a conservative approach such as distal ureteral resection with reimplantation including a psoas hitch or Boari flap, or segmental resection of the upper or mid ureter. Besides simple excision, a number of endourologic treatment options are also available for conservative management of urothelial carcinomas. Ureteroscopic fulguration or resection of ureteral tumors may be performed using a traditional electric-coagulation source or using laser probes (Nd:YAG or argon). This may represent the optimal treatment for patients with low-grade, low-stage tumors of the distal ureter. However, patients with higher-grade or higher-stage tumors or with tumors of the renal pelvis or upper or middle ureter are best served by nephroureterectomy. The possibility of undergrading or understaging must also be considered in planning surgical intervention.

As in other urothelial tumors, chemotherapeutic and immunologic agents may also be used locally (topically) in the treatment of urothelial carcinomas. Direct instillation of BCG or mitomycin C into the collecting system has been applied through percutaneous nephrostomy tubes or by retrograde instillation using an indwelling catheter.

Periodic surveillance is crucial following therapy for urothelial carcinomas. Regular cystoscopy and examination of urine cytology specimens should be performed in all patients. Imaging studies of the collecting system, cytology of ureteral saline barbotage, and periodic ureteroscopy with biopsy are indicated on a regular basis. The frequency of these procedures will depend on the stage and grade of the lesion. The results of adjuvant radiation therapy or chemotherapy are similar to those reported for bladder cancer. Radiation therapy may decrease local recurrence rates but has little apparent effect on overall survival[79]. Chemotherapeutic regimens [methotrexate, vinblastine, Adriamycin, and cisplatin (M-VAC) or newer, less toxic regimens] are similar to those employed for advanced transitional cell cancer of the bladder and the long-term efficacy of these regimen remain to be defined.

Secondary malignant urothelial tumors

Hematogenous spread or direct extension of tumors from other organs may affect the renal pelvis or ureters secondarily. The most common primary site is the breast, followed by the stomach, bladder, colon, cervix, and prostate. Most cases are asymptomatic and are discovered at autopsy, but low back pain, hematuria, and renal insufficiency due to obstructive nephropathy may be present. Bilateral obstruction is noted in approximately 30% of cases and usually occurs in the lower third of the ureter. Palliative treatment (indwelling ureteral stent placement or percutaneous nephrostomy) may be performed to alleviate the obstruction and symptoms, improving the renal function for future adjuvant therapy. More aggressive surgical intervention is discouraged in light of the overall guarded prognosis usually associated with widespread metastases.

REFERENCES

1. Harris RP. An analytical examination of 100 cases of extirpations of the kidney. Am J Med Sci. 1882;84:109.

2. Glenn JF. Renal tumors. In: Harrison JH, Gittes RF, Perlmutter AD, et al., eds. Campbell's urology, 4th edn. Philadelphia: WB Saunders; 1980.

3. Deming CL, Harvard BM. Tumors of the kidney. In: Campbell MF, Harrison JH, eds. Urology, vol. 2, 3rd edn. Philadelphia: WB Saunders; 1970:884.

4. Carson WJ. Tumors of the kidney: Histologic study. Trans Sect Urol AMA. 1928.

5. Presti JC, Rao PH, Chen Q, et al. Histopathological, cytogenetic, and molecular characterization of renal cortical tumors. Cancer Res. 1991;51:1544.

6. O'Toole KM, Brown M, Hoffmann P. Pathology of benign and malignant kidney tumors. Urol Clin North Am. 1993;20:193.

7. Lieber MM. Renal oncocytoma. Urol Clin North Am. 1993;20:355.

8. Zerban H, Nogueira E, Riedasch G, Bannasch P. Renal oncocytoma: origin from the collecting duct. Virchows Arch. 1987;52:375.

9. Nogueira E, Bannasch P. Cellular origin of rat renal oncocytoma. Lab Invest. 1988;59:337.

10. Bonavita JA, Pollack HM, Banner MP. Renal oncocytoma: further observations and literature review. Urol Radiol. 1981;2:229.

11. Davidson AJ, Hayes WS, Hartman DS, et al. Renal oncocytoma and carcinoma: failure of differentiation with CT. Radiology. 1993;186:693.

12. Crotty TB, Lawrence KM, Moertel CA, et al. Cytogenetic analysis of six renal oncocytomas and a chromophobe cell renal carcinoma: evidence that Y, I may be a characteristic anomaly in renal oncocytomas. Cancer Genet Cytogenet. 1992;61:61.

13. Dobin SM, Harris CP, Reynolds JA, et al. Cytogenetic abnormalities in renal oncocytic neoplasms. Genes Chromosomes Cancer. 1992, 4:25.

14. Licht MR, Novick AC, Tubbs RR, et al. Renal oncocytoma: clinical and biological correlates. J Urol. 1993;150:1380.

15. Lieber MM. Renal oncocytoma. Urol Clin North Am. 1993;20:355.

16. McCullough DL, Scott R Jr, Seybold HM. Renal angiomyelolipoma (hamartoma of retroperitoneal tumors with large vena caval thrombi. Ann Surg.): review of the literature and report of 7 cases. J Urol. 1971;105:32.1990;212:472.

17. Stillwell TJ, Gomez MR, Kelalis PP. Renal lesions in tuberous sclerosis. J Urol. 1987, 138:477.

18. Steiner MS, Goldman SM, Fishman EK, et al. The natural history of renal angiomyolipoma. J Urol. 1993;150:1782.

19. Taylor RS, Joseph DB, Kohaut EC, et al. Renal angiomyolipoma associated with lymph node involvement and renal cell carcinoma in patients with tuberous sclerosis. J Urol. 1989;141:930.

20. Colvin RB, Dickersin GR. Pathology of renal tumors. In: Skinner DG, deKernion JB, eds. Genitourinary cancer. Philadelphia: WB Saunders; 1978:84.

21. Bosniak MA, Megibow AJ, Huluick DH, et al. CT diagnosis of renal angiomyolipoma: the importance of detecting small amounts of fat. AJR. 1988;151:497.

22. Blute ML, Malek RS, Segura JW. Angiomyolipoma: Clinical metamorphosis and concepts for management. J Urol. 1988;139:20.

23. Glover SD, Buck AC. Renal medullary fibroma: a case report. J Urol. 1982;127:758.

24. Orjauvik OS, Aas M, Fauchald P, et al. Renin-secreting renal tumor with severe hypertension. Acta Med Scand. 1975;197:329.

25. Wingo PA, Tong T, Bolden S. Cancer statistics. CA. 1995;45:8.

26. Lauritsen JG. Lindau's disease: A study of one family through six generations. Acta Chir Scand. 1975;139:482.

27. Colvin RB, Dickersin GR. Pathology of renal tumors. In: Skinner DG, deKernion JB, eds. Genitourinary cancer. Philadelphia: WB Saunders; 1978:84.

28. Kantor AF. Current concepts in the epidemiology and etiology of primary renal cell carcinoma. J Urol. 1977;117(4):415–7.

29. Wallace AC, Nairn RC. Renal tubular antigens in kidney tumors. Cancer. 1972;29(4):977–81.

30. Sargent ER, Gomella LG, Belldegrun A, Linehan WM, Kasid A. Epidermal growth factor receptor gene expression in normal human kidney and renal cell carcinoma. J Urol. 1989;142(5):1364–8.

31. Zbar B, Lerman M. Inherited carcinomas of the kidney. Adv Cancer Res. 1998;75:163–201.

32. Gnarra JR, Tory K, Weng Y, et al. Mutations of the VHL tumour suppressor gene in renal carcinoma. Nat Genet. 1994;7:85–90.

33. Kakehi Y, Kanamaru H, Yoshida O, et al. Measurement of multidrug-resistance messenger RNA in urogenital cancers; elevated expression in renal cell carcinoma is associated with intrinsic drug resistance. J Urol. 1988;139:862–5.

34. Kloppel G, Knofel WT, Baisch H, Otto U. Prognosis of renal cell carcinoma related to nuclear grade, DNA content and Robson stage. Eur Urol. 1986;12:426–31.

35. Sufrin G, Chasan S, Golio A, Murphy GP. Paraneoplastic and serologic syndromes of renal adenocarcinoma. Semin Urol. 1989;7:158–71.

36. Janik, 1993 Stewart RR, Dunnick NR. Imaging renal neoplasms. Prob Urol. 1990;4:175.

37. Amendola MA, Bree RL, Pollack HM, et al. Small renal cell carcinomas: resolving a diagnostic dilemma. Radiology. 1988;166:637.

38. Skinner DG, Pfister RF, Colvin R. Extension of renal cell carcinoma into the vena cava: the rationale for aggressive surgical management. J Urol. 1972;107:711.

39. Swierzewski DJ, Swierzewski MJ, Libertino JA. Radical nephrectomy in patients with renal cell carcinoma with venous, vena caval, and atrial extension. Am J Surg. 1994;168:205.

40. Pollack HM, Banner MP, Amendola MA. Other malignant neoplasms of the renal parenchyma. Semin Roentgenol. 1987;22:260.

41. Medeiros LJ, Gelb AB, Weiss LM. Renal cell carcinoma: prognostic significance of morphologic parameters in 121 cases. Cancer. 1988;61:1639.

42. Guinan PD, Vogelzang NJ, Fremgen AM, et al. Renal cell carcinoma: Tumor stage, size and survival. J Urol. 1995;153:901.

43. Maldazys JD, deKernion JB. Prognostic factors in metastatic renal carcinoma. J Urol. 1986;136:376.

44. Robey EL, Schellhammer PF. The adrenal gland and renal cell carcinoma: is ipsilateral adrenalectomy a necessary component of radical nephrectomy? J Urol. 1986;135:453.

45. Giuliani L, Giberti C, Martorama G, et al. Radical extensive surgery for renal cell carcinoma: long term results and prognostic factors. J Urol. 1990;143:468.

46. Chute R, Soutter L, Kerr W. The value of thoracoabdominal incision in the removal of kidney tumors. N Engl J Med. 1949;241:951.

47. DeKernion JB, Huland H. The operable renal cell carcinoma: summary and conclusions. Eur Urol. 1990;18(suppl. 2):48.

48. Robson CJ, Churchill BM, Anderson W. The results of radical nephrectomy for renal cell carcinoma. Trans Am Assoc Genitourin Surg. 1968;60:122.

49. McNichols DW, Segura JW, deWeerd JH. Renal cell carcinoma: long-term survival and late recurrence. J Urol. 1981;126:17.

50. Licht MR, Novick AC. Nephron sparing surgery for renal cell carcinoma. J Urol. 1993;149:1–7.

51. Morgan WR, Zincke H. Progression and survival after renal conserving surgery for renal cell carcinoma: experience in 104 patients and extended follow up. J Urol. 1990;144:852.

52. Campbell SC, Novick AC, Streem S, et al. Complications of nephron-sparing surgery for renal tumors. J Urol. 1994;151:1177.

53. Marshall FF, Holdford SS, Hamper UM. Intraoperative sonography of renal tumors. J Urol. 1992;148:1393.

54. Levy DA, Slaton JW, Swanson DA, Dinney CP. Stage specific guidelines for surveillance after radical nephrectomy for local renal cell carcinoma. J Urol. 1998;159:1163–7.

55. Giuliani L, Giberti C, Martorana G, Rovida S. Radical extensive surgery for renal cell carcinoma: long-term results and prognostic factors. J Urol. 1990;143(3):468–73; discussion 473–4.

56. Herrlinger A, Schrott KM, Schott G, Sigel A. What are the benefits of extended dissection of the regional renal lymph nodes in the therapy of renal cell carcinoma? J Urol. 1991 Nov;146(5):1224–7.

57. Golimbu M, Al-Askari S, Tessler A, Morales P. Aggressive treatment of metastatic renal cancer. J Urol. 1986;136(4):805–7.

58. Finney R. The value of radiotherapy in the treatment of hypernephroma – a clinical trial. Br J Urol. 1973;45:258.

59. Waters WB, Richie JP. Aggressive surgical approach to renal cell carcinoma: review of 130 cases. J Urol. 1979;122:306–9.

60. Maulard-Durdux C, Dufour B, Hennequin C, et al. Postoperative radiation therapy in 26 patients with invasive transitional cell carcinoma of the upper urinary tract: no impact on survival? J Urol. 1996;155(1):115–7.

61. Sella A, Zukiwski A, Robinson E, et al. Interleukin-2 with interferon-or and 5-fluorouracil in patients with metastatic renal cell cancer (abstract). Proc Am Soc Clin Oncol. 1994;13:237.

62. Spencer WF, Linehan WM, Walther MM, et al. Immunotherapy with interleukin-2 and α-interferon in patients with metastatic renal cell cancer with in situ primary cancers: a pilot study. J Urol. 1992;147:24.

63. Montie JE, Bukowski RM, James RE, et al. A critical review of immunotherapy of disseminated renal adenocarcinoma. J Surg Oncol. 1982;21:5.

64. Morales A, Wilson JL, Pater JL, Loeb M. Cytoreductive surgery and systemic bacillus Calmette–Guérin therapy in metastatic renal cancer: a phase II trial. J Urol. 1982;127:230.

65. McMannis JD, Fisher RI, Creekmore SP, Braun DP, Harris JE, Ellis TM. In vivo effects of recombinant IL-2. I. Isolation of circulating Leu-19+ lymphokine-activated killer effector cells from cancer patients receiving recombinant IL-2. J Immunol. 1988;140:1335–40.

66. Kaufmann Y, Levanon M, Davidsohn J, Ramot B. Interleukin 2 induces human acute lymphocytic leukemia cells to manifest lymphokine-activated-killer (LAK) cytotoxicity. J Immunol. 1987;139:977–82.

67. Flanigan RC. The failure of infarction and/or nephrectomy in stage IV renal cell cancer to influence survival or metastatic regression. Urol Clin North Am. 1987;14:757.

68. Spellman JE Jr, Driscoll DL, Huben RP. Primary renal sarcoma. Am Surg. 1995;61:456.

69. Pollack HM, Banner MP, Amendola MA. Other malignant neoplasms of the renal parenchyma. Semin Roentgenol. 1987;22:260.

70. Karakousis CP, Gerstenbluth R, Kontzoglou K, Driscoll DL. Retroperitoneal sarcomas and their management. Arch Surg. 1995;130:1104.

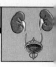
71. Heiken JP, Gold RP, Schaur MJ, et al. Computed tomography of renal lymphoma with ultrasound correlation. J Comput Assist Tomogr. 1983;7:245.

72. Flanigan RC. The failure of infarction and/or nephrectomy in stage IV renal cell cancer to influence survival or metastatic regression. Urol Clin North Am. 1987;14:757.

73. Flanigan RC. Role of surgery in metastatic renal cell carcinoma. Semin Urol. 1989;7:191.

74. Babaian RJ, Johnson DE, Chan RC Combination nephroureterectomy and postoperative radiotherapy for infiltrative ureteral carcinoma. Int J Radiat Oncol Biol Phys. 1980;6:1229–32.

75. Fraley EE, Lange PH, Hakala TR. Recent studies on the immunobiology and biology of human urothelial tumors. Urol Clin North Am. 1976;3:31.

76. Anderstrom C, Johansson SL, von Schultz L. Primary adenocarcinoma of the urinary: A clinicopathologic and prognostic study. Cancer. 1983, 52:1273.

77. Radovanovic Z, Krajinovic S, Jankovic S, Hall PW, Petkovic S. Family history of cancer among cases of upper urothelial tumours in a Balkan nephropathy area. J Cancer Res Clin Oncol. 1985;110(2):181–3.

78. Bloom NA, Vidone RA, Lytton B. Primary carcinoma of the ureter: a report of 102 cases. J Urol. 1970;103:590.

79. Cozad SC, Smalley SR, Austenfeld M. Adjuvant radiotherapy in high stage transitional cell carcinoma of the renal pelvis and ureter. J Radiat Oncol Biol Phys. 1992;24:743.

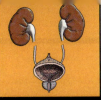

Chapter 25

Superficial Bladder Cancer

D Michael A Wallace

KEY POINTS

- In the developed world smoking is responsible for 40% of bladder cancers.
- Stromal invasion and tumor grade remain the best indicators of progression.
- Approximately 50% of pT1G3 tumors will progress.
- Best treatment occurs when accurate staging results from close liasion between urologist and pathologist.
- Intravesical BGG is the initial treatment of choice for carcinoma in situ.
- Prospective trials are required to determine the efficacy and cost-effectiveness of new urine tests for bladder cancer.

INTRODUCTION

Superficial bladder cancer is a stage grouping of three distinct tumors – papillary and noninvasive (pTa), tumors invading into lamina propria only (pT1) and carcinoma in situ (CIS). They are grouped together for the simple practical reason that they can all be managed endoscopically and with intravesical therapy. Their prognosis varies widely as the stromal invasion has a significant impact on survival with high-grade T1 tumors having a survival as poor as some muscle-invasive tumors if managed by endoscopic means alone.

The management of patients with superficial bladder tumors is a long-term commitment. These patients are usually under urologic surveillance for at least 7 years and many will be followed up for life. Most cases will be undemanding and routine, but a small proportion are destined to progress, when disease becomes life-threatening. These high-risk patients must be identified and selected for more aggressive curative therapy. Too often, however, these cases progress to invasion of muscle and metastasize while under urologic care. The reasons for treatment failure for superficial bladder cancer can be summarized as follows:

- inadequate initial assessment, usually providing insufficient material for a proper pathologic assessment;
- failure to act when high risk factors identified such as the pT1G3 tumor;
- inappropriate delegation of follow-up to junior or inexperienced staff;
- inappropriate treatment such as using radiotherapy when recurrent superficial tumors cannot be controlled endoscopically;

- prolonged attempts to conserve the bladder using intravesical therapy that is not controlling the disease; and
- failure to detect extravesical disease in the prostatic ducts, urethra, and upper tracts.

ETIOLOGY

Bladder cancer is almost always caused by urine-borne carcinogens. The main exception is when ionizing radiation is used, for instance for the treatment of cervical cancer (Fig. 25.1). The urothelial carcinogens are mainly specific aromatic amines or nitrosamines (Fig. 25.2). The aromatic amines are easily absorbed through skin or mucous membranes, are metabolized in the liver and are excreted in the urine. Individuals vary in their ability to inactivate these carcinogens with liver enzyme systems such as N-acetyl transferase and glutathione transferase (Fig. 25.3). Nitrosamines can be produced in the bladder by the action of bacteria on urinary amines and nitrates, such as can occur in long-term catheterized paraplegic patients and patients with bilharzia of the bladder.

Cigarette smoking is the main etiologic factor in most developed countries and probably accounts for over 40% of bladder cancers. Cigarette smoke contains known urothelial carcinogens such as 2-naphthylamine and 4-aminobiphenyl. DNA and hemoglobin adducts of these compounds can be demonstrated in the bladder and blood after exposure to cigarette smoke. The risk is

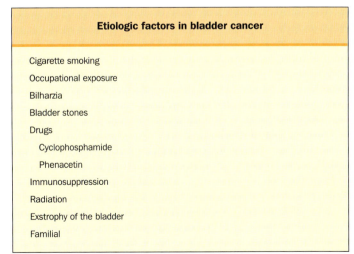

Etiologic factors in bladder cancer

Cigarette smoking

Occupational exposure

Bilharzia

Bladder stones

Drugs
   Cyclophosphamide
   Phenacetin

Immunosuppression

Radiation

Exstrophy of the bladder

Familial

Figure 25.1 Etiologic factors in bladder cancer.

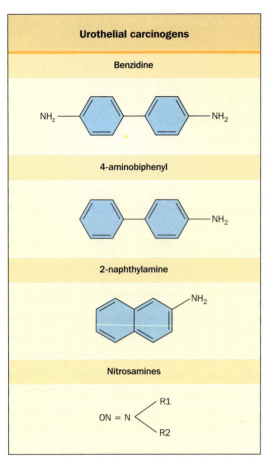

Figure 25.2 Urothelial carcinogens.

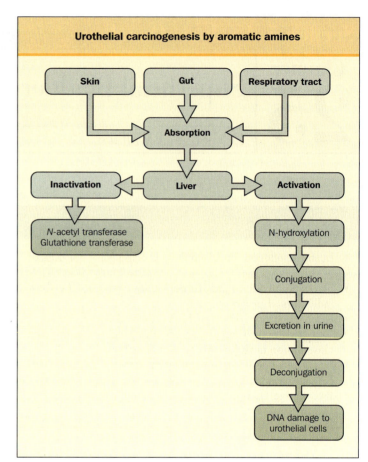

Figure 25.3 Urothelial carcinogenesis by aromatic amines.

related to the type of tobacco and the duration and intensity of exposure. What is not clearly established is the benefit that a smoker with bladder cancer may gain from giving up smoking at diagnosis. It is likely that over the patient's follow-up period the risk of recurrence or progression may be reduced and the opportunity should not be lost for counseling the patient on the benefit to the bladder of giving up smoking. Cessation of smoking gradually reduces the risk of developing a bladder cancer, but over a 20-year period[1].

The second commonest cause of bladder cancer is occupational exposure to urothelial carcinogens. Most industries have now got rid of the main carcinogens and working practices have much improved. Also, the workforces are now much smaller, which makes it very much more difficult to identify where small excesses of bladder cancers are occurring[2,3]. Patients should be questioned about possible occupational exposure, particularly for any known local industries. Certain patients may be eligible for state benefits and very rarely patients may be advised to pursue a claim for compensation, but only if it is likely that exposure, causation and negligence can be established[4].

Age

The median age for presentation with bladder cancer is 69–70. Bladder tumors occur from the third decade onwards although most of the tumors below the age of 40 years are low-grade and noninvasive. The age-specific registration rate rises steadily with age.

Sex

The male:female ratio is around 3:1 in most countries. Cigarette smoking and occupational exposure can only partly account for this difference. We may expect this sex ratio to fall with the decrease in men smoking and the lack of change in smoking by younger women. The sex ratio in the UK has now fallen to 2.5:1[5]. Hormonal effects and differences in bladder function and metabolism of carcinogens may account for some of the sex differences.

THE DEVELOPMENT OF BLADDER CANCER

There is a very long latent period between exposure to carcinogen and the development of a tumor, usually 20–25 years although the range is 1–40 years. One reason for this may be that urothelium, being highly specialized, has a very slow turnover, yet is capable of rapid proliferation in response to injury. Urothelial cancer is an example of multistage carcinogenesis, with initiation causing a number of specific changes to the genome and nonspecific factors causing proliferation to produce the tumor growth.

A large number of chromosomal abnormalities have so far been described in urothelial cancer. The most common are deletions on chromosome 9, which may be the initiating event[6], whilst also a number of chromosomal deletions or mutations have now been associated with the disease. A pattern is emerging of certain

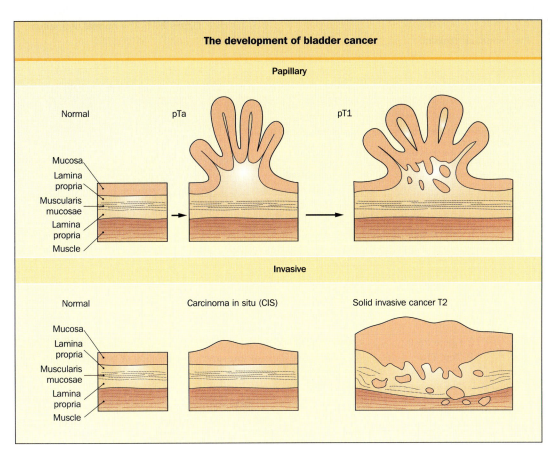

chromosomes that are not involved and others that may be, particularly with the development of invasion, such as chromosome 17 and *p53* mutations.

There are two main pathways along which bladder tumors develop – the papillary and the invasive (Fig. 25.4). In the papillary pathway the urothelium may show a number of premalignant changes that are not easily recognized, such as hyperplasia and degrees of atypia. As proliferation occurs, papillary structures form to give the characteristic tumors. The majority of these will remain noninvasive but a minority may go on to break down the basement membrane and then start to infiltrate into the lamina propria, and then on to muscle invasion and metastasis.

In the invasive pathway the premalignant changes are well recognized because of the high degree of anaplasia that is known as carcinoma in situ. When carcinoma in situ progresses it usually infiltrates from the start to form a solid, invasive tumor with a high risk of metastasizing. Over 70% of tumors will develop along the papillary pathway and the majority of muscle-invasive tumors do not have a preceding history of papillary tumors.

PATHOLOGY

The dominant cell type of bladder tumors is the urothelial or transitional cell. Over 90% of bladder cancers are urothelial but this may vary with geography depending on the prevalence of bilharzia, where squamous cell cancers are more common. Urothelial cancers may have some degree of squamous metaplasia but pure squamous cancer accounts for approximately 5% of

tumors. Adenocarcinoma is rare and must be distinguished from extravesical tumors such as those of the prostate and large bowel by the use of immunohistochemistry.

Grade and presence of invasion are the two most important prognostic factors in superficial bladder cancer and these are both subject to significant variation between pathologists, particularly when reporting the premalignant changes[7,8]. Grading is a subjective assessment based on the degree of anaplasia and mitotic activity. No two pathologists will always agree but there should not be variation by more than one grade. Only the World Health Organization (WHO) grading system should be used and the urologist should be wary of the intermediate gradings such as I/II and II/III. These should either be reviewed or graded as the higher grade.

Invasion of the lamina propria should be an objective assessment but in practice this is often very difficult because of the interpretation of the papillary structure of the tumor and the sectioning of the specimen. Even special staining of the basement membrane is not always helpful. Also, within the lamina propria are small filaments of smooth muscle, the muscularis mucosae (Fig. 25.5). This forms an incomplete layer roughly dividing the lamina propria. It should not be confused with detrusor muscle invasion. What is important for the urologist to know is the extent and confidence of the diagnosis of lamina propria invasion (Fig. 25.6). This has been subdivided into T1a and T1b categories. Focal invasion of the papillary stalks has a much lower risk of progression than when there is widespread infiltration of the lamina propria right up to detrusor muscle but not actually invading it, yet both may be reported as T1 tumors[9].

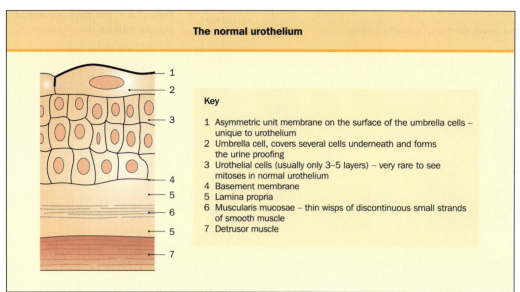

Figure 25.5 The normal urothelium.

The normal urothelium

Key

1 Asymmetric unit membrane on the surface of the umbrella cells – unique to urothelium
2 Umbrella cell, covers several cells underneath and forms the urine proofing
3 Urothelial cells (usually only 3–5 layers) – very rare to see mitoses in normal urothelium
4 Basement membrane
5 Lamina propria
6 Muscularis mucosae – thin wisps of discontinuous small strands of smooth muscle
7 Detrusor muscle

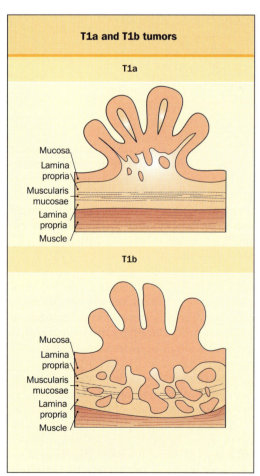

T1a and T1b tumors

T1a

Mucosa
Lamina propria
Muscularis mucosae
Lamina propria
Muscle

T1b

Mucosa
Lamina propria
Muscularis mucosae
Lamina propria
Muscle

Figure 25.6 (Top) T1a and (bottom) T1b tumors. The importance of accurate pathologic description.

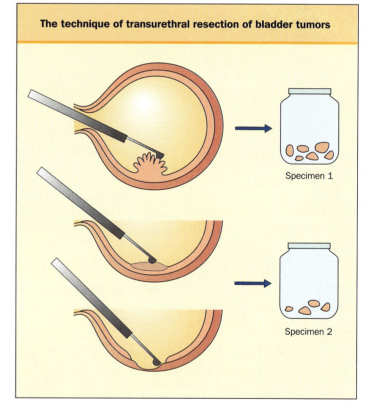

The technique of transurethral resection of bladder tumors

Specimen 1

Specimen 2

Figure 25.7 The technique of transurethral resection of bladder tumors. For large tumors the pathologist may not be able to section all of the tumor. Therefore, resect the exophytic part first and then resect into muscle so that the pathologist can concentrate on sectioning the deeper part of the tumor. Some pathologists prefer deep cold cup biopsies to avoid diathermy artefact.

The urologist must make sure than the pathologist receives detrusor muscle in the specimen and the pathologist must make sure that the presence or absence of muscle is reported (Fig. 25.7). Without muscle in the specimen pathologic staging is unreliable and an early repeat resection is indicated for T1 tumors (Fig. 25.8).

Urologists managing bladder cancer must meet with their pathologists and review sections together. This is particularly important for high-risk cases, where management is often dependent on the accuracy of the pathology.

Early repeat transurethral resection
Indications
No muscle in tumor specimen
High-grade tumors
Concomitant CIS in specimen and no mucosal biopsies taken
Resection incomplete
Original resection done elsewhere or by inexperienced urologist
Practice of early repeat TUR
Should be done by senior, experienced urologist
Resect into muscle
Take mucosal biopsies, including prostatic urethra
Careful bimanual exam

Figure 25.8 Early repeat transurethral resection (TUR). CIS, carcinoma in situ.

DIAGNOSIS

Hematuria is the cardinal sign of malignant disease in the urinary tract. All urologic departments must have a rapid and efficient system for the investigation of hematuria that includes upper tract imaging and flexible cystoscopy. The choice of imaging for the upper tract in cases of hematuria is a matter of department choice between ultrasound and intravenous urography. When bladder cancer has been diagnosed, then the greater anatomic detail of the upper tracts shown by urography is a great advantage in excluding upper tract tumors or minor degrees of obstruction.

The investigation of microscopic hematuria is a problem for most busy departments and also for primary care. The prevalence of microhematuria in the population would overwhelm most urologists if all cases were referred for urologic investigation. Most published series have looked at selected populations and the pickup rate for urologic cancers varies from 0% to 11%. A rational approach to this should be developed between urologists, nephrologists and general practitioners. Patients under 40 years are very unlikely to have malignant disease and should be referred to a nephrologist first if they have confirmed microhematuria or if they have proteinuria, hypertension or renal impairment. Older patients, even with a single positive test, should be investigated urologically unless the hematuria was in the presence of a confirmed urinary infection and no blood is present on repeat testing after treatment[10].

Population screening using stick testing for microhematuria has been studied and if used in selected populations has a yield of tumors that may make this cost-effective[11]. The categories where population screening may be effective are males, smokers or ex-smokers, ages 55–75 and those with an occupational history of exposure to urothelial carcinogens. However, patients with defined occupational exposures should have regular urine cytology rather than just stick testing for hematuria. Urine cytology has a high rate of false negatives in patients with superficial bladder tumors, which are mostly of low grade, but for high-grade lesions, especially carcinoma in situ, the sensitivity is of the order of 90%. Urine cytology is the most important method of detecting carcinoma in situ, which can easily be missed even on flexible cystoscopy and all patients over 40 years with unexplained irritative symptoms must have urine cytology to exclude such pathology.

ENDOSCOPIC ASSESSMENT

When carrying out the initial diagnostic cystoscopy it is necessary to document what is seen and what is done in the bladder. The following should be noted:

Tumor:	Size
	Number
	Position
	Growth pattern (papillary or solid).
Mucosa:	Normal, red areas or areas of red, irregular mucosa.
Lower tract:	The urethra
	The prostate.
Bimanual exam:	Is there a mass before resection?
	Is there a mass or induration after resection?
	Size of mass and mobility.

TRANSURETHRAL RESECTION

Transurethral resection (TUR) is both the main treatment and the staging procedure for superficial bladder cancers. Simple biopsy under local anesthesia gives an inadequate sample of the tumor and should only be used when the patient is unfit for any procedure under general or regional anesthesia. Before commencing resection the urologist should make an assessment as to whether the tumor is likely to be in the extraperitoneal or peritoneal part of the bladder and also the probable thickness of the bladder wall (Fig. 25.9). Tumors should be resected with great care if they are in the peritoneal part of the bladder, whereas if they are in the extraperitoneal part then perforations into the perivesical fat do not usually cause major morbidity.

The resection should aim to remove the tumor by resecting down to and into the detrusor muscle. If there is any question of the tumor invading into the wall of the bladder, then resection should be continued into perivesical fat provided this is in the extraperitoneal part. For small tumors the pathologist will block out all the tissue but with larger tumors it is helpful to send the

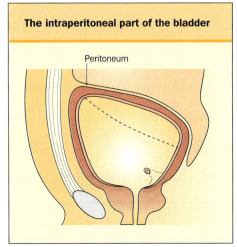

The intraperitoneal part of the bladder

Peritoneum

**Figure 25.9
The intraperitoneal part of the bladder.**

exophytic part of the tumor as one specimen, which may not be completely blocked out, and then send the base of the tumor separately.

Care should be taken when resecting near the obturator nerve. This should be anticipated when resecting above and lateral to the ureteric orifice. An unexpected kick can result in a deep perforation which can often be prevented by a short-acting muscle relaxant given in advance.

MUCOSAL BIOPSIES

Routine sampling of the normal-looking mucosa is not indicated in all cases as it will very rarely change management and generates unnecessary work[12]. Any red areas or abnormal-looking mucosa, however, should be sampled with cold cup biopsy forceps. If the patient is known to have high-grade malignant cells on urine cytology then s/he is likely to have a high grade tumor and more likely to have concomitant carcinoma in situ. If mucosal biopsies are being taken because of a high risk of carcinoma in situ then the prostatic urethra should be included by taking two deep samples with the resectoscope to include the prostatic ducts.

Early repeat transurethral resection

If the staging information is not adequate or the tumor is high-grade and showing stromal invasion then the patient should be considered for early repeat resection. Any T1 tumor where muscle has not been identified in the specimen should have an early repeat resection and this should be done after an interval of 4–6 weeks. The original tumor site should be resected well into muscle and mucosal biopsies will usually be indicated in these cases. A significant proportion of cases will be found to have residual tumor and some may be upstaged[13].

STAGING OF BLADDER CANCER

The purpose of having a uniform and widely accepted staging system for any cancer is to:
- aid planning of treatment;
- indicate prognosis;
- assist in evaluating the results of treatment;
- facilitate the exchange of information;
- contribute to the investigation of human cancer.

The International Union Against Cancer (UICC) TNM (tumor, nodes, and metastasis) system is widely used for most cancer sites (Fig. 25.10). For superficial bladder cancer (as opposed to invasive disease) the classification has remained unchanged for the last 20 years and should be used for all cases. For bladder cancer it is important to use correctly the clinical and pathologic classifications. If definitive surgical treatment has been used and the pathologist has the whole specimen then a pathologic assessment can be given. For bladder cancer this means an adequate resection into and including muscle for pTa and pT1 tumors and for muscle-invasive tumors a cystectomy specimen is required. The pathologic classification is denoted by the prefix 'p'[14].

ASSESSMENT OF RISK OF PROGRESSION OR RECURRENCE

Some 70–88% of Ta and T1 tumors will recur after endoscopic treatment[15,16]. Management of recurrent tumors is a major

The TNM classification of bladder tumors	
Tis	Carcinoma in situ
Tis pu	Carcinoma in situ in prostatic urethra
Tis pd	Carcinoma in situ in prostatic ducts
Ta	Noninvasive papillary carcinoma
T1	Tumor invades subepithelial connective tissue
T2	Tumor invades muscle
T2a	Tumor invades superficial muscle (inner half)
T2b	Tumor invades deep muscle (outer half)
T3	Tumor invades perivesical tissue
T3a	Microscopically
T3b	Macroscopically (extravesical mass)
T4	Tumor invades any of the following: prostate, uterus, vagina, pelvic wall, abdominal wall
T4a	Tumor invades prostate, uterus or vagina
T4b	Tumor invades pelvic wall or abdominal wall

Figure 25.10 The TNM (tumor, nodes, and metastasis) classification of bladder tumors.

MRC prognostic groups for superficial bladder tumors	
Group 1	Single tumor with no recurrence at 3-month cystoscopy
Group 2	Multiple tumors and no recurrence at 3-month cystoscopy
OR	
	Single tumor with recurrence at 3-month cystoscopy
Group 3	Multiple tumors with recurrence at 3-month cystoscopy

Figure 25.11 Medical Research Council (MRC) prognostic groups for superficial bladder tumors[17].

workload for most urologic departments and the follow-up requirements are a burden for the patient. Progression, on the other hand, is likely to be life-threatening and will require more radical therapy. Stromal invasion and grade of tumor are the most useful predictors of progression. In studies selecting predominantly Ta, T1 G1–2 patients the progression rates were 5–8%. For T1 tumors overall the progression rate is 29–39% but for the pT1G3 tumor the progression rate is of the order of 50%. Neither grade nor T category is a good predictor of tumor recurrence.

Parmar et al.[17] used the number of tumors at diagnosis and the presence of tumor recurrences at the first check cystoscopy at 3 months to divide patients into three groups (Fig. 25.11). Group 1 consists of patients with a single tumor at presentation and no recurrence at first cystoscopy; these tumors have a low risk of recurrence. Such patients can have a less intense follow-up schedule of cystoscopies and go straight on to annual cystoscopies[18]. Group 3 patients have multiple tumors at presentation and recurrences at first cystoscopy; these patients have a very high risk of further recurrences and will need additional intravesical chemotherapy to reduce the recurrence rate (Fig. 25.12).

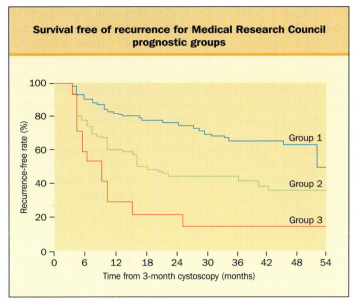

Figure 25.12 Survival free of recurrence for Medical Research Council prognostic groups[17].

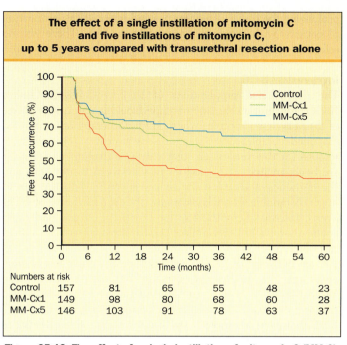

Figure 25.13 The effect of a single instillation of mitomycin C (MM-C) and five instillations of mitomycin C up to 5 years compared with transurethral resection alone[22].

INTRAVESICAL THERAPY FOR Ta AND T1 TUMORS

Intravesical therapy can be used in two ways. It can be widely applied to almost all cases using just a single instillation in order to reduce recurrences with minimal cost and morbidity, or it can be used in courses for those at high risk of progression and recurrence. Where prolonged therapy is required the choice is between intravesical cytotoxics and bacillus Calmette–Guérin (BCG).

Most chemotherapeutic agents have been tried in the bladder but only a few have found a routine place. Mitomycin C, adriamycin and epirubicin have established themselves as being the most useful agents because of their efficacy and low toxicity. In studies with marker lesions these drugs can produce complete responses in 50–60% of tumors treated[19]. Systemic toxicity is minimal because these drugs have a high molecular weight and very little of the drug gets absorbed, even if it is being used just after a transurethral resection[20].

Intravesical chemotherapy is effective because the Ta and T1 tumors and the preoplastic mucosa have a very large surface area and the drugs used can penetrate the mucosa with very little being absorbed systemically. The cytotoxic effect depends on the concentration, not the total dose, of the drug and the time in the bladder.

At the time of resection of a tumor the bladder contains a suspension of malignant cells from the tumor and raw surfaces on the bladder suitable for implantation. Two studies have used a single instillation of chemotherapy at the time of resection and both showed a reduction in recurrences that was sustained (Figs 25.13 & 25.14)[21,22]. The single instillation has minimal cost, very little morbidity and little inconvenience for the patient. It is likely that this prevents some tumor implantation and should be considered in all resections for superficial tumors[18].

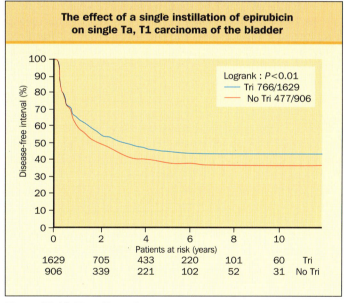

Figure 25.14 The effect of a single instillation of epirubicin on single Ta, T1 carcinoma of the bladder[21].

Many large-scale, multicenter, randomized studies have been carried out on the effect of adjuvant intravesical chemotherapy following transurethral resection of superficial bladder cancers. A combined analysis of the randomized trials conducted by the Medical Research Council (MRC) and European Organization for Research and Treatment of Cancer (EORTC) groups showed a statistically significant effect of adjuvant treatment in

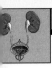

prolonging the disease-free interval and reduced the proportion of patients with recurrence from 53% to 47%. There was no effect on progression to invasive disease, metastases, or survival[23].

Intravesical BCG

The use of live preparations of bacillus Calmette–Guérin (BGG) for immunotherapy for superficial bladder cancer is one of the very few examples where immunotherapy has produced sustained complete remissions for early cancer. The probable reasons for this success are that very small volumes of disease are being treated with good contact between tumor cells and the immunogen and that the cancer is confined to the parent organ. A number of trials have now shown superiority of BCG over cytotoxic chemotherapy for carcinoma in situ and high-grade tumors and BCG, unlike the cytotoxics, has been shown to reduce progression[24-26]. Some studies have not shown a difference between BCG and cytotoxic agents and these differences may be due to the selection of cases, especially the proportion of high-grade tumors and those with carcinoma in situ, the strain of BCG used or the chemotherapy regimen used. BCG, however, has more toxicity and systemic side effects can be life-threatening. In general, cytotoxics can be used initially where the objective of treatment is to reduce recurrences and BCG treatment should be used for the higher-risk cases where the main objective is to prevent progression.

BCG is administered directly into the bladder at weekly intervals for an initial course of 6–8 weeks. Greater reduction in recurrences can be obtained by using maintenance courses of three instillations at 3-, then 6-monthly intervals, but this has greater toxicity and many patients drop out because of it[27]. After BCG there may be quite marked inflammatory changes in the bladder with noncaseating granulomas in the mucosa. The results of BCG usually need to be assessed by repeat biopsies.

Cytotoxic chemotherapy can be given safely within 24–48 hours of resection without significant toxicity but BCG is hazardous in the presence of a recent resection or when there has been trauma to the urethra on catheterization. It is important that any doctor looking after a patient undergoing BCG therapy understands that severe, life-threatening systemic infection can occur and that this needs to be treated promptly with appropriate antibiotics, usually triple therapy as for tuberculosis.

HIGH-RISK SUPERFICIAL BLADDER CANCER

Much of the management of superficial bladder cancer is concerned with the detection and treatment of noninvasive recurrences so it is easy to overlook the threat of some of these tumors becoming invasive and metastasizing as this occurs relatively infrequently. There is also a reluctance to employ radical treatments for disease that is 'only superficial' unless it is fully appreciated that this superficial disease carries a risk of death from bladder cancer if inadequately treated. The established risk factors for progression of superficial bladder cancer are the presence of stromal invasion (T1), high grade (grade 3), and carcinoma in situ.

pT1G3 tumors

The pT1G3 tumor carries almost as high a risk of progression and metastases as a muscle-invasive tumor and is an invasive cancer that is inappropriately classified with the superficial tumors. This tumor has a high recurrence rate, as expected, but has a progression rate of over 40%[28]. These account for approximately 10% of all superficial tumors and frequently have concomitant carcinoma in situ. On receiving such a pathology report the urologist should first consider an early repeat TUR. This is to check that the tumor has not been understaged and is muscle-invasive, and also to look for residual tumors and for carcinoma in situ, especially if cystectomy and orthotopic bladder substitution are being considered. In these cases the prostatic urethra should be biopsied.

Unless the patient is elderly and frail the options to be considered for the patient with a pT1G3 tumor are:
- intravesical BCG
- radiotherapy, or
- cystectomy with bladder substitution or ileal conduit.

Intravesical chemotherapy with cytotoxics may reduce recurrences but will not have an effect on progression. Intravesical BCG offers the patient the possibility of clearing the disease and preserving normal bladder function. Radical radiotherapy may be effective for this tumor as it is treating a high-grade cancer of early stage that is likely to be very small in volume[29]. However, a randomized trial comparing radiotherapy to intravesical therapy or TUR alone is ongoing and needs to be completed. Radical cystectomy for pT1G3 disease will get excellent control of the disease but at a high price. However, the possibility of having a bladder substitution, rather than an ileal conduit, has made this a very much more attractive option for the patient to consider. Randomized studies should be carried out comparing BCG with cystectomy for pT1G3 disease but are unlikely to be completed because of the problem that patients will have in giving informed consent between a radical surgical and a conservative treatment option. Comparing nonrandomized treatment series is always going to be affected by bias in selection of cases, especially from tertiary referral centers with a single treatment policy for these tumors.

CARCINOMA IN SITU

Unlike premalignant changes in the urothelium, carcinoma in situ has a good consensus among pathologists as the term is applied to high-grade lesions of the urothelium without invasion of the basement membrane or papillary growth (Fig. 25.15). Some confusion inevitably surrounds discussion of carcinoma in situ when the pathologic descriptive term is used as a clinical entity. The most useful classification of carcinoma in situ is primary, concomitant, and secondary (Fig. 25.16). Primary carcinoma in situ accounts for between 1% and 5% of all new bladder cancers. It can be missed easily and must be suspected in patients presenting with irritative bladder symptoms and bladder or urethral pain, especially if there is microscopic hematuria. The key to diagnosis is a high index of suspicion. Urine should be sent for cytology in all suspected cases and on cystoscopy all areas of mucosal change should be biopsied. Concomitant or secondary carcinoma in situ should be suspected in high-grade lesions and where cytology is positive. These lesions can be made to fluoresce by prior treatment with 5-amino levulinic acid. This technique can be used for the photodynamic detection of carcinoma in situ and tumors and can also be used for photodynamic

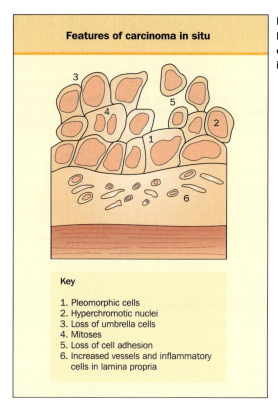

Figure 25.15
Features of
carcinoma
in situ.

Features of carcinoma in situ

Key

1. Pleomorphic cells
2. Hyperchromotic nuclei
3. Loss of umbrella cells
4. Mitoses
5. Loss of cell adhesion
6. Increased vessels and inflammatory cells in lamina propria

Classification of carcinoma in situ of the bladder

Primary	No previous or concomitant tumor
Concomitant	Occurs in the presence of a tumor
Secondary	Occurs when there has been a previous tumor

Symptomatic or asymptomatic

Focal or widespread

Confined to bladder or with extravesical CIS in urethra, prostatic ducts, or ureters

Figure 25.16 Classification of carcinoma in situ (CIS) of the bladder.

therapy whereby tumor cells are destroyed by the release of singlet oxygen by light of the critical wavelength[30].

Primary carcinoma in situ has a high risk of progressing to a muscle-invasive tumor within a few months. Aggressive treatment is justified, especially if the disease can be seen to be widespread within the bladder and symptomatic. Intravesical BCG is the treatment of choice with the prospect of sustained, complete remission in up to 70% of cases. If intravesical BCG fails or cannot be tolerated then radical cystectourethrectomy should be offered[31,32].

FOLLOW-UP

Cystoscopy

The standard follow-up for the detection of recurrent superficial tumors is to carry out flexible cystoscopy. This procedure allows regular inspection of the whole bladder and urethra, and

Urine tests for the detection of bladder tumors

Urine cytology, voided or bladder washings

BTA stat test – measures complement factor H-related proteins in urine

BTA track test – quantitative immunoassay using monoclonal antibody

NMP22 – measures nuclear matrix proteins quantitatively

TRAP assay – measure telomerase activity in the urine using fluorescein-labeled polymerase chain reaction technique

Figure 25.17 Urine tests for the detection of bladder tumors.

has very low morbidity and low cost. With experience and good equipment very small lesions can be detected reliably. Small tumors, however, can be overlooked and interpretation of flat mucosal changes can be very difficult.

In the group at low risk of recurrence the interval between cystoscopies can be yearly after the first cystoscopy at 3 months. For all other groups the intervals should be 3-monthly initially, gradually increasing to annually when the patient has been recurrence-free for 3 years. There is no clear consensus on when follow-up cystoscopies can cease. After 7–10 years recurrence-free the risk of a further tumor developing is about 1% and the burden of a check cystoscopy in an elderly patient may not be justified. Detection of microscopic hematuria in these patients should be an indication for early full reassessment.

Urine testing

A number of urine tests have now been developed for the detection of bladder cancer (Fig. 25.17)[33]. Some are simple office tests and others still require to be sent to a reference laboratory. Much interest has been shown in these tests because of the shortcomings of urine cytology in the detection of low-grade tumors and the expense of a subjective test dependent on training, skill, and experience. A number of important questions must be addressed before these tests can be adopted as standard practice.

- Does the test have sufficient sensitivity to allow flexible cystoscopy to be omitted in a patient at risk of having a new or recurrent bladder cancer?
- Will the test replace urine cytology (i.e. be cheaper) or will it become an adjunct to cytology (i.e. be more expensive)?
- Is the false-positive rate low enough to justify the unnecessary investigation of these patients and its costs?
- If these tests are adopted will this have a detrimental effect on the quality of urine cytology?

All the tests require further detailed prospective study, including urine cytology, and they are further discussed in Chapter 26. It is reasonable to reduce the burden of follow-up flexible cystoscopy for both the patient and the health service. The most important objective for superficial bladder cancer remains the accurate prediction of those patients at risk of progression who require early radical therapy.

Upper tract imaging

In treating urothelial cancer it is important to remember that this has usually been caused by urine-borne carcinogens; hence

<table>
<tr><th colspan="2">Indications for upper tract imaging in the follow-up of superficial bladder cancer</th></tr>
</table>

Positive cytology or hematuria in the absence of tumor in the bladder

Recurrent tumors occurring around the ureteric orifice

When the intramural ureter has been resected and there is a risk of scarring

When planning cystectomy for uncontrolled disease

Figure 25.18 Indications for upper tract imaging in the follow-up of superficial bladder cancer.

the whole urothelium has been exposed from the calix down to the urethra and further tumors can occur anywhere in the urinary tract over a long period of time. With superficial tumors, upper tract recurrence is relatively rare and does not justify regular upper tract imaging. There are certain circumstances where upper tract pathology is more likely and imaging, usually with intravenous urography, is justified (Fig. 25.18).

REFERENCES

1. Cholerton S, Hall RR. Smoking and bladder cancer. In: Clinical management of bladder cancer. London: Arnold; 1999:337.
2. Wallace DMA. Occupational urothelial cancer. Br J Urol. 1988;61:175
3. Sorahan T, Hamilton L, Wallace DMA, et al. Occupational urothelial tumours: a regional case-control study. Br J Urol. 1998;82:25.
4. British Association of Urological Surgeons Subcommittee on Industrial Bladder Cancer. Occupational bladder cancer: a guide for clinicians. Br J Urol. 1988;61:183.
5. Office of National Statistics. Monitor MB1 98/2 July 1998. London: Office of National Statistics.
6. Cairns P, Shaw ME, Knowles MA. Preliminary mapping of the deleted region of chromosome 9 in bladder cancer. Can Res. 1993; 53:1230.
7. Ooms ECM, Anderson WAD, Allons CL, et al. Analysis of the performance of pathologists in the grading of bladder tumours. Human Path. 1983;14:140
8. Richards B, Parmar MKB, Anderson CK, et al. Interpretation of biopsies of 'normal' urothelium in patients with superficial bladder cancer. Br J Urol. 1991;6:369.
9. Younes M, Sussman J, True LD. The usefulness of the level of the muscularis mucosae in the staging of invasive transitional cell carcinoma of the urinary bladder. Cancer. 1990;66:543.
10. Lynch TH, Waymont B, Dunn JA, et al. Repeat testing for haematuria and underlying urological pathology. Br J Urol. 1994;74:730.
11. Messing EM, Young TB, Hunt VB, et al. Comparison of bladder cancer outcome in men undergoing haematuria home screening versus those with standard clinical presentation. Urology. 1995;45:387.
12. Kiemeney LALM, Witjes JA, Heijbroek RP, et al. Should random urothelial biopsies be taken from patients with primary superficial bladder cancer? A decision analysis. Br J Urol. 1994;73:163.
13. Klan R, Loy V, Huland H. Residual tumor discovered in the routine transurethral resection in patients with stage T1 transitional cell carcinoma of the bladder. J Urol. 1991;146:316.
14. Haukaas S, Daehlin L, Maartman-Moe H, Ulvik NM. The long term outcome in patients with superficial transitional cell carcinoma of the bladder: a single institution experience. BJU Int. 1999;83:957.
15. Sobin LH, Wittekind C, eds. UICC TNM classification of malignant tumors. New York: Wiley-Liss; 1997.
16. Lamm DL, Griffiths JG. Intravesical therapy: does it affect the natural history of superficial bladder cancer. Sem Urol. 1992;10:39.
17. Parmar MKD, Freidman LS, Hargreave TB, Tolley DA. Prognostic factors for recurrence and follow-up policies in the treatment of superficial bladder cancer. A report from the Medical Research Council Subgroup on superficial bladder cancer. J Urol. 1989;142:284
18. Hall RR, Parmar MKB, Richards AB, Smith PH. Proposals for change in cystoscopic follow-up of patients with bladder cancer and adjuvant intravesical chemotherapy. Br Med J. 1994;308:257.
19. Bouffioux C, van der Meijden A, Kurth K, Sylvester R. Objective response criteria to intravesical chemotherapy: the marker lesion. In: Pagano F, Fair WR, eds. Superficial bladder cancer. Oxford: Isis Medical Media; 1997:90.
20. Bouffioux C, Kurth KH, Bono A, et al. Intravesical adjuvant chemotherapy for superficial transitional cell carcinoma: results of two European Organisation for Research and Treatment of Cancer randomised trials with Mitomycin C and Doxorubicin comparing early versus delayed instillations and short term versus long term treatment. J Urol. 1995;153:934.
21. Oosterlink W, Kurth KH, Schroder F, et al. A prospective European Organisation for Research and Treatment of Cancer Genitourinary Group randomised trial comparing transurethral resection followed by a single intravesical instillation of epirubicin or water in single, stage Ta,T1 papillary carcinoma of the bladder. J Urol. 1993;149:749.
22. Tolley DA, Parmar MKB, Grigor KM, et al. The effect of intravesical mitomycin C on the recurrence of newly diagnosed superficial bladder cancer: a further report with 7 years follow-up. J Urol. 1996;155:1233.
23. Pawinski A, Sylvester R, Kurth KH, et al. A combined analysis of the European Organisation for Research and Treatment of Cancer and Medical Research Council randomised clinical trials for the prophylactic treatment of Ta, T1 bladder cancer. J Urol. 1996;156:1934.
24. Herr HW, Laudrone VP, Badalment RA. Bacillus Calmette–Guérin therapy alters the progression of superficial bladder cancer. J Clin Oncol. 1988;6:1450
25. Lamm DL, Crissman J, Blumenstein BA, et al. Adriamycin versus BCG in superficial bladder cancer: a Southwest Oncology Group study. Proc Clin Biol Res. 1989;310:263
26. Pagano F, Bassi P, Milani C, et al. A low dose Bacillus Calmette–Guérin regimen for superficial bladder cancer therapy. Is it effective? J Urol. 1991;146:32.
27. Lamm DL, Blumenstein BA, Sarosdy MF, et al. Significant long term patient benefit with BCG maintenance therapy: a Southwest Oncology Group Study. J Urol. 1997;157(Suppl 213):abstract 831.
28. Birch BRP, Harland SJ. The pT1 G3 bladder tumour. Br J Urol. 1989;64:109.
29. Quilty PM, Duncan W. Treatment of superficial (T1) tumours of the bladder by radical radiotherapy. Br J Urol. 196;58:147.
30. Kreigmair M, Baumgartner R, Kneckel R, et al. Detection of early bladder cancer by 5-aminolevulinic acid induced porphyrin fluorescence. J Urol. 1996;155:105.
31. Herr HW, Pinsky CM, Whitmore WF, et al. Long term effects of intravesical Bacillus Calmette–Guérin on flat carcinoma in situ of the bladder. J Urol. 1986;135:265.
32. Jakse G, Putz A, Feichtinger J. Cystectomy: the treatment of choice inpatients with carcinoma in situ of the urinary bladder? Eur J Surg Oncol. 1989;15:211.
33. Landeman J, Chang Y, Kavaler E, et al. Sensitivity and specificity of NMP22, telomerase and BTA in the detection of human bladder cancer. Urology. 1998;52:398.

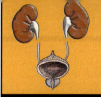

Section 5 Urologic Oncology

Chapter 26

Invasive Bladder Cancer

Gary D Grossfeld and Peter R Carroll

KEY POINTS

- The clinical utility of recent diagnostic urine tests remains unproved.
- Accurate staging is crucial to treatment planning and comparison of results.
- Radical surgery in appropriate patients appears to offer the best chance of survival at 5 years.
- Lesser procedures in compromised patients may produce favorable medium-term results.

INTRODUCTION

It has been estimated that the number of new cases of bladder cancer diagnosed in 2000 will be 53,200, leading to 12,200 deaths from this disease[1]. Hence bladder cancer is the fifth most commonly diagnosed noncutaneous solid malignancy, and second most commonly diagnosed genitourinary malignancy among people living in the United States. Bladder cancer is approximately three times more common in men than in women, and the disease is diagnosed more often in Caucasian patients than in African–Americans. There is a positive social class gradient for bladder cancer incidence in both sexes, as reflected in the distribution of bladder cancer by occupational category; incidence rates are highest among 'white collar' occupations and lowest among 'blue collar' workers[2].

At the time of diagnosis, approximately 70–75% of patients with bladder cancer present with superficial disease limited to the mucosal lining of the bladder[3]. In such patients, the risk of distant disease is low, and the natural history of bladder cancer is based on two separate, but related, processes – tumor recurrence and progression to a higher stage of disease. Overall, tumor recurrence occurs in 50–70% of patients with superficial bladder cancer[4], while progression to a higher stage of disease occurs in only 10–15% of these patients[3]. This high recurrence rate in areas distant from the primary tumor suggests that bladder cancer represents a 'field defect' in which the entire urothelium may be altered by exposure to a chemical carcinogen. Risk factors for recurrence and progression include high tumor grade, tumor stage (Ta versus T1), the number of tumors at presentation, the presence of atypia or carcinoma in situ (CIS) adjacent to the primary tumor or on random mucosal biopsies, and the presence of tumor at the first follow-up cystoscopy (3 months after resection)[4]. For example, a patient who presents with a single, low-grade, stage Ta tumor is at

'good' risk with respect to tumor recurrence and has a low risk of disease progression (<5%). Conversely, a patient who presents with a high-grade, stage T1 tumor has a much greater risk of disease progression (as high as 30%). For details see Chapter 25.

Invasive bladder cancers include tumors that invade into or through the muscular wall of the bladder. These tumors may be confined to the bladder (stage T2) or they may extend through the bladder to involve the perivesical fat (stage T3) or adjacent organs (stage T4). Fortunately, a minority of newly diagnosed bladder tumors present with muscle invasion. In contrast to superficial bladder tumors, invasive bladder tumors demonstrate an aggressive pattern of growth that often results in systemic spread of disease. Consequently, treatment of invasive tumors needs to be directed at aggressive local disease control as well as prevention or treatment of metastatic disease. Although disease may appear to be limited to the bladder at the time of presentation, as many as 50% of patients with newly diagnosed muscle invasive bladder cancer may have micrometastatic disease at the time of presentation[5]. Thus, invasive bladder cancer represents a high-risk disease that may prove fatal to the host unless aggressively treated.

The purpose of this chapter is to address important issues with respect to the diagnosis, staging, and treatment of patients with newly diagnosed muscle invasive bladder cancer. Hypotheses regarding the etiology and pathogenesis of this disease are also explored. New advances in molecular staging and prognostic markers are summarized, as the application of these novel techniques may soon allow clinicians to select patients appropriately for one of the various local treatment options.

ETIOLOGY

The etiology of invasive bladder cancer is outlined in Figure 26.1.

Cigarette smoking

An association between cigarette smoking and bladder cancer was first reported in 1956[6]. Since that time, numerous studies have identified a positive association between cigarette smoking and bladder cancer that appears to be dose related[2,7]. Most case control studies report a relative risk of approximately 2.0 for smokers as compared to nonsmokers, and nearly all studies demonstrate a progressively higher risk with increased cigarette consumption. Former smokers appear to have a relative risk of developing bladder cancer that lies somewhere between those of current smokers and nonsmokers. Interestingly, pipe and cigar smokers are only weakly associated with the development of bladder cancer, while smokeless tobacco is not associated with development of the disease.

The mechanism by which cigarette smoking leads to the development of bladder cancer is unclear, but it likely involves carcinogens that are present in cigarette smoke. These carcinogens, which include the aromatic amines α- and β-naphthylamine, appear in the urine of smokers. In addition, certain cyclic *N*-nitrosamines derived from tobacco smoke are known bladder-specific chemical carcinogens in animals[2].

Industrial exposure

Industrial chemical exposure may account for 15–35% of bladder cancer cases in men and 1–6% of cases in women[7]. Arylamines are the class of chemicals most strongly related to the development of bladder cancer. These chemicals were initially used in the textile dye industry in the mid 1800s, and the first case of bladder cancer in a dye worker was reported in 1895. Other occupations with exposures associated with the development of bladder cancer include those in the rubber tire industry, hairdressers (from hair dyes), painters (from paint pigment), metal workers, and those in the leather industry.

Other risk factors

Although a variety of other potential etiologic agents have been associated with the development of bladder cancer, sufficient epidemiologic evidence is lacking in most cases. Animal studies suggest that artificial sweeteners, such as saccharin, may cause bladder cancer in rodents[2]. However, studies in humans do not confirm this association. Bladder cancer has also been associated with the heavy use of analgesics, especially those that contain phenacetin, as well as with coffee drinking. Patients treated with cyclophosphamide for the management of various other malignancies also appear to be at increased risk for the development of bladder cancer. Finally, physical trauma to the urothelium, such as infection, instrumentation, prolonged catheterization, and calculi appear to be risk factors for the development of squamous cell carcinoma of the bladder.

PATHOGENESIS

Transitional cell carcinoma is a heterogeneous disease. Although the histologic appearance of transitional cell carcinoma suggests a continuum of disease that begins with dysplasia and CIS, progresses to superficial carcinoma, and ultimately ends up as muscle invasive disease, the natural history of bladder cancer does not support this orderly progression[8]. Most patients diagnosed with bladder cancer initially present with superficial disease. The natural history of these tumors is recurrence, and only 10–15% of patients progress to a higher stage disease[4]. By comparison, over 80% of patients who present with invasive transitional cell carcinoma have no previous history of superficial disease[8]. These observations suggest that superficial and muscle invasive transitional cell carcinomas may represent separate, but related disease processes.

In contrast to superficial bladder cancer, urothelial dysplasia and CIS may truly represent preinvasive lesions. Although confined to the mucosal layer of the bladder, CIS carries a worse prognosis than superficial disease. Without treatment, such lesions may progress to invasive bladder cancer in as many as 80% of patients[9]. In 20–30% of CIS cases, microinvasion into the muscular wall can be identified[10]. Moreover, up to 60% of

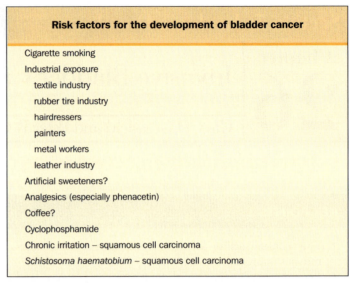

Risk factors for the development of bladder cancer

Cigarette smoking
Industrial exposure
   textile industry
   rubber tire industry
   hairdressers
   painters
   metal workers
   leather industry
Artificial sweeteners?
Analgesics (especially phenacetin)
Coffee?
Cyclophosphamide
Chronic irritation – squamous cell carcinoma
Schistosoma haematobium – squamous cell carcinoma

Figure 26.1 Risk factors for the development of bladder cancer.

patients with CIS only at the time of clinical staging may have muscle invasive disease at the time of radical cystectomy[11].

It has been suggested that multiple genetic alterations are necessary for epithelial cells to progress from normal to malignant cells. The nature of these genetic alterations is not well defined for any malignancy, including bladder cancer. However, a large body of research has focused on determining specific mutations that may be necessary for bladder cancer progression (Fig. 26.2). Multiple genetic changes, which include the activation of oncogenes and inactivation of tumor suppressor genes, have been described for patients with bladder cancer. Early studies that examined genetic changes in bladder cancer identified the loss of genetic material on chromosome 9 as a unique and consistent finding in patients with bladder cancer[12,13]. Such changes are seen in both low-grade, low-stage disease and high-grade, high-stage disease, which suggests that loss of heterozygosity of chromosome 9 may be an early event in bladder cancer development. Loss of chromosome 9 in multiple tumors from an individual patient supports the concept that genetic changes in bladder cancer represent a 'field defect' that may occur throughout the urothelium.

Additional genetic changes specific for invasive bladder tumors have been described. Chromosome 11p contains the c-Ha-ras proto-oncogene. This chromosome is deleted in approximately 40% of bladder cancers[8]. Increased expression of the c-Ha-ras protein product, p21, has been detected in dysplastic and high-grade tumors, but not in low-grade bladder cancers. Deletions of chromosome 17p have also been detected in over 60% of all invasive bladder cancers, while 17p deletions have not been described in superficial tumors. This finding is noteworthy because the p53 tumor suppressor gene maps to chromosome 17p. Alterations of p53 represent the most commonly identified genetic abnormality in human cancers, which makes deletion of this chromosome an important finding in muscle invasive bladder cancer. Furthermore, p53 status has been associated with outcome in patients who undergo radical cystectomy for muscle invasive bladder cancer[14].

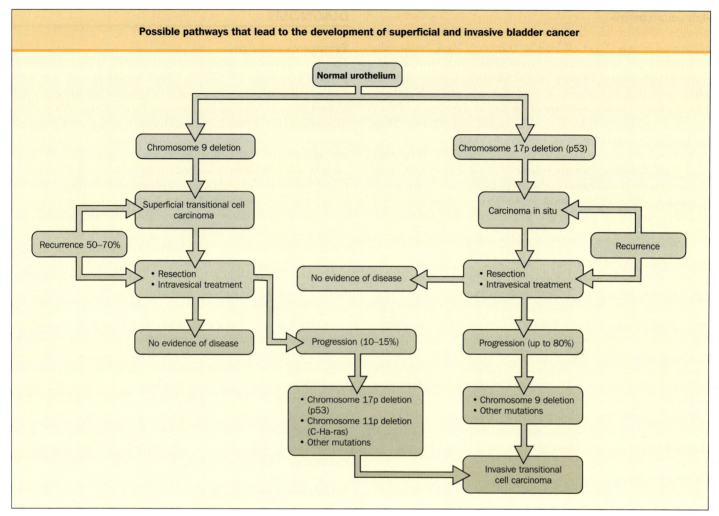

Figure 26.2 Possible pathways that lead to the development of superficial and invasive bladder cancer.

Genetic changes in CIS lesions are more characteristic of invasive than superficial bladder cancer. Previous studies demonstrated that CIS lesions express p53 mutations, but they do not demonstrate a high frequency of chromosome 9 alterations[15]. These data support the concept that CIS precedes the development of invasive bladder cancer in some patients.

HISTOLOGY

Transitional cell carcinoma

Approximately 90% of all bladder cancers are transitional cell carcinomas (Fig. 26.3)[3]. Invasive transitional cell tumors commonly appear as sessile lesions, while superficial tumors are papillary and exophytic. Although no grading system is universally accepted, carcinomas are usually grouped into three or four categories (grades) that progress from well-differentiated, grade 1 tumors to poorly differentiated (anaplastic) grade 3 or 4 tumors. Grading is based on urothelial architecture and cytologic characteristics, such as cell size, degree of pleomorphism, nuclear anaplasia, and hyperchromatism, and the number of mitoses[16,17]. A precursor to invasive transitional cell carcinoma is considered to be CIS. Grossly, it may be recognized as a

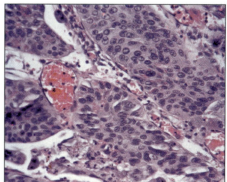

Figure 26.3 Transitional cell carcinoma of the bladder. The nests of intermediate-sized epithelial cells have large, atypical nuclei. Well and moderately differentiated transitional cell carcinomas infiltrate into the underlying tissue as nests of cells. This pattern is lost in poorly differentiated, higher grade tumors, which infiltrate as single cells.

flat, erythematous, velvety patch in the bladder mucosa. Microscopically, cells are large with prominent nucleoli, and the urothelium lacks normal cellular polarity. These lesions may occur in association with either exophytic or sessile tumors, or (less commonly) they may occur as focal or diffuse lesions in patients with no grossly identifiable tumors.

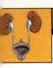

Adenocarcinoma

Primary adenocarcinoma of the bladder (Fig. 26.4) is rare, and accounts for only 2% of all bladder tumors[18]. More commonly, transitional cell carcinoma may be associated with areas of glandular differentiation. Primary vesical adenocarcinomas are most often located at the trigone or posterior wall of the bladder[18]. Histologically, these tumors are often mucus secreting, and they may have either glandular, colloid, or signet-ring patterns. They are usually preceded by a long history of cystitis.

Urachal adenocarcinomas are located at the dome or anterior wall of the bladder. They are primarily intramural in that there is usually little or no change in the overlying mucosa[18]. Although adenocarcinomas are often localized to the bladder at the time of diagnosis, muscle invasion is usually present and the tumor may be locally extensive.

Squamous cell carcinoma

Squamous cell carcinoma (Fig. 26.5) is often associated with chronic irritation of the bladder mucosa. In the United States, this histologic subtype accounts for only 3–7% of all bladder cancers[3]. Risk factors include a history of chronic infection, bladder calculi, chronic instrumentation, or prolonged catheterization.

Squamous cell carcinoma is also associated with bilharzial infection secondary to *Schistosoma haematobium*. This histologic subtype represents the most commonly diagnosed bladder tumor in the Middle East (especially Egypt) and in parts of Africa. In these areas, squamous cell carcinoma may account for up to 60% of all bladder tumors[7]. Tumors are often invasive at the time of diagnosis.

Miscellaneous

Sarcomas account for only 2% of all bladder tumors[3]. Approximately 4–6% of all bladder cancers are mixed carcinomas, composed of transitional, glandular, squamous, or undifferentiated patterns. Undifferentiated carcinomas contain no mature epithelial elements and include a type of small cell carcinoma that histologically resembles those seen in the lung[19]. Other rare tumors include villous adenomas, carcinoid tumors, carcinosarcomas, melanomas, pheochromocytomas, lymphomas, and choriocarcinomas[7]. Tumors of the prostate, cervix, and rectum may involve the bladder by direct extension, while melanoma, lymphoma, stomach cancer, breast cancer, renal cell carcinoma, and lung cancer may metastasize to the bladder.

DIAGNOSIS

Symptoms and signs

The most common presenting symptom of bladder cancer is painless hematuria (Fig. 26.6), which occurs in approximately 85% of patients[3]. Hematuria may be gross or microscopic, and it is usually intermittent in character. Patients may also present with symptoms of bladder irritability, such as urinary frequency, urgency, or dysuria. Such irritative voiding symptoms may indicate the presence of CIS. Patients with advanced disease may present with flank pain secondary to ureteral obstruction, a pelvic mass, or constitutional symptoms such as weight loss or bone pain. It is emphasized that all patients with gross hematuria, as well as those patients with persistent microscopic hematuria for which a cause cannot be identified, must undergo a complete evaluation to exclude bladder cancer.

Patient history should not only focus on pertinent symptoms, but also patients should be questioned about potential risk factors for bladder cancer, including cigarette smoking and occupational exposures.

A thorough physical examination should include a complete abdominal examination as well as a digital rectal examination and bimanual examination to rule out any obvious pelvic mass. Patients with invasive tumors may demonstrate a palpable mass, especially when the examination is carried out under anesthetic. When a mass is detected, mobility or fixation should be determined. The presence of a fixed mass suggests invasion of contiguous organs or the pelvic sidewall. Other pertinent physical findings include hepatomegaly or supraclavicular lymphadenopathy suggestive of metastatic disease.

Laboratory investigations

Laboratory examination for patients suspected of having bladder cancer requires a complete blood count, a serum chemistry panel that includes an assessment of renal function, alkaline phosphatase level, a urinalysis and a urine culture (Fig. 26.6). Patients may demonstrate anemia secondary to hematuria, bone marrow metastases, or anemia of chronic disease. The serum chemistry panel may demonstrate evidence of renal insufficiency secondary to ureteral obstruction by tumor. Serum alkaline phosphatase may be elevated because of liver or bone metastases. Urinalysis usually demonstrates hematuria, and a urine culture excludes infection as a cause for blood in the urine.

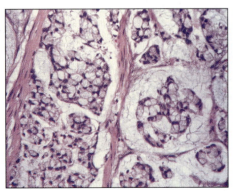

Figure 26.4 Mucinous adenocarcinoma of the bladder. Clusters of cells, some with a signet-ring morphology, are located within a pool of mucin. Adenocarcinoma of the bladder may also appear as a well-differentiated, glandular pattern of cells reminiscent of intestinal adenocarcinoma.

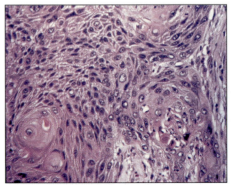

Figure 26.5 Squamous cell carcinoma of the bladder. The cytologically atypical cells have clear cytoplasmic borders and intercellular bridges (desmosomes). These cells have ample eosinophilic (pink) cytoplasm. Also present is extracellular keratin, which appears in a 'whorl-like' pattern (bottom left).

Initial evaluation of patients with bladder cancer

History – symptoms

Painless hematuria – microscopic or gross
Bladder irritability – urgency, frequency, dysuria
Flank pain
Weight loss
Bone pain

Physical signs

Pelvic mass
Hepatomegaly
Supraclavicular adenopathy

Laboratory

Complete blood count
Serum chemistry panel
Blood urea nitrogen and serum creatinine
Alkaline phosphatase
Urinalysis and urine culture
Urinary cytology

Figure 26.6 Initial evaluation of patients with bladder cancer: history, physical examination and laboratory evaluation.

Malignant transitional cells may be detected on microscopic evaluation of the urine sediment or bladder washings (urine cytologic examination). Urothelial cells are exfoliated into the voided urine from both normal patients and patients with bladder cancer. These cells can be identified and analyzed after fixation and staining. To increase the number of exfoliated cells, the bladder can be irrigated gently with isotonic saline, either through a catheter or a cystoscope (bladder wash). The sensitivity of voided urinary cytology varies between 40% and 76%, depending upon the grade of the tumor (increased sensitivity with higher grade disease)[20,21]. Consequently, urine cytology may be of limited value in patients with low-grade disease, although high-grade invasive tumors are detected commonly. Sensitivity of urinary cytology can be improved with multiple voided specimens or bladder washing[20]. In addition, urine cytology may be combined with flow cytometry to detect malignant cells with abnormal DNA content[7].

In response to the limitations of urinary cytology, newer diagnostic tests have been developed that detect tumor-specific antigens in voided urine. These tests are currently being evaluated, and their results with respect to bladder cancer detection are being compared with those of urinary cytology. These tests detect the presence of antigens that have been isolated and characterized from the urine of patients with bladder cancer, urinary nuclear matrix proteins, Lewis X antigen expression on exfoliated urothelial cells and expression of telomerase activity in exfoliated cells (Fig. 26.7). The clinical utility of these newer tests, however, has not yet been established. Thus, at present no test can reliably substitute for cystoscopy (endoscopic examination of the bladder) in the evaluation of patients suspected of having bladder cancer.

Cystoscopy and tumor resection (transurethral resection of bladder tumor)

All patients who are suspected of having a bladder tumor, including those with gross and persistent microscopic hematuria, need to undergo a thorough cystoscopic examination of the bladder. Initial diagnostic cystoscopy, if carried out under local anesthetic, can be achieved safely with a flexible cystoscope. This is associated with less discomfort to the patient than is rigid cystoscopy. Superficial, low-grade lesions usually appear as single or multiple papillary lesions. Higher grade, invasive lesions are often larger and sessile. If an invasive tumor is suspected from diagnostic cystoscopy, cross-sectional imaging tests, such as computed tomography (CT), should be scheduled prior to transurethral resection. This is so that local tissue changes after transurethral resection are not confused with extravesical disease extension. In addition, upper tract imaging is carried out prior to resection so that retrograde pyelography can be performed during the same anesthetic if an upper tract lesion is identified.

When a bladder tumor is detected cystoscopically, initial local staging and treatment consists of a transurethral (cystoscopic) resection of the bladder tumor (TURBT). After induction of either general or regional anesthetic, the patient is placed in the lithotomy position and a thorough bimanual examination is carried out with the patient under anesthetic. This allows the clinician to determine the position, size, and degree of fixation of any pelvic mass that is detected. The bimanual examination should also be performed following tumor resection to note changes in the character of the mass. The disappearance of a

Marker	Sensitivity (%)	Specificity (%)	Positive predictive value (%)	Negative predictive value (%)
BTA[22–30]	28–70	73–96	33–80	52–94
NMP22[24,31–37]	48–100	61–99	29–65	60–100
BTA Stat[31,36,38,39]	57–83	33–95	20–56	70–95
BTA Trak[37,40]	62–72	73–98	62	73
Lewis X antigen[41–43]	80–97	73–86	72–81	83–98
Telomerase[24,36,44]	62–80	80–99	84	89
Fibrin/fibrinogen degradation products[26,36]	52–81	75–91	79	78
Cytokeratin 20[45]	91	85	95	76
CD44 variant[46]	77	100	100	76

Sensitivity, specificity, and positive and negative predictive values of voided urinary markers in the detection of primary and recurrent bladder cancer

Figure 26.7 Sensitivity, specificity, and positive and negative predictive values of voided urinary markers in the detection of primary and recurrent bladder cancer.

mass after transurethral resection suggests a large minimally invasive tumor, while a persistent mass suggests residual, locally extensive, muscle invasive disease.

Before proceeding with tumor resection, a complete cystoscopic evaluation of the bladder is carried out with both a 30° and a 70° lens. The urethra and prostate are evaluated for any evidence of tumor. Examination of the bladder is comprehensive and methodic, as multiple areas of the urothelium may be involved with bladder cancer. The number, size, and location of all tumors is noted. Erythematous areas, consistent with the presence of CIS, are also recorded. Random biopsies of grossly uninvolved bladder mucosa are often recommended for patients who present with their first bladder tumor. Such biopsies can document CIS or dysplasia at sites adjacent to, or distant from, the primary tumor, which may predict an increased likelihood of tumor recurrence and/or progression[7].

All visible tumor should be resected if possible. Resection continues to the base of the tumor, at which a portion of the muscularis propria of the bladder wall should be resected for pathologic examination. This procedure enables a complete local tumor staging. Complete resection is critical for superficial tumors, as it may be the only treatment necessary. For patients with muscle invasive disease, complete resection is carried out if possible. However, if technically difficult, a biopsy to confirm muscle invasion may be appropriate as additional treatment is necessary. Such patients may be at increased risk for perforation and dissemination of tumor cells.

STAGING

Once the diagnosis of bladder cancer has been established, the depth of tumor invasion must be determined. Such a determination is based primarily on tissue obtained at the time of TURBT. However, physical examination and radiologic imaging can provide complimentary information. Bladder tumor treatment, prognosis, and the likelihood of metastatic disease are strongly associated with the depth of primary tumor invasion. The first staging system, described by Jewett and Strong in 1946[47], was based on the relationship between the depth of tumor invasion into the bladder wall and the likelihood of lymph node or distant metastatic disease. This system was subsequently modified by Marshall[48]. In the Jewett–Strong–Marshall system, no patient with disease confined to the mucosa (Stage A) was found to have metastatic disease, while 13% of patients with disease that involved the muscularis (Stage B) and 74% of patients with perivesical disease extension (Stage C) had metastatic disease.

Currently, bladder tumors are staged according to the TNM (tumor, nodes, and metastasis) system[49,50], which enables precise and simultaneous description of primary tumor extent (T), status of the lymph nodes (N), and extent of metastatic disease (M). This system was modified recently, in 1997[50]. Figure 26.8 demonstrates the relationship between the Jewett–Strong–Marshall staging system and the two TNM systems most often cited in the literature.

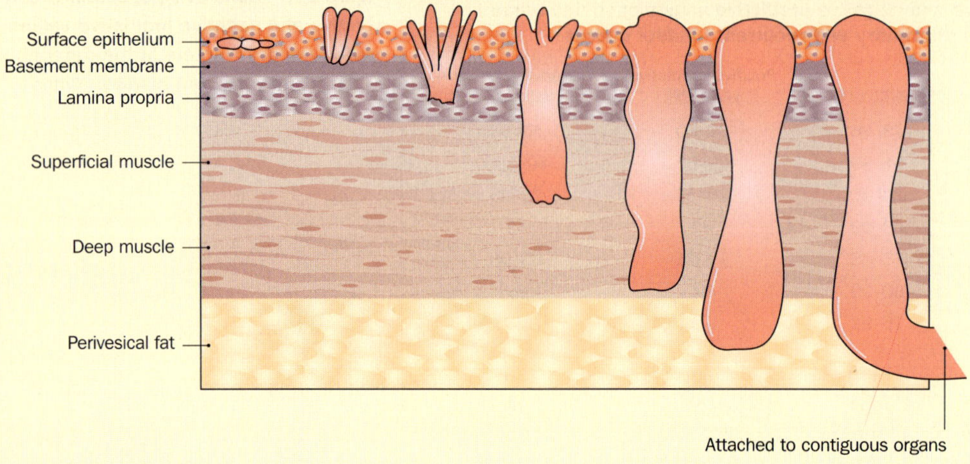

Figure 26.8 Comparison of the staging systems most commonly used for bladder cancer. TNM, tumor, nodes, and metastasis.

Comparison of the staging systems most commonly used for bladder cancer

Staging system	Stages						
Jewett–Strong–Marshall	0	0	A	B1	B2	C	D1
TNM 1987	TIS	Ta	T1	T2	T3a	T3b	T4
TNM 1997	TIS	Ta	T1	T2a	T2b	T3 T3a – microscopic extension into fat T3b – microscopic extension into fat	T4
Penetration	Epithelial membrane intact	Urothelium only	To lamina propria	Superfical muscle	Deep muscle	To perivesical fat	organs

Surface epithelium
Basement membrane
Lamina propria

Superficial muscle

Deep muscle

Perivesical fat

Attached to contiguous organs

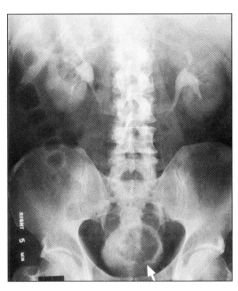

Figure 26.9 Filling defect in the bladder. Intravenous urographic appearance of bladder cancer. Note the large filling defect in the bladder (arrow) without concomitant hydronephrosis.

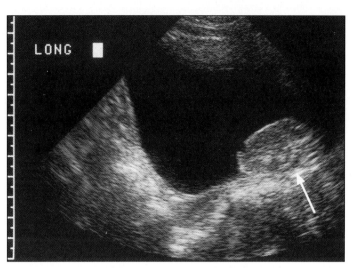

Figure 26.10 Ultrasonographic appearance of bladder cancer. A large intraluminal mass (arrow) is present within the well-distended bladder.

All patients with Stage T2 disease and above are considered to have invasive bladder cancer. The natural history of such invasive tumors appears to be much more aggressive than that of tumors confined to the urothelial lining of the bladder. Thus, invasion into the muscularis propria of the bladder wall carries important implications, with respect to both prognosis and treatment. The depth of tumor invasion is associated strongly with both the likelihood of lymph node metastasis and the outcome after treatment. For example, regional lymph node metastases are seen in 20–30% of patients with organ-confined (pT2, pT3a) disease and in as many as 30–66% of patients with extravesical disease extension (pT3b or greater)[5].

RADIOLOGIC IMAGING

Bladder cancer can be detected by a variety of imaging techniques. However, the diagnosis of bladder cancer can be confirmed by cystoscopy and transurethral resection only. Bladder tumors may appear as filling defects on an intravenous urogram (IVU; Fig. 26.9), or they may be detected by ultrasonographic evaluation of an adequately distended bladder (Fig. 26.10). Detection of bladder tumors using these imaging modalities depends not only on the size of the lesion, but also on the degree to which the bladder is distended. Even though the data are limited, the literature suggests an advantage of ultrasound over IVU in the detection of bladder tumors[51]. With respect to cross-sectional imaging (Fig. 26.11), no data in the literature show the detection rate of previously undiagnosed bladder tumors using either CT or magnetic resonance imaging (MRI). Thus, the role of diagnostic imaging in the detection of bladder tumors is limited. Nevertheless, imaging remains an important part of the evaluation of patients with newly diagnosed muscle invasive bladder cancer. In this setting, imaging serves three purposes:

- evaluate the upper urinary tracts;
- determine the extent of local disease; and
- exclude the presence of distant metastases.

Imaging the upper urinary tracts

Most patients with bladder cancer initially present with hematuria. As hematuria can originate from any point along the

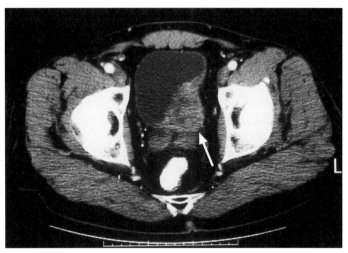

Figure 26.11 Recurrent bladder cancer. The computed tomography scan shows a large mass on the left lateral wall of the bladder (arrow). This mass represented a large recurrent bladder tumor.

urinary tract, upper tract imaging is an important component of the hematuria evaluation. In such patients, upper tract imaging can detect either solid parenchymal renal lesions (renal cell carcinoma) or lesions in the renal pelvis and ureter caused by transitional cell carcinoma. Renal pelvic tumors account for only 5–10% of all upper tract tumors, while ureteral tumors are even less common than those in the renal pelvis[3]. However, in patients with known bladder cancer, exclusion of upper tract transitional cell carcinoma is necessary, given that transitional cell carcinoma may represent a 'field defect' in the entire urothelium. Upper tract transitional cell carcinomas may occur in 2–4% of such patients[3].

Upper tract imaging may also detect the presence of hydronephrosis, which is indicative of muscle invasive bladder cancer. The presence of hydronephrosis in patients with invasive bladder cancer (especially bilateral hydronephrosis) correlates with poor outcome after both radical cystectomy[52] and definitive chemoradiation[53].

Traditionally, an IVU was recommended to evaluate the upper urinary tracts, as it provides complete visualization of the kidneys, collecting systems, and ureters. More recently, ultrasound has been advocated as a less invasive and less costly method to screen the upper tracts[51,54,55]. However, ultrasound does not provide the same anatomic detail of the collecting systems and ureters as does IVU. An advantage of CT over both IVU and ultrasound is that cross-sectional images of the entire abdomen and pelvis can be obtained. Thus, CT can image the kidneys and collecting systems, and it can be used to determine the extent of local and systemic disease.

Currently, no reported studies have compared the performance of the various diagnostic imaging modalities in the detection of upper tract transitional cell carcinomas. Traditionally, IVU was used as the 'gold standard' to detect these lesions, given the complete visualization of the upper tracts. However, renal pelvic tumors can often be diagnosed by ultrasound or CT[56,57], as can the obstruction that is often associated with a lesion in the ureter[54]. Furthermore, CT can detect soft-tissue lesions in the ureter. Buckley et al.[58] detected 31 of 31 renal transitional cell carcinomas using contrast-enhanced CT scans. Igarashi et al.[59] demonstrated 18 of 19 renal transitional cell carcinomas by ultrasound and 8 of 8 by contrast-enhanced CT. Although further studies are needed, it is clear that ultrasound and CT can be used to evaluate the upper urinary tracts of patients with bladder cancer.

Evaluation of local disease extent

Both CT and MRI can be used to assess the extent of bladder wall invasion by tumor prior to transurethral resection. The overall accuracy of such cross-sectional imaging modalities is 40–85%[60–64]. With respect to assessment of the depth of tumor invasion, these imaging modalities are limited by their inability to recognize microscopic disease extension and their dependence on the disruption of normal tissue planes to identify invasion.[10] Consequently, cross-sectional imaging has limited ability to distinguish muscle invasive from superficial disease, which results in overstaging in as many as two-thirds of patients with superficial disease and understaging in up to 30% of patients with muscle invasive disease. Recent reports suggest improved sensitivity and specificity of gadolinium-enhanced MRI in the detection of muscle invasion by tumor, with a sensitivity of 96% and a specificity of 83%[65].

One of the main advantages of CT and MRI is in distinguishing extravesical disease from organ-confined disease. If possible, patients with suspected muscle invasive disease undergo cross-sectional imaging prior to transurethral resection to avoid local tissue artifact that may be caused by the resection. The sensitivity of CT in the detection of extravesical disease ranges from 60% to 96%, while the specificity ranges from 66% to 93%[66]. In this regard, MRI has several theoretic advantages over CT, which include the ability to obtain images in multiple planes, better differentiation of tumor from normal bladder tissue, and better demonstration of the perivesical fat planes and boundaries between the bladder and the prostate and seminal vesicles. However, both the sensitivity and specificity of MRI for extravesical disease extension is similar to that of CT, in the range of 60–100%[67,68]. Obviously, neither CT nor MRI can detect microscopic extension of disease into the perivesical tissue.

Both CT and MRI rely on size criteria to detect regional lymphadenopathy. Lymph nodes larger than 1cm in size are considered suspicious for metastatic disease. Again, microscopic spread of disease into the lymph nodes cannot be identified with these cross-sectional imaging modalities. The overall staging accuracy for lymph node involvement using CT or MRI ranges from 50% to 90%[60–64].

Determination of metastatic disease

Patients with muscle invasive bladder cancer should undergo a complete staging evaluation to exclude the presence of metastatic disease. The most common sites of metastasis for invasive bladder cancer include the regional lymph nodes, liver, lung, and bone[3]. Consequently, a complete metastatic work-up includes a CT scan of the abdomen and pelvis, a chest radiograph or CT scan of the chest, liver function studies, and a serum alkaline phosphatase level. A bone scan is carried out if the history and/or physical examination suggest the possibility of bone metastases or if the serum alkaline phosphatase level is elevated[69].

TREATMENT OF INVASIVE BLADDER CANCER

Radical cystectomy

Radical cystectomy involves removal of the anterior pelvic organs. In men, this includes removal of the bladder (with its surrounding fat and peritoneal attachments), the prostate, and the seminal vesicles. In women, the bladder (with its surrounding fat and peritoneal attachments), the cervix, uterus, anterior vagina, urethra, ovaries, and fallopian tubes are removed. In appropriate female candidates for orthotopic urinary diversion, the anterior vaginal wall and urethra may be preserved.

Radical cystectomy remains the 'gold standard' of treatment for patients with muscle invasive disease for several important reasons. First, the natural history of invasive bladder cancer is to invade progressively through the bladder wall, which allows tumor cells to invade adjacent structures and gain access to the lymphatic and vascular systems[70]. Radical cystectomy involves wide local resection designed to provide negative surgical margins and remove all local disease. Second, invasive transitional cell carcinoma of the bladder is resistant to other local treatments such as radiation. As a result, radical cystectomy provides for the best local control of disease, with local, recurrence-free survival expected in approximately 90–95% of patients following surgery[71]. Finally, radical cystectomy provides accurate pathologic staging of disease. Clinical staging can be inaccurate in as many as 60% of patients, of whom 20% are clinically overstaged and 40% clinically understaged[11]. Accurate pathologic staging provides important information with respect to prognosis and allows for the appropriate selection of patients for adjuvant treatment protocols. Thus, radical cystectomy should be considered for all patients with invasive bladder cancer in whom disease is confined to the pelvis.

Radical cystectomy is usually accompanied by an extended pelvic lymph node dissection. When bladder cancer metastasizes to the lymph nodes, the obturator, hypogastric, and external iliac chains are most commonly involved with disease[70]. Thus, these nodal chains are removed during the lymph node dissection. Lymph node metastases are detected in approximately 15–25% of patients who undergo radical cystectomy[72]. Patients with more advanced primary tumor stage are most likely to have pelvic lymph nodal metastases. The rationale for including bilateral pelvic lymph node dissection with radical cystectomy is based on the following observations[72]:

- even though some patients with invasive bladder cancer have pelvic lymph node metastases, preoperative staging is not sufficiently accurate to detect nodal metastases in many of these patients prior to surgery;
- pelvic lymph node dissection does not significantly add to the morbidity of radical cystectomy, while it provides important prognostic information; and
- some patients with minimal nodal disease may derive a therapeutic benefit from undergoing pelvic lymph node dissection (see below).

When reviewing the results of radical cystectomy for patients with invasive bladder cancer, it must be recognized that early series (prior to 1980) demonstrated poor results, with operative mortality rates as high as 15–40%[5]. With improvements in surgical technique and perioperative care, mortality after radical cystectomy is currently <2%[70,71,73–75]. In addition, the incidence of perioperative complications significantly decreased between 1970 and the end of the century. Advances in surgical technique have also led to improvements in quality of life after radical cystectomy. While the ileal conduit was previously the only choice for urinary diversion following cystectomy, many patients are now appropriate candidates for orthotopic urinary diversion that allows for volitional voiding per urethra (see Chapter 35). This has led patients to opt for cystectomy at an earlier point in their disease process[76], a possible contribution to improved outcomes in contemporary series.

Before 1984, a short course of preoperative radiation was routinely given to patients with invasive bladder cancer prior to radical cystectomy. The rationale for such combination therapy was based on the belief that preoperative radiation could potentially decrease the incidence of local tumor recurrence in the pelvis and decrease the incidence of tumor dissemination at the time of surgery. Skinner and colleagues compared the outcome of patients who underwent preoperative radiation followed by radical cystectomy to that of patients who underwent radical cystectomy alone[71]. When stratified by pathologic tumor stage, no difference in outcome was seen between the two groups. Consequently, preoperative radiation is no longer routinely given prior to radical cystectomy.

Contemporary series that report disease-free survival for patients with lymph node negative muscle invasive bladder cancer treated by radical cystectomy are summarized in Figure 26.12. It is evident that the outcome in these patients is associated with the extent of the primary tumor. Disease-free 5-year survival can be expected in up to 90% of patients with stage pT2N0 disease, 77% of patients with stage pT3aN0 disease, and 62% of patients with stage pT3bN0 disease. In a recent update of their experience, Stein et al. reported disease-free and overall survival for 994 patients treated with radical cystectomy between 1971 and 1997[73]. Median follow-up in this group of patients was 8.2 years after surgery, and perioperative mortality was 2%. When stratifying patients by stage, 5- and 10-year recurrence-free survival rates were 90% and 87% for patients with pT2N0 disease, 77% and 74% for patients with stage pT3aN0 disease, 62% and 60% for patients with stage pT3bN0 disease, and 50% and 44% for patients with stage pT4N0 disease, respectively. These data indicate that radical cystectomy is an effective treatment modality for patients with muscle invasive bladder cancer. Furthermore, if patients are destined to fail after such treatment, recurrence is usually seen within the first 5 years of surgery.

Figure 26.13 summarizes contemporary series that report disease-free survival for patients with lymph node positive muscle invasive bladder cancer treated by radical cystectomy. Survival 5 years after surgery is approximately 30% in these studies. In all of these series, patients with fewer nodal metastases demonstrate better outcome than patients with extensive nodal disease[72–74,79,80]. Furthermore, the extent of the primary tumor also has an impact on outcome. Patients with a primary bladder tumor that is organ confined (pT2 or pT3a) have a better prognosis than patients with extravesical disease (pT3b or pT4). For example, in the series by Lerner et al.[72], patients with less than six lymph nodes involved with tumor fared significantly better than patients with six or more positive lymph nodes. In addition, while 50% of the patients with positive lymph nodes and organ-confined primary tumors survived for 5 years after surgery, only 18% of patients with positive lymph nodes and extravesical disease extension were alive 5 years after surgery[72].

Vieweg et al. demonstrated that patients with a single positive lymph node and organ-confined disease have an identical disease-specific 5-year survival as patients with node negative, organ-confined disease[80]. However, patients with organ-confined disease and more than one positive lymph node have poor outcome despite

Disease-specific 5-year survival for patients with lymph node negative, invasive bladder cancer treated by radical cystectomy (contemporary series)						
				Five year disease specific survival		
Author	Number	Year	All patients (%)	Stage pT2 (5)	Stage pT3a (%)	Stage pT3b (%)
Freiha[77]	–	1990	–	83*	–	47
Pagano et al.[75]	261	1991	55	63	50	15
Frazier et al.[78]	531	1993	59	64	39†	–
Soloway et al.[11]	130	1994	65	–	–	–
Stein et al.[73]	994	1998	–	90%	77%	62%

*Includes both pT2 and pT3a patients.
† Includes both pT3a and pT3b patients.

Figure 26.12 Disease-specific 5-year survival for patients with lymph node negative, invasive bladder cancer treated by radical cystectomy (contemporary series).

Disease-specific 5-year survival for patients with lymph node positive, invasive bladder cancer treated by radical cystectomy (contemporary series)							
			Five year disease specific survival				
Author	Number	Year	All patients (%)	Overall (%)	Organ-confined (%)	Extravesical disease extension (%)	Follow-up (years)
Roehrborn et al.[74]	42	1991	15	27*	–	–	–
Lerner et al.[72]	132	1993	22	29	50	18	5.5
Vieweg et al.[79]	193	1999	28	31	58	22	7.7
Stein et al.[73]	238	1998	22	33	44	25	8.19
*3-Year follow-up.							

Figure 26.13 Disease-specific 5-year survival for patients with lymph node positive, invasive bladder cancer treated by radical cystectomy (contemporary series).

surgery. In patients with extravesical disease extension, poor outcome was seen irrespective of the status of the lymph nodes, even though patients with extravesical disease extension and positive lymph nodes fared significantly worse than those with extravesical disease and negative lymph nodes. These patients are at high risk, presumably because of the presence of microscopic hematogenous spread at the time of diagnosis. Taken together, these data suggest that the patients most likely to benefit from pelvic lymph node dissection at the time of radical cystectomy are those with limited nodal disease and organ-confined tumors. Lymph node dissection may be curative in many of these patients.

Indications for urethrectomy

Urethrectomy traditionally has been carried out in all women who undergo radical cystectomy, and it has been selectively used in men who undergo the procedure. In men with a retained urethra after cystectomy, the risk of urethral recurrence has been estimated at 10%[81]. Indications for urethrectomy in men have included involvement of the prostatic stroma or prostatic urethra with cancer or CIS. Hardeman and Soloway reported anterior urethral recurrences in 37% of patients with prostatic stromal involvement by tumor and in only 4% of patients without prostatic stromal involvement[82].

With the advent of orthotopic urinary diversion, the indications for urethrectomy have been reevaluated. Risk factors for urethral involvement by tumor in women include the presence of tumor at the bladder neck and tumor invasion of the anterior vaginal wall[83,84]. Women without such features appear to be at low risk for urethral tumor involvement. Consequently, these patients may be spared urethrectomy and can be considered candidates for orthotopic urinary diversion. Current data also suggest that prostatic stromal invasion by tumor may not be an absolute indication for urethrectomy in male patients who undergo radical cystectomy. Freeman et al. analyzed the risk of urethral recurrence in men treated by radical cystectomy who underwent urinary diversion with either an ileal conduit or an orthotopic neobladder[81]. In this group of patients, tumor invasion of the prostate significantly increased the risk of urethral tumor recurrence. However, the risk of urethral recurrence was significantly lower in men with prostatic involvement who underwent orthotopic urinary diversion compared to similar men who underwent urinary diversion with an ileal conduit. In those men with prostatic stromal involvement, none of the nine patients who underwent orthotopic diversion experienced a urethral recurrence.

These data have led some investigators to propose a modification to the indications for urethrectomy. Urethrectomy may only be necessary in those patients who have a positive distal urethral margin at the time of radical cystectomy[85]. Thus, male and female patients with a negative distal urethral margin, which includes men with prostatic stromal involvement, may still be appropriate candidates for orthotopic urinary diversion. In patients who are spared urethrectomy, follow-up must be vigilant and include a wash cytology of the urethra and urethroscopy when indicated (positive cytology, bloody urethral discharge, urethral pain).

Outcome predictors

Traditional predictors of outcome after radical cystectomy included tumor grade and stage. The frequency of transitional cell carcinoma tumor invasion, as well as survival after treatment, is strongly associated with tumor grade. In patients with superficial tumors, progression to more advanced disease has been reported to occur in 10–20% of grade 1 tumors, 19–37% of grade 2 tumors, and 33–67% of grade 3 tumors[86,87]. Similarly, cancer-specific survival after radical cystectomy is associated with tumor grade, since patients with high-grade tumors tend to have a poorer outcome after surgery[78,88].

Prognosis after cystectomy is also significantly associated with tumor stage. Numerous studies demonstrated that overall survival correlates better with pathologic tumor stage than with clinical tumor stage – not surprising given the inaccuracy of clinical staging[11]. In patients with organ-confined disease, the presence of pelvic lymph node metastases appears to be the most important prognostic factor. For patients with extravesical disease extension, poor survival rates only partially result from the presence of lymph node metastases. This may result from the higher probability of systemic disease spread in patients with extravesical disease extension. Prostatic stromal involvement also appears to be a poor prognostic factor for patients who undergo radical cystectomy[70,78]. For patients with prostatic stromal invasion, 5-year survival has been reported to be only 20%. For patients with CIS of the prostatic urethra only (i.e. no stromal invasion), survival depends on the stage of the primary tumor.

In addition to tumor grade and stage, the presence of hydronephrosis prior to surgery also appears to be a poor prognostic factor. It has been reported recently that hydronephrosis prior to surgery is significantly correlated with increased primary tumor stage and decreased overall survival[52]. Moreover, bilateral hydronephrosis appears to be a more ominous sign than unilateral hydronephrosis.

Molecular markers of tumor progression

Conventional histopathologic analysis of bladder tumors, which includes determination of tumor grade and stage, is inadequate to predict the behavior of an individual invasive bladder tumor, because tumor heterogeneity, even within the same clinical grade and stage stratum, prevents accurate determination of a bladder tumor's true biologic potential. Our understanding of tumor biology and the molecular predictors of tumor progression has evolved rapidly over the past several years. This understanding coupled with advances in molecular biology and immunology have made available several techniques that may help to better characterize the true biologic potential of a tumor. These techniques, most notably immunohistochemistry, have been extensively applied to invasive bladder tumors to determine which molecular markers are useful in predicting disease progression and overall survival in patients treated by radical cystectomy. The markers that have been studied are summarized in Figure 26.14.

Blood group antigens

Antigens related to blood group are carbohydrate determinants present on membrane lipids and proteins[90]. These antigens, including the ABH and Lewis antigens (Le[a,b,x,y]), were first described on the cell surface of erythrocytes; subsequently, they have been identified on various epithelial tissues, including transitional urothelium. Loss of ABH antigens has been associated with increased recurrence rates and progression to muscle invasive disease for patients with superficial bladder cancer[91-93]. However, certain difficulties have been encountered that preclude routine clinical use of these blood group antigens. Most notably, the secretory status of the individual must be considered when interpreting blood group antigen status. Although the majority of normal urothelium is rich in A, B, H, Le[b], and Le[y] blood group antigens (secretors), 20% of individuals with normal urothelium lack expression of these antigens (nonsecretors). Thus, loss of ABH antigen expression can be reliably determined only in secretory individuals.

The focus of research into blood group antigens has shifted to the evaluation of the Le[x] antigen. Immunohistochemical evaluations of Le[x] on fresh frozen and formalin-fixed bladder tissues demonstrated that most tumors (90%) express this blood group antigen while only an occasional umbrella cell of normal urothelium express this antigen[94]. Current data suggest that immunocytologic evaluation of Le[x] antigen expression on exfoliated bladder cells may not only enhance the detection of low-grade and low-stage cancers, but Le[x] may also be a useful clinical marker for the prediction of tumor recurrence or progression in patients with superficial bladder cancer who are at high risk for disease progression[95].

Cellular proliferation

The growth fraction of a tumor (percentage of proliferating cells) is an important prognostic marker for many malignancies as it helps to define the biologic potential of a given tumor. Several markers have been used to quantify cellular proliferation, but the two most promising immunohistochemical markers of cellular proliferation are Ki-67 and PCNA. Increased expression of these antigens indicates higher proliferative activity of tumor cells and is associated with an increased propensity for tumor progression and metastasis[96].

Predictors of outcome after radical cystectomy for patients with invasive bladder cancer	
Traditional	**Blood group antigens**
Tumor grade	ABH
Tumor stage	Lewis antigens – a, b, x, y
Hydronephrosis	
Tumor associated antigens	**Proliferating antigens**
M344	Mitotic count
19A211	Silver-stained nucleolar organizer regions
T138	Ki-67
	PCNA
Oncogenes	**Epidermal growth factor receptor Peptide growth factors**
c-H-ras	Epidermal growth factor
c-myc	Fibroblast growth factor
mdm2	Transforming growth factors α and β
c-erbB2	
Cellular adhesion molecules	**Tumor angiogenesis and angiogenesis inhibitors (thrombospondin-1) Cell cycle regulatory proteins**
E-Cadherin	Retinoblastoma gene
Integrins	p53
	p21

Figure 26.14 Predictors of outcome after radical cystectomy for patients with invasive bladder cancer[89].

An antibody that reacts with a nuclear antigen expressed in proliferating cells, Ki-67 has been studied extensively in patients with bladder cancer. Okamura et al. found a correlation between increased Ki-67 expression and tumor grade and stage[97]. Other studies not only confirmed this relationship, but also demonstrated a significant association between tumor recurrence and increased Ki-67 immunoreactivity in patients with bladder cancer[98-103]. Evidence to date suggests that the cellular proliferative fraction of a tumor, as determined by the Ki-67 labeling index, may supplement the routine use of histologic grade and stage in the assessment of a bladder tumor's aggressiveness and metastatic potential.

Cellular adhesion molecules

Cellular adhesion molecules participate in cell-to-cell interactions and interactions between cells and components of the extracellular matrix. For bladder cancer cells to invade and/or metastasize, they must first be released from the urothelial lining of the bladder and either penetrate into the muscular layer of the bladder or gain access to the blood or lymphatic circulation. This mechanism presumably involves the loss of cell–cell adhesion, and thus cellular adhesion molecules are likely participants in the processes that lead to invasion and metastasis.

E-Cadherin is the most extensively studied cellular adhesion molecule in bladder cancer. It belongs to a family of transmembrane glycoproteins involved in calcium-dependent cell-to-cell adhesion. The cadherins are crucial to establish and maintain intercellular connections[104]. They associate with proteins of the cytoskeleton through their interactions with a group of cytoplasmic proteins known as the catenins (specifically α, β, and γ catenins), which function to link the intracellular portion of the cadherins to the cytoskeleton[104]. In addition to their involvement in cellular adhesion, the regulated expression of cadherins also appears to control cell polarity, cell-sorting, and tissue morphology.

E-Cadherin expression has been reported abnormal in a variety of solid tumors, and hence the hypothesis that E-cadherin may function as an invasion (tumor) suppressor molecule. Studies to examine E-cadherin expression in bladder cancer uniformly demonstrate a significant association between the level of E-cadherin expression (as determined by immunohistochemistry) and tumor grade and stage[105–110]. Decreased levels of E-cadherin expression are associated with high-grade, high-stage cancers. In addition, E-cadherin expression appears to be significantly associated with prognosis in patients with bladder cancer. These data suggest that E-cadherin may be a useful prognostic marker in patients with bladder cancer.

Tumor angiogenesis

Tumor growth and metastasis requires the growth of new blood vessels. Such a response has been labeled tumor angiogenesis. New vessel growth is tightly regulated by both angiogenic stimulators, such as fibroblastic growth factors and the vascular endothelial growth factor, and angiogenic inhibitors, such as thrombospondin-1 and angiostatin. These factors may be produced by the tumor cells themselves, they may be released from the surrounding extracellular matrix or the tumor-associated stromal cells, or they may be products of inflammatory cells that infiltrate into the tumor. Immunohistochemical methods have been developed to quantify the neovascular response induced by a given tumor. This is achieved by measuring a tumor's microvessel density. In addition, expression of certain angiogenesis inhibitors and stimulators can also be determined using immunohistochemical techniques.

Microvessel density is a useful prognostic indicator for a variety of human malignancies, which include melanoma, breast cancer, and prostate cancer. Increased microvessel density counts are associated consistently with tumor progression and decreased overall survival. The relationship between microvessel density and tumor progression has also been studied extensively in patients with invasive bladder cancer, and the results confirm its role as a prognostic indicator in patients with this disease[111–113]. Microvessel density is associated with lymph node metastases, disease progression, and overall survival in patients with invasive bladder cancer treated by radical cystectomy[111–113]. Furthermore, immunohistochemical expression of an inhibitor of angiogenesis, thrombospondin-1, is reported to be associated significantly with both tumor recurrence and overall survival in a group of 163 patients with invasive bladder cancer who were treated by radical cystectomy[114].

Cell-cycle regulatory proteins

Malignancy is characterized by uncontrolled cell growth. Normal cellular proliferation occurs as a result of an orderly progression through the cell cycle (Fig. 26.15). Protein complexes (composed of cyclins and cyclin-dependent kinases) associated with the cell cycle tightly regulate this progression[115]. These

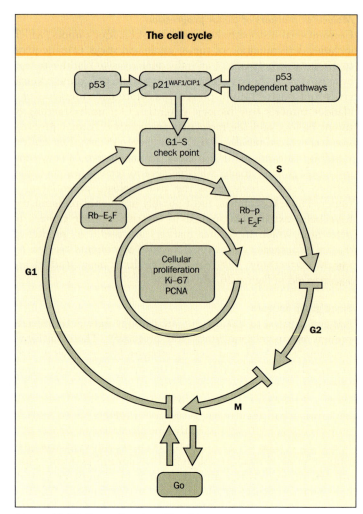

Figure 26.15 The cell cycle. p53, p21, and Rb are crucial to maintain cell-cycle control at the G1–S check point.

complexes phosphorylate key proteins involved in cell-cycle transition points, including the protein encoded by the retinoblastoma gene (pRb) and the p53 gene. Loss of cell-cycle control may be an early step in the development of carcinogenesis. Recent studies have examined several genes involved in cell cycle regulation, and their protein products, to determine their prognostic significance in bladder cancer progression.

The most extensively characterized molecular marker in patients with invasive bladder cancer is p53 expression. The p53 gene is a tumor suppressor gene that plays a vital role in regulation of the cell cycle[116], and mutations in the p53 gene are the most common genetic defect in human tumors. When DNA damage occurs, the level of p53 protein increases, which causes cell cycle arrest. This enables the repair of DNA and prevents propagation of the DNA defect. Mutations in the p53 gene result in the production of an abnormal and usually dysfunctional protein product, which allows cells with damaged DNA to continue through the cell cycle. The altered p53 protein has a prolonged half-life compared to the wild-type protein. This abnormal protein accumulates in the cell nucleus, and so it can be detected by standard immunohistochemical techniques.

It has been shown that p53 alteration, as determined by immunohistochemical techniques, is an important prognostic indicator for bladder cancer progression[14,117–119]. Increased nuclear reactivity for p53 has been found in high-grade and high-stage bladder cancers. Patients with altered p53 expression by immunohistochemistry (indicating possible mutation of the p53 gene) appear to have an increased risk for disease recurrence and a lower disease-specific survival when compared to patients with normal p53 expression. Esrig et al. examined a group of 243 bladder cancer patients, all treated by radical cystectomy[14]. Disease recurrence 5 years after surgery was detected in approximately 75% of patients with p53 positive (altered) tumors, but in only 30% of patients with p53 negative (wild-type) tumors. Such data led to a recent clinical trial in which patients were assigned to adjuvant treatment after radical cystectomy based upon the p53 status of their tumor.

One way in which p53 acts as a tumor suppressor is through the upregulation of p21$^{WAF1/CIP1}$ expression (Fig. 26.15)[115]. Alterations in p53 result in decreased p21 expression, which leads to loss of cell-cycle control and unregulated cell growth. However, p21 expression may also be mediated through p53-independent pathways[120–122]. In some instances, these pathways may allow cells in p53 altered tumors to maintain p21 expression, and thereby preserve cell-cycle control. Recent data support this hypothesis, as patients with p53-altered transitional cell carcinomas with no p21 expression demonstrated a significantly higher probability of recurrence and a significantly decreased probability of survival than patients with p53-altered tumors that maintained expression of p21[123].

The retinoblastoma (Rb) tumor suppressor gene was the first tumor suppressor gene to be identified. Although initially discovered in patients with inherited retinoblastoma, altered Rb gene expression has been reported in a number of human tumors, including transitional cell carcinoma of the bladder. When hypophosphorylated, pRb inhibits cell-cycle progression at the G1–S check-point by binding to a number of cellular proteins that include the transcription factor E2F[124,125]. With entry into the S phase, pRb becomes phosphorylated.

Similar to p53, inactivation of the Rb gene appears to be involved in bladder cancer progression. As determined by immunohistochemistry, Rb alteration is associated with high-grade, high-stage bladder cancers. In addition, Rb alteration appears to be associated significantly with decreased survival in patients with invasive bladder cancer[126,127]. Cordon-Cardo et al. reported 5-year survival in 85% of bladder cancer patients with normal Rb expression, but in only 15% of bladder cancer patients with altered expression of the Rb protein[127]. Studies in which both p53 and Rb were examined in patients with invasive bladder cancer suggest that bladder tumors with alterations in both p53 and Rb have a poorer prognosis and decreased overall survival when compared to tumors with wild-type p53 and wild-type Rb. Tumors with an alteration in only one of these genes behave in an intermediate fashion[128,129].

Further investigation

The above data demonstrate the potential importance of molecular markers to predict bladder cancer progression. Although remarkable advances have been made in our understanding of tumor biology, further investigation is necessary before any of these markers can be used in routine clinical practice to determine the proper course of treatment for a given patient with

Adjuvant and neoadjuvant chemotherapy		
Chemotherapy	Advantages	Disadvantage
Adjuvant	Pathologic staging allows appropriate selection of patients for additional treatment Patients at low risk for recurrence spared toxicity of additional treatment	Patients unwilling or unable to tolerate additional treatment after surgery
Neoadjuvant	Early administration of chemotherapy to patients at high risk for occult metastatic disease Render unresectable patients surgical candidates In vivo test of chemosensitivity May be able to select patients for bladder preservation	Low risk patients receive unnecessary treatment with high toxicity Inaccuracy of clinical staging makes determination of benefit difficult Patients with complete response to treatment may continue to have invasive disease No proved benefit with respect to survival

Figure 26.16   Adjuvant and neoadjuvant chemotherapy: advantages and disadvantages.

invasive bladder cancer. Nevertheless, it is important to be aware of these tumor markers as they will undoubtedly become more important in the prognostic and therapeutic evaluation of patients with this disease.

Adjuvant and neoadjuvant chemotherapy

Chemotherapy for bladder cancer is covered in detail in Chapter 46. However, as chemotherapy may be given either after radical cystectomy (so-called adjuvant chemotherapy) or immediately prior to radical cystectomy (so-called neoadjuvant chemotherapy), some discussion of this topic is warranted here (Fig. 26.16).

Adjuvant chemotherapy

Adjuvant chemotherapy may be given to patients at high risk for disease recurrence after radical cystectomy. The primary advantage of chemotherapy in this setting is that pathologic analysis of the cystectomy specimen allows the identification of patients with extravesical disease extension (pT3b, pT4) and/or positive lymph nodes, who are truly at high risk for recurrence. Thus, patients at low risk are spared the toxicity of chemotherapy. The disadvantage of chemotherapy in this setting is that some patients may be unable to tolerate additional treatment after an extensive postoperative recovery period. In addition, some patients may refuse additional treatment after major surgery.

Three randomized trials using contemporary chemotherapeutic regimens have examined the benefit of adjuvant chemotherapy after radical cystectomy[130–132]. Skinner et al. randomized 91 patients with pathologic stages pT3 or pT4, or lymph node positive disease, to adjuvant chemotherapy or observation after radical cystectomy[131]. Chemotherapy was planned as four cycles of cisplatin, doxorubicin, and cyclophosphamide. These authors reported a significant delay in time to progression in treated patients as compared to those patients who were observed only. Median survival was 4.3 years in the treatment group and

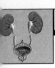

2.4 years in the observation group. The number of involved lymph nodes was the single most important variable to predict outcome, as no benefit was seen with chemotherapy for those patients with two or more lymph nodes involved with tumor.

The two other randomized studies that examined adjuvant chemotherapy for bladder cancer were reported by Freiha et al. and Stockle et al.[130,132] In these studies, 50 and 49 patients, respectively, were randomized to either chemotherapy or observation after surgery. Chemotherapy consisted of either methotrexate, vinblastine, doxorubicin (adriamycin), and cisplatin (MVAC) or methotrexate, vinblastine, epirubicin, and cisplatin (MVEC) in the study reported by Stockle et al.[132], while Freiha et al.[130] used CMV (cisplatin, methotrexate, and vinblastine) in the treatment group. The study by Stockle et al.[132] was closed early because an interim analysis demonstrated a significant advantage to the treatment group when compared to the observation group. Similarly, Freiha et al.[130] also reported a delay in the interval to progression in these high-risk patients treated with chemotherapy after cystectomy.

Neoadjuvant chemotherapy

Chemotherapy may also be given prior to radical cystectomy (so-called neoadjuvant chemotherapy). Treatment failure after radical cystectomy is more often the result of unrecognized metastatic disease than of persistent local disease. Thus, early administration of chemotherapy to such patients can be beneficial in that the primary local lesion is treated as well as any occult micrometastatic deposits. Theoretically, this may lead to improved disease-specific survival for patients with invasive bladder cancer.

Neoadjuvant chemotherapy has other potential advantages when compared with adjuvant treatment:

- patients with clinically unresectable lesions who respond to treatment may eventually become surgical candidates;
- neoadjuvant chemotherapy represents an in-vivo test of chemosensitivity, as the response of the primary bladder lesion can be followed endoscopically; and
- in select patients with a clinically complete response to treatment, bladder preservation protocols may be considered.

Neoadjuvant chemotherapy also has several disadvantages:

- all patients (both high and low risk) receive chemotherapy with its associated toxicity, and so patients at low risk for disease recurrence receive potentially unnecessary treatment;
- inaccuracy of clinical staging prior to cystectomy makes determination of response to treatment difficult; and
- even if patients demonstrate a clinically complete response to chemotherapy, a significant percentage continue to have invasive disease at the time of surgery.

Studies in which the use of neoadjuvant chemotherapy prior to radical cystectomy was examined demonstrate downstaging of disease in a significant proportion of patients. Overall, 23–31% of patients who undergo radical cystectomy after neoadjuvant chemotherapy exhibit no evidence of disease (pT0) on the final cystectomy specimen[133–135]. However, these patients cannot be identified reliably using the currently available clinical staging modalities. Clinical staging after neoadjuvant chemotherapy often includes repeat cystoscopy and biopsy, cytology, radiologic imaging, and physical examination. A clinically complete response (no evidence of residual tumor on all clinical staging modalities) may be seen in 20–24% of patients after neoadjuvant chemotherapy, while a clinically partial response is seen in approximately 40% of such patients[134,135].

Of those patients with no evidence of tumor at the time of cystoscopy and biopsy, 34–52% demonstrate residual tumor in the radical cystectomy specimen, and most of these patients harbor muscle invasive disease[134,135]. Furthermore, approximately 25% of patients with a clinically complete response (no evidence of tumor by biopsy, imaging, cytology, and physical examination), and over 80% of patients with a partial clinical response are found to have residual tumor at the time of radical cystectomy[134,135]. Thus, additional treatment after neoadjuvant chemotherapy remains indicated because of the high incidence of residual muscle invasive disease. With respect to overall survival, it is currently unknown whether the combination of neoadjuvant chemotherapy and radical cystectomy offers a benefit when compared to radical cystectomy alone. This may become clear upon the completion of a Southwest Oncology Group randomized trial to compare three cycles of neoadjuvant chemotherapy plus cystectomy to cystectomy alone.

Bladder-sparing treatments
Radical transurethral resection of bladder tumor

The role of TURBT in the diagnosis and staging of bladder cancer is well recognized. Such a procedure is often sufficient treatment for patients with disease limited to the urothelial lining and lamina propria of the bladder (stages Ta, TIS, T1). In a select group of patients with minimally invasive bladder cancer, TURBT alone may also be appropriate initial treatment.

When TURBT alone is chosen for definitive local therapy, an extensive (or so-called 'radical') TURBT is carried out by an experienced urologist. Follow-up in these patients must be vigilant and frequent because of the high local recurrence rate. Although hospitalization is short and the bladder is preserved, this type of conservative treatment is appropriate only for a very limited, highly selected patient population with minimally invasive bladder cancer.

Figure 26.17 summarizes the results of TURBT alone for selected patients with clinical stages T2 and T3 bladder cancer. Of 217 patients diagnosed with muscle invasive bladder cancer over a 4-year period, Herr analyzed 45 patients (21%) who were managed with TURBT alone[136]. In these patients, restaging TURBT demonstrated either no additional cancer, CIS, stage T1 disease, or localized stage T2 cancer. With a median follow-up of 5.1 years, 30 of these 45 patients (67%) were either free of disease with no additional treatment or they required repeat TURBT and intravesical therapy only. Of the 15 failures, 11 required cystectomy and four demonstrated metastatic disease. Thus, two-thirds of these highly selected patients were alive with an intact bladder 5 years after radical TURBT. Solsona et al. examined 133 patients treated with radical TURBT who had negative biopsies of the muscle bed of the tumor after resection[142]. With a mean follow-up of 81.6 months, 46% of patients did not experience disease recurrence, 26% had disease recurrence only, and 28% experienced disease progression. Bladder preservation was achieved in 83% of patients with a minimum of 5 years of follow-up.

Although these studies demonstrate the feasibility of radical TURBT for a subset of carefully selected patients with muscle invasive bladder cancer, certain caveats must be emphasized.

Five-year survival for patients with invasive bladder cancer treated by radical transurethral resection of bladder tumor alone			
Author	Number	Year	5-year survival (%)
Flocks[137]	142	1951	47
Milner[138]	88	1954	53
Barnes et al.[139]	75	1967	31
O'Flynn et al.[140]	123	1975	52
Herr[136]	45	1987	82
Henry et al.[141]	43	1988	55
Solsona et al.[142]	133	1998	44
Mean			52

Figure 26.17 Five-year survival for patients with invasive bladder cancer treated by radical transurethral resection of bladder tumor alone.

First, local recurrence is common in these patients, in the range 54–71%[136,142]. Consequently, follow-up must be vigilant and frequent since to withhold definitive local therapy in these patients may result in poor outcome. Moreover, it is impossible to distinguish patients destined to benefit from radical TURBT from those who are destined to fail. The studies by Herr et al. and Solsona et al. suggest that patients with either no residual disease or minimal disease only at restaging TURBT are the most appropriate candidates for conservative treatment[136,142]. Factors such as the presence of a single small tumor, increased age, significant comorbidities, and tumor location (away from the dome, anterior bladder neck, and prostatic urethra) may help to select patients for TURBT alone[5,136,137].

Partial cystectomy

Partial cystectomy as single modality treatment is indicated rarely for patients with muscle invasive bladder cancer. The goal of partial cystectomy is to remove all local disease with adequate (2cm) margins and to leave enough bladder volume to maintain a functional urinary reservoir. Potential advantages of partial over radical cystectomy include preservation of normal bladder function as well as preservation of potency in male patients. Possible indications include:
- solitary tumor in a location amenable to obtaining clear surgical margins;
- tumor within a diverticulum; or
- patients considered to be at poor surgical risk secondary to comorbid medical conditions or advanced age.

Tumor locations amenable to partial cystectomy include the posterolateral bladder wall and the bladder dome. Tumors located at the trigone are usually not appropriate for partial cystectomy. Concomitant CIS and/or atypia at sites away from the primary tumor are absolute contraindications to this procedure, and such findings must be excluded by random biopsy prior to the procedure. In addition, partial cystectomy is not well suited for patients with multiple tumors or male patients with tumor involvement of the prostatic urethra. Given these indications and contraindications, no more than 5–10% of all patients with muscle invasive bladder cancer can be considered appropriate candidates for partial cystectomy[143,145].

Overall 5-year survival and local recurrence rates for patients who undergo partial cystectomy for muscle invasive bladder cancer are summarized in Figure 26.18. The 5-year survival rates range from 29% to 80% for patients with organ-confined disease and from 6% to 33% for patients with extravesical disease extension. Herr and Scher examined 26 patients with invasive bladder cancer who received four courses of MVAC chemotherapy prior to partial cystectomy[147]. Even in this highly selected patient population that received neoadjuvant systemic chemotherapy, only 65% were alive beyond 5 years while 46% developed bladder recurrences. Overall, survival with an intact, functioning bladder at 5 years was 54%.

Local recurrences after partial cystectomy are high (Fig. 26.18), and most occur within 2 years of surgery[146,149,153]. Recurrence rates are higher in those patients with a prior history of bladder cancer; hence partial cystectomy is most appropriate for patients diagnosed with their first bladder tumor[5]. On

Figure 26.18 Overall 5-year survival for patients with invasive bladder cancer treated by partial cystectomy.

Overall 5-year survival for patients with invasive bladder cancer treated by partial cystectomy					
		5-year survival			
Author	Year	Overall (%)*	Organ confined disease (%)	Extravesical disease extension (%)	Local recurrence (%)
Novick and Stewart[143]	1976	–	53	20	50
Kaneti[144]	1986	48	40	33	38
Utz et al.[145]	1973	43	40	29	50
Resnick and O'Connor[146]	1973	35	77/19†	12.5	75
Herr and Scher‡[147]	1994	65	–	–	46
Schoborg et al.[148]	1979	43	29/50†	12	70
Faysal et al.[149]	1979	40	29/32†	7	78
Brannan et al.[150]	1978	58	54/62†	33	–
Cummings et al.[151]	1978	60	80/45†	6	49
Merrell et al.[152]	1979	48	57	25	30

*May include some patients with superficial disease at the time of surgery.
†Stage B1/Stage B2 (T2/T3a).
‡All patients treated with preoperative methotrexate, vinblastine, doxorubicin (adriamycin), and cisplatin chemotherapy.

average, approximately 8% of patients initially treated with partial cystectomy eventually undergo radical cystectomy because of local failure[153].

Wound implantation with tumor is a potential complication of partial cystectomy. With good surgical technique, which includes isolation of the bladder and irrigation of the field with distilled water, implantation rates are low[143,145]. Additional measures that can be utilized to decrease wound implantation include local preoperative radiation, intravesical chemotherapy prior to entering the bladder, or bladder irrigation with sterile water or silver nitrate.

Predictors of failure in patients with invasive bladder cancer who undergo partial cystectomy include multiple tumors, large tumors, and positive surgical margins[5]. As a result of the high local recurrence rate after partial cystectomy, it is important to follow the patients aggressively and vigilantly with cystoscopy and urinary cytology at regular intervals.

Radiotherapy

Radiation has been used as a single modality treatment for patients with invasive bladder cancer. The total dose delivered for definitive local therapy is usually 55–65Gy. Radiotherapy as a single modality treatment for invasive disease is generally well tolerated, but the majority of patients experience some side effects related to the lower gastrointestinal and urinary tract during treatment[154]. The severity of these acute symptoms depends on the location and extent of the tumor; tumors that invade the trigone and/or bladder neck are most likely to be associated with irritative voiding symptoms. Late toxicity, although rare, may include hematuria, urinary frequency, and (in the most severe cases) intractable bleeding or a contracted bladder[154].

For stages T2–T4 bladder cancer treated with radiotherapy, 5-year survival ranges from 23% to 40%[155]. Unfortunately, local recurrence is common; it occurs in approximately 55–65% of patients[155]. Consequently, radiation as monotherapy is usually offered only to those patients who are poor surgical candidates because of advanced age or significant comorbid medical problems.

Chemotherapy followed by radiation

Chemotherapy alone is unlikely to render patients with invasive bladder cancer free of disease. However, such therapy can be administered prior to radiation in an attempt to cure local disease and preserve bladder function. To this end, several investigators have reported on bladder-sparing treatment approaches for selected patients with muscle invasive bladder cancer using combination chemoradiation.

The rationale for combined chemoradiation in patients with invasive bladder cancer is based on studies that analyzed neoadjuvant chemotherapy prior to radical cystectomy. These studies demonstrated that approximately 30% of patients who receive chemotherapy prior to radical cystectomy have no evidence of residual cancer in the cystectomy specimen (pT0)[134]. Furthermore, if radiation and chemotherapy are both administered prior to radical cystectomy, an even higher percentage of patients may be pT0 at the time of surgery[156].

Patients who are candidates for chemoradiation should first undergo a thorough TURBT during which all visible bladder tumors are resected completely. After this initial complete TURBT, patients are given combination systemic chemotherapy followed by radiation treatments (Fig. 26.19). Cisplatin is usually given at the time of radiation to act as a radiation sensitizer, known as the induction phase of treatment. Following induction, urologic evaluation is carried out to determine response. This evaluation may include physical examination, cystoscopy, biopsy, cytology, and/or radiologic imaging. Patients who do not respond to the induction treatment, as well as those who develop invasive local recurrences, subsequently undergo radical cystectomy. Patients who respond to induction treatment are given consolidation therapy with additional radiation. Patients may drop out of such protocols at any time because of unacceptable toxicity (Fig. 26.20).

Results of trials to analyze combination chemoradiation for patients with invasive bladder cancer are summarized in Figure 26.21. Initial complete response rates to chemoradiation may be as high as 50–70%. Overall 5-year survival rates in these trials approach 50–60%. However, local recurrence is common, and exceeds 50% in many of these studies. As a result of invasive local recurrences, only 18–44% of patients are alive with an intact bladder 5 years after chemoradiation. Predictors of poor outcome after combined chemoradiation for invasive bladder cancer include hydronephrosis at presentation, advanced clinical T-stage (T3), inability to complete the treatment protocol, and poor

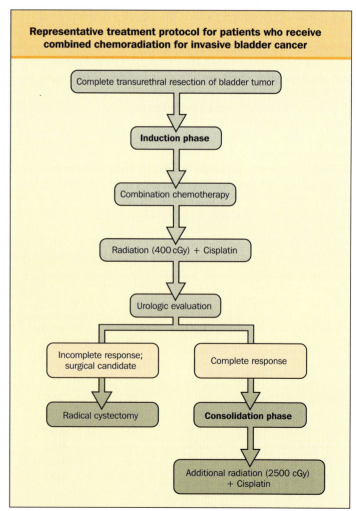

Representative treatment protocol for patients who receive combined chemoradiation for invasive bladder cancer

- Complete transurethral resection of bladder tumor
- **Induction phase**
- Combination chemotherapy
- Radiation (400 cGy) + Cisplatin
- Urologic evaluation
  - Incomplete response; surgical candidate → Radical cystectomy
  - Complete response → **Consolidation phase** → Additional radiation (2500 cGy) + Cisplatin

Figure 26.19. Representative treatment protocol for patients who receive combined chemoradiation for invasive bladder cancer.

Toxicity of combined chemoradiation for patients with invasive bladder cancer	
Effect	**Percent affected**
Cardiopulmonary (pulmonary embolus, myocardial infarction)	5
Renal dysfunction	Not specified
Sepsis/leukopenia	34 (including four deaths)
Nausea and/or vomiting	44
'Bladder irritation'	40
Diarrhea	34
Hematuria	10
Fatigue/anorexia	Not specified
Erectile dysfunction	30

Figure 26.20. Toxicity of combined chemoradiation for patients with invasive bladder cancer[53].

performance status. A recent study suggests that chemoradiation may also be inappropriate for patients with bladder tumors that are p53 positive[163].

Tester et al. reported the results of a phase II trial of chemoradiation for patients with stages T2M0–T4aM0 bladder cancer[161]. The 91 patients suitable for radical cystectomy received two courses of methotrexate, cisplatin, and vinblastine followed by radiotherapy and concurrent cisplatin. After treatment 85 patients underwent complete urologic evaluation, and a complete response was noted in 68%. Of 70 patients treated with chemotherapy followed by cisplatin–radiotherapy, 36 developed bladder recurrences, 23 of which were invasive. Also, 37 patients underwent cystectomy. The 4-year risk of invasive local failure was 43%, distant metastasis 22%, survival 62%, and survival with the bladder intact 44%. Acute toxicity was common and delayed complications occurred in 12 patients.

Given et al. reported complete responses in 53 (56%) of 94 patients treated with neoadjuvant chemotherapy followed by radiotherapy[159]. Of these 53 patients, 30 (57%) developed a local recurrence. Only 18% of the original 94 patients were alive with an intact bladder at last follow-up.

When considering the results of the above studies it must be recognized that follow-up is limited in many of these trials, local recurrence after initial complete response is not uncommon, and that no study to date has documented adequately the function of the remaining bladder after such treatment. Although bladder-sparing regimens remain an option for the treatment of patients with muscle invasive bladder cancer, long-term follow-up of larger patient populations treated in this fashion is necessary before such regimens can be recommended routinely.

Results of combined chemoradiation for patients with invasive bladder cancer						
Author	**Number**	**Year**	**Complete response (%)**	**Overall 5-year survival (%)**	**5-year survival with bladder intact (%)**	**Local recurrence (%)**	**Percent undergoing cystectomy**
Cervek et al.[157]	105	1998	52	58	45	31	35
Srougi and Simon[158]	36	1994	47	53	20	71	80
Given et al.[159]	94	1995	63	51	18	57	47
Chauvet et al.[160]	109	1996	70	42	37	30	17
Tester et al.[161]	91	1996	68	62	44	43	40
Kachnic et al.[53]	106	1997	66	52	43	32	34
Serretta et al.[162]	40	1998	68	35	55	30	7.5

Figure 26.21. Results of combined chemoradiation for patients with invasive bladder cancer.

REFERENCES

1. American Cancer Society – Cancer Facts and Figures 2000. http://www.cancer.org

2. Ross RK, Paganini-Hill A, Henderson BE. Epidemiology of bladder cancer. In: Skinner DG, Lieskovsky G, eds. Diagnosis and management of genitourinary cancer. Philadelphia: WB Saunders; 1988:23–32.

3. Catalona WJ. Urothelial tumors of the urinary tract. In: Walsh PC, Retik AB, Stamey TA, Vaughan ED Jr, eds. Campbell's urology, Vol. 2. Philadelphia: WB Saunders; 1992:1094–158.

4. Grossman HB. Superficial bladder cancer: decreasing the risk of recurrence. Oncology. 1996;10:1617–24.

5. Pressler LB, Petrylak DP, Olsson CA. Invasive transitional cell carcinoma of the bladder: prognosis and management. In: Oesterling JE, Richie JP, eds. Urologic oncology. Philadelphia: WB Saunders; 1997:275–91.

6. Lilienfeld AM, Levin ML, Moore GE. The association of smoking with cancer of the urinary bladder in humans. Arch Intern Med. 1956;98:129–35.

7. Carroll PR. Urothelial carcinoma: cancers of the bladder, ureter and renal pelvis. In: Tanagho EA, McAninch JW, eds. Smith's general urology. Norwalk: Appleton and Lange; 1995:353–71.

8. Olumi AF, Skinner EC, Tsai YC, Jones PA. Molecular analysis of human bladder cancer. Semin Urol. 1990;8:270–7.

9. Utz DC, Hanash KA, Farrow GM. The plight of the patient with carcinoma in situ of the bladder. J Urol. 1970;103:160–4.

10. Droller MJ. Diagnosis and staging of bladder cancer. In: Oesterling JE, Richie JP, eds. Urologic oncology. Philadelphia: WB Saunders; 1997:245–55.

11. Soloway MS, Lopez AE, Patel J, Lu Y. Results of radical cystectomy for transitional cell carcinoma of the bladder and the effect of chemotherapy. Cancer. 1994;73:1926–31.

12. Tsai YC, Nichols PW, Hiti AL, Williams Z, Skinner DG, Jones PA. Allelic losses of chromosomes 9, 11, and 17 in human bladder cancer. Cancer Res. 1990;50:44–7.

13. Miyao N, Tsai YC, Lerner SP, et al. Role of chromosome 9 in human bladder cancer. Cancer Res. 1993;53:4066–70.

14. Esrig D, Elmajian D, Groshen S, et al. Accumulation of nuclear p53 and tumor progression in bladder cancer. N Engl J Med. 1994;331:1259–64.

15. Spruck CH 3rd, Ohneseit PF, Gonzalez-Zulueta M, et al. Two molecular pathways to transitional cell carcinoma of the bladder. Cancer Res. 1994;54:784–8.

16. Bergkvist A, Ljungqvist A, Moberger G. Classification of bladder tumours based on the cellular pattern. Preliminary report of a clinical–pathological study of 300 cases with a minimum follow-up of eight years. Acta Chir Scand. 1965;130:371–8.

17. Mostofi FK, Sobin LH, Torloni H. Histological typing of urinary bladder tumors (International Histologic Classification of Tumors, No. 10). Geneva: World Health Organization, 1973.

18. Mostofi FK, Davis CJ, Sesterhenn IA. Pathology of tumors of the urinary tract. In: Skinner DG, Lieskovsky G, eds. Diagnosis and management of genitourinary cancer. Philadelphia: WB Saunders; 1988:83–117.

19. Mills SE, Wolfe JTD, Weiss MA, et al. Small cell undifferentiated carcinoma of the urinary bladder. A light-microscopic, immunocyto-chemical, and ultrastructural study of 12 cases. Am J Surg Pathol. 1987;11:606–17.

20. Badalament RA, Hermansen DK, Kimmel M, et al. The sensitivity of bladder wash flow cytometry, bladder wash cytology, and voided cytology in the detection of bladder carcinoma. Cancer. 1987;60:1423–7.

21. Badalament RA, Kimmel M, Gay H, et al. The sensitivity of flow cytometry compared with conventional cytology in the detection of superficial bladder carcinoma. Cancer. 1987;59:2078–85.

22. Leyh H, Mazeman E. Bard BTA test compared with voided urine cytology in the diagnosis of recurrent bladder cancer. Eur Urol. 1997;32:425–8.

23. Leyh H, Hall R, Mazeman E, Blumenstein BA. Comparison of the Bard BTA test with voided urine and bladder wash cytology in the diagnosis and management of cancer of the bladder. Urology. 1997;50:49–53.

24. Landman J, Chang Y, Kavaler E, Droller MJ, Liu BC. Sensitivity and specificity of NMP-22, telomerase, and BTA in the detection of human bladder cancer. Urology. 1998;52:398–402.

25. Ianari A, Sternberg CN, Rossetti A, et al. Results of Bard BTA test in monitoring patients with a history of transitional cell cancer of the bladder. Urology. 1997;49:786–9.

26. Johnston B, Morales A, Emerson L, Lundie M. Rapid detection of bladder cancer: a comparative study of point of care tests. J Urol. 1997;158:2098–101.

27. D'Hallewin MA, Baert L. Initial evaluation of the bladder tumor antigen test in superficial bladder cancer. J Urol. 1996;155:475–6.

28. Murphy WM, Rivera-Ramirez I, Medina CA, Wright NJ, Wajsman Z. The bladder tumor antigen (BTA) test compared to voided urine cytology in the detection of bladder neoplasms. J Urol. 1997;158:2102–6.

29. Sarosdy MF, deVere White RW, Soloway MS, et al. Results of a multicenter trial using the BTA test to monitor for and diagnose recurrent bladder cancer. J Urol. 1995;154:379–83.

30. Van der Poel HG, Van Balken MR, Schamhart DH, et al. Bladder wash cytology, quantitative cytology, and the qualitative BTA test in patients with superficial bladder cancer. Urology. 1998;51:44–50.

31. Wiener HG, Mian C, Haitel A, Pycha A, Schatzl G, Marberger M. Can urine bound diagnostic tests replace cystoscopy in the management of bladder cancer? J Urol. 1998;159:1876–80.

32. Zippe C, Pandrangi L, Agarwal A. NMP22 is a sensitive, cost-effective test in patients at risk for bladder cancer. J Urol. 1999;161:62–5.

33. Stampfer DS, Carpinito GA, Rodriguez-Villanueva J, et al. Evaluation of NMP22 in the detection of transitional cell carcinoma of the bladder. J Urol. 1998;159:394–8.

34. Soloway MS, Briggman V, Carpinito GA, et al. Use of a new tumor marker, urinary NMP22, in the detection of occult or rapidly recurring transitional cell carcinoma of the urinary tract following surgical treatment. J Urol. 1996;156:363–7.

35. Serretta V, Lo Presti D, Vasile P, Gange E, Esposito E, Menozzi I. Urinary NMP22 for the detection of recurrence after transurethral resection of transitional cell carcinoma of the bladder: experience on 137 patients. Urology. 1998;52:793–6.

36. Ramakumar S, Bhuiyan J, Besse JA, et al. Comparison of screening methods in the detection of bladder cancer. J Urol. 1999;161:388–94.

37. Abbate I, D'Introno A, Cardo G, et al. Comparison of nuclear matrix protein 22 and bladder tumor antigen in urine of patients with bladder cancer. Anticancer Res. 1998;18:3803–5.

38. Sarosdy MF, Hudson MA, Ellis WJ, et al. Improved detection of recurrent bladder cancer using the Bard BTA stat Test. Urology. 1997;50:349–53.

39. Pode D, Shapiro A, Wald M, Nativ O, Laufer M, Kaver I. Noninvasive detection of bladder cancer with the BTA stat test. J Urol. 1999;161:443–6.

40. Ellis WJ, Blumenstein BA, Ishak LM, Enfield DL. Clinical evaluation of the BTA TRAK assay and comparison to voided urine cytology and the Bard BTA test in patients with recurrent bladder tumors. The Multi Center Study Group. Urology. 1997;50:882–7.

41. Golijanin D, Sherman Y, Shapiro A, Pode D. Detection of bladder tumors by immunostaining of the Lewis X antigen in cells from voided urine. Urology. 1995;46:173–7.

42. Planz B, Striepecke E, Jakse G, Bocking A. Use of Lewis X antigen and deoxyribonucleic acid image cytometry to increase sensitivity of urinary cytology in transitional cell carcinoma of the bladder. J Urol. 1998;159:384–7.

43. Pode D, Golijanin D, Sherman Y, Lebensart P, Shapiro A. Immunostaining of Lewis X in cells from voided urine, cytopathology and ultrasound for noninvasive detection of bladder tumors. J Urol. 1998;159:389–92 (discussion 393).

44. Yoshida K, Sugino T, Tahara H, et al. Telomerase activity in bladder carcinoma and its implication for noninvasive diagnosis by detection of exfoliated cancer cells in urine. Cancer. 1997;79:362–9.

45. Buchumensky V, Klein A, Zemer R, Kessler OJ, Zimlichman S, Nissenkorn I. Cytokeratin 20: a new marker for early detection of bladder cell carcinoma? J Urol. 1998;160:1971–4.

46. Miyake H, Hara I, Gohji K, Yamanaka K, Arakawa S, Kamidono S. Urinary cytology and competitive reverse transcriptase–polymerase chain reaction analysis of a specific CD44 variant to detect and monitor bladder cancer. J Urol. 1998;160:2004–8.

47. Jewett HJ, Strong GH. Infiltrating carcinoma of the bladder: relation of the depth of penetration of the bladder wall to incidence of local extension and metastasis. J Urol. 1946;55:366–72.

48. Marshall VF. The relation of the preoperative estimate to the pathologic demonstration of the extent of vesical neoplasms. J Urol. 1952;68:714–23.

49. UICC–International Union Against Cancer TNM classification of malignant tumors. In: Hermanek P, Sobin LH, eds. Heidelberg: Springer-Verlag, 1987.

50. Urinary bladder. In: Fleming ID, Cooper JS, Henson DE, et al., eds. AJCC cancer staging manual. Philadelphia: Lippincott–Raven; 1997:241–3.

51. Spencer J, Lindsell D, Mastorakou I. Ultrasonography compared with intravenous urography in the investigation of adults with haematuria. Br Med J. 1990;301:1074–6.

52. Haleblian GE, Skinner EC, Dickinson MG, Lieskovsky G, Boyd SD, Skinner DG. Hydronephrosis as a prognostic indicator in bladder cancer patients. J Urol. 1998;160:2011–4.

53. Kachnic LA, Kaufman DS, Heney NM, et al. Bladder preservation by combined modality therapy for invasive bladder cancer. J Clin Oncol. 1997;15:1022–9.

54. Corwin HL, Silverstein MD. The diagnosis of neoplasia in patients with asymptomatic microscopic hematuria: a decision analysis. J Urol. 1988;139:1002–6.

55. Aslaksen A, Gadeholt G, Gothlin JH. Ultrasonography versus intravenous urography in the evaluation of patients with microscopic haematuria. Br J Urol. 1990;66:144–7.

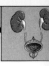
56. Aslaksen A, Halvorsen OJ, Gothlin JH. Detection of renal and renal pelvic tumours with urography and ultrasonography. Eur J Radiol. 1990;11:54–8.

57. Pitts WR Jr, Kazam E, Gershowitz M, Muecke EC. A review of 100 renal and perinephric sonograms with anatomic diagnoses. J Urol. 1975;114:21–6.

58. Buckley JA, Urban BA, Soyer P, Scherrer A, Fishman EK. Transitional cell carcinoma of the renal pelvis: a retrospective look at CT staging with pathologic correlation. Radiology. 1996;201:194–8.

59. Igarashi T, Muakami S, Shichijo Y, Matsuzaki O, Isaka S, Shimazaki J. Clinical and radiological aspects of infiltrating transitional cell carcinoma of the kidney. Urol Int. 1994;52:181–4.

60. Amendola MA, Glazer GM, Grossman HB, Aisen AM, Francis IR. Staging of bladder carcinoma: MRI–CT–surgical correlation. AJR Am J Roentgenol. 1986;146:1179–83.

61. Fisher MR, Hricak H, Tanagho EA. Urinary bladder MR imaging. Part II. Neoplasm. Radiology. 1985;157:471–7.

62. Husband JE, Olliff JF, Williams MP, Heron CW, Cherryman GR. Bladder cancer: staging with CT and MR imaging. Radiology. 1989;173:435–40.

63. Koss JC, Arger PH, Coleman BG, Mulhern CB Jr, Pollack HM, Wein AJ. CT staging of bladder carcinoma. AJR Am J Roentgenol. 1981;137:359–62.

64. Wood DP Jr, Lorig R, Pontes JE, Montie JE. The role of magnetic resonance imaging in the staging of bladder carcinoma. J Urol. 1988;140:741–4.

65. Tanimoto A, Yuasa Y, Imai Y, et al. Bladder tumor staging: comparison of conventional and gadolinium-enhanced dynamic MR imaging and CT. Radiology. 1992;185:741–7.

66. Bryan PJ, Butler HE, LiPuma JP, Resnick MI, Kursh ED. CT and MR imaging in staging bladder neoplasms. J Comput Assist Tomogr. 1987;11:96–101.

67. Nishimura K, Hida S, Nishio Y, et al. The validity of magnetic resonance imaging (MRI) in the staging of bladder cancer: comparison with computed tomography (CT) and transurethral ultrasonography (US). Jpn J Clin Oncol. 1988;18:217–26.

68. See WA, Fuller JR. Staging of advanced bladder cancer. Current concepts and pitfalls. Urol Clin North Am. 1992;19:663–83.

69. Berger GL, Sadlowski RW, Sharpe JR, Finney RP. Lack of value of routine preoperative bone and liver scans in cystectomy candidates. J Urol. 1981;125:637–9.

70. Lerner SP, Skinner E, Skinner DG. Radical cystectomy in regionally advanced bladder cancer. Urol Clin North Am. 1992;19:713–23.

71. Skinner DG, Lieskovsky G. Contemporary cystectomy with pelvic node dissection compared to preoperative radiation therapy plus cystectomy in management of invasive bladder cancer. J Urol. 1984;131:1069–72.

72. Lerner SP, Skinner DG, Lieskovsky G, et al. The rationale for en bloc pelvic lymph node dissection for bladder cancer patients with nodal metastases: long-term results. J Urol. 1993;149:758–64 (discussion 764–5).

73. Stein JP, Freeman JA, Boyd SD, et al. Radical cystectomy in the treatment of invasive bladder cancer: long-term results in a large group of patients. J Urol. 1998;159:213 (abstract 823).

74. Roehrborn CG, Sagalowsky AI, Peters PC. Long-term patient survival after cystectomy for regional metastatic transitional cell carcinoma of the bladder. J Urol. 1991;146:36–9.

75. Pagano F, Bassi P, Galetti TP, et al. Results of contemporary radical cystectomy for invasive bladder cancer: a clinicopathological study with an emphasis on the inadequacy of the tumor, nodes and metastases classification. J Urol. 1991;145:45–50.

76. Hautmann RE, Paiss T. Does the option of the ileal neobladder stimulate patient and physician decision toward earlier cystectomy? J Urol. 1998;159:1845–50.

77. Freiha FS. Open bladder surgery. In: Walsh PC, Retik AB, Stamey TA, Vaughan ED Jr, eds. Campbell's urology, Vol. 3. Philadelphia: WB Saunders; 1992:2750–74.

78. Frazier HA, Robertson JE, Dodge RK, Paulson DF. The value of pathologic factors in predicting cancer-specific survival among patients treated with radical cystectomy for transitional cell carcinoma of the bladder and prostate. Cancer. 1993;71:3993–4001.

79. Vieweg J, Gschwend JE, Herr HW, Fair WR. Pelvic lymph node dissection can be curative in patients with node positive bladder cancer. J Urol. 1999;161:449–54.

80. Vieweg J, Gshwend JE, Herr HW, Fair WR. Impact of primary stage on survival in patients with lymph node positive bladder cancer. J Urol. 1999;161:72–6.

81. Freeman JA, Tarter TA, Esrig D, et al. Urethral recurrence in patients with orthotopic ileal neobladders. J Urol. 1996;156:1615–9.

82. Hardeman SW, Soloway MS. Urethral recurrence following radical cystectomy. J Urol. 1990;144:666–9.

83. Stein JP, Cote RJ, Freeman JA, et al. Indications for lower urinary tract reconstruction in women after cystectomy for bladder cancer: a pathological review of female cystectomy specimens. J Urol. 1995;154:1329–33.

84. Stenzl A, Draxl H, Posch B, Colleselli K, Falk M, Bartsch G. The risk of urethral tumors in female bladder cancer: can the urethra be used for orthotopic reconstruction of the lower urinary tract? J Urol. 1995;153:950–5.

85. Stein JP, Esrig D, Freeman JA, et al. Prospective pathologic analysis of female cystectomy specimens: risk factors for orthotopic diversion in women. Urology. 1998;51:951–5.

86. Lutzeyer W, Rubben H, Dahm H. Prognostic parameters in superficial bladder cancer: an analysis of 315 cases. J Urol. 1982;127:250–2.

87. Torti FM, Lum BL, Aston D, et al. Superficial bladder cancer: the primacy of grade in the development of invasive disease. J Clin Oncol. 1987;5:125–30.

88. Thrasher JB, Frazier HA, Robertson JE, Dodge RK, Paulson DF. Clinical variables which serve as predictors of cancer-specific survival among patients treated with radical cystectomy for transitional cell carcinoma of the bladder and prostate. Cancer. 1994;73:1708–15.

89. Stein JP, Grossfeld GD, Ginsberg DA, et al. Prognostic markers in bladder cancer: a contemporary review of the literature. J Urol. 1998;160:645–59.

90. Lloyd KO. Philip Levine award lecture. Blood group antigens as markers for normal differentiation and malignant change in human tissues. Am J Clin Pathol. 1987;87:129–39.

91. Decenzo JM, Howard P, Irish CE. Antigenic deletion and prognosis of patients with stage A transitional cell bladder carcinoma. J Urol. 1975;114:874–8.

92. Newman AJ Jr, Carlton CE Jr, Johnson S. Cell surface A, B, or O(H) blood group antigens as an indicator of malignant potential in stage A bladder carcinoma. J Urol. 1980;124:27–9.

93. Weinstein RS, Alroy J, Farrow GM, Miller AWD, Davidsohn I. Blood group isoantigen deletion in carcinoma in situ of the urinary bladder. Cancer. 1979;43:661–8.

94. Cordon-Cardo C, Reuter VE, Lloyd KO, et al. Blood group-related antigens in human urothelium: enhanced expression of precursor, LeX, and LeY determinants in urothelial carcinoma. Cancer Res. 1988;48:4113–20.

95. Sheinfeld J, Reuter VE, Melamed MR, et al. Enhanced bladder cancer detection with the Lewis X antigen as a marker of neoplastic transformation. J Urol. 1990;143:285–8.

96. Fradet Y, Cordon-Cardo C. Critical appraisal of tumor markers in bladder cancer. Semin Urol. 1993;11:145–53.

97. Okamura K, Miyake K, Koshikawa T, Asai J. Growth fractions of transitional cell carcinomas of the bladder defined by the monoclonal antibody Ki-67. J Urol. 1990;144:875–8.

98. Fontana D, Bellina M, Gubetta L, et al. Monoclonal antibody Ki-67 in the study of the proliferative activity of bladder carcinoma. J Urol. 1992;148:1149–51.

99. Cohen MB, Waldman FM, Carroll PR, Kerschmann R, Chew K, Mayall BH. Comparison of five histopathologic methods to assess cellular proliferation in transitional cell carcinoma of the urinary bladder. Hum Pathol. 1993;24:772–8.

100. Tsujihashi H, Nakanishi A, Matsuda H, Uejima S, Kurita T. Cell proliferation of human bladder tumors determined by BrdUrd and Ki-67 immunostaining. J Urol. 1991;145:846–9.

101. Mulder AH, Van Hootegem JC, Sylvester R, et al. Prognostic factors in bladder carcinoma: histologic parameters and expression of a cell cycle-related nuclear antigen (Ki-67). J Pathol. 1992;166:37–43.

102. King ED, Matteson J, Jacobs SC, Kyprianou N. Incidence of apoptosis, cell proliferation and bcl-2 expression in transitional cell carcinoma of the bladder: association with tumor progression. J Urol. 1996;155:316–20.

103. Bush C, Price P, Norton J, et al. Proliferation in human bladder carcinoma measured by Ki-67 antibody labelling: its potential clinical importance. Br J Cancer. 1991;64:357–60.

104. Takeichi M. Cadherin cell adhesion receptors as a morphogenetic regulator. Science. 1991;251:1451–5.

105. Bringuier PP, Umbas R, Schaafsma HE, Karthaus HF, Debruyne FM, Schalken JA. Decreased E-cadherin immunoreactivity correlates with poor survival in patients with bladder tumors. Cancer Res. 1993;53:3241–5.

106. Otto T, Birchmeier W, Schmidt U, et al. Inverse relation of E-cadherin and autocrine motility factor receptor expression as a prognostic factor in patients with bladder carcinomas. Cancer Res. 1994;54:3120–3.

107. Lipponen PK, Eskelinen MJ. Reduced expression of E-cadherin is related to invasive disease and frequent recurrence in bladder cancer. J Cancer Res Clin Oncol. 1995;121:303–8.

108. Syrigos KN, Krausz T, Waxman J, et al. E-Cadherin expression in bladder cancer using formalin-fixed, paraffin-embedded tissues: correlation with histopathological grade, tumour stage and survival. Int J Cancer. 1995;64:367–70.

109. Ross JS, del Rosario AD, Figge HL, Sheehan C, Fisher HA, Bui HX. E-Cadherin expression in papillary transitional cell carcinoma of the urinary bladder. Hum Pathol. 1995;26:940–4.

110. Giroldi LA, Bringuier PP, Schalken JA. Defective E-cadherin function in urological cancers: clinical implications and molecular mechanisms. Invasion Metastasis 1994;14:71–81.

111. Jaeger TM, Weidner N, Chew K, et al. Tumor angiogenesis correlates with lymph node metastases in invasive bladder cancer. J Urol. 1995;154:69–71.

112. Dickinson AJ, Fox SB, Persad RA, Hollyer J, Sibley GN, Harris AL. Quantification of angiogenesis as an independent predictor of prognosis in invasive bladder carcinomas. Br J Urol. 1994;74:762–6.

113. Bochner BH, Cote RJ, Weidner N, et al. Angiogenesis in bladder cancer: relationship between microvessel density and tumor prognosis. J Natl Cancer Inst. 1995;87:1603–12.

114. Grossfeld GD, Ginsberg DA, Stein JP, et al. Thrombospondin-1 expression in bladder cancer: association with p53 alterations, tumor angiogenesis, and tumor progression. J Natl Cancer Inst. 1997;89:219–27.

115. Cordon-Cardo C. Mutations of cell cycle regulators. Biological and clinical implications for human neoplasia. Am J Pathol. 1995;147:545–60.

116. Lane DP. Cancer. p53, guardian of the genome. Nature. 1992;358:15–6.

117. Cordon-Cardo C, Dalbagni G, Saez GT, et al. p53 mutations in human bladder cancer: genotypic versus phenotypic patterns. Int J Cancer. 1994;56:347–53.

118. Lipponen PK. Over-expression of p53 nuclear oncoprotein in transitional-cell bladder cancer and its prognostic value. Int J Cancer. 1993;53:365–70.

119. Sarkis AS, Dalbagni G, Cordon-Cardo C, et al. Nuclear overexpression of p53 protein in transitional cell bladder carcinoma: a marker for disease progression. J Natl Cancer Inst. 1993;85:53–9.

120. Bond JA, Blaydes JP, Rowson J, et al. Mutant p53 rescues human diploid cells from senescence without inhibiting the induction of SDI1/WAF1. Cancer Res. 1995;55:2404–9.

121. Michieli P, Chedid M, Lin D, Pierce JH, Mercer WE, Givol D. Induction of WAF1/CIP1 by a p53-independent pathway. Cancer Res. 1994;54:3391–5.

122. Parker SB, Eichele G, Zhang P, et al. p53-independent expression of p21Cip1 in muscle and other terminally differentiating cells. Science. 1995;267:1024–7.

123. Stein JP, Ginsberg DA, Grossfeld GD, et al. Effect of p21WAF1/CIP1 expression on tumor progression in bladder cancer. J Natl Cancer Inst. 1998;90:1072–9.

124. Bagchi S, Weinmann R, Raychaudhuri P. The retinoblastoma protein copurifies with E2F-I, an E1A-regulated inhibitor of the transcription factor E2F. Cell. 1991;65:1063–72.

125. Wang JY, Knudsen ES, Welch PJ. The retinoblastoma tumor suppressor protein. Adv Cancer Res. 1994;64:25–85.

126. Logothetis CJ, Xu HJ, Ro JY, et al. Altered expression of retinoblastoma protein and known prognostic variables in locally advanced bladder cancer. J Natl Cancer Inst. 1992;84:1256–61.

127. Cordon-Cardo C, Wartinger D, Petrylak D, et al. Altered expression of the retinoblastoma gene product: prognostic indicator in bladder cancer. J Natl Cancer Inst. 1992;84:1251–6.

128. Esrig D, Shi SR, Bochner B, et al. Prognostic importance of p53 and Rb alterations in transitional cell carcinoma of the bladder. J Urol. 1995;153:362A (abstract 536).

129. Lerner SP, Linn D, Chakraborty S, et al. Correlation of p53 and retinoblastoma protein expression with established pathologic prognostic features in radical cystoprostatectomy specimens. J Urol. 1995;153:353A (abstract 537).

130. Freiha F, Reese J, Torti FM. A randomized trial of radical cystectomy versus radical cystectomy plus cisplatin, vinblastine and methotrexate chemotherapy for muscle invasive bladder cancer. J Urol. 1996;155:495–9 (discussion 499–500).

131. Skinner DG, Daniels JR, Russell CA, et al. The role of adjuvant chemotherapy following cystectomy for invasive bladder cancer: a prospective comparative trial. J Urol. 1991;145:459–64.

132. Stockle M, Meyenburg W, Wellek S, et al. Advanced bladder cancer (stages pT3b, pT4a, pN1 and pN2): improved survival after radical cystectomy and 3 adjuvant cycles of chemotherapy. Results of a controlled prospective study. J Urol. 1992;148:302–6.

133. Schultz PK, Herr HW, Zhang ZF, et al. Neoadjuvant chemotherapy for invasive bladder cancer: prognostic factors for survival of patients treated with M-VAC with 5-year follow-up. J Clin Oncol. 1994;12:1394–401.

134. Scher HI, Yagoda A, Herr HW, et al. Neoadjuvant M-VAC (methotrexate, vinblastine, doxorubicin and cisplatin) effect on the primary bladder lesion. J Urol. 1988;139:470–4.

135. Fair WR, Scher H, Herr H, et al. Neoadjuvant chemotherapy for bladder cancer: the MSKCC experience. Semin Urol. 1990;8:190–6.

136. Herr HW. Conservative management of muscle-infiltrating bladder cancer: prospective experience. J Urol. 1987;138:1162–3.

137. Flocks RH. Treatment of patients with carcinoma of the bladder. JAMA. 1951;145:295–301.

138. Milner WA. The role of conservative surgery in the treatment of bladder tumors. Br J Urol. 1954;26:375–86.

139. Barnes RW, Bergman RT, Hadley HL, Love D. Control of bladder tumors by endoscopic surgery. J Urol. 1967;97:864–8.

140. O'Flynn JD, Smith JM, Hanson JS. Transurethral resection for the assessment and treatment of vesical neoplasms: a review of 840 consecutive cases. Eur Urol. 1975;1:38–40.

141. Henry K, Miller J, Mori M, Loening S, Fallon B. Comparison of transurethral resection to radical therapies for stage B bladder tumors. J Urol. 1988;140:964–7.

142. Solsona E, Iborra I, Ricos JV, Monros JL, Casanova J, Calabuig C. Feasibility of transurethral resection for muscle infiltrating carcinoma of the bladder: long-term followup of a prospective study. J Urol. 1998;159:95–8.

143. Novick AC, Stewart BH. Partial cystectomy in the treatment of primary and secondary carcinoma of the bladder. J Urol. 1976;116:570–4.

144. Kaneti J. Partial cystectomy in the management of bladder carcinoma. Eur Urol. 1986;12:249–52.

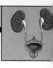

145. Utz DC, Schmitz SE, Fugelso PD, Farrow GM. Proceedings: a clinicopathologic evaluation of partial cystectomy for carcinoma of the urinary bladder. Cancer. 1973;32:1075–7.

146. Resnick MI, O'Conor VJ Jr. Segmental resection for carcinoma of the bladder: review of 102 patients. J Urol. 1973;109:1007–10.

147. Herr HW, Scher HI. Neoadjuvant chemotherapy and partial cystectomy for invasive bladder cancer. J Clin Oncol. 1994;12:975–80.

148. Schoborg TW, Sapolsky JL, Lewis CW Jr. Carcinoma of the bladder treated by segmental resection. J Urol. 1979;122:473–5.

149. Faysal MH, Freiha FS. Evaluation of partial cystectomy for carcinoma of bladder. Urology. 1979;14:352–6.

150. Brannan W, Ochsner MG, Fuselier HA Jr, Landry GR. Partial cystectomy in the treatment of transitional cell carcinoma of the bladder. J Urol. 1978;119:213–5.

151. Cummings KB, Mason JT, Correa RJ Jr, Gibbons RP. Segmental resection in the management of bladder carcinoma. J Urol. 1978;119:56–8.

152. Merrell RW, Brown HE, Rose JF. Bladder carcinoma treated by partial cystectomy: a review of 54 cases. J Urol. 1979;122:471–2.

153. Sweeney P, Kursh ED, Resnick MI. Partial cystectomy. Urol Clin North Am. 1992;19:701–11.

154. Gospodarowicz MK, Warde P. The role of radiation therapy in the management of transitional cell carcinoma of the bladder. Hematol Oncol Clin North Am. 1992;6:147–68.

155. Shipley WU, Zietman AL, Kaufman DS, Althausen AF, Heney NM. Invasive bladder cancer: treatment strategies using transurethral surgery, chemotherapy and radiation therapy with selection for bladder conservation. Int J Radiat Oncol Biol Phys. 1997;39:937–43.

156. Housset M, Maulard C, Chretien Y, et al. Combined radiation and chemotherapy for invasive transitional-cell carcinoma of the bladder: a prospective study. J Clin Oncol. 1993;11:2150–7.

157. Cervek J, Cufer T, Zakotnik B, et al. Invasive bladder cancer: our experience with bladder sparing approach. Int J Radiat Oncol Biol Phys. 1998;41:273–8.

158. Srougi M, Simon SD. Primary methotrexate, vinblastine, doxorubicin and cisplatin chemotherapy and bladder preservation in locally invasive bladder cancer: a 5-year followup. J Urol. 1994;151:593–7.

159. Given RW, Parsons JT, McCarley D, Wajsman Z. Bladder-sparing multimodality treatment of muscle-invasive bladder cancer: a five-year follow-up. Urology. 1995;46:499–504.

160. Chauvet B, Brewer Y, Felix-Faure C, Davin JL, Choquenet C, Reboul F. Concurrent cisplatin and radiotherapy for patients with muscle invasive bladder cancer who are not candidates for radical cystectomy. J Urol. 1996;156:1258–62.

161. Tester W, Caplan R, Heaney J, et al. Neoadjuvant combined modality program with selective organ preservation for invasive bladder cancer: results of Radiation Therapy Oncology Group phase II trial 8802. J Clin Oncol. 1996;14:119–26.

162. Serretta V, Lo Greco G, Pavone C, Pavone-Macaluso M. The fate of patients with locally advanced bladder cancer treated conservatively with neoadjuvant chemotherapy, extensive transurethral resection and radiotherapy: 10-year experience. J Urol. 1998;159:1187–91.

163. Herr HW, Bajorin DF, Scher HI, Cordon-Cardo C, Reuter VE. Can p53 help select patients with invasive bladder cancer for bladder preservation? J Urol. 1999;161:20–23.

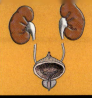

Chapter 27

Early Prostate Cancer

Roger Kirby

INTRODUCTION

Every year, in almost all countries, more cases of prostate cancer are diagnosed than in the previous year. Throughout the developed world prostate cancer is an increasing health problem. The disease mainly affects men beyond middle age, and often results in significant morbidity and mortality. In 1990, prostate cancer was the third most common cancer in men in the European Community, with 86,925 new cases per annum[1]. In the USA it is currently the most common cancer in men; the number of new cases in 1997 was 334,000, and the number of deaths from the disease was 41,800 in 1997[2,3]. Although prostate cancer mortality has remained relatively constant over time, the incidence of prostate cancer continues to rise in most regions of the world[4,5]. A quarter of a million cases were diagnosed worldwide in 1986[6], and the number of cases is expected to rise to at least half a million in the early years of the twenty-first century[7]. The cost of prostate cancer treatment in the year 2001 in the USA alone (diagnosis or terminal care not included) is forecast to be $2–$4 billion per year[8].

The reason for this continuous increase in the prevalence of prostate cancer is not entirely clear. Possible contributory factors include:
- increasing longevity of the population in the West;
- greater awareness of the disease, by both the general public and medical professionals;
- improved diagnostic techniques, such as prostate-specific antigen (PSA), transrectal ultrasound (TRUS), and the development of automatic biopsy devices[9]; and
- especially the increased use of PSA as a screening procedure[10].

It is also possible, although not proved, that carcinogens or other factors may be present in the environment in larger concentrations or that an excess of saturated fat in the diet may predispose toward the malignant transformation of prostate epithelial cells[9].

It is apparent that improved diagnosis, the use of PSA screening, and increased patient awareness account for the current rise in the number of patients who present with earlier stages of disease (i.e. prostate cancer with no demonstrable distant metastases)[11,12].

The early detection of prostate cancer is considered important by most urologists, mainly because of the opportunity to use therapy of curative intent, which improves the prognosis compared with that of patients detected with later stages of disease. Indeed, it is claimed that screening could reduce the number of prostate cancer deaths in the USA by 31%[13]. Despite this, the value of actively screening for prostate cancer is unclear, and many articles cover this ongoing debate[8,11,14,15]. There have been concerns expressed that screening may lead to considerable overdiagnosis and hence overtreatment[15]. Other reasons for caution include increased medical expenditure[8], treatment morbidity, and anxiety to patients and their relatives[11].

Traditionally, younger, fitter patients are generally offered radical treatment for their early stage prostate cancer (either prostatectomy or radiation therapy). Ongoing improvements in both of these techniques have been achieved over recent years. In addition, new treatment options for early prostate cancer are becoming available; these include various forms of hormonal therapy, cryotherapy, interstitial seed implantation, and laser therapy. Another option is watchful waiting without primary intervention (often referred to as expectant or conservative management), especially in older men.

The focus in this chapter is on the possible management options for patients with early prostate cancer in the light of recent therapeutic advances; highlighted are the dilemmas posed for both clinicians and patients in the choice of appropriate therapy for the individual patient.

DIAGNOSIS

The diagnosis of localized prostate cancer requires a history, examination, and some special investigations. As small prostate cancers seldom cause symptoms, patient history may be unrewarding, but a family history may be relevant. Around 9% of prostate cancers are judged to be familial; thus, if one or more first-degree family members have suffered from the disease, suspicion of this diagnosis is raised.

Inquiries are also made about lower urinary tract symptoms suggestive of bladder outflow obstruction and hematuria. The cornerstone of the physical examination is digital rectal examination (DRE). Induration or nodularity of the gland is an important physical sign. Other rectal pathologies also need to be excluded.

Investigations include an estimation of serum PSA, a glycoprotein protease secreted exclusively from the epithelial cells that line the acini of the prostate (Figs 27.1 & 27.2). Elevation of this marker above 4ng/mL carries a 22% probability of cancer; an

increase above 10ng/mL raises the risk of cancer to 63%[16]. In general, prostate cancers that present when the PSA is <10ng/mL are still confined to the gland and therefore potentially surgically curable.

In men with a life expectancy in excess of 10 years, a raised PSA usually prompts a TRUS-guided prostate biopsy (Fig. 27.3). Histologic examination of the tissue removed either confirms or excludes prostate cancer (Fig. 27.4). The Gleason score of the lesion also provides important prognostic and staging information. Recently, Partin used a combination of the clinical grade, PSA value, and Gleason score to provide an estimate of the probability of extraprostatic extension of cancer (Fig. 27.5)[17].

Other staging information can be gleaned from radionuclide bone scans, as well as computed tomography (CT) and magnetic

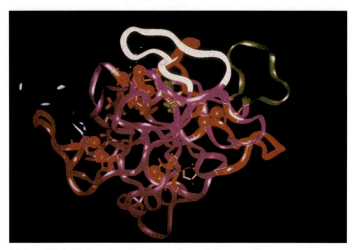

Figure 27.1 Molecular structure of prostate-specific antigen, a 34kDa glycoprotein molecule.

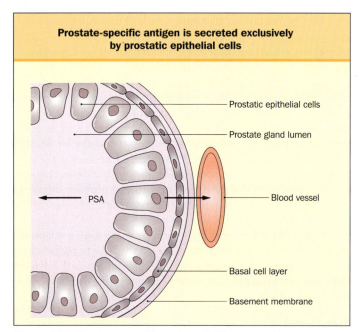

Figure 27.2 Prostate-specific antigen (PSA) secreted is exclusively by prostatic epithelial cells. Most is secreted into the lumen of prostatic acini, but a proportion is absorbed into the blood stream in which it can be measured by radioimmunoassay.

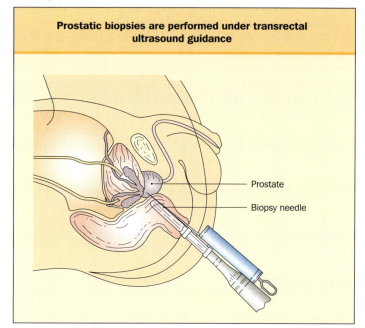

Figure 27.3 Prostatic biopsies are performed under transrectal ultrasound guidance.

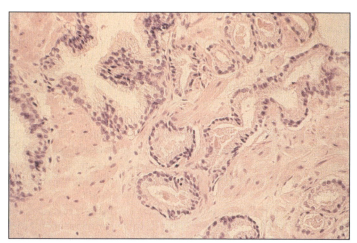

Figure 27.4 Histology from a biopsy guided by transrectal ultrasound confirms the presence of adenocarcinoma of the prostate.

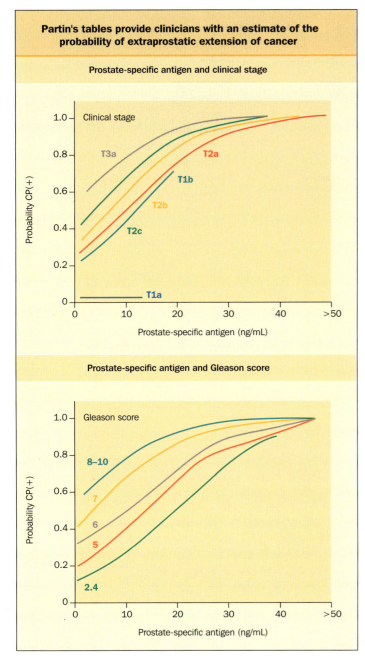

Figure 27.5 Partin's tables provide clinicians with an estimate of the probability of extraprostatic extension of cancer. (Top) Based on prostate-specific antigen and clinical stage, and (bottom) based on prostate-specific antigen and Gleason score.

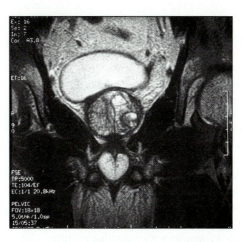

Figure 27.6 Magnetic resonance imaging of the prostate provides some information about the probability of capsular penetration and lymph node metastases.

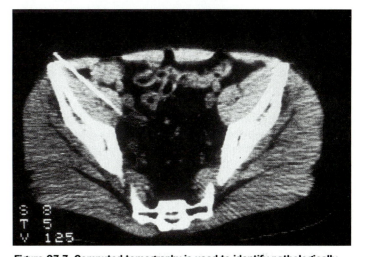

Figure 27.7 Computed tomography is used to identify pathologically enlarged lymph nodes. Under computed tomography guidance, enlarged nodes can be biopsied to provide histologic confirmation of their involvement.

resonance imaging (MRI) of the pelvis (Fig. 27.6). The sensitivity and specificity of the latter two imaging modalities in terms of their ability to identify accurately either lymph node metastases or extraprostatic extension of cancer is unfortunately suboptimal. As a consequence many urologists no longer request these scans for patients with biopsy-proved cancer and low (<10g/mL) PSA values. When the PSA is higher, however, CT can be used to accomplish skinny needle aspiration of enlarged lymph nodes to confirm their involvement with prostate cancer (Fig. 27.7). Magnetic resonance imaging or ultrasound-guided biopsy can also confirm seminal vesicle involvement.

MANAGEMENT

Watchful waiting

Watchful waiting as a policy for patients with early prostate cancer involves careful observation and PSA monitoring at regular intervals (e.g. 3 monthly), with no specific treatment initiated until the cancer begins to cause symptoms or PSA values rise above an arbitrarily defined cut-off point.

Deferred conservative treatment generally has been considered a valid option only for patients older than 70 years with low-stage, clinically localized prostate cancers (stage T1a) and life expectancies <10 years. Such cancers are not uncommonly discovered at the time of transurethral prostatectomy (TURP) for benign prostatic hyperplasia. These cancers only progress in 10–25% of patients within 10 years, and seldom advance significantly within 5 years[18,19]. As these low grade prostate cancers often grow and spread slowly, many of these older men may not require any treatment within the span of their natural life and can be reassured accordingly, but carefully monitored with regular PSA estimation.

A number of arguments favor watchful waiting. The morbidity of any active treatment can be significant (e.g. the possibility of urinary incontinence and erectile dysfunction with radical prostatectomy – see later), especially in older men. Although early treatment is expected to reduce mortality, to date no firm evidence is available that proves this is the case – no prospective randomized trial has yet documented clear therapeutic benefit of radical treatment over expectant management. Retrospective studies with 5–10 years of follow-up question the need for a radical approach to stage T1 disease[20-30]. A Swedish study by Johansson et al. observed 223 patients (mean age 72 years) with early prostate cancer (stage T0–T2NXM0) who were untreated until symptomatic disease progression occurred, at which time hormonal therapy was administered[31]. After a mean of 15 years follow-up, the disease-specific survival rate was 81%, comparable to the rate for men who received treatment after diagnosis. The authors concluded that many patients with localized prostate cancer have a favorable prognosis with watchful waiting.

However, at least as many arguments count against watchful waiting in men with cancer detected at a very early stage. Aus et al. found that in patients with nonmetastatic disease at diagnosis who survived for more than 10 years, 63% eventually died from prostate cancer[30]. Results of an ongoing European study of current screening techniques in Rotterdam by Schröder and colleagues suggest that very few patients who have truly latent disease are identified[32]. It has been postulated that survival and progression curves for early 'screen-detected' cancers can be expected to be similar to those for clinically localized prostate cancer[32]. Furthermore, it is evident that younger men with T2 disease who are managed conservatively have a considerable risk that they will develop metastases and eventually die from their disease[30,33]; for example in a multicenter pooled analysis of disease progression in over 800 patients 42% of patients with moderately differentiated cancers had developed distant metastases by 10 years[29]. It is also evident that for cancers that do progress, many are found to be pathologically (after radical prostatectomy) of a much higher grade and stage than that expected from clinical findings[32]. Importantly, any local or distant cancer progression is likely to result in significant morbidity and consequently an increased financial burden.

The concept of watchful waiting remains controversial and the majority of physicians in Europe and the USA continue to offer active treatment. For example, in a recent European survey only 20% of urologists offered watchful waiting to their early prostate cancer patients[33]. This view is reinforced by recent evidence from a US population-based study that suggests benefits of radical local therapies, notably prostatectomy, over conservative management, particularly in poorly differentiated tumors[34]. Currently, two large prospective randomized trials are underway to compare expectant management with radical prostatectomy in patients with clinically localized prostate cancer. One of these, by the Scandinavian Prostatic Cancer Group, started in 1989 and involves over 500 patients. More recently, the US Prostate Cancer Intervention versus Observation Trial (PIVOT) trial commenced and plans to recruit over 1000 patients[35]. Both these studies highlight the difficulties with randomization of patients into studies with arms as different as watchful waiting and radical surgery, and account for the failure of the Medical Research Council study to recruit sufficient patients into its own attempted, and now abandoned, comparable study.

Active interventions that can be employed in patients with early prostate cancer are listed in Figure 27.8. At present the

Active treatments for early prostate cancer	
Therapy type	**Treatment**
Radical	Prostatectomy:
	perineal
	retropubic
	Radiation therapy:
	external beam radiation therapy
	interstitial (brachytherapy)
Hormonal	Primary therapy (early or delayed):
	orchiectomy
	estrogens
	luteinizing hormone-releasing hormone analogs
	steroidal antiandrogens
	nonsteroidal antiandrogens
	castration plus antiandrogen
	Neoadjuvant therapy
	Adjuvant therapy
Other	Cryotherapy

Figure 27.8 Active treatments for early prostate cancer.

main alternatives to watchful waiting are radical retropubic prostatectomy and radiation therapy.

Radical prostatectomy

In the USA, radical prostatectomy has become increasingly the first-line treatment option. A study in Wisconsin indicated that the proportion of newly diagnosed prostate cancer cases treated with surgery doubled between 1989 and 1991 (from 12 to 25% of cases)[36]. A nationwide survey further indicated that 95% of American urologists recommended radical prostatectomy to men aged 70 years or less with clinically localized disease[37]. In a similar, smaller survey in the UK 29% of urologists said that radical prostatectomy was their preferred management for pathologically aggressive T1 disease and 44% said that it was their preferred management for less poorly differentiated T1 disease[38]. In general, however, surgery is not performed in older (>70 years) patients or those with comorbidity who are not fit enough for a major operation.

When carried out on men with localized prostate cancer and a life expectancy of 15 years or more, radical prostatectomy is considered an acceptable and effective treatment. The benefit relates to the extent of disease at the time of detection. Generally, over 70% of properly selected cases remain tumor free over 7–10 years[39]. For stage T2 tumors, the probability that they remain progression-free (based on PSA determinations) can be as high as 90% in patients with no evidence of positive margins, as evident from several large series[40].

Two main techniques are used for radical prostatectomy, the retropubic and perineal approaches[41,42]. Both techniques appear to offer similar cure rates in terms of tumor progression, cause-specific survival, or positive surgical margins[42-44]. Reportedly, with the retropubic approach the rate of positive apical margins is greater, and with the perineal approach the rate of positive anterior margins is greater[44], but whether this has any clinical significance is currently unclear.

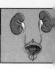

The pros and cons of each approach have been extensively discussed[41–43,45,46]. One of the main advantages of the perineal approach (Fig. 27.9) is that it avoids an abdominal incision, which reduces ileus, postoperative pain, and the length of hospitalization; its main disadvantages are the risk of rectal injury, difficulty in visualization of the neurovascular bundles, and occasional difficulty in dissection of the seminal vesicles[41]. The main advantages of the retropubic approach (Fig. 27.10) are that bilateral pelvic lymphadenectomy can be carried out easily during the operation, and that the neurovascular bundles are more readily visualized, which thereby allows preservation of autonomic innervation to maintain potency. The main disadvantage of retropubic prostatectomy is that an abdominal incision is necessary and so the patient's stay in hospital is usually longer than that for the perineal approach[42]. The final choice depends on the preference of the urologist (based on their own training, experience, and skill) and the needs and preferences of the particular patient.

Whether the retropubic or perineal approach is used, radical prostatectomy is advantageous because it is a 'one-off' procedure that does not involve repeated interventions. However, radical prostatectomy must still be viewed as major surgery – a major disadvantage particularly if the patient has significant comorbidity. Some experts can complete the operation routinely in <2 hours; however, the operation may sometimes take much longer, particularly for less experienced surgeons and if complications such as bleeding occur during the procedure. In the past, blood transfusions frequently accompanied radical retropubic prostatectomy. The occurrence is now less because of improvements in techniques to reduce blood loss[47], mainly by careful control of the dorsal vein complex at the apex of the prostate gland. Blood loss has not been a problem for the perineal approach, which is carried out below the dorsal venous complex. Today, blood transfusions are infrequent for either approach when performed by experienced urologic surgeons.

Radical prostatectomy can now be carried out with minimal mortality and acceptable morbidity. Indeed, several trials indicate perioperative mortality rates below 1%[48,49], but perioperative mortality rates can range from 1 to 4.6%[33,50,51], depending on patient age. In a recent series of almost 500 consecutive radical prostatectomies, the overall preoperative mortality was 2 (0.4%); however, both deaths occurred in older men (69 and 72 years of age) who had an American Society of Anesthesiologist's classification of 3[52]. One of the main complications of radical prostatectomy is erectile dysfunction, which affects from 30 to 100% of patients, depending on patient age and whether nerve-sparing techniques are used or not[53,54]. The other main complication is incontinence, which occurs in 2–18% of patients, with mild stress incontinence in up to 27.5%[48,53,55–58]. Not surprisingly, when patients are asked directly about these problems, the incidence rates are even higher. In a survey of over 750 patients after radical prostatectomy, only 11% had an erection sufficient for intercourse and as many as 47% dripped at least some urine daily[59]. Erectile dysfunction and incontinence rates have been reduced recently by using other operative refinements, such as maintenance of a longer length of distal urethra and preservation of the bladder neck and both neurovascular bundles. Recent advances in the management of erectile dysfunction, which include intraurethral and intracorporeal prostaglandins, and new oral agents such as the phosphodiesterase type-5 inhibitor

sildenafil, now offer safe and effective treatments of post-prostatectomy impotence.

As alluded to earlier, after surgery the cancer is often upstaged (pathologically); reports indicate that this is the case in 30–40% of patients[33]. In these patients progression rates are much higher than those in localized disease at surgery. Moreover, in a review of over 7500 patients treated with radical prostatectomy, the positive surgical margin rate ranged from 14 to 41%[60]. In patients with positive surgical margins and an undetectable PSA, subsequent adjuvant therapy may be necessary[60].

In summary, it has to be appreciated that with radical prostatectomy a potential survival benefit must be balanced against possible loss in quality of life. Until the results of a definitive trial (e.g. PIVOT) are available, the cost of surgery and its associated morbidity (in terms of cost per quality-adjusted life year) need to be considered carefully on the basis of both the individual patient and the surgeon performing the procedure.

Radiation therapy

External beam radiation therapy (EBRT) is an alternative radical approach widely used to treat early prostate cancer, especially outside the USA. Candidates for radiotherapy tend to be patients with localized cancer and a life expectancy of 7–10 years or more, in whom surgery is either not suitable or not desired.

Radiotherapy does not actually remove the prostate, so new cancers can occur in the future. Results from 1245 Californian patients with no evidence of distant metastases indicated a median survival of 10 years postradiotherapy, compared with 15 years for an age-matched cohort, irrespective of the stage, histopathologic grade, or lymph node status of the primary prostate tumor. The best results were found in patients with stage T1 or T2a disease and histologically proved negative lymph nodes, with a 53% survival rate at 15 years, equivalent to the survival rate of an age-matched cohort[61]. Studies of 15-year outcome by the Patterns of Care Study and the Radiation Therapy Oncology Group (RTOG) indicated that patients with stage T1 prostate cancer are in many cases cured by radiotherapy and approximately half are cured with stage T2 cancer[62]. Indeed, T stage and pretreatment PSA are predictors of treatment failure. However, the most important independent predictor of outcome is the nadir PSA[63], for which a level that indicates a potential cure after radiotherapy was established in a study that involved 660 men with T1–T2N0 disease[64]. In that study Critz et al. defined a cure as the achievement and maintenance of a PSA nadir <0.5ng/mL[64].

Most of the studies described above were carried out using EBRT. More recently, interstitial radiation therapy (also termed brachytherapy or seed implant therapy) has become increasingly popular. Long-term data in 122 men with T1–T2 disease treated by a group in Seattle suggest that biochemical outcomes are comparable with those that result from radical prostatectomy and EBRT[65]; the 7-year actuarial disease-free survival (defined as a PSA <0.5ng/mL) was 79% and the overall 7-year survival was 77%, with no deaths from prostate cancer. Also, a Dutch group recently presented their results using this approach in 90 men with T1–T3 prostate cancer and a median follow-up of 54 months. Survival was 69%, but only 7% of the men died from their disease. Most of the patients (eight out of nine) with

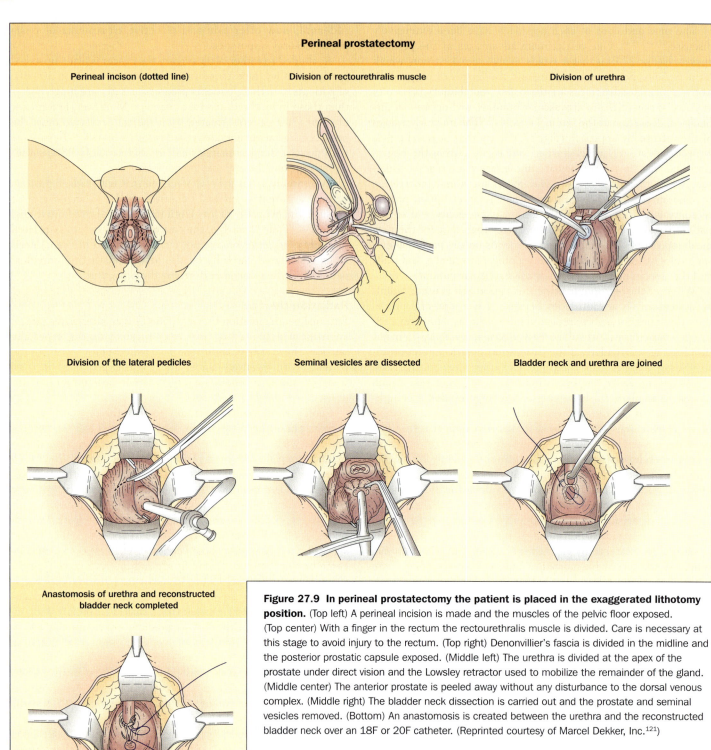

Perineal prostatectomy

Perineal incison (dotted line)	Division of rectourethralis muscle	Division of urethra

Division of the lateral pedicles	Seminal vesicles are dissected	Bladder neck and urethra are joined

Anastomosis of urethra and reconstructed bladder neck completed

Figure 27.9 In perineal prostatectomy the patient is placed in the exaggerated lithotomy position. (Top left) A perineal incision is made and the muscles of the pelvic floor exposed. (Top center) With a finger in the rectum the rectourethralis muscle is divided. Care is necessary at this stage to avoid injury to the rectum. (Top right) Denonvillier's fascia is divided in the midline and the posterior prostatic capsule exposed. (Middle left) The urethra is divided at the apex of the prostate under direct vision and the Lowsley retractor used to mobilize the remainder of the gland. (Middle center) The anterior prostate is peeled away without any disturbance to the dorsal venous complex. (Middle right) The bladder neck dissection is carried out and the prostate and seminal vesicles removed. (Bottom) An anastomosis is created between the urethra and the reconstructed bladder neck over an 18F or 20F catheter. (Reprinted courtesy of Marcel Dekker, Inc.[121])

progression had a nadir PSA >1.5ng/mL[66]. Short-term efficacy results from the Memorial Sloan–Kettering Cancer Center in New York are also encouraging[67].

The two main radiotherapy techniques differ in a number of ways. With EBRT, electron beams are generated from linear accelerators, and treatment is given for 5 days per week over a 5–7 week period. The actual dose only takes minutes to administer, but its intensity can be varied according to how aggressive the cancer is. Typically, around 6000–7000cGy is directed to the prostate for low-grade cancers and for high-grade cancers

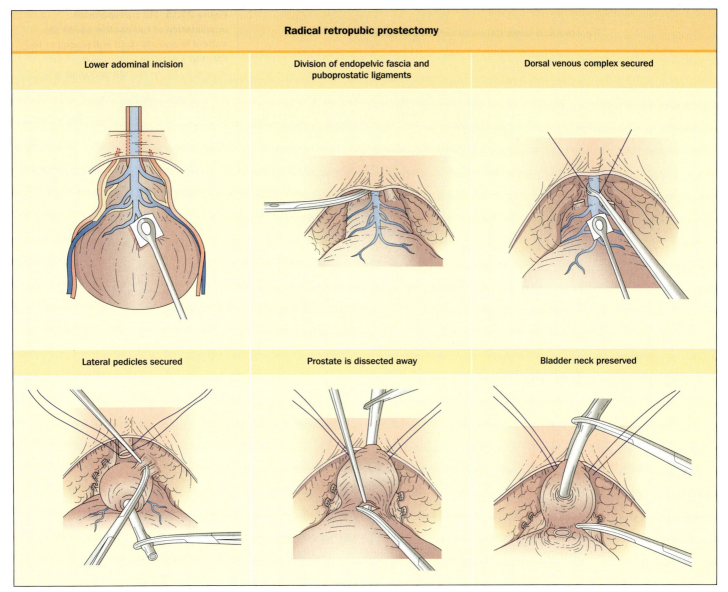

Radical retropubic prostectomy

Lower adominal incision	Division of endopelvic fascia and puboprostatic ligaments	Dorsal venous complex secured
Lateral pedicles secured	Prostate is dissected away	Bladder neck preserved

Figure 27.10 Radical retropubic prostatectomy. (Top left) A lower abdominal incision is made and the retropubic space developed. (Top center) The endopelvic fascia and puboprostatic ligaments are divided on both sides to mobilize the prostate. (Top right) The dorsal venous complex is secured. (Bottom left) The urethra is divided as it enters the apex of the prostate. (Bottom center) With or without preservation of the neurovascular bundles the prostate is dissected away from the bladder neck and removed. (Bottom right) Subsequently, a urethrovesical anastomosis is created.

approximately 7000cGy is delivered to the prostate with an additional 5000cGy to the surrounding pelvic area[68]. Interstitial radiation therapy involves the surgical implantation of small radioactive pellets or 'seeds' into the prostate gland, under local or general anesthetic. The seed implants are generally inserted using the perineal approach and are often permanently left *in situ* (Figs 27.11–27.13). Recently, a stereotactic transgluteal CT-guided conformal technique of brachytherapy that is not limited by prostate size, bone, or TURP defects has been described[69]. This approach was said to decrease the likelihood of seed placement in the urethra, rectum, or bladder. Currently, the most frequently used isotopes are iodine-125 and palladium-103, while iridium-192 is also being investigated[70–72]. Initial results appear promising (Figs 27.14 and 27.15)[73].

The main advantage of radiotherapy is that, unlike radical prostatectomy, the patient avoids major surgery. Each treatment for EBRT is painless, takes only a few minutes, and can be carried out in an outpatient center.

One of the main disadvantages with EBRT is the frequent number of hospital visits required. Side effects that can occur during the course of EBRT include mild symptoms of urinary frequency or urgency, nocturia, and diarrhea. In a 30-year prostate study (Stanford) that involved over 900 patients, these complications were reported in up to 50% of patients, with some degree of erectile dysfunction also reported in 14% of patients 15 months after therapy[74]. Other reports indicate that erectile dysfunction can occur in 40–60% of patients[75,76]. Additional side effects that may become chronic in some patients include cystitis (8%),

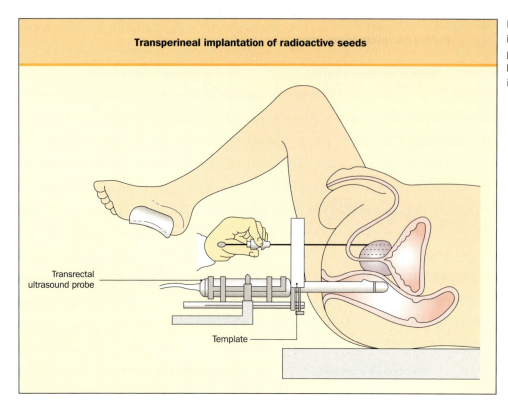

Transperineal implantation of radioactive seeds

Transrectal ultrasound probe

Template

Figure 27.11 For transperineal implantation of radioactive seeds the patient is anesthetized and placed in the lithotomy position. The prostate is then imaged by transrectal ultrasonography.

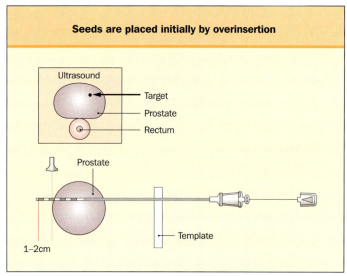

Seeds are placed initially by overinsertion

Ultrasound

Target
Prostate
Rectum

Prostate

Template

1–2cm

Figure 27.12 Seeds are placed initially by overinsertion.

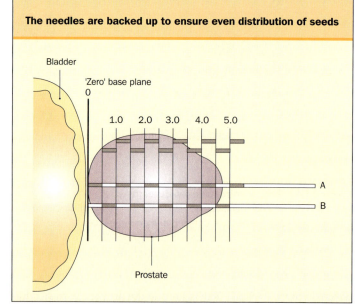

The needles are backed up to ensure even distribution of seeds

Bladder

'Zero' base plane
0

1.0   2.0   3.0   4.0   5.0

A

B

Prostate

Figure 27.13 The needles are backed up to ensure even distribution of seeds.

urethral stricture (4%), enteritis (3%), proctitis (2%), and (rarely) diarrhea, incontinence, and edema[77]. Hospitalization as a result of side effects is required in 5–6% of patients and surgery in 2%[77]. The main postoperative side effects with interstitial radiation therapy include urinary voiding symptoms (12% of patients), impotence (10%), rectal discomfort (3%), and edema (3%)[77].

Recent advances in radiation therapy include conformal therapy with three-dimensional planning, a relatively new form of EBRT, which allows the beam to be focused accurately on the prostate itself. The opportunities for increased doses and reduced morbidity offer the potential for improved outcomes[62,78]. Conformal radiotherapy is becoming more popular; a national

UK trial of the conformal approach is underway. A number of treatment techniques can be used for three-dimensional conformal therapy. For example, in the USA four, six, or eight coplanar fields are used, whereas in the UK it is only three or four. However, differences between these treatment techniques appear to be small and are unlikely to be clinically significant[79].

Selection of patients for whom radiotherapy is as appropriate a therapeutic option as surgery is extremely important[80]. Direct comparisons between patients treated with radiation after clinical

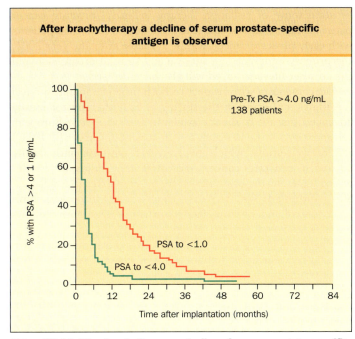

Figure 27.14 After brachytherapy a decline of serum prostate-specific antigen is observed.

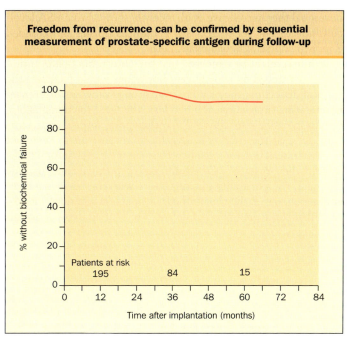

Figure 27.15 Freedom from recurrence can be confirmed by sequential measurement of prostate-specific antigen during follow-up.

staging to those treated with prostatectomy and pathologic staging are often difficult. It is clear, however, that biochemical relapse rates, as determined by PSA levels, tend to be higher with radiotherapy than radical prostatectomy (unless lymph node or seminal vesicle involvement is apparent at the time of surgery)[80–83].

In conclusion, as with surgery, radiotherapy is generally considered effective but can also result in considerable morbidity, which can add significantly to the initial cost of treatment. Careful follow-up is mandatory, as PSA relapse may occur at any time after treatment. If the PSA starts to rise after radiotherapy, further treatment is likely to be necessary.

Neoadjuvant therapy

Whichever active intervention is selected, prostate cancer progresses in a proportion of patients in spite of treatment. For this reason, neoadjuvant therapy is actively under investigation as a means to improve success rates. With radical prostatectomy it s apparent that while very good survival rates are achieved in patients with organ-confined prostate cancer, in those patients with seminal vesicle invasion, positive surgical margins, or disease that extends beyond the prostatic capsule, the prognosis is very much less favourable[84,85]. This problem is compounded because many men believed to have organ-confined disease at diagnosis are found to have more advanced disease at surgery; this appears to be the case for around 30% of patients[86]. In many of these patients the cancer cannot be totally removed by surgery, so the surgical procedure is of limited value. It has been hypothesized that neoadjuvant therapy should improve the success rate of surgery in a number of ways (Fig. 27.16), and ultimately improve survival.

Pretreatment of radical prostatectomy candidates with hormonal therapies, either complete androgen blockade (CAB) or antiandrogen monotherapy, is being investigated by several groups. Following encouraging results from a neoadjuvant pilot study using

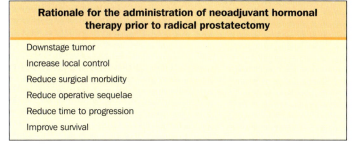

Figure 27.16 Rationale for the administration of neoadjuvant hormonal therapy prior to radical prostatectomy.

DES, the Memorial Sloan–Kettering Cancer Center initiated a randomized study using 3-months of CAB followed by radical prostatectomy versus radical prostatectomy alone in patients with clinically localized prostate cancer[86]. Rates of extracapsular penetration and positive surgical margins were significantly decreased in the neoadjuvant arm, but at a mean follow-up of 28.6 months no significant difference was found with respect to PSA progression. The group also hopes to identify specific patients whose tumors might respond optimally to neoadjuvant hormonal therapy. Similarly, although several other investigators have found a reduction in positive surgical margins with neoadjuvant therapy, follow-up data at 2–3 years suggest that this may not translate into improvements in PSA progression[87–90]. Only one study, in which 126 patents with T1b–T3a disease underwent immediate prostatectomy or were pretreated with triptorelin, has shown a significant difference in terms of time to PSA progression (10.9 versus 22.9 months; $p = 0.03$)[91]. Sufficient follow-up information is not available from any of these studies to establish if there is any clinical benefit for patients with localized disease in terms of survival. The optimum duration of neoadjuvant therapy has yet to be defined; while most studies have utilized a 3-month course of hormonal therapy, Gleave et al. recently showed that PSA levels continue to fall between 3 and 8 months during an extended 8 month course of neoadjuvant CAB[92].

While it might be expected that the clear reduction in tumor volume achieved by neoadjuvant hormones would facilitate the surgical dissection, the results of two groups show no differences in operating time, surgical blood loss, the need for transfusions, or perioperative morbidity[88–93]. Furthermore, some investigators consider that the surgery is actually more difficult to carry out after hormonal therapy, mainly because of increased fibrotic tissue around the prostate[94]. Disadvantages of pretreatment include costs and the possibility of side effects with the hormonal therapy, depending on the choice of components. In addition, it is possible that some patients may not wish to wait an extra 3 months for surgery[95].

While survival data with neoadjuvant therapy are awaited, one of the groups currently studying this approach conducted a multivariate analysis of their patients to establish those unlikely to benefit[96]. Their results suggest further clinical gains are unlikely in patients with clinically localized, well or moderately differentiated cancer, and a PSA ≤ 4ng/mL.

Neoadjuvant therapy has also been evaluated prior to radiotherapy; an advantage of hormonal therapy in this setting is a potential reduction in radiation-associated morbidity[97]. In a randomized study in 471 men with T2–4NXM0 disease, neoadjuvant maximum androgen blockade (MAB; goserelin plus flutamide) given for 2 months before and during radiotherapy significantly reduced local progression at 5 years, although no significant effect on overall survival is yet apparent[97]. Data from Canada indicate that the nadir PSA is reached more rapidly with neoadjuvant MAB and that PSA measurements remain lower over 3 years of follow-up[98]. Adjuvant MAB for 6 months after radiotherapy conferred further benefits. The neoadjuvant approach may be particularly valuable in patients with unfavorable locoregional disease, and result in significant improvements in local control compared to treatment with radiation or hormonal therapy alone[99,100].

Adjuvant therapy

Adjuvant hormonal therapy has had a highly significant effect on both tumor recurrence and mortality in localized breast cancer[101]. Extrapolation of these results to the analogous setting of hormonally sensitive prostate cancer provides a rationale for the use of adjuvant therapy after radical prostatectomy in patients with positive surgical margins or in whom PSA levels do not become undetectable[102]. Patients with pathologically organ-confined and margin-negative disease, with preoperative PSA levels >10ng/mL, and/or a pathologic Gleason score ≥ 7 may also benefit[103]. A number of hormonal adjuvant treatment options are possible, including luteinizing hormone–releasing hormone (LHRH) monotherapy, antiandrogen monotherapy, and possibly finasteride[62,104,105]. Adjuvant treatment, in the form of orchiectomy or radiotherapy, increased local and systemic progression in patients with pT3, N0, M0 prostate cancer who had been treated with radical retropubic prostatectomy[106]. However, no improvement was seen in cause-specific or crude survival. A large placebo-controlled study that involved over 8000 patients is now underway to assess the possible benefits of bicalutamide monotherapy (150mg daily) in postradical prostatectomy or radiation therapy in 'early' prostate cancer patients. The results of this study, the largest to date in patients with early prostate cancer, will be available after the year 2001; the primary endpoints are survival and time to progression and the cost per life-year saved will also be addressed.

Outcome data with respect to both progression and survival for adjuvant therapy in the setting of radiotherapy for locally advanced disease is already available[106,107]. A recent European Organization for the Research and Treatment of Cancer (EORTC) randomized study, which involved 415 patients with locally advanced prostate cancer, indicated that adjuvant LHRH analog (goserelin depot) started at the onset of external irradiation, and continued for 3 years, significantly improved both local control and survival after a median of 45 months follow-up[107]. The 5-year Kaplan–Meier estimates for survival were 79% for the adjuvant arm and 62% for the radiotherapy alone arm ($p = 0.001$). For bulky tumors, adjuvant therapy with a goserelin depot after radiation therapy has been shown by radiotherapy and oncology groups (RTOG) to be beneficial in terms of treatment outcome (time to PSA relapse and time to progression); longer follow-up is necessary to examine any effect on survival[108]. Outcome improvements have also been noted for locally advanced prostate cancer treated by radiation therapy and adjuvant hormonal therapy with either combined androgen deprivation or monotherapy[62,109].

In summary, adjuvant hormonal therapy is a promising approach and is undergoing extensive clinical evaluation at present. Survival outcome appears to be improved when applied postradiotherapy, but the effects on survival postprostatectomy have yet to be determined. As with any adjuvant therapy, basic criteria must be met for the choice of hormonal therapy, such as good efficacy and tolerability, maintenance of quality of life (particularly sexual interest and function), a convenient route of administration, and a dosing regimen to aid compliance.

SUMMARY

Tumor stage, patients' age, and general medical condition have an important impact on the selection of the appropriate treatment for early prostate cancer. In selected groups of patients with clinically localized prostate cancer, many of the available treatments result in rates of survival comparable to the expected survival rate for the general population[77]. These good results arise from a number of factors, which include the:
- favorable natural history of indolent cancers (especially those detected at TURP);
- detection and effective treatment of aggressive cancers;
- confounding effects of competing causes of death; and
- balancing effect of hormonal therapy for relapses.

With the advent of PSA screening in some countries, it is important to establish whether we are detecting clinically significant prostate cancers and whether it is justifiable to offer a radical prostatectomy to the majority of patients. Available evidence shows that the majority of screen-detected patients do have clinically significant prostate cancer[110]. However, screening still remains a controversial issue[111]; in spite of this the American Cancer Society Guidelines recommend that the PSA test and DRE should be offered annually to men of 50 years of age onward and that they should be provided with information on

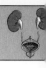

the potential risks and benefits of screening[112]. In the USA the recent decrease in incidence and mortality rate of prostate cancer, together with an observed shift in stage, may arise from annual screening using PSA and DRE[113]. There is an urgent need for more randomized controlled studies and public policy guidelines about screening and treatment. The American Urologic Association Prostate Cancer Clinical Guidelines Panel has recently identified the advantages and disadvantages of the main treatments, and recommended that newly diagnosed, clinically localized prostate cancer patients should be informed of all the commonly accepted options[114].

Decision analysis modeling, based on a number of clinical assumptions, was used to assess alternative treatment strategies for clinically localized prostate cancer – radical prostatectomy, EBRT, and watchful waiting with delayed hormonal therapy[115]. This analysis indicates that for the most part 'the potential benefits of therapy are small enough that the choice of therapy is sensitive to the patient's preferences for various outcomes.' The analysis further indicates that radical prostatectomy and radiation therapy may benefit specific patients, particularly younger patients with high-grade tumors. Watchful waiting is suggested as a suitable alternative to radical treatment for many men, particularly those with significant comorbidity[115]. However, it has been suggested that for accurate decision making, effects on quality of life should also be taken into account; studies in this area are clearly needed[116].

The cost effectiveness of the various treatment options must also be fully considered; preferably the cost per quality-adjusted life year, as this measures the cost implications of morbidity and impact on quality of life. Few studies have so far addressed this important area. Though increasingly popular in many countries, radical prostatectomy is relatively expensive compared with the alternatives. In the USA, for example, radical prostatectomy has been estimated to be twice as expensive as radiotherapy ($18,140 versus $9,800)[117]. Insurance industry figures estimate that 60,000–70,000 radical prostatectomies are carried out annually at significant total cost[118]. A true cost:effectiveness ratio for this procedure needs to be established, including the costs of managing the complications.

In summary, because we do not know precisely how the tumor will behave, the tendency is to treat the patient surgically rather than with less invasive therapies. Radical prostatectomies are often used in men with clinically localized disease who are under 75 years of age and have a life expectancy of more than 10 years. Time itself and randomized studies will show whether such therapy in patients with locally confined prostate cancer leads to a decrease in mortality from prostate cancer.

In the meantime, less aggressive options such as hormonal therapy and watchful waiting should be considered in selected patients, especially those with a life expectancy <10 years. Antiandrogens are likely to play an increasing role in the treatment of early stages of prostate cancer and the current early prostate cancer trial of bicalutamide versus placebo will play an important part in determining this role. In the selection of appropriate anti-androgen therapy, urologists must consider factors, with respect to tolerability and dosing regimen, that may encourage compliance. Neoadjuvant treatment in the setting of radiotherapy is also likely to assume more importance, whereas in the surgical setting further data on survival outcome is needed before neoadjuvant hormones can be used routinely. Radiofrequency interstitial tumor ablation and high-intensity focused ultrasound are other new techniques that are undergoing preliminary investigation[119,120]. Other treatments that are generating interest include cryotherapy, laser therapy with photodynamic enhancers, and brachytherapy. All of these need to be fully assessed in terms of long-term outcome.

Future research is likely to focus increasingly on the role of growth factors, oncogenes, tumor-suppressor genes, and inducers of apoptosis. This, together with the clinical studies that are underway and/or planned in the treatment of early prostate cancer, should provide not only novel treatments, but also answers to some of the existing controversies that surround the management of early prostate cancer.

REFERENCES

1. Black RJ, Bray F, Ferlay J, Parkin DM. Cancer incidence and mortality in the European Union: cancer registry data and estimates of national incidence for 1990. Eur J Cancer. 1997;33:1075–107.

2. Parker SL, Tong T, Bolden S, Wingo PA. Cancer statistics 1997. CA Cancer J Clin. 1997;47:5–27.

3. Wingo PA, Tong T, Bolden S. An adjustment to the 1997 estimate for new prostate cancer cases. CA Cancer J Clin. 1997;47:239–42.

4. Alexander FE, Boyle P. The rise in prostate cancer: myth or reality? In: Garraway MJ, ed. The epidemiology of prostate disease. Berlin: Springer; 1995:192–202.

5. Boyle P, Maisonneuve P, Napalkov P. Incidence of prostate cancer mortality will double by the year 2030: the argument for. Eur Urol. 1996;29(Suppl 2):3–9.

6. Parkin DM, Pisani P, Ferlay J. Estimates of the worldwide incidence of 18 major cancers in 1985. Int J Cancer. 1993;55:891–903.

7. Boyle P. Prostate cancer 2000: evolution of an epidemic of unknown origin. In: Denis L, ed. Prostate cancer 2000. Heidelberg: Springer-Verlag; 1994:5–11.

8. Mayer FJ. Future trends in incidence and management of prostate cancer. West J Med. 1994;160:380–1.

9. Haas GP. Epidemiology of early prostate cancer. In Vivo. 1994;8:403–6.

10. Woolf HS. Public health perspective: the health policy implications of screening for prostate cancer. J Urol. 1994;152:1685–8.

11. Dearnaley DP. Cancer of the prostate. Br Med J. 1994;308:780–4.

12. Hall RR. Screening and early detection of prostate cancer will decrease morbidity and mortality from prostate cancer: the argument against. Eur Urol. 1996;29(Suppl 2):24–6.

13. Labrie F, Cusan L, Gomez J-L, Diamond F, Candas B. Combination of screening and pre-operative endocrine therapy: the potential for an important decrease in prostate cancer mortality. J Clin Endocrinol Metab. 1995;80:2002–13.

14. Mandelson MT, Wagner EH, Thompson RS. PSA screening: a public health dilemma. Annu Rev Public Health. 1995;16:283–306.

15. Iversen P, Adolfsson J, Johansson J-E, Torp-Pedersen S. Localised prostate cancer – a Scandinavian view. Monogr Urol. 1994;15:93–112.

16. Catalona WJ, Smith DS, Ratliff TL, et al. Measurement of prostate-specific antigen in serum as a screening test for prostate cancer. N Engl J Med. 1991;324:1156–61.

17. Partin AW, Subong ENP, Walsh PC, et al. Combination of prostate-specific antigen, clinical stage, and Gleason score to predict pathological stage of prostate cancer. JAMA. 1997;277:1445–51.

18. Blute ML, Zincke H, Farrow GM. Long-term follow up of young patients with stage A adenocarcinoma of the prostate. J Urol. 1986;136:840–3.

19. Epstein JI, Paull G, Eggleston JC, Walsh PC. Prognosis of untreated stage A1 prostatic carcinoma: a study of 94 cases with extended follow up. J Urol. 1986;136:837–9.

20. Newling DW, Hall RR, Richards B. The natural history of prostatic cancer, the argument for a no treatment policy. In: Pavone-Macaluso M, ed. Testicular cancer and other tumours of the genito-urinary tract. New York: Plenum Publications; 1985:443–9.

21. Moskovitz B, Nitecki A, Richter Levin D. Cancer of the prostate: is there a need for aggressive treatment? Urol Int. 1987;42:49–52.

22. George NJR. Natural history of localized prostatic cancer managed by conservative therapy alone. Lancet. 1988;i:494–7.

23. Goodman CM, Busuttil A, Chisholm GD. Age, and stage and grade of tumour predict prognosis in incidentally diagnosed carcinoma of the prostate. Br J Urol. 1988;62:576–80.

24. Handley R, Carr TW, Travis D, Powell PH, Hall RR. Deferred treatment for prostate cancer. Br J Urol. 1988;62:249–53.

25. Orestano F. Problems of the wait-and-see policy in incidental carcinoma of the prostate. In: Altwein JE, Faul P, Schneider W, ed. Incidental carcinoma of the prostate. Berlin: Springer; 1991:163–6.

26. Whitmore WF Jr, Warner JA, Thompson IM. Expectant management of localized prostatic cancer. Cancer. 1991;67:1091–6.

27. Adolfsson J, Carstensen J, Lowhagen T. Deferred treatment in clinically localized prostatic carcinoma. Br J Urol. 1992;69:183–7.

28. Jones GW. Prospective, conservative management of localized prostate cancer. Cancer. 1992;70(Suppl):307–10.

29. Chodak GW, Thisted RA, Gerber GS, et al. Results of conservative management of clinically localized prostate cancer. N Engl J Med. 1994;330:242–8.

30. Aus G, Hugosson J, Norlen L. Long-term survival and mortality in prostate cancer treated with noncurative intent. J Urol. 1995;154:460–5.

31. Johansson J-E, Holmberg L, Johansson S, Bergstrom R, Adami H-O. Fifteen-year survival in prostate cancer: a prospective, population-based study in Sweden. N Engl J Med. 1997;277:467–71.

32. George N. Natural history of localized prostate cancer managed by conservative therapy alone. Lancet. 1988;1:494–7.

33. Brausi M, Palladini PD, Latini A. 'Watchful waiting' for clinically localized prostate cancer: long term results. Eur Urol. 1996;30(Suppl 2):225 (Abs 833).

34. Lu-Yao GL, Yao S-L. Population-based study of long-term survival in patients with clinically localised prostate cancer. Lancet. 1997;349:906–10.

35. Wilt TJ, Brawer MK. The Prostate Cancer Intervention versus Observation Trial (PIVOT). Oncol (Huntingt). 1997;11:1133–9.

36. Pezzinio G, Remington PL, Anderson HA, et al. Trends in the surgical treatment of prostate cancer in Wisconsin 1989–1991. J Natl Cancer Inst. 1994;86:1083–6.

37. Gee WF, Holtgrewe HL, Albertsen PC, et al. Practice trends in the diagnosis and management of prostate cancer in the United States. J Urol. 1995;154:207–8.

38. Savage P, Bates C, Abel P, Waxman J. British urological surgery practice. 1. Prostate cancer. Br J Urol. 1997;79:749–55.

39. Epstein JI, Pizov G, Walsh PC. Correlation of pathologic findings with progression after radical retropubic prostatectomy. Cancer. 1993;71:3582–93.

40. Huland H. The risks outweigh the benefits of radical prostatectomy in localised prostate cancer: the argument against. Eur Urol. 1996;29(Suppl 2):31–3.

41. Resnick MI. Radical prostatectomy: the perineal approach. Urology. 1996;47:457–9.

42. Oesterling JE. Radical prostatectomy: the retropubic approach. Urology. 1996;47:460–2.

43. Frazier HA, Robertson JE, Paulson DF. Radical prostatectomy: the pros and cons of the perineal versus retropubic approach. J Urol. 1992;147:888–90.

44. Weldon VE, Tavel FR, Neuwirth H, Cohen R. Patterns of positive specimen margins and detectable prostate-specific antigen after radical perineal prostatectomy. J Urol. 1995;153:1565–9.

45. Walther PJ. Radical perineal vs. retropubic prostatectomy: a review of optimal application and technical considerations in the utilization of these exposures. Eur Urol. 1993;24(Suppl 2):34–8.

46. Walsh PC. Radical retropubic prostatectomy: indication, technique, and long-term results. In: Oesterling JE, Richie JP, eds. Urologic oncology. Philadelphia: WB Saunders; 1997:147–61.

47. Reiner WG, Walsh PC. An anatomical approach to the surgical management of the dorsal vein and Santorini's plexus during radical retropubic surgery. J Urol. 1979;121:198–200.

48. Pedersen KV, Herder A. Radical retropubic prostatectomy for localized prostatic carcinoma: a clinical and pathological study of 201 cases. Scand J Urol Nephrol. 1992;26:235–9.

49. Davidson PJT, van den Ouden D, Schröder FH. Radical prostatectomy: prospective assessment of mortality and morbidity. Eur Urol. 1996;29:168–73.

50. Lu-Yao GL, McLerran D, Wasson J, Wennberg JE, Patient Outcomes Research Team. An assessment of radical prostatectomy. Time trends, geographic variation, and outcomes. JAMA. 1993;269:2633–6.

51. Zincke H, Bergstralh EJ, Blute ML, et al. Radical prostatectomy for clinically localized prostate cancer: long-term results of 1,143 patients from a single institution. J Clin Oncol. 1994;12:2254–63.

52. Dillioglugil O, Leibman BD, Leibman NS, Kattan MW, Rosas AL, Scardino PT. Risk factors for complications and morbidity after radical retropubic prostatectomy. J Urol. 1997;157:1760–7.

53. Gibbons RP, Correa RJ, Brannen GE, Mason JT. Total prostatectomy for localized prostate cancer. J Urol. 1984;131:73–6.

54. Walsh PC. Radical prostatectomy, preservation of sexual function, cancer control. Urol Clin North Am. 1987;14:663–73.

55. Lindner A, deKernion JB, Smith RB, Katske FA. Risk of urinary incontinence following radical prostatectomy. J Urol. 1983;129:1007–8.

56. Middleton RG, Smith JA, Melzer RB, Hamilton PE. Patients' survival and local recurrence rate following radical prostatectomy for prostatic carcinoma. J Urol. 1986;136:422–4.

57. Igel TC, Barrett DM, Segyra JW, Benson RC Jr, Rife CC. Perioperative and postoperative complications from bilateral pelvic lymphadenectomy and radical retropubic prostatectomy. J Urol. 1987;137:1189–91.

58. Catalona WJ, Bigg SW. Nerve-sparing radical prostatectomy: evaluation of results after 250 patients. J Urol. 1990;143:538–44.

59. Fowler FJ, Roman A, Bary MJ, Wasson J, Lu-Yang G, Wennberg JE. Patient-reported complications and follow-up treatment after radical prostatectomy. The National Medicare Experience, 1988–1990 (updated June 1993). Urology. 1993;42:622–9.

60. Scardino PT. Surgical treatment of clinically localized prostate cancer: the role of combination therapy. 32nd AUA Annual Meeting May 18–21, 1996. Philadelphia: Educational Book; 230–6.

61. Bagshaw MA, Cox RS, Hancock SL. Control of prostate cancer with radiotherapy: long-term results. J Urol. 1994;152:1781–5.

62. Hanks GE, Hanlon A, Schultheiss T, Corn B, Shipley WU, Lee WR. Early prostate cancer: the national results of radiation treatment from the Patterns of Care and Radiation Therapy Oncology Group studies with prospects for improvement with conformal radiation and adjuvant androgen deprivation. J Urol. 1994;152:1775–80.

63. Crook JM, Bahadur YA, Bociek RG, Perry GA, Robertson SJ, Esche BA. Radiotherapy for localized prostate cancer. Cancer. 1997;79:328–36.

64. Critz FA, Levinson AK, Williams WH, Holladay DA, Holladay CT. The PSA nadir that indicates potential cure after radiotherapy for prostate cancer. Urology. 1997;49:322–6.

65. Ragde H, Blasko JC, Grimm PD, et al. Interstitial iodine-125 radiation without adjuvant therapy in the treatment of clinically localized prostate carcinoma? Cancer. 1997;80:442–53.

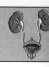
66. Schipper RA, van Andel G, de Reijke TM, Kurth KH. Prostate carcinoma treated by brachytherapy with I-125: is cure possible? Br J Urol. 1997;80(Suppl 2):239 (Abs 937).

67. Wallner K, Roy J, Harrison L. Tumor control and morbidity following transperineal iodine 125 implantation for stage T1/2 prostatic carcinoma. J Clin Oncol. 1996;14:449–453.

68. Bostwick DG, MacLennan GT, Larson TR, The American Cancer Society. Prostate cancer: what every man – and his family – needs to know. New York: Villard Books; 1996.

69. Koutrouvelis PG, Schwartz DT, Mondalek P, Pan J, Bondy HE, Mostofi K. Stereotactic transgluteal CT-guided conformal brachytherapy of prostate cancer is not limited by prostate size, bone or urinary obstruction, or TURP defects. J Urol. 1997;80(Suppl 2):268 (Abs 1054).

70. Koprowski CD, Berkenstock KG, Borofski AM, Ziegler JC, Lightfoot DA, Brady LW. External beam irradiation versus 125 iodine implant in the definitive treatment of prostate carcinoma. Int J Radiat Oncol Biol Phys. 1991;21:955–60.

71. Brosman SA, Tokita K. Transrectal ultrasound-guided interstitial radiation therapy for localized prostate cancer. Urology. 1991;38:372–6.

72. Marinelli D, Shanberg AM, Tansey LA, Sawyer DE, Syed N, Puthawala A. Follow-up prostate biopsy in patients with carcinoma of the prostate treated by 192 iridium template irradiation plus supplemental external beam radiation. J Urol. 1992;147:922–5.

73. Ragde H, Elgamal AA, Snow PB et al. Ten-year disease free survival after transperineal sonography-guided Iodine^{-125} brachytherapy with or without 45-gray external beam irradiation in the treatment of patients with clinically localized, low to high Gleasor grade prostate carcinoma. Cancer 1998;83:989–1001.

74. Bagshaw MA, Cox RS, Ray GR. Status of radiation treatment of prostate cancer at Stanford University. NCI Monogr. 1988;7:47–60.

75. Paulson DF, Moul JW, Robertson JE, Walther PJ. Postoperative radiotherapy of the prostate for patients undergoing radical prostatectomy with positive margins, seminal vesicle involvement and/or penetration through the capsule. J Urol. 1990;1143:1178–82.

76. Shipley WU, Prout GR Jr, Coachman NM, et al. Radiation therapy for localized prostate carcinoma: experience at the Massachusetts General Hospital (1973–1981). In Wittes RE: Consensus Development Conference on the Management of Clinically Localized Prostate Cancer. NCI Monographs No. 7 (NIH publication No 88–3005). Washington: Government Printing Office; 1988:67–73.

77. Catalona WJ. Management of cancer of the prostate. N Engl J Med. 1994;331:996–1004.

78. Soffen EM, Hanks GE, Hunt MA, Epstein BE. Conformal static field radiation therapy treatment of early prostate cancer versus non-conformal techniques: a reduction in acute morbidity. Int J Radiat Oncol Biol Phys. 1992;24:485–8.

79. Neal AJ, Oldham M, Dearnaley DP. Comparison of treatment techniques for conformal radiotherapy of the prostate using dose–volume histograms and normal tissue complication probabilities. Radiother Oncol. 1995;37:29–34.

80. Kaplan ID, Cox RS, Bagshaw MA. Radiotherapy for prostatic cancer: patient selection and the impact of local control. Urology. 1994;43:634–9.

81. Bigg SW, Kavoussi LR, Catalona WJ. Role of nerve-sparing radical prostatectomy for clinical stage B2 prostate cancer. J Urol. 1990;144:1420–4.

82. Stamey TA, Villers AA, McNeal JE, Link PC, Freiha FS. Positive surgical margins at radical prostatectomy: importance of the apical dissection. J Urol. 1990;142:1166–73.

83. Stein A, deKernion JB, Smith RB, Dorey F, Patel H. Prostate-specific antigen levels after radical prostatectomy in patients with organ confined and locally extensive prostate cancer. J Urol. 1992;147:942–6.

84. Frazier HA, Robertson JE, Humphrey PA, Paulson DF. Is prostate-specific antigen of clinical importance in evaluating outcome after radical prostatectomy? J Urol. 1993;149:516–8.

85. Paulson DF, Moul JW, Walther PJ. Radical prostatectomy for clinical stage T1–2N0M0 prostatic adenocarcinoma: longterm results. J Urol. 1990;144:1180–4.

86. Kirby RS. Treatment options for early prostate cancer. Urology. 1998;52:948–62.

87. Fair WR, Cookson MS, Stroumbakis N, et al. The indications rationale and results of neoadjuvant androgen deprivation in the treatment of prostate cancer. Memorial Sloan–Kettering Cancer results. Urology. 1997;49(Suppl 3A):46–55.

88. Cookson MS, Sogani PC, Russo P, et al. Pathological staging and biochemical recurrence after neoadjuvant androgen deprivation therapy in combination with radical prostatectomy in clinically localised prostate cancer: results of a phase II study. Br J Urol. 1997;79:432–8.

89. Schulman CC, Debruyne FMJ, Forster G, van Cangh PJ, Witjes WPJ. Neoadjuvant combined androgen deprivation therapy in locally confined prostatic carcinoma. Three years of follow up of a European multicentric randomised study. Br J Urol. 1997;80(Suppl 2):259.

90. Soloway MS, Shairifi R, Wajsman Z, McLeod D, Wood DP, Puras-Baez A. Radical prostatectomy alone vs radical prostatectomy preceded by androgen blockade in cT2b prostate cancer – 24 month results. Br J Urol. 1997;80:(Suppl 2):259.

91. Klotz LH, Goldenberg SL, Bullock M, et al. Neoadjuvant androgen ablation prior to radical prostectomy (CUOG P-92): 24 month post-treatment PSA results. Br J Urol. 1997;80(Suppl 2):266 (Abs 1045).

92. Aus G, Hugosson J, Abrahamsson P-A, et al. Pretreatment with triptorelin before radical prostatectomy – a 3 year follow-up. J Urol. 1997;157:393 (Abs 1540).

93. Gleave M, Goldenberg SL, Jones E, Bruchovsky N, Sullivan L. Biochemical and pathological effects of 8 months of neoadjuvant hormonal therapy – an update on 125 consecutive patients. Br J Urol. 1997;80(Suppl 2):259 (Abs 1016).

94. Aso Y, Homma Y, Sakamoto A, Ohasi Y. A randomized prospective study on radical prostatectomy alone versus radical prostatectomy preceded by androgen deprivation. Eur Urol. 1996;30(Suppl 2):210 (Abs 776).

95. Soloway MS, Shairifi R, Wajsman Z, McLeod D, Wood DP, Puras-Baez A. Randomized prospective study comparing radical prostatectomy alone versus radical prostatectomy preceded by androgen blockade in clinical stage B2 (T2bNxM0) prostate cancer. J Urol. 1995;154:424–8.

96. Klein EA. Hormone therapy for prostate cancer: a topical perspective. Urology. 1996;47(Suppl 1A):3–12.

97. Rabbani F, Sullivan LD, Goldenberg SL, Stothers L. Neoadjuvant androgen deprivation therapy before radical prostatectomy: who is unlikely to benefit? Br J Urol. 1997;79:221–5.

98. Zelefsky MJ, Harrison A. Neoadjuvant androgen ablation prior to radiotherapy for prostate cancer: reducing the potential morbidity of therapy. Urology. 1997;49(Suppl 3A):38–45.

99. Pilepich MV, Krall JM, Al-Sarraf M, et al. Androgen deprivation with radiation therapy compared with radiation therapy alone for locally advanced prostatic carcinoma: a randomized comparative trial of the Radiation Therapy Oncology Group. Urology. 1995;45:616–23.

100. Candas B, Gomes JL, Cusan L, Diamond P, Laverdiere J, Labrie F. Effects of neoadjuvant and adjuvant combined androgen blockade associated to radiation therapy on serum PSA. Br J Urol. 1997;80(Suppl 2):259 (Abs 1017).

101. Zagars GK, Pollack A, von Eschenbach AC. Management of unfavorable locoregional prostate carcinoma with radiation and androgen ablation. Cancer. 1997;80:764–75.

102. Early Breast Cancer Trialists' Collaborative Group: systemic treatment of early breast cancer by hormonal, cytotoxic, or immune therapy. Lancet. 1992;339:1–15.

103. Zincke H, Utz DC, Taylor WF. Bilateral pelvic lymphadenectomy and radical prostatectomy for clinical stage C prostatic cancer: role of adjuvant treatment for residual cancer and in disease progression. J Urol. 1986;135:1199–205.

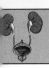

104. D'Amico AV, Whittington R, Malkowicz B, Schulktz D, Tomaszewski JE, Wein A. Prostate-specific antigen failure despite pathologically organ-confined and margin-negative prostate cancer: the basis for an adjuvant therapy trial. J Clin Oncol. 1997;15:1465–69.

105. Andriole G, Lieber M, Smith J, et al. Treatment with finasteride following radical prostatectomy for prostate cancer. Urology. 1995;45:491–7.

106. Cheng WS, Frydenberg M, Bergstralh EJ, Larson-Keller JJ, Zincke H. Radical prostatectomy for pathological stage C prostate cancer: influence of pathological variables and adjuvant treatment on disease outcome. Urology. 1993;42:283–91.

107. Bolla M, Gonzalez D, Warde P, et al. Improved survival in patients with locally advanced prostate cancer treated with radiotherapy and goserelin. N Engl J Med. 1997;337:295–300.

108. Pilepich MV, Caplan R, Byhardt RW, et al. Phase III trial of androgen suppression using goserelin in unfavorable prognosis of carcinoma of the prostate treated with definitive radiotherapy (report of RTOG Protocol 85–31). Proc Am Soc Clin Oncol. 1995;14:239–45.

109. Pollack A, Zagars GK, Kopplin RN. Radiotherapy and androgen ablation for clinically localized high-risk prostate cancer. Int J Radiat Oncol Biol Phys. 1995;32:13–20.

110. Catalona WJ, Smith DS, Ratliff TL, Basler JW. Detection of organ-confined prostate cancer is increased through prostate-specific antigen-based screening. JAMA. 1993;270:948–54.

111. Mandelson MT, Wagner EH, Thompson RS. PSA screening: a public health dilemma. Annu Rev Public Health. 1995;16:283–306.

112. von Eschenbach A, Ho R, Murphy GP, Cunningham M, Lins N. American Cancer Society guidelines for the early detection of prostate cancer. Update, June 10, 1997. Cancer. 1997;80:1805–7.

113. Stephenson RA, Stanford JL. Population-based prostate cancer trends in the United States: patterns of change in the era of prostate-specific antigen. World J Urol. 1997;15:331–5.

114. Middleton RG, Thompson IM, Austenfeld IM. Prostate cancer clinical guidelines panel summary report on the management of clinically localized prostate cancer. J Urol. 1995;154:2144–8.

115. Fleming C, Wasson JH, Albertsen PC, Barry MJ, Wennberg JE, for the Prostate Patient Outcomes Research Team. A decision analysis of alternative treatment strategies for clinically localized prostate cancer. JAMA. 1993;269:2650–8.

116. Beck JR, Kattan MW, Miles BJ. A critique of the decision analysis for clinically localized prostate cancer. J Urol. 1994;152:1894–9.

117. Sperduto P, Rose M, Jolitz G, Koering S. The cost-effectiveness of alternative treatment in prostate cancer. J Radiat Oncol Biol Phys. 1994;30:220–4.

118. National Inpatient Profile, October 1992–September 1993. HCIA; 1994:1–16.

119. Gelet A, Chapelon JY, Bouvier R, et al. Treatment of prostate cancer with transrectal focused ultrasound: first clinical experience. Br J Urol. 1997;80(Suppl 2):265 (Abs 1041).

120. Schulman CC, Zlotta AR, Wildschutz T, et al. A new modality of treatment of localized prostate cancer: initial experience with radiofrequency interstitial tumor ablation (RITA) through a transperineal ultrasound-guided approach. Br J Urol. 1997;80(Suppl 2):267 (Abs 1049).

121. Weldon VE. Radical perineal prostatectomy. In: Das S, Crawford ED (eds). Cancer of the Prostate. New York: Marcel Dekker;1993, pp225–226.

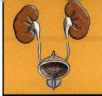

Chapter 28

Locally Advanced and Late Prostate Cancer

John W Colberg

KEY POINTS

- With the advent of prostate-specific antigen (PSA)-based screening, fewer men present with locally-advanced or late prostate cancer.
- The use of PSA in combination with clinical stage based on digital rectal examination and Gleason score improves the ability to predict pathological stage.
- Imaging for locally-advanced prostate cancer is imprecise in determining the extent of extracapsular disease.
- Radiotherapy has been the mainstay of treatment for locally-advanced prostate cancer. Neoadjuvant androgen deprivation may improve survival.
- Androgen deprivation therapy, either surgical or medical, has been the gold standard for treatment of late prostate cancer.
- Maximum androgen blockade does not appear to show significant benefit for men with late prostate cancer.
- The management of hormone refractory prostate cancer continues to be a major dilemma with the majority of men dying within 12 months.

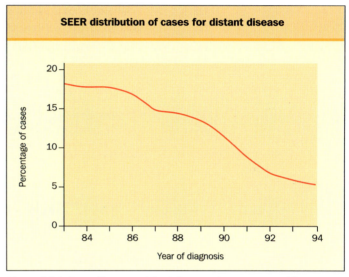

Figure 28.1 Surveillance, epidemiology, and end results (SEER) distribution of cases for distant disease. Annual distribution of cases for distant disease. (From Stephenson RA. Population-based prostate cancer trends in the PSA era: data from the surveillance, epidemiology, and end results (SEER) program. Monographs in Urology. 1998 1998; 19:14.)

INTRODUCTION

By definition, locally advanced and late prostate cancer is considered incurable by most patients and physicians. Historically, the majority of prostate cancers at the time of diagnosis were either locally advanced or metastatic. However, with the advent of prostate-specific antigen (PSA)-based screening and increased public awareness of prostate cancer, there has been a progressive downward migration in stage at time of diagnosis (Fig. 28.1). This has translated into fewer men presenting with advanced prostate cancer. However, worldwide, considerable numbers of men still present or eventually develop locally advanced and late disease.

The term 'locally advanced prostate cancer' implies that there is extracapsular spread of prostate cancer but no evidence of metastasis to regional lymph nodes or distant sites. Late prostate cancer has traditionally been defined by the presence of bony and/or soft tissue metastases. This chapter will review the current concepts in the diagnosis and management of locally advanced and late prostate cancer.

STAGING SYSTEMS

Two staging systems, an ABCD (Whitmore–Jewett) system and a tumor, nodes, and metastasis (TNM) system are currently used for prostate cancer (Fig. 28.2). There is considerable overlap between the two systems. Locally advanced prostate cancers are considered clinical stage C or T3N0M0. Late prostate cancers are considered clinical stage D or T3N+M+.

INVESTIGATION AND DIAGNOSIS

Digital rectal examination, prostate-specific antigen, and Gleason score

The digital rectal examination (DRE) is the most useful means of diagnosing clinical stage T3 or higher disease (Fig. 28.3). Typically the DRE is remarkable for an irregular, stony, hard, or markedly indurated or nodular area with distortion of the normal prostate outline, loss of the median sulcus, lateral extension of the disease process, extension into the seminal vesicles, and in higher stages fixation to adjacent structures.

PSA correlates with clinical and more closely with pathological stage[1]. However, there is considerable overlap within any

Staging systems for prostate cancer		
Whitmore–Jewett	TNM 1992	Description
Incidental finding; no tumor palpable		
A1	T1a	Tumor found by chance in <5% of excised tissue
A2	T1b	Tumor found by chance in >5% of excised tissue
	T1c	Tumor confirmed by needle biopsy (raised PSA)
	Tx	Local tumor cannot be evaluated
	To	No local tumor detectable
Intracapsular palpable tumor		
B1	T2a	Tumor limited to half of one lobe or less
B2	T2b	Tumor has spread to half of one lobe but not to both
B3	T2c	Tumor has spread into both lobes
Extracapsular tumor		
C1	T3a	Unilateral extracapsular spread
C2	T3b	Bilateral extracapsular spread
	T3c	Tumor has spread one or both seminal vesicles
	T4	Tumor is attached to or has invaded adjacent structures other than the seminal vesicles
Disseminated tumor		
D1	Nx	Loco-regional lymph nodes cannot be evaluated
	N0	No lymph node involvement
	N1	Lymph node ≤ 2cm in diameter
	N2	One node only >2cm or ≤ 5cm; multiple ≤ 5cm
D2	Mx	Distant metastases can not be evaluated
	M0	No distant metastases
	M1	Distant metastases present a=lymph nodes other than regional nodes b=skeletal c=other sites
D3 resistant to hormonal therapy		

Figure 28.2 Staging systems for prostate cancer. Comparison of Whitmore–Jewett and tumor, nodes, and metastasis (TNM) staging systems. (Reproduced with permission from Kirby RS, Christmas TJ, Brawer MK. Prostate cancer. London: Mosby; 1996.)

Local staging of prostate cancer	
T3	T4

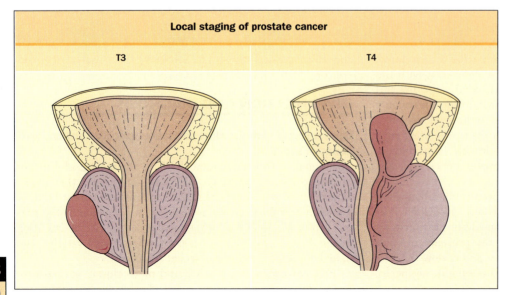

Figure 28.3 Local staging of prostate cancer. T3 and T4 disease.

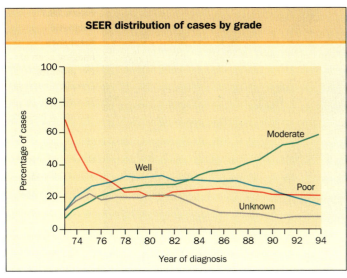

Figure 28.4 Surveillance epidemiology, and end results (SEER) distribution of cases by grade. (From Stephenson RA. Population-based prostate cancer trends in the PSA era: data from the surveillance, epidemiology, and end results (SEER) program. Monographs in Urology. 1998 1998; 19:8.)

one stage, making PSA a poor predictor of pathologic stage for an individual patient. PSA is directly related to the volume of cancer present[2]. Other variables, including benign prostatic hyperplasia (BPH) and infection, can affect the overall PSA level. In general, if the PSA level is less than 10ng/mL lymph node or bony metastasis is rare. If the PSA level is greater than 50ng/ml two thirds of patients have microscopic lymph node metastasis and 90% have extracapsular disease. Recently, measurement of the percentage of free PSA has been shown to improve the ability to predict postoperative pathological stage[3].

A high Gleason score (8–10) is predictive of locally advanced disease but the majority of currently diagnosed cases of prostate cancer are moderately differentiated Gleason score (5–7; Fig. 28.4)[4].

The use of PSA in combination with clinical stage based on DRE and Gleason score has been shown to improve the ability to predict pathological stage[5]. Nomograms have been devised to predict pathological stage (Fig. 28.5). This is now commonly being used to help predict the presence of extracapsular disease, lymph node involvement, or seminal vesicle involvement.

Nomogram for prediction of final pathological stage

Gleason Score	PSA 0.0–4.0ng/mL Clinical stage							PSA 4.1–10.0ng/mL Clinical stage							PSA 10.1–20.0ng/mL Clinical stage							PSA > 20.0ng/mL Clinical stage						
	T1a	T1b	T1c	T2a	T2b	T2c	T3a	T1a	T1b	T1c	T2a	T2b	T2c	T3a	T1a	T1b	T1c	T2a	T2b	T2c	T3a	T1a	T1b	T1c	T2a	T2b	T2c	T3a
Organ-confined disease																												
2–4	90	80	89	81	72	77	...	84	70	83	71	61	66	43	76	58	75	60	48	53	...	...	38	58	41	29	...	...
5	82	66	81	68	57	62	40	72	53	71	55	43	49	27	61	40	60	43	32	36	18	...	23	40	26	17	19	8
6	78	61	78	64	52	57	35	67	47	67	51	38	43	23	...	33	55	38	26	31	14	...	17	35	22	13	15	6
7	...	43	63	47	34	38	19	49	29	49	33	22	25	11	33	17	35	22	13	15	6	...	...	18	10	5	6	2
8–10	...	31	52	36	24	27	...	35	18	37	23	14	15	6	...	9	23	14	7	8	3	...	3	10	5	3	3	1
Established capsular penetration																												
2–4	9	19	10	18	25	21	...	14	27	15	26	35	29	44	20	36	22	35	43	37	...	...	47	34	48	52	...	...
5	17	32	18	30	40	34	51	25	42	27	41	50	43	57	33	50	35	50	57	51	59	...	57	48	60	61	55	54
6	19	35	21	34	43	37	53	27	44	30	44	52	46	57	...	49	38	52	57	50	54	...	51	49	60	57	51	40
7	...	44	31	45	51	45	52	36	48	40	52	54	48	48	38	46	45	55	51	45	40	...	...	46	51	43	37	2
8–10	...	43	34	47	48	42	...	34	42	40	49	46	40	34	...	33	40	46	38	33	26	...	24	34	37	28	23	17
Seminal vesicle involvement																												
2–4	0	1	1	1	2	2	...	1	2	1	2	4	5	10	2	4	2	4	7	8	...	...	9	7	10	14	...	...
5	1	2	1	2	3	3	7	2	3	2	3	5	6	12	3	5	3	5	8	9	15	...	10	9	11	15	19	26
6	1	2	1	2	3	4	7	2	3	2	3	5	6	11	...	4	4	5	7	9	14	...	8	8	10	13	17	21
7	...	6	4	6	10	12	19	6	9	8	10	15	18	26	8	11	12	14	18	22	28	...	...	22	24	27	32	36
8–10	...	11	9	12	17	21	...	10	15	15	19	24	28	35	...	15	20	22	25	30	34	...	20	31	33	33	38	40
Lymph node involvement																												
2–4	0	0	0	0	0	0	...	0	1	0	0	1	1	1	0	2	0	1	1	1	...	...	4	1	1	3	...	...
5	0	1	0	0	1	1	2	1	2	0	1	2	2	3	3	5	1	2	4	4	7	...	10	3	3	7	7	11
6	1	2	0	1	2	2	5	3	5	1	2	4	4	9	...	13	3	4	10	10	18	...	23	7	8	16	17	26
7	...	6	1	2	5	5	9	8	12	3	4	9	9	15	18	24	8	9	17	18	26	...	...	14	14	25	25	32
8–10	...	14	4	5	10	10	...	18	23	8	9	16	17	24	...	40	16	17	29	29	37	...	51	24	24	36	35	42

Figure 28.5 Nomogram for prediction of final pathological stage. The use of PSA, clinical stage, and Gleason score to predict pathological stage. Numbers represent the percentage predictive probability (95% confidence interval) of the patient having a given final pathological stage based on a multinomial log-linear regression of all three variables combined. (Reproduced from Partin AW, Kazan MW, Subong EN, et al. Combination of prostate-specific antigen, clinical stage and Gleason score to predict pathological stage of localized prostate cancer: a multi-institutional update. JAMA. 1997;227: 1445–51 © American Medical Association.)

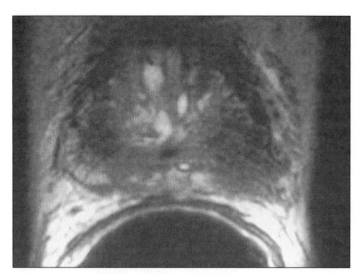

Figure 28.6 Magnetic resonance imaging scan of the prostate.
T2-weighted endorectal magnetic resonance imaging of the prostate showing cancer infiltrating the right neurovascular bundle.

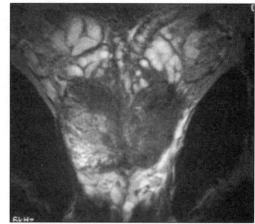

Figure 28.7 Magnetic resonance imaging scan of the prostate. Coronal, T2-weighted endorectal magnetic resonance imaging of the prostate showing cancer invading the right seminal vesicle.

Imaging for locally advanced and late prostate cancer

For locally advanced prostate cancer the use of radiographic methods has proved to be imprecise in determining the extent of extracapsular disease. It often adds little additional information over DRE alone. However, the presentation of clinical stage T3 disease has changed. Cases of bulky, palpable T3 disease are uncommon. A larger number of men with microscopic penetration or positive surgical margins of the prostate capsule (pT3) are now being detected after surgery. Transrectal ultrasound (TRUS), computed tomography (CT) scans, and magnetic resonance imaging (MRI) scans in their current state have all been disappointing in detecting minimal involvement of the prostatic capsule preoperatively. MRI scanning using an endorectal coil has shown the most promise in visualizing prostate cancer involving the neurovascular bundles, seminal vesicles, or prostatic capsule (Figs 28.6 & 28.7)[6–8].

For the evaluation of lymph node and bony metastasis, radiographic studies may be warranted in men at higher risk of metastases [elevated PSA levels (>20ng/mL), the presence of locally advanced disease on DRE (cT3), or a poorly differentiated tumor

on prostate biopsy (Gleason 8–10)]. Several modalities are available to investigate nodal involvement and bony metastasis:
- computed tomography of the pelvis;
- magnetic resonance imaging of the pelvis;
- radionuclide bone scan;
- bone radiographs; and
- immunoscintigraphy with indium-111 capromab pendetide.

Computed tomography
Computed tomography scanning can detect relatively large-volume lymph node metastasis in men with large primary tumors (Fig. 28.8). However, CT scanning can often fail to detect minimal or microscopic disease. It is only 40–50% accurate in identifying metastatic involvement of pelvic lymph nodes[9]. However if enlarged, suspicious lymph nodes are detected, needle biopsy or aspiration can easily be performed with CT scanning guidance.

Magnetic resonance imaging
As with CT scanning, MRI relies upon size criteria in the detection of enlarged pelvic lymph nodes (Fig. 28.9). At present there is no evidence that MRI is superior to CT scanning in the detection of pelvic lymph node metastases.

Radionuclide bone scan
The radionuclide bone scan is the most sensitive imaging technique to detect skeletal metastases (Fig. 28.10). The isotope

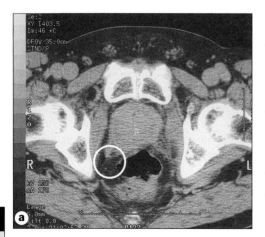

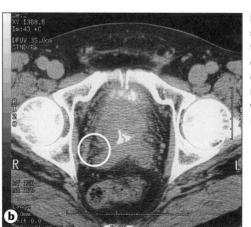

Figure 28.8 Computed tomography scan of the pelvis. (a) Computed tomography scan of the pelvis demonstrating local extension of prostate cancer (circled). (b) Lymph node metastases from prostate cancer (circled) visualized on computed tomography scan (right pelvic region).

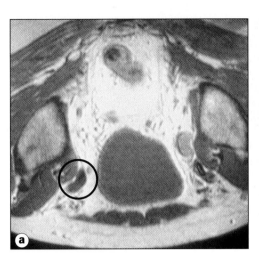

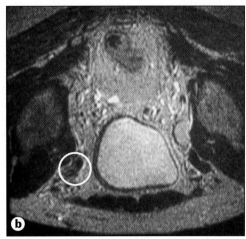

Figure 28.9 Magnetic resonance imaging scan of the pelvis. (a) T1 weighted magnetic resonance imaging scan revealing enlarged right pelvic lymph node from prostate cancer (circled). (b) T2-weighted magnetic resonance imaging scan of same region.

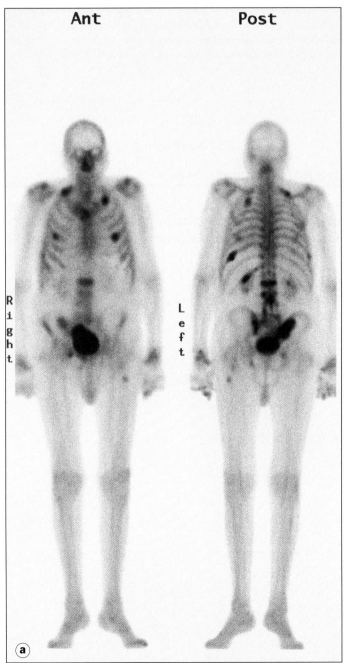

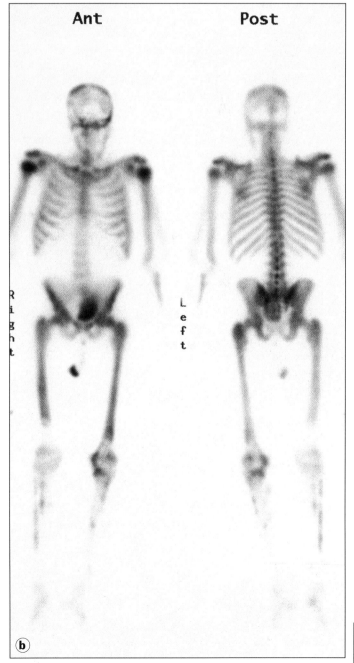

Figure 28.10 Radionuclide bone scan. (a) Widely metastatic bone scan in a patient with prostate cancer: ribs, cervical spine, and pelvis.

(b) Diffuse uptake throughout skeleton – superscan. Notice absence of renal imaging.

used most commonly today is technetium. A number of other bone lesions, including Paget's disease, trauma (healing bone fractures), arthritis, degenerative joint disease, osteomyelitis, metabolic bone disease, and other malignant or benign bone lesions, may result in a positive radionuclide scan. Confirmation on routine or tomographic radiographs, CT scan or MRI studies, or bone biopsy is occasionally necessary.

Prostate-specific antigen testing has resulted in the elimination of routine radionuclide bone scanning in all but a select group of patients[10]. Patients who are asymptomatic (no bone pain) with PSA levels of less than 10ng/mL do not routinely require radionuclide bone scans. However, a negative bone scan can provide a valuable baseline study to compare after treatment in men who later develop bone pain. Whether the cost of performing bone scans in men with lower PSA levels is justified remains controversial.

Bone radiographs
The majority of patients with prostate cancer in whom bone films demonstrate metastatic involvement have osteoblastic lesions (Fig. 28.11). Mixed osteoblastic–osteolytic and osteolytic lesions occur less commonly. The role of bone radiographs is presently limited to further investigating areas of the body that reveal equivocal areas on radionuclide bone scanning.

Indium-111 capromab pendetide
Indium-111 capromab pendetide has recently been approved as diagnostic imaging agent in patients with prostate cancer who are at a high risk of pelvic lymph node metastases (Figs 28.12 & 28.13). This radiolabeled monoclonal antibody targets a

membrane-associated antigen of prostate cells that is more highly expressed in malignant cells. Preliminary data suggests that immunoscintigraphy may be useful in identifying possible sites of disease before therapy and in patients with biochemical evidence of recurrent or residual disease postoperatively[11-12]. Imaging techniques and interpretation of the images are challenging and require specific training and experience.

Laparoscopic pelvic lymphadenectomy
The ability of noninvasive imaging techniques to detect involvement of pelvic lymph nodes is poor. In the past, pelvic lymph node staging has been accomplished with an open operation as a separate procedure before radiotherapy or radical perineal prostatectomy or as part of radical retropubic prostatectomy. Laparoscopic pelvic lymph node dissection offers a minimally invasive, less morbid option for the evaluation of a patient's node status. However, this procedure should be reserved for patients who might benefit from curative therapy but who have larger-volume, higher-stage tumors and negative noninvasive pelvic imaging. Recent clinical selection criteria for laparoscopic pelvic lymph node dissection include[13]:

PSA ≥50ng/mL
or
PSA ≥ 20ng/mL and Gleason score ≥ 7
or
PSA ≥ 10ng/mL and Gleason score ≥ 8.

THERAPEUTIC OPTIONS

The treatment of locally advanced and late prostate cancer is controversial. The results of definitive treatment for clinical stage T3 disease are poor. The currently available treatment options for locally advanced and late prostate cancer are discussed below.

Surgery
Radical prostatectomy for clinical stage T3 disease is generally considered unjustified. Up to 50% of patients have lymph node

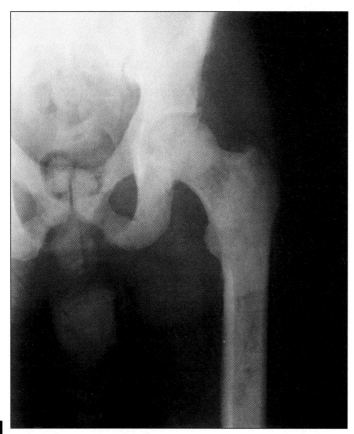

Figure 28.11 Bone radiograph. Osteoblastic skeletal metastases from prostate cancer involving left proximal femur and pelvis.

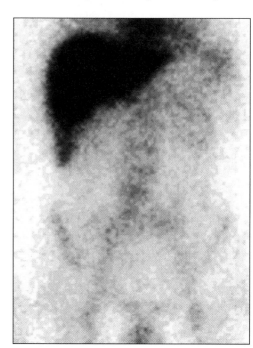

Figure 28.12 Indium-111 capromab pendetide scan. Normal planar single photon emission computed tomography image of indium-111 capromab pendetide scan in a patient with prostate cancer.

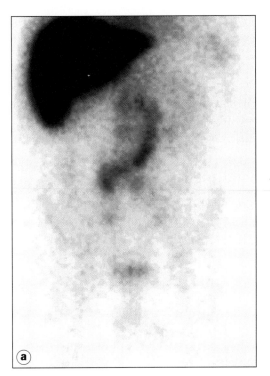

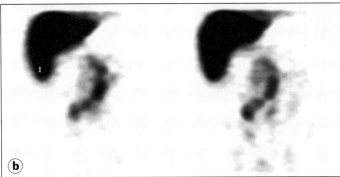

Figure 28.13 Indium-111 capromab pendetide scan. (a) Planar single photon emission computed tomography image of indium-111 capromab pendetide scan demonstrating extensive uptake in lymph nodes in para-aortic region. (b) Coronal single photon emission computed tomography images of same patient.

metastases[14]. Only 30% of patients will have an undetectable PSA level at 5 years[15]. Patients with clinical stage T3 disease will die of disseminated disease despite local control[16–17].

In an attempt to improve survival rates in clinical stage T3 prostate cancer, the use of neoadjuvant androgen deprivation therapy has been proposed. The use of hormonal therapy before radical prostatectomy was described over 50 years ago. However, this approach did not gain acceptance until the development of reversible, better tolerated forms of androgen deprivation therapy became available. In patients with clinical stage T3 disease, the use of preoperative 'hormonal downstaging' with androgen deprivation has resulted in an overall rate of organ-confined disease of 28%, which is similar to the 24% for control groups[18–30]. The overall positive margin rate of 43% with androgen deprivation therapy was lower than the 52% for surgery alone. However, many of the studies were not randomized and different androgen

deprivation therapy regimens were used, making comparisons difficult. More importantly, few studies have reported biochemical relapse rates. The longest followup reported a 24% actuarial PSA relapse-rate survival at 3 years[27]. Neoadjuvant androgen deprivation does not seem to alter long-term recurrence rate in men with clinical stage T3 disease.

Radiotherapy

External beam radiation therapy has been the mainstay of treatment for clinical stage T3 disease. The 10-year survival rate using standard doses is approximately 15–30%[31–32]. Failure of radiotherapy to effectively treat locally advanced prostate cancer may be related to the sheer bulk or volume of tumor present and the high probability of pre-existing nodal disease.

Modifications of radiotherapy to improve local control and survival for clinical stage T3 disease have been undertaken. These strategies include dose escalation without conformal field tailoring, dose escalation with conformal field tailoring, and androgen deprivation before radiotherapy.

One can increase the dose the tumor receives by conforming the beam shape by the integration of three-dimensional planning (conformal external beam radiation therapy). It is possible to deliver higher doses of radiation therapy to the prostate tumor without additional toxicity to the normal surrounding tissues. Doses above 7,000cGy have been given with results suggesting an improvement in local control[33–34].

Neoadjuvant androgen deprivation before radiotherapy has also been studied in an attempt to improve local control and survival in clinical stage T3 disease. Neoadjuvant androgen deprivation reduces the prostate volume and optimizes the geometry of the prostate volume in relation to the surrounding normal structures. Two randomized trials have compared neoadjuvant androgen deprivation before radiotherapy with radiotherapy alone[35–36]. Local control and disease-free survival rates at 5 years were superior in the neoadjuvant androgen deprivation group. More recently, results of the European Organization for Research and Treatment of Cancer (EORTC) trial examined the use of radiation and an luteinizing hormone-releasing hormone (LHRH) agonist (goserelin) starting on the first day of radiation and continuing for 3 years versus radiation therapy alone[37]. The 5-year actuarial rates with and without androgen deprivation therapy were 79% versus 63% for overall survival, 85% versus 48% for disease-free survival, and 97% versus 77% for local control.

The lack of an androgen deprivation therapy arm, relatively short followup, imprecise definitions of assessing local control, and PSA failures make interpretation of these studies difficult. Nonetheless, neoadjuvant androgen deprivation plus radiotherapy may be the preferential way to administer radiation therapy in locally advanced prostate cancer.

Androgen deprivation therapy

In patients suffering from late prostate cancer, androgen deprivation in the form of surgical castration has been the gold standard since Huggins and Hodges demonstrated the cancer's androgen dependence[38]. A favorable clinical response rate of 70–80% is expected after treatment. However, the time to clinical progression and death in patients with metastases is between 18 and 36 months.

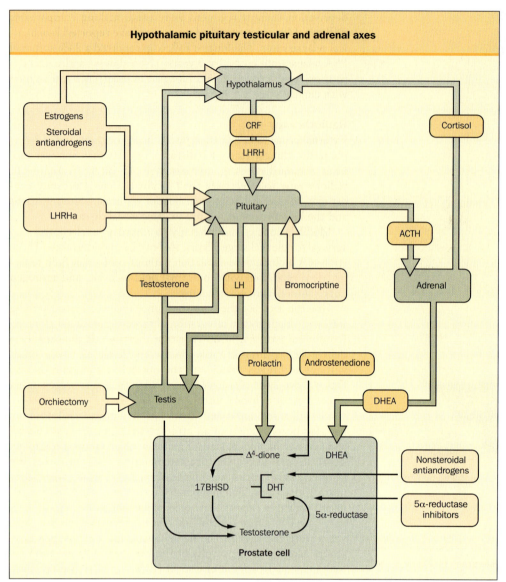

Figure 28.14 Hypothalamic pituitary testicular and adrenal axes. Regulation of testicular testosterone production and adrenal androgen secretion. ACTH, adrenocorticotrophic hormone; CRF, corticotrophin-releasing hormone; DHEA, dehydroepiandrosterone; DHT, dihydrotestosterone; LHRH, luteinizing hormone-releasing hormone. (Reproduced from Crawford ED. Changing paradigms in the treatment of prostate cancer. Adv Oncol. 1996;12:14–21 © Cliggott Communications.)

The major source of androgens in males is the Leydig cells located in the testes. These account for 90% of circulating testosterone. The remaining testosterone is derived from adrenal androgens, which may be metabolized to testosterone and 5α-dihydrotestosterone. The production of testosterone is governed by the hypothalamic–pituitary–testicular–adrenal axis (Fig. 28.14). There are several possible ways in which androgen deprivation therapy can be achieved (Fig. 28.15):

- Surgical castration (bilateral orchiectomy)
- Medical castration: estrogens, LHRH agonists
- Androgen blockade at target cells: pure antiandrogens, steroidal antiandrogens
- Maximal androgen blockade
- 5α-reductase inhibitor

Luteinizing hormone-releasing hormone agonist

Luteinizing hormone-releasing hormone agonist causes an initial stimulation of luteinizing hormone (LH) and follicle stimulating hormone (FSH) production with a rise in serum testosterone. Within 2 weeks, however, they cause an inhibition of LH and FSH release, resulting in castrate levels of testosterone. During the first 2–3 weeks of administration a biochemical flare that can accompany the initial rise in plasma testosterone may occur. This may manifest itself by a worsening of clinical symptoms such as bone pain or obstructive voiding symptoms. An antiandrogen should be given before or at the time of initiation of LHRH agonist treatment. Other side-effects are similar to those of surgical castration including loss of libido, erectile dysfunction, 'hot flashes', and loss of body hair.

Antiandrogens

Antiandrogens may be either steroidal or nonsteroidal. Steroidal antiandrogens, because of their progesteronal properties, act by suppressing gonadotrophins, thereby lowering plasma testosterone. Nonsteroidal antiandrogens do not have any antigonadotrophic effects. Antiandrogens interfere with androgen action by competitively binding to the androgen receptor.

5α-reductase inhibitors

5α-reductase inhibitors are a steroid competitor of 5α reductase, which is the enzyme that converts testosterone to dihydrotestosterone (DHT) within the prostate. The drug alone

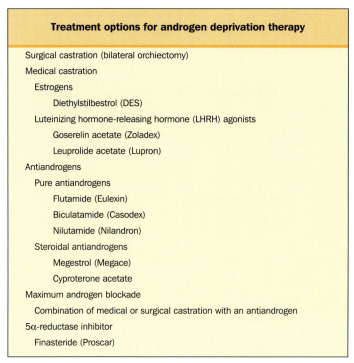

Treatment options for androgen deprivation therapy

Surgical castration (bilateral orchiectomy)

Medical castration

  Estrogens

    Diethylstilbestrol (DES)

  Luteinizing hormone-releasing hormone (LHRH) agonists

    Goserelin acetate (Zoladex)

    Leuprolide acetate (Lupron)

Antiandrogens

  Pure antiandrogens

    Flutamide (Eulexin)

    Biculatamide (Casodex)

    Nilutamide (Nilandron)

  Steroidal antiandrogens

    Megestrol (Megace)

    Cyproterone acetate

Maximum androgen blockade

  Combination of medical or surgical castration with an antiandrogen

5α-reductase inhibitor

  Finasteride (Proscar)

Figure 28.15 Treatment options for androgen deprivation therapy.

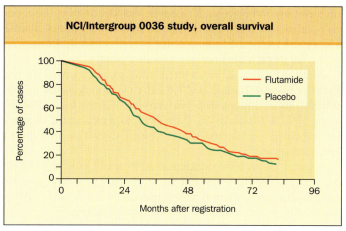

Figure 28.16 National Cancer Institute (NCI)/Intergroup 0036 study, overall survival[43]. Luteinizing hormone-releasing hormone agonist (leuprolide) and placebo versus luteinizing hormone-releasing hormone agonist and anti-androgen (flutamide).

has minimal activity in late prostate cancer, but may work in combination with antiandrogens. The potential advantage of the use of 5α-reductase inhibitors is the preservation of libido and potency.

Although androgen therapy is standard treatment for many locally advanced and all late prostate cancer patients, there is intense debate regarding the optimal regimen and timing of androgen deprivation therapy. These issues include the use of maximum androgen blockade (MAB); early versus delayed androgen deprivation therapy, and intermittent androgen suppression (IAS).

Maximum androgen blockade

Maximum androgen blockade is the simultaneous suppression of both testicular and adrenal androgens as initial treatment for prostate cancer. The role of adrenal androgens in the progression of prostate cancer was recognized in the 1940s[39]. Bilateral adrenalectomy was performed in attempts to treat patients who had progressed after orchiectomy. However, because of the morbidity associated with this procedure, orchiectomy alone remained the treatment of choice until the development of androgen receptor blockers (antiandrogens).

Adrenal androgens are converted to DHT in the prostate gland by the action of 5α-reductase. DHT is four to five times more active than testosterone as a mitogen for prostate cell growth[40]. Studies have confirmed increased levels of DHT in prostate tissue in 20% of patients castrated for prostate cancer[41]. Thus, the addition of an antiandrogen with an LHRH agonist or following orchiectomy may block the stimulating effect of DHT and improve survival. Further evidence was furnished by results of a phase II clinical trial[42]. A marked improvement in response and survival rate was noted when an antiandrogen (flutamide) was combined with medical or surgical castration. However, this

nonrandomized study did not enroll a large population and employed weak criteria by which response to therapy was defined.

A large number of randomized, controlled trials demonstrate mixed results with MAB. Comparing and analyzing these trials is difficult because of the different types of castration used (surgical versus medical), type of antiandrogen administered (steroidal versus nonsteroidal), randomization procedures, assessment of treatment outcomes, and study design.

Support for MAB is based on several randomized trials. The National Cancer Institute (NCI) Intergroup 0036 study randomized patients with untreated stage D2 prostate cancer to treatment with LHRH agonist (leuprolide) in combination with either placebo or an antiandrogen (flutamide)[43]. The MAB arm demonstrated a longer progression-free survival (16.5 versus 13.9 months) and an increase in median survival (35.6 versus 28.3 months) (Fig. 28.16). Subset analysis of patients with minimal disease demonstrated a longer median survival in the MAB arm (51.9 months versus 39.6 months). Similarly, the EORTC 30853 trial comparing an LHRH agonist (goserelin) and an antiandrogen (flutamide) with orchiectomy alone has shown an increase in duration of survival (34.4 weeks versus 27.1 weeks) with MAB[44]. An international study comparing orchiectomy in combination with either placebo or an antiandrogen (nilutamide) demonstrated an increased time to progression (20.9 months versus 14.9 months) and an increase in median survival (37 months versus 30 months) in the MAB arm[45].

Other well-designed studies have failed to show a benefit for MAB. The National Cancer Institute (NCI) Intergroup Study 0105 compared overall and progression-free survival in patients with previously untreated stage D2 prostate cancer treated with bilateral orchiectomy and an antiandrogen (flutamide) versus orchiectomy and placebo[46]. The study was designed to eliminate issues of adverse outcome caused by disease flare, which may have confounded the NCI Intergroup Study 0036. Preliminary analysis failed to identify a benefit in overall survival of progression-free (31 months versus 30 months) or progression-free survival (52 months versus 51 months) with MAB compared to orchiectomy and placebo. No benefit was identified in the good-risk patients with good performance status and minimal disease (52 months versus 51 months for overall survival; 49 months versus 36 months for progression-free survival).

Meta-analysis of 22 randomized trials evaluating MAB by the Prostate Cancer Trialists' Collaborative Group revealed no significant improvement in 5-year survival (22.8% for castration versus 26.2% for MAB)[47]. There was no significant difference among subgroups according to type of castration or type of antiandrogen used.

Overall, the available studies addressing the issue of MAB do not show a significant benefit for men with stage D2 prostate cancer. Currently, there is no compelling evidence that MAB is superior to conventional medical or surgical castration.

Early versus delayed androgen deprivation therapy in N+(D1) disease

The question of whether early or delayed androgen deprivation may improve overall survival remains controversial. Traditionally, patients with late prostate cancer have had deferred treatment with androgen deprivation therapy, often waiting until symptoms appeared before treatment. This deferred approach was based on the findings from Study I of the Veterans Administration Cooperative Urological Research Group (VACURG)[48]. This study reported that delayed androgen deprivation therapy was as effective as early therapy. However, re-analysis identified men with stage D2 disease and younger men with high-grade disease as having a survival advantage with early therapy[49].

The Medical Research Council Prostate Cancer Working Group Investigators Group randomized patients into either immediate treatment (orchiectomy or LHRH agonist) or to the same treatment deferred until an indication occurred[50]. In the deferred treatment group, pathological fracture, spinal cord compression, ureteral obstruction, and the development of extraskeletal metastases were twice as common. Progression from M0 to M1 disease and the development of pain caused by metastases occurred more rapidly in the deferred group. While overall survival rates were not significantly different in M1 or MX disease, the differences were significant in M0 disease. Younger patients receiving deferred treatment were less likely to die of other causes.

The EORTC protocol 30846 compared immediate with delayed androgen deprivation in patients with N+ disease without distant metastases. An interim analysis revealed a significant difference in time to progression, favoring early therapy[51].

A recent study comparing observation after radical prostatectomy in men with node-positive prostate cancer with immediate androgen deprivation improved survival and reduced the risk of recurrence (Fig. 28.17)[52]. After a median of 7.1 years follow-up, 77% of men in the immediate-treatment group versus 18% for the observation group were alive without evidence of recurrent disease, including an undetectable PSA level. Previous retrospective studies have also confirmed these findings.

Early androgen deprivation may offer a survival advantage over delayed treatment, particularly when the tumor burden is minimal. However, the prevention of catastrophic complications of late prostate cancer may be an added benefit of early androgen deprivation.

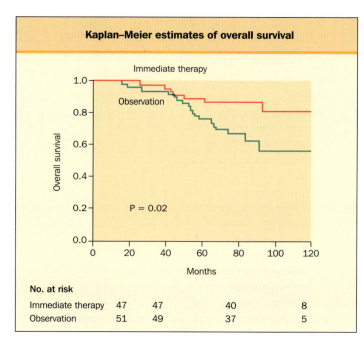

Kaplan–Meier estimates of overall survival

No. at risk				
Immediate therapy	47	47	40	8
Observation	51	49	37	5

Figure 28.17 Kaplan–Meier estimates of overall survival. Immediate hormonal therapy compared with observation after radical prostatectomy in men with node-positive prostate cancer[52].

Intermittent androgen suppression

The concept of intermittent androgen suppression (IAS) involves the initiation of androgen deprivation and then halting therapy upon a predefined clinical response (serum PSA level). The concept of IAS was devised in an attempt to delay the progression to the androgen-independent state. Studies have demonstrated that consecutive cycles of androgen withdrawal and replacement result in the maintenance of apoptotic potential in both animal models and human prostate cancer cell lines[53–54]. IAS seems to delay progression to an androgen-independent state but does not prevent it.

Typically, patients are treated for a minimum of 6 months with MAB until a PSA nadir is achieved. If the PSA level remains above 4.0ng/mL it has been found that the median survival time is much worse as compared to patients with a PSA level of below 4.0ng/mL (18 months versus 40 months). Only those patients whose serum PSA levels have reached a stable or decreasing value of below 4.0ng/mL should be considered as candidates for IAS. Therapy is withdrawn until the serum PSA level reaches pretreatment levels (if pretreatment PSA <20ng/mL) or 20ng/mL (if pretreatment PSA level >20ng/mL), at which time therapy is reinstituted. This cycle is continuous until progression to androgen independence is detected. Results reveal that patients were off therapy for a mean of 41% and 45% of the time over the first two cycles[55]. Mean and median times to progression were 128 weeks and 108 weeks. Mean overall survival was 52 months.

It appears that IAS results in improved quality of life when the patient is off therapy, reduces toxicity and cost of treatment, and possibly delays tumor progression. However, this approach remains experimental until benefits of survival are confirmed in a prospective, randomized trial.

HORMONE REFRACTORY PROSTATE CANCER

The management of hormone refractory prostate cancer (HRPC) continues to be a major dilemma, with the majority of patients dying within 12 months. Their clinical course is characterized by progressive debilitation, pain, and other complications of late prostate cancer. There is no consensus about the best systemic treatment for HRPC. The treatment is palliative and all patients can expect to die of their disease.

With the widespread use of serum PSA testing the definition of HRPC has changed. HRPC can be defined as a consecutive series of increasing PSA levels following the PSA nadir experienced by androgen deprivation therapy.

A variety of regimens have been examined in clinical trials for the treatment of HRPC (Fig. 28.18)[56]. These include:

- antiandrogen therapy;
- antiandrogen withdrawal;
- second antiandrogens;
- adrenal androgen inhibitors;
- estrogens and antiestrogens;
- chemotherapy agents;
- growth factors;
- angiogenesis inhibition; and
- gene therapy.

Antiandrogen therapy/antiandrogen withdrawal/second antiandrogens

For patients managed initially by orchiectomy or LHRH analogs alone, the addition of an antiandrogen to eliminate the adrenal androgens after evidence of PSA failure has been recommended. However, this usually has few beneficial long-term effects.

Regardless of whether the therapy initially used was maximum androgen blockade or whether antiandrogens were subsequently added, the withdrawal of the antiandrogen is the first line of treatment after failure of androgen deprivation therapy. This antiandrogen withdrawal phenomenon was first reported in 1993[57]. Both clinical and serum PSA response were seen in 21% of patients after discontinuation of the antiandrogen (flutamide). The median response duration of response was 5 months. Later reports have confirmed this response with other antiandrogens (biculatamide)[58].

Second-line antiandrogens have been used in patients who have previously received and subsequently failed therapy with other antiandrogens. In pilot studies the use of the antiandrogen biculatamide has been shown to decrease serum PSA levels in 25% of patients for 2 months or longer[59]. Responses seem to be limited to patients who have been treated with long-term flutamide as opposed to patients treated with androgen deprivation without flutamide (response rate 43% versus 6%).

Adrenal androgen inhibitors

A variety of therapeutic agents can suppress adrenal secretion of androgens. The most commonly used are aminoglutethamide, ketoconazole, and corticosteroids.

Aminoglutetamide blocks the conversion of cholesterol into pregnenolone. It inhibits the production of testicular and adrenal androgens, aldosterone, cortisol, and estrogens. Replacement glucosteroids must be given with aminoglutethamide to avoid

Treatment options in hormone-refractory prostate cancer
Antiandrogen therapy (if not already instituted)
Antiandrogen withdrawal
Second antiandrogen therapy
Adrenal androgen inhibitors
Aminoglutethimide
Ketoconazole
Corticosteroids
Estrogens and antiestrogens
Tamoxifen
Diethylstilbestrol (DES)
Chemotherapy
Estramustine
Mitozantrone
Taxanes
Paclitaxel (Taxol)
Docetaxel (Taxotere)
Growth factor inhibitors
Suramin
HER-2/neu antibodies (herceptin)
Angiogenesis inhibitors
Thalidomide
TNP-470
Immunotherapy
Interleukin-2
Granulocyte–macrophage colony stimulating factor
Vaccines

Figure 28.18 Treatment options in hormone refractory prostate cancer.

cortisol insufficiency. Studies report a 10% overall response rate in patients who have HRPC[60]. This drug is associated with significant side effects, including fatigue, rash, drowsiness, orthostatic hypertension, and ataxia.

A less toxic agent, ketoconazole is a synthetic compound that effects the C17–20 lyase biosynthesis in the adrenals.[61] It suppresses both adrenal and testicular androgen production. In HRPC patients, ketoconazole and replacement hydrocortisone has resulted in objective response rates in 15% of patients[62]. In patients who progressed despite androgen withdrawal (flutamide), PSA decreases of 50% were seen in 75% of patients. Nausea and fatigue are major side-effects reported.

Low-dose corticosteroids (prednisone) inhibit hypothalamic secretion of adrenocorticotrophic hormone (ACTH) by negative feedback mechanisms. This results in diminished adrenal androgen production. Corticosteroids with or without other agents have resulted in PSA decreases of 50% in 20% of patients[63].

Estrogens and antiestrogens

Estrogen receptors may be unregulated after androgen deprivation therapy. Mutant androgen receptors have been isolated in HRPC. However, the response rate with the use of antiestrogens (tamoxifen) in prostate cancer has been poor (0–10%).

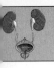

Alternatively, high-dose estrogens (diethylstilbestrol (DES)) have had an overall response rate of 43%[64].

Chemotherapy

Estramustine is a combination of estrogen and nitrogen mustard. Its mechanism of action involves disruption of cytoplasmic microtubules, inhibition of nuclear matrix assembly and inhibits the multidrug resistance transporter p-glycoprotein. Estramustine alone accounted for only a 19% objective response rate. However, the combination of estramustine with vinblastine demonstrated a decrease in PSA of 50% of patients. These treatment benefits lasted approximately 7 months[65].

Taxanes are a new type of cytotoxic drug that polymerize tubulin into stable microtubules, leading to mitotic arrest and cell death. Initial single-agent trials in HRPC had a response rate of only 4.3%[66]. However, more encouraging results have been seen in trials using taxanes in combination with estramustine and etoposide (VP-16)[67].

Mitozantrone, structurally related to doxorubicin, an anthracycline antibiotic, is a topoisomerase II inhibitor. Clinical trials have demonstrated the combination of mitozantrone and corticosteroids to be superior over corticosteroid therapy alone in alleviating bone pain[68]. No difference in survival was noted in any of the trials. Time to treatment failure and disease failure was improved by 1.4 months. Quality of life indexes were better in the combination therapy, particularly for pain control[63]. Based on these studies, the Food and Drug Administration approved mitozantrone for palliation of symptomatic bone pain in men with HRPC.

To date, no single agent or combination therapy has proven to improve survival in patients with HRPC.

Growth factor inhibitors

Growth factors are important in the regulation of cell proliferation. These processes are also important in tumorigenesis. Suramin, used initially for the treatment of trypanosomiasis, has been used in the treatment of HRPC. Its activity is mediated through inhibiting binding of growth factors to their receptors. Early studies reported a response rate as high as a 77%[69]. More recent studies showed only a 20% PSA response rate[70].

Overexpression of a human-epidermal-growth-factor-like receptor (HER-2/neu) has been common finding in several human tumors[71]. HER-2/neu has been expressed in 42% of prostate cancers. Trials have begun using specific antibodies (herceptin) to the extracellular domain of the membrane-based protein product of the *HER-2/neu* oncogene to inhibit the growth of tumors that overexpress the gene.

Angiogenesis inhibitors

The formation of new blood vessels is essential for solid tumors to survive. Targeting tumor growth by inhibiting factors that promote tumor blood supply is the mechanism behind angiogenesis inhibitors. Thalidomide and TNP-470 are presently being evaluated in ongoing studies.

Immunotherapy

Gene therapy approaches for HRPC relies on the induction of specific immune responses by the patient. Nonspecific immunostimulatory agents used have included interleukin-2 and granulocyte–macrophage colony stimulating factor. Newer approaches have targeted the molecule PSA. Vaccines consisting of liposome-encapsulated recombinant PSA and lipid A have been used in early pilot studies[72]. Infusions of autologous dendritic cells and two human histocompatability antigen (HLA-A2)-specific prostate-specific membrane antigen (PSMA) peptides have also been used in clinical trials for HRPC[73].

COMPLICATIONS OF LATE PROSTATE CANCER

The benefits of androgen deprivation are often short-lived. Unfortunately, there is no cure for these patients. The focus of treatment shifts to palliation of symptoms and to ensure the highest possible quality of life. Troublesome symptoms associated with late hormone-resistant prostate cancer include bone pain, spinal cord compression, urinary tract obstruction, and anemia.

Bone pain

The most common symptom in patient with late prostate cancer is bone pain. Frequent sites affected include the lumbar spine and pelvis but prostate cancer can be seen in any bone in the skeletal system. Bony metastases can lead to pathological fractures. The neck of the femur is a common site for this to occur. Surgical stabilization is necessary not only in pathological fractures but also in impending fractures where more than 50% of the cortical bone is destroyed.

Treatment of bone pain is of critical importance in maintaining quality of life. Several treatment options are currently available to patients with late prostate cancer for pain management. These include the use of irradiation and bisphosphonates.

Irradiation

Irradiation is an effective method for the control of pain associated with tumor growth. For specific sites external beam irradiation provides pain relief in approximately 75% of patients for up to 6 months[74]. It is usually delivered either as a single dose or more commonly as a short 2–3 week course (3,000cGy in 10 divided doses). When multiple sites are involved, local therapy is less effective. However, intravenous radiopharmaceuticals including strontium-89 and samarium-153 are alternatives that can deliver radiation directly to multiple metastatic sites throughout the body[75]. Pain improvement has been noted in approximately 50% of patients but the duration of response has been disappointing. Side effects include thrombocytopenia and leukopenia, which often limits the use of more aggressive chemotherapy. Selection criteria for the use radiopharmaceuticals include:
- multiple sites of painful skeletal metastases;
- White blood cells count $>3000 \times 10^9$/L;
- platelet count $>60,000 \times 10^9$/L; and
- life expectancy >3 months.

Bisphosphonates

Bisphosphonates are pyrophosphate analogs (clodronate or pamidronate) that are known to suppress bone resorption and mineralization by direct inhibitory effects on osteoclast activity. Their clinical use has been shown to be effective in Paget's disease, in multiple myeloma, and in breast cancer patients with lytic bone lesions. Although most bony metastasis from prostate cancer are osteoblastic, there tends to be an increase in bone

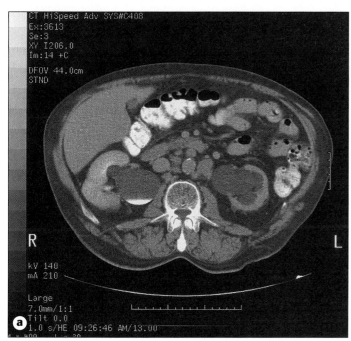 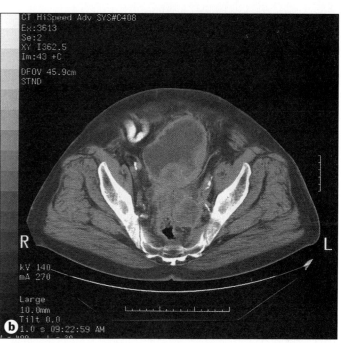

Figure 28.19 Bilateral ureteral obstruction due to extrinsic compression by pelvic lymph nodes. (a) Bilateral hydronephrosis with cortical thinning of left renal cortex. (b) Enlarged pelvic lymph nodes obstructing both ureters with invasion of the posterior wall of the bladder.

turnover at these sites and an increase in osteoclastic activity. In androgen-deprived patients there is an increase risk of bone demineralization. The use of bisphosphonates may be of added benefit in this group of patients[76].

Spinal cord compression
Spinal cord compression occurs most often in the thoracic or upper lumbar regions of the spine. This can result either from vertebral collapse caused by tumor invasion or from extradural tumor growth. Common symptoms include radicular pain, motor weakness, sensory deficits, and bladder dysfunction. The process may be indolent or acute with rapid progression to paraplegia.

Spinal cord compression is a medical emergency. Immediate androgen deprivation is required if previously untreated with hormones. Magnetic resonance imaging provides the best detail of the involved region, including the exact level and extent of the tumor compression[77].

Successful treatment of spinal cord compression requires prompt diagnosis and therapy. Steroid administration should begin immediately. The next step in management includes either surgical decompression in combination with radiation therapy or radiation therapy alone. In most cases, radiation therapy will be effective and surgery can be avoided. Retrospective studies fail to show any clear advantage of one therapeutic approach[78–79]. Both treatments provide pain relief in two thirds of patients. Improvement in symptoms occurs in over 50% of patients. Complete paraplegia before treatment rarely sees a return of normal function.

Urinary tract obstruction
Bladder obstruction
Acute or chronic bladder outlet obstruction is another common complication of late prostate cancer. Androgen deprivation

results in resolution of bladder outlet obstruction in up to two thirds of patients[80–81]. However, prolonged catheter drainage or intermittent self-catheterization may be required for up to 3 months before return of spontaneous voiding. Transurethral prostatectomy (TURP) can be performed for relief of obstruction in patients failing androgen deprivation therapy. TURP may also be helpful in patients with gross hematuria from tumor infiltration of the prostatic urethra or bladder base. Caution must be exercised in these patients because there is a higher incidence of urinary incontinence.

Ureteral obstruction
Unilateral or bilateral ureteral obstruction may also occur in late prostate cancer. This may be caused by direct extension of the prostate cancer at the bladder base or by extrinsic compression by enlarged retroperitoneal or pelvic lymph node metastases (Fig. 28.19). Ureteral obstruction may present with symptoms of azotemia, flank pain, sepsis, or asymptomatic hydronephrosis.

Management of ureteral obstruction is guided by the patient's overall status. Asymptomatic unilateral hydronephrosis with preserved renal function may be appropriately observed. Retrograde ureteral stent placement is technically impossible if the trigone and bladder base are involved because of difficulties in visualizing the ureteral orifices. Alternatively, percutaneous nephrostomy tube placement can be performed under ultrasonic or fluoroscopic guidance (Fig. 28.20). Internalization of the system can be performed through the nephrostomy site. The use of percutaneous nephrostomy placement and ureteral stenting has made cutaneous diversion rarely necessary.

Anemia
Patients with late prostate cancer commonly develop anemia. Several factors contribute, including involvement of metastatic

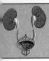

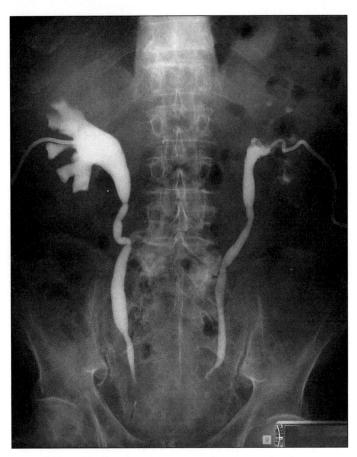

Figure 28.20 Bilateral percutaneous nephrostomy tube placement.
Antegrade nephrostomy tube demonstrating bilateral ureteral obstruction
due to extrinsic compression by pelvic lymph nodes.

disease in significant sites of red blood cell production (pelvis, long bones, and vertebral bodies). Malaise and anorexia may result in iron deficiency caused by lack of dietary factors. There is also the anemia of chronic disease and malignancy. The anemia of late prostate cancer is often of insidious onset. Patients tend to tolerate profound anemia surprisingly well. However, many patients do become symptomatic, requiring treatment. The use of iron and vitamin supplements and bone marrow stimulants (erythropoietin) may be useful. Transfusion dependency usually emerges as the disease process progresses. Blood transfusion can improve overall strength and performance status of many patients.

REFERENCES

1. Partin AW, Yoo JK, Carter HB, et al. The use of prostate-specific antigen, clinical stage, and Gleason score to predict pathological stage in men with localized prostate cancer. J Urol. 1993c;150:110–4.
2. Catalona WJ, Smith DS, Ratliff TL, et al. The measurement of prostate-specific antigen in serum as a screening test for prostate cancer. N Engl J Med. 1991;324:1156–61.
3. Stamey TA, Yang N, Hay AR, et al. Prostate-specific antigen as a serum marker for adenocarcinoma of the prostate. N Engl J Med. 1987;317:909–16.
4. Southwick PC, Catalona WJ, Partin AW, et al. Prediction of post-radical prostatectomy pathological outcome for stage T1c prostate cancer with percent free prostate specific antigen: a prospective multicenter clinical trial. J Urol. 1999;162:1346–51.
5. Partin AW, Kazan MW, Subong EN, et al. Combination of prostate-specific antigen, clinical stage, and Gleason score to predict pathological stage of localized prostate cancer: a multi-institutional update. JAMA. 1997;277:1445–551.
6. Elici S, Ozen M, Agildere A, et al. A comparison of transrectal ultrasonography and endorectal magnetic resonance imaging in the local staging of prostatic carcinoma. BJU Int. 1999;83:796–800.
7. Rifkin MD, Xerhouni EA, Gatsonis CA, et al. Comparison of magnetic resonance imaging and ultrasonography in staging early prostate cancer: results of a multi-institutional cooperative trial. New Engl J Med. 1990;323:621–6.
8. Tempany CM, Zhou X, Zerhouni EA, et al. Staging of prostate cancer: results of Radiology Diagnostic Oncology Group project comparison of three MR imaging techniques. Radiology. 1994;192:47–54.
9. Platt JF, Bree RL, and Schwab RE. The accuracy of CT in the staging of carcinoma of the prostate. Am J Radiol. 1987;149:315–8.
10. Chybowski FM, Larson Keller JJ, Bergstralh EJ, et al. Predicting radionucleotide bone scan findings in patients with newly diagnosed untreated prostate cancer: prostate specific antigen is superior to all other parameters. J Urol. 1991;145:313–8.
11. Manyak MJ, Hinkle GH, Olsen JO, et al. Immunoscintigraphy with indium-111-capromab pendetide: evaluation before definitive therapy in patients with prostate cancer. Urology. 1999;54:1058–63.
12. Hinkle GH, Burgers JK, Neal CE, et al. Multicenter radio-immunoscintigraphic evaluation of patients with prostate carcinoma using indium-111-capromab pendetide. Cancer. 1998;83:739–747.
13. Wolf JS Jr, Andriole GL. The selection of patients for cross-sectional imaging and pelvic lymphadenectomy before radical prostatectomy. AUA Update Ser. 1997;16 (15):113–9.
14. Gervasi LA, Mata J, Easley JD, et al. Prognostic significance of lymph node metastases in prostate cancer. J Urol. 1989;142:332–6.
15. Eastham JA, Scardino PT. Radical prostatectomy. In: Walsh PC, Retik AB, Vaughan ED Jr, et al. eds. Campbell's urology, vol 3. Philadelphia: WB Saunders; 1998:2547–64.

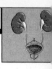
16. Morgan WR, Bergstrahl EJ, Zinke H. Long term evaluation of radical prostatectomy as treatment for clinical stage C (T3) prostate cancer. Urology. 1993;41:113–20.

17. Epstein JI, Hanks GE. Prostate cancer: evaluation and radiotherapeutic management. Cancer J Clin. 1992;42;223–40.

18. Schulman CC, Sassine AM. Neoadjuvant hormone deprivation before radical prostatectomy. Clin Invest Med. 1993;16:523–31.

19. Aprikian AG, Fair WR, Reuter VE, et al. Experience with neoadjuvant diethylstilbestrol and radical prostatectomy in patients with locally advanced prostate cancer. Br J Urol. 1994;74:630–6.

20. MacFarlane MT, Abi-Aad A, Stein A, et al. Neoadjuvant hormonal deprivation in patients with locally advanced prostate cancer. J Urol. 1993;150:132–4.

21. Van Poppel H, de Ridder D, Elgamal AA, et al. Neoadjuvant hormonal therapy before radical prostatectomy decreases the number of positive surgical margins in stage T2 prostate cancer: interim results of a prospective randomized trial. J Urol. 1995;154:429–34.

22. Labrie F, Cusan L, Gomez JL, et al. Downstaging of early stage prostate cancer before radical prostatectomy: the first randomized trial of neoadjuvant combination therapy with flutamide and a luteinizing hormone-releasing hormone agonist. Urology Symp. 1994;44(6A):29–37.

23. Oesterling JE, Andrews PE, Suman VJ, et al. Preoperative androgen deprivation therapy: artificial lowering of serum prostate specific antigen without downstaging the tumor. J Urol. 1993;149:779–82.

24. Witjes WP, Schulman CC, Dubruyne FM. Preliminary result of a prospective randomized study comparing radical prostatectomy versus radical prostatectomy associated with neoadjuvant hormonal combination therapy in T2-3 N0M0 prostatic carcinoma; the European Study Group of Prostate Cancer. Urology. 1997;499(Suppl):65–9.

25. Kennedy TJ, Sonneland AM, Marlett MM, et al. Luteinizing hormone-releasing hormone downstaging of clinical stage C prostate cancer. J Urol. 1192;147:891–3.

26. Van Popped HV, Ameba F, Yen R, et al. Radical prostatectomy for localized prostate cancer. Eur J Surg Oncol. 1992;18:460–2.

27. Gomella LG, Liberaman SN, Mulholland SG, et al. Induction androgen deprivation plus prostatectomy for stage T3 disease: failure to achieve prostate-specific antigen-based freedom from disease status in a phase II trial. Urology. 1996;47:870–7.

28. Pummer K, Crawford ED, Daneshgari F, et al. Hormonal pretreatment does not affect the final pathological stage in locally advanced prostate cancer. Urology Symp. 1994;44(6A):38–42.

29. Solomon MH, McHugh TA, Dorr RP, et al. Hormone ablation therapy as neoadjuvant treatment to radical prostatectomy. Clin Invest Med. 1993;16:532–8.

30. Soloway MS, Hachiya T, Civantos F, et al. Androgen deprivation prior to radical prostatectomy for T2b and T3 prostate cancer. Urology. 1994;43(Suppl):52–6.

31. Crook J, Robertson S, Collin G, et al. Clinical relevance of transrectal ultrasound biopsy, and serum prostate-specific antigen following external beam radiotherapy for carcinoma of the prostate. Int J Oncol Biol Phys. 1993;27:31–7.

32. Perez CA, Pilepich MV, Garcia D, et al. Definitive radiation therapy in carcinoma of the prostate localized to the pelvis: experience at the Mallinckrodt Institute of Radiology. NCI Monogr. 1988;7:85–94.

33. Forman JD, Orton C, Ezzell G, et al. Preliminary results of a hyperfractionated dose escalation study for locally advanced adenocarcinoma of the prostate. Radiother Oncol. 1993;27:203–8.

34. Leibel SA, Heimann R, Kutcher GJ, et al. Three-dimensional conformal radiation therapy in locally advanced carcinoma of the prostate: preliminary results of phase-I dose escalation study. Int J Radiat Biol Phys. 1993;28:55–65.

35. Pilepich MV, Krall JM, Al-Sarraff M, et al. Androgen deprivation with radiation therapy compared with radiation therapy alone for locally advanced prostatic carcinoma: a randomized comparative trial of the Radiation Therapy Oncology Group. Urology. 1995;45:616–23.

36. Lavediere J, Gomez JL, Cusan L, et al. Beneficial effect of combination hormonal therapy administered prior to and following external beam radiation therapy in localized prostate cancer. Int J Radiat Oncol Biol Phys. 1997;37:247–52.

37. Bolla M, Gonzalez D, Warde P, et al. Improved survival in patients with locally advanced prostate cancer treated with radiotherapy and goserelin. N Engl J Med. 1997;337:295–300.

38. Huggins C, Hodges CV. Studies on prostatic cancer: I. The effect of castration, of estrogen and of androgen injection on serum phosphatases in metastatic carcinoma of the prostate. Cancer Res. 1941;1:293–7.

39. Huggins C, Scott WW. Bilateral adrenalectomy in prostate cancer. Ann Surg. 1945;122:1031–41.

40. Wilbert DM, Griffin JE, Wilson JD. Characterization of the cytosol androgen receptor of the human prostate. J Clin Endocrinol Metab. 1983;56:113–20

41. Geller J, Albert J, Nachtsheim DA, et al. Comparison of prostate cancer tissue, dihydrotesterone levels at the time of relapse following orchiectomy or estrogen therapy. J Urol. 1984;132:693–6.

42. Labrie F, Dupont A, Belanger A, et al. Combination therapy with flutamide and castration (LHRH agonist or orchiectomy) in advanced prostate cancer: a marked improvement in response and survival. J Steroid Biochem. 1985;23:833–42.

43. Crawford ED, Eisenberger MA, McLeod DG, et al. A controlled trial of leuprolide with and without flutamide in prostatic carcinoma. N Engl J Med. 1989;321:419–24.

44. Denis LJ, Carnelro de Moura JL, Bono A, et al. Goserelin acetate and flutamide versus bilateral orchiectomy: a phase III EORTC trial (30853). Urology. 1993;42:119–30.

45. Janknegt RA, Abbou CC, Bartoletti R, et al. Orchiectomy and nilutamide or placebo as treatment of metastatic prostatic cancer in a multinational double-blind randomized trial. J Urol. 1993;149:77–83.

46. Crawford ED, Eisenberger MA, McLeod DG, et al. Comparison of bilateral orchiectomy with or without flutamide for the treatment of patients with stage D2 adenocarcinoma of the prostate: results of NCI Intergroup Study 0105 (SWOG and ECOG). J Urol. 1997;157:336. Abstract 1311.

47. Prostate Cancer Trialists' Collaborative Group. Maximum androgen blockade in advanced prostate cancer: an overview of 22 randomized trials with 3283 deaths in 5710 patients. Lancet. 1995;346:265–9.

48. Mellinger GT. Veterans Administration Cooperative Urological Research Group. Carcinoma of the prostate; a continuing co-operative study. J Urol. 1964;91:590–4.

49. Byar DP and Corle D. Hormone therapy for prostate cancer: results of the Veterans Administration Cooperative Urological Research Group's studies of the prostate. Cancer. 1973;32:1126–30.

50. Medical Research Council Prostate Cancer Working Party Investigators Group. Immediate versus deferred treatment for advanced prostatic cancer: initial results of the Medical Research Council trial. Br J Urol. 1997;79:235–46.

51. Van den Ouden D, Tribukait B, Blom JHM, et al. Deoxyribonucleic acid ploidy of core biopsies and metastatic lymph nodes of prostate cancer patients: impact on time to progression. The European Organization for Research and Treatment of Cancer Genitourinary Group. J Urol. 1993;150:400–6.

52. Messing EM, Manola J, Sarodsy M, et al. Immediate hormonal therapy compared with observation after radical prostatectomy and pelvic lymphadenectomy in men with node-positive prostate cancer. N Engl J Med. 1999;341:1781–88.

53. Sato N, Gleave ME, Bruchovsky N, et al. Intermittent androgen suppression delays progression to androgen-independent regulation of prostate-specific antigen gene in the LNCaP prostate tumor model. J Steroid Biochem Molec Biol. 1996;58:139–46.

54. Klotz LH, Herr HW, Morse MJ, et al. Intermittent endocrine therapy for advanced prostate cancer. Cancer. 1986;58:2546–50.

55. Goldenberg SI, Bruchovsky N, Gleave ME, et al. Intermittent androgen suppression in the treatment of prostate cancer: a preliminary report. Urology.1995;45:839–44.

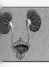

56. Oh WK and Kantoff PW. Management of hormone refractory prostate cancer: current standards and future prospects. J Urol. 1998;160:1220–9.

57. Kelly WK and Scher HI. Prostate specific antigen decline after anti-androgen withdrawal: the flutamide withdrawal syndrome. J Urol. 1993;149:607–9.

58. Schellhammer PF, Venner P, Haas GP, et al. Prostate specific antigen decreases after withdrawal of antiandrogen therapy with biculatamide or flutamide in patients receiving combined androgen blockade. J Urol. 1997;157:1731–5.

59. Scher HI, Liebertz C, Kelly WK, et al. Biculatamide for advanced prostate cancer: the natural versus treated history of disease. J Clin Oncol. 1997;15:2928–38.

60. Dawson NA. Treatment of progressive metastatic prostate cancer. Oncology. 1993;7:17–24.

61. Mahler C, Berhelst J, Denis L. Ketoconazole and liazorole in the treatment of advanced prostate cancer. Cancer. 1993;71:1068–73.

62. Small EJ, Bavon AD, Fippin L, et al. Ketoconazole retains activity in advanced prostate cancer patients despite flutamide withdrawal. J Urol. 1997;157:1204–7.

63. Kantoff PW, Conaway M, Winer E. Hydrocortisone with and without mitozantrone in patients with hormone refractory prostate cancer: preliminary results from a prospective randomized cancer and leukemia group B (9182) trial comparing chemotherapy to best supportive care. Proc Am Soc Clin Oncol. 1996;14:1748.

64. Smith DC, Redman BG, Flaherty LE, et al. A phase II trial of oral diethystilbesterol as a second-line hormonal agent in advanced prostate cancer. Urology. 1998;52:257–60.

65. Seidman AD, Scher HI, Petrylak D, et al. Estramustine and vinblastine: use of PSA as a clinical trial end point in hormone refractory prostate cancer. J Urol. 1992;147:931–7.

66. Roth BJ, Yeap BY, Wilding, et al. Taxol in advanced, hormone-refractory carcinoma of the prostate: a phase II trial of the Eastern Oncology Group. Cancer. 1993;72 (8):2457–60.

67. Smith DC and Pienta KJ. Paclitaxel in the treatment of hormone refractory prostate cancer. Semin Oncol. 1999;261(1 Suppl 2):109–11.

68. Tannock IF, Osoba D, Stockler MR, et al. Chemotherapy with mitoxantrone plus prednisone or prednisone alone for symptomatic hormone-resistant prostate cancer: a Canadian randomized trial with palliative end points. J Clin Oncol. 1996;14:1756–64.

69. Dawson NA, Cooper MR, Figg WD, et al. Antitumor activity of suramin in hormone-refractory prostate cancer controlling for hydrocortisone treatment and flutamide withdrawal as potentially confounding variables. Cancer. 1995;76:453–62.

70. Kelly WK, Curley T, Leibertz C, et al. Prospective evaluation of hydrocortisone and suramin in patients with androgen-independent prostate cancer. J Clin Oncol. 1995;13:2208–13.

71. Stancovski I, Dela M, Yarden Y. Molecular and clinical aspects of the neu/erbB-2 receptor tyrosine kinase. Cancer Treatment Res. 1994;71:161–91.

72. Harris DT, Matyas GR, Gomella LG, et al. Immunologic approaches to the treatment of prostate cancer. Semin Oncol. 1999;26(4);439–47.

73. Tjoa BA, Simmons SJ, Elgamal A, et al. Follow-up evaluation of a phase II prostate cancer vaccine trial. Prostate. 1999;40(2):125–9.

74. Benson RC Jr, Hasa SM, Jones AG. External beam radiotherapy for palliation of multiple of pain form metastatic carcinoma of the prostate. J Urol. 1981;127:69–71.

75. Ben-Josef E, Porter AT. Radioisotopes in the treatment of bone metastases. Ann Med. 1997;29:31–5.

76. Adami S. Bisphosphonates in prostate carcinoma. Cancer. 1997;80(Suppl 8):1674–9.

77. Modic MT, Masaryk T, Paushter D. Magnetic resonance imaging of the spine. Radiol Clin North Am. 1986;24:229–45.

78. Young FR, Post EM, King GA. Treatment of spinal epidural metastases. J Neurosurg. 1980;53:741–8.

79. Constans JP, de Divitiis E, Donzelli R, et al. Spinal metastases with neurological manifestations. J Neurosurg. 1983;59;111–8.

80. Fleischmann JD, Catalona WJ. Endocrine therapy for bladder outlet obstruction from carcinoma of the prostate. J Urol. 1985;134:498–500.

81. Varenhorst E, Alund G. Urethral obstruction secondary to carcinoma of the prostate: response to endocrine treatment. Urology. 1985;25:354–6.

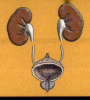

Chapter 29

Testicular Tumors

Graeme S Steele and Jerome P Richie

KEY POINTS

- Effective platinum-based chemotherapy has dramatically improved the prognosis of patients with germ cell tumours.
- Predictable pathways of lymphatic spread have important implications for surgical management.
- 30–50% of patients with stage 1 non-seminomatous germ cell tumor may have occult metastatic disease.
- Optimal results for patients with testicular tumours will only be achieved in specialist tertiary referral centres.

INTRODUCTION

The management of germ cell tumors (GCT) of the testis has proved to be a model of success among solid tumors. This is due to tremendous advances during the past two decades, which have changed the once dismal prognosis for patients with advanced disease[1].

Testicular cancer, has in fact become one of the most curable of all solid neoplasms. Thirty years ago testicular cancer accounted for 11.4% of all cancer deaths in the 25–34-year age group, with an overall 5-year survival rate of 64%[2]. The most recent 5-year survival rates for GCT of the testis in the USA were recently reported as being in excess of 90%[3].

Improved prospects for cure and long-term disease-free survival rates are related to a better understanding of the natural history of testicular tumors, improved staging methods and surgical techniques, as well as to the introduction of effective platinum-based combination chemotherapy[4].

High cure rates associated with modern treatment regimens for early-stage testis cancer have resulted in a shift in focus towards reducing morbidity of potentially toxic treatment regimens. This concept is especially relevant to preservation of reproductive function as well as reduction in pulmonary, neural, and renal toxicity associated with chemotherapeutic agents.

Although there is little dispute that chemotherapy is appropriate as the initial therapy in patients with advanced GCT, there is ongoing controversy regarding the management of patients who present with low-stage GCT. Essentially the controversies center on attempts to refine therapy without compromising survival in low-stage disease.

Although the prognosis for low-stage GCT is generally good, approximately 20% of patients who present with metastatic GCT

eventually die of their disease[5]. On the basis of predicted response to therapy, patients with advanced disease are divided into two groups: good risk and poor risk GCT[6–9]. While patients with good risk GCT are likely to achieve a complete response to therapy, patients with poor risk GCT disease are unlikely to achieve a complete response to therapy and are therefore the focus of ongoing clinical trials[10–12].

At present there are a number of challenges facing physicians who are responsible for care of patients with testis tumors. Furthermore, ongoing developments in the field of molecular biology are likely to enhance our understanding of the etiology and pathogenesis of testis tumors in the future, and hopefully the prevention of these fascinating tumors in the new millennium.

ANATOMICAL PRINCIPLES OF TESTICULAR CANCER SURGERY

Testicular anatomy
Testicular tunics
The testis is covered by a series of tunics acquired during testicular descent that include the tunica vaginalis, internal and external spermatic fascia, and the cremasteric fascia. The tunica albuginea, a dense fascial structure, gives rise to numerous septae posteriorly at the mediastinum testis that divide the testis into lobules within which the seminiferous tubules are arranged. The seminiferous tubules converge at the mediastinum testis and drain into 20–30 tubuli rectae, which in turn enter the mediastinum to form the rete testis, a collection of anastomosing ducts. After leaving the rete testis the efferent ductules traverse the tunica albuginea and enter the globus epididymidis (Fig. 29.1).

Cell populations
The seminiferous tubules contain two cell populations, supporting Sertoli cells and spermatogenic cells called spermatogonia. The connective tissue stroma surrounding seminiferous tubules contains the interstitial cells of Leydig, which are androgen-producing cells essential to spermatogenesis.

Tumors may arise from spermatogenic cells, in which case they are known as GCT, as well as from the supporting and interstitial cells. In addition, tumors may arise from the rete testis, epididymis, and cord structures (Figs 29.2 & 29.3).

The American Joint Committee on Cancer (AJCC) TNM (tumor, nodes, and metastasis) staging system defines tumors confined to the tunica albuginea as pT1t, while tumors invading through the tunica albuginea are pT2 and are associated with an increased risk of metastatic disease. Spermatic cord and scrotal involvement constitute pT3 and pT4 tumors respectively (Fig. 29.4).

Structure of the testis and epididymis

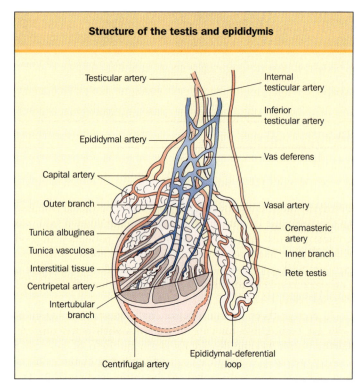

Figure 29.1 Structure of the testis and epididymis.

Revised World Health Organization classification of germ cell tumors of the testis

A. Precursor lesion

B. Tumors of one histologic type
1. Seminoma
2. Spermatocytic seminoma
3. Embryonal carcinoma
4. Yolk sac tumor
5. Polyembryoma
6. Trophoblastic tumors

    Choriocarcinoma
    a. Pure
    b. Mixed
    c. Placental site implantation tumor
7. Teratoma
    a. Mature teratoma
    b. Immature teratoma
    c. Teratoma with malignant areas

C. Tumors of more than one histologic type

All the components should be listed in the diagnosis and the volume estimated

Figure 29.2 Revised World Health Organization classification of germ cell tumors of the testis.

Revised World Health Organization classification of non-germ-cell tumors of the testis

Sex cord and stromal tumors
1. Leydig cell tumors
2 Sertoli cell tumors

    Large-cell calcifying Sertoli cell tumor
3. Granulosa cell tumors

    Adult

    Juvenile
4. Theca cell tumor
5. Undifferentiated
6. Mixed

Tumors and tumorlike lesions containing both germ cells and sex cord stromal cells
1. Gonadoblastoma
2. Mixed germ-cell–gonadal stromal tumors

Miscellaneous tumors
1. Gonadal hamartomas
2. Carcinoid
3. Others

Lymphoid and hematopoietic tumors

Secondary tumors

Figure 29.3 Revised World Health Organization classification of non-germ-cell tumors of the testis.

Testicular blood supply

The testis is supplied by three vessels:
- the testicular artery, a branch of the aorta;
- the vasal artery, a branch of the superior vesical artery; and
- the cremasteric artery, a branch of the inferior epigastric artery.

Abundant anastomoses between these arteries usually allow for division of the testicular artery when necessary in orchiopexy.

The vascular supply to the testis separates from the vascular supply to the epididymis well above the area of dissection for epididymectomy. Nevertheless, it is important to remember that injury to testicular vessels can be avoided by dissecting close to the epididymis, especially on the medial aspect where testicular vessels course (Fig. 29.1).

Lymphatic drainage of the testis and sites of metastases
Retroperitoneal lymph nodes

The principles that underlie the modern surgical treatment of GCT of the testis are based on the fact that testis cancer spreads in a predictable and stepwise fashion, with the notable exception of choriocarcinoma. The spermatic cord contains four to eight lymphatic channels, which ascend into the retroperitoneum and fan out medially into the retroperitoneal lymph node chain. The first echelon of lymph nodes draining the right testis is located within the interaortocaval nodes, at the level of the second vertebral body. The first echelon of nodes draining the left testis is located in the para-aortic region in an area bounded by the renal vein superiorly, aorta medially, ureter laterally, and the origin of the inferior mesenteric artery inferiorly. Following spread to either the left or right primary echelon of nodes, subsequent spread may occur in a retrograde fashion to the common external and inguinal nodes, or cephalad via the cysterna chyli, thoracic duct and supraclavicular nodes (Fig. 29.5).

In a review of 104 consecutive cases of stage II non-seminomatous germ cell tumor (NSGCT), the Indiana group made a number of important observations confirming the predictability of lymphatic spread in testicular cancer[13]. They reported that suprahilar lymph node spread was rare in stage IIA disease; on the

Boden/Gibb Stage	Memorial Sloan–Kettering Cancer Center	Royal Marsden Hospital	American Joint Committee	
A (I)) Tumor confined to testis	A	1	TX	Unknown status
			T0	No evidence of primary
			T1	Confined to testis
			T2	Extending through tunica
			T3	Invasion of spermatic cord
			T4	Invasion of scrotum
B(II)	B1 ≤ 5 cm	IIA ≤ 2 cm	N1	Single ≤ 2 cm
	B2 > 5 cm	IIB > 2, ≤ 5 cm	N2	Single >2 cm ≤5 cm
	B3 > 10 cm (bulky)	IIC > 5 cm	N3	>5 cm
C(III) Spread beyond retroperitoneal nodes	C	III Supraclavicular (SCN) or mediastinal involvement	M	Spread beyond regional nodes
		IV Extralymphatic metastasis		

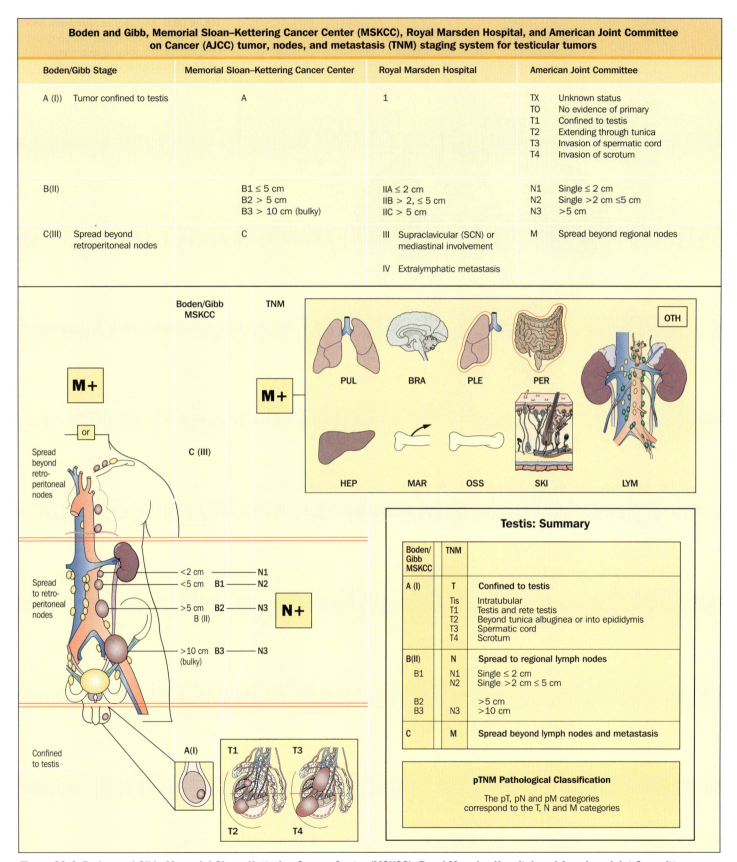

Figure 29.4 Boden and Gibb, Memorial Sloan–Kettering Cancer Center (MSKCC), Royal Marsden Hospital, and American Joint Committee on Cancer (AJCC) tumor, nodes, and metastasis (TNM) staging system for testicular tumors. (Top) staging nomenclature; (bottom) graphical illustration of staging systems.

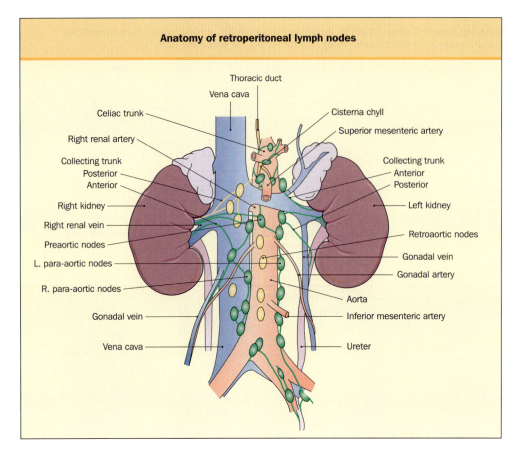

Anatomy of retroperitoneal lymph nodes

Figure 29.5 Anatomy of retroperitoneal lymph nodes. (Reproduced with permission from Hinman F Jr. Atlas of urosurgical anatomy. London: WB Saunders; 1993.)

other hand, suprahilar spread was not uncommon in stage IIB disease. In low-stage disease the absence of contralateral node involvement was noted. Cross-metastases occur more commonly in patients with right-sided tumors, because of lymphatic drainage from right to left. These observations obviously have important implications for the surgical management of testis cancer (Fig. 29.6).

Pelvic and inguinal lymph nodes
Lymphatics of the epididymis drain into the external iliac chain; therefore, in locally extensive disease, epididymal involvement may be associated with positive pelvic nodes. Testis cancer that involves the scrotum may result in inguinal node metastases; in addition prior scrotal surgery or retrograde spread from extensive retroperitoneal involvement may result in inguinal metastases. Scrotal violation in the setting of orchiectomy for testis cancer has generally been condemned as compromising patient prognosis. However, recent studies have shown that this may not necessarily be the case[14].

Distant spread
Despite the predictability of lymph node metastasis in testis cancer, there is a failure rate of 5% with distant metastasis following node-negative retroperitoneal lymph node dissection (RPLND)[15]. This is probably due to the fact that testicular lymphatics may very occasionally bypass retroperitoneal lymph nodes altogether and communicate directly with the thoracic duct. Distant spread of testis cancer occurs most commonly to the pulmonary region, with intraparenchymal pulmonary involvement. Subsequent spread is to the liver, viscera, brain,

and bone, with bony secondaries being encountered late in the course of the disease.

In summary, with the notable exception of choriocarcinoma, testicular cancer generally spreads in a predictable pattern. This predictability has led to the development of new surgical techniques, which provide accurate pathological staging while at the same time providing therapeutic benefit. These techniques are also associated with reduced morbidity when compared to the classic full RPLND.

Neuroanatomy of emission and ejaculation
Antegrade propulsion of semen through the urethra occurs as a result of emission and ejaculation.

Emission is the movement of semen into the posterior urethra immediately prior to ejaculation. Emission is a sympathetic response, mediated by sympathetic nerves from spinal segments T12 to L3 and effected by contractions of the vas deferens, prostate, and seminal vesicles.

Ejaculation is the process whereby semen passes distally through the urethra and results from tightening of the normally closed bladder neck (sympathetic reflex), relaxation of the external sphincter (parasympathetic reflex), and contraction of the bulbocavernosus muscle (pudendal nerve). The spinal reflex centers for ejaculation are in the upper sacral and lower lumbar segments of the spinal cord, and the motor pathways traverse the first to third sacral roots and the internal pudendal nerves.

The sympathetic nerves responsible for emission and bladder neck closure during ejaculation leave the spinal cord with the ventral roots of the 12th thoracic (T12) to the third lumbar (L3) spinal nerves. These nerves pass via white rami communicantes

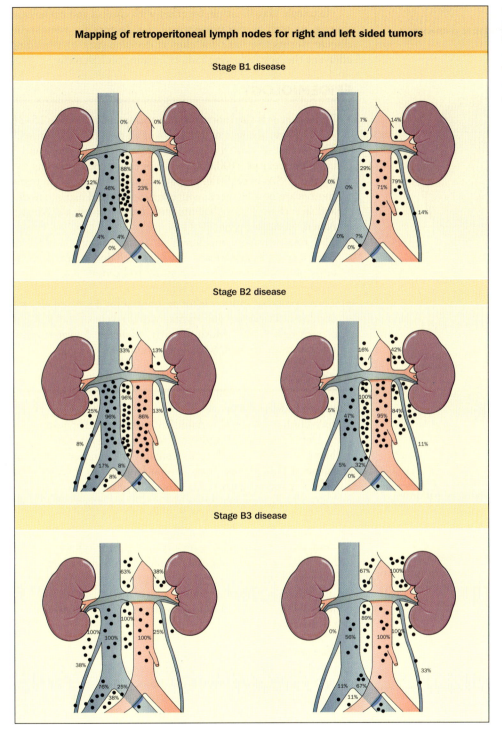

Figure 29.6 Mapping of retroperitoneal lymph nodes for right and left sided tumors. Circles represent patient with positive node(s) in zone. (Reproduced with permission from Gillenwater JT, Grayhack JT, Howard SS, Duckett JW. Adult and pediatric urology, 3rd edn. London: Mosby International; 1995.)

to the paravertebral sympathetic ganglion chain, located beneath the medial edges of the vena cava on the right and the aorta on the left, lying in the gutter between the vertebral bodies and the psoas muscle. There, most of them end on cell bodies of postganglionic neurons, the axons of which travel to organs of emission and ejaculation.

The sympathetic fibers that mediate emission and bladder neck closure (T12 to L3) travel via the retroperitoneum to the superior hypogastric plexus, situated in front of the body of the fifth lumbar vertebra and the bifurcation of the abdominal aorta, and behind the left common iliac vein. From the superior hypogastric plexus, two nerves, the right and left hypogastric nerves, pass down into the pelvic plexuses. In the male each pelvic plexus is situated on either side of the rectum, seminal vesicles, bladder, and prostate (Figs 29.7 & 29.8).

Investigators generally agree that resection of the superior hypogastric plexus results in failure of emission and antegrade ejaculation[16]. Therefore, RPLND for low-stage disease can prevent both failure of emission and ejaculation by avoiding injury to

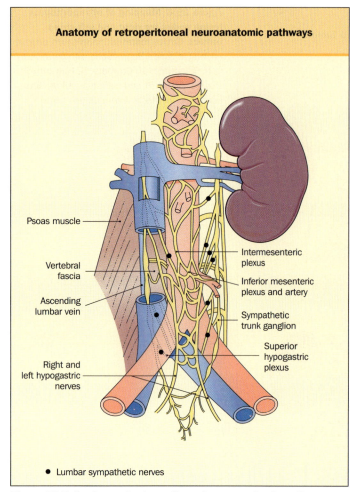

Anatomy of retroperitoneal neuroanatomic pathways

Psoas muscle

Vertebral fascia

Ascending lumbar vein

Right and left hypogastric nerves

Intermesenteric plexus

Inferior mesenteric plexus and artery

Sympathetic trunk ganglion

Superior hypogastric plexus

• Lumbar sympathetic nerves

Figure 29.7 Anatomy of retroperitoneal neuroanatomic pathways.

both the sympathetic chains, their visceral branches and the superior hypogastric plexus. This principle underpins both template RPLND, in which the dissection is limited by the inferior mesenteric artery on the contralateral side, and nerve-sparing dissections, in which lumbar postganglionic nerves are prospectively identified and preserved[17,18].

HISTOLOGIC CLASSIFICATION OF TESTIS TUMORS

Germ cell tumors that arise from germ cell elements within the seminiferous tubules account for 90–95% of all testicular tumors (Fig. 29.9). Non-GCTs include neoplasms arising from gonadal stroma and mesenchymal structures in addition to other miscellaneous lesions (Fig. 29.10). Metastases to the testis are extremely rare; malignant lymphoma, however, has been reported to be the most common testis tumor in patients over the age of 50 years[19].

Carcinoma in situ (CIS), defined as the occurrence of intratubular germ cells that are atypical in nature, has more recently been included in the histologic classification of testis tumors because it is now recognized that CIS may predispose some patients to 'invasive' disease[20]. A summary of testicular CIS is included at the end of this chapter.

Histologic classification, together with clinical and pathologic staging, as well as the presence of risk factors for metastatic disease, forms the basis for clinical decision-making regarding adjuvant therapy following radical inguinal orchiectomy.

EPIDEMIOLOGY

- Testis cancer is the most common malignancy in males 15–35 years of age, accounting for 1–2% of all neoplasms in males.
- The incidence, which is generally quoted as between 2 and 3 cases per year per 100,000 men, appears to be increasing[20].
- In the USA over 90% of patients presenting with testis tumors are non-Hispanic white males, 5% are Hispanic males and less than 3% of patients with testis cancer are African American males[20] (Fig. 29.11).
- The relatively low incidence of testis tumors in African Americans, and in Africans, has been well documented previously, and was shown in one study to be due to a very low incidence of seminoma and teratoma[21].
- Thirty years ago testis cancer accounted for 11.4% of all cancer deaths in young adult males, with a 5-year overall survival rate of only 64%[22]. More recently, however, 5-year survival rates of more than 90% have been reported.

ETIOLOGY

Cryptorchidism

Cryptorchidism is a well-established risk factor for testis cancer[23]. Data from several series indicate that even after successful orchiopexy the affected testis remains at significant risk of malignancy. Pooled data from several large series indicate that 7–10% of patients with testis cancer have a history of cryptorchidism[24]. The estimated incidence of tumorigenesis in men with a history of cryptorchidism is calculated to be 48 times higher than in men with normally descended testes[25]. Between 5% and 10% of men with a history of cryptorchidism develop malignancy in the contralateral normally descended testis.

The general consensus of opinion at present is that orchiopexy should be performed between the ages of 1 and 2 years and that patients should be taught how to perform self-examination at an appropriate age.

Endocrine factors

Elevated gonadotrophins have been reported in a significant percentage of patients with GCT[26]. In addition, elevated levels of follicle-stimulating hormone (FSH) have been shown to be predictive of an increased risk of developing a tumor in the contralateral testis[27].

Trauma

A history of trauma has been postulated as a risk factor for testis cancer. Reports have indicated a history of trauma in 8–25% of patients with testis cancer[28]. More recently, however, epidemiologic studies have failed to show an increased risk for cancer following testis trauma[29,30].

CLINICAL SIGNS AND SYMPTOMS

Scrotal swelling is the most common symptom associated with testis tumors. In addition, scrotal heaviness, a sensation of scrotal

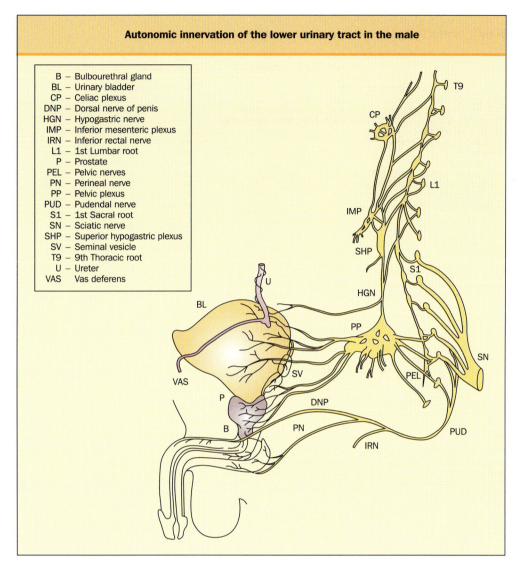

Autonomic innervation of the lower urinary tract in the male

B – Bulbourethral gland
BL – Urinary bladder
CP – Celiac plexus
DNP – Dorsal nerve of penis
HGN – Hypogastric nerve
IMP – Inferior mesenteric plexus
IRN – Inferior rectal nerve
L1 – 1st Lumbar root
P – Prostate
PEL – Pelvic nerves
PN – Perineal nerve
PP – Pelvic plexus
PUD – Pudendal nerve
S1 – 1st Sacral root
SN – Sciatic nerve
SHP – Superior hypogastric plexus
SV – Seminal vesicle
T9 – 9th Thoracic root
U – Ureter
VAS Vas deferens

Figure 29.8 Autonomic innervation of the lower urinary tract in the male. (Reproduced with permission from Gillenwater JT, Grayhack JT, Howard SS, Duckett JW. Adult and pediatric urology, 3rd edn. London: Mosby International; 1995.)

fullness and sometimes even pain can also be presenting features of testis tumors. Rarely, the patient may manifest features of metastatic disease such as chronic cough and hemoptysis in pulmonary involvement or palpable masses in the neck, abdomen, or groin. In a small subset of patients gynecomastia may be the presenting feature, caused either by secretion of β-human chorionic gonadotrophin (β-hCG) or by increased estrogen production.

Delay to time of definitive diagnosis is usually caused by an erroneous diagnosis of epididymitis, which may be treated with a prolonged coarse of antibiotics, or occurs in cases where a secondary hydrocele obscures the testicular mass. These scenarios can be avoided by attaching a high index of suspicion to any young adult male with scrotal symptoms, as well as by ensuring careful followup in any patient managed conservatively.

DIAGNOSIS OF GERM CELL TUMORS

Tumor markers
Tumor markers in GCT have well established roles in the diagnosis and followup of GCT. In addition, degree of elevation of tumor markers at time of diagnosis is now recognized as a prognostic indicator.[9]

α-fetoprotein
α-fetoprotein (AFP) has proved to be a very useful tumor marker in both hepatocellular carcinoma and GCT, where it is produced by the yolk sac cells. AFP may also be elevated in some patients with pancreatic, biliary, gastric, and bronchial cancers. AFP is an important protein of gestation; levels peak at 12–14 weeks of gestation but begin to decline by week 16 and are undetectable after the first year of life (see also Fig. 16.22).

The half life of AFP is 5–7 days.

Human chorionic gonadotrophin
Human chorionic gonadotrophin (hCG) is a glycoprotein with an α and a β subunit secreted by placental syncytiotrophoblasts. Generally the β subunit is measured because it exhibits less homology with other hormones, which can result in false-positive measurements. However, some GCT can produce forms of β-hCG that are not detected by routine antibodies used in radioimmunoassay testing, giving rise to false-negative readings[31].

β-hCG is elevated in pregnancy and in a variety of tumors: breast, kidney, bladder, stomach, liver, biliary tract, hydatidiform mole, and NSGCT as well as a small percentage of seminomas that contain syncytiotrophoblasts.

The half life of β-hCG is 24 hours.

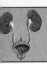

\multicolumn{5}{c}{**Germ cell tumor type, relative incidence, pathology, tumor markers and presentation**}				
GCT	**%**	**Pathology**	**Serum tumor markers**	**Presentation**
Seminoma • Classic • Anaplastic • Spermatocytic	35–70	Classic seminoma – solitary homogeneous tumor with distinct borders. Uniform cells with clear cytoplasm and well defined borders. Lymphocytic infiltrate present. Nuclei are spherical and hyperchromatic with 1–2 enlarged nucleoli. Mitoses are infrequent Anaplastic seminoma – characterized by 3 or more mitotic figures per high power field Lymphocytic infiltrate absent Prognosis not necessarily worse than classic seminoma	PLAP – 90% hCG – <10% (produced by syncytiotrophoblasts found in small numbers of seminomas)	Typically enlarged painless testis (can be 10× normal) Testis is normal or decreased in size in 15% Age range 35–55 years for classic and anaplastic seminomas and >60 years for spermatocytic seminomas Extragonadal sites include mediastinum, pituitary and pineal gland Spermatocytic seminoma – comprises 9% of seminomas, occurs most frequently in men > 40 years of age. In men >65 years this tumor is the most common germ cell tumor. Generally behaves in a benign fashion, very rarely may be associated with a sarcoma, which may metastasize
Embryonal carcinoma (EC)	3–6%	Asymmetric heterogeneous mass Glycogen containing pleomorphic cells with less distinct cell membranes and increased numbers of mitoses Over 40% of GCT of the testis contain embryonal elements Smallest of the germ cell tumors – 40% are less than 2cm in diameter and often in close proximity to the rete testis Vascular and lymphatic invasion may be noted and represent a risk factor for metastatic disease Presence of more than 40% embryonal cell carcinoma in mixed GCT (more than one histologic entity) represents a risk factor for metastatic disease	hCG elevation not due to EC cells but rather to syncytiotrophoblastic cells, which may be present in the stroma hCG elevation does not occur in pure embryonal carcinoma, which does not contain syncytiotrophoblastic cells AFP rarely elevated in pure embryonal carcinoma AFP elevation usually due to yolk sac elements	Hard irregular testis, often normal size. Age range 25–35 years
Teratoma • Mature • Immature • With malignant transformation Simple epidermoid cysts	3% in adults 38% in childhood	By definition composed of two or more embryonic germ cell layers which may be both mature or immature • Endoderm – mucus secreting glands (may degenerate into adenocarcinoma) • Mesoderm – cartilage, bone, muscle or lymphoid tissue • Ectoderm – stratified squamous epithelium and neural tissue Tumor very heterogeneous with both solid and cystic components Divided into three subsets: 1. Mature: well differentiated ecto, meso or endodermal tissues 2. Immature: incompletely differentiated tissues 3. Teratoma with areas of malignant degeneration: sarcoma, squamous carcinoma, adenocarcinoma Simple epidermoid cysts – keratinizing, stratified squamous cell lined cysts supported by fibrous tissue are therefore not strictly teratomas because only one germ cell layer is present	AFP in 20–25%; seen in areas with mucinous glands and areas of hepatoid differentiation	Age range – first, second, and third decades Mature and immature forms have metastatic potential in adults but in children are uniformly benign Enlarged testis with both solid and cystic components Epidermoid cysts have a uniformly benign course Vascular and lymphatic vessel invasion imparts worse prognosis Metastatic GCT containing teratoma is generally resistant to chemotherapy
Choriocarcinoma	1–2%	Occurs as either pure choriocarcinoma or in tumors with more than one histologic type (mixed GCT) *Pure choriocarcinoma*: hemorrhagic mass with viable tumor at the periphery *Mixed GCT*: hemorrhagic foci with viable tumor in association with other cell types, e.g. embryonal carcinoma Two cells types – *Syncytiotrophoblasts*: large mutinucleated giant cells with multiple irregular nuclei *Cytotrophoblasts*: medium sized closely packed cells with single uniform nucleus	hCG >99%;	Age range second and third decades Testis usually not enlarged Patient may present with manifestations of metastatic disease such as pulmonary insufficiency or features of brain secondaries
Mixed tumors – tumors of more than one histologic type	60%	Cell types may occur in any combination Most frequent mixed tumor is: embryonal cell, yolk sac, teratoma and syncytiotrophoblasts Cell types and their relative contributions to tumor volume should be documented	Depends on the cell types; usually AFP due to yolk sac elements and hCG due to syncytiotrophoblasts	Age range second and third decades

Figure 29.9 Germ cell tumor type, relative incidence, pathology, tumor markers, and presentation. AFP, α-fetoprotein; GCT, germ cell tumor; hCG, human chorionic gonadotrophin; PLAP, placental alkaline phosphate.

Non-germ cell tumor type, relative incidence, pathology, tumor markers, presentation and treatment			
Tumor type	Pathology	Presentation	Treatment
Sex cord and stromal tumors			
Leydig cell tumor (1–3% of testis tumors)	Homogeneous well-circumscribed tumor characterized by hexagonal cells with pathognomonic cigar-shaped crystals in the cytoplasm – Reinke crystals – found in 40% of tumors 10% are malignant – necrosis and hemorrhage should raise this suspicion; most malignant tumors are 6–10cm	In adults clinical features of both excessive androgen or estrogen production may be present; gynecomastia may be present before a testicular mass is palpable All children with Leydig cell tumors manifest signs and symptoms of excessive androgen production	Radical inguinal orchiectomy is the initial treatment of choice; if there are histopathologic features of malignancy then RPLND is an option Virilizing and feminizing features may take a while to resolve and therefore initial persistence is not an indication of metastatic disease
Sertoli cell tumor (less than 1% of testis tumors)	Homogeneous tumor, medium-sized cells, round nuclei and distinct nuclear membrane Essential diagnostic feature: epithelial cells representing Sertoli cells, and varying amounts of stroma 10–20% are malignant – vascular invasion	Most often in patients under the age of 40 years; vary in size from 1cm to 20 cm Metastases to both retroperitoneal lymph nodes and viscera occur	Radical inguinal orchiectomy is the initial treatment of choice and cures 80–90% of patients If there are histopathologic features of malignancy, then RPLND may have therapeutic benefit
Mixed germ cell and stromal tumor			
Gonadoblastoma (less than 0.5% of testis tumors)	Mixed tumor containing large germ cells similar to seminoma and small cells similar to Sertoli cells; Leydig cells may also be present	Associated with dysgenetic gonads – either a streak gonad or testis; 80% of patients are phenotypic females – usually present with primary amenorrhea and sometimes with a lower abdominal mass High incidence of bilaterality	Radical inguinal orchiectomy and contralateral orchiectomy when gonadal dysgenesis is present on that side

Figure 29.10 Non-germ cell tumor type, relative incidence, pathology, tumor markers, and presentation.

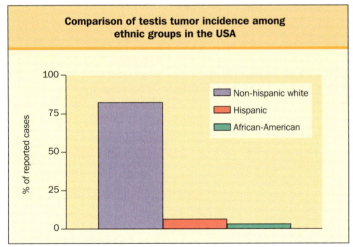

Figure 29.11 Comparison of testis tumor incidence among ethnic groups in the USA.

Lactate dehydrogenase

Lactate dehydrogenase (LDH), which is expressed in numerous organs, has four subtypes, of which LDH-1 is the most frequently measured. Although LDH is elevated in some patients with seminoma, the sensitivity is limited, as a result of which, clinical usefulness with respect to decision making is unfortunately also limited. LDH does, however, correlate with bulk of disease[32].

Placental alkaline phosphatase

Although placental alkaline phosphatase (PLAP) was initially thought to be a useful tumor marker in seminomas, enthusiasm for it has waned. PLAP may be elevated in low- and high-stage seminomas but the sensitivity is low because of false positives, which occur in other tumors such as breast, lung, and ovary as well as in cigarette smokers.

Other tumor markers

There are a number of other tumor markers such as carcino-embryonic antigen (CEA) and neuron-specific enolase, which, although raised in some patients with GCT, have proved to be unreliable in terms of clinical decision making.

STAGING AND IMAGING OF TESTIS CANCER

Testis cancer is generally staged clinically and radiologically, and frequently by surgical means as well. Clinical staging is associated with a degree of error whereby patients may be understaged.

Clinical staging

Clinical staging includes local and regional examination as well as a thorough general examination for metastatic disease, which should always include careful palpation of the supraclavicular fossae. Scrotal examination provides information regarding both the size and local extent of the primary tumor, especially with respect to spread through the tunica albuginea into epididymis, spermatic cord, or scrotal wall, in which case inguinal lymph nodes should be carefully palpated.

Imaging in testis cancer
Ultrasound

Scrotal ultrasound (US) has now become an extension of the physical examination but should never be considered a substitute for it. Scrotal US can distinguish with a very high degree of accuracy intra- from extratesticular lesions, and furthermore can detect intratesticular lesions as small as 1–2mm in diameter. While seminomas are characterized as well-defined hypoechoeic lesions without cystic areas, NSGCT are more typically inhomogeneous, with calcification, cystic areas, and indistinct margins[33]. Because the tunica albuginea is difficult to discern with US, local T staging has proved to be unreliable with this technique[34].

Magnetic resonance imaging

In contrast to US, the tunica albuginea can easily be distinguished by magnetic resonance imaging (MRI), which therefore offers improved local T staging. If performed, MRI demonstrates a mass that is relatively isointense on T1-weighted images and hypointense on T2-weighted images with brisk and early enhancement after intravenous gadolinium. High-resolution MRI with surface coils may provide useful information in selected patients with atypical masses, especially in those patients where US proves inconclusive[35].

Computed tomography scanning

Computed tomography (CT) scanning is the imaging modality of choice for the retroperitoneum, although there is a significant false-negative rate caused by the fact that CT cannot detect micrometastases. False-negative rates of up to 44% have been reported[36]. Furthermore, the cutoff value used to determine an abnormal node also has an important bearing on clinical decision making. Higher cutoffs (>15mm) yield higher false negatives, thus unnecessarily delaying therapy, while lower cutoffs (<5mm) subject some patients to unnecessary therapy[37]. This problem has far-reaching implications with respect to patients placed on surveillance protocols.

Chest X-ray

Accurate staging of the chest is essential in testis cancer patients because the chest is the most common site of involvement after the retroperitoneal lymph nodes. A variety of imaging studies have been used to evaluate the chest, including chest X-ray, whole lung tomography, and CT scanning. While intuitively it would seem that CT scanning would be more accurate than chest X-ray in terms of detecting metastatic disease, this has in fact been shown not to be the case. For this reason, chest X-ray is still considered the imaging technique of choice for evaluating pulmonary metastases in testis tumors[38].

Surgical staging
Orchiectomy and RPLND

Following orchiectomy, evaluation of the primary tumor and radiologic staging of the retroperitoneum, a subset of patients with low-stage NSGCT (T1–3 N0–2 M0) undergo RPLND, which is still the gold standard for providing accurate pathologic staging of the retroperitoneum. Currently available clinical staging techniques are associated with a 15–30% error rate, and therefore RPLND remains the only reliable means of identifying the subset of patients with micrometastases in retroperitoneal lymph nodes.

Staging systems

Although numerous staging systems are currently employed, the majority are a variation on the system employed by Boden and Gibb in 1951[39]. For clinical purposes patients with testis tumors are generally referred to as having either low-stage or advanced-stage disease (Fig. 29.12).

Low-stage disease:
- Disease confined to the testis, epididymis or spermatic cord (T1–T3).
- Minimal retroperitoneal lymph node involvement (N1 and N2).

Changes in staging for stage I testicular tumors: 1997 AJCC staging system				
Primary tumor (pT)				
pTX	Primary tumor cannot be assesed (if no radical orchiectomy has been performed, TX is used)			
pT0	No evidence of primary tumor (e.g. histologic scar in testis)			
pTis	Intratubular germ cell neoplasia (carcinoma-in-situ)			
pT1	Tumor limited to the testis and epididymis without vascular/lymphatic invasion; tumor may invade into the tunica albuginea but not the tunica vaginalis			
pT2	Tumor limited to the testis and epididymis with vascular/lymphatic invasion, or tumor extending through the tunica albuginea with involvement of tunica vaginalis			
pT3	Tumor invades the spermatic cord with or without vascular/lymphatic invasion			
pT4	Tumor invades the scrotum with or without vascular/lymphatic invasion			
Serum tumor markers (S)				
SX	Marker studies not performed			
S0	Markers normal			
S1	LDH <1.5× normal *and* hCG <5,000mIU/mL *and* AFP <1,000ng/mL			
S2	LDH 1.5–10× normal *or* hCG =5,000–50,000mIU/mL *or* AFP =1,000–10,000ng/mL			
S3	LDH >10× normal *or* hCG >50,000mIU/mL *or* AFP >10,000ng/mL			
Stage grouping for stage I testicular cancer				
Stage I	pT1–4	N0	M0	SX
Stage IA	pT1	N0	M0	S0
Stage IB	pT2–4	N0	M0	S0
Stage IS	Any T	N0	M0	S1–3

Figure 29.12 Changes in staging for stage I testicular tumors: 1997 American Joint Committee on Cancer (AJCC) staging system. AFP, α-fetoprotein; hCG, human chronic gonadotrophin, LDH, lactate dehydrogenase. (From Fleming ID, et al. AJCC cancer staging manual, 5th edn. Philadelphia; Lippincott-Raven; 1997.)

Advanced-stage disease:
- Disease involving the scrotal wall (T4).
- High-volume retroperitoneal lymph node disease (N3).
- Presence of visceral metastases (M1).

PREDICTION OF METASTATIC POTENTIAL

Nonseminomatous germ cell tumors

Most patients with NSGCT present with clinical stage I disease. However, it is well known that 30–50% of this subset of patients may have clinically undetectable metastatic disease, and for this reason predictors of occult metastatic disease have been developed to offer the patient the highest chance of cure with the lowest possible morbidity[40]. There are a number of important factors that predict likelihood of relapse in retroperitoneal nodes, or of late recurrence in clinical stage I NSGCT:
- vascular or lymphatic invasion;
- extent of primary tumor – T stage;
- embryonal carcinoma – 30–40% of total tumor volume;
- absence of yolk sac tumor.

In one study the presence of three risk factors correlated with a 58% relapse rate at 2 years followup[41]. Treatment decisions can be individualized based on these risk factors: in other words, patients with low risk of metastatic disease may undergo surveillance while patients with significant risk of occult metastatic disease may be given the option of undergoing either RPLND or chemotherapy.

However, despite the prognostic criteria, it is still not possible to establish highly accurate distinctions between high- and low-risk patients with clinical stage I NSGCT. Moreover, the patients with high-risk stage I disease constitute less than 25% of patients with testicular cancer and account for less than half of relapses[41].

Seminomas

Surveillance studies in stage I seminoma patients report a 4-year actuarial rate of relapse after orchiectomy alone of approximately 20% of patients[42]. A number of risk factors for relapse in low-stage seminomas have been reported:

- tumor size
- vascular and lymphatic invasion
- elevated β-hCG.

Univariate analysis revealed that tumor size, histologic subtype, presence of necrosis, and invasion of rete testis were predictive of recurrence, but only tumor size was a statistically significant predictor on multivariate analysis[42]. In this study 36% of patients with tumors larger than 6cm in diameter relapsed[42]. Other risk factors such as vascular invasion and elevated β-hCG have also been shown to be risk factors for relapse[43,44].

FERTILITY IN PATIENTS WITH TESTIS CANCER

- Testis cancer affects young adult men; therefore, fertility becomes an important issue.
- Approximately 25% of patients have defects in spermatogenesis at the time of presentation[45].
- Higher concentrations of antisperm antibodies are present in the serum of patients with testis cancer than in the normal population[45].
- Approximately 50% of patients are at least temporarily hypofertile postorchiectomy prior to any adjuvant therapy. This may be caused by a variety of factors, such as stress, hormone production by the tumor, and surgical trauma to one testicle that may have an adverse effect on the contralateral testicle.
- Fertility can be further impaired by adjuvant therapy (RPLND, radiation therapy (RT), and chemotherapy).
- Some 50% of patients who receive chemotherapy experience return of normal sperm counts by 2 years, while 25% continue to remain azoospermic after chemotherapy.
- The best measurement of fertility is pregnancy. One study reported that only 35% of patients achieved paternity following chemotherapy. On the other hand, the Indiana group reported a 76% paternity rate following RPLND for clinical stage I NSGCT[46,47].
- Cryopreservation of semen is therefore applicable to patients who undergo chemotherapy. Recent developments such as intracytoplasmic sperm injection, however, may make sperm banking less relevant in the future.

PRINCIPLES OF TREATING TESTIS CANCER

Radical inguinal orchiectomy

The decision to proceed to radical inguinal orchiectomy is taken after careful consideration of all the available data, including the clinical findings, imaging studies and tumor markers. This procedure should be performed through an inguinal approach without scrotal violation, which may preclude a patient from a surveillance protocol. In those patients with elevated serum tumor markers prior to radical orchiectomy, tumor markers should be checked on a weekly basis in the postoperative period to document the postorchiectomy decline in levels of tumor markers. In some patients, persistence of tumor markers after the period during which normalization is expected to occur may be the only evidence of persistent occult disease.

We generally do not delay radical orchiectomy in patients with clinically advanced disease, for two reasons: first, the testis has been shown to be a privileged site with respect to its ability to harbor viable tumor despite chemotherapy; and second, chemotherapy in our experience does not impair wound healing following radical orchiectomy.

Principles of surveillance in stage I testis cancer

Surveillance protocols require a strong commitment from both patient and physician alike. Although the optimal followup protocol for patients on surveillance has not been determined, various protocols have developed over time:

- **First 3 years**: patient seen at 4-monthly intervals for:
  - Physical examination
  - CT scan abdomen and pelvis
  - Chest X-ray
  - Tumor markers
- **Years 4–7**: patient seen at 6-monthly intervals for:
  - Physical examination
  - CT scan abdomen and pelvis
  - Chest X-ray.

Seminoma

Postorchiectomy treatment options in patients with seminoma include adjuvant RT and surveillance. Currently, adjuvant RT remains the treatment of choice, despite the fact that majority of seminoma patients present with clinical stage I disease. However, the success of surveillance protocols for low-stage NSGCT have encouraged the use of surveillance protocols in stage I seminoma patients as well. In addition, although acute morbidity from low-dose adjuvant therapy is minimal, reports of long-term side-effects such as infertility and gastrointestinal complications, and the possible induction of second malignancies, have prompted a review of the approach that subjects all stage I seminoma patients to adjuvant RT[42,48-50].

The available data from surveillance and adjuvant RT series suggest that almost 100% of patients with stage I seminoma are cured, whichever approach is selected postorchiectomy. Surveillance is advantageous both in terms of reducing short- and long-term morbidity as well as because survival appears not to be compromised. To date, only 4 deaths have been reported among 826 patients in surveillance studies with stage I seminoma. Nevertheless, surveillance protocols mandate careful and long-term followup, and seminoma patients are disadvantaged by the fact that a reliable serum tumor marker does not exist for this disease.

More work needs to be done in the area of developing risk factors for relapse, which should enable more physicians to feel comfortable with this option[51,52]. Meantime, it seems appropriate for patients with tumors less than 6cm in diameter, absence of vascular invasion, and normal β-hCG levels to be given the option of surveillance. With further research it may be possible to refine treatment options for individual patients on the basis of highly reliable prognostic factors for relapse

Non-seminomatous germ cell tumor

Ultimate patient survival in NSGCT appears to be slightly less in patients who undergo surveillance than those who elect RPLND. Despite this, centers in the USA generally advocate either surveillance or RPLND.

Surveillance is appropriate in patients with clinical stage I disease, without any risk factors for relapse, who are motivated to rigidly adhere to a surveillance protocol and who fully understand the risks of failure to comply with the followup schedule. In general, the relapse rate with surveillance is 28% and most relapses occur at a median of 6 months. However, relapses beyond 2 years have been described, something that needs to be borne in mind when planning the duration of surveillance protocols. Patients with poor prognostic features have relapse rates on surveillance of around 50%.

ADJUVANT THERAPY FOLLOWING RADICAL ORCHIECTOMY

- Surgery – RPLND
- RT
- Chemotherapy.

Principles of retroperitoneal lymph node dissection in germ cell tumor of the testis
Retroperitoneal lymph node dissection-I

This operation is advocated in patients with NSGCT who have at least one risk factor for micrometastases in retroperitoneal lymph nodes (vascular invasion, embryonal carcinoma [volume >40%], T2 or T3 stage), with no radiological features of spread to the retroperitoneum. In addition, at the time of exploratory laparotomy there must be no evidence of retroperitoneal lymph node involvement. In other words, RPLND-I is confined to patients with clinical stage I disease, only if clinical staging is confirmed intraoperatively. The surgical technique employed is either a template or nerve-sparing technique (Figs 29.13 & 29.14). Therefore, sympathetic nerves responsible for emission and antegrade ejaculation are preserved in the vast majority of patients undergoing this dissection.

Reported survival rates for patients with stage I NSGCT disease (confined to the testis) who undergo RPLND approach 100%, even though the relapse rate is 6–14%[53,17]. Relapses following a well-performed RPLND-I almost always occur outside the retroperitoneum and these patients are invariably salvaged by chemotherapy. For this reason pathologic stage I disease does require post-RPLND surveillance (CT scan abdomen and pelvis once a year for 3 years), albeit far less intense than in those patients who undergo surveillance following radical orchiectomy alone.

Template dissections rely on the predictable stepwise fashion in which GCTs metastasize to the retroperitoneum. For right-sided tumors, the dissection encompasses the right renal hilar

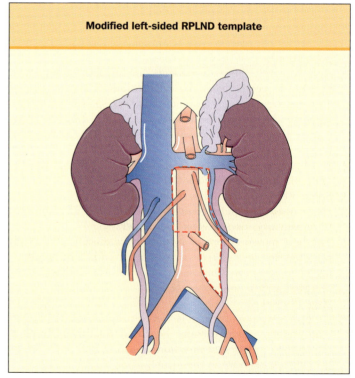

Modified right-sided RPLND template

Figure 29.13 Modified right-sided retroperitoneal lymph node dissection (RPLND) template. The dissection is complete above the level of the inferior mesenteric artery but is limited to the ipsilateral side below the level of the inferior artery.

Modified left-sided RPLND template

Figure 29.14 Modified left-sided retroperitoneal lymph node dissection (RPLND) template.

area, extends inferiorly medial to the ureter to the level of the common iliac artery, then superomedially initially on the anterior surface of the common iliac artery, then on the aorta (sparing the origin of the inferior mesenteric artery), to the level of the left renal vein; the dissection is completed by closing the template superiorly by skeletonizing the left renal vein and right renal artery proximally. To gain access to nodes anterior to the anterior spinous ligament, both lumbar arteries and veins are carefully ligated and divided where necessary to enhance exposure posteriorly. It is important to bear in mind that 30% of all positive nodes are posterior to the great vessels and therefore no dissection is complete without removing all tissue in this region. In stage I and IIA disease, suprahilar spread is rare but can occur in up to 30% of patients with stage IIB disease, especially in left-sided tumors.

For left-sided tumors, the template does not cross the midline because left-to-right spread is rare (unlike right-to-left spread); instead, the margin of dissection passes inferiorly down the right anterolateral aspect of the aorta then medially to skirt the origin of the inferior mesenteric artery, inferolaterally along the anterior aspect of the common iliac artery to the ureter, then superiorly along the medial edge of the ureter. Just as with right-sided tumors, lumbar vessels are ligated where necessary to excise all tissue within the template behind the great vessels.

Nerve-sparing dissections employ a technique whereby postganglionic sympathetic fibers within the template of dissection are prospectively identified and preserved while nodal tissue is teased out from around these delicate structures. Template dissections spare the contralateral sympathetic fibers while nerve-sparing dissections spare both ipsi- and contralateral postganglionic sympathetic fibers.

Therefore, in both template and nerve sparing dissections, sympathetic nerves responsible for emission and antegrade ejaculation are preserved in the vast majority of patients[19].

Reported survival rates for patients with pathologic stage I NSGCT disease who undergo RPLND approach 100%, even though the relapse rate is 6–14%[54]. Relapses following a well-performed RPLND-I almost always occur outside the retroperitoneum and these patients are invariably salvaged by chemotherapy. For this reason, pathologic stage I disease does require post-RPLND surveillance, albeit far less intense than in those patients who undergo surveillance following radical orchiectomy alone.

Retroperitoneal lymph node dissection-II

This operation is performed in patients with low-volume NSGCT with clinically demonstrable disease or visible disease at the time of surgery, i.e. clinical stage IIA or IIB disease. Pathologic stage II disease is found in 25–30% of patients who undergo RPLND for clinical stage I disease.

The surgical boundaries are wider than in RPL-I, usually bilateral, both above the renal arteries and below the inferior mesenteric artery. Every attempt is made to preserve both the lumbar sympathetics and the hypogastric plexus, resulting in preservation of normal ejaculation, in experienced hands, in the majority of patients undergoing RPLND-II (Figs 29.15 & 29.16).

The risk of relapse following RPLND-II approaches 30% and depends on the volume of involved retroperitoneal lymph nodes. Once again, relapse usually occurs outside the retroperitoneum when RPLND-II is well performed.

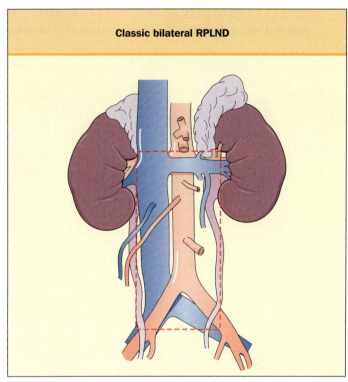

Classic bilateral RPLND

Figure 29.15 Classic bilateral retroperitoneal lymph node dissection (RPLND). See text for details.

Laparoscopic retroperitoneal lymph node dissection

Although laparoscopic RPLND has been shown to be an effective staging procedure, its role as a therapeutic operation is currently unknown[55]. This procedure may have a role in low-stage disease; however, in its present form it appears to have little if any role for residual disease following chemotherapy[56].

Advantages of retroperitoneal lymph node dissection for low-stage non-seminomatous germ cell tumor

- RPLND provides accurate pathologic staging.
- RPLND has proven therapeutic benefit: Donohue reviewed 464 patients who underwent RPLND for low-stage NSGCT. The majority of patients with retroperitoneal lymph node involvement did not relapse[57].
- Patient followup after RPLND involves only tumor markers and chest X-rays; relapse is rare and usually curable with chemotherapy.
- Adjuvant chemotherapy for stage II disease consists of only two cycles of chemotherapy as opposed to 3 or 4 cycles given to patients who elect primary chemotherapy for clinical stage II NSGCT.
- RPLND in experienced hands is associated with extremely low morbidity, both in the short and long term[58].

Principles of surgical management of advanced germ cell tumor

Retroperitoneal lymph node dissection-III

Approximately 30% of patients with advanced NSGCT will experience only a partial remission (defined as normal tumor markers in combination with radiographic evidence of disease in the chest, abdomen, mediastinum, neck, or elsewhere),

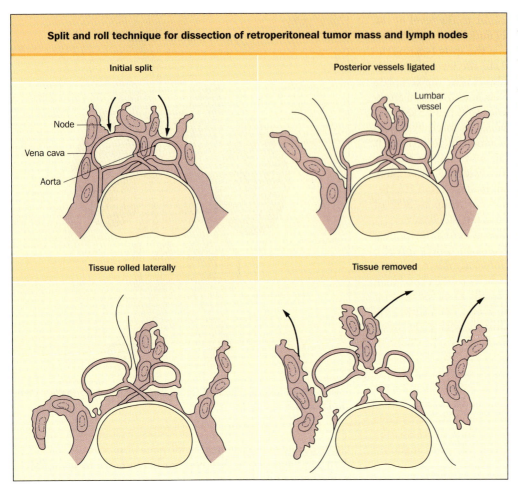

Split and roll technique for dissection of retroperitoneal tumor mass and lymph nodes

Initial split	Posterior vessels ligated

Node
Vena cava
Aorta

Lumbar vessel

Tissue rolled laterally	Tissue removed

Figure 29.16 Split and roll technique for dissection of retroperitoneal tumor mass and lymph nodes. (Top left) the tissue overlying the great vessels is split in longitudinal fashion. (Top right) the lumbar veins and arteries where necessary are ligated to improve exposure and to obtain access to the tissue overlying the anterior spinous ligament. (Bottom left) The tissue is rolled laterally. (Bottom right) En bloc removal of right, left and central tissue bundles. (Reproduced with permission from Gillenwater JT, Grayhack JT, Howard SS, Duckett JW. Adult and pediatric urology, 3rd edn. London: Mosby International; 1995.)

following cisplatin-based chemotherapy. These patients are therefore candidates for resection of residual disease, in addition to those patients who experience retroperitoneal recurrence following incomplete RPLND for low-stage disease. This subset of patients may also have pulmonary, mediastinal, brain, and other residual lesions following chemotherapy and are therefore candidates for surgical extirpation of residual disease in these areas as well[59,60].

RPLND-III is performed in both seminoma and NSGCT patients who have failed primary therapy, either primary chemotherapy or primary retroperitoneal node dissection, and who have either retroperitoneal recurrences or a persistent retroperitoneal mass detected radiographically (usually by CT scan).

Essentially, RPLND-III involves both resection of residual mass and bilateral RPLND. On occasion, suprahilar dissection of residual disease is necessary and may even involve dissecting as high as the mediastinum. In some patients, resection of the infrarenal vena cava is sometimes necessary, and in addition, aortic tube grafts may be required to replace aortic segments that are surrounded by tumor or damaged by subadventitial dissection[61]. Needless to say, RPL-III is neither for the inexperienced surgeon nor the faint-hearted, especially in view of the fact that incomplete excision may expose the patient to further resections in the future (Fig. 29.17).

Advantages of retroperitoneal lymph node dissection-III for low-stage non-seminomatous germ cell tumor
- Evaluates the response to chemotherapy.
- Removes viable GCT teratoma and therefore improves chances for cure.
- Provides essential information for the future management of the patient.

Persistent or recurrent retroperitoneal mass: histopathology and implications
Early retrospective studies revealed that RPLND-III defines three subsets of patients based on histopathologic analysis of the resected specimen:
- 40% – necrosis/fibrosis;
- 40% – adult teratoma;
- 20% – residual NSGCT[62,63].

Therefore, approximately 60% of patients with evidence of a residual mass on postchemotherapy imaging studies will have either viable cancer or teratoma. A more recent study showed that the likelihood of malignancy in postchemotherapy resected tumor was 13%, with the remainder of tumor specimens containing teratoma or necrosis[64].

The finding of only necrotic/fibrotic tissue implies that no further treatment is required, while patients with viable GCT require additional chemotherapy[65].

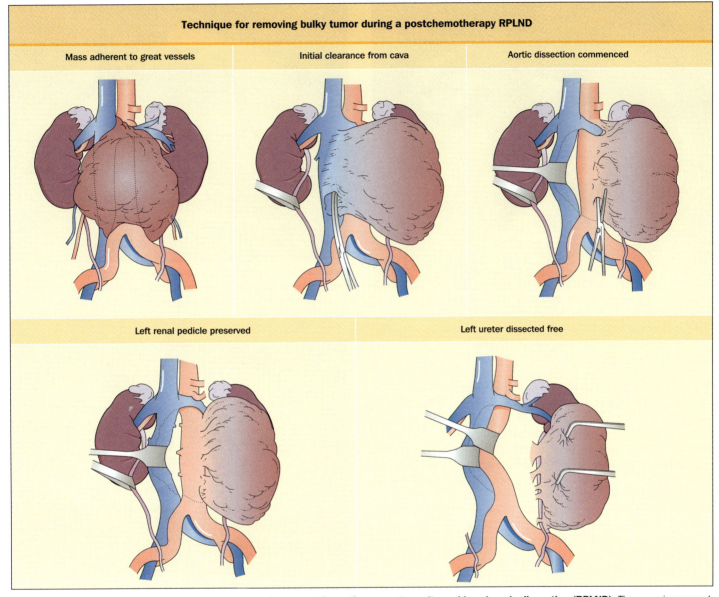

Figure 29.17 Technique for removing bulky tumor during a postchemotherapy retroperitoneal lymph node dissection (RPLND). The mass is removed by separating it anterior to the great vessels and ureters. Once the mass has been resected a standard full bilateral RPLND is performed. (Reproduced with permission from Gillenwater JT, Grayhack JT, Howard SS, Duckett JW. Adult and pediatric urology, 3rd edn. London: Mosby International; 1995.)

The rationale to resect residual teratoma is multifactorial:
- Growing teratoma syndrome – indolent teratoma growth may compromise vital organ function[66] (Fig. 29.18).
- Malignant transformation of mature teratoma to sarcoma and adenocarcinoma which is resistant to chemotherapy has been well described[67].
- Embryonal carcinoma – viable GCT has been described in both mature and immature[68].
- Chemotherapy and radiotherapy are ineffective against benign or malignant teratoma.

Indications for retroperitoneal lymph node dissection-III
Seminoma
Fortunately, the occurrence of residual mass after chemotherapy for pure seminoma is rare. There are generally two presentations of a residual mass in seminoma patients after chemotherapy.

First, the tumor has an appearance of a sheet of tissue around the great vessels obliterating radiographic and surgical planes[69]. This form of residual disease merges with the great vessels, psoas muscles, and other retroperitoneal structures, usually represents fibrosis, and is often unresectable[70]. Second, some masses are well delineated and distinct from surrounding structures, and usually resectable. Surgery is justifiable in this setting because these may represent residual seminoma[66]. Current recommendations are that well-delineated postchemotherapy retroperitoneal masses (detected by CT scan) in seminoma patients should be resected if the diameter is more than 3cm.

Non-seminomatous germ cell tumor
Despite the well-described hazards of residual viable GCT in the retroperitoneum following chemotherapy, as well as recurrent retroperitoneal GCT following RPLND-I or RPLND-II, the

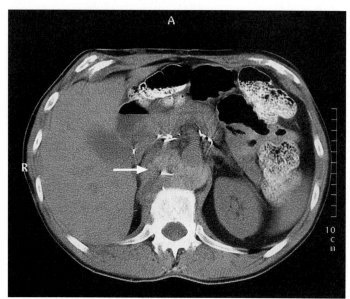

Figure 29.18 Retroperitoneal teratoma. Abdominal computed tomography scan showing large retroperitoneal teratoma extending from the diaphragmatic hiatus to the level of L2 (arrow), the mass is confluent with the aorta and the inferior vena cava. Aortic resection was required to excise this mass completely.

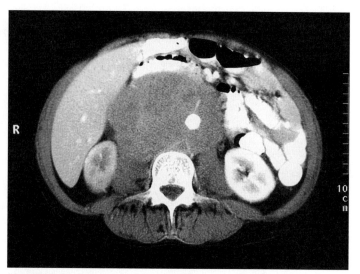

Figure 29.19 Retroperitoneal teratoma. Abdominal computed tomography scan showing a large retroperitoneal mass in a patient with advanced mixed non-seminomatous germ cell tumor.

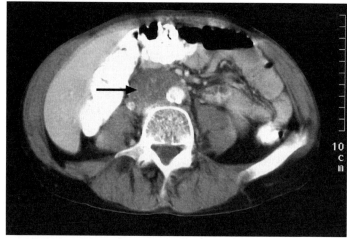

Figure 29.20 Retroperitoneal teratoma. Abdominal computed tomography in the same patient 6 weeks after 3 cycles of bleomycin, etoposide and cisplatin. Note the extent to which the mass has been reduced in size. The vena cava (arrow) is attenuated and compressed against the anterior aspect of the vertebral bodies, and required resection at the time of RPLND-III.

indications for RPLND-III are controversial and there are no clear guidelines. The presence of elevated tumor markers, however, remains the only generally accepted contraindication to adjunctive surgery in patients after chemotherapy[71].

The management of patients whose tumor markers have normalized following chemotherapy ranges from observation, irrespective of the results of imaging studies, to surgery for all patients. A residual mass is usually detected by CT scan following chemotherapy; however, the definition of a normal CT scan differs from one institution to another. Definitions include: no visible mass, lymph nodes no larger than 1cm, and lymph nodes less than 1.5–2cm in diameter[59,72,73].

In view of the well-described complications related to RPLND-III, patient selection plays an important role in excluding those patients who are unlikely to have viable disease (Figs 29.19 & 29.20). Donohue found that, in cases where no teratomatous elements were detected in the primary tumor and a greater than 90% decrease was seen in the volume of retroperitoneal disease by sequential CT scans, viable germ cell tumor or teratoma was not seen in the resected specimen[74,75]. However other reports indicate that predicting the presence or absence of residual viable GCT or teratoma with any degree of accuracy is not possible with currently available technology[59].

In general, despite careful patient evaluation the risk of a false-negative prediction is approximately 20%.

Principles of adjuvant radiation therapy
Seminoma – low stage
Radiation therapy (RT) has long been the standard adjuvant treatment for low-stage seminoma, which is very sensitive to low-dose RT (2,500–3500cGy) and, when given over a 3 week period to the periaortic and ipsilateral inguinopelvic nodes, results in 5-year survival rates of 95% in patients with stage I disease. For patients with stage IIA (retroperitoneal nodal disease <2cm), IIB (retroperitoneal nodal disease 2–5cm) and IIC (retroperitoneal nodal disease >5cm) seminoma, the 5-year relapse rates have been reported as 10%, 18%, and 38% respectively[76].

Therefore seminoma patients who are candidates for RT include patients with stages I, IIA, and IIB disease. Prophylactic treatment of the mediastinum or supraclavicular region is not recommended.

Seminoma – advanced stage
In advanced seminoma, adjuvant RT is sometimes used for patients with residual disease after chemotherapy, especially in patients whose disease appears radiographically to be unresectable.

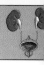

Non-seminomatous germ cell tumor
Relatively higher doses (4,000–5,000cGy) are necessary to treat patients with NSGCT. The attendant long-term morbidity associated with these doses, combined with the fact that NSGCTs are chemotherapy sensitive, has resulted in adjuvant RT falling out of favor as first-line adjuvant therapy for low- and high-stage NSGCT.

Principles of adjuvant chemotherapy
Seminoma – low stage
The success of chemotherapy for high-stage seminoma has led investigators to examine its use in low-stage disease. The role of single-agent carboplatin in stage I disease has been evaluated[77]. The efficacy of this approach has been found to compare favorably with adjuvant RT for low-stage disease. A retrospective comparison of patients' quality of life following adjuvant RT versus adjuvant chemotherapy revealed only minor differences. Therefore, on the basis of this data, a single course of carboplatin as adjuvant therapy for low-stage seminoma patients may in the future gain wider acceptance.

Seminoma – advanced stage
Combination chemotherapy in the form of cisplatin, vinblastine, and bleomycin has proved to be very effective in patients with advanced seminoma. More than 90% of patients who present with stage III disease achieve complete response to chemotherapy alone, and approximately 90% of responders remain disease-free during followup evaluation to 4 years[78,79].

Non-seminomatous germ cell tumor – primary chemotherapy in low-stage disease
A number of published reports have indicated that survival in patients who receive two cycles of bleomycin, etoposide, and cisplatin (BEP) for low-stage NSGCT is between 95% and 100%. None of these studies, however, were randomized against RPLND and selection criteria were not standardized in terms of prognostic risk factors (T stage, vascular invasion, and embryonal carcinoma volume). Nevertheless, survival appears to be comparable to RPLND, and some patients may choose adjuvant chemotherapy over RPLND, especially in those centers where the necessary expertise required to perform RPLND is unavailable. However, the long-term effects in young adults who receive chemotherapy are unclear and for the time being remain a real concern. Chronic toxicity related to chemotherapy generally falls into six categories[80]:
- **Nephrotoxicity**: *cis*-platinum may cause an acute deterioration in renal function, which may persist for up to 1 year and in some cases may prove to be irreversible[81].
- **Cardiovascular**: bleomycin alone or in combination with vinblastine can lead to Raynaud's phenomenon, which is reported in 20–40% of patients. In addition, vascular occlusive disease and alterations in blood lipids have also been described[77].
- **Neurotoxicity**: cisplatin and vinblastine may cause both chronic peripheral neuropathy and impaired auditory function[77].
- **Pulmonary**: bleomycin may cause pneumonitis, which can progress to pulmonary fibrosis. This can be fatal in up to 1–2% of patients, and is of particular concern during surgical procedures under general anesthetic because these patients are sensitive to increases in intravascular volume[82].
- **Second malignancies**: Both second GCT and non-germ-cell malignancies have been described in patients who have undergone therapy for testis cancer. The risk in patients who have received chemotherapy alone is low, while the risk for patients who have undergone chemotherapy and radiotherapy has been reported to be significantly increased over the general population[83].
- **Fertility**: While oligospermia is invariable in young adults receiving chemotherapy, azoospermia has been reported in up to 27% of patients[84]. Although the trend is towards recovery with time, paternity rates have been shown to be adversely affected; in one report only 30% of men were successful[85].

Non-seminomatous germ cell tumor – adjuvant chemotherapy in low-stage disease
Recurrence rates following RPLND for low-stage NSGCT are higher among patients with advanced nodal stage but invariably occur outside the retroperitoneum. In one series 60% of patients with nodal disease greater than 2cm in diameter relapsed[86]. Richie, however, reported a relapse rate of only 8% following RPLND-II, indicating that results from institutions where RPLND is performed frequently may not parallel results form co-operative multicenter trials[87].

There is considerable debate in the literature regarding management of patients with pathologic stage II disease. Patients who undergo surveillance post-RPLND require frequent followup visits, imaging, and laboratory studies. However, fewer than 50% of patients with pathologic stage II disease eventually relapse following RPLND. Therefore a considerable subset of these patients do not require adjuvant chemotherapy[17, 83].

A rational approach to pathologic stage II disease is as follows:
- Low-volume pathologic stage II disease – fewer than six positive nodes all less than 2cm in diameter: surveillance protocol for up to 5 years. Patients who relapse usually require either 4 cycles of EP or 3 cycles of BEP, with salvage rates approximating 100%.
- Higher-volume pathologic stage II disease – more than six positive nodes; any node greater than 2cm in diameter: adjuvant chemotherapy, i.e. 2 cycles of BEP. The relapse rate with this protocol is less than 2%.

In summary, chemotherapy for low-stage NSGCT has been shown to be an effective option but concerns regarding long-term morbidity remain.

Non-seminomatous germ cell tumor – advanced stage
While chemotherapeutic trials were being conducted, it became clear that prognosis varied and that patients should therefore be divided into low (good) risk and high (poor) risk categories. For those patients predicted to have a more favorable outcome, i.e. good risk, the goals have been to maintain high cure rates while reducing treatment-related toxicity[88]. On the other hand, the goal of treating poor-risk patients has been to improve the proportion of patients achieving a complete response, while at the same time achieving tolerable treatment side effects.

The International Germ Cell Cancer Collaborative Group developed a classification of independent prognostic variables following analysis of data from over 5,000 GCT patients[89] (Fig. 29.21). The variables in the model included the number of metastatic sites as well as levels of serum tumor markers β-hCG and LDH. Good and intermediate prognosis disease is also referred to as good-risk disease.

Hopefully the widespread use of a standardized prognostic model will result in more patients benefiting from chemotherapeutic regimens with fewer side effects.

Advanced non-seminomatous germ cell tumor – good risk

Patients with advanced good-risk disease, generally receive either 4 cycles of EP or 3 cycles of BEP. Bleomycin is essential in the treatment of good-risk disease if only 3 cycles of chemotherapy are given. These protocols yield disease-free rates approaching 80–90%[90].

Advanced Non-seminomatous germ cell tumor – poor risk (Fig. 29.21)

The International Germ Cell Consensus Classification of poor prognosis NSGCT includes primary mediastinal site, nonpulmonary metastases, and poor risk markers. These unfortunate patients represent around 10% of NSGCT, and experience a 5-year progression-free survival rate of approximately 40% and an overall 5-year survival rate of 48%. A series of phase III trials examining conventional chemotherapeutic approaches has failed to demonstrate an increase in number of cures[91]. More recently, however, the application of high-dose chemotherapy with autologous bone marrow transplantation (ABMT) or stem cell support has yielded more promising results. Studies have looked at the value of high-dose chemotherapy in patients predicted to fail conventional therapy by prolonged decay of markers[92]. Patients in this latter study received 4 cycles of BEP and then an additional 2 cycles of etoposide and carboplatin with ABMT. Almost 50% of patients were disease free at a median followup of 31 months.

Germ cell consensus classification of good, intermediate, and poor prognosis disease	
Good prognosis	Primary tumor – testis or retroperitoneal and No nonpulmonary visceral metastases and Good markers – all of: AFP <1,000ng/mL, and hCG <5,000IU/L, and LDH <1.5× upper limit of normal
Intermediate prognosis	Primary tumor – testis or retroperitoneal and No nonpulmonary visceral metastases and Intermediate markers – any of: AFP >1,000 and <10,000ng/mL, or hCG >5,000 and <50,000IU/L, or LDH >1.5× and <10× upper limit of normal
Poor prognosis	Mediastinal primary or Nonpulmonary visceral metastases or Poor markers – any of: AFP >10,000ng/mL, or hCG >50,000IU/L, or LDH >10× upper limit of normal

Figure 29.21 Germ cell consensus classification of good, intermediate, and poor prognosis disease. AFP, α-fetoprotein; hCG, human chorionic gonadotrophin; LDH, lactate dehydrogenase.

In addition, peripheral blood stem cell support has been used in combination with high-dose chemotherapy. In a study involving 77 poor-risk patients, dose escalation of chemotherapy was combined with granulocyte–macrophage colony stimulating factor (GM-CSF). Overall 67% of patients achieved progression-free survival[93].

In summary, there is no regimen based on conventional chemotherapy that has been shown to significantly improve survival of patients with poor-risk GCT. Current trials involving 2 cycles of BEP followed by 2 cycles of high dose chemotherapy, with stem cell or ABMT rescue, are eagerly awaited[94].

Pathology presentation and treatment of carcinoma-in-situ of the testis			
Preinvasive GCT	**Pathology**	**Presentation**	**Treatment**
Carcinoma in situ (CIS)	CIS cells are located on the basement membrane of the seminiferous tubule and possess morphologic features of malignancy – large irregular nucleus, coarse chromatin, and abundant cytoplasm Typically only one layer of CIS cells is seen, but occasionally the whole tubule is filled with CIS cells, which may represent an early stage in progression to GCT	Risk factors for CIS include: • Contralateral gonad in men with unilateral testis cancer – incidence ranges from 2% to 38% • Cryptorchidism • Infertility – infertile men have an incidence of 0.4–1% • Extragonadal GCT – 35–50% incidence of CIS in one or both testes • Intersex individuals with Y chromosome karyotype Testis may be atrophic but is usually normal to palpation Testis biopsy reliably diagnoses CIS because the CIS is almost always found throughout the testis Progression of CIS to invasive disease may take 15 years	Theoretically, with long enough followup, CIS will progress to invasive disease Treatment options include • Orchiectomy • Radiation • Chemotherapy • Observation while observation may be complicated by delayed diagnosis of GCT Low dose radiation is currently being investigated Chemotherapy so far appears to be ineffective against CIS

Figure 29.22 Pathology presentation and treatment of carcinoma-in-situ of the testis. GCT, germ cell tumor.

Chemotherapy for relapsed testis cancer

For the 20–30% of patients who do not achieve complete response to first-line chemotherapy, second-line salvage chemotherapy remains an option. The current standard chemotherapy that serves as a basis for comparison is vinblastine, ifosfamide, and cisplatin (VeIP). Approximately 40% of patients achieve a complete response with ifosfamide-based regimens, which has been found to be durable in approximately 50% of patients[95]. In view of this, ifosfamide is generally considered to be a standard first-line salvage therapy.

Favorable pretreatment prognostic factors for survival to treatment with conventional dose salvage therapy include a prior complete response to cisplatin-based chemotherapy and a testicular primary site.

Prognostic factors that predict an inferior long-term disease-free survival include an initial incomplete response to cisplatin-based chemotherapy and a primary mediastinal site of disease. These factors predict a very poor outcome and the role of standard chemotherapy is thus limited. Aggressive surgery may offer a reasonable alternative, as may radiotherapy, in to addition high-dose chemotherapeutic regimens with ABMT rescue.

Summary pathologies of more unusual testicular tumors are covered in Figures 29.22–29.24. Summary algorithms for the diagnosis and treatment of seminoma and non-seminomatons germ cell tumors are shown in Figures 29.25–29.28.

Pathology, tumor markers, presentation and treatment of yolk sac tumors			
Tumor type	**Pathology**	**Presentation**	**Treatment**
Yolk sac carcinoma (embryonal cell carcinoma of infants and children)	Gross appearance similar to embryonal cell carcinoma; yolk sac elements are found in one third of mixed adult GCT Approximately 75% of pure yolk sac tumors are malignant Four microscopic patterns: • Microcystic and myxomatous-honeycomb appearance • Endodermal sinus – perivascular formations known as Schiller Duval bodies • Solid cellular – small polygonal cells, clear cytoplasm, frequent mitoses	Most common testis tumor in pre pubertal boys. Presentation – slow growing scrotal mass in a young boy. Hydrocele present in 25% of cases AFP is elevated in > 90%	Over 80% of yolk sac tumors are confined to the testis at the time of diagnosis and are cured by radical inguinal orchiectomy Radiographic evidence of low-volume retroperitoneal lymph node involvement best treated by RPLND Advanced disease – chemotherapy Radiotherapy can be used for residual disease that has failed to respond to chemotherapy Overall prognosis good – mean survival is 87% for all stages of disease

Figure 29.23 Pathology, tumor markers, presentation and treatment of yolk sac tumors. AFP, α-fetoprotein; GCT, germ cell tumor; RPLND, retroperitoneal lymph node dissection.

Pathology, presentation and treatment of testicular lymphoma, testicular secondary tumors, adnexal tumors			
Tumor type	**Pathology**	**Presentation**	**Treatment**
Hematopoietic tumors			
Lymphoma	Large homogeneous tumor with marked intertubular and interstitial infiltration with lymphoma cells	Most common testis in men over the age of 50 years Most common secondary neoplasm of the testis Tumors may be primary (cured by radical orchiectomy alone) or secondary and may be unilateral or bilateral	Orchiectomy for primary disease Chemotherapy for secondary lymphoma
Secondary tumors			
Malignant melanoma, lung, skin, gastrointestinal, thyroid, prostate (most common)	Depends on the primary tumor	Depends on stage and site of primary tumor	Depends on stage and site of primary tumor
Tumors of testicular adnexa			
Adenomatoid tumor (most common paratesticular tumor)	Benign tumor, consisting of cells that may resemble endothelium, epithelium, or mesothelium; tumor cells characterized by vacuoles Smooth muscle may be present	Epididymis is most frequent location Within the epididymis globus minor is most frequent site Well-circumscribed 0.5–4cm mass, usually asymptomatic These tumors behave in a benign fashion: metastases have never been reported	Surgical excision
Primary malignant tumors of epididymis Tumors of spermatic cord structures	Sarcomas more common than carcinomas; rhabdomyosarcoma account for >50% Majority are sarcomas – rhabdomyosarcoma accounts for 40% of all paratesticular tumors	Poor prognosis Tumors are distal i.e close to the epididymis and testis and can therefore be difficult to distinguish from primary testicular or epididymal tumors	Surgical excision Combination of surgery, radiotherapy and chemotherapy, depending on stage of disease
Rete testis tumor	Adenocarcinoma	Scrotal mass or scrotal pain; tumor may be concealed by hydrocele	Surgical excision

Figure 29.24 Pathology, presentation and treatment of testicular lymphoma, testicular secondary tumors, adnexal tumors.

Algorithm for treatment of low- and high-stage seminoma

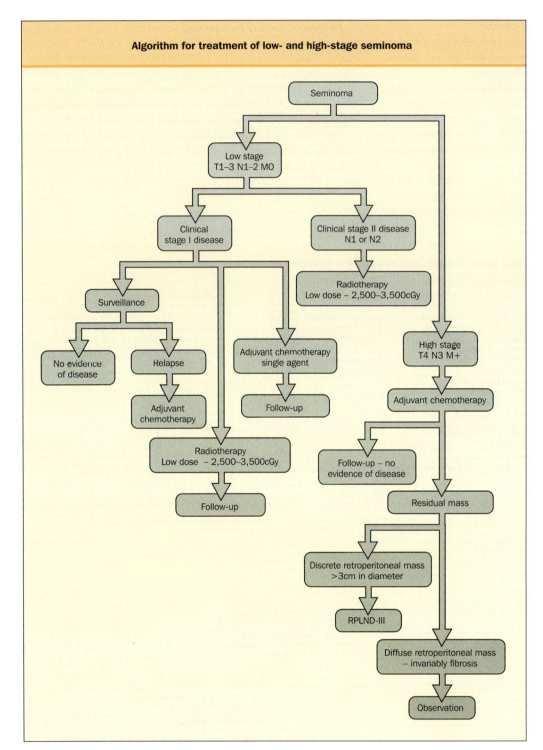

Figure 29.25 Algorithm for treatment of low- and high-stage seminoma.

Algorithm for clinical stage I NSGCT

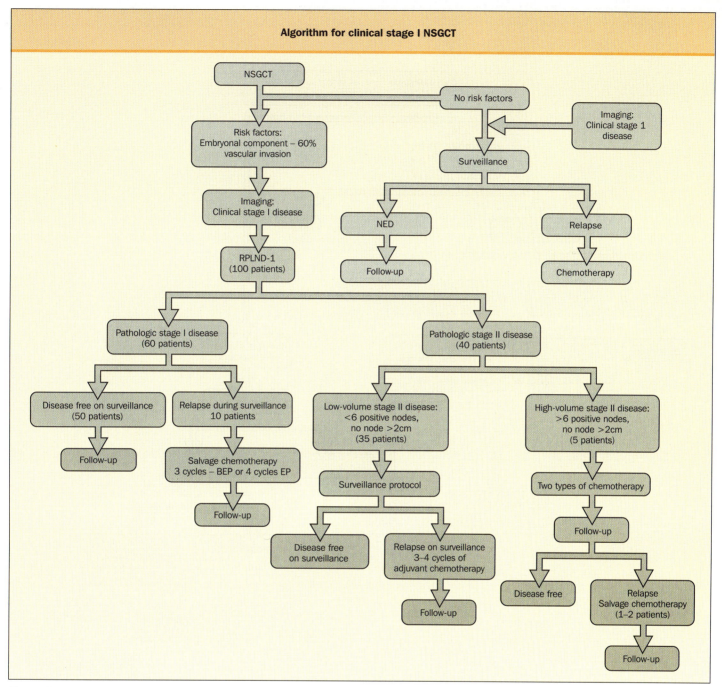

Figure 29.26 Algorithm for clinical stage I non-seminomatous germ cell tumor (NSGCT). BEP, bleomycin, etoposide, and cisplatin; EP, etoposide; NED, no evidence of disease.

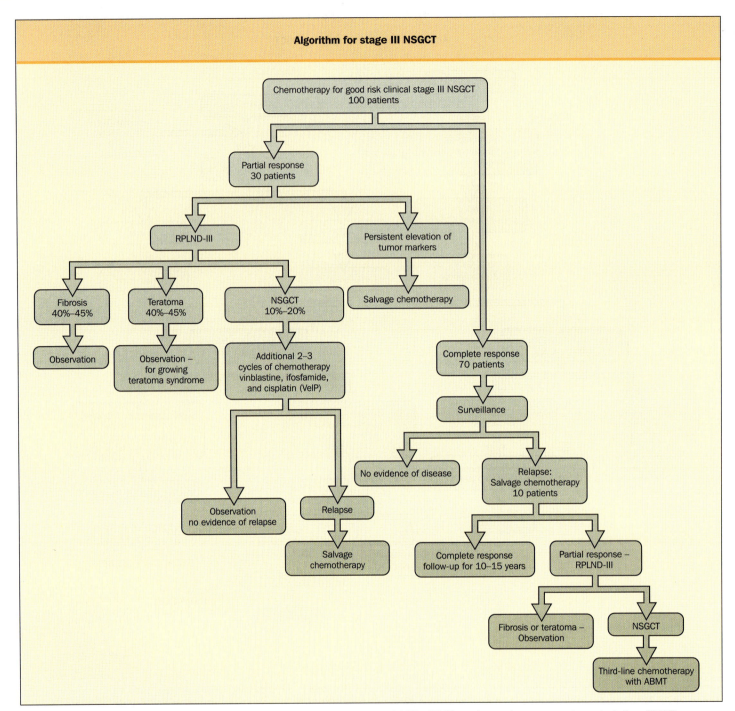

Figure 29.27. Algorithm for stage III non-seminomatous germ cell tumors (NSGCT). ABMT, antologuns bone marrow transplantation; RPLND, retroperitoneal lymph node dissection.

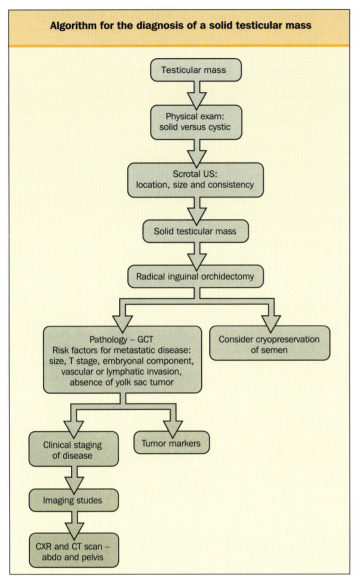

Algorithm for the diagnosis of a solid testicular mass

Figure 29.28 Algorithm for the diagnosis and workup of a solid testicular mass. CT, computed tomography; CXR, chest X-ray; GCT, germ cell tumor; US, ultrasound.

REFERENCES

1.   Einhorn LH. Treatment of testicular cancer: a new and improved model. J Clin Oncol. 1990;8:1777.

2.   Oliver RTD. Clues from the natural history and results of treatment supporting the monoclonal origin of germ cell tumors. Cancer Surv. 1990;9:333.

3.   Bosl GJ, Motzer RJ. Testicular germ cell cancer. N Engl J Med. 1997;337:242.

4.   Levin M. Prognostic features of primary and secondary germ cell tumors. Urol Clin North Am. 1993;20:39.

5.   McCaffrey JA, Bajorin D, Motzer J. Risk assessment for metastatic testis cancer. Urol Clin North Am. 1998;25(3):389–95.

6.   Foster RS, Donohue JP. Can retroperitoneal lymphadenectomy be omitted in some patients after chemotherapy. Urol Clin North Am. 1998;25(3):479–84.

7.   Ong RR, Oliver RT, Badendoch DF, Fowler CG, Hendry WF. Surgery as salvage therapy in chemotherapy-resistant nonseminomatous germ cell tumors. Br J Urol. 1998;81(6):884–8.

8.   Herr HW, Sheinfeld J, Puc HS, et al. Surgery for a post-chemotherapy residual mass in seminoma. J Urol. 1997;157(3):860–2.

9.   International Germ Cell Consensus Classification. A prognostic factor-based staging system for metastatic germ cell cancers. International germ cell cancer collaborative group. J Clin Oncol. 1997;15(2):549.

10. Bajorin DF, Sarosdy MF, Pfister DG, et al. Randomized trial of etoposide and cisplatin versus etoposide and carboplatin in patients with good risk germ cell tumors: a multi-institutional study. J Clin Oncol. 1993;11:598.

11. Bosl GJ, Geller NL, Cirrincione C, Vogelzang NJ, Bosl GJ. Multivariate analysis of prognostic variables in patients with metastatic testicular cancer. Cancer Res. 1983;43:3403.

12. Chevreau C, Droz JP, Pico JL, et al. Early intensified chemotherapy with autologous bone marrow transplantation in first line treatment of poor risk nonseminomatous germ cell tumors. Eur Urol. 1993;23:213.

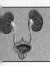

13. Donohue JP, Zachary JM, Maynard BR. Distribution of nodal metastases in nonseminomatous testis cancer. J Urol. 1982;128(2):315–20.

14. Capelouto CC, Clark PE, Ransil BJ, Loughlin KR. A review of scrotal violation in testicular cancer: is adjuvant local therapy necessary? J Urol. 1995;153:981–5.

15. Whitemore WF Jr. Germinal tumors of the testis. In: Proceedings of the Swedish National Cancer Conference. Philadelphia: JB Lippincott; 1973:485.

16. Narayan P, Lange PH, Fraley EE. Ejaculation and fertility after extended retroperitoneal lymph node dissection for testicular cancer. J Urol. 1982;127:685–8.

17. Richie JP. Clinical stage I testicular cancer: the role of modified RPLND. J Urol. 1990;144:1160–3.

18. Donohue JP, Foster RS, Rowland Bihrle R, Jones J, Geier G. Nerve-sparing retroperitoneal lymphadenectomy with preservation of ejaculation. J Urol. 1990;144(2):287–91; discussion 291–2.

19. Gowing NFC. Malignant lymphoma of the testis. In: Pugh RCB, ed. Pathology of the testis. Philadelphia: JB Lippincott; 1976:334–40.

20. Skakkebaek NE. Carcinoma in situ of the testis: frequency in relation to invasive tumors in infertile men. Histopathology. 1978;2:157–62.

21. Templeton CA. Testicular neoplasms in Ugandan Africans. Afr J Med Sci. 1972;3:157–60.

22. Oliver RTD. Clues form the natural history and results of treatment supporting the monoclonal origin of germ cell tumors. Cancer Surv. 1990;9:333–68.

23. Chivlers C, Dudley NE, Gough MH. Undescended testis: the effect of treatment on subsequent risk of subfertility and malignancy. J Pediatr Surg. 1986;21:691–6.

24. Whitaker RH. Management of undescended testis. Br J Hosp Med. 1970;4:25–9.

25. Gilbert JB, Hamilton JB. Studies in malignant testis tumors. Incidence and nature of tumors in ectopic testis. Surg Gynecol Obstet. 1940;71:731–4.

26. Hansen PV, Hansen SW. Gonadal function in men with testicular germ cell cancer: the influence of cis-platin based chemotherapy. Eur Urol. 1993;23(1):153–6.

27. Hoff Wanderas E, Fossa SD, Heilo A, Stenwig AE, Norman N. Serum follicle stimulating hormone – predictor of cancer in the remaining testis in patients with unilateral testis cancer. Br J Cancer. 1990;66:315–7.

28. Parker RG, Holyoke JB. Tumors of the testis. AJR. 1960;83:457–60.

29. Swerdlow AJ, Huttly SRA, Smith PG. Is the incidence of testis cancer related to trauma or temperature? Br J Urol. 1988;61:518–21.

30. Oliver RTD. Atrophy, hormones, genes and viruses in etiology of germ cell tumors. Cancer Surv. 1990;9:263–8.

31. Karman A. Cole LA. Polypeptide nicks cause erroneous results in assays of human chorionic gonadotrophin free beta subunit. Clin Chem. 1992;38:26–30.

32. Klein EA. Tumor markers in testis cancer. Urol Clin North Am. 1993;29:67–73.

33. Benson CB. The role of ultrasound in diagnosing and staging of testis cancer. Semin Urol. 1988;6:189–202.

34. Marth D, Scheidegger J, Studer UE. Ultrasonography of testicular tumors. Urol Int. 1990;45:237–40.

35. Coakley FV, Hedvick H, Presti JC Jr. Imaging and management of atypical testicular masses. Urol Clin North Am. 1998;25(3):375–88.

36. Richie JP, Granick MB, Finberg H. Computerized tomography: how accurate for abdominal staging of testis tumors? J Urol. 1982;127:715–7.

37. Socinski MA, Stomper PC. Radiologic evaluation of nonseminomatous germ cell tumor of the testis. Semin Urol. 1988;6:203–15.

38. Jochelson MS, Garnick MB, Balikian JP, Richie JP. The efficacy of whole lung tomography in germ cell tumors. Cancer. 1984;54:1007–9.

39. Boden G, Gibb R. Radiotherapy and testicular neoplasms. Cancer. 1951;2:1195.

40. Levin M. Prognostic features of primary and metastatic germ cell tumors. Urol Clin North Am. 1993;20(1):39–53.

41. Freedman LS, Parkinson MC, Jones WG, et al. Histopathology in the prediction of relapse of patients with stage I testicular teratoma treated by orchidectomy alone. Lancet. 1987;2(8554):294–8.

42. Von der Maase H, Specht L, Jacobsen GK, et al. Surveillance following orchidectomy for stage I seminoma of the testis. Eur J Cancer. 1993;29A(14):1931–4.

43. Dosmann MA, Zagars GK. Post orchiectomy radiotherapy for stages II and II testicular seminoma. Int J Radiat Oncol Biol Phys. 1993l26:381–90.

44. Marks LB, Rutgers JL, Shipley WU, et al. Testicular seminoma: clinical and pathological features that may predict para-aortic lymph node metastases. J Urol. 1990;143(3):524–7.

45. Lange PH, Chang WY, Fraley EE. Fertility issues in the therapy of non-seminomatous testicular tumors. Urol Clin North Am. 1987;14:731–4.

46. Mansen SW, Berthelsen JG, Von Der Mease H. Long term fertility and Leydig cell function in patients treated for germ cell cancer with cisplatin, vinblastin, bleomycin versus surveillance. J Clin Oncol. 1990;10:1695–9.

47. Foster RS, McNulty A, Rubin LR. The fertility of patients with clinical stage I testis cancer managed by nerve sparing retroperitoneal lymph node dissection. J Urol. 1994;152(4):1139–11.

48. Mason M, Jones W. Treatment of stage I seminoma: more choices, more dilemmas. Clin Oncol. 1997;9:210–2.

49. Van Leeuwen FE, Stiggelbout AM, van den Belt-Dusebout AW, et al. Second cancer risk following testicular cancer: a follow-up study of 1,909 patients. Clin Oncol. 1993;11(3):415–24.

50. Warde PR, Gospodarowicz MK, Goodman PJ, et al. Results of a policy of surveillance in stage I testicular seminoma. Int J Radiat Oncol Biol Phys. 1993;27(1):11–5.

51. Warde P, Jewett MAS. Surveillance for stage I testicular seminoma. Is it a good option? Urol Clin North Am. 1998;25(3):425–33.

52. Fiveash J, Sandler HM. Controversies in the management of stage I seminoma. Oncology. 1998;12(8):1203–21.

53. Pizzocaro G, Salvioni R, Zanoni F. Unilateral lymphadenectomy in intraoperative stage I nonseminomatous germinal testis cancer. Urol. 1985;134(3):485–9.

54. Pizzocaro G, Salvioni R, Zanoni F. Unilateral lymphadenectomy in intraoperative stage I nonseminomatous germinal testis cancer. J Urol. 1985;134(3):485–9.

55. Winfield HN. Laparoscopic retroperitoneal lymphadenectomy for cancer of the testis. Urol Clin North Am. 1998;25(3):469–78.

56. Rassweiler JJ, Seemann O, Henkel TO. Laparoscopic lymph node dissection for nonseminomatous germ cell tumors: indications and limitations. J Urol. 1996;156:1108–13.

57. Donohue JP, Thornhill JA, Foster RS, Rowland RG, Bihrle R. Primary retroperitoneal lymph node dissection in clinical stage A non-seminomatous germ cell testis cancer. Review of the Indiana University experience 1965–1989. Br J Urol. 1993;71(3):326–35.

58. Baniel J, Foster RS, Rowland RG, Bihrle R, Donohue JG. Complications of primary retroperitoneal lymph node dissection. J Urol. 1994;152:424–7.

59. Liu D, Abolhoda A, Burt ME, et al. Pulmonary metastasectomy for testicular germ cell tumors: a 28-year experience. Ann Thorac Surg. 1998;66(5):1709–14.

60. Mahalati K, Bilen CY, Ozen H, Aki FT, Kendi S. The management of brain metastasis in nonseminomatous germ cell tumours. Br J Urol Int. 1999;83(4):45761.

61. Donohue JP, Thornhill JA, Foster RS, Bihrle R. Vascular considerations in post chemotherapy retroperitoneal lymph node dissection: part I – vena cava. World J Urol. 1994;12:182–6.

62. Einhorn LH, Williams SD, Mandelbaum I, Donohue JP. Surgical resection in disseminated testicular cancer following cytoreduction. Cancer. 1981;48: 904–8.

63. Toner G, Panicek DM, Heelan RT, et al. Adjunctive surgery after chemotherapy for nonseminomatous germ cell tumors: recommendations for patient selection. J Clin Oncol. 1990;8:1638–94.

64. Law TM, Motzer RJ, Bajorin DF, Bosl GJ. The management of patients with advanced germ cell tumors. Urol Clin North Am. 1994;24:773.

65. Loehrer PJ, Mui S, Majdu SI. Teratoma following cisplatin based chemotherapy for nonseminomatous germ cell tumors. A clinico-pathologic correlation. J Urol. 1986;135:1189.

66. Logothesis CJ, Samuels ML, Trindade A, Johnson DE. The growing teratoma syndrome. Cancer. 1982;50:1629.

67. Herr HW, LaQuaglia MP. Management of teratoma. Urol Clin North Am. 1993;20:145.

68. Bajorin DF, Herr HW, Motzer RJ, Bosl GJ. Current perspectives on the role of adjunctive surgery in combined modality treatment of patient with germ cell tumors. Semin Oncol. 1992;19:145–58.

69. Friedman EL, Garnick MB, Stomper PC, Much PM, Harrington DP, Richie JP. Therapeutic guidelines and results in advanced seminoma. J Clin Oncol. 1985;3(10):1325–32.

70. Herr HW, Sheinfeld J, Puc HS, et al. Surgery for a post-chemotherapy residual mass in seminoma. J Urol. 1997;157(3):860–2.

71. Levitt MD, Reynolds PM, Steiner M. Nonseminomatous germ cell testicular tumors: residual masses after chemotherapy. Br J Surg. 1985;72:1902.

72. Fossa SD, Ous S, Lien HH, Steinwig AE. Post-chemotherapy lymph node histology in radiologically normal patients with metastatic non-seminomatous testicular cancer. J Urol. 1989;141:557–9.

73. Donohue JP, Foster RS. Management of retroperitoneal recurrences: seminoma and nonseminoma. Urol Clin North Am. 1993;21(4):761–72.

74. Steyerberg EW, Keizer HJ, Fossa SD. Prediction of residual retroperitoneal mass histology after chemotherapy for metastatic NSGCT: multi variate analysis of individual patient data from six study groups. J Clin Oncol. 1995;13:1177.

75. Debono DJ, Heilman DK, Einhorn LH, Donohue JP. Decision analysis for avoiding postchemotherapy surgery in patients with disseminated nonseminomatous germ cell tumors. J Clin Oncol. 1997;15(4):1455–64.

76. Peckham MJ, Barrett A, McElwain TG, Hendry WF, Raghavan D. Non-seminoma germ cell tumours (malignant teratoma) of the testis. Results of treatment and an analysis of prognostic factors. Br J Urol. 1981;53(2):162–72.

77. Krege S, Kalund G, Otto T, Goepel M, Rubben H. Phase II study: adjuvant single-agent carboplatin therapy for clinical stage I seminoma. Eur Urol. 1997;31(4):405–7.

78. Mencel PJ, Motzer RJ, Mazumdar M, Vlamis V, Bajorin DF, Bosl GJ. Advanced seminoma: treatment results, survival, and prognostic factors in 142 patients. J Clin Oncol. 1994;12(1):120–6.

79. Fossa SD, Droz JP, Stoter G, Kaye SB, Vermeylen K, Sylvester R. Cisplatin, vincristine and ifosphamide combination chemotherapy of metastatic seminoma: results of EORTC trial 30874. EORTC GU Group. Br J Cancer. 1995;71(3):619–24.

80. Grossfeld GD, Small EJ. Long-term side effects of treatment for testis cancer. Urol Clin North Am. 1998;25(3):503–15.

81. Boyer M, Raghavan D. Toxicity of treatment of germ cell tumors. Semin Oncol. 1992;19(2):128–42.

82. Donat SM, Levy DA. Bleomycin associated pulmonary toxicity: is perioperative oxygen restriction necessary? J Urol. 1998;160(4):1347–52.

83. Kaldor JM, Day NE, Band P, et al. Second malignancies following testicular cancer, ovarian cancer and Hodgkin's disease: an international collaborative study among cancer registries. Int J Cancer. 1987;39(5):571–85.

84. Nijman JM, Schraffordt Koops H, Kremer J, Sleijfer DT. Gonadal function after surgery and chemotherapy in men with stage II and III nonseminomatous testicular tumors. J Clin Oncol. 1987;5(4):651–6.

85. Hansen SW, Berthelsen JG, von der Maase H. Long-term fertility and Leydig cell function in patients treated for germ cell cancer with cisplatin, vinblastine, and bleomycin versus surveillance. J Clin Oncol. 1990;8(10):1695–8.

86. Williams SD, Stablein DM, Einhorn LH, et al. Immediate adjuvant chemotherapy versus observation with treatment at relapse in pathological stage II testicular cancer. N Engl J Med. 1987;317(23):1433–8.

87. Richie JP, Kantoff PW. Is adjuvant chemotherapy necessary for patients with stage B1 testicular cancer? J Clin Oncol. 1991;9(8):1393–6.

88. Law TM, Motzer RJ, Bajorin DF, Bosl, GJ. The management of patients with advanced germ cell tumors. Urol Clin North Am. 1994;21(4):773–83.

89. Mead GM, Stenning SP. The International Germ Cell Consensus Classification: a new prognostic factor-based staging classification for metastatic germ cell tumours. Clin Oncol (Coll Radiol). 1997;9(4):207–9.

90. Loehrer PJ, Einhorn LH, Elson P. Phase three study of cisplatin (P) plus etoposide (VP-16) with either bleomycin (B) or ifosfamide (I) in advanced stage germ cell tumors (GCT): an intergroup trial. Proc Am Soc Clin Oncol. 1993;12:831.

91. De Wit R, Stoter G, Sleijfer DT, et al. Four cycles of BEP versus an alternating regime of PVB and BEP in patients with poor-prognosis metastatic testicular non-seminoma; a randomized study of the EORTC Genitourinary Tract Cancer Cooperative Group. Br J Cancer. 1995;71(6):1311–4.

92. Motzer RJ, Mazumdar M, Bajorin DF, Bosl GJ, Lyn P, Vlamis V. High-dose carboplatin, etoposide, and cyclophosphamide with autologous bone marrow transplantation in first-line therapy for patients with poor-risk germ cell tumors. J Clin Oncol. 1997;15(7):2546–52.

93. Schmoll HJ, Bokemeyer C. Sequential intermediate high-dose chemotherapy in the primary treatment of poor risk testicular cancer. Bone Marrow Transplant. 1996;18(Suppl 1):S48–9.

94. Dodd PM, Motzer RJ, Bajorin DF. Poor-risk germ cell tumors. Recent developments. Urol Clin North Am. 1998;25(3):485–93.

95. Nichols CR, Tricot G, Williams SD, et al. Dose intensive chemotherapy in refractory germ cell cancer: a phase I/II trial of high dose carboplatin and etoposide with autologous bone marrow transplantation. J Clin Oncol. 1989;7:932.

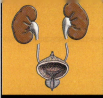

Section 6 Benign Conditions of the Lower Urinary Tract

Chapter 30

Benign Prostatic Hypertrophy and Lower Urinary Tract Dysfunction

D Andrew Jones

KEY POINTS

- Benign prostatic hypertrophy (BPH) is part of the normal male aging process.
- Bladder outflow obstruction (BOO), benign prostatic hypertrophy, and lower urinary tract symptoms are different entities, but may coexist.
- Assessment of lower urinary tract symptoms aims to identify the patient with BOO, who may benefit from treatment to his BPH.
- The majority of patients with BOO caused by BPH are uncomplicated and require symptomatic treatment or no treatment.
- Patients with complicated BOO, such as chronic retention, require surgical treatment of their BPH.
- Transurethral prostatectomy is the 'gold standard' option in cases that require such treatment.

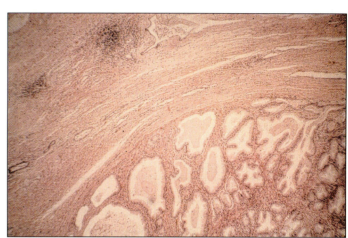

Figure 30.1 Histologic appearances of benign prostatic hypertrophy. Note both glandular and fibromuscular components.

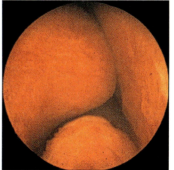

Figure 30.2 Benign prostatic hypertrophy as seen through the cystoscope. Note the enlargement of the lateral lobes that encroach into the prostatic urethra. Verumontanum at six o'clock.

DEFINITIONS

Benign prostatic hypertrophy

The diagnosis of benign prostatic hypertrophy (BPH) is based on histopathology. Prostatic enlargement consists of both glandular and fibromuscular hyperplasia in proportions that vary (Fig. 30.1). The fibromuscular component is innervated by α_1-type adrenergic autonomic nerves[1]. The glandular component is thought to be controlled hormonally[2]. BPH does not occur in the small number of men who have congenital deficiency of the enzyme 5-α-reductase, which is responsible for the conversion within the prostate cell of testosterone into its active metabolite, dihydrotestosterone.

Development of BPH is part of the normal aging process. The transitional zone of the postpubertal prostate slowly enlarges under the influence of the normal male hormonal environment and continues to do so throughout adult life. Approximately 10% of men in their fourth decade and over 90% of those aged 80 years or more have detectable BPH. This can be identified as an enlarged prostate gland on digital rectal examination (DRE), by transrectal ultrasound, or by urethroscopy (Fig. 30.2).

The presence of BPH does not necessarily indicate that bladder outflow obstruction (BOO) is present or that it is the cause of lower urinary tract symptoms.

Bladder outflow obstruction

The diagnosis of BOO requires urodynamic validation. It is present when the relationship between the detrusor pressure during voiding and the urine flow rate indicates impaired transport of urine out of the bladder because of increased outflow resistance. Classically, this produces a high-pressure, low-flow urodynamic situation (Fig. 30.3).

Lower urinary tract symptoms

Bladder outflow obstruction may cause lower urinary tract symptoms, but BOO can also be asymptomatic. Equally, lower urinary tract symptoms may have an alternative cause that coexists with BOO.

Lower urinary tract symptoms are the initial complaint of the patient. They may suggest various diagnoses, and are not specific for BOO or BPH. Indeed, they are present with similar prevalence

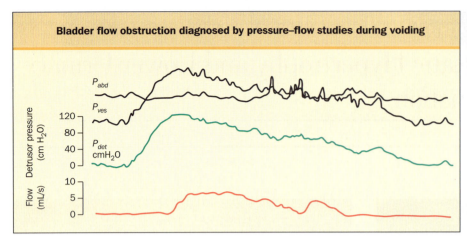

Bladder flow obstruction diagnosed by pressure–flow studies during voiding

Figure 30.3 Bladder outflow obstruction diagnosed by pressure–flow studies during voiding. Note the high detrusor pressure (green) and the low urine flow rate (red). P_{abd}, abdominal pressure; P_{det}, detrusor pressure; P_{ves}, intravesical pressure.

in both sexes. They are very common, and affect one-third and one-half of men over 55 and over 65 years of age, respectively.

Thus, the relationship between BPH, BOO, and lower urinary tract symptoms is complex. Each may exist separately or in combination with either or both of the others (Fig. 30.4).

PATIENT ASSESSMENT

Patients present with lower urinary tract symptoms. Evaluation is designed to ascertain which patients have BOO and, of these, which patients have complicated disease that requires surgical treatment of their BPH. Evaluation must also identify urologic causes other than BOO and/or BPH, that account for lower urinary tract symptoms, such as bladder tumors and prostatic carcinomas. Nonurologic causes of lower urinary tract symptoms should also be sought and appropriate management initiated.

History and examination

Figure 30.5 indicates the important features to ascertain from the patient history. Symptom score sheets, such as the International Prostate Symptom Score (IPSS) or the American Urologic Association symptom score, are valuable ways to assess lower urinary tract symptoms objectively (Fig. 30.6)[3]. These are used to assess both obstructive-type symptoms, such as hesitancy and poor urine flow, and irritative symptoms, such as frequency, urgency, and incontinence. Each is assigned a score that can give valuable information with regard to both symptom severity and to changes over time on sequential testing. It is important that the assessment includes a quality-of-life score to help judge the impact of a patient's lower urinary tract symptoms.

Questions with respect to other urinary symptoms are essential because these may indicate the need for assessment in a different way (e.g. hematuria requires evaluation to exclude malignant disease).

A history of previous pelvic surgery or a neurologic condition may suggest the presence of a neuropathic bladder. Many elderly people are on drugs that have an effect on the urinary tract. Diuretics are a common cause of urinary frequency. Cardiac conditions may result in fluid retention; the fluid is subsequently excreted by the kidneys on becoming supine at night leading to nocturnal polyuria. Diabetes results in thirst and urinary frequency.

A formal written urine diary or frequency volume chart is invaluable in the assessment of urinary frequency. It often reveals

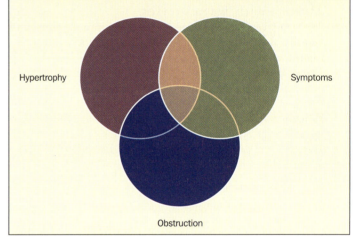

The relationship between benign prostatic hypertrophy, lower urinary tract symptoms, and bladder outflow obstruction

Hypertrophy

Symptoms

Obstruction

Figure 30.4 The relationship between benign prostatic hypertrophy, lower urinary tract symptoms, and bladder outflow obstruction. Each circle represents the total population of men exhibiting each parameter. Thus each can exist alone or in combination with the others (after Tag Hald).

Essential information from the patient's history

Lower urinary tract symptoms (including quality-of-life score)

Other urinary symptoms (e.g. hematuria, dysuria)

Previous pelvic surgery (e.g. anterior resection)

Neuropathy (e.g. Parkinson's disease, multiple system atrophy, cerebrovascular accident)

Cardiac problems

Diabetes mellitus or insipidus

Fluid intake and output (frequency–volume charts)

Figure 30.5 Essential information from the patient's history.

excessive fluid intake or the loss of the nocturnal reduction in urine output, which results in primary nocturnal polyuria[4] commonly seen in the elderly (Fig. 30.7).

International Prostate Symptom Score

Question	Not at all	Less than one time in five	Less than half the time	About half the time	More than half the time	Almost always
Over the past month, how often have you had a sensation of not emptying your bladder completely after you finished urinating?	0	1	2	3	4	5
Over the past month, how often have you had to urinate again less than 2 hours after you finished urinating?	0	1	2	3	4	5
Over the past month, how often have you stopped and started again several times when you urinated?	0	1	2	3	4	5
Over the past month, how often have you found it difficult to postpone urination?	0	1	2	3	4	5
Over the past month, how often have you had a weak urine stream?	0	1	2	3	4	5
Over the past month, how often have you had to push or strain to begin urination?	0	1	2	3	4	5
	None	Once	Twice	Three times	Four times	Five or more times
Over the past month, how many times most typically did you get up to urinate from the time you went to bed at night until the time you got up in the morning?	0	1	2	3	4	5
					Total IPSS, S =	

Quality of life as a result of urinary symptoms

	Delighted	Pleased	Mostly satisfied	Mixed about equally satisfied and dissatisfied	Mostly dissatisfied	Unhappy	Terrible
If you were to spend the rest of your life with your urinary condition, just the way it is now, how would you feel about that?							

Figure 30.6 The International Prostate Symptom Score (IPPS) sheet. Questions relate to obstructive and irritative symptoms, as well as quality of life.

Figure 30.8a indicates the important features to confirm on physical examination. A palpable bladder is uncommon. A tense palpable bladder of uterine consistency (Fig. 30.8b) suggests high-pressure chronic retention (HPCR) of urine, whereas a softer, more difficult to determine bladder indicates a low-pressure bladder (see below).

A prostate that feels malignant requires appropriate further evaluation and the size of the gland may indicate the choice of treatment options. (See also Chapters 27 & 28.)

Measurement of blood pressure and evaluation of fluid retention are important in HPCR and a targeted neurologic examination is required for cases in whom neuropathy is suspected.

Investigations

Investigations are listed in Figure 30.9. Initial investigations should exclude unsuspected diabetes, hematuria, and urine infection, which require further evaluation in their own right. Plasma creatinine gives an indication of major renal impairment.

A request for prostate-specific antigen (PSA) measurement is a complex subject, but PSA should be measured in men who present with lower urinary tract symptoms and in whom radical therapy for prostatic carcinoma would be considered, should the diagnosis be made (see Chapter 27). Furthermore, if the prostate on digital rectal examination feels malignant, PSA should be measured.

Measurements of urine flow rate and postvoid bladder residual urine are the cornerstone of the assessment of lower urinary tract symptoms for BOO caused by BPH. Measurements vary somewhat and ideally should be repeated more than once before conclusions are drawn. If these values are normal (see below), BOO is unlikely and therapy designed to treat BPH is unlikely to be of benefit.

Interpretation of urine flow rates

Peak urine flow rate (PFR), voided volume, and the shape of the flow trace are all important measurements. They cannot replace complete pressure–flow studies in the diagnosis of BOO,

Frequency volume charts				
Nocturnal polyuria in a 78-year-old man				
	Daytime (when you are awake, up and about)		**Night time (in bed)**	
Day	**Time**	**Volume (mL)**	**Time**	**Volume (mL)**
Monday	08.00	150	01.00	250
	10.00	200	02.30	300
	13.00	150	04.00	300
	16.30	150	05.30	350
	20.45	200	07.00	200
	23.30	150		
Tuesday	08.30	150	00.30	250
	11.00	150	02.00	300
	14.30	150	03.00	250
	20.30	200	04.30	300
	23.45	100	06.00	350
Early morning diuretic tablets in a 69-year-old man				
	Daytime (when you are awake, up and about)		**Night time (in bed)**	
Day	**Time**	**Volume (mL)**	**Time**	**Volume (mL)**
Monday	07.00	400	02.15	200
	08.00	100		
	08.30	200		
	09.15	150		
	11.00	200		
	12.00	150		
	14.00	200		
	16.00	150		
	19.00	200		
	21.30	150		
	23.30	100		
Tuesday	07.15	350	02.00	200
	08.00	100		
	08.30	170		
	09.00	200		
	10.00	150		
	10.45	150		
	12.00	200		
	14.30	200		
	17.00	150		
	19.45	170		
	20.30	150		

Figure 30.7 Frequency volume charts. (Top) These demonstrate nocturnal polyuria (more than 50% of the daily urine output is at night) and (bottom) increased urinary frequency after a morning diuretic tablet.

but they do provide a useful guide to diagnosis and management in everyday clinical practice. Formal urodynamic tests are not practical in every patient who presents with lower urinary tract symptoms.

Various shapes of the flow curve can be identified (Fig. 30.10). Flow rates are dependent on the voided volume. Too large or too small a volume and the detrusor contracts inefficiently, and so

Important features of the physical examination		
Examination	**Finding**	**Suggestion**
Bladder	Palpable, tense, uterine consistency	High-pressure chronic retention
	Soft, more difficult to feel	Low-pressure chronic retention
Genitalia	Phimosis or meatal stenosis	
Digital rectal examination of prostate	Consistency Benign or malignant	
Blood pressure	Raised	High-pressure chronic retention
Jugular venous pressure	Raised	High-pressure chronic retention
Ankle	Edema	High-pressure chronic retention
Neurologic assessment	Abnormal	Neuropathic bladder

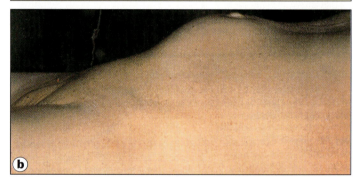

(a)

(b)

Figure 30.8 Clinical examination. (a) Features to seek on clinical examination. (b) High-pressure chronic retention bladder is visible and tense to palpation, but painless.

produces an unrepresentative flow pattern. A volume of 150–200mL is optimal for assessment, although smaller volumes can still be useful if that is the normal voided volume for the individual in question[5]. Nomograms are available to help interpret PFRs at various volumes (Fig. 30.11)[6].

A rough guide to PFR interpretation is that with a voided volume of 150mL or more, a PFR >15mL/s represents non-obstruction 80% of the time. A PFR <10mL/s suggests BOO (positive predictive value, 70%) and a PFR between 10 and 15mL/s is equivocal. A patient whose normal voided volume is <150mL still has approximately a 70% chance of BOO when formally assessed by full urodynamic studies[5].

Significance of residual urine

A residual urine volume consistently >300mL generally is considered to represent chronic retention of urine with the potential for upper tract obstruction in HPCR. Thus, any patient who exhibits more than 200mL residual volume on at least two separate measurements should have their upper urinary tracts assessed, ideally with ultrasound at the same time as the initial lower tract assessment. Smaller volumes of residual urine may still be significant in terms of a cause of symptoms, susceptibility to urine infections, and as a contribution to a diagnosis of BOO.

Essential investigations in the assessment of lower urinary tract symptoms

Urine dipstix for sugar and blood

Midstream urine for culture to exclude infection

Blood for plasma creatinine

Blood for prostate-specific antigen in patients of 40–75 years of age or if physical examination suggests malignancy

Urine flow rate

Ultrasound to measure postvoid residual urine

Figure 30.9 Essential investigations in the assessment of lower urinary tract symptoms.

Urinary flow rate curves

Normal and abnormal flow traces

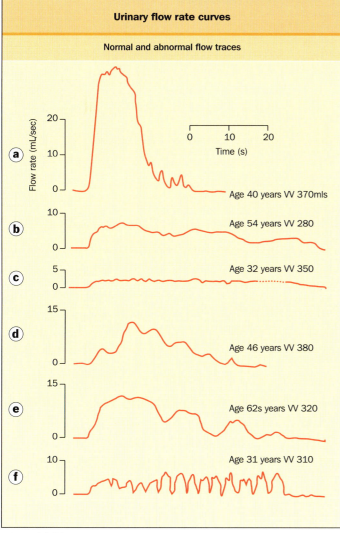

Figure 30.10 Urine flow rate curves. Note how the pattern of the curve is a useful adjunct to making a diagnosis. (a) Normal flow rate, (b) high-pressure low flow rate caused by bladder neck obstruction, (c) urethral stricture, (d, e) low-pressure low flow rates differing patterns, (f) straining to void. VV, voided volume.

The majority of patients who undergo assessment for lower urinary tract symptoms have negligible residual urine (<50mL). Hence, even if obstruction is present it can often be

---

Urine flow rate nomograms

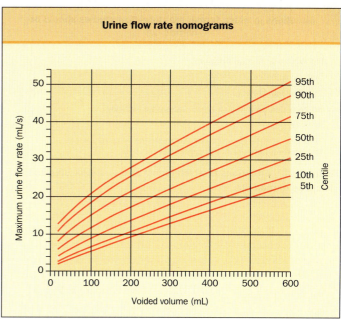

Figure 30.11 Urine flow rate nomograms. Flow rates vary with voided volume and age as well as the underlying pathologic processes. (Adapted with permission from Haylen et al.[6])

considered uncomplicated and potentially suitable for nonsurgical management.

Urodynamic assessment

The purpose of an urodynamic investigation in lower urinary tract symptoms and /or BPH is to determine which patients have BOO and whether or not there is associated detrusor instability. This is an important concept because patients who have therapy, particularly transurethral resection of the prostate (TURP), directed at the treatment of BPH generally do well if they have proven BOO but have a relatively poor postoperative result if they are not obstructed. In those patients in whom detrusor instability is associated with BOO, about 70% become stable after TURP[7]. In the group with relatively poor detrusor contractility (see below) the outcome after bladder outlet surgery is variable. It is useful to obtain such information prior to surgery so that the patient can be counseled as to possible outcomes rather than be disappointed with a poor result. Indeed, some investigators advocate the routine use of pressure–flow studies prior to bladder outflow surgery, although in a busy practice this is not practical and selective use needs to be made of the investigation. Patients with predominantly irritative symptoms, those with equivocal flow rates (in which the shape of the flow curve suggests poor detrusor contractility), and younger (<55 years of age) patients in whom the potential adverse effects of surgery are likely to have the most impact should all be considered for formal urodynamic tests prior to outflow surgery (Fig. 30.12).

Technique – filling phase

The patient is asked to void immediately prior to the study, after which bladder filling at approximately 30mL/minute is commenced on top of any residual urine. The volume of residual urine can be estimated ultrasonically or from the radiographic

Situations in which formal pressure–flow studies should be carried out
Predominantly irritative symptoms
Urge incontinence
Equivocal flow studies
Shape of flow curve that suggests underactive detrusor
Age <55 years
Neuropathy suspected (e.g. post abdominoperineal rectal surgery, Parkinson's disease, spinal surgery, etc.)

Figure 30.12 Situations in which formal pressure–flow studies should be carried out.

images if concurrent screening is available. The subtracted detrusor pressure at the beginning of the study (i.e. the end-void pressure) should be noted if significant residual urine is present (see below). Poor compliance and/or detrusor instability during filling is recorded (Fig. 30.13). (See also Chapter 6.)

Technique – voiding phase

The void should be voluntary, and not induced by an unstable wave. Instability that does result in uncontrolled bladder emptying, particularly if concurrent radiography shows no anatomic restriction to the bladder outflow tract, is good evidence that BOO does not exist and TURP should be avoided.

Classically, a high voiding pressure combined with poor urine flow is diagnostic of obstruction (see Fig. 30.3). Most investigators consider a maximum voiding pressure (MVP) over 80cmH$_2$O to indicate obstruction. However, not all studies fall into such a distinct group. More complex pressure–flow relationships can be calculated[8]. The ICS nomogram is widely used to help determine those patients who are truly obstructed (Fig. 30.14)[9].

An underactive detrusor is diagnosed by the classic low-pressure low-flow urodynamic test. A maximum detrusor pressure <50cmH$_2$O together with a rather undulating pressure and flow curve is typical of an underactive detrusor (Fig. 30.15).

Bladder outlet surgery in these nonobstructed patient groups must be approached with caution. If significant anatomic restriction (radiography during voiding is again useful here) is present, TURP may improve the situation by allowing the detrusor to contract against less resistance, although the result is inevitably less dramatic than if the detrusor were more powerful. Patients in this category with large residual urine volumes may have particularly poor outcomes from surgery (see below)[10].

When these studies are carried out it is not uncommon to encounter a patient who has great problems voiding as required 'on screen'. It used to be thought that such patients were typically those who had an underactive detrusor. However, if these men are studied with ambulatory urodynamics a significant number can be shown to be obstructed. Thus, in these patients it is important to obtain a voiding study whenever possible. For voiding detail, see also Chapter 6.

Ambulatory urodynamics

Results obtained during natural bladder filling and ambulatory recording are somewhat different to those obtained from conventional urodynamics[11]. In patients without chronic urinary retention, end-void resting detrusor pressures are low and

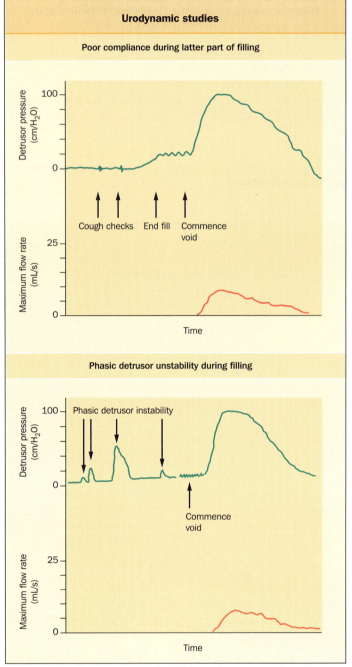

Figure 30.13 Urodynamic studies. Schematic representation of (top) moderately poor compliance during the latter stages of filling and (bottom) phasic detrusor instability during filling. In both cases high-pressure low-flow voiding also occurs, which indicates bladder outflow obstruction.

approximately equal with both techniques. End-fill pressures, however, tend to be somewhat lower during ambulatory studies. With voiding, maximum detrusor pressures tend to be higher with ambulatory recordings than with conventional studies. These differences probably reflect the detrusor reaction to differing filling rates. The faster fill of conventional urodynamics induces a less compliant fill and a suboptimal detrusor contraction. Ambulatory studies consume significantly more urologic resources and in the diagnosis of BOO have no real advantage

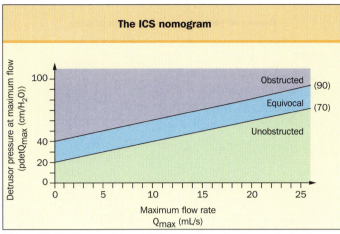

Figure 30.14 The provisional ICS nomogram for the analysis of voiding. Patients are divided into three classes, according to the bladder outflow obstruction index (BOOI) pdetQ$_{max}$–20$_{max}$). Purple, obstructed (BOOI $\geq$ 40); blue, equivocal (BOOI = 20–40); green, unobstructed (BOOI $\leq$ 20)[9].

over conventional studies, with the exception of the patient who simply cannot void in the unnatural surroundings of the urodynamic room.

Anatomic variants of bladder outlet obstruction

In the majority of men BPH is the cause of BOO. In some (particularly younger) patients, a prominent bladder neck with no significant lateral lobe enlargement results in bladder neck obstruction. Obstruction in these men actually arises from a detrusor bladder neck dyssynergia, in which the ring of muscle at the bladder neck fails to relax when voiding is initiated. This produces typical bladder neck nipping on radiography and can paradoxically produce a flow rate curve in which the peak flow is toward the end of the void as detrusor contraction starts to fade.

Urethral strictures are the third common cause of BOO, and are usually identified from the typical flow rate curve. Urethral catheterization for urodynamics is not usually possible; however, if obtained, it shows not only the level of stricture, but also the reactive bladder neck hypertrophy that may occur (Fig. 30.16).

CLINICAL MANIFESTATIONS

Uncomplicated bladder outlet obstruction

The majority (approximately 70%) of men with BOO have an impaired flow rate, a residual urine volume <150mL, a negative urine culture, no bladder stones or other intravesical abnormalities, and a benign prostate. If urodynamics are carried out they show normal bladder-filling characteristics and typical high-pressure low-flow voiding. These men are said to have uncomplicated BOO. Their symptom scores may indicate any severity of lower urinary tract symptoms and impact on quality of life, but frequently the symptoms are moderate or minor with an equivocal or little impact on lifestyle. The management of this group of patients is determined by patient preference after a discussion of the relative merits of TURP, medical therapy, watchful waiting, and alternative therapies (see below and Chapter 31).

The unstable bladder

Urodynamic tests, particularly in those patients with predominantly irritative lower urinary tract symptoms, often show detrusor instability, with or without BOO. If there is no evidence of BOO, TURP should not be considered as it would make the patient more prone to urge incontinence. These men often respond to anticholinergic medication.

In those patients with combined detrusor instability and BOO, 70% resolve with TURP[7], although it can take up to 1 year for optimal improvement. However, the 30% who have persistent instability can be difficult to manage. Thus, it is worth considering nonsurgical treatment in this group (see below and Chapter 31).

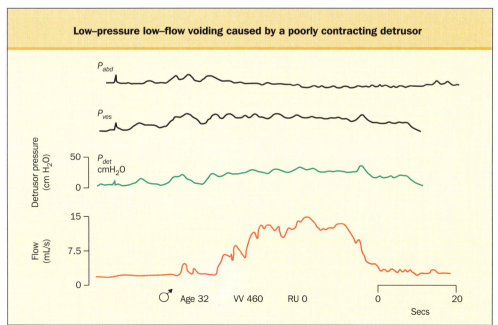

Figure 30.15 Low-pressure low-flow voiding caused by a poorly contracting detrusor. Detrusor pressure shown in green and flow rate in red. P$_{abd}$, abdominal pressure; P$_{det}$, detrusor pressure; P$_{ves}$, intravesical pressure; RU, residual urine; VV, voided volume.

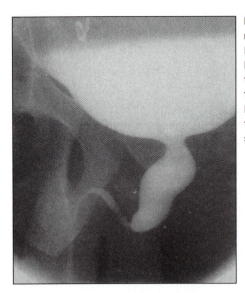

Figure 30.16 Bladder neck obstruction.
Note the hypertrophied bladder neck muscle that produces the typical nipping at the bladder outlet due, in this case, to urethral stricture.

Causes of postoperative retention of urine
General
Drugs (central and local actions)
Immobility
Constipation
Pain
Local
Edema
Neuropraxia (central or peripheral)
Neurotemesis
Preexisting bladder outflow obstruction

Figure 30.17 Causes of postoperative retention of urine.

Bladder outlet obstruction and diverticula formation

The formation of solitary or multiple diverticula is a recognized complication of BOO. It is thought to occur as a result of high intravesical pressures during voiding, which force mucosal pouches or saccules out through highly trabeculated detrusor muscle bundles. In the majority of cases, treatment of BOO alone results in satisfactory emptying and no further treatment is required (unless the diverticulum develops a complication, such as tumor or stone). Occasionally, a diverticulum fills from the bladder proper during voiding and, when voiding is complete, slowly reempties into the bladder to produce a 'delayed residual urine'. Double micturition, in which the patient is instructed to void again about 10 minutes afterward, usually helps. Rarely, the diverticulum has to be excised.

Acute painful retention of urine

Typically, the patient who presents urgently to the emergency service with a rapid onset of inability to void despite a strong desire to do so and has associated significant lower abdominal and urethral pain. It is frequently induced by the combination of large volume of fluid intake and delayed micturition, which causes detrusor overdistention and impaired contractility. Intravesical pressures are raised to about 50cmH$_2$O and upper tract drainage is impaired, which produces early dilatation on imaging[12]. However, this is a short-lived phenomenon and is relieved by the bladder catheterization that the pain demands.

Some of these patients give a history of preceding lower urinary tract symptoms that suggest BOO; this together with a residual volume of over 800mL is considered a relative indication for proceeding straight to TURP. Conservative treatment in this group often fails. However, it is common for painful retention to occur in the absence of these factors, in which case a trial of voiding after a brief period of detrusor rest often results in successful reestablishment of the normal voiding pattern. This can be helped by the correction of any adverse factors (such as constipation), the withdrawal of drugs with inappropriate lower urinary tract effects, and the temporary addition of α-adrenergic-blocking drugs to reduce urethral resistance.

Acute painless retention

The rapid onset of painless urine retention suggests a neuropathic etiology and should prompt neurologic assessment. The patient may have obvious acute lumbar pain and neurologic signs in the lower limbs, which suggest acute disc prolapse, but this is not always the case. Urgent neurologic assessment, which includes sensory tests of the saddle area, should be carried out; magnetic resonance imaging of the lumbosacral spine and expert neurologic or neurosurgical help may be required.

Postoperative retention

Many factors can adversely affect the ability of the bladder to empty satisfactorily in the immediate postoperative period (Fig. 30.17). Urodynamic studies show that actual BOO is a rare cause of retention in these circumstances[13]. Patients are generally managed with an indwelling catheter or, if possible, taught clean intermittent self-catheterization (CISC). Normal voiding is often reestablished once the immediate adverse factors have resolved. For patients in whom neurologic impairment is possible (e.g. pelvic surgery, such as anterior resection of rectum, or spinal surgery), institution of CISC and formal urodynamic tests are undertaken if micturition is not reestablished by 6 weeks postoperatively. Sometimes BOO is demonstrated. This is inferred by the ability to generate a high-pressure detrusor contraction without effective bladder emptying. In such cases, TURP results in effective voiding. Frequently, however, the cause is impaired detrusor function from neurologic impairment, in which case CISC is the preferred long-term management option. Effective voiding may become reestablished, but can take up to 12 months. Not infrequently, however, the impairment is permanent.

Chronic retention

Chronic retention is the painless retention of more than 300mL of residual urine. It can broadly be subdivided into two groups, high-pressure chronic retention (HPCR) and low-pressure chronic retention (LPCR), in which 'high' and 'low' refer to the intravesical pressure at the end of micturition, i.e., the beginning of the next filling phase. While HPCR is associated with bilateral hydronephrosis, LPCR does not result in upper tract dilatation.

Pressure cycle in high–pressure chronic retention

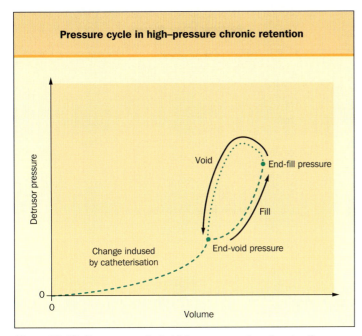

Figure 30.18 Pressure cycle in high-pressure chronic retention.
Note intravesical pressure remains elevated throughout both phases of the micturition cycle. It is the abnormally raised pressure during bladder filling which differs from other kinds of bladder outflow obstruction. Pressure drops if bladder is catheterized.

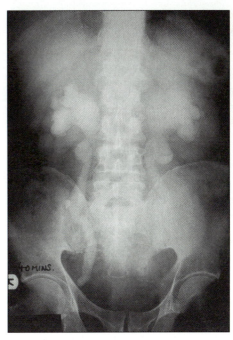

Figure 30.19 Bilateral hydroureteronephrosis in high-pressure chronic retention. Note ureters visible to ureterovesical junction no bladder filling has occurred.

High-pressure chronic retention

In HPCR, the residual urine volume remains at a pressure higher than the intra-abdominal pressure immediately after micturition[14]. This is the cornerstone of the diagnosis. During subsequent bladder filling, poor compliance results in high end-fill pressures and, because BOO exists, the detrusor pressure during voiding is also high, with associated impaired flow rates. Thus, intravesical pressures remain high throughout the entire micturition cycle (Fig. 30.18). It is this constantly raised pressure during both the filling and voiding phase that creates an effective obstruction to upper tract drainage and results in bilateral hydronephrosis (Fig. 30.19).

Ambulatory urodynamic studies in HPCR show that the reduced compliance seen on conventional studies is replaced by abnormal phasic detrusor activity. The frequency, duration, and magnitude of this activity can be quantified in the so called 'A20' value, which represents the area under the pressure–volume curve in the 20 minutes prior to micturition. Once again, high values correlate with upper tract impairment[15].

Lower urinary tract symptoms often are minimal in HPCR. The symptom that typically causes the patient to present is late-onset nocturnal enuresis, which occurs because during sleep urethral resistance falls slightly and so the high intravesical pressure results in urine leakage (often inaccurately referred to as overflow incontinence).

Upper tract pressures are low at rest, but the combination of diuresis and bladder filling causes upper tract pressures to rise and results in dilatation and obstructive renal impairment[16]. Once the ureters become dilated, coaptive peristalsis is lost and ureteric drainage becomes dependent on gravity. Thus, the hydrostatic pressure of $25cmH_2O$ generated by the column of urine between the renal pelvis and bladder is critical. Upper tract drainage only occurs in the erect posture (Fig. 30.20)[17]. Prolonged recumbency results in renal deterioration. Once end-void detrusor pressure rises above $25cmH_2O$, rapid deterioration in renal function ensues (Fig. 30.21). (See also 'Leak pressure', Chapter 6.)

Renal function changes

Renal impairment secondary to obstructive uropathy typically leads to sodium and water retention. Clinically, HPCR is associated with hypertension in 50% of cases and signs of peripheral edema and congestive cardiac failure in 20%[18]. Indeed, HPCR is the most common cause of surgically reversible hypertension. Any elderly male who presents with congestive heart failure should have HPCR excluded as an easily treatable cause.

Postobstructive diuresis

Bladder catheterization leads to both hematuria (mucosal congestion) and relief of obstruction in cases of HPCR, which is followed by a postobstructive diuresis (POD)[19]. This consists of an increased excretion of salt and water and occurs in all cases, although it may be recognized clinically only when the diuresis is marked. In the majority of cases the salt and water excreted is that retained during the period of obstruction; in such patients POD is of clinical benefit, and results in normalization of blood pressure and reversal of signs of fluid overload (Fig. 30.22).

In approximately 10% of cases the diuresis is excessive and requires fluid-replacement therapy. In <1% of cases the diuresis can be prolonged and life threatening. POD thus needs to be monitored carefully. Erect and supine blood pressures reflect circulating intravascular volume. The most accurate clinical method to measure fluid loss is change in daily weight. Daily assessment of jugular venous pressure, edema, and signs of congestive cardiac failure are all important. Urine output should be monitored, but not slavishly replaced because this perpetuates the diuresis in the 90% of cases in which it is of clinical benefit and self-limiting. The 'at-risk' patient usually can be identified by

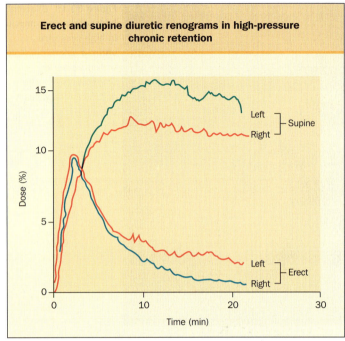

Figure 30.20 Superimposed erect and supine diuretic renograms in high-pressure chronic retention. Note that in the supine position the curves continue to rise, which indicates a lack of upper tract emptying. When the patient is placed erect, isotope washout indicates upper tract drainage. (Adapted with permission from George et al.[17])

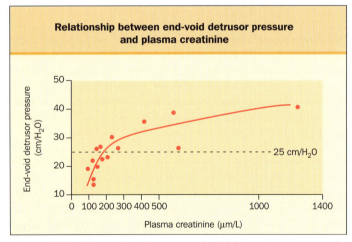

Figure 30.21 Relationship between end-void detrusor pressure and plasma creatinine. Once intravesical pressure consistently exceeds 25cmH$_2$O ureteric emptying caused by hydrostatic pressure can no longer take place and renal function rapidly deteriorates. (Adapted with permission from George et al.[14])

a urine output consistently in excess of 200mL/hour for the first 12 hours (after drainage of the initial residual urine). These patients need to be monitored carefully and may well require fluid-replacement therapy.

Plasma potassium also must be monitored carefully. High potassium levels are typical of renal impairment. After relief of obstruction and with improving renal function, potassium levels in plasma usually fall. Occasionally, however, they may rise, which is thought to be caused by hyporesponsiveness of the distal nephron to aldosterone. High potassium levels can be particularly

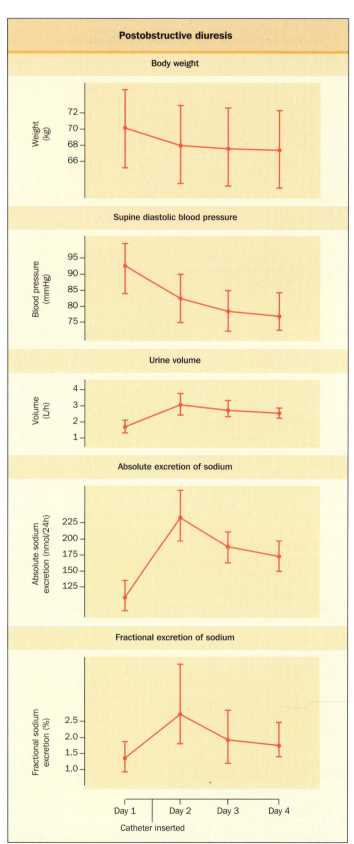

Figure 30.22 Postobstructive diuresis. Mean, with 95% confidence limits, body weight, supine diastolic blood pressure, urine volume, absolute and fractional excretion of sodium before catheterization (day 1) and for 3 days after catheterization (days 2, 3, and 4), measured in 21 patients with high-pressure chronic retention. No further significant changes were seen at 2 weeks. (© The Lancet Ltd, 1987[18].)

troublesome in patients who take potassium-sparing diuretics or potassium supplements. It usually stabilizes as the nephrons continue to recover normal function.

The POD changes are inevitable and the practice once advocated, of slow decompression to lessen hematuria (usually settles in 24–72 hours) is no longer indicated. Slow or intermittent drainage does not prevent the POD but only serves to confuse the management of this important physiologic event.

Prostatectomy is required for definitive treatment and the question arises as to whether preoperative catheterization is essential whilst attendant risks of infection and preoperative bladder shrinkage. Signs of clinical salt and water retention or significant renal failure clearly demands catheterization, monitoring, and optimization of the patient preoperatively. This usually takes 3–7 days, although occasionally it can take up to 2 weeks (Chapter 23). However, with only mild impairment of renal function and no clinical signs of fluid overload, the POD changes are likely to be minor and TURP without prior catheterization can be considered.

Long-term recovery

In HPCR, TURP with effective relief of BOO is usually successful[20]. Not all patients void and completely empty their bladder immediately, but given time the vast majority do so (in contrast to LPCR – see below). Immediately post-TURP, when the catheter is first removed, it is not uncommon for voiding to be delayed for a number of hours, but then begins with associated significant residual urine. If the patient has no symptoms, the urine is sterile, and renal function is stable over the subsequent few days and/or weeks, bladder emptying usually improves with no need for recatheterization. Sometimes CISC or indwelling catheterization needs to be reinstituted for approximately 6 weeks, after which the majority of patients void and empty satisfactorily.

There are reports of recurrent BOO and renal failure after TURP for HPCR, and so it is vital to ensure that the urine is sterile and residual urine minimal (<100mL) before the patients can be discharged from follow-up.

Low pressure chronic retention

The bladder-filling phase pressures in this condition are low[10]. The bladder is highly compliant, and thus upper tract obstruction

does not occur because the bladder 'exists' at a low pressure (i.e. equal to intra-abdominal pressure) throughout its filling phase. During voiding two different patterns may be seen. The high-pressure, low-flow void is typical of 'straightforward' BOO with significant residual urine (but rarely more than a few hundred milliliters). The more common group are those patients with low-pressure low-flow voiding (see Fig. 30.15) and large residual urines, not infrequently of 2–3 liters or more. This group develops retention because of detrusor failure – there simply is not enough power to overcome urethral resistance and effect bladder emptying. Although TURP may reduce urethral resistance somewhat, it is common for these patients to fail to void even after prolonged periods of catheterization and 'detrusor rest'. The best method to achieve emptying in these men is CISC.

Many patients with LPCR void but do not empty, have very few troublesome lower urinary tract symptoms, and by definition no upper tract impairment. If the urine is sterile these patients can be managed conservatively, as their residual urine is stored 'safely' at low pressure.

TREATMENT OF BLADDER OUTLET OBSTRUCTION

Treatment depends initially on whether the patient has uncomplicated or complicated BOO (Figs 30.23 & 30.24).

Prostatectomy

In the UK approximately 60% of prostatectomies are carried out for complicated BOO[22]. The aim of prostatectomy, be it transurethral electrosurgical resection (Fig. 30.25; the norm in >95% of cases) or an open transvesical or retropubic operation (Fig. 30.26; when the gland exceeds approximately 80–100g), is to remove all of the adenomatous tissue and thus reduce urethral resistance and relieve BOO. Flow rates often improve up to 20mL/s, and it is the only treatment option whereby BOO is consistently relieved.

With modern equipment, hospital stay is only 2 or 3 days, transfusion rates are approximately 5%, and the previously fit patient can return to normal activity almost immediately, although most surgeons advise a 2 week 'take it easy' period to minimize the risk of secondary hemorrhage. Patient satisfaction rates that exceed 90% can be achieved when the patients are selected appropriately, using objective assessment criteria as outlined above, and the likely benefits and limitations are discussed with them. Thus, TURP is considered the 'gold standard ' treatment option.

Complicated and uncomplicated bladder outflow obstruction		
Type	**Signs**	**Treatment**
Uncomplicated bladder outflow obstruction caused by benign prostatic hypertrophy	Residual urine <150mL Sterile urine No stones	Treat for symptoms only
Complicated bladder outflow obstruction caused by benign prostatic hypertrophy	High-pressure chronic retention	Prostatectomy indicated
	Low-pressure chronic retention	Prostatectomy indicated
	Acute retention	Prostatectomy indicated
	Recurrent urinary tract infection with residual urine	Prostatectomy indicated
	Vesical calculus	Prostatectomy indicated

Figure 30.23 Complicated and uncomplicated bladder outflow obstruction.

Treatment options for uncomplicated bladder outflow obstruction
Watchful waiting

Drugs
    α-blockers
    5α-Reductase inhibitors

Prostatectomy
    Transurethral
    Open

Alternative Therapies

Figure 30.24 Treatment options for uncomplicated bladder outflow obstruction.

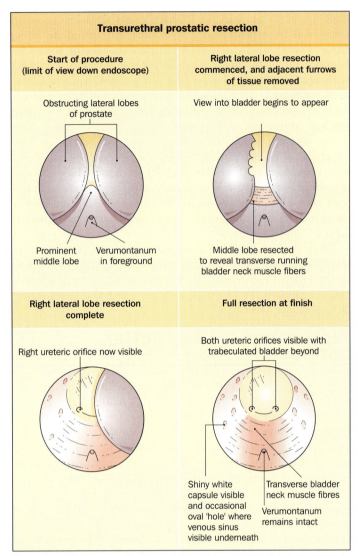

Figure 30.25 Transurethral prostatic resection. The tissue is removed in 'chips' by repeated passes through the gland of a wire loop. An electric current is passed through the loop to produce the cutting effect.

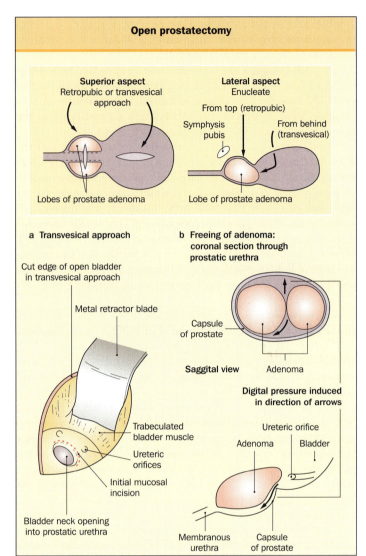

Figure 30.26 Open prostatectomy: surgical technique. The adenoma may be approached either transvesically through the bladder (a), or retropubically directly through the prostatic capsule. In either case enucleation is required as in coronal and sagittal views (b).

However, TURP does have associated problems. Retrograde ejaculation occurs in the majority and impotence in approximately 10% of patients[23]. Reoperation rates of 1–2% per year because of prostatic regrowth or stricture are reported. There is a small incidence of sphincter weakness incontinence (<1%). Adverse cardiac effects from the impact of irrigation fluid absorption and body cooling are also recognized[24]. Mortality is <1%, but it is a particular risk with large, prolonged resections in the group over 80 years of age. These problems all serve to discourage men who only may have moderate-to-minor lower urinary tract symptoms and no complications that necessitate surgery. All of these factors must be discussed with the patient preoperatively and it is good practice to provide written information for the patient to peruse prior to making an informed decision about treatment.

Bladder neck incision (for bladder neck obstruction; Fig. 30.27) or transurethral incision of the prostate (TUIP; for glands less than approximately 30g) are associated with a much lower adverse occurrence rate and are as effective as TURP in the short term[25].

There is a worry that long-term results with TUIP may not be as good because the bulk of obstructing tissue is not removed[26].

Drug therapy

Two types of drugs are commonly used to treat BOO caused by BPH. The α-blockers, which relax prostatic smooth muscle and thus inhibit the dynamic component of BOO, and the 5α-reductase inhibitors, which reduce prostate volume. Both produce worthwhile symptomatic improvement.

The α-blockers onset of action is rapid; generally, if they have not produced a significant benefit by 4 weeks, they are unlikely to do so. They do improve urine flow rates, although rarely out of the obstructed range[27]. Residual urine may diminish, but not enough to render them effective treatment in chronic retention. Their effect is in the region of 25% of that expected with TURP. Side effects are related primarily to their action on vascular smooth muscle, which produces dizziness, although with the newer 'uroselective' agents this is minimal. Retrograde ejaculation does occur,

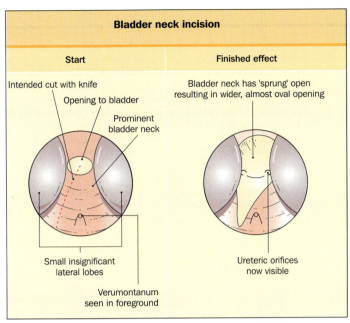

Bladder neck incision	
Start	**Finished effect**
Intended cut with knife Opening to bladder Prominent bladder neck Small insignificant lateral lobes Verumontanum seen in foreground	Bladder neck has 'sprung' open resulting in wider, almost oval opening Ureteric orifices now visible

Figure 30.27 Bladder neck incision is carried out in similar manner to Transurethral prostatic resection (see Fig. 30.25). A single cut is made through the full thickness of the hypertrophied bladder neck muscle.

Symptoms that may not resolve with treatment of bladder outflow obstruction	
Dominant symptom	**Approach**
Nocturia	Is it polyuria, age, or cardiac related?
	Frequency/volume charts essential
	Consider desmopressin[21]
Urgency and/or urge incontinence	Urodynamics essential
	Avoid transurethral resection of the prostate (TURP) in the unstable non-obstructed patient
Postmicturition dribble (PMD)	Difficult to distinguish from terminal dribble caused by prolonged voiding time
	True PMD responds poorly to TURP
	May result from poor bulbospongiosis muscle tone

Figure 30.28 Symptoms that may not resolve with treatment of bladder outflow obstruction.

but is reversible on stopping the medication. Despite concerns to the contrary, they do seem to be safe in patients who take other cardiac and vascular-acting drugs, but they must be used with caution[28]. Initiation of therapy prior to retiring to bed and dose reduction are sensible precautions in the elderly.

The 5α-reductase inhibitors have a long period before onset of action (anything up to 6 months), which has limited their popularity. Recent evidence suggests that they may be more effective in the larger gland (>40g) and in one study were shown to reduce the acute retention rate from 7% to 3% in patients managed with watchful waiting[29]. They can sometimes cause impotence and do cause serum PSA levels to fall, which can mask the early detection of prostate cancer.

Watchful waiting

Patients with BPH and/or BOO do not necessarily deteriorate if not treated. Approximately 30% of patients have surgery because of symptomatic deterioration or the development of a complication[30]; the rest either remain much the same, and some even improve with time. Symptoms often wax and wane in severity. Long-term urodynamic studies in those who are untreated show that symptomatic change is often related to the development of detrusor instability with advancing age rather than to progression of obstruction. The risks of developing acute retention are relatively small, approximately 1–2% per year.

Many men are unwilling to risk the potential side effects of TURP and are apprehensive about the safety of long-term drug therapy. Thus, watchful waiting is an attractive and perfectly reasonable management for the majority of men whose symptoms are not particularly bothersome and do not unduly impair their quality of life.

HOW TO AVOID THE UNHAPPY PATIENT

Some symptoms are particularly bothersome to patients (Fig. 30.28). They may be caused by BOO, but frequently are not. Mixed causes of lower urinary tract symptoms are common in the elderly: BOO and/or BPH, cardiac problems, polypharmacy, and nocturnal polyuria all frequently coexist. It is particularly important to counsel such patients about the improvements that might be achieved by treatment of BPH, especially if surgery is considered. A TURP that produces an excellent flow rate and relieves obstruction may still be considered a failure by the uninformed patient who still has to rise four times a night to void because of nocturnal polyuria.

Section 6

Benign Conditions of the Lower Urinary Tract

REFERENCES

1. Kirby RS, Pool JL. Alpha adrenoceptor blockade in the treatment of benign prostatic hyperplasia: past, present and future. Br J Urol. 1997;80:521–32.
2. Diokno AC. Benign changes in the prostate with aging. Br J Urol. 1998;82(Suppl. 1):44–6.
3. Barry MJ, Fowler FJ Jr, O'Leary MP, et al. and the Measurement Committee of the American Urological Association. Correlation of the American Urological Association symptom index with self administered versions of the Madsen Iverson, Boyarsky and Maine medical assessment program symptom indexes. J Urol. 1992;148:1558–63.
4. Saito M, Kondo A, Kato T, et al. Frequency–volume charts: comparison of frequency between elderly and adult patients. Br J Urol. 1993;72:38–41.
5. Reynard JM, Yang Q, Donovan JL, et al. The ICS–'BPH' study: uroflowmetry, lower urinary tract symptoms and bladder outlet obstruction. Br J Urol. 1998;82:619–23.
6. Haylen BT, Ashby D, Sutherst JR, et al. Maximum and average urine flow rates in normal male and female populations – the Liverpool nomograms. Br J Urol. 1989;64:30–8.
7. Abrams PH, Farrar DJ, Turner-Warwick R, et al. The results of prostatectomy: a symptomatic and urodynamic analysis of 152 patients. J Urol. 1979;121:640–5.
8. Schafer W. Principles and clinical application of advanced urodynamic analysis of voiding function. Urol Clin North Am. 1990;17;553–66.
9. Abrams P. Bladder outlet obstruction index, bladder contractility index and bladder voiding efficiency: three simple indices to define bladder voiding function. BJU International. 1999;84:14–15.
10. George NJR, Feneley RCL, Roberts JBM. Identification of the poor risk patient with 'prostatism' and detrusor failure. Br J Urol. 1986;58:290–5.
11. Webb RJ, Griffiths CJ, Ramsden PD, et al. Measurement of voiding pressures on ambulatory monitoring: comparison with conventional cystometry. Br J Urol. 1990;65:152–4.
12. Murray K, Massey A, Feneley RCL. Acute urinary retention – a urodynamic assessment. Br J Urol. 1984;56:468–73.
13. Anderson JB, Grant JBF. Postoperative retention of urine: a prospective urodynamic study. Br Med J. 1991;302:894–6.
14. George NJR, O'Reilly PH, Barnard RJ, et al. High pressure chronic retention. Br Med J. 1983;286:1780–3.
15. Styles RA, Neal DE, Griffiths CJ, et al. Long term monitoring of bladder pressure in chronic retention of urine: the relationship between detrusor activity and upper tract dilatation. J Urol. 1988;140:330–4.
16. Jones DA, Holden D, George NJR. Mechanism of upper tract dilatation in patients with thick walled bladders, chronic retention of urine and associated hydroureteronephrosis. J Urol. 1988;140:326–9.
17. George NJR, O'Reilly PH, Barnard RJ, et al. Practical management of patients with dilated upper tracts and chronic retention of urine. Br J Urol. 1984;56:9–12.
18. Jones DA, George NJR, O'Reilly PH, et al. Reversible hypertension associated with unrecognised high pressure chronic retention of urine. Lancet. 1987;i:1052–4.
19. Jones DA, George NJR, O'Reilly PH, et al. The biphasic nature of renal functional recovery following relief of chronic obstructive uropathy. Br J Urol. 1988;61:192–7.
20. Jones DA, Gilpin SA, Holden D, et al. Relationship between bladder morphology and long term outcome of treatment in patients with high pressure chronic retention of urine. Br J Urol. 1991;67:280–5.
21. Asplund R, Sundberg B, Bengtsson P. Desmopressin for the treatment of nocturnal polyuria in the elderly: a dose titration study. Br J Urol. 1998;82:642–6.
22. Emberton M, Neal DE, Black N, et al. The national prostatectomy audit: the clinical management of patients during hospital admission. Br J Urol. 1995;75:301–16.
23. Hanbury DC, Sethia KK. Erectile function following transurethral prostatectomy. Br J Urol. 1995;75:12–3.
24. Evans JW, Singer M, Coppinger SW, et al. Cardiovascular performance and core temperature during transurethral prostatectomy. J Urol. 1994;152:2025–9.
25. Orandi A. Transurethral incision of prostate (TUIP) compared with transurethral resection of prostate (TURP) in 100 matched cases. J Urol. 1985;133:198A.
26. Jahnson S, Dalen M, Gustavsson G, et al. Transurethral incision versus resection of the prostate for small to medium benign prostatic hyperplasia. Br J Urol. 1998;81:276–81.
27. Jardin A, Bensadoun H, Delauche-Cavallier MC, et al. Long term treatment of benign prostatic hyperplasia with alfuzosin: a 24–30 month survey. Br J Urol. 1994;74:579–84.
28. Kaplan SA, Te AE, Ikeguchi E, et al. The treatment of benign prostatic hyperplasia with alpha blockers in men over the age of 80 years. Br J Urol. 1997;80:875–9.
29. McConnell JD, Bruskewitz R, Walsh P, et al. The effect of finasteride on the risk of acute urinary retention and the need for surgical treatment among men with benign prostatic hyperplasia. N Engl J Med. 1998;338:557–63.
30. Girman CJ. Population based studies of the epidemiology of benign prostatic hyperplasia. Br J Urol. 1998;82(Suppl. 1):34–43.

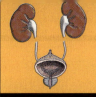

Section 6 Benign Conditions of the Lower Urinary Tract

Chapter 31 Nonsurgical Management of Benign Prostatic Hyperplasia

Nicholas J Hegarty and John M Fitzpatrick

KEY POINTS

- Surgery remains the most effective treatment for complicated or severe symptomatic benign prostatic hyperplasia (BPH). Its invasive nature and potential side effects has led to the search for nonsurgical alternatives.
- α-blockers continue to evolve. Refinements are aimed at achieving reduced frequency dosage and achieving preferential side effects, while maintaining clinical efficacy.
- 5α-reductase inhibitors show the greatest benefit in large prostates. Finasteride has also been applied to the treatment of prostatic bleeding and may positively effect the natural history of clinical BPH.
- The popularity of phytotherapeutic agents and relative lack of information into their safety profiles, mode of action and clinical efficacy suggests this to be an area with tremendous potential for study.
- Heat-based treatments are being explored with the aim of developing durable office-based alternatives to surgery.

INTRODUCTION

Benign prostatic hyperplasia (BPH) is the most common neoplasm that occurs in men. The relationship between BPH and bladder outlet obstruction, or lower urinary tract symptoms[1], is complex. It is well known that a small prostate can cause more obstruction than an enlarged prostate, and a number of other factors contribute to lower urinary tract symptoms, such as increased tone of the bladder neck and reduced bladder compliance[2]. Nevertheless, an enlarged prostate is associated with a more than three-fold increase in the risk of developing moderate-to-severe symptoms[3], and the improvement achieved following prostate surgery implicates the prostate and bladder neck in the development of lower urinary tract symptoms. The incidence of BPH increases with age and previously a 50-year-old man was estimated to have a 20–25% chance of requiring a prostatectomy during his lifetime[4]. Although the recent increase in medical treatment of BPH has altered this figure, the treatment for BPH is a significant public health issue as a large number of men will be exposed to the morbidity associated with BPH and its various treatment modalities.

CURRENT SURGICAL OPTIONS

The surgical management of BPH was a central element in the development of urology as a specialty and continues to constitute a significant portion of the urologist's workload. Prior to the most recent 10–15 years, the choice of treatment for BPH was largely between watchful waiting, transurethral resection of the prostate (TURP), and open surgery (Fig. 31.1). However, recently a tremendous expansion has occurred in the number and variety of modalities available for the treatment of BPH.

Open prostatectomy

As absorption of irrigation fluids and the dilutional hyponatremia from absorption of irrigation fluid (TUR syndrome) limit resection time to 40–60 minutes, which equates to a prostate size of 80–100g for most resectionists, open prostatectomy is the standard treatment for very large obstructing prostate glands.

Transurethral resection of prostate

Currently, TURP remains the 'gold standard' for the surgical management of BPH and it is against this that newer modalities of treatment must be compared[5]. Although TURP has been in use for over 60 years refinements in the technique continue to be made. There are on-going advances in optics, resection loops

Surgical therapy for benign prostatic hyperplasia	
Surgical therapy	**Outline**
Transurethral resection of the prostate (TURP)	'Gold standard' and gives symptomatic relief in 93% of cases
	Requires general or regional anesthetic and hospital stay
	Significant morbidity
Transurethral vaporization of the prostate	Similar to TURP, but employs vaporization rather than a cutting loop
Transurethral incision of the prostate	Prostates <30g
	Laser incision may obviate the need for catheterization
Laser prostatectomy	Reduced risk of bleeding compared to TURP
	Can be carried out under local anesthetic in selected case
Open prostatectomy	Treatment of choice for prostates >100g
	Also used in cases for which urethral instrumentation not possible

Figure 31.1 Surgical therapy for benign prostatic hyperplasia.

(resection and vaporization[6]), irrigation fluids[7], and perioperative care that contribute to the changing outcomes for this procedure. Improvements in preoperative assessment help to identify those patients who are likely to gain the most benefit from surgery, although it is still difficult in many cases to differentiate BPH from other causes of lower urinary tract symptoms. This difficulty prompts the use of urodynamics, particularly in patients with suspected neurologic disease, in young patients, or in patients in whom symptoms are complex or vague[8]. Some investigators even recommend an almost routine application of urodynamics in the preoperative work-up[9].

Transurethral incision of the prostate

Another operative technique that has evolved to complement TURP and open prostatectomy is transurethral incision of the prostate (TUIP). No tissue is resected, but rather the prostate is incised using a single or two lateral incisions[10,11], classically from below the ureteral orifices to the verumontanum at 4 and 7 o'clock. The incision is made through the substance of the prostate down to the prostate capsule, and can be achieved using a Collings knife, resection loop, or laser; a urethral catheter is inserted for 24 hours after the procedure. The best results are obtained when the procedure is used to treat bladder neck strictures or prostates <30g in size[12]. Low rates of retrograde ejaculation are seen with preservation of the supramontanal 1cm of prostatic urethra[13]. Laser incision allows TUIP to be carried out with no need for a catheter[14].

Transurethral ultrasound-guided laser prostatectomy and endoscopic laser ablation of the prostate

Laser resection also has evolved as a surgical option from transurethral ultrasound-guided laser prostatectomy to endoscopic laser ablation of the prostate, and to contact, noncontact, and interstitial fibers. Often laser resection is classified as a minimally invasive procedure as in many cases it can be carried out under local anesthetic. It has been performed safely on patients with bleeding disorders or who are on anticoagulants. Results at 1 year approach those of TURP[15], but postoperative irritative symptoms may persist for weeks and require prolonged postoperative catheterization.

The need for nonsurgical treatments

To date no treatment has surpassed TURP or open surgery in the ability to relieve obstruction. TURP is generally recommended in cases of complicated BPH, such as those with associated bladder calculus formation, bladder decompensation, renal failure, recurrent hematuria, or recurrent urinary retention[16]. Studies prior to the use of symptom scores, peak urinary flow, postvoid residual volumes, and pressure flow measurements showed symptomatic relief in 80% of patients who undergo TURP[17]. More recently symptomatic benefit has been demonstrated in 93% of patients who present with severe symptoms[18]. However, TURP does require hospital admission, the use of regional or general anesthetic, and postoperative catheterization for 24–72 hours. Mortality from TURP is low, but finite, and other forms of morbidity, which include the need for transfusion, urinary tract infection (UTI), urethral stricture, and incontinence (<1%), occur in 18% of patients[17]. Also, TURP may have profound effects on sexual function. Retrograde ejaculation occurs

Medical management of benign prostatic hyperplasia	
Medical therapy	**Outline**
Adrenergic antagonists	Effective in glands of all sizes
	Main action is to reduce the dynamic component of bladder outlet obstruction
	May act on voiding and prostate cell biology
5α-reductase inhibitors	Most effective in glands >40g
	May reduce the incidence of acute urinary retention and surgery
Combined therapy	Early studies show little benefit over monotherapy[52]
Plant extracts	In widespread use
	Efficacy and mode of action not clearly defined
	Source of considerable potential for clinical study

Figure 31.2 Medical management of benign prostatic hyperplasia.

in two-thirds of patients[19] and new-onset erectile dysfunction in 4–14%. The results of surgery are durable in the majority of patients, but reoperation is required in up to 10% within 8 years[20]. These reasons account for the interest in the development of less invasive therapies for the treatment of lower urinary tract symptoms, albeit (in most incidences) with reduced efficacy. Patient acceptance of the less invasive therapies has been high, especially in those with milder symptoms or with particular concerns about potency and fertility, and in those unfit for or unlikely to derive great benefit from surgery.

MEDICAL MANAGEMENT

A number of medical strategies have been attempted to treat BPH (Fig. 31.2), but only two have achieved widespread acceptance:
- suppression of androgen stimulation of prostatic growth; and
- inhibition of sympathetic tone in the prostate and bladder neck.

These treatments have become widespread in their application over the past decade. Thus the treatment of BPH, formerly almost the sole preserve of the urologist, has shifted to involve other health care professionals.

As the majority of patients with lower urinary tract symptoms remain symptomatic for life, it is likely that medical treatments will be required for long-term use. It is therefore encouraging that a number of medical agents have been shown to maintain their safety profile and efficacy at a 5-year follow-up. Although BPH remains static or progresses in the majority of patients, symptomatic improvement does occur in a sizeable minority of patients who do not receive any active management. Furthermore, the administration of many treatments is accompanied by a placebo effect, which must be accounted for when the impact of a new therapy is assessed.

α-Blockers

Studies of cellular changes that occur in BPH suggest that prostate enlargement is related predominantly to stromal proliferation[21], which leads to outflow obstruction in two different ways:

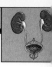

- static obstruction from increased tissue mass; and
- dynamic obstruction from contraction of the bladder neck, prostatic fibromuscular stroma, and capsule.

It is estimated that this latter sympathetic-mediated contraction may be responsible for up to 40% of the bladder outflow obstructive effect of BPH[22], which provides the rationale for the development and use of α-blockers in BPH. The first adrenergic agent to be employed in the treatment of BPH was the α-antagonist phenoxybenzamine[23]. Use of this drug, which has both α_1- and α_2-adrenergic antagonist activity, lowered intraurethral pressure and improved voiding function through inhibition of adrenergic tone.

Further studies showed a similar effect with prazosin, which has predominantly α_1-activity[24] and fewer side effects than phenoxybenzamine. Its rapid onset of action, however, is associated with a number of side effects, which include 'first-dose' hypotension and syncope (because of the dual action of venous and arterial vasodilatation). A short half-life also requires frequent daily doses. The other short acting α_1-agent currently in clinical use is alfuzosin. This initially required dosage three times a day, but slow release forms that enable a single daily dose are now available. Longer acting agents, such as terazosin, doxazosin, and tamsulosin also enable a single daily dose. Despite a number of slight differences in the actions and side effects of these agents, in general symptomatic and flow-rate improvements occur in 70% of patients[25]. The side effects include dizziness, headache, asthenia, peripheral edema, postural hypotension, and syncope; they are thought to be mediated by both peripheral and central actions, especially dizziness.

Originally, cloning of cDNA sequences of the α-adrenergic receptors showed at least three subtypes – α_{1a}, α_{1b}, and α_{1c}. Pharmacologic studies of the α-adrenergic receptor also showed the presence of receptors with different pharmacologic activities, termed α_{1A} and α_{1B}. A degree of confusion as to nomenclature arose as it was found that the pharmacologic α_{1A}-receptor corresponded to the cloned α_{1c}-receptor, and α_{1B} corresponded to α_{1b}. These receptors are now termed α_{1A}, α_{1B}, and α_{1D}[26] (more recently a fourth subtype was postulated, α_{1L}). Of the adrenoreceptors in the prostate, 70% are of the α_{1A}-subtype[27,28], while the α_{1B}-subtype is implicated in the constriction of large vessels[29]; thus, considerable interest was created in the development of adrenoreceptor antagonists with α_{1A}-specificity. These agents have the theoretic advantage that they retain the ability to reduce intraurethral pressure, but have few peripheral vascular side-effects. Tamsulosin was shown to have an 8–38 times greater affinity for the α_{1A}-receptor than for other adrenergic receptors. Its efficacy and safety have been demonstrated in clinical trials[30], and side effects occur in 21% of patients; the most common of these are dizziness and abnormal ejaculation, with a very low incidence of headache, postural hypotension, syncope, asthenia and rhinitis[31]. Maximum improvement in flow rates occurs within 4–8 hours of the first dose, and the maximum improvement in symptom score at 8 weeks[32]. Blood pressure and pulse rate show no significant change[30] and tamsulosin has been used safely in conjunction with antihypertensive medications[33].

The subdivision of α-receptors into their various subtypes has resulted in discussion on the uroselectivity of these agents. Uroselectivity can be seen to embrace pharmacological, physiological components and, most importantly, clinical uroselectivity[34].

The pharmacokinetics are also important, as they define tissue distribution and appropriate dosing, and influence clinical effects as well as central and peripheral side effects[35]. Evidence is accruing to suggest that improvement in voiding is not exclusively the result of relaxation of the prostatic capsule and fibromuscular stroma. α-Adrenergic pathways also influence voiding, both at the spinal level[36] and at the level of efferent discharges to the bladder[37]. Agents with high specificity for α_{1A}-receptors may lack some of these activities. The ability of doxazosin to induce apoptosis in both glandular and smooth muscle cells in patients with BPH[38] suggests another mechanism by which α-blockers might act. Apoptosis seems to increase with duration of treatment; as many investigators believe that the basic cellular defect in BPH is a decrease in the rate of apoptosis, rather than an increase in cellular proliferation, apoptosis may be an important mechanism by which α-blockers exert their clinical effect. Doxazosin also lowers cholesterol levels, which also may help to relieve lower urinary tract symptoms.

Hormonal strategies

The development of BPH is probably multifactorial, but two of the primary conditions required are the presence of a functioning testis and aging. Men castrated before puberty do not develop BPH. Castration after the onset of the disease process also may interrupt the process[39,40]. That androgens may not only be responsible for the initiation, but also for the maintenance of BPH, has led to the investigation of hormone manipulation for the treatment of BPH. The most potent androgen with activity in the prostate is dihydrotestosterone (DHT)[41], which is formed from testosterone by the enzyme 5α-reductase. There are two known isoenzymes:

- type 2 is the form found predominantly in the prostate[42]; whereas
- type 1 is found in extraprostatic tissues.

In congenital deficiency of type 2 5α-reductase, individuals have a 46XY karyotype, with ambiguity of the external genitalia. In these individuals at puberty, a normal surge in testosterone leads to external virilization and normal muscle growth, but prostate development is absent[43]. Efforts to find a selective inhibitor led to the development of finasteride (a competitive 5α-reductase type 2 inhibitor), which has been extensively investigated in the clinical setting.

Finasteride treatment reduces serum DHT levels by 80–90%[44]. Reduction in mean prostate size of 19–24% is seen at 12 months[45,46], and the time to onset of maximal clinical effect is typically 6–12 weeks[45]. The degree of benefit attained has been related to the pretreatment prostate size. Superior improvement compared to placebo is seen in glands >40mL in volume[47]. A concern with all forms of minimally invasive treatments is the durability of effect. The improvements seen with finasteride therapy have been maintained at 5 years[48]. Finasteride also reduces the incidence of acute urinary retention and decreases the need for surgery[49,50].

Side effects of finasteride include reduced libido in 6% and erectile dysfunction in 5% of patients. These side effects are generally reversible within weeks of discontinuing treatment. Prostate size and symptoms also return to pretreatment values on discontinuation of therapy. Finasteride decreases prostate-specific antigen (PSA) levels in both benign and malignant

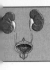

prostate disease. It is therefore recommended that the appropriate level for a patient on finasteride should be double the measured value, to give an estimated normal PSA in the range of 0–2ng/mL.

Other hormonal strategies explored in the management of symptomatic BPH include luteinizing hormone-releasing hormone (LHRH) analogs. The cost, compared to other forms of medical management and their side effects (hot flushes, asthenia, decreased libido, etc.), has limited their application. Empirically, LHRH analogs have been used in a small subset of patients who experienced rapid regrowth of tissue after surgery and required resection on an almost annual basis. Antiandrogens show a similar profile of efficacy, but these too are limited by their side-effect profile and cost constraints.

In summary, finasteride appears to produce symptomatic improvement in approximately one-third of patients; the effects are more pronounced in those patients with large prostates. Safety and durability of results have been shown after several years of treatment and it appears that finasteride treatment reduces the incidence of acute urinary retention and the need for surgery.

Combined therapy

As the aim of hormonally based treatments is to reduce the volume of glandular tissue and that of adrenoreceptor blockade is to decrease tone in the stromal and capsular tissues, the concept of combining these agents to attain an increased clinical benefit has obvious appeal. With the tolerability and safety of both forms of treatment established, a number of studies examined these therapies in combination. Initially terazosin was combined with the antiandrogen flutamide[51]. Almost 50% of patients withdrew because of adverse side effects and many of the remainder required reduction in the dose of flutamide. Neither peak urinary flow rates nor symptom scores improved significantly overall, but 25% of the patients did exhibit a moderate symptomatic improvement after the addition of flutamide.

For the combination of terazosin and finasteride, no statistically significant benefit was attained in comparison to terazosin alone[52]. Analysis of the benefit in patients with pre-treatment prostate volume >50mL showed a trend toward improved flow rates and decreased symptom scores in the dual therapy group, but this was not of statistical significance[52]. It appears from these early data that any benefit of combination over single-agent treatment is slight and probably outweighed by side effects and cost factors; however, a number of ongoing trials are likely to provide further information.

Plant extracts

Phytotherapeutic agents have been used for centuries throughout Europe for the treatment of lower urinary tract symptoms and are readily available over the counter in many countries. The safety of these agents is probably confirmed by their widespread and long-term use. As there is considerable doubt as to whether these agents possess clinical efficacy outside of the well-documented placebo effect of medications and the variation in the natural history of BPH, it is now opportune to subject these therapies to the same rigorous testing as applied to medical treatments. Agents have been classified as[53]:

- phytotherapeutic;
- cholesterol lowering;
- amino acid complexes; and
- organ extracts.

There is considerable overlap between groups.

Phytotherapeutic agents include the roots of *Hypoxis rooperi* and *Echinacea purpurea*, the fruit of *Sabal serulata* (*Serenoa repens*), the bark of *Pygeum africanum*, pollen extract, *Cucurbita pepo* seeds, and the leaves of the trembling poplar. The mode of action of these agents is unknown. Laboratory findings reveal a number of properties, which include:

- antiandrogenic and antiestrogenic effects;
- decrease in sex hormone-binding globulin;
- inhibition of production of growth factors (fibroblast growth factor and epidermal growth factor)[54]; and
- anti-inflammatory effects through interference with metabolism of prostaglandins.

Prostate secretions and the substance of the prostate gland contain an abundance of cholesterol. In addition, hyperplastic prostate tissue contains twice as much cholesterol as normal prostate; it is by reducing this that cholesterol-lowering agents, such as sitosterol, are postulated to reduce prostate size.

The mode of action of amino acid complexes, such as Balometan and Paraprostin, has not been fully elucidated. Similarly prostate extracts, such as Raveron, have been applied to clinical use without a full description of the rationale for their use.

The availability and safety of plant extracts account for their appeal as potential treatments for BPH. However, the mode of action of many of these agents needs to be elucidated. Similarly, accurate assessment of their clinical effect needs to be established using symptom scores (other than assessments of global well-being) and objective measures, such as flow rate, residual volume, and pressure flow studies. Preliminary studies suggest[55] objective improvements in symptom score and flow rates over controls. It will be interesting to see if these results are confirmed by subsequent studies.

NONMEDICAL ALTERNATIVE THERAPIES

Balloon dilation

The enthusiasm that greeted the arrival of balloon dilation reflects the desire to provide an alternative treatment to prostatectomy (Fig. 31.3). Claims that it might completely replace TURP have failed to be realized. Dilation is achieved using a modification of an Amplatz cardiology catheter. A 90–105F balloon is positioned in the prostatic urethra, 1cm proximal to the external sphincter. Placement can be carried out either cystoscopically or fluoroscopically. The balloon is maintained in position by a small low-pressure balloon just distal to the dilating balloon. The cardiac catheter balloon is inflated to 404kPa (4atm) and this maintained for 10 minutes. A 22F urethral catheter is inserted for 72 hours postoperatively.

The treatment achieves its effect by splitting the anterior and posterior commissures of the prostate. Other postulated mechanisms of action include pressure atrophy of the prostate from the inflated balloon or stretch and loss of elasticity of the prostate capsule. Balloon dilation of the prostate is a safe procedure, which can in many cases be performed under local anesthetic. Symptomatic improvement has been demonstrated in up to

Nonsurgical Management of Benign Prostatic Hyperplasia

Balloon dilation

Obstructive enlargement

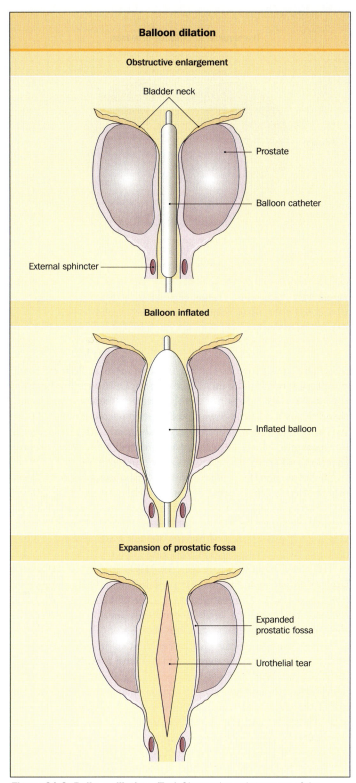

Figure 31.3 Balloon dilation. (Top) Obstructive enlargement of the prostate is achieved with the balloon catheter placed in the prostatic fossa; (center) the balloon is inflated; (bottom) following dilation, the prostatic fossa expands with breach of the mucosa.

two-thirds of patients[56], but with little improvement in flow rates; it has largely been superseded by other forms of minimally invasive treatment.

Heat-based treatments

| High-intensity focused ultrasound |
| Transurethral needle ablation |
| Microwave treatment |

Figure 31.4 Heat-based treatments.

Heat-based treatments

The prostate and surrounding tissues can survive temperatures up to 42.5°C (108.5°F) for 90 minutes[57], which must be exceeded to produce tissue destruction. This ability to survive slight elevations in temperature is termed thermal tolerance and is associated with the production of heat-shock proteins. It is postulated that these may even confer on the cell an improved ability to survive in the face of noxious stimuli. When the temperature is elevated above 42.5°C (108.5°F) for an hour, an increase in the rate of cell death occurs. Elevation in tissue temperature to 42–45°C (108–113°F) is termed hyperthermia; these are the temperatures typically observed in low-energy microwave therapy. Treatments that cause elevation of tissue temperatures above 45°C (113°F) are termed thermotherapy, while elevations above 60°C (140°F) lead to thermoablation (Fig. 31.4).

High-intensity focused ultrasound

High-intensity focused ultrasound (HIFU) is one such treatment and possesses a number of interesting properties. Its ability to cause tissue ablation has been known for some time[58], and it has been explored in the fields of neurosurgery[59] and ophthalmology[60], as well as in the treatment of liver tumors[61]. More recently, it has been applied to the canine prostate[62,63] and to the human[64,65] prostate for the treatment of BPH.

The HIFU procedure can be carried out transrectally or transabdominally. The transrectal approach is generally preferred, as in the transabdominal route the bony pelvis prevents access to treat the entire gland. The probe focal length employed varies with the size of the gland (3, 3.5, 4, or 4.5cm). The probe is introduced into the rectum and the covering sheath is inflated with degassed water to ensure air-free contact with the rectal wall. Imaging is used to map out the treatment area and the probe is then fixed in position with the multiarticulated arm (Fig. 31.5). Treatment settings comprise 4 seconds of heat with an ultrasound intensity of about 1.68kW/cm² to obtain tissue temperatures of 80–100°C (176–212°F). The tissue is allowed to cool for 12 seconds, during which dissipation of heat occurs, to prevent damage to surrounding tissues and to allow imaging to be carried out throughout the treatment. Each treatment cycle covers an area of 2 × 2 × 10mm (40mm³) in a horizontal plane of the periurethral prostate. Further lesions are created as the focus of treatment is advanced from the bladder neck to the verumontanum (Fig. 31.6). After completion, this process is repeated to create a further 6–8 tracts in a circumferential manner (Fig. 31.7). A suprapubic catheter is introduced routinely, as earlier studies showed a high rate of postoperative retention[66]. A combination of local and sedoanalgesia has been employed successfully[66], but general or regional anesthetic is often required because of excessive patient movement or discomfort.

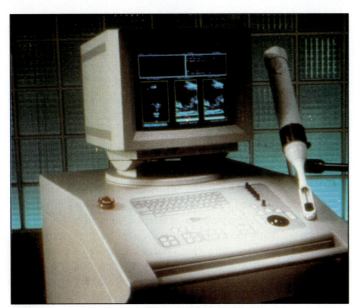

Figure 31.5 High-intensity focused ultrasound.

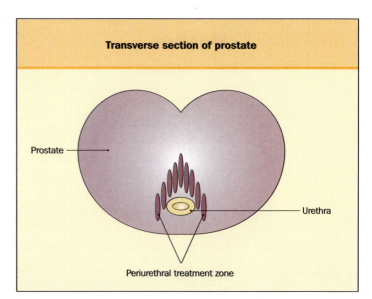

Transverse section of prostate

Prostate

Urethra

Periurethral treatment zone

Figure 31.7 Transverse section of prostate. High-intensity focused ultrasound creates tissue ablation tracts circumferentially in the periurethral tissue.

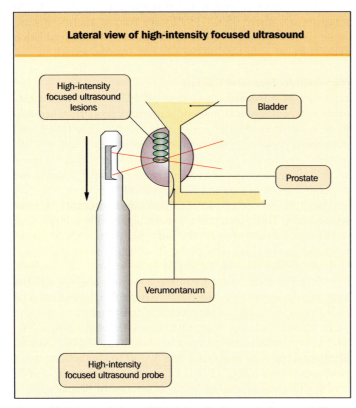

Lateral view of high-intensity focused ultrasound

High-intensity focused ultrasound lesions

Bladder

Prostate

Verumontanum

High-intensity focused ultrasound probe

Figure 31.6 Lateral view of high-intensity focused ultrasound. The rectal high-intensity focused ultrasound probe is used to create focal lesions that overlap in the periurethral tissue, commencing at the bladder neck and continued to the level of the verumontanum.

Treatment results show a mean improvement in International Prostate Symptom Score (IPSS) from 23 to 5, with best results at 6 and 12 months. Mean flow rates improve by over 50%, but these return to pretreatment rates after 2 years. Patients, however, still maintain symptomatic improvement and reduced postvoid residual volume[65]. Inclusion of the bladder neck in the treatment area provides further improvement in flow rates and symptom scores[67]. The incidence of postoperative complications is low. As HIFU does not involve intraurethral manipulation, theoretically it carries a lower likelihood of postoperative UTI and stricture. Bleeding is generally not associated with HIFU, as the intraprostatic blood vessels are coagulated. Effects on erectile function and antegrade ejaculation are uncommon.

Disproportionate improvement in symptomatic score has been reported with other forms of thermal ablation and may arise in part from thermal injury to bladder neck innervation and consequent reduced sensation in this area. Such improvement also may result from a reduction in the work required of the detrusor, with no increase in flow rate.

Prostates deemed unsuitable for HIFU include those with a large middle lobe and those that contain calculi (which attenuate the ultrasound). The initial set-up cost of HIFU is high, as it requires the purchase of dedicated equipment. However, the short duration of hospital stay and the use of only a few disposables per case reduce the cost per patient treated. The true cost of the procedure can be evaluated only with a study of the long-term efficacy and the requirement for other treatments. The need for postoperative catheterization may be overcome by the use of biodegradable stents [as in transurethral microwave therapy (TUMT)], and the use of prostate block or sedoanalgesic means that general anesthetic requirements can be reduced. More recently, HIFU showed promise in the ablation of urologic tumors and its application in renal, testicular, and prostate tumors, as well as the reduced morbidity in the treatment of BPH, may lead to the broader acceptance and use of HIFU for the management of benign and malignant urologic conditions (Fig. 31.8).

Transurethral needle ablation

The transurethral needle ablation (TUNA) device consists of a modified 22F urethral catheter. At its distal end are two retractile needles, which advance perpendicular to the urethra into the substance of the prostate, to form a 40° angle with one another

Advantages and disadvantages of high-intensity focused ultrasound	
Advantages	**Disadvantages**
Noncontact	Expense of dedicated probe (offset by subsequent low equipment cost per patient)
No radiation	General or regional anesthetic often required
No intraurethral manipulation	Postoperative catheterization required
Area of maximum energy intensity can be focused deep in the prostate	
Potential application to other treatments (e.g. tumors)	

Figure 31.8 Advantages and disadvantages of high-intensity focused ultrasound.

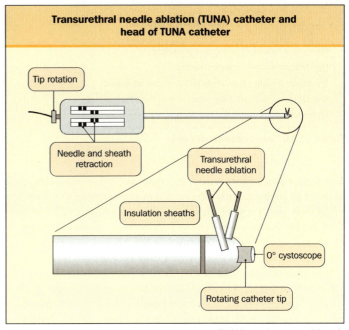

Figure 31.9 Transurethral needle ablation (TUNA) catheter and head of TUNA catheter.

(Fig. 31.9). The head of the catheter can be rotated to access the entire prostate, and it is positioned in the prostatic urethra under direct vision, via a 0° cystoscope introduced through the center of the TUNA catheter. The volume of the prostate is determined prior to the procedure using transrectal ultrasound, and the needles are advanced into the prostate to a depth of 5–6mm from the prostatic capsule. The insulation sheaths are retracted to within 5–6mm of the prostatic urethra to enable treatment of the substance of the prostate and yet protect the prostatic urethra. Low-level radiofrequency (460kHz) generates temperatures in excess of 100°C (212°F) at the tip of the needles, and creates lesions within 3–5 minutes. Thermosensors at the urethra automatically interrupt treatment delivery when the temperature exceeds 47°C (116°F) or when tissue impedance reaches 500 ohms or more. Treatment is commenced 1cm distal to the bladder neck and is continued down to 1cm proximal to the verumontanum. Thus, the number of areas treated and the overall duration of treatment depend on the length of the prostatic urethra. Treatment times are about 30–50 minutes. Treatment can be carried out under local anesthetic, but patient comfort is often facilitated by the use of intravenous sedation.

Histologic examination of patients who undergo TUNA prior to radical prostatectomy showed a necrotic area of treatment with sharp demarcation from the surrounding untreated tissue[68]. In this study, the size of the lesion varied from 12 × 7mm up to 18 × 12mm with treatment times of 3 and 5 minutes (and needle deployment of 10mm), respectively. Transrectal ultrasound and MRI may show a cavity defect, but this occurs only in a few cases and an overall reduction in prostate size is not usually seen. As in HIFU, thermoablation by TUNA is likely to cause decreased bladder neck sensation, and therefore decreased symptoms and reduced bladder neck tone. The results at a 12-month follow-up showed that TUNA produces a modest, but significant, improvement in flow rates (from 8.71mL/s to 11.64mL/s), IPSS symptom score (from 22.0 to 7.5), quality of life from (4 to 2.0) and postvoid residual urine volume (from 91.7mL to 53.6mL)[69]. At 2 year follow-up, improvements in symptom score and flow rates are maintained[70]. Complications, which include retention, dysuria, and prostatitis, are transient and are generally resolved by 30 days. When compared to TURP, both treatments show equivalent improvements in indices of bother and quality of life at 12 months. Symptom score improvement is seen in 78% of TUNA patients versus 91% of the TURP group, and a 50%

increase in flow rate is seen in 62.5% of TUNA patients versus 81.8% of those who undergo TURP[71].

As the safety of this procedure continues to be established, further modifications may be possible, such as a flexible scope to improve patient comfort and the use of longer needle deployment and more powerful machines to speed up the procedure[72].

Microwave treatment
The delivery of microwave treatment to the prostate can be either by the transrectal or transurethral route (Fig. 31.10). Both procedures are carried out on a day-case basis, without the need for general or regional anesthetic. A major disadvantage of both transrectal and transurethral microwave treatments is that the most intense delivery of energy is experienced in the tissue closest to the probe, which renders the rectum and urethra, respectively, susceptible to injury. This places a limit on the duration and intensity of treatment. To address these problems cooling sheaths were designed to cool the surface with simultaneous delivery of high-intensity energy to the deeper tissues. Rectal and urethral temperature probes are employed to reduce microwave output when a rectal temperature of 42°C (107°F) [or 43.5°C (110°F) on high-intensity settings] or a urethral temperature of 45°C (113°F) is attained. A rapid dissipation of energy occurs in the prostate, with a 1°C (1.8°F) decrease in temperature per 3mm distance from the temperature applicator[73]. Thus only tissue penetration distances of approximately 2cm can be attained per treatment, and hence the need for multiple treatment sessions. Also, transrectal microwave therapy preferentially treats the peripheral portion of the prostate, while the predominant sites for BPH are the central and intermediate zones treated by the transurethral approach.

The initial studies employed treatment temperatures of 42–45°C (107–113°F; hyperthermia). Comparison between hyperthermia transrectally and transurethrally showed a higher degree

Microwave treatment

Day-patient procedure under local anesthetic

High retreatment rate in earlier studies

Transurethral route has superseded transrectal microwave

Thermotherapy appears more effective than hyperthermia

Higher side-effect profile occurs with high energy settings

Figure 31.10 Microwave treatment.

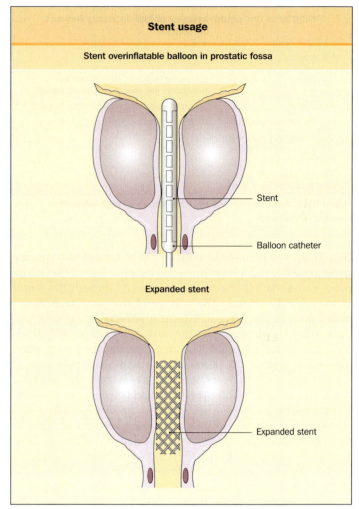

Stent usage

Stent overinflatable balloon in prostatic fossa

Stent

Balloon catheter

Expanded stent

Expanded stent

Figure 31.11 Stent usage. (Top) Stent overinflatable balloon in prostatic fossa; (bottom) expanded stent.

of symptomatic improvement at 3 months (79% versus 41%) and number of patients with a reduction in prostate size (79% versus 45%), but also a higher incidence of complications (27% versus 8%) in the transurethral group[74]. A greater response is seen in those patients for whom treatment is for a longer duration and at higher intensity[75]. It is likely that a large proportion of this group had treatment that might be classified as thermotherapy [i.e. tissue temperature >45°C (113°F)]. Indeed, many of the earlier studies in which hyperthermia was used tended to show improvements in symptom scores with little change in flow rates[76]. The sharp rise in PSA witnessed in other heat treatments is not seen in microwave hyperthermia, which suggests only modest, if any, thermal injury.

More recently, software has become available to deliver TUMT at a higher intensity. Such treatments allow thermotherapy [temperatures >45°C (>113°F), often >60°C (>140°F)] to be carried out rather than hyperthermia. Short-term results show this to provide a more pronounced effect than low-intensity treatment, but the associated morbidity also increases. There also is an associated increase in treatment discomfort and an increased need for analgesic and sedation[77].

In comparison with TURP, TUMT is equally effective at reducing symptom score at 6 months, but has far less effect on objective indices of obstruction [maximum flow rate (Q_{max}), detrusor pressure, and postvoid residual volume][78].

The role of TUMT and the appropriate treatment settings are currently under review; a balance is needed between increased efficacy of higher power versus the increased invasiveness and higher side-effect profile.

Stents

Experience in the field of cardiology in particular has been applied to the development of expandable intraurethral endoprostheses. The initial indication was intractable urinary retention in poor-risk surgical patients, in whom the other options were permanent indwelling or intermittent catheterization[79]. Patients almost universally regained the ability to void after the insertion of the stent (Fig. 31.11). The indication for stents was extended to those patients with moderate-to-severe symptoms, who again were considered poor candidates for surgery; in this group mean peak flow rates improved by almost 50%[80].

Many patients experience irritative symptoms postinsertion, but these tend to improve within a few months. With long-term follow-up, 13–40%[80,81] of patients require removal of the stent, in most cases cystoscopically. The principal indications for removal are detrusor instability, stent migration, and encrustation. Other troublesome side effects include recurrent UTI, prostatitis, epididymitis, and hematuria. Use of more biocompatible materials, such as titanium[82], has resulted in similar rates of stent

removal. Most of the original stents were cylindric in shape, which did not conform exactly to the prostatic urethra and so allowed urine to collect behind the stent, which resulted in postmicturition dribbling. Other materials have been developed subsequently to reduce this problem, including nitinol which expands at body temperature to the cavity of the prostatic urethra.

Temporary stents continue to be reviewed; although the initial success rates do not appear to be quite as high as those of permanent stents, the overall function appears comparable. The division between permanent and temporary is somewhat artificial, in that many of the temporary stents are left in place for several years – indeed a number of patients die of comorbid illness with these in place. It is clear that the ideal combination of stent design and material has yet to be defined and their use is best limited to those patients in whom the only other choice is indwelling or intermittent catheterization. An area of stent design that holds considerable promise is that of dissolvable stents. Galactide spirals are resorbed over a period of 6–12 months and maintain urethral patency. These have potential application in treatments associated with a high rate of post-treatment retention, as in a number of heat treatments of the prostate. They have been used with TUMT[83] and are being explored in combination with other treatment modalities.

FUTURE DIRECTIONS

The number of men who seek and receive treatment for lower urinary tract symptoms continues to increase. A number of factors are likely to contribute to this increase, including an increase in the aged male population and an increased awareness and desire for treatment of lower urinary tract symptoms. The development of a number of minimally invasive treatments and, in particular, the widespread acceptance of the safety and efficacy of medical treatments also contribute to this increase. Similarly, improvements in overall patient selection and facilities for patient care are likely to lead to further improvements in outcome.

For the treatment of complicated BPH, TURP remains the gold standard, but many of these patients are keen to try a less invasive treatment to avoid or defer surgery. It seems appropriate that surgical options be compared to TURP as well as to placebo or sham treatment groups. However, the profile of patients who receive treatment continues to expand and the role of minimally invasive treatments in some instances might be regarded as complementary to rather than competitive with TURP in the management of BPH. Thus, in these circumstances it is appropriate that the value of these treatments be assessed by direct comparison with one another and with respect to medical management. As TURP continues to be reassessed and refined, the standard set for competing modalities to achieve continues to rise. Indeed, there are reports emerging of TURP being carried out on a day-case basis[84]. Similarly, as competing medical and minimally invasive therapies continue to be developed a number of modalities, such as balloon dilation and transrectal microwave hyperthermia, are almost relegated to the realms of history.

Medical management is likely to continue to play a central role in the management of BPH, with increased understanding of bladder neck and voiding physiology. Thermotherapy and thermal ablation are likely to be improved by the use of removable or biodegradable stents to bypass the edematous prostate after thermal ablation. There is likely to be further refinement in the intensity and duration of treatment of contact and interstitial laser and microwave therapies, as are developments in flexibility according to prostate characteristics, all to help achieve maximum improvement and maintain tolerability, and cost and side-effect profiles. Future trials of available technology should focus on establishing the long-term efficacy and the type of patient who would gain most benefit from such therapy[85]. Further approaches to treatment are likely to emerge – enzymatic digestion of the prostate has been carried out in the experimental animal with promising results[86] and application to the human is a distinct possibility.

It is likely that the health care professional who treats BPH in the near future will require familiarity with surgery, a medical agent, and a minimally invasive technique to provide a comprehensive service to the patient. New technologies will continue to emerge and accepted treatments will continue to be refined. Each must be closely assessed with regard to efficacy and the potential role they might play in the armamentarium for the treatment of BPH.

REFERENCES

1. Abrams P. New words for old: lower urinary tract symptoms for 'prostatism'. Br Med J. 1994;308:929–30.
2. Ohnishi K, Watanabe H, Ohe H. Development of benign prostatic hyperplasia estimated from ultrasonic measurement with long-term follow-up. J Exp Med. 1987;151:51–6
3. Girman C, Jacobsen S, Guess H, et al. Natural history of prostatism: relationship among symptoms, prostate volume and peak urinary flow rate. J Urol. 1995;153:1510–5.
4. Birkhoff J. Natural history of benign prostatic hyperplasia. In: Hinman F, ed. Benign prostatic hypertrophy. New York: Springer-Verlag; 1983.
5. Fitzpatrick JM. A critical evaluation of technological innovations in the treatment of symptomatic benign prostatic hyperplasia. Br J Urol. 1998;81(Suppl 1):56–63.
6. Thomas K, Cornaby A, Hammadeh M, Philp T, Matthews P. Transurethral vaporization of the prostate: a promising new technique. Br J Urol. 1997;79:186–9.
7. Hahn R, Sandfeldt L, Nyman C. Double-blind randomized study of symptoms associated with absorption of glycine 1.5% or mannitol 3% during transurethral resection of the prostate. J Urol. 1998;160:397–401.
8. McConnell J. Why pressure flow studies should be optional and not mandatory studies for evaluating men with benign prostatic hyperplasia. Urology. 1994;44:156–8.
9. Abrams PH. In support of pressure-flow studies for evaluating men with lower urinary tract symptoms. Urology. 1994;44:153–5.
10. Orandi A. Transurethral incision of the prostate compared with transurethral resection of the prostate in 132 matching cases. J Urol. 1987;138:810–5.
11. Orandi A. Incision of the prostate (TUIP): 646 cases in 15 years – a chronological appraisal. Br J Urol. 1985;57:703–7.
12. Edwards L, Powell C. An objective comparison of transurethral resection and bladder neck incision in the treatment of prostatic hypertrophy. J Urol. 1982;128:325–7.
13. Ronzoni G, De Vecchis M. Preservation of anterograde ejaculation after transurethral resection of both prostate and bladder neck. Br J Urol. 1998;81:830–3.
14. Cornford C, Biyani C, Powell C. Transurethral incision of the prostate using the holmium:YAG laser: a catheterless procedure. J Urol. 1998;159:1229–31.
15. Carter A, Speakman M, O'Boyle P. A prospective randomised controlled trial comparing hybrid KTP/Nd:YAG laser treatment of the prostate with TURP. Br J Urol. 1997;80(S2):224–7.
16. Kaplan S, Goluboff E, Olsson C, Deverka P, Chmiel J. Effect of demographic factors, urinary peak flow rates, and Boyarsky symptom scores on patient treatment choice in benign prostatic hyperplasia. Urology. 1995;45:398–405.
17. Mebust W, Holtgrave H, Cockett A. Transurethral prostatectomy: immediate and postoperative complications. A cooperative study of 13 participating institutions evaluating 3855 patients. J Urol. 1989;141:243–7.

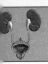

18. Fowler F, Wennberg J, Timothy R, Barry M, Mulley A, Hanley D. Symptom status and quality of life following prostatectomy. JAMA. 1988;259:3018–22.

19. Libman E, Fichten C. Prostatectomy and sexual function. Urology. 1987;29:467–78.

20. Roos N, Wennberg J, Malenka D, et al. Mortality and reoperation after transurethral resection of the prostate for benign prostatic hyperplasia. N Eng J Med. 1989;320:1120–4.

21. Bartsch G, Muller H, Boerholzer M, Rohr H. Light microscopic stereological analysis of the normal human prostate and benign prostatic hyperplasia. J Urol. 1979;122:487–91.

22. Furuya S, Kumamoto Y, Yokoyama E. α-adrenergic activity and urethral pressure in prostatic zone in benign prostatic hypertrophy. J Urol. 1982;128:836–9.

23. Caine M, Pfau A, Perlberg S. The use of α-adrenergic blockers in benign prostatic hyperplasia. Br J Urol. 1976;48:255–63.

24. Kirby R, Coppinger S, Corcoran M, Chapple C, Flannigan M, Milroy E. Prazosin in the treatment of prostatic obstruction. Br J Urol. 1987;60:136–42.

25. Lepor H. The treatment of benign prostatic hyperplasia with α-1 blockers. Curr Opin Urol. 1992;4:16–21.

26. Bylund D, Eikenberg D, Hieble J, et al. International Union of Pharmacology nomenclature of adrenoreceptors. Pharmacol Rev. 1994;46:121–36.

27. Forray C, Bard J, Wetzel J, et al. The α_1-adrenergic receptor that mediates smooth muscle contraction in the prostate has the pharmacological properties of the cloned human α_{1C} subtype. Mol Pharmacol. 1994;45:703–8.

28. Lepor H, Tang R, Meretyk S, Shapiro E. α-1 adrenoreceptor subtypes in the human prostate. J Urol. 1993;149:640–2.

29. Hatano A, Takahashi H, Tamaki M, Komeyama T, Koizumi T, Takeda M. Pharmacological evidence of distinct α-1 adrenoreceptor subtypes mediating the contraction of human prostatic urethra and peripheral artery. Br J Pharmacol. 1994;113:723–8.

30. Schulman C, Cortvriend J, Jonas U, et al. The first prostate-selective α-1A adrenoreceptor antagonist. Analysis of a multinational, multicentre, open-label study assessing the long-term efficacy and safety in patients with benign prostatic obstruction (symptomatic BPH). Eur Urol. 1996;29:145–54.

31. Beduschi M, Beduschi R, Oesterling J. α-blockade therapy for benign prostatic hyperplasia: from a nonselective to a more selective α1A-adrenergic antagonist. Urology. 1998;51:861–72.

32. Michel M, Grubbel B, Taguchi K, Verfurth F. Drugs for treatment of benign prostatic hyperplasia: affinity comparison at cloned α-1 adrenoreceptor subtypes and in human prostate. J Auto Pharmacol. 1996;16:21–8.

33. Lowe F. Coadministration of tamsulosin and three antihypertensive agents in patients with benign prostatic hyperplasia: pharmacodynamic effect. Clin Ther. 1997;19:730–42.

34. Andersson K, Lepor H, Wylie M. Prostatic α 1-adenoreceptors and uroselectivity. Prostate. 1997;30:3202–15.

35. Chapple C. Pharmacotherapy for benign prostatic hyperplasia – the potential for α1-adrenorecptor subtype-specific blockade. Br J Urol. 1998;81(Suppl 1):34–47.

36. Ishizuka O, Persson K, Mattiasson A, Naylor A, Wyllie M, Andersson K. Micturition in conscious rats with and without outlet obstruction: role of spinal α-1 adrenoreceptors. Br J Pharmacol. 1996;117:962–6.

37. Ramage A, Wyllie M. Effects of doxazosin and terazosin on inferior mesenteric nerve activity, spontaneous bladder contraction and blood pressure in anaesthetised cats. Br J Pharmacol. 1994;112:526P.

38. Kyprianou N, Litvak J, Borkowski A, Alexander R, Jacobs S. Induction of prostate apoptosis by doxazosin in benign prostatic hyperplasia. J Urol. 1998;159:1810–5.

39. White J. The results of double castration in hypertrophy of the prostate. Ann Surg. 1895;22:1–80.

40. Schroder F. Medical treatment of benign prostatic hyperplasia: the effect of surgical or medical castration. Prog Clin Biol Res. 1994;386:191–6.

41. Wilson J. The pathogenesis of benign prostatic hyperplasia. Am J Med. 1980;68:745–56.

42. Silver R, Wiley E, Thigpen A. Cell type specific expression of steroid 5α reductase 2. J Urol. 1994;152:438–42.

43. Imperato-McGinley J, Guerrero L, Gautier T, Peterson R. Steroid 5α reductase deficiency in man: an inherited form of male pseudo-hermaphroditism. Science. 1974;186:1213–5.

44. McConnell J, Wilson J, George F. Finasteride, an inhibitor of 5α reductase, suppresses prostatic dihydrotestosterone in men with benign prostatic hyperplasia. J Clin Endocrin Metab. 1992; 74:505–8.

45. Gormley G, Stoner E, Bruskewitz R, et al. The effect of finasteride in men with benign prostatic hyperplasia. N Eng J Med. 1992;327:1185–91.

46. The Finasteride Study Group. Finasteride in the treatment of benign prostatic hyperplasia. Prostate. 1993;22:291–9.

47. Boyle P, Gould A, Roehrborn C. Prostate volume predicts outcome of treatment of benign prostatic hyperplasia with finasteride: meta-analysis of randomized clinical trials. Urology. 1996; 48:398–405.

48. Geller J. Five year follow-up of patients with benign prostatic hyperplasia treated with finasteride. Eur Urol. 1995;21:267–73.

49. Andersen J, Nickel J, Marshall V, Schulman C, Boyle P. Finasteride significantly reduces acute urinary retention and the need for surgery in patients with symptomatic benign prostatic hyperplasia. Urology. 1997;49:839–45.

50. McConnell J, Bruskewitz R, Walsh P, et al. The effect of finasteride on the risk of acute urinary retention and the need for surgical treatment among men with benign prostatic hyperplasia. N Eng J Med. 1998;338:557–63.

51. Lepor H, Machi G. The relative efficacy of terazosin versus terazosin and flutamide for the treatment of symptomatic BPH. Prostate. 1992;20:89–95.

52. Lepor H, Williford W, Barry M, et al. The efficacy of terazosin, finasteride, or both in benign prostatic hyperplasia. Veterans Affairs Cooperative Studies Benign Prostatic Hyperplasia Study Group. N Engl J Med. 1996;335:533–9.

53. Fitzpatrick JM, Lynch TH. Phytotherapeutic agents in the management of symptomatic benign prostatic hyperplasia. Urol Clin North Am. 1995;22:407–12.

54. Habib F, Ross M, Buck A. In vitro evaluation of pollen extract, cernitin T-60, in the regulation of prostate cell growth. Br J Urol. 1990;66:393–7.

55. Berges R, Windeler J, Trampisch H, Senge T. Randomised, placebo-controlled, double-blind clinical trial of α-sitosterol in patients with benign prostatic hyperplasia. Lancet. 1995;345:1529–32.

56. McLoughlin J, Keane P, Jager R, Gill K, Machann L, Williams G. Dilation of the prostatic urethra with a 35mm balloon. Br J Urol. 1991;67:177–81.

57. Lieb Z, Rothem A, Lev A, Servadio C. Histopathological observations in the canine prostate treated by local hyperthermia. Prostate. 1986;8:93–102.

58. Wood R, Loomis A. The physical and biological effect of high frequency sound waves of great intensity. London J Sci. 1927; 4:417–36.

59. Fry W, Mosberg W, Barnard J, Fry FJ. Production of focal destructive lesions in the central nervous system with ultrasonics. J Neurosurg. 1954;11:471–8.

60. Coleman D, Lizzi F, Driller J, et al. Therapeutic ultrasound in the treatment of glaucoma. I. Experimental model. Ophthalmology. 1985;92:339–46.

61. ter Haar G, Sinnett D, Rivens I. High intensity focused ultrasound – a surgical technique for the treatment of discrete liver tumours. Phys Med Biol. 1989;34:1743–50.

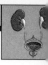

62. Foster R, Bihrle R, Sanghvi N, et al. Production of prostatic lesions in canines using transrectally administered high-intensity focused ultrasound. Eur Urol. 1993;23:330–6.

63. Gelet A, Chapelon J, Morgonari J, et al. Prostatic tissue destruction by high intensity focused ultrasound: experimentation on canine prostate. J Endourol. 1993;7:249–53.

64. Foster RS, Bihrle R, Fry FJ, Donohue JP. Transrectal focused ultrasound ablation of the prostate: the first fifteen patients. J Urol. 1994;147:237A.

65. Mulligan ED, Lynch TH, Mulvin D, Greene D, Smith JM, Fitzpatrick JM. High-intensity focused ultrasound in the treatment of benign prostatic hyperplasia. Br J Urol. 1997;79:177–80.

66. Bihrle R, Foster R, Sanghvi N, Donohue J, Hood P. High intensity focused ultrasound for the treatment of benign prostatic hyperplasia: early United States clinical experience. J Urol. 1994;151:1271–5.

67. Sullivan LD, McLoughlin MG, Goldenberg LG, Gleave ME, Marich KW. Early experience with high-intensity focused ultrasound for the treatment of benign prostatic hypertrophy. Br J Urol. 1997;79:172–6.

68. Schulman C, Zlotta A, Rasor J, Hourriez J, Noel J, Edwards S. Transurethral needle ablation (TUNA): safety feasibility and tolerance of a new office procedure for treatment of benign prostatic hyperplasia. Eur Urol. 1993;24:415–23.

69. Ramon J, Lynch TH, Eardley I, et al. Transurethral needle ablation of the prostate for the treatment of benign prostatic hyperplasia: a collaborative multicentre study. Br J Urol. 1997;80:128–35.

70. Schulman C, Zlotta A. Transurethal needle ablation (TUNA) of the prostate: clinical experience with two years' follow-up in patients with benign prostatic hyperplasia. Eur Urol. 1996;30:985–90.

71. Bruskewitz R, Issa M, Roehrborn C, et al. A prospective, randomized 1-year clinical trial comparing transurethral needle ablation to transurethral resection of the prostate for the treatment of symptomatic benign prostatic hyperplasia. J Urol. 1998;159:1588–94.

72. Lepor H. Editorial comment. J Urol. 1998;159:1588–94.

73. Roehrborn C, Krongrad A, McConnell J. Temperature mapping in the canine prostate during transurethrally applied local microwave hyperthermia. Prostate. 1992;20:97–104. `

74. Stawarz B, Szmigielski S, Ogrodnik J, Astrahan M, Petrovich Z. A comparison of transurethral and transrectal microwave hyperthermia in poor surgical risk benign prostatic hyperplasia patients. J Urol. 1991;146:353–7.

75. Devonec M, Ogden C, Perrin P, St. Clair Carter S. Clinical response to transurethral microwave thermotherapy is thermal dose dependent. Eur Urol. 1993;23:267–74.

76. Abbou C. Transrectal and transurethral hyperthermia versus sham to treat benign prostatic hyperplasia: a double blind randomized multicenter study. J Urol. 1994;151:761A.

77. Djavan B, Shariat S, Schafer B, Marberger M. Tolerability of high energy transurethral microwave thermotherapy with topical urethral anesthesia: results of a randomized, single-blinded clinical trial. J Urol. 1998;160:772–6.

78. Ahmed M, Bell T, Lawrence W, Ward J, Watson G. Transurethral microwave thermotherapy (ProstatronTM version 2.5) compared with transurethral resection of the prostate for the treatment of benign prostatic hyperplasia: a randomized, controlled, parallel study. Br J Urol. 1997;79:181–5.

79. Fabian K. Der intraprostatische 'Partielle Katheter' (Urologische Spirale). Urologe A. 1980;19:236–8.

80. Oesterling J, Kaplan S, Epstein H, Defalco A, Reddy P, Chancellor M. The North American experience with the UroLume endoprosthesis as a treatment for benign prostatic hyperplasia: long term results. Urology. 1994;44:353–62.

81. Anjum M, Chari R, Shetty A, Keen M, Palmer J. Long-term clinical results and quality of life after insertion of a self-expanding endourethral prosthesis. Br J Urol. 1997;80:885–8.

82. Kaplan S, Merrill D, Mosely W, et al. The titanium intraprostatic stent: the United States experience. J Urol. 1993;150:1624–9.

83. Dahlstrand T, Grundtman S, Pettersson S. High-energy transurethral microwave thermotherapy for large severely obstructing prostates and the use of biodegradable stents to avoid catheterisation after treatment. Br J Urol. 1997;79:907–9.

84. Gordon N. Catheter-free same day surgery transurethral resection of the prostate. J Urol. 1998;160:1709–12.

85. Fitzpatrick JM. Editorial: benign prostatic hyperplasia – further lessons, further problems? J Urol. 1998;160:1707–8.

86. Harmon W, Barrett D, Qian J, Lauvetz R, Bostwick D, Gocken M. Transurethral enzymatic ablation of the prostate: canine model. Urology. 1996;48:229–33.

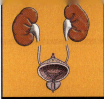

Chapter 32

Female Urology and Incontinence

Harris E Foster Jr

KEY POINTS

- Urinary incontinence is most frequently related to bladder and/or urethral dysfunction. Characteristics that promote continence include maintenance of normal bladder pressure–volume relations, absence of uninhibited bladder contractions, reasonable bladder emptying, satisfactory intrinsic closure capabilities of the urethra, and functional support structures that maintain the urethra in its normal retropubic position.

- Urgency urinary incontinence resulting from involuntary bladder contractions during the storage phase can be treated by behavioral modification, pharmacotherapy with anticholinergic and tricyclic antidepressants, and, where necessary, surgical procedures such as subtrigonal rhizolysis, sacral nerve stimulation, and augmentation cystoplasty.

- Stress urinary incontinence resulting from failure to maintain the normal retropubic position of the bladder neck and proximal urethra during increases in abdominal pressure and/or an impaired internal sphincter mechanism can be treated by behavioral modification, pharmacotherapy with α-adrenergic agonists, tricyclic antidepressants and estrogens, and surgical procedures such as bladder neck suspension procedures, an artificial urinary sphincter, and intraurethral bulking agents.

Common female urologic disorders
Urinary incontinence
Urinary fistulae
Urinary tract infection
Interstitial cystitis/urethral syndrome
Urethral diverticulum
Urethral/vaginal mass
Urethral caruncle
Bartholin's duct cyst
Skene's gland cyst
Pelvic prolapse

Figure 32.1 Common female urologic disorders.

INTRODUCTION

The discipline entitled female urology has only recently become one of the recognized urologic subspecialties. Urology has traditionally been viewed as a specialty that focused primarily on genitourinary diseases in the male. Although any urologic disorder that occurs in the female patient (i.e. neoplasia, calculus disease, urinary tract infection (UTI), and obstruction) could technically be deemed female urology, this subspecialty has generally involved the evaluation and management of urologic disorders that frequently, if not exclusively, occur in the female. Common genitourinary abnormalities found in the female include urinary incontinence with or without pelvic prolapse; urethral diverticula, caruncles and prolapse; vaginal wall cysts; UTI; ureteral and vesicovaginal fistulae; and interstitial cystitis (Fig. 32.1). Although many of these disorders are also treated by gynecologists, it is the urologist who has usually taken the

lead in their management. Consequently, it is imperative that urologists have a thorough understanding of the pathophysiology, diagnosis and treatment of these problems since they will often be the first specialist consulted. Finally, female urology has attained true subspecialty status in the field of urology as many fellowship programs exist and most major urology departments have a faculty member with a dedicated interest in this area. The goal of this chapter will be to address the typical female urologic entities, with a particular focus on incontinence, with the exception of those (interstitial cystitis, UTI, and fistulae) that are addressed elsewhere in this text.

URINARY INCONTINENCE

Epidemiology

Urinary incontinence (UI) is a multifactorial disease process known to affect an astounding number of men and women. It has recently been estimated that the prevalence of UI in the population between 15 and 64 years of age ranges from 1.5% to 5% in men and 10% to 25% in women. Thomas et al. reported an overall prevalence of 8.5% in English women and 16% in those above the age of 75[1]. Some 26% of women will experience some form of urinary incontinence in their adult life[2]. Diokno and colleagues found that 37.6% of women above the age of 60 admitted to some form of UI[3]. The incidence of UI clearly increases with age, as prevalence rates in the elderly range from 48% to 55%[4,5]. Furthermore, of those patients institutionalized, more than 50% experience regular episodes of UI, often several times per day. It is not unreasonable to assume that many of these estimates may be conservative, as there can be a significant underreporting of incontinence by patients, their families, and caregivers.

The consequences exacted upon patients with UI can take a toll on their health, financial status, social and behavioral capabilities, and psychologic stability. Common health problems in those who are incontinent include skin breakdown from chronic dampness, and falls resulting from frequent trips to the bathroom. Many studies have demonstrated the social impact of UI in affected patients. It has been shown that patients who have UI are more likely to suffer from depression and decreased life satisfaction[6]. Wyman et al. reviewed a number of reports which demonstrated that social behaviors such as participation in out of home functions and sexual activity were reduced in patients with UI[7]. To complicate matters, many patients become frustrated with a sometimes unsympathetic medical profession notwithstanding the fact that most (86%) women will see their physician at least once for the evaluation of UI[8]. Finally, cost estimates of managing UI in the community and nursing homes exceeds $10 billion dollars per year in 1987 dollars[9]. Estimated consumer cost for urinary incontinence pads was $365 million early in the 1990s, increasing to $600 million in 1997. Clearly, the social and financial impact of UI on our society can be quite significant.

Pathophysiology of urinary incontinence

The etiology of UI can usually be divided into causes related to bladder and/or urethral dysfunction (Fig. 32.2). Another useful method for characterizing UI involves determining if the underlying abnormality is related to a failure in bladder emptying or storage. Characteristics of bladder function that promote continence include maintenance of the normal pressure–volume relationship, which accommodates increasing volumes of urine with minimal pressure changes (high compliance), and an absence of uninhibited bladder contractions, which when present result in the involuntary loss of urine (urge incontinence). Furthermore, bladder emptying needs to be reasonably complete to prevent detrusor storage pressures at high volumes from exceeding urethral resistance (overflow incontinence). Finally, dysfunction in either the intrinsic closure capabilities of the urethra or a defect in the support structures that maintain its normal retropubic position will prevent maintenance of urinary continence in the face of transient increases in intra-abdominal pressure (stress incontinence). A detailed discussion of the normal physiology of lower urinary tract function can be found in Chapter 6.

Bladder dysfunction

Urgency urinary incontinence

The most common cause of UI secondary to bladder dysfunction is the presence of involuntary bladder contractions during the storage phase, which results in the clinical symptom of urgency urinary incontinence (UUI). Any noxious stimulus to the bladder has the capability of triggering an involuntary bladder contraction. The potential causative mechanisms are varied and include infection, inflammation, obstruction, calculi, neoplasia, urethral hypermobility, and neurologic diseases. Although probably secondary to a subclinical neurologic abnormality (i.e. peripheral denervation or changes in sensory nerve fibers), many patients, particularly the elderly, are deemed to have an idiopathic origin. The end result, however, is the same – an uninhibited detrusor contraction, usually associated with co-ordinated relaxation of the external urethral sphincter, resulting in urinary incontinence.

Etiology of urinary incontinence
Bladder dysfunction
Urethral dysfunction
Mixed (bladder and urethral) dysfunction
Others (fistulae, ectopic ureters, etc.)

Figure 32.2 Etiology of urinary incontinence.

Different terminology has been used to describe situations in which involuntary bladder contractions occur. When associated with a known neurologic disorder it is called detrusor hyperreflexia, whereas when no obvious neurologic disease can be identified it is labeled detrusor instability[10]. The presence or absence of documented involuntary bladder contractions during urodynamic evaluation has also been used to separate those with UUI into motor and sensory types respectively. The clinical significance of this differentiation is questionable; however, the former tends to respond better to pharmacologic therapy than does the latter.

The typical clinical presentation of UUI is an uncontrolled desire to urinate that cannot be suppressed prior to reaching a socially acceptable location. Since many patients fail to experience urgency prior to the incontinent episode despite similar pathophysiology, the term urgency incontinence is technically a misnomer. Nevertheless, this term has gained the acceptance of the urodynamic community and those who treat UI regularly. Precipitating events include such situations as hearing running water, assuming a standing position from recumbency, and rapid changes in environmental temperature. Other irritative voiding symptoms often accompany UUI such as frequency, urgency, and nocturia. Some patients will also suffer from nocturnal enuresis, which coincidentally is often related to an involuntary bladder contraction in conjunction with either a sleep disturbance or neurologic abnormality. Entrance of urine into the proximal urethra because of a failure in its closure mechanism during transient increases in intra-abdominal pressure can also trigger UUI (stress-induced UUI).

Evaluation of the patient with UUI first requires understanding that it is not a disease but rather a manifestation of some underlying urologic disorder, notwithstanding the presence of an idiopathic variant. It therefore is incumbent upon the clinician to thoroughly search for any causative disorder that when treated could eradicate the symptom. The history, physical examination, and laboratory studies should all be directed at determining if a treatable etiology exists. Voiding diaries can be an important component of the history as they allow a detailed representation of the patient's voiding pattern, functional bladder capacity, and frequency of incontinent episodes. Urinalysis should always be performed in an attempt to rule out urinary tract infection and neoplasia, with urine culture and cytology obtained when clinically indicated. A measurement of the postvoid residual volume (determined by ultrasound or urethral catheterization) gives a crude estimation of lower urinary tract function since some abnormality in bladder contractility and/or outlet resistance must by definition exist if it is elevated.

Urodynamic testing can provide useful information in the evaluation of UUI. The classic study is the cystometrogram

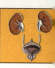

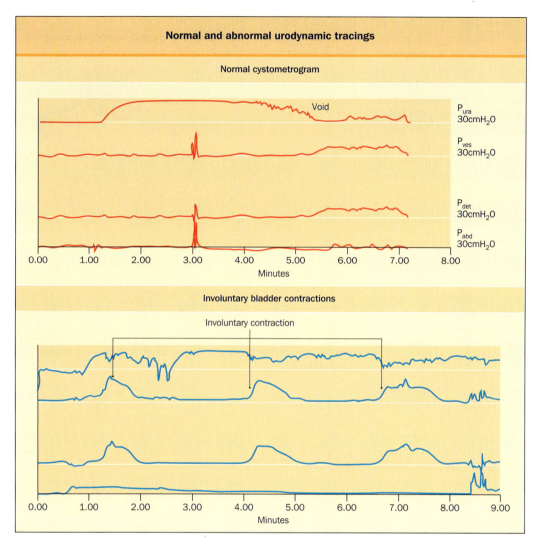

Normal and abnormal urodynamic tracings

Normal cystometrogram

Void

P_{ura}
30cmH$_2$O

P_{ves}
30cmH$_2$O

P_{det}
30cmH$_2$O

P_{abd}
30cmH$_2$O

Minutes

Involuntary bladder contractions

Involuntary contraction

Minutes

Figure 32.3 Normal and abnormal urodynamic tracings. Normal urodynamic study (upper tracing) with absence of involuntary bladder contractions until patient is asked to void. Note co-ordinated relaxation of external urinary sphincter as indicated by reduction in maximum urethral pressure. Patient with urgency urinary incontinence demonstrating multiple involuntary bladder contractions during the cystometrogram (lower tracing). P_{ura}, maximum urethral pressure; P_{ves}, intravesical pressure; P_{det}, subtracted detrusor pressure $P_{ves} - P_{abd}$; P_{abd}, abdominal pressure measured by intrarectal probe.

(CMG), which assesses the relationship between pressure and volume in the bladder primarily during the filling phase. Parameters such as first sensation, cystometric capacity, bladder compliance, and the presence or absence of involuntary contractions provide the most useful information when this study is performed. Although gas can be used as the filling medium, liquid is preferred because of its ability to mimic the normal physiologic milieu. A medium fill rate (approximately 50mL/min) is generally chosen and, although supraphysiologic, usually results in reproducible findings. The International Continence Society has defined an involuntary bladder contraction as a transient increase in the detrusor pressure of more than 15cmH$_2$O during the filling phase[10] (Fig. 32.3). Other urodynamic studies such as noninvasive uroflowmetry, pressure-flow analyses, electromyography, urethral profilometry, and those performed with the addition of fluoroscopy, can also provide useful information regarding the etiology of involuntary bladder contractions such as the presence of bladder outlet obstruction, urethral instability, detrusor external sphincter dyssynergia, and stress incontinence anatomy.

The treatment of UUI mandates a search for specific disease processes (i.e. infection, obstruction, calculus, neoplasia, and neurologic abnormality) that require therapy, unlike that typically used for UUI secondary to untreatable neurologic conditions or the idiopathic variant (Fig. 32.4). When a treatable cause has

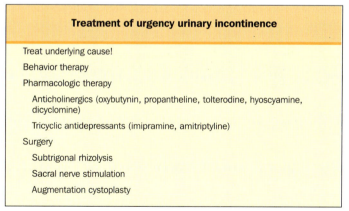

Treatment of urgency urinary incontinence

Treat underlying cause!

Behavior therapy

Pharmacologic therapy

   Anticholinergics (oxybutynin, propantheline, tolterodine, hyoscyamine, dicyclomine)

   Tricyclic antidepressants (imipramine, amitriptyline)

Surgery

   Subtrigonal rhizolysis

   Sacral nerve stimulation

   Augmentation cystoplasty

Figure 32.4 Treatment of urgency urinary incontinence.

been defined, therapy should be directed appropriately. Conversely, if an obvious underlying cause is elusive or nonexistent, behavioral modification, pharmacologic therapy, and surgery are the mainstays of treatment. Timed voiding, a conscious emptying of the bladder on a regular schedule despite the absence of urgency (usually every 2–3 hours), is generally the first line of treatment when the patient does not suffer from extreme urinary frequency and bladder emptying is relatively complete. The goal of this therapy is to empty the bladder frequently prior to the development of urgency, which is often impossible to suppress. This is particularly useful in patients with decreased mobility such as the elderly[11]. When urinary frequency coexists with urgency incontinence, a gradual increase in the interval between voiding, termed bladder retraining, can also be potentially helpful, although long-term results can be disappointing[12]. The addition of pelvic floor exercises to these regimens has been reported to reduce incontinence by 50% or more in up to 75% of patients[13]. Finally, biofeedback and electrical stimulation have been found by some to be a useful adjunct[14,15].

More often than not, behavior modification alone is insufficient to control UUI. Successful treatment generally requires the addition of pharmacotherapy. Although it would be expected that sympathomimetics could suppress involuntary bladder contractions via stimulation of the β_2-adrenoceptors located in the detrusor, these have not demonstrated particular efficacy. The muscarinic cholinergic antagonists have proved to be the most efficacious for the treatment of UUI. Multiple agents exist (i.e. oxybutynin, propantheline, tolterodine, hyoscyamine, and dicyclomine) that can be used successfully alone or in combination. Side effects are not uncommon and include dry mouth, constipation, blurred vision, and exacerbation of narrow-angle glaucoma. Although not technically muscarinic antagonists, the family of tricyclic antidepressants have demonstrated an ability to improve the symptoms of patients with UUI because of their known anticholinergic side effects. Imipramine, nortriptyline, and amitriptyline are the most common drugs used from this family. Combinations of behavior modification and the aforementioned pharmacologic agents generally provide most patients with UUI with significant improvement or cure.

Surgical management of UUI primarily involves procedures that alter the innervation of the bladder or physically enlarge its capacity, except when it exists concomitantly with SUI. In this situation, surgical correction of SUI can often eradicate the UUI by preventing entrance of urine into the posterior urethra during increases in intra-abdominal pressure[16]. Since the base of the female bladder is accessible via the anterior vaginal wall, attempts have been made to denervate it by either chemical injection or surgical lysis. Phenol injections have been used with limited success[17], but McGuire and colleagues reported better results with the Ingleman–Sundberg subtrigonal rhizolysis in those patients who responded to an office injection of bupivacaine[18]. A simple deep dissection of the anterior vaginal wall off the undersurface of the bladder is apparently all that is necessary to achieve sufficient denervation using this technique. Sacral nerve stimulation via its bony foramen has recently demonstrated efficacy in the treatment of UUI following a successful office test procedure (Fig. 32.5). Cure/significantly improved rates have been reported to be approximately 75%[19]. The therapeutic mechanism by which this mode of treatment exerts its beneficial effect is thought to be stimulation of the sacral sensory fibers, which have the ability to inhibit the sacral parasympathetic neurons responsible for detrusor contractility. Typical problems following this procedure include lead migration, pain, and technical difficulties with the hardware. Surgical enlargement of the bladder (augmentation cystoplasty) has proved to be one of the most reliable treatments for refractory UUI. Although practically any segment of bowel

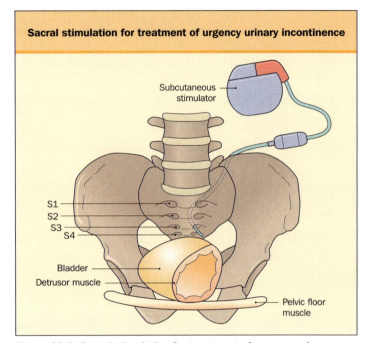

Sacral stimulation for treatment of urgency urinary incontinence

Subcutaneous stimulator

S1
S2
S3
S4

Bladder
Detrusor muscle

Pelvic floor muscle

Figure 32.5 Sacral stimulation for treatment of urgency urinary incontinence.

can be used for augmentation of the bladder, the ileum has remained the most popular because of its favorable location and absorptive characteristics[20,21] (Fig. 32.6). The price of increased storage capability, however, is often paid by a reduction in bladder emptying, thereby necessitating intermittent catheterization. Furthermore, the possibility of future carcinoma has led some to have a less than favorable view of this procedure. Autoaugmentation, sometimes termed detrusor myomectomy, is another alternative for surgically enlarging the bladder capacity[22]. Many questions have arisen regarding its long-term efficacy, which ultimately needs to be established in future clinical trials.

Overflow incontinence

Less prevalent types of bladder dysfunction that result in UI are detrusor areflexia with or without the loss of normal compliance. Detrusor areflexia can present initially as overflow incontinence and is often seen in patients with conditions that impair detrusor contractility, such as diabetes mellitus, tabes dorsalis, and spinal cord injury. Decreased detrusor compliance, classically seen in children with myelodysplasia, results in elevated detrusor pressures at low to moderate volumes, unrelated to a detrusor contraction, which exceed urethral resistance. Although not the focus of this chapter, loss of compliance can ultimately cause diminution of upper urinary tract function. The mainstay of therapy for detrusor areflexia is intermittent catheterization since effective pharmacologic and surgical therapies to augment bladder contractility are elusive. Early data from sacral stimulation, however, suggest a possible role for this technique in the management of detrusor areflexia and nonobstructive incomplete bladder emptying. In a similar way to UUI, management of decreased bladder compliance involves the use of oral anticholinergic agents, augmentation cystoplasty, and intermittent catheterization when necessary.

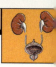

Augmentation ileocystoplasty

Ileal segment opened along antimesenteric border	Medial segments have been sutured and configured into a patch	Ileal patch anastomosed to a bivalved bladder

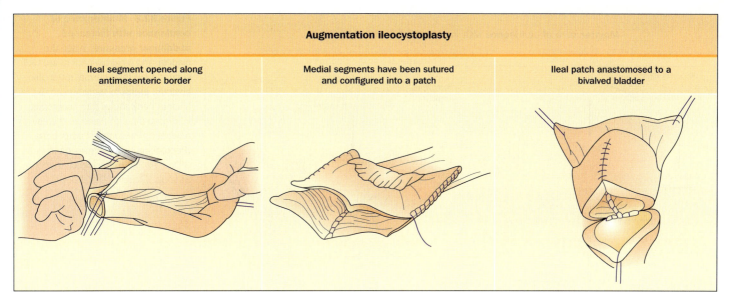

Figure 32.6 Augmentation ileocystoplasty. (Left) Ileal segment opened along antimesenteric border as initial step for detubularization. (Center) Medial segments have been sutured and configured into a patch. (Right) Ileal patch anastomosed to a bivalved bladder. (Reproduced with permission from Hinman F Jr. Atlas of urologic surgery, 2nd edn. London: WB Saunders; 1998.)

Urethral dysfunction – stress urinary incontinence

Urinary incontinence secondary to urethral dysfunction presents as a loss of urine following increases in intra-abdominal pressure, and is generally referred to as stress urinary incontinence (SUI). As a result of its partial intraperitoneal position, transient increases in abdominal pressure are directly transmitted to the bladder, requiring a properly functioning urethra that can counteract these forces, allowing maintenance of continence. Normal urethral function mandates a coapted bladder neck (internal sphincter) and maintenance of its normal retropubic position during increases in intra-abdominal pressure. Failure of either mechanism will generally lead to SUI. The more common type of SUI, termed genuine SUI (GSUI), is related to a transient loss of the normal retropubic position of the bladder neck and proximal urethra during increases in abdominal pressure. Intrinsic sphincter deficiency (ISD), a less common variant of SUI, results from a poorly or nonfunctioning internal sphincter mechanism. In contrast to UI secondary to detrusor dysfunction, de novo SUI primarily occurs in the female population.

Etiology of stress urinary incontinence

The main mechanism of support in the normal female urethra is via the pubourethral ligaments, which extend from the inferior portion of the os pubis to the mid-urethra. In addition, the levator ani musculature, particularly the pubourethralis portion, functions as a hammock in continuity with the endopelvic fascia and provides support to both the bladder base and the urethra. The perineal musculature and fascia provide additional support (Fig. 32.7). These support mechanisms all function to avert abnormal downward and posterior rotational displacement of the urethra in response to increases in intra-abdominal pressure. By maintaining its normal retropubic position, adequate transmission of intra-abdominal pressure to the proximal urethra allows it to counteract the passive expulsory pressures occurring in the bladder, preventing involuntary loss of urine (Fig. 32.8). At the same time, this hammock mechanism provides rigid support to the posterior wall of the urethra such that increases in

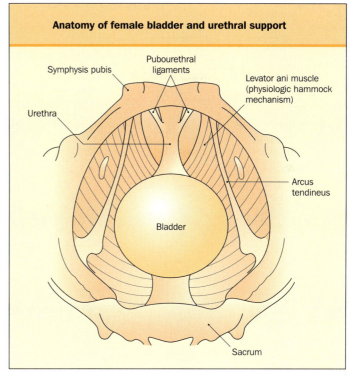

Anatomy of female bladder and urethral support

Figure 32.7 Anatomy of female bladder and urethral support. Note the strong pubourethral ligaments extending from the posterior surface of the symphysis pubis to the urethra and the physiologic hammock formed by the levator ani muscle.

abdominal pressure force the anterior portion of the urethra inferiorly, thereby increasing outlet resistance. Disturbances in this urethral support mechanism compromise the ability of the urethra to efficiently counteract these transient increases in intra-abdominal pressure, subsequently resulting in SUI (Fig. 32.9). Typical causes of abnormal urethral support include congenital weakness and shortness of the vagina, difficult labor,

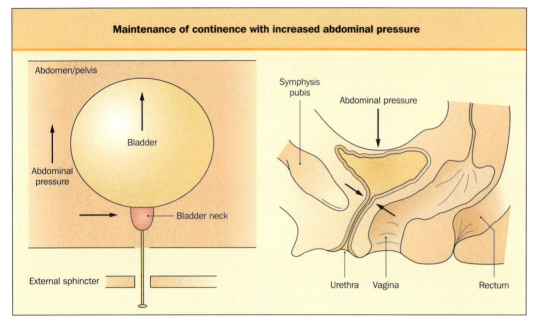

Figure 32.8 Maintenance of continence with increased abdominal pressure. When the bladder and proximal urethra are well supported in their normal retropubic position, pressure transmission to the bladder neck allows it to counteract increased bladder pressure thereby preventing involuntary loss of urine. (Reproduced with permission from O'Donnell PD. Urinary incontinence. St Louis: Mosby; 1997.)

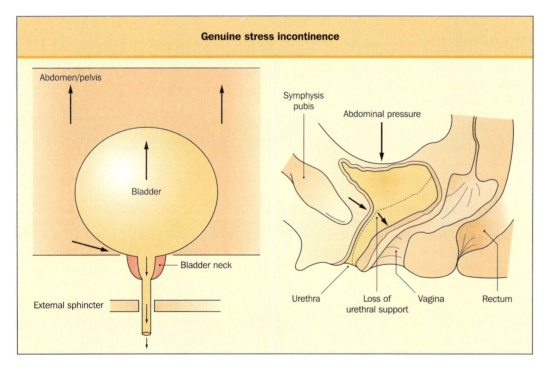

Figure 32.9 Genuine stress incontinence. When pelvic support of the urethra is deficient, allowing abnormal descent or loss of the physiologic hammock mechanism, it loses its mechanical advantage during increases in abdominal pressure allowing loss of urine. The resting cystogram (left) reveals a closed bladder neck and good position of the bladder base. During a Valsalva maneuver (right), the bladder base and urethra descend, allowing opening of the bladder neck. (Reproduced with permission from O'Donnell PD. Urinary incontinence. St Louis: Mosby; 1997.)

multiparity, and menopause. Iatrogenic causes include radical or simple hysterectomy and other types of extensive pelvic surgery.

Another arguably more important aspect of urethral function is its ability to provide a mucosal seal at the level of the bladder neck and proximal urethra. This is in part related to the plasticity of the mucosa and the vascular supply of the submucosa. Estrogens are known to play a major role in the maintenance of this pliability and estrogen deficiency, as occurs with menopause can result in SUI. Furthermore, other processes that promote the development of less pliable chronic inflammatory tissue, such as previous surgical procedures and radiation therapy, can also compromise this essential urethral closure mechanism. In addition to pliable mucosa and submucosa, maintenance of adequate urethral closure pressure requires functioning smooth muscle in the

bladder neck and proximal urethra. This musculature, named the internal urethral sphincter, is innervated by the sympathetic nervous system via the hypogastric nerve, supplied by neurons at the T10–L2 levels of the spinal cord. A deficiency in either of the above mechanisms – the mucosal pliability or functioning internal sphincter smooth musculature – can result in SUI despite adequate urethral support. This type of SUI, intrinsic sphincter deficiency (ISD), is less common than GSUI and represents one of the major causes of surgical failure in the management of SUI (Fig. 32.10).

The external sphincter is not generally considered an important mechanism in the maintenance of urethral resistance following increases in intra-abdominal pressure but is able to compensate for mild deficiencies in either urethral support

Intrinsic sphincter deficiency

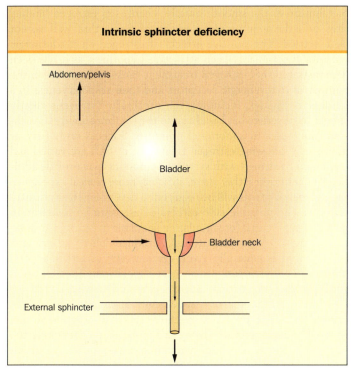

Figure 32.10 Intrinsic sphincter deficiency. When the internal sphincter is nonfunctional, loss of urine with increases in abdominal pressure can occur even in the presence of adequate urethral support. Note open bladder neck in the resting cystogram of a patient with intrinsic sphincter deficiency.

Treatment of female stress urinary incontinence

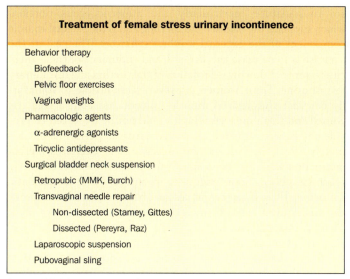

Behavior therapy
  Biofeedback
  Pelvic floor exercises
  Vaginal weights
Pharmacologic agents
  α-adrenergic agonists
  Tricyclic antidepressants
Surgical bladder neck suspension
  Retropubic (MMK, Burch)
  Transvaginal needle repair
    Non-dissected (Stamey, Gittes)
    Dissected (Pereyra, Raz)
  Laparoscopic suspension
  Pubovaginal sling

Figure 32.11 Treatment of female stress urinary incontinence. MMK, Marshall–Marchetti–Kranz.

or proximal urethral function. This complex consists of a rhabdosphincter, mostly circularly arranged small-diameter slow twitch fibers designed to generate constant tonus, and the periurethral striated muscle, which is an extension of the pubourethralis portion of the levator ani. Contraction of the latter muscle via fast twitch fibers occurs in response to increases in abdominal pressure (cough reflex).

Evaluation and classification of stress urinary incontinence

Patients with SUI usually present with the classic symptoms of involuntary loss of urine associated with increases in intra-abdominal pressure such as coughing, sneezing, laughing, and exercising. The history should search for other processes that could explain the SUI such as prior childbirth, previous pelvic surgery, or neurologic disease. Physical examination will generally reveal descent of the anterior vaginal wall following Valsalva maneuver with loss of urine when the bladder is partially full. Eradication of this incontinence by digital elevation (not compression) of the urethrovesical junction suggests that surgical treatment by simple bladder neck suspension would be adequate. Other types of pelvic prolapse should also be assessed at the time of this examination. Routine tests such as urinalysis and postvoid residual should be performed. The value of urodynamics for the simple case of SUI is debatable but certainly should be considered when the type of incontinence is unclear or there are historical factors present that would suggest other potential diagnoses. Cystometry is useful to rule out involuntary bladder contractions as a cause for the incontinence. Valsalva leak point pressures and fluoroscopy are the most helpful in

assessing SUI. Static urethral pressure profilometry is difficult to perform and provides results that correlate poorly with the clinical situation, leading to its abandonment by most in the field.

Stress urinary incontinence can be classified based on the underlying abnormality in the continence mechanism. Blaivas and Olsson separated SUI secondary to urethral hypermobility into two types depending on the amount of bladder neck descent[23]. Type I SUI referred to patients with less than 2cm descent of the urethrovesical angle during performance of a Valsalva maneuver. More significant descent (>2cm) was designated as type II. A variant of SUI occurs when the internal sphincter fails to function correctly, which has been termed ISD or type III[24]. The use of urodynamically obtained Valsalva leak point pressures has greatly simplified the diagnosis of ISD, as values less than 60cmH$_2$O are predictive of its presence[24]. It was previously thought that differentiation between types I and II was important in determining the appropriate treatment for SUI. Since the differences involve only the extent of bladder neck descent, and the treatment is similar, most now refer to it as genuine SUI (GSUI). Conversely, the ability to recognize ISD is important because standard treatments for GSUI are generally inadequate at treating this variant.

Treatment of stress urinary incontinence

The treatment of SUI varies depending upon its severity, patient expectation, and experience of the treating physician. The three major treatment categories include behavior modification, pharmacotherapy, and surgery (Fig. 32.11). In general, the least invasive measures are attempted first, gradually progressing to more aggressive treatments based on response and desire for dryness. Many patients are inclined to avoid surgery because of its invasiveness and complication rates.

When SUI results from hypermobility of the bladder neck and proximal urethra, or loss of the posterior urethral support mechanism, behavioral techniques can be used to strengthen the pelvic floor musculature. First described in 1948, these have been referred to as Kegel's exercises. Specifically, the exercise involves the voluntary contraction and relaxation of the levator ani musculature, particularly the pubococcygeus portion, which supports the bladder and urethra, and is the skeletal muscle component of the external urethral sphincter. The goal of the exercise is to increase the strength and endurance of these muscles to prevent downward rotation of the urethra and involuntary loss of urine. Some women, however, seem unable to voluntarily contract the desired muscles, oftentimes contracting the gluteal and thigh muscles which would not be expected to provide any benefit. It is felt that these errors in performance ultimately affect the success rate of pelvic floor exercises. Verbal instruction alone has been shown to be insufficient at correctly teaching pelvic floor exercises in up to 40% of patients. Consequently, various techniques have been employed to improve the ability of affected women to exercise the correct muscles. These techniques vary from vaginal examination during the exercise, use of successively increasing vaginal weights, vaginal electrical stimulation, and biofeedback. Vaginal cones of identical size and shape but increasing weight require a sustained contraction of the pelvic muscles to retain their position. Electrical stimulation has mainly been used to modify bladder sensation to promote bladder storage but stimulation of the pelvic floor muscles to increase tone may be accomplished in certain situations. Biofeedback uses electrical instrumentation that measure electromyographic and manometric indices that relay information back to the patient about pelvic and abdominal muscle activity. In theory, this allows increased control of the appropriate muscles so that exercises can be performed more accurately. Improvement in incontinence has been shown to exceed that in patients where only verbal feedback was given. Although behavioral techniques provide a noninvasive opportunity to improve incontinence, the effort is often time-consuming, labor intensive, and not curative for most patients.

The pharmacologic treatment of SUI is primarily based upon the presence of high concentrations of α_1-adrenergic receptors in the bladder neck and proximal urethra. Stimulation of the α-receptors in the proximal urethra with oral administration of α-adrenergic agonists has been shown to cause smooth muscle contraction and an increase in the maximum urethral closing pressure[25]. The most common oral agents used in the treatment of SUI have been ephedrine and phenylpropanolamine. Ephedrine, which is a noncatecholamine sympathomimetic, increases the release of norepinephrine (noradrenaline) from peripheral sympathetic nerves. Norepinephrine subsequently stimulates both α- and β-adrenergic receptors. Phenylpropanolamine has similar pharmacologic effects to ephedrine but has less central stimulation. In general, cure rates using oral sympathomimetic agents have been low but many demonstrate significant improvement in 19–60% of patients[26]. Potential side effects of sympathomimetic agents can include hypertension, anxiety, insomnia, headache, tremor, weakness, palpitations, cardiac arrhythmia, and respiratory difficulties. Significant increases in blood pressure do not occur in most normotensive patients but care needs to be taken when administering these agents to patients with a history of hypertension, hyperthyroidism, cardiac arrhythmia, and angina.

Estrogens are another category of pharmacologic agents used to treat SUI. The clinical effects of estrogen on the human female urethra are not completely understood. Whether this effect is related to changes in the autonomic innervation, receptor content,

metabolism of the smooth muscle, changes in estrogen binding sites, or in the nonmuscular elements of the urethral wall has not been settled. The positive effects of estrogen on α-adrenergic receptor functionality is an attractive hypothesis as it has been demonstrated that estrogen treatment causes an increase in the number of α-adrenergic receptors and their responsiveness in a number of tissues, including the urethra[27]. Estrogens clearly appear to be somewhat beneficial to the urethra's ability to withstand increases in abdominal pressure. Success rates (dry or improved) following estrogen treatment of SUI are varied and combined treatment with sympathomimetics may provide additional benefit over either alone, although more clinical experience and prospective trials will be required to determine their ultimate efficacy. The possible side effects of estrogen administration involve the potential for stimulating neoplasia in estrogen-responsive organs (i.e. breast and uterus). Although delivery of estrogen replacement is generally given systemically as either an oral preparation or skin patch, when used specifically for SUI, local administration as a vaginal cream is often sufficient.

Tricyclic antidepressants, specifically imipramine, have been used to treat SUI. By inhibiting the reuptake of norepinephrine, an α-adrenergic agonist effect can be obtained, mimicking the response to the more typical sympathomimetic agents. An advantage over the pure α-agonists are their anticholinergic effects, which can simultaneously suppress uninhibited bladder activity in those patients with mixed stress and urge incontinence.

Surgical treatment of genuine stress urinary incontinence

When the cause of SUI is hypermobility of the bladder neck and proximal urethra or loss of the posterior urethral support mechanism (GSUI), the classic treatment has been surgical bladder neck suspension. There are many techniques to perform bladder neck suspension, including anterior colporrhaphies; retropubic, laparoscopic, and needle suspensions; and sling procedures. The goal of each is universal: to return the bladder neck and proximal urethra to their normal retropubic position. Maintenance of this position allows proper transmission of pressure to the bladder neck and urethra, preventing SUI. They differ only in the method by which the bladder neck is accessed and the structures to which it is attached.

The classic bladder neck suspensions include the Marshall–Marchetti–Krantz (MMK) and Burch procedures[28,29]. The bladder neck is approached retropubically in these procedures, oftentimes via a Pfannenstiel incision, with the suspending sutures attached to the symphysis pubis and Cooper's ligament in the MMK and Burch operation respectively (Fig. 32.12). The retropubic suspensions are very effective at correcting SUI. With followup of at least 5 years, success rates approaching 80% can be expected following these procedures[30]. An additional advantage of the Burch procedure is its ability to correct small cystoceles by the placement of the suspending sutures more laterally into the paravaginal tissues. Complications are relatively uncommon with these approaches and include urinary tract infection, urinary retention, wound infection, detrusor instability, and suprapubic pain.

In an attempt to reduce the morbidity and hospital stay associated with the traditional bladder neck suspensions, modifications have been made to allow its performance via a predominantly transvaginal approach. In these techniques, the bladder neck is accessed through an anterior vaginal wall incision

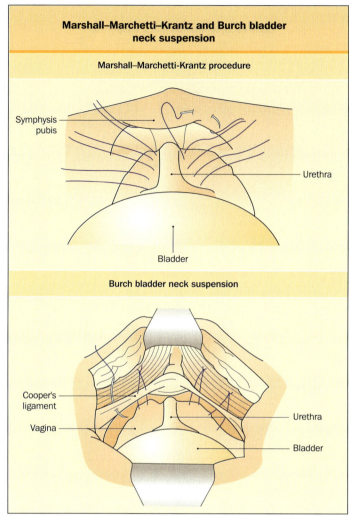

Figure 32.12 Marshall–Marchetti–Krantz (MMK) and Burch bladder neck suspension. In both procedures, the bladder neck is approached retropubically. In the MMK procedure (top), the suspension sutures are placed just lateral to the urethra and bladder neck and are attached to the symphysis pubis. In the Burch procedure (bottom), the suspension sutures are placed into the paravaginal tissue and attached to Cooper's ligament. (Reproduced with permission from Hinman F Jr. Atlas of urologic surgery, 2nd edn. London: WB Saunders; 1998.)

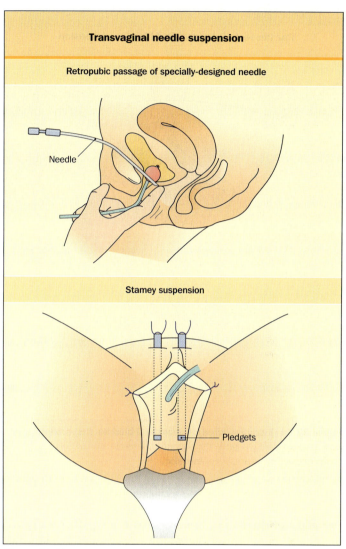

Figure 32.13 Transvaginal needle suspension. (Top) Retropubic passage of specially designed needle via a small suprapubic incision to allow transference of bladder neck suspension sutures. (Bottom) Stamey (nondissected) transvaginal bladder neck suspension. (Reproduced with permission from O'Donnell PD. Urinary incontinence. St Louis: Mosby; 1997.)

with transference of the suspending sutures by a specially designed needle to a small suprapubic incision, where they are tied over the anterior rectus fascia (Fig. 32.13 top panel). Many variations exist of this original concept, including the mechanism by which the sutures attach to the bladder neck (i.e. direct suture placement or use of pledgets) and the structures to which they are attached. Some employ minimal to no dissection of the bladder neck and urethra (nondissected techniques) and others require a relatively extensive dissection (dissected techniques). Classic nondissected techniques include the Stamey and Gittes bladder neck suspensions[31,32]. The former employs the use of synthetic pledgets to suspend the proximal urethra and bladder neck whereas the latter involves full-thickness penetration of the vaginal wall by a nonabsorbable suture, which is then reinforced in a helical fashion prior to its passage suprapubically (Fig. 32.13 bottom panel). The dissected techniques require a more

extensive separation of the vaginal wall from the underlying periurethral and perivesical fascia followed by placement of the suspension sutures, which are passed suprapubically. The first of these techniques was described by Pereyra and later modified by Raz[33,34] (Fig. 32.14). With all these procedures, the sutures are passed suprapubically using a specially designed needle and tied over the rectus fascia. Recent modifications of these techniques have involved the use of bone anchors into the symphysis pubis with the goal of improving the long-term success rates and minimizing postoperative morbidity such as hospital stay and urinary retention. Whether or not these goals will ultimately be accomplished requires further study.

Early success rates with transvaginal needle suspensions have been favorable. Raz and colleagues reported a success rate of 90% in 206 patients (mean follow-up of 15 months) who underwent his previously reported technique[35]. Unfortunately, these

Raz (dissected) transvaginal bladder suspension

Figure 32.14 Raz (dissected) transvaginal bladder suspension.
Helical sutures are placed in the pubocervical fascia and passed
suprapubically by needle for suspension.

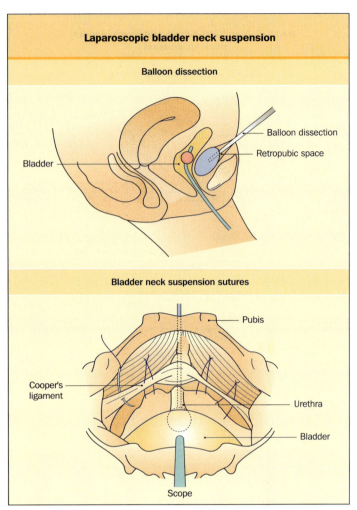

Figure 32.15 Laparoscopic bladder neck suspension. (Top) Balloon
dissection of retropubic space. (Bottom) Placement of bladder neck
suspension sutures laparoscopically to paravaginal tissue and Cooper's
ligament. (Balloon dissection reproduced from Smith AD, et al. Smith's
textbook of endourology. St Louis: Quality Medical Publishing Inc; 1996.)

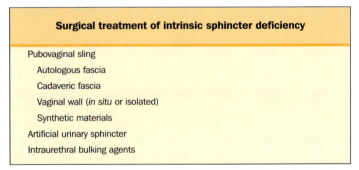

Figure 32.16 Surgical treatment of intrinsic sphincter deficiency.

procedures have not fared quite as well over the long term,
prompting various modifications to the technique. Trockman et
al. reported a disappointing 20% success rate with an average
followup of almost 10 years[36]. Risk factors related to poor success
rates for the transvaginal needle procedures have been reported
to be the presence of detrusor instability, low urethral pressure
profile, a fibrotic urethra, neurogenic incontinence, and a negative Q tip test (minimal urethral movement with Valsalva), many
of which suggest the presence of ISD.

The technique of laparoscopy has allowed many procedures to
be performed in a minimally invasive manner, including bladder
neck suspension. Both transperitoneal and extraperitoneal
approaches have been used to perform bladder neck suspension
laparoscopically. Most prefer the extraperitoneal route after
balloon development of the retropubic space (Fig. 32.15). The
urethrovesical junction is usually suspended by attachment to
Cooper's ligament, similar to the Burch colposuspension, using
nonabsorbable suture or mesh with staples (Fig. 32.15).
Advantages of the laparoscopic approach include decreased
hospital stay, postoperative convalescence, and pain. Early continence rates following the laparoscopic suspensions have generally
been comparable to the open procedures; however, more extensive followup has revealed success rates inferior to their open
counterparts[37,38]. In summary, some skepticism must remain
about the durability of these procedures until more long-term
data become available.

Treatment of intrinsic sphincter deficiency
Treatment of SUI secondary to ISD requires procedures that
coapt the urethral mucosa at the level of the bladder neck
and proximal urethra (Fig. 32.16). The aforementioned procedures when correctly performed do not accomplish this goal as
they only return the bladder neck and urethra to their normal
retropubic position. Surgical procedures to manage ISD include

suburethral slings, intraurethral injection of bulking agents, and insertion of an artificial urinary sphincter. Suburethral slings have been used most commonly to correct female ISD.

The suburethral sling used most often to treat ISD has been the pubovaginal sling (PVS) popularized by McGuire and Lytton, which incorporates anterior rectus fascia[39] (Fig. 32.17). Recent modifications to the original technique include the use of synthetic material, in situ or isolated vaginal wall, and cadaveric tensor fascia lata as the suburethral sling in an attempt to avoid the morbidity of harvesting rectus fascia. Synthetic materials have become less popular because of the risk of infection and erosion, whereas the long-term infectious safety of cadaveric tissue is in question. Nevertheless, these modifications have allowed greater options for the surgeon. More recently, the ability to insert bone anchors via a transvaginal route has allowed the PVS to be performed without an abdominal incision when material other than autologous fascia is used. Ultimately, PVS may become a purely outpatient procedure.

Similar to the previously mentioned surgical bladder neck suspensions, the early results of PVS have been quite favorable. The long-term efficacy of PVS, however, is clearly superior. Although primarily used to treat ISD, the long-term success rates have been excellent, approximating 80–90% at 3 years[40,41]. Data from a recent series of 251 patients with fascial slings indicated that 92% were cured or improved with a median followup of 3 years, and in those that had been followed for at least 10 years, 95% had no SUI[42].

Advantages of the PVS include similar morbidity to transvaginal needle suspensions and an ability to simultaneously coapt the proximal urethral mucosa and suspend the bladder neck. Therefore, if urethral hypermobility and/or ISD exist, PVS would appear to be the ideal surgical procedure, since it could correct either. This would theoretically increase early success rates of surgical bladder neck suspension since unrecognized ISD would be treated and probably produce better long-term results. Zaragoza described his experience using PVS for both types of SUI and reported a 95% success rate at 25 months[43].

The main concern about PVS has been the rate of urethral obstruction. Unlike the surgical bladder neck suspensions, suburethral slings have a higher propensity for compressing the urethra and therefore overcorrecting the urethrovesical angle. This usually presents as urinary retention or poor bladder emptying, but very often is manifested by irritative voiding symptoms secondary to the effects of obstruction on the detrusor. This complication can be minimized by applying almost no tension when tying the suspension sutures over the rectus fascia. As mentioned above, synthetic material used as the sling can erode into the urethra or vagina, requiring its removal.

The artificial sphincter has also been proposed as a surgical alternative for the treatment of ISD in females. First introduced by Scott et al. in 1973, the device underwent a major modification in 1983 with subsequent minor modifications made at later times[44]. The device is manufactured by American Medical Systems (AMS) and the most current model is the AMS800.

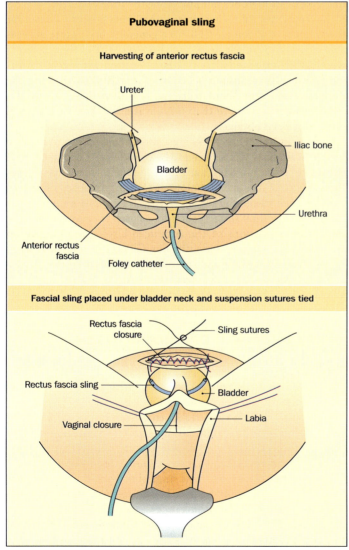

Figure 32.17 Pubovaginal sling. Sling using autologous anterior rectus fascia. (Top) Harvesting of anterior rectus fascia through Pfannenstiel incision. (Bottom) Fascial sling placed under bladder neck and suspension sutures tied loosely over the closed anterior rectus fascia.

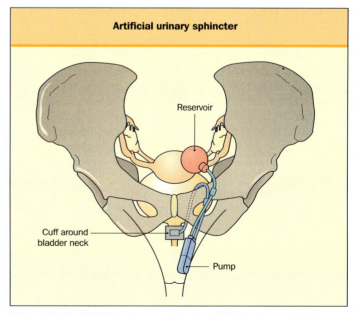

Figure 32.18 Artificial urinary sphincter. Artificial urinary sphincter placed around female bladder neck.

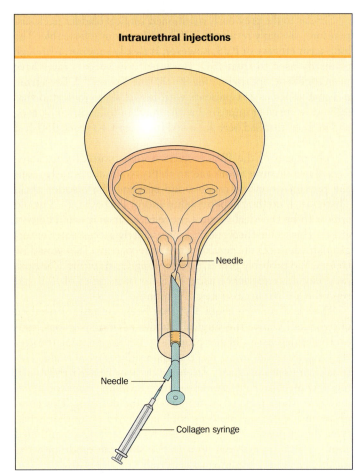

Intraurethral injections

Needle

Needle

Collagen syringe

Figure 32.19 Intraurethral injections. Cystoscopic injection of periurethral bulking agent.

It consists of a cuff, pump, and pressure-regulating reservoir, and is made of a wear-resistant biocompatible silicone elastomer. In females, the cuff is placed around the bladder neck, the reservoir in the space of Retzius, and the pump in one of the labia (Fig. 32.18). Reasonable success rates have been reported by some authors when used to treat female ISD[45]. Nevertheless, it is generally accepted that the infection, erosion, and mechanical failure rates, which all necessitate reoperation, and the technical difficulties associated with its insertion in the female, result in this procedure being much less preferable than some of the other techniques used to correct ISD (i.e. PVS and periurethral injections). It has, however, proved to be invaluable for the treatment of severe sphincteric incontinence in men such as follows prostatectomy.

Intraurethral bulking agents
Intraurethral injection of bulking agents has proved to be a very attractive and successful method to treat SUI in a particular subset of patients (Fig. 32.19). Ideally it is suitable for those with pure ISD in the absence of urethral hypermobility. Intraurethral injections only increase proximal urethral coaptation without affecting periurethral support, such that those patients with hypermobility generally experience minimal benefit. Some authors, however, have reported success in patients with minimal (type I) and more significant hypermobility (type II)[46,47].

Polytetrafluorethylene was one of the earlier agents used for injection and generally produced good clinical results[48]. The size of the micropolymer particles and subsequent reports in the literature demonstrating its ability to migrate to other areas of the body led to increasing concern and a decrease in its use[49]. Presently, the most common injectable substance and the only one approved by the Food and Drug Administration in the USA is glutaraldehyde cross-linked bovine collagen[50]. The cross-linking is felt to improve the consistency of the material, thereby facilitating injection and delaying its destruction by collagenases. Although as originally described the collagen was injected into its submucosal position via a periurethral route, with the development of specialized cystoscopes similar if not better success rates can be obtained by transurethral injection. Furthermore, smaller amounts of collagen are needed, resulting in decreased expense. Other substances have been used or are presently being investigated. Injection of autologous fat has the advantage of lower cost and increased biocompatibility but is absorbed much quicker than collagen[51]. Clinical trials are presently under way evaluating larger-sized silicone microparticles in hopes of eliminating the migration risk.

Success rates following intraurethral injection of collagen for the treatment of female SUI have generally been quite acceptable. Cross and colleagues found that over 90% of their patients were dry or improved after collagen injection with most requiring two or less treatment sessions[52]. Consistent with some the durability concerns about collagen, 11% of patients required a 'booster injection' more than 6 months after their final clinical result had been obtained.

In conclusion, when choosing a surgical procedure to manage female SUI, many factors need to be considered. The type of SUI should be determined with as much certainty as possible. If urethral hypermobility is the etiology of the incontinence, a standard bladder neck suspension of any type can be performed or some form of suburethral sling. It should be noted that, on the basis of the recommendations of the American Urological Association Female Stress Urinary Incontinence Clinical Guidelines Panel, retropubic suspensions and suburethral sling procedures appear to be the most efficacious procedures for long-term success[53]. When pure ISD is present, periurethral injection of bulking agents can be considered as an alternative to PVS.

OTHER UROLOGIC DISORDERS IN FEMALES

Pelvic prolapse
In addition to SUI, pelvic floor weakening in the female can result in the prolapse of organs that abut the vagina (Fig. 32.20). These organs include the urethra (urethrocele), bladder (cystocele), uterus (uterine prolapse), intestine (enterocele), and rectum (rectocele). Total vaginal prolapse can also occur, which is termed procidentia. Although an extensive discussion of the various types of prolapse and their surgical treatment is not possible in this chapter, it should be noted that urologists should develop a basic understanding of these processes, since they often coexist with SUI. Furthermore, appropriate surgical management of SUI often requires that these entities also be addressed.

Prolapse of the anterior vaginal wall generally includes a cystocele or urethrocele. The bladder base protrudes through a weakened pubocervical fascia (medial edges of the levator muscles) or may result from a tearing of the vaginal wall from its bony

Pelvic prolapse

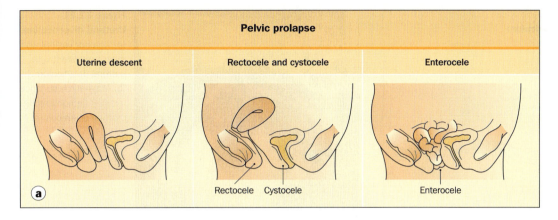

| Uterine descent | Rectocele and cystocele | Enterocele |

(a)

Rectocele   Cystocele

Enterocele

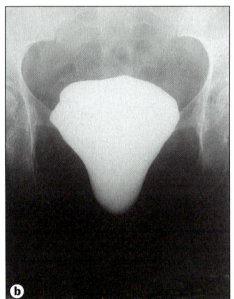

(b)

Figure 32.20 Pelvic prolapse. (a) Different consequences of pelvic prolapse. (b) Upright cystogram revealing cystocele. [Part (a) reproduced with permission from O'Donnell PD. Urinary incontinence. St Louis: Mosby; 1997.]

support in the pelvis. Descent of the vaginal apex and uterus can also cause what is termed a traction cystocele and will often require simultaneous hysterectomy at the time of surgical correction. Symptoms of a cystocele include vaginal pressure and bulging, incomplete bladder emptying, and urinary incontinence. It is extremely important to realize that the presence of a large cystocele can mask the effects of urethral hypermobility. The prolapsing bladder base will accept the transmission of intra-abdominal pressure, allowing maintenance of continence despite poor urethral support. If the cystocele only is repaired in this situation, postoperative SUI can ensue. To prevent this complication, patients should undergo careful physical examination and urodynamics with the cystocele in its prolapsed position and when reduced to assess for evidence of urethral hypermobility and SUI. It is also recommended that moderate cystoceles be repaired at the time of bladder neck suspension to prevent a worsening of the cystocele caused by correction of only urethral descent.

Rectocele results from prolapse of the rectum into the vagina secondary to a weakened perineal body and rectovaginal septum. Although many women present with no symptoms, they will sometimes complain of perineal pressure, difficulty with bowel movements, and fecal soiling. Repair of the symptomatic rectocele is well accepted; however, there is considerable debate about

performing this procedure in the asymptomatic patient. An enterocele occurs when bowel (usually small intestine) protrudes into the vagina near its proximal junction with the rectum. Enteroceles can result from significant uterine descent or prior pelvic surgery such as hysterectomy or bladder neck suspension (retropubic or transvaginal). They can often be difficult to separate from high rectoceles and therefore require careful rectal and pelvic examination. Enteroceles can generally be repaired via the transvaginal route but sometimes require transabdominal correction.

Urethral diverticulum

The first description of a female urethral diverticulum was in the early 19th century, followed by sporadic reports in the literature until a larger series was published in 1952[54]. Urethral diverticula have been reported to occur in approximately 1–6% of the adult female population with a racial predilection favoring African–Americans[55]. The detection rate will vary depending on the diagnostic method used, radiographic methods far exceeding endoscopic evaluation. Ages of affected women range from 20 to 60 with a mean of 40 years[55].

There is considerable debate regarding the origin of urethral diverticula. Much of the disagreement involves deciding whether or not there is a congenital or acquired etiology. Many theories exist, the most popular one being infection and obstruction of the periurethral glands resulting in the formation of suburethral cysts. Initial infection of the periurethral glands is thought to be secondary to vaginal flora, sexually transmitted disease (particularly gonorrhea), and some of the more typical enteric bacteria such as *Escherichia coli*. These infected cysts eventually rupture into the urethra, establishing a communication with the lumen, allowing urine to enter and pool. This cavity then epithelializes over time, gradually enlarging as voided urine accumulates. Other potential etiologies include congenital development, traumatic childbirth, aborted attempts at urethral duplication, remnants of Gartner's ducts, urethral instrumentation, and complications from anterior vaginal wall surgery.

The typical presenting symptoms of patients with a urethral diverticulum are related to an accumulation of infected urine in this structure (Fig. 32.21a). In addition to pain from the presence of a cystic anterior vaginal wall mass are other symptoms such as a purulent urethral discharge, dyspareunia, postvoid dribbling and recurrent lower urinary tract infections. Urethral diverticula should be high in the differential diagnosis when urinary tract infections recur despite prophylactic antibiotic treatment. Other less common symptoms include urinary retention, chronic pelvic

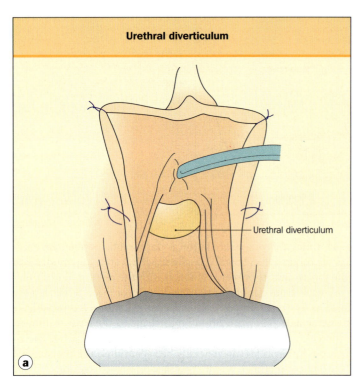

Urethral diverticulum

Urethral diverticulum

(a)

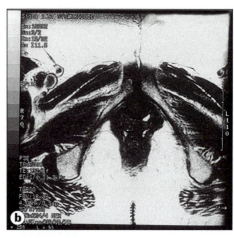

**Figure 32.21
Urethral diverticulum.**
(a) Anterior vaginal wall mass consistent with urethral diverticulum. (b) Magnetic resonance imaging demonstrating urethral diverticulum.

pain, and pain with ambulation. The symptoms do not appear to be related to the size of the diverticulum. In rare cases, carcinoma has been identified within the diverticular sac[56].

The diagnosis of urethral diverticula requires a high index of suspicion. The usual symptoms can often be elicited in the medical history with confirmatory studies including physical examination, cystoscopy, urethrography, or more recently magnetic resonance imaging. Vaginal examination frequently demonstrates a suburethral mass that is tender to palpation. Upon compression, purulent material can be expressed from the urethral meatus. At times, the mass can feel firm or hard, suggesting concomitant calculus or neoplastic disease.

Cystourethroscopy can sometimes be useful in identifying urethral diverticula, particularly when purulent material can be seen exiting from its intraurethral orifice. Use of zero degree lens and compression of the meatus can provide better visualization because of the relatively short female urethra. It is not uncommon, however, for the orifice to go unnoticed as a consequence of its small size or concealment by inflammation. Frequently, additional radiologic studies are required to confirm the diagnosis. Contrast studies such as voiding cystourethrogram (VCUG) and double-balloon urethrography (DBU) have been most popular. VCUG distends the urethra poorly such that filling of the diverticulum is inconsistent. DBU allows better urethral distention and has a reported sensitivity of approximately 90%[57]. It can be difficult to perform DBU because of catheter positioning and patient discomfort so that its ability to diagnose a diverticulum is diminished. MRI has been found to be superior to DBU in demonstrating urethral diverticula, prompting some to suggest it as the gold standard, assuming the costs are not prohibitive[58] (Fig. 32.21b).

The primary treatment of a symptomatic urethral diverticulum is by surgical excision although some have advocated urethrotomy or marsupialization[59]. Excision of a female urethral

diverticulum can be performed almost exclusively through a vaginal incision. Sometimes it is helpful to cannulate the orifice with a balloon catheter cystoscopically allowing easier identification. Through a transverse or horizontal incision, the vaginal wall is dissected off the underlying periurethral fascia. This fascia is then entered through an incision perpendicular to the original incision allowing identification of the urethral diverticulum. The diverticulum is resected followed by closure of the urethra and the other layers separately. The urine is usually diverted with a urethral and/or suprapubic catheter for 10–14 days. Since infected urine secondary to urinary stasis commonly coexists with urethral diverticula, preoperative clearance will improve healing and reduce the likelihood of recurrence. Finally, the presence of concomitant stress urinary incontinence does not preclude its correction at the time of diverticulum excision with either a transvaginal needle suspension or suburethral sling; however, the latter is felt to be more appropriate.

Other vaginal wall masses
The urologist is often faced with vaginal/urethral masses of unclear origin. A common finding in elderly women is a beefy red mass protruding from the urethral meatus. This most likely represents a urethral caruncle, which is a protrusion of inflamed and friable urethral mucosa. Urethral caruncles can cause a number of symptoms such as bleeding, pain, obstructive symptoms, and recurrent urinary tract infections. It is important to recognize that this is not a neoplastic mass, although it often requires excision. Cystoscopic evaluation of the urethra can be helpful to demonstrate a normal proximal urethra and to rule out neoplasia. Many women do not need treatment if the diagnosis is clear and the symptoms are either minimal or nonexistent. Conservative measures such as warm sitz baths or local application of estrogen cream should precede surgical management, since symptom abatement is common.

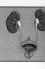

When surgical management is necessary, complete excision of the inflamed mucosa with reapproximation of the remaining urethral mucosa and vaginal wall epithelium provides excellent results.

Cysts and/or infection can develop in Bartholin's duct or in Skene's gland, which can often be problematic. Presenting symptoms include dyspareunia, vaginal discomfort, voiding difficulties, recurrent urinary tract infection, and purulent drainage. Bartholin duct cysts are usually located inside the labia minora just adjacent to the introitus, whereas Skene's gland cysts are positioned closer to the urethral meatus in an inferolateral position. Palpation of an infected Skene's gland cyst will often result in a purulent discharge from the urethral meatus because of its communication with the urethra. Medical treatment with antibiotics is often sufficient to eradicate the infection, followed by obliteration of the cavity by scarring. If this form of treatment is unsuccessful or if symptoms persist, surgical resection or marsupialization may be required for Bartholin's duct cysts and excision alone for the Skene's gland cysts.

REFERENCES

1. Thomas TM, Plymat DR, Blannin J, Meade TW. Prevalence of urinary incontinence. Br Med J. 1980;281:1243–5.
2. Elving LB, Foldspang A, Lam GW. Descriptive epidemiology of urinary incontinence in 3,100 women age 30–59. Scand J Urol Nephrol. 1989;125(Suppl):37–43.
3. Diokno AC, Brock BM, Brown MB, Herzog AR. Prevalence of urinary incontinence and other urological symptoms in the non-institutionalized elderly. J Urol. 1986;136:1022–5.
4. Wells T, Brink C. Urinary incontinence: assessment and management. In: Burnside M, ed. Nursing and the aged. New York: McGraw-Hill; 1981:519–48.
5. Department of Health, Education, and Welfare. Long-Term Care Facility Improvement Study. Washington, DC: US Government Printing Office; 1975.
6. Herzog AR, Fultz NG, Brock BM, Brown MB. Urinary incontinence and psychological distress among older adults. Psychol Aging. 1988;3:115–21.
7. Wyman JF, Harkins SW, Fantl JA. Psychosocial impact of urinary incontinence in the community-dwelling population. J Am Geriatr Soc. 1990;38:282–8.
8. Jeter KF, Verdell LL. Consumer focus '93: a survey of community-dwelling incontinent people. Union, SC: Help for Incontinent People; 1993.
9. Hu TW. Impact of urinary incontinence on health care costs. J Amer Geriat Soc. 1990;38:292–5.
10. Abrams P, Blaivas JG, Stanton SL, Andersen JT. The standardisation of terminology of lower urinary tract function. Scand J Urol. Nephrol. 1988;114(Suppl):5–19.
11. McClish DK, Fantl JA, Wyman JF, Pisani G, Bump RC. Bladder training in older women with urinary incontinence: relationship between outcome and changes in urodynamic observation. Obstet Gynecol. 1991;77:281–6.
12. Holmes DM, Stone AR, Bary PR, Richards CJ, Stephenson TP. Bladder retraining: 3 years on. Br J Urol. 1983;55:660–4.
13. Fantl JA, Wyman JF, McClish DK, et al. Efficacy of bladder training in older women with urinary incontinence. JAMA 1991;265:609–13.
14. Appell RA. Electrical stimulation for the treatment of urinary incontinence. Urology. 1998;51:24–6.
15. Burgio KL, Locher JL, Goode PS, et al. Behavioral vs. drug treatment for urge urinary incontinence in older women: a randomized controlled trial. JAMA. 1998;280:1995–2000.
16. McGuire EJ, Savastano JA. Stress incontinence and detrusor instability/urge incontinence. Neurourol Urodyn. 1985;4:313–6.
17. Chapple CR, Hampson SJ, Turner-Warwick RT, Worth PH. Subtrigonal phenol injection: how safe and effective is it? Br J Urol. 1991;68:483–6.
18. Cespedes RD, Cross CA, McGuire EJ. Modified Ingelman-Sundberg bladder denervation procedure for intractable urge incontinence. J Urol. 1996;156:1744–7.
19. Shaker HS, Hassouna M. Sacral nerve root neuromodulation: an effective treatment for refractory urge incontinence. J Urol. 1998;159:1516–9.
20. Flood HD, Malhotra SJ, O'Connell HE, Ritchey MJ, Bloom DA, McGuire EJ. Long-term results and complications using augmentation cystoplasty in reconstructive urology. Neurourol Urodyn. 1995;14:297–309.
21. Mundy AR, Stephenson TP. 'Clam' ileocystoplasty for the treatment of refractory urge incontinence. Br J Urol. 1985;57:641–6.
22. Cartwright PC, Snow BW. Bladder auto-augmentation: partial detrusor excision to augment the bladder without use of bowel. J Urol. 1989;142:1050–3.
23. Blaivas JG, Olsson CA. Stress incontinence: classification and surgical approach. J Urol. 1988;139:727–31.
24. McGuire EJ, Fitzpatrick CC, Wan J, et al. Clinical assessment of urethral function. J Urol. 1993;158:1452–7.
25. Wein AJ, Levin RM, Barrett DM. Voiding function: relevant anatomy, physiology, pharmacology. In: Gillenwater JY, Grayhack JT, Howards SS, et al, eds. Adult and pediatric urology. Chicago: Year Book; 1987:863–962.
26. Urinary Incontinence Guideline Panel. Urinary incontinence in adults: clinical practice guideline. AHCPR Pub No. 92–0038. Rockville, MD: Agency for Health Care Policy and Research, Public Health Service, US Department of Health and Human Services; 1992.
27. Larsson B, Andersson KE, Batra S, Mattiason A, Sjögren C. Effects of estradiol on norepinephrine-induced contraction, alpha adrenoceptor number and norepinephrine content in the female rabbit urethra. J Pharmacol Exp Ther. 1984;229:557–63.
28. Marshall VF, Marchetti AA, Krantz KE. The correction of stress incontinence by simple vesicourethral suspension. Surg Gynecol Obstet. 1949;88:509–18.
29. Burch JC. Urethrovaginal fixation to Cooper's ligament for correction of stress incontinence, cystocele, and prolapse. Am J Obstet Gynecol. 1961;81:281–90.
30. Feyereisl J, Dreher E, Haenggi W, Zikmund J, Schneider H. Long-term results after Burch colposuspension. Am J Obstet Gynecol. 1994;171:647–52.
31. Stamey TA. Endoscopic suspension of the vesical neck for urinary incontinence. Surg Gynecol Obstet. 1987;136:547–54.
32. Gittes RF, Loughlin DR. No-incision pubovaginal suspension for stress incontinence. J Urol. 1987;138:568–70.
33. Pereyra AJ. A simplified surgical procedure for correction of stress incontinence in women. West J Surg Obstet Gynecol. 1959;67:223.
34. Raz S. Modified bladder neck suspension for female stress incontinence. Urology. 1981;17:82–5.
35. Raz S, Sussman EM, Erickson DB, Bregg KJ, Nitti VW. The Raz bladder neck suspension: results in 206 patients. J Urol. 1992;148:845–50.

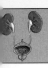

Section 6

Benign Conditions of the Lower Urinary Tract

36. Trockman BA, Leach GE, Hamilton J, Sakamoto M, Santiago L, Zimmern PE. Modified Pereyra bladder neck suspension: 10-year mean follow-up using outcome analysis in 125 patients. J Urol. 1995;154:1841–7.

37. Kung RC, Lie K, Lee P, Drutz HP. The cost-effectiveness of laparoscopic abdominal Burch procedures in women with urinary stress incontinence J Am Assoc Gynecol Laparosc. 1996;3:537–44.

38. Lobel RW, Davis GD. Long-term results of laparoscopic Burch urethropexy. J Am Assoc Gynecol Laparosc. 1997;4:341–5.

39. McGuire EJ, Lytton B. Pubovaginal sling for stress incontinence. J Urol. 1978;119:82–4.

40. McGuire EJ, Bennett CJ, Konnak JA, et al. Experience with pubovaginal sling for urinary incontinence at the University of Michigan. J Urol. 1987;138:525–6.

41. Blaivas JG, Jacobs BZ. Pubovaginal fascial sling for the treatment of complicated stress urinary incontinence. J Urol. 1991;145:1214–8.

42. Chaikin DC, Rosenthal J, Blaivas JG. Pubovaginal fascial sling for all types of stress urinary incontinence: long-term analysis. J Urol. 1998;160:1312–6.

43. Zaragoza MR. Expanded indications for the pubovaginal sling: treatment of type 2 or 3 stress incontinence. J Urol. 1996;156:1620–2.

44. Scott FB, Bradley WE, Timm GW. Treatment of urinary incontinence by implantable prosthetic sphincter. Urology. 1973;1:252–9.

45. Webster GD, Perez LM, Khoury JM, Simmons SL. Management of type III stress urinary incontinence using artificial urinary sphincter. Urology. 1992;39:499–503.

46. Faerber GJ. Endoscopic collagen injection therapy in elderly women with type I stress urinary incontinence. J Urol. 1996;155:512–4.

47. Hershorn S, Radomski SB, Steele DJ. Early experience with intraurethral collagen injections for urinary incontinence. J Urol. 1992;148:1797–800.

48. Politano V. Periurethral polytetrafluorethylene injection for urinary incontinence. J Urol. 1982;127:439–42.

49. Malizia AA Jr, Reiman HM, Myers RP, et al. Migration and granulomatous reaction after periurethral injection of Polytef (Teflon). JAMA. 1984;251:3277–81.

50. McGuire EJ, Appell RA. Transurethral collagen injection for urinary incontinence. Urology. 1994;43:413–5.

51. Santarosa RP, Blaivas JG. Periurethral injection of autologous fat for the treatment of sphincteric incontinence J Urol. 1994;151:607–11.

52. Cross CA, English SF, Cespedes RD, McGuire EJ. A follow-up on transurethral collagen injection therapy for urinary incontinence. J Urol. 1998;159:106–8.

53. Leach GE, Dmochowski RR, Appell RA, et al. Female stress urinary incontinence clinical guidelines panel summary report on surgical management of female stress urinary incontinence. J Urol. 1997;158:875–80.

54. Davis HJ, TeLinde RW. Urethral diverticula: an assay of 121 cases. J Urol. 1958;80:4.

55. Young GPH, Wahle GR, Raz S. Female urethral diverticulum. In: Raz S, ed. Female urology. Philadelphia: WB Saunders; 1996.

56. Rajan N, Tucci P, Mallouh C, Choudhury M. Carcinoma in female urethral diverticulum: case reports and review of management. J Urol. 1993;150:1911–4.

57. Kohorn EI, Glickman MG. Technical aids in investigation and management of urethral diverticula in the female. Urology. 1992;40:322–5.

58. Neitlich JD, Foster HE Jr, Glickman MG, Smith RC. Detection of urethral diverticula using a high resolution fast spin echo technique: comparison with double balloon urethrography. J Urol. 1998;159:408–10.

59. Spence HM, Duckett JW. Diverticulum of the female urethra: clinical aspects and presentation of a simple operative technique for cure. J Urol. 1970;104:432–7.

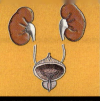

Chapter 33

Interstitial Cystitis

C Lowell Parsons

KEY POINTS

- Interstitial cystitis is best defined by the clinical symptoms of urinary urgency, frequency, and/or pelvic pain in a patient with no other definable pathology, such as urinary tract infection, carcinoma, and radiation- or medication-induced cystitis.
- Interstitial cystitis pathogenesis may involve an impairment in the regulatory role of mucus in reducing bladder epithelial permeability and once impaired, high levels of urinary potassium result in increased interstitial levels in the bladder that induce sensory nerves to depolarize, which causes pain and urgency, and may result in tissue destruction.
- Interstitial cystitis therapies include, bladder hydrodistension, dimethyl sulfoxide, pentosanpolysulfate, intravesical heparin, antidepressants, sodium oxycholorosene (Clorpactin), intravesical silver nitrate, BCG, antihistamines, and L-arginine.

INTRODUCTION

Perhaps one of the main problem areas in working with the syndrome interstitial cystitis (IC) is to recognize the patient population that actually has the disease complex. Historically, the diagnosis was limited to only those patients with the severe symptom complex of urinary urgency, frequency, pelvic, and perineal pain. However, this traditional concept recognizes only those patients with end-stage disease and probably only represents 5% or less of the people who are actually afflicted with IC. This syndrome has been and continues to be misdiagnosed as recurrent bladder infections, urethral syndrome, and perhaps even prostatitis in men. In the gynecologic realm it is probably misdiagnosed as pelvic pain and confused with endometriosis, or various types of vaginitis or vulvodynia. Often the disease is confused with either problems associated with bladder outlet obstruction (BOO) from prostate enlargement or prostatitis.

In this chapter, in part, an attempt is made to define more appropriately the patient population that actually has IC. While IC was traditionally thought to be quite rare, actually it may be quite common. Part of the confusion with recognition of IC in its early phases is that frequently the patients' complaints are intermittent and confused with other bladder disorders such as bacterial cystitis. It seems to progress slowly and intermittently, but

until the symptoms become more continuous, it is likely that the patient will not be diagnosed as having IC.

Other areas in which much progress has been made in the understanding of IC are in the new concepts of pathogenesis as well as the new methods to treat and manage patients successfully.

DEFINITION

Definition may be one of the most confusing parts of IC, because it changes drastically as we understand better the patient population that has the disease, the progression of IC, and the factors that provoke it. Little progress was made in the definition of this patient population until 1987, when a group of interested researchers met at the National Institutes of Health (NIH) and established the National Institute of Diabetes and Digestive and Kidney Diseases (NIDDKD) clinical criteria to characterize the IC syndrome patient for research studies[1]. For incorporation of patients into research, it was agreed that the criteria should represent those patients with sufficiently advanced and persistent disease such that their pathologic changes be sufficient for abnormalities to be recognized. These criteria were not developed to define or diagnose the patient population, since the researchers had all agreed that the criteria defined the very advanced patient. More recent studies show that these criteria only represent a small percentage of the patients with IC. Indeed, most of the patients (75%) who were diagnosed with IC sufficient to participate in an NIH-sponsored IC Database did not meet the criteria[2]. An attempt to better define the patient population is undertaken herein, but substantial changes will continue to occur in the future as our understanding improves with regard to the manner in which the disease presents itself.

For practical purposes we believe that the main problem in IC definition is that this remains a clinical syndrome with no distinct pathologic tissue or serum changes to indicate IC. Importantly, the symptoms that may actually be present depend upon the state of the disease, whether it is in the early phase (i.e. a milder version of the symptom complex) or in a more advanced later stage (as seen in older patients). In general, the disease is best defined by the clinical symptoms of urinary urgency, frequency, and/or pelvic pain present in a patient with no other definable pathology, such as urinary infection, carcinoma, and radiation- or medication-induced cystitis. It may well be that the syndrome encompasses a number of different etiologies, but with a bladder insult that ultimately results in urinary frequency and urgency or pain that is essentially the only clinical response to noxious stimuli. Also important is that pain may be the only component of the syndrome in some

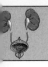

people, and perhaps this patient population is most likely to present to the gynecologist rather than the urologist.

Data are presented herein to establish clinical parameters that help define the disease. The clinician must be aware that some significant variance may occur in patients depending upon how severe patients' symptoms are when they are seen and how long the disease process has been present. Most important, perhaps, is to use a broad definition of the syndrome and to recognize that the disease is significantly underdiagnosed[3]. As a result, many patients with milder forms of the disease could receive substantial benefit if the diagnosis is considered and treatment initiated, as such patients respond readily to therapy and thus do not advance to the more severe end-stage disease.

PATHOGENESIS

Substantial progress has been made in our understanding of the etiology of IC, and a number of mechanisms probably lead to the production of symptoms in the individual patient. Several factors have slowed acquisition of new knowledge in IC. In most people, IC starts out with mild, intermittent flares of symptoms, and so it is difficult at this stage of the disease to quantify and study abnormalities. Thus, historically, the focus of studies was only the end-stage patient with very severe and advanced disease. However, the number of severe patients is not large, so it is difficult to conduct research; nevertheless, substantial progress has been made. The many suggested etiologies include lymphatic and chronic infection, neurologic, psychologic, and autoimmune disorders, and vasculitis[4-11]. Most of the proposed etiologies are still hypothetic in nature, with not much data to define the role of these mechanisms. For example, Oravisto[10] suggested that the number of antinuclear antibodies present in patients with IC is increased, which appears to be true. However, it is difficult to know the relevance of this, because mild elevations in autoimmune antibodies may be present in many chronic diseases and may only represent a secondary phenomenon. Also, there is no obvious association of the IC syndrome in most patients with autoimmune phenomena.

A number of discoveries have helped to put some of the IC puzzle pieces in place. One of the more widely accepted theories is that of a defective bladder epithelium in which loss of the 'blood urine barrier' results in a leaky membrane[12,13]. An epithelium permeable to small molecules could explain the induction of symptoms, especially if the diffusing substances stimulate depolarization of sensory nerves[14,15]. In particular, it has been shown that diffusion of potassium across the bladder epithelium could trigger the sensory nerve endings and result not only in symptoms, but also in disease progression because of tissue injury from toxic levels of this cation[16]. Other factors seem to be important in IC, such as mast cells and their degranulation, vascular problems (such as reflex sympathetic dystrophy), and probably neuroinflammation from upregulation of sensory nerves.

Inflammation and interstitial cystitis

For long it has been stated in the literature that IC is primarily an inflammatory disease, but this is probably not true and has not been substantiated by any data. Indeed, the role of inflammation and inflammatory mediators in IC is not known. Several points support the notion that inflammation plays little role in most IC patients. First, biopsy specimens show almost no

inflammation. Second, no systemic signs are found (e.g. no leucocytosis)[17]. And third, neither inflammatory mediators[18] nor white blood cells are found in the urine of these patients. Furthermore, patients with IC do not suffer from generalized inflammatory diseases such as collagen vascular diseases[4,8]. Mild inflammation in the bladder wall may be secondary to the diffusion of urinary solutes (potassium) and not the cause of the problem. Perhaps it is best to consider IC as a long-term chronic disease with so gradual a destruction of bladder tissue over time that minimal or no inflammation occurs.

Mast cells are a prominent feature in perhaps one third of patients and may be important in the provocation of symptoms, especially in atopic people[19-28]. In addition, animal models of mast-cell stimulation also suggest that these cells may provoke abnormalities in both smooth muscle activity and epithelial permeability[29,30]. In our experience, it is important to control allergies in patients with IC as they can often provoke the induction of significant symptom flares. Consequently, mast-cell aggravation may be very relevant and important to recognize for therapy and suggests that combinations of treatment are necessary to control the disease.

Vascular insufficiency

Reduction of vascular perfusion may negatively affect mucosal, muscle, and nerve nutrition and initiate a cascade of events that cause symptoms. Radiation is known to impair blood supply by injury to the microvasculature of organs and, certainly in the case of the urinary bladder, leads to a syndrome that is basically IC with urgency, frequency, and altered epithelial permeability[31]. Other profusion abnormalities, such as reflex sympathetic dystrophy[32], may result in a secondary decrease in blood flow that also triggers events leading to symptoms in the IC syndrome. Vascular injury could be accelerated because of reduced epithelial permeability regulation that results in potassium leak into the bladder interstitial space. This potassium is directly toxic to the small blood supply of the subepithelial tissues and results in further bladder destruction.

Epithelial leak

A widely held theory on IC pathogenesis is that of an epithelial leak. The hypothesis is that the permeability regulatory mechanism of the superficial epithelial cells is impaired, which results in solute migration across the epithelium. Initially, little data supported the concept that such a leak existed[12]. An early observation was that both normal individuals and IC patients had abnormal findings in their tight junctions relative to ruthenium-red penetration. However, a well-controlled study of 56 patients provided data to support the hypothesis that the bladder surface in many IC patients may indeed leak solute[13]. These data are supported by subsequent investigations that employed an even more sensitive 'leak assay' to screen individual patients for potential permeability aberrations. From these studies it is estimated that about 70–75% of IC patients could have a leaky epithelium[31,33]. The caveat here is that there are false negative responses to the test (probably not false positives) and epithelial problems may be present in even more patients. In addition, the study group was a slightly skewed population, as patients who have a nonleaky epithelium are more difficult to treat and thus more likely to present to a tertiary care center.

The hypothesis of an epithelial leak is further supported by other investigators who found similar responses to the potassium test[34,35], and found that that up to 90% of IC patients have a leaky epithelium to potassium. These studies also suggest that there is a small proportion of this patient population that does not have a detectable epithelial leak (by current technologies) and may represent some other problem such as neurologic inflammation. These data also suggest that perhaps a method is now available to at least stratify the IC patients into two groups, those who appear to be epithelial leakers and those who are nonleakers. The test also is a good aid in diagnosis.

Glycosaminoglycans: the blood–urine barrier

The transitional epithelium is one of the most impermeable in the body. The regulation of epithelial permeability traditionally has been ascribed to tight junctions and ion pumps as well as to the actual membranes[12,36–41]. Many of these concepts are still hypothetic and not completely validated physiologically. More recently, it was discovered that the surface mucus, which contains proteoglycans and glycoproteins, may be another critical component by which the epithelium maintains a barrier between the bladder wall and urine, an important part of the so-called blood–urine barrier[13–15]. These studies suggest that perhaps the tight junctions (which are present in most epithelia), the bilipid membranes, and the ion pumps are all important in the process of permeability regulation. However, the initial contact for the solute is the mucus, which may be the one barrier that excludes most of the urinary solutes, and thus prevents them from reaching the membrane and the other secondary controllers of permeability.

Surface mucus [glycosaminoglycan (GAG), proteoglycans] appears to have multiple protective roles in the bladder; these include antiadherence (relative to bacteria and crystalloid) and regulation of transepithelial solute movement[15,42–44]. The transitional cell's external surface polysaccharides are able to prevent the adherence of bacteria, crystals, proteins, and ions; this function is lost when this layer is removed with a dilute acid or detergent[42–45], but is restored when mucus is replaced by exogenous polysaccharides such as heparin or pentosanpolysulfate (PPS)[42,46,47]. The oxygen atom present on the sulfated polysaccharides in the mucus is charged negatively and has a high affinity to bond ionically with water. This results in exclusion of urinary ionic solutes by a Donnan effect[48]. When GAGs are present at a surface (the bladder), in effect it binds water molecules tightly to the oxygen of the sulfate groups in these molecules, in preference to calcium, barium, and even hydrogen ions[49–51]. Water molecules become trapped and interposed at the boundary between the cell surface (bladder) and the environment (urine), as illustrated in Figure 33.1. This bound molecular layer of water acts as a physical barrier so that urinary solutes, such as urea and calcium[15,42], are not able to reach the underlying cell membrane, adhere to it, or move across it.

Quaternary amines, however, have a high affinity for sulfated polysaccharides and displace the water that is bound to the oxygen groups to form a salt[46,52,53]. In support of this concept is that the chemical reaction of GAG with quaternary amines results in increased entropy to reflect the loss of order of water molecules around the sulfate groups[48,54]. This interaction is the basis of the clinical use of protamine sulfate (a highly charged

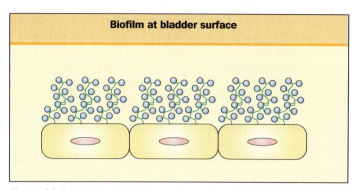

Figure 33.1 Biofilm at bladder surface drawn to demonstrate the location of trapped water at the surface. Circles represent bound water and wavy lines are protein backbone.

proteinaceous group of amines with quaternary amines) to precipitate and inactivate the anticoagulant effects of heparin. It has been demonstrated both in animal and human models that protamine sulfate inactivates native cell surface polysaccharides and results in increased epithelial permeability. Such damage to the transitional cells can be reversed by the addition of an exogenous GAG such as heparin or PPS[14,15].

Based on these concepts, Parsons et al.[13] hypothesized that the surface polysaccharide is functionally defective (not absent) in some patients with IC. Possible causes for the deficiency include reduced sulfation of the polysaccharides, diminished density or thickness of the polysaccharide, or the presence of a compound, such as a urinary quaternary amine, that could bind to it and inactivate it. It is known that normal individuals who have their bladder surface challenged by protamine lose the impermeability of the epithelium. The permeability to urea in normal individuals increases from 5% to 25%[14]. When the blood–urine barrier is lost because of protamine treatment, normal subjects experience urgency, frequency, and in some cases bladder pain (the symptoms of IC). These symptoms can be reversed with heparin.

These data are supported additionally by the fact that a semisynthetic polysaccharide (PPS) similar to heparin ameliorates the symptoms of IC[55–58]. To test the hypothesis that some patients with IC have a permeable transitional-cell layer, Parsons et al. measured the permeability of the normal bladder epithelium to a concentrated solution of urea and compared it to the permeability of the epithelium obtained from patients with IC[13]. In the test, 29 normal individuals absorbed approximately 5% of the urea, whereas 56 patients with IC absorbed 25% (these differences were statistically significant, $p < 0.01$). Recent evidence from Buffington and Woodworth provides further support to an epithelial permeability dysfunction in IC[59]. Controls and IC patients were given oral fluorescein. The IC patients maintained significantly higher serum levels and took longer to clear the fluorescein from their blood than did the normal controls. The authors concluded that IC patients 'reabsorbed' the fluorescein from their bladder, which resulted in recycling and prolonged clearance from the blood stream. As a result of the increased epithelial permeability, a leak of urinary solutes in IC results in the symptoms of urgency, frequency, and pain.

In another study a small group of patients were examined for ^{99m}Tc-diethylenetriamine pentaacetic acid (^{99m}Tc-DTPA) absorption across the bladder; an 80% increase in DTPA absorption was found in IC patients with respect to normal individuals.[59a] However, the numbers involved were not sufficient – the difference between normal individuals and controls only just approaching statistical significance, with a *p* value of 0.07. Nonetheless, these data also support the concept of epithelial dysfunction in IC patients.

Role of urinary potassium in the pathogenesis and diagnosis of interstitial cystitis

One of the most important aspects of the IC puzzle is to identify the toxic substance in urine that leaks across the epithelium and provokes the symptoms of IC. It has been proposed by Parsons.[33] that the principal toxic substance in urine is potassium. In essence, it is rather an obvious toxin in that urine levels in humans range between 30 and 150mmol/L (mEq/L) with an average of about 75mmol/L, a concentration long known to be toxic to all mammalian cells. In addition, potassium levels of approximately 15mmol/L depolarize sensory nerves and muscle. Since the kidneys are the main route of excretion of dietary potassium, the bladder had to develop a method to handle these very toxic levels. It may well be that the most important role of the relatively impermeable bladder epithelium is to prevent the diffusion of potassium into the bladder interstitium and subsequent destruction of the tissue.

The role of the transitional epithelium in potassium regulation is summarized in Figure 33.2. If urinary potassium should excessively leak into the bladder interstitium, there may be another secondary defense mechanism. The rich supply of subepithelial lymphatics and blood vessels could resorb this cation and restore the normal equilibrium[60]. However, the diffusion of potassium at excessive rates may lead to the destruction of these blood and lymphatic vessels, and result in the acceleration and progression of the disease process. The sequence of events may explain both the symptoms and the gradual progression of disease in most patients.

Toxic levels of interstitial potassium could also induce other neurologically active agents, such as substance P, and lead to upregulation of pain fibers, which may be an important feature of IC[25–28]. The potassium hypothesis also explains the lack of any significant inflammatory response in most patients with IC, either in the urine or bladder interstitium[21].

Based on the above concepts, two components may be important in the paradigm of IC pathogenesis:
- the regulatory role of mucus in reducing permeability is impaired (for reasons unknown); and
- once impaired, the high levels of urinary potassium result in increased interstitial levels in the bladder that induce sensory nerves (and muscle) to depolarize, which causes pain and urgency and may destroy tissue, and hence the progression of the disease.

These concepts are supported by data from Hohlbrugger and colleagues[16,61]. Incorporated into the progression may be the upregulation of nerve fibers, mast cells, and an ever-increasing neurogenic inflammation, which may become an important and perhaps driving force of the disease that also must be dealt with in terms of therapy. In effect, as the disease progresses, patients become both solute and volume sensitive.

To test the hypothesis that potassium induces symptoms in IC, Parsons et al. tested normal individuals and patients with a

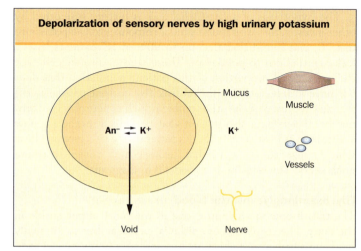

Figure 33.2 Role of the epithelial mucus layer in protecting the bladder from urinary solutes such as potassium. The high levels of potassium in normal urine are more than sufficient to depolarize sensory nerves and muscle if a dysfunctional epithelium allows the potassium to diffuse into the subepithelial area. Excessive leakage of potassium could overwhelm a secondary bladder defense mechanism, the capacity of subepithelial lymphatics and blood vessels to resorb the potassium and restore tissue levels of potassium to normal. An, anion.

variety of bladder sensory disorders for sensitivity to a solution of intravesical potassium (Fig. 33.3).

As can be seen, IC patients reacted strongly to the potassium solution but normal individuals did not. Patients with acute urinary tract infection and radiation cystitis were found to be potassium sensitive also, whereas benign prostatic hyperplasia (BPH) patients and most detrusor instability patients were not provoked. Last, to test the hypothesis we compared sodium (which should not depolarize nerves) to potassium. Sodium chloride did not cause symptoms in the normal subjects who were evaluated while potassium did (Fig. 33.4). Individual potassium sensitivity may be a useful diagnostic tool, especially in patients with milder forms of IC.

Mast cells and nerve fibers

The role of mast cells in this disorder is unclear. A number of investigators have reported the presence of mast cells in IC bladders, but other data suggest that they also are present in non-IC bladders[9,11,19,62–65]. The main dilemma is whether or not mast cells play a causative or secondary role. Do they degranulate and produce the symptoms or are they a response to the actual cause of IC (e.g. an epithelial leak) and so a type of defense mechanism that may ultimately become part of the problem by degranulating and causing a 'leak'?

Regardless of how the data are viewed, most clinical IC researchers believe that mast cells play an important role in IC. Clinical impressions are supported by data derived from animal models. Saban and colleagues showed that mast-cell activation in guinea pig bladders results in an increase in epithelial permeability[29]. Add to this our observations, as well as that of other investigators, that active allergies can exacerbate IC symptoms and the mast cell takes on added significance, especially in terms of therapy.

Mast cells also interact with sensory nerves and release transmitters that activate pain; Sant and other workers obtained data

Results of stimulation of sensory urgency or pain in various groups using potassium chloride				
Group	N	Positive* to potassium chloride (%)	p value†	Positive to water (%)
Normal individuals	41	4	–	0
Interstitial cystitis (meeting National Institutes of Health criteria)	92	74	<0.001‡	10
Interstitial cystitis (not cystoscoped)	139	76	<0.001‡	10
Radiation cystitis§	5	100	0.001	0
Benign prostatic hyperplasia	29	3	1.0	3
Urinary tract infection, acute#	4	100	0.01	0
Urinary tract infection, uninfected¶	5	0	1.0	0
Detrusor instability	16	25	0.03	0

*At least 2 point change in visual analog scale
†Fisher's exact test employed to compare group with controls
‡Chi square analysis
§Parsons, et al.[31]
#Test performed when infected
¶Test performed when uninfected

Figure 33.3 Results of stimulation of sensory urgency or pain in various groups using potassium chloride.

to reveal the regulation of nerves and neurotransmitters with IC[17,18,25–28,63,65–68]. This is relevant when therapy is reviewed because suppression of mast cells seems important.

Pyschosomatic factors

It has been suggested that psychosomatic factors initiate IC, but this is rarely true. Most patients (especially those with chronic pain) are secondarily affected by their disease and as a result may show signs of mild or moderate chronic depression. Those who suffer from severe nocturia exhibit even more profound depression because of sleep deprivation. In the author's experience, essentially no-one has been cured of IC by psychotherapy. Earlier researchers reported similar findings[5]. Importantly, the treatment of depression can result in an overall sense of well-being for patients and help them to cope with their disease, but it does not cure IC or reduce the number of daily voids. Although acute stress does flare IC symptoms and stress reduction improves them, the patient still has IC. Stress factors that aggravate symptoms also may be physical (such as viral infections, exercise, surgery, travel in a car or plane, or jogging) and, of course, the stress also could be emotional. It is important to the rapport between physician and patient for the physician to make it clear that IC is not a psychologic disorder.

INCIDENCE AND EPIDEMIOLOGY

Although IC was first identified in 1907 by Nitze, few epidemiologic studies have been reported[71]. Oravisto, in a Finnish study of 103 people with IC, estimated an annual incidence of 1.2 cases per 100,000 and a prevalence of about 10–11 per 100,000[72]. Held et al. estimated that there are about 44,000 cases in the US[73]; the author's estimate extrapolated from San Diego County data is placed at 40–60,000. Held also estimated a worst case scenario in the US of 450,000[74]. These are the traditional reported incidences of IC. However, they are probably not even close to the actual number of individuals who may have this disease.

Sodium versus potassium provocation in interstitial cystitis subjects*			
Treatment arm	Urgency $\frac{1}{M}$ sodium (%)	Urgency $\frac{1}{M}$ potassium (%)	p value
Control	0/10 (0%)	0/11 (0%)	–
Protamine	1/10 (10%)	10/11 (90%)	<0.001
Heparin	1/10 (10%)	5/11 (54%)	0.035*

*Parsons, et al.[33]

Figure 33.4 Sodium versus potassium provocation in interstitial cystitis subjects.

More recently, Jones and Nyberg[3] reported a prevalence of 500,000 to 1,000,000 people with IC in the US. Further, it was estimated in 1966 that 4–6% of premenopausal females in the US have bladder infections every year, but this has not been documented by clinical experience or data reported in the literature. In fact, in a large study in England of 1000 successive patients who presented to outpatient centers for a clinical trial, 50% of those with signs and symptoms of a urinary tract infection (urgency and/or frequency) had negative cultures[75]. It was concluded that these patients had 'the urethral syndrome', which was defined as signs and symptoms of infection with negative cultures. It is likely that such patients have a mild form of IC, which very gradually escalates over the years; once symptoms become severe enough, the diagnosis becomes 'classic' IC.

It is best to think of IC as a gradually progressive disease process, intermittent in the beginning and more persistent as IC advances. A time line (Fig. 33.5) can be associated with IC. The younger patient has mild intermittent urgency and/or frequency that is diagnosed as recurrent bladder infections. After persistent negative cultures in spite of symptoms, perhaps the next diagnosis for these patients is urethral syndrome. As their disease progresses further and they become continuously symptomatic, they may reach the so-called NIH criteria for IC. Ultimately, as

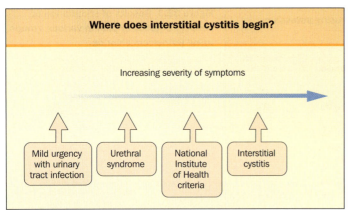

Figure 33.5 Where does interstitial cystitis begin? In most people, interstitial cystitis appears to be a slowly and insidiously progressive disease. Symptoms are mild and intermittent early on. As the disease progresses, different diagnoses are applied to the patient. It is not until near the end-stage that patients are diagnosed with 'classic' interstitial cystitis. Its spectrum of severity is broad.

the disease continues to destroy the bladder, primarily in older patients, a diagnosis of 'classic' IC is made. In all likelihood, all patients represent the same disease process but are early or late in disease development and receive a diagnosis relative to where they are on this time line. Generally, the disease appears to incubate slowly over years, with a progressive increase in symptomatology and decrease in bladder function as the disease takes its toll.

Demographic factors

The female:male ratio of patients with IC is about 9:1[73,76–78]. However, if males are being misdiagnosed with prostatitis or benign prostatic hyperplasia (BPH), this ratio may change substantially. Age also is a risk factor, with the disease generally limited to those over 18 years of age, although cases in younger people have been reported[79–82]. The median age of diagnosis is between 40–46 years of age, and the disease symptoms appear on average 3–4 years earlier[73,76,83]. The advanced age of patients with IC may reflect the slow disease progression. Race and ethnicity appear to be risk factors, as IC occurs mostly in Caucasians[84–86], although IC has been reported in African–Americans[87]. However, these numbers probably do not reflect an accurate picture since many patients with milder forms of the disease are misdiagnosed.

In a review of 300 cases at the University of California, San Diego, it was observed that those without diabetes seemed to be at a greater risk[83]. Furthermore, a 400% higher incidence was seen in Jewish people. These values are similar to those of inflammatory bowel diseases[76,88–92]. The bottom line is that IC is not rare, but common, with a frequency as high as 1–2% of females. The male incidence also may be grossly underestimated, with misdiagnosis as prostatitis or BPH.

PATHOLOGY

That IC is a continuously progressive disease is important. The 19-year-old with early disease has significant sensory nerve activation, but no real damage to the bladder. As the disease progresses over 10–20 years, the female may develop some

significant secondary changes of the bladder (such as an alteration of epithelial mucus and adhesion molecules, basement membrane changes, muscle loss, and nerve upregulation), but no translational clinical pathologic changes. Consequently, routine pathologic processing of tissue yields no pathognomonic changes in IC.

As methods are developed to identify proteins, GAG, etc., methods also may be developed to aid in the clinical diagnosis of IC. It must be remembered, however, that in early disease no anatomic changes of IC may occur. Early phases represent 75% of IC patients. The physiologic changes may be dramatic (e.g. epithelial leak of potassium) and functional tests of nerve function (not anatomic) may be important to the diagnosis. Various descriptions have been proposed, but unfortunately nothing pathognomonic of IC occurs in bladder biopsy specimens. The mast-cell controversy is reviewed above; approximately one-third of patients have an increased bladder wall and mucosa mast-cell infiltration. Light microscopy generally reveals a urothelium that is thinned, readily detached, and nearly absent in many areas.

Unlike the normal epithelium of thickness six or seven layer, the bladder mucosa of IC patients is frequently only 2–4 cell layers thick. These changes are consistent with a dysfunctional epithelium[13]. A generalized pancystitis[62,87,93,94] with infiltration of the lamina propria by mononuclear and chronic inflammatory cells is seen in some patients, but the caveat is that biopsies are only carried out for more advanced disease. Most physicians biopsy after the hydrodistention and perhaps many of the observed histologic changes are artifacts.

The distribution of collagen within the bladder wall is unclear[95]. One hypothesis suggests that, as the disorder progresses, a fibrotic small bladder of the end-stage type develops. As yet, little or no data supports this theory. The author believes that this is not the process, but that frequent low-volume voiding, coupled with possible epithelial solute leaks, leads to a thinned epithelium with destruction of smooth muscle bundles; the net result is a small bladder. Furthermore, the only scarring present in the bladder wall is probably iatrogenic (from prior biopsies), since many of these patients undergo multiple biopsies over the years[95]. As the bladder shrinks from frequent low-volume voiding, a disproportionate part of the bladder wall becomes scar tissue. In the author's experience (over 500 biopsies), scarring is not identified when biopsies are obtained from an area of the bladder not previously biopsied.

At our institution, cystectomy has been carried out for 35 patients with IC. Of these patients, 80% had only epithelium and a few blood vessels and muscle bundles left in the urinary bladder. Also, perivesical fat is severely wasted. Perhaps the urinary solutes (potassium) leak through the thin (perhaps 3–4mm) bladder wall and lead to destruction and atrophy of the perivesical fat. This may help to explain the increasingly diffuse lower abdominal pain experienced by these patients. Medial thigh pain may result from provocation of the obturator nerves through this process.

Bladder biopsy is useless in IC as it is not diagnostic, although some changes (as mentioned above) are associated with IC. While it is rare for these patients to be confused with those who have carcinoma in situ of the bladder, a biopsy may be necessary to rule out cancer[96]. A combination of cytologic evaluation of the urine and bladder washings plus biopsy is necessary to exclude malignancy. In over 3000 patients evaluated by the author, no cancers have been diagnosed at presentation but one male developed a transitional cell tumor 8 years after the initial diagnosis of IC. An additional male with suspicious cytologies at presentation had a second bladder biopsy after 6 months that was positive for cancer. Thus, it is always necessary to screen and perhaps monitor at-risk patients (i.e. males over 40 and females over 45 years of age, and people with hematuria).

SIGNS AND SYMPTOMS

The principal symptoms of IC are the presence of abnormal sensory urgency and pain (Fig. 33.6). Sensory urgency leads to urinary frequency. In addition, most patients have associated bladder pain, but some patients have pelvic pain and no urgency. One study of over 200 patients[83] showed that of those who present with IC, approximately 15% have little or no bladder pain while 85% of patients have significant pain. It is important to determine whether the pain is of bladder origin. The patient is asked if the pain (despite being constantly present) worsens if the bladder is not emptied and improves (not disappears) with voiding. This is helpful information, but some patients have pain that is not affected by bladder volume. Bladder pain of IC is experienced suprapubically, in the perineum, in the vulva and vagina, in the low back, or even in the medial thighs[5]. One-third of patients experience dysuria. Men may experience pain in the scrotum.

Nocturia is variable, but in general 90% of patients complain of voiding at least 1–2 times per night, but some patients have no nocturia[83]. Nocturia increases with the severity and duration of the disease. The average patient voids approximately 16 times/day; a minimum for diagnostic purposes is considered to be eight voids per day[1]. The average voided volume is 75mL. Between 85–90% of individuals with IC are female. Of those who are sexually active, the majority (75%) complain of an exacerbation of the symptom complex associated with sexual intercourse[83]. The increase in symptoms may be felt during sexual activity, immediately after, or within 24 hours. In addition, most women who are still menstruating complain of a flare of symptoms several days to a week before the onset of the menstrual cycle[53,83].

EVALUATION

The NIDDKD criteria were a practical attempt to quantitate findings in IC[1]. In part they were based on a study reported by Parsons et al. in which the symptoms of over 200 IC patients had been measured and analyzed[83]. From Parsons' data each variable was examined; the value that included 90% of the patients was the number taken for the NIDDKD criteria. For example, 90% of IC patients were found to void at least 1–2 times at night, complained of eight or more voidings during the day, and had moderate urinary urgency. The presence of bladder pain was variable. The data upon which these criteria were based are given in Figure 33.6.

The duration of symptoms helps to distinguish patients with IC from those with the milder form of IC, often called the urgency–frequency syndrome (UFS; Fig. 33.7). The diagnosis of IC is more likely if the individual has suffered continuous symptoms for at least 6 months. Clinically, to separate IC from UFS

Symptom	Value	Number of times	Number of patients	Percentage of patients
Nocturia	Mean	4.7		
	90% cut-off level[†]	1.5 (1–2 voidings)		
	Range	0–13		
		1–2	41	18
		2–4	90	40
		4.5–8	63	28
Daytime frequency	Mean	16.0		
	90% cut-off level	7		
	Range	5.5–40		
Urgency	Mild		8	3.5
	Moderate		63	28
	Moderate–severe		35	15.5
	Severe		119	53
Pain	None		41	18
	Mild		16	7
	Moderate		82	36
	Severe		86	39

*Parsons[83]
[†]Present in 90% of patients

Figure 33.6 Symptoms reported in 225 patients, with frequency distributions for symptom severity.

Changes in voiding measurements over time in patients with interstitial cystitis*		
	Average value for patients with symptoms for 1 year	Average value for patients with symptoms for >7 years
Number of patients	34	42
Voidings	15.2	17.3
Voided volume (mL)	128	105
Anesthetic bladder capacity (mL)	711	518

*Parsons[83]

Figure 33.7 Changes in voiding measurements with time in patients with interstitial cystitis.

(even though they are probably the same disease) is worthwhile as UFS may need little or no therapy and the prognosis for the patient is good.

Voiding log

An accurate assessment of number of daily voidings and average volume can be determined from a 2-day voiding log for which each voiding is measured and recorded by the patient at home. From such data it was found that the average patient voids 16 times per day with a capacity of 73mL[1]. The voiding profile is a useful method to help establish the diagnosis of IC, and may be used to create a therapeutic plan and to determine progress in

Voiding profiles of patients with interstitial cystitis and normal individuals				
Patient	Parameter	Number of voidings/day	Voided volume (mL)	Nocturia
Interstitial cystitis (145 patients)	Average	16.4	73	4.7
	90%* confidence limit	9	100	
	Range	6–39	26–235	
Normal (48)	Average	6.5	270	
	90%* confidence limit	7	150†	
	Range	3–13	100–600	

*90% of subjects had at least this level
†90% of patients above this level

Figure 33.8 Voiding profiles of patients with interstitial cystitis and normal individuals.

therapy. It is recommended that the clinician obtain one initially and at subsequent visits. Patients with a longer disease history have a smaller functional bladder capacity, as reflected in the average voided volume and number of daily voidings (Fig. 33.8).

Physical examination

On physical examination, over 95% of patients complain of a tender bladder base during the pelvic examination. This discomfort is easily demonstrated by palpation of the anterior vaginal wall. Urine analysis and cultures on voided specimens are not useful in these patients as their low voided volumes make midstream collection impossible. A catheterized specimen examined under the microscope should show no bacteria, and most show no red or white blood cells. Urine should be sent for cytologic evaluation to rule out the possibility of carcinoma, but a positive cytology has not been found at our center. Patients who present with hematuria are rare, but require a full genitourinary work-up to exclude malignancy. All men and women over 40 years of age probably deserve at least an initial screening (cytology and office cystoscopy) to rule out malignancy.

Urodynamics

The cystometrogram (CMG) is a valuable study to carry out in patients with this syndrome, as a normal study essentially excludes the diagnosis of IC. Recent published data by the NIH Interstitial Cystitis Database Study Group demonstrated that for diagnosis urodynamics could be substituted for cystoscopy[97]. Together with the voiding log and the potassium test, the CMG is quite helpful in IC diagnosis. Significant urinary urgency can usually be documented with cystometry. If gas is employed, IC patients have a sensation of significant urgency at $<125cm^3$ and with water at $<150mL$. If this portion of the CMG is normal, they may not have IC or only a mild form.

In 75 IC patients with CMGs reported by Parsons[83], the average bladder capacity was $220cm^3$ and over 90% of the patients had a functional volume of $<350cm^3$. In general, patients should have the bladder discomfort they experience provoked by the CMG, although (as noted previously) some patients' bladder pain is not provoked by volume. However, there is an important caveat relative to maximum bladder capacity. A small group (about 5%) of

patients with significant IC develop detrusor myopathy, but muscle dysfunction is seen in most patients with advanced disease[83,98]. Individuals with this complication have large atonic bladders with little muscle present. They have moderate-to-severe sensory urgency, large bladder capacities ($>1L$), and usually carry residual urine ($>100mL$). Detrusor function is poor or absent. Many patients with IC have poor muscle function as the disease gradually destroys their bladder and hence they empty their bladders only with difficulty. Since most of the patients are female, they are able to void but primarily with a valsalva maneuver. As a result of the generalized atrophy of bladder muscle with this disease, males with low voiding pressure may require clean intermittent self catheterization (CISC) as part of their treatment. Urodynamics may help differentiate men with IC from those with symptoms secondary to BOO. If the patient has increased sensory urgency, and a low volume bladder with low flow rates and low intravesical pressure, the diagnosis is more likely IC than BPH.

Cystoscopic evaluation

Cystoscopic evaluation of the bladder under anesthetic is primarily important as a therapeutic maneuver. Examination under local anesthetic is not appropriate for IC diagnosis[97], since it offers little help and causes the patient severe discomfort. It may be used to exclude carcinoma in high-risk groups (males and females over 40 years of age, or if hematuria is present). Cystoscopy for therapy should be carried out under anesthetic. Most patients do not need this unless severe symptoms are present. It is best to omit cystoscopy for milder patients and proceed with the therapies discussed below.

Cystoscopy under anesthesia, when appropriate, is carried out in a manner to both diagnose and treat. The diagnosis depends on the discovery of one of two findings – a Hunner's ulcer or the presence of glomerulations or petechial hemorrhages. However, not all patients show these changes, so their absence does not exclude the diagnosis.

Potassium test

A simple method has been devised by Parsons (the Parsons Test) to measure epithelial permeability. The test is based on the hypothesis that if a solution of potassium chloride is placed into a normal bladder, it provokes no symptoms of urgency or pain. However, if the solution is placed into a bladder of which the mechanism to maintain the impermeable epithelium is impaired, the potassium diffuses across the transitional cells and depolarizes sensory nerves, which causes urgency or pain (Fig. 33.9).

Cystoscopy for therapy

A report by Bumpus in 1930 that bladder hydrodistention improved the symptoms of IC has resulted in this procedure being a mainstay of therapy[99]. Few investigators question that hydrodistention ameliorates the symptoms in 60% of IC patients. The procedure must be carried out under anesthetic, as it is not possible to dilate a painful bladder without it. The procedure for hydrodistention is described below. Pressure dilation of the bladder using a syringe should not be attempted as it can result in bladder rupture.

The cystoscopy is carried out in two phases. In phase one, the initial inspection, the physician obtains specimens for cytology and urine for both routine and tuberculosis culture (the latter is

Potassium protocol	
Patient type	**Treatment with best response**
Potassium positive*	Dilation
	Dimethyl sulfoxide
	Heparin
	Pentosanpolysulfate
	Polycitra
Potassium negative	Antidepressants
	Possibly pentosanpolysulfate
*Add hydroxyzine if allergies are present	

Figure 33.9 Potassium protocol.

optional as it is very rarely diagnosed). Visual examination of the bladder may reveal a true Hunner's ulcer (patch). The patch, which is velvety red and present in only 6–8% of patients[83], is very similar in appearance to carcinoma in-situ. However, it is not actually a true ulcer, only a red patch. A biopsy is not taken at this part of the cystoscopy. Prior biopsy site scars, which are frequently mistaken for ulcers, also may be seen[95]. Bladders with IC appear to heal poorly, and biopsy scars are frequently large, but recognizable by the spoke-wheel blood vessels that radiate from the central scarred portion. These scars frequently tear and bleed after distention and account for most so-called epithelial disruptions. Parsons reported that as many as 75% of ulcers described at previous cystoscopy by other urologists were biopsy site scars[83].

The second phase of the cystoscopic procedure is hydrodistention to demonstrate glomerulations. Hydrodistention also induces a disease remission in 60% of patients. Hydrodistention is achieved by filling the bladder slowly up to a pressure of 80–100cmH$_2$O (7.8–9.8kPa). The urethra of the female is manually compressed over the cystoscope to prevent leakage of fluid. After several minutes, the bladder is emptied, and the volume measured and recorded. The last part of the effluent is usually bloody if glomerulations or ulcers are present. When the bladder is reexamined, glomerulations should be visible, diffusely located around the bladder and at least 10–20 per field of vision. Hemorrhages on the trigone or posterior bladder wall are irrelevant and do not constitute a positive finding as they probably represent cystoscope trauma.

What constitutes an abnormal bladder capacity under anesthetic may be a surprise to many physicians. A normal female bladder holds well over 1000mL, while the IC bladder usually holds <850mL. The average anesthetic capacity for moderate to advanced IC patients is between 550 and 650mL. Patients with a longer history of symptoms have smaller bladder capacities, which suggests the disease is slowly progressive[83]. Other factors also suggestive of a slowly progressive disease are that patients with Hunner's ulcers are the oldest, have the worst symptoms, the smallest bladder capacities, and the greatest problem with loss of epithelial impermeability[13,83].

The mechanism by which hydrodistention improves symptoms is unknown; several theories have been postulated. Neuropraxis induced by mechanical trauma may occur in some individuals. However, few patients awaken with decreased pain, which does not support the neuropraxis concept. Rather, most (90%) recover from anesthetic with significantly worse pain that slowly improves over 2–3 weeks. This pain usually requires narcotic analgesia, and remission occurs over several weeks.

As a result of the increased pain, it is recommended that all patients receive belladonna and opium rectal suppositories immediately in the recovery room or, better yet, that 10mL of 2% viscous lidocaine (lignocaine) be instilled into the bladder at the end of hydrodistention. In addition, patients are discharged with medication (narcotic) to control the increased pain.

As most patients' symptoms are exacerbated by hydrodistention, we believe epithelial damage from the mechanical trauma is responsible. Disruption in the integrity of the mucosal cells increases the epithelial leak of potassium, which causes symptoms to flare. Healing may occur over several weeks posthydrodistention, which correlates with the time of clinical remission. Perhaps the epithelium regenerates and for a period of time is 'healthy' and impermeable, and/or perhaps there is a delayed neuropraxis from nerve injury secondary to the increased epithelial permeability. If so, whatever events initiate the disease continue and relapse usually occurs.

Remission may persist between 4–12 months, and hydrodistention may be repeated as needed. If no remission is obtained, the dilation is repeated at least twice more as frequently patients respond to this. Unfortunately, symptom remission decreases in duration and response as the disease progresses and many patients become resistant to it.

Biopsy

The final part of the cystoscopic procedure is the biopsy. A biopsy must not be taken before hydrodistention, as the bladder could tear at the biopsy site and produce a significant bladder rupture. If a caustic agent is used for therapy, the biopsy must not occur before the solution is placed in the bladder. Should the solution extravasate through the biopsy site, severe tissue damage may result.

The biopsy itself is not diagnostic for IC, but can rule out other diseases such as carcinoma in-situ. The findings on pathologic examination include the presence of mast cells (demonstrated by toluidine blue staining)[63,64], inflammatory cells, and a thinned mucosa. A normal biopsy does not exclude IC and biopsy should not be utilized in diagnosis. Conversely, no pathologic findings specifically make a diagnosis of IC.

While diagnosis of IC depends in part on abnormal cystoscopic findings, the disease cannot be arbitrarily ruled out purely by endoscopic findings. Many patients who have IC show no such findings and benefit from therapy. The physician needs to remember that this disease is complex and primarily manifested by significant urinary urgency or frequency, with perhaps few or no other findings.

At the end of the cystoscopy, 10mL of 2% viscous lidocaine jelly is placed into the bladder, to aid control during the anesthetic recovery period.

THERAPY

Therapy for IC continues to evolve, with better treatments emerging. The most important considerations are multiple therapies (polytherapy) and time. A number of drugs have been employed to treat IC, but most have been used empirically and only a few have been tested in controlled trials. Basically, therapy for IC can be divided into three major categories:

- Drugs that alter nerve function directly or indirectly, such as narcotics, antidepressants, antihistamines, anti-inflammatories, anticholinergics, antispasmodics, and analgesics.
- Cytodestructive techniques that destroy the umbrella cells of the bladder, which causes a regeneration, a new bladder surface, and a period of remission. In general, they cause symptoms of flare before the repair process is completed and the symptoms resolve. These techniques include dimethyl sulfoxide (DMSO), hydrodistention, sodium oxychlorosene (Clorpactin), silver nitrate, and more recently bacillus Calmette–Guérin (BCG).
- Cytoprotective techniques involve medications, primarily polysaccharides, that can 'coat' the bladder and help reestablish or protect the bladder surface mucus. These include heparin, PPS, and possibly hyaluronic acid.

When therapy is discussed with the individual patient, it is important for the physician to emphasize that if the symptoms have been present for more than a year, no particular therapy is likely to be curative. In such circumstances, the disease is chronic and requires chronic therapy. While the patient may have a significant remission of symptoms, in all probability, relapse will occur. If patients are prepared for this eventuality, they are much less distressed when symptoms return and cope better with their disease. The physician–patient relationship is strengthened in terms of credibility if this area is addressed prior to the initiation of treatment. Patients readily accept this explanation and overall appear to adjust to their disorder when their outlook is realistic, and so persist with their treatment regimen. Otherwise many patients stop therapy too quickly, even though they would benefit from it.

Pharmacotherapy

Antidepressant therapy

Chronic pain and sleep loss cause depression. Thus, it is valuable to place most IC patients with moderate or severe symptoms on antidepressant medications (Fig. 33.10). Tricyclic antidepressants have several modes of action that are beneficial. Their side-effects are drowsiness (aids sleep), increased pain thresholds, and elevation of mood. If tricyclic antidepressants are used, start with low doses and warn patients that they will be tired (for 12–15 hours per day) for the first 2–3 weeks of therapy. Once they become tolerant to this side effect, the dose is increased, if needed. Amitriptyline[100] or imipramine can be prescribed in doses of 25mg (or even 10mg) 1 hour before bedtime.

In an uncontrolled trial, amitriptyline was reported by Hanno et al.[100] to ameliorate the symptoms of IC. Patients were treated with 25mg of amitriptyline 1 hour before bedtime for 1 week; the dose was then increased weekly by 25mg to 75mg; 50% of patients responded to this medication. The exact mechanism of amitriptyline is unknown, although it may block H_1-histamine receptors and perhaps mast cell degranulation. More likely the drug raises pain tolerance through its antidepressant activity.

If fluoxetine is selected, the dose is 20mg per day, increased if needed to 40mg. Sertraline is another well-tolerated antidepressant, which can be used at 50mg per day and increased to 100mg if needed.

Antidepressant therapy
Mild patients
Dimethyl sulfoxide for 3 months may induce long remission* Pentosanpolysulfate
Moderate–severe patients
Antidepressant plus pentosanpolysulfate and/or daily intravesical heparin*† Dimethyl sulfoxide (When improved, slowly taper off heparin)
Severe patients
Antidepressant plus pentosanpolysulfate and/or daily intravesical heparin*† Dimethyl sulfoxide (When improved, slowly taper off heparin)
*Add hydroxyzine if food or pollen allergies †Add Polycitra

Figure 33.10 Antidepressant therapy.

Antidepressant therapy is an important adjunct to treatment. It does not cure IC, but patients function much better with their disabling symptoms if they are not depressed. In essence, they 'feel better' even if they still void 20 times per day.

Surprisingly, many patients (about 25–30%) improve dramatically with antidepressant therapy only. No matter what other therapy has been initiated, we place all moderately or severely symptomatic patients on antidepressants and remove these if the patient improves or is being successfully managed with some other treatment (e.g. heparin or PPS).

Dimethyl sulfoxide

On the basis of uncontrolled trials, DMSO was approved for use in IC in 1977[101]. Perez-Marrero[102] carried out one small controlled clinical trial with DMSO, which does appear to induce remission in 34–40% of the patients. The difficulty with DMSO is that it may induce an excellent remission in the first one to three cycles of therapy, but as an individual relapses and requires subsequent treatment, progressive resistance to its beneficial effects occurs in almost all patients, for reasons unknown.

For treatment, instill 50mL of 50% DMSO into the bladder for 5–10 minutes. Longer periods are unnecessary as DMSO rapidly absorbs into the bloodstream. Instillation is an outpatient procedure, or patients are taught to carry it out themselves. The author recommends that patients receive 6–8 weekly treatments to determine whether a therapeutic response is achieved. It usually requires 2–3 months to obtain a good clinical response. If the patient has moderate or severe symptoms, the therapy is continued for an additional 4–6 months once every other week. Importantly, once DMSO is stopped, the patient is likely to become resistant to its use. Some patients experience a flare of symptoms when DMSO is placed into the bladder. This phenomenon most likely results from a detergent-like activity in which DMSO destroys the superficial bladder umbrella cells and causes a significant increase in the epithelial leak. Nonetheless, DMSO may treat these patients very effectively. Should a patient experience pain with DMSO, he or she should receive intravesically 10mL of 2% viscous lidocaine jelly 15 minutes before placement of DMSO. If this is not successful, an injectable narcotic (ketorolac 60mg) or intramuscular meperidine is used before the intravesical instillation. The flare of symptoms associated with DMSO usually disappears over 24 hours. As these patients receive subsequent treatments, the pain tends to diminish.

Patients also may receive indefinite therapy using DMSO. As originally reported by Stewart et al.[101], patients have used DMSO weekly for several years without problems. Although DMSO has been associated with cataracts in animals, this complication has not been reported in humans. It seems reasonable, if the patient is on chronic therapy, to carry out a slit-lamp evaluation at 6–12 month intervals, but we have not found this to be necessary and rarely do it.

Antihistamines

Antihistamines are critical to the management of IC patients with hay fever, sinusitis, or food allergies. Patients in good control of their symptoms suffer setbacks in the allergy season. Antihistamines have been tried in IC, but without controlled studies. They were chosen because of the possible role of mast cells in IC[64,87,103,104]. While most patients may not respond to antihistamines, subsets of patients seem to benefit significantly, especially when the antihistamine is combined with other therapy. Patients with allergies, in particular, benefit from hydroxyzine 25–50mg at bedtime[105]. This is an extremely effective way to manage allergies when the medication is used chronically. Beneficial effects appear 2–3 months after the start of treatment and patients are urged to stay on medication for at least 3 months to determine the effectiveness. Hydroxyzine is the only antihistamine that, when used chronically, inhibits mast cell function[105]. We use it routinely in 50–60% of the patients that we see.

Corticosteroids

As a result of the assumption that inflammation plays a role in this disorder, patients have been given corticosteroids. Badenoch[106] found significant improvement in 19 of 25 patients treated with prednisone. However, all were treated after hydrodistention under anesthetic, which may have been responsible for most of the benefit. In the author's experience, corticosteroids do not ameliorate the symptoms of this complex. As with most drugs, no controlled clinical trials have been conducted on the efficacy of corticosteroids in the treatment of IC.

Intravesical silver nitrate

Intravesical silver nitrate was first reported in 1926 by Dodson[107]. Pool[84] fashioned a treatment regimen in which bladder irrigations in a 1:5000 concentration were begun under anesthetic. This was followed by gradually increasing the concentrations on a daily basis, until ultimately a 1% solution was employed. Again, the setting was uncontrolled and patients had been given dilation of the bladder under anesthetic. Pool reported good results in 89% of patients[84]. Other uncontrolled studies have reported that this compound is helpful, but it is not very widely used today. One caution is vital in the use of silver nitrate – do not instill it into the bladder after biopsy. If there is a perforation and this solution is placed into the bladder, intra- and extraperitoneal extravasation could occur and result in major tissue damage.

Intravesical sodium oxychlorosene (Clorpactin WCS-90)

Clorpactin, a modified derivative of hypochlorous acid in a buffered base, is a highly reactive chemical compound. Its activity is dependent on the liberation of hypochlorous acid and its resultant oxidizing effects and detergency[108]. Wishard et al. treated 20 patients with five weekly instillations of 0.2% Clorpactin WCS-90 under local anesthetic[108]. Improvement was reported in 14 of the 20 patients, but follow-up was brief. Messing and Stamey[78] treated 38 patients with 0.4% Clorpactin and reported significant improvement in 72%. Ureteral reflux is a contraindication to the use of Clorpactin. It is recommended that the compound be used under anesthetic.

Urinary alkalinizers

Polycitra is an agent that not only alkalinizes the urine, but also binds potassium. Both effects may be beneficial in IC and it is recommended that patients receive a trial of therapy for 3–6 months. The use of two doses a day appears to be sufficient. In general, this drug is combined with other treatments, such as heparin, PPS, or amitriptyline to obtain the best effect. The best-tolerated salt of Polycitra is potassium. When Polycitra is absorbed and excreted in the urine, it helps chelate urinary potassium, so the original salt does not pose a problem for the bladder.

Bacillus Calmette–Guérin therapy

In a recent study in which BCG therapy was employed for IC, efficacy was demonstrated. As BCG causes intense desquamation of the mucosa theoretically it should be active. Its desquamating ability places it in the class of cytodestructive techniques, similar to DMSO and dilation. As a consequence of its infectious side-effects, it is recommended that DMSO and dilation be employed before BCG therapy is used.

L-Arginine

Smith and associates[109] reported the use of L-arginine for patients with IC. It was used in a limited open-phase study and its true activity is unknown. It is nontoxic.

Heparinoid therapy

A major breakthrough in therapy is the use of heparin-like drugs (heparin, PPS). When effective, these reverse the course of the disease (Fig. 33.11). Patients rarely become resistant to their use.

Heparin

Heparin, when given by injection, was reported to alleviate the symptoms of IC[110], but this study was uncontrolled. Chronic systemic heparin therapy cannot be employed in most individuals as it results in osteoporosis in 100% of patients who use it for 26 weeks. In our experience, intravesical heparin has significant activity in approximately 50% of patients[111], but again the data were obtained in an uncontrolled investigation.

The technique uses 40,000 units of heparin in 20cm^3 of saline, and the solution is instilled intravesically, initially daily; after 3–4 months this is reduced to 3–4 times per week if the patient has improved. This treatment can be carried on indefinitely. It takes 2–4 months before improvements begin, but therapy must be encouraged and urged for at least 9–12 months before it is abandoned. The best improvements are noted after 1–2 years. Long-term therapy is recommended for patients with moderate or severe disease who respond to its use. Serum prothrombin time and partial prothrombin time are monitored for several weeks after therapy begins to rule out the formation of any unusual

Heparinoid therapy		
Drug*	**Dose**	**Route**
Heparin	20–40,000 units daily	Intravesical and self-administered
Pentosanpolysulfate	100–200mg 8q24†	Oral
*Drugs work best after 6–12 months of chronic use †Males and severely affected females should receive 200mg 8q24		

Figure 33.11 Heparinoid therapy.

antibody to heparin or of systemic absorption (heparin should not be absorbed across the bladder mucosa). Patients are instructed in self-catheterization so that this therapy can be performed at home.

Pentosanpolysulfate

Parsons and colleagues[55,56] first reported that PPS actively ameliorated the symptoms of IC. Since PPS is a sulfated polysaccharide, theoretically it may augment the bladder surface defense mechanism or detoxify urine agents that have a capacity to attack the bladder surface (e.g. quaternary amines).

In a controlled clinical study, 42% of patients were shown to have their symptoms controlled, versus 20% for placebo[55]. Similar results were obtained in several subsequent studies, including a five-center trial in which 28% of patients on PPS improved versus 13% on placebo[56] and a seven-center study of 150 patients in which 32% of patients on PPS improved versus 15% on placebo[112]. Additionally, an English–Danish study also found a significant reduction of pain in patients on drug compared to those on placebo[19].

An oral dose of 100mg of PPS three times per day is used. In patients with moderate disease, the drug appears to have about 40–50% activity. In the controlled clinical trials that were undertaken on patients with severe disease, its activity was lower. In an open trial when the drug was used for more than 6 months, 74% of the patients responded to treatment[113]. Continued use of PPS for several years leads to long-term disease control. Long-term success has not been reported previously with any other therapy except heparin. A response to therapy is first seen in milder IC patients after 6–10 weeks, but it may take 6–12 months (or longer) to work in severe IC patients.

Male and female patients with more severe disease may need 200mg 8q24 to control their disease. It takes 3–12 months to obtain a good response and so the medication should be used for at least 9–12 months before its use is abandoned. We currently see about a 60% efficacy rate when it is used for longer periods and at larger doses. The primary side effects are gastrointestinal and can frequently be reduced if the medication is taken with a small snack or is taken out of the capsule and dissolved in 28mL (1 ounce) of water. Hair loss is reported in about 1–2% of people, but this is completely reversible even when the medication is continued. The oral form of PPS has no detectable anticoagulant activity.

Surgery

Approximately 2% of patients who present with IC to the University of California, San Diego Medical Center ultimately undergo surgery for disease that is severe and refractory to all treatment. The question is the type of surgery to be carried out.

Cystolysis

Attempts at surgical ablation of the bladder innervation by cystolysis are discouraged as most patients fail this and develop a neurogenic bladder with significant urinary pain and frequency, and may require ICP.

Bladder augmentation

A concept exists that such patients have small bladders and thus void frequently. Actually, the reverse is true. They have sensory urgency, void frequently, and subsequently develop a small bladder. Hence, attempts to augment the bladder with a patch of bowel are likely to fail. Patients are left with a capacity that is perhaps too large and have more difficulty emptying it (and usually require ICP), but they still retain all the sensory urgency and pain[114].

Urinary diversion alone

No controlled studies have been used to evaluate diversion alone, but other studies suggest it is not effective[115]. The author has taken out two bladders in patients who had urinary diversions alone with persistent pelvic pain. The pain was eliminated by removal of the bladder. In counseling, the patients must be told that diversion alone may not be sufficient to control their pain and they may subsequently require a cystectomy. The patient can then decide whether or not they want the risk of more than one surgery. It is the author's experience that almost no-one elects for the potential of two surgeries.

Cystectomy and diversion

Cystectomy and diversion is the mainstay of therapy for patients with 'end-stage bladder'. It is successful, especially in today's environment in which continent diversions are carried out. Pelvic pain presents after the procedure in 5% of patients. In general, if the patients have classic bladder pain that is associated with filling and relieved or partially relieved by emptying, urinary frequency and urgency, and the usual stigmata of IC under anesthetic, they are likely to have relief of their symptoms by cystectomy. Those individuals with severe pelvic pain that is not associated with the classic parameters of IC and particularly that is not exacerbated by bladder filling are less likely to have their pain alleviated.

When continent diversion is carried out, 40–50% of patients develop pouch pain 6–36 months after surgery. This can be managed successfully by the patient who instills 10,000 units of heparin in 10mL water into the pouch after each catheterization. To prevent development of pouch pain, we now routinely place all patients on PPS 300mg orally and daily heparin.

BLADDER TRAINING

Whatever therapy successfully alleviates the pain and sensory urgency of IC, the individual afflicted with the chronic form of the disorder has a small capacity bladder that is in part based on sensory urgency and in part on frequent low-volume voiding. In controlled clinical trials, it has been reported that even with good remission of pain and urgency, almost no change in urinary frequency occurs over a 12-week period[55,56,110]. This issue must be addressed to obtain a functional recovery of the bladder.

Persistent urinary frequency from a small bladder can be reversed after therapy has controlled the urgency and pain. This is accomplished by training the patients to undergo a program to progressively hold their urine to increase their bladder capacity[114]. Such therapy can be directed by a urologic nurse. To begin this treatment, a 3-day voiding profile is obtained from the patient (to include time of voiding and a measurement of volume). The average time interval between voids is determined, and this interval is gradually increased monthly. For example, if the patient voids every hour, it is recommended that he or she attempt to void every hour and a quarter and at the end of 1 month increase that to an hour and a half.

The patient must not try to progress too quickly as they may become discouraged and quit. It takes 3–5 months of this protocol before good results develop. At the end of 3–4 months, the bladder capacity increases by approximately twofold and there is a corresponding reduction in urgency and number of voids per day.

We also discovered that in patients who have minimal or no pain associated with their urinary frequency, bladder training may be the only therapy required for improvement and sometimes the only therapy that is effective[116].

CONCLUSION

The majority of patients can now be treated for IC successfully. With early diagnosis of IC and the institution of treatment before the bladder is severely damaged, patients do better in general. It is urged that the old time diagnostic criteria be abandoned and a more liberal view of diagnosis be adopted, as presented herein. Treatment in the earlier phases of the disease is often effective and, hopefully, will prevent advancement to disease. The disease IC is easy to diagnose, far more common than originally thought, and responds well to current therapies.

REFERENCES

1. Gillenwater JY, Wein AJ. Summary of the National Institute of Arthritis, Diabetes, Digestive and Kidney Diseases Workshop on Interstitial Cystitis, National Institutes of Health, Bethesda, Maryland, August 28–29, 1987. J Urol. 1988;140:203–6.

2. Hanno PM, Landis JR, Matthews-Cook Y, Kusek J, Nyberg Jr L and the Interstitial Cystitis Database Study Group. The diagnosis of interstitial cystitis revisited: lessons learned from the National Institutes of Health Interstitial Cystitis Database Study. J Urol. 1999;161:553–7.

3. Jones CA, Nyberg L. Epidemiology of interstitial cystitis. Urology. 1997;49(Suppl 5A):2–9.

4. Oravisto KJ, Alfthan OS, Jokinen EJ. Interstitial cystitis. Clinical and immunological findings. Scand J Urol Nephrol. 1970;4:37–42.

5. Hand JR. Interstitial cystitis, a report of 223 cases. J Urol. 1949;61:291–310.

6. Hanash KA, Pool TL. Interstitial and hemorrhagic cystitis: viral, bacterial and fungal studies. J Urol. 1970;104:705–6.

7. Oravisto KJ, Alfthan OS. Treatment of interstitial cystitis with immunosuppression and chloroquine derivatives. Eur Urol. 1976;2:82–4.

8. Silk MR. Bladder antibodies in interstitial cystitis. J Urol. 1970;103:307–9.

9. Holm-Bentzen M, Lose G. Pathology and pathogenesis of interstitial cystitis. Urology. 1987;29(4 Suppl):8–13.

10. Oravisto KJ. Interstitial cystitis as an autoimmune disease. A review. Eur Urol. 1980;6:10–3.

11. Weaver RG, Dougherty TF, Natoli C. Recent concepts of interstitial cystitis. J Urol. 1963;89:377–83.

12. Eldrup J, Thorup J, Nielsen SL, Hald T, Hainau B. Permeability and ultrastructure of human bladder epithelium. Br J Urol. 1983;55:488–92.

13. Parsons CL, Lilly JD, Stein P. Epithelial dysfunction in nonbacterial cystitis (interstitial cystitis). J Urol. 1991;145:732–5.

14. Lilly JD, Parsons CL. Bladder surface glycosaminoglycans is a human epithelial permeability barrier. Surg Gynecol Obstet. 1990;171:493–6.

15. Parsons CL, Boychuk D, Jones S, Hurst R, Callahan H. Bladder surface glycosaminoglycans: an epithelial permeability barrier. J Urol. 1990;143:139–42.

16. Hohlbrugger G, Lentsch P. Intravesical ions, osmolality and pH influence the volume pressure response in the normal rat bladder, and this is more pronounced after DMSO exposure. Eur Urol. 1985;11:127–30.

17. MacDermott JP, Miller CH, Levy N, Stone AR: Cellular immunity in interstitial cystitis. J Urol. 145: 274–278, 1991.

18. Felsen D, Frye S, Bavendam T, Trimble L, Vaughan ED Jr Interleukin-6 activity in the urine of interstitial cystitis (IC) patients. J Urol. 147: 460A, 1992.

19. Holm-Bentzen M, Jacobsen F, Nerstrom B, et al. Painful bladder disease: clinical and pathoanatomical differences in 115 patients. J Urol. 1987;138:500–2.

20. Lotz M, Villiger PM, Hugli T, Koziol J, Zuraw BL. Interleukin-6 and interstitial cystitis. J Urol. 1994;152:869–73.

21. Holm-Bentzen J, Sondergaard I, Hald T. Urinary excretion of a metabolite of histamine (1,4-methylimidazole-acetic acid) in painful bladder disease. Br J Urol. 1987;59:230–3.

22. Kastrup J, Hald T, Larsen S, Nielsen VG. Histamine content and mast cell count of detrusor muscle in patients with interstitial cystitis and other types of chronic cystitis. Br J Urol. 1983;55:495–500.

23. Sant GR. Interstitial cystitis: pathophysiology, clinical evaluation and treatment. Ann Urol. 1989;3:172–9.

24. Sant GR, Kalaru P, Ucci AA Jr. Mucosal mast cell (MMC) contribution to bladder mastocytosis in interstitial cystitis. J Urol. 1988;139:276A.

25. Spanos C, Pang X, Ligris K, et al. Stress-induced bladder mast cell activation: implications for interstitial cystitis. J Urol. 1997;157:669–72.

26. Pang X, Boucher W, Triadafilopoulos G, Sant GR, Theoharides TC. Mast cell and substance P-positive nerve involvement in a patient with both irritable bowel syndrome and interstitial cystitis. Urology. 1996;47:436–8.

27. Letourneau R, Pang X, Sant GR, Theoharides TC. Intragranular activation of bladder mast cells and their association with nerve processes in interstitial cystitis. Br J Urol. 1996;77:41–54.

28. Spanos C, El-Mansoury M, Letourneau R, et al. Carbachol-induced bladder mast cell activation: augmentation by estradiol and implications for interstitial cystitis. Urology. 1996;48:809–16.

29. Bjorling DE, Saban MR, Zine MJ, Haak-Frendscho M, Graziano FM, Saban R. In vitro passive sensitization of guinea pig, rhesus monkey and human bladders as a model of noninfectious cystitis. J Urol. 1994;152:1603–8.

30. Saban R, Christensen M, Keith I, et al. Experimental model for the study of bladder mast cell degranulation and smooth muscle contraction. Semin Urol. 1991;9:88–101.

31. Parsons CL, Stein PC, Bidair M, Lebow D. Abnormal sensitivity to intravesical potassium in interstitial cystitis and radiation cystitis. Neurol Urodyn. 1994;13:515–20.

32. Galloway N, Gabale D, Irwin P. Interstitial cystitis or reflex sympathetic dystrophy of the bladder? Semin Urol. 1991;9:148–53.

33. Parsons CL, Greenberger M, Gabal L, Bidair M, Barme G. The role of urinary potassium in the pathogenesis and diagnosis of interstitial cystitis. J Urol. 1998;159:1862–7.

34. Payne CK, Browning S. Graded potassium chloride testing in interstitial cystitis. J Urol. 1996;155:438A.

35. Teichman JMH, Nielsen-Omeis BJ, McIver BD. Modified urodynamics for interstitial cystitis. J Urol. 1996;155:433A.

36. Englund SE. Observation on the migration of some labeled substances between the urinary bladder and blood in rabbits. Acta Radiol. 1956;135(Suppl):9–13.

37. Fellows GJ, Marshall DH. The permeability of human bladder epithelium to water and sodium. Invest Urol. 1972;9:339–44.

38. Hicks RM. The permeability of rat transitional epithelium. J Cell Biol. 1966;28:21–31.

39. Hicks RM, Ketterer B, Warren RC. The ultrastructure and chemistry of the luminal plasma membrane of the mammalian urinary bladder: a structure with low permeability to water and ions. Phil Trans R Soc Lond B. 1974;268:23–38.

40. Staehelin LA, Chlapowski FJ, Bonneville MA. Luminal plasma membrane of the urinary bladder. J Cell Biol. 1972;53:73–91.

41. Lewis SA, Diamond JM. Na+ transport by rabbit urinary bladder, a tight epithelium. J Membr Biol. 1976;28:1–40.

42. Parsons CL, Stauffer C, Schmidt J. Bladder surface glycosaminoglycans: an efficient mechanism of environmental adaptation. Science. 1980;208:605–7.

43. Parsons CL, Greenspan C, Mulholland SG. The primary antibacterial defense mechanism of the bladder. Invest Urol. 1975;13:72–6.

44. Parsons CL, Greenspan C, Moore SW, Mulholland SG. Role of surface mucin in primary antibacterial defense of bladder. Urology. 1977;9:48–52.

45. Gill WB, Jones KW, Ruggiero KJ. Protective effects of heparin and other sulfated glycosaminoglycans on crystal adhesion to urothelium. J Urol. 1982;127:152–4.

46. Hanno PM, Parsons CL, Shrom SH, Fritz R, Mulholland SG. The protective effect of heparin in experimental bladder infection. J Surg Res. 1978;25:324–9.

47. Parsons CL, Mulholland S, Anwar H. Antibacterial activity of bladder surface mucin duplicated by exogenous glycosaminoglycan (heparin). Infect Immun. 1979;24:552–7.

48. Menter JM, Hurst RE, Nakamura N, West SS. Thermodynamics of mucopolysaccharide-dye binding. III. Thermodynamic and cooperatively parameters of acridine orange–heparin system. Biopolymers. 1979;18:493–505.

49. Gryte CC, Gregor HP. Poly-(styrene sulfonic acid)-poly-(vinylidene fluoride) interpolymer ion–exchange membranes. J Polymer Sci. 1976;14:1839–54.

50. Gregor HP. Anticoagulant activity of sulfonate polymers and copolymers. In: Gregor HP, ed. Polymer science and technology, vol. 5. New York: Plenum Press. 1975;51–6.

51. Gregor HP. Fixed charge ultrafiltration membranes. In: Selegny E, ed. Charged gels and membranes, Part I. Holland: D Reider; 1976:235.

52. Hurst RE, Rhodes SW, Adamson PB, Parsons CL, Roy JB. Functional and structural characteristics of the glycosaminoglycans of the bladder luminal surface. J Urol. 1987;138:433–7.

53. Bekturov EA, Bakauova Kh, eds. Synthetic water-soluble polymers in solution. Basel: Hüthig & Wepf; 1986:38–54.

54. Hurst RE. Thermodynamics of the partition of chondroitin sulfate–hexadecylpyridinium complexes in butanol/aqueous salt biphasic solutions. Biopolymers. 1978;17:2601–8.

55. Parsons CL, Mulholland S. Successful therapy of interstitial cystitis with pentosanpolysulfate. J Urol. 1987;138:513–6.

56. Mulholland SG, Hanno P, Parsons CL, Sant GR, Staskin DR. Pentosanpolysulfate sodium for therapy of interstitial cystitis: A double-blind placebo-controlled clinical study. Urology. 1990;35:552–8.

57. Fritjofsson A, Fall M, Juhlin R, et al. Treatment of ulcer and nonulcer interstitial cystitis with sodium pentosanpolysulfate: a multicenter trial. J Urol. 1987;138:508–12.

58. Holm-Bentzen M, Jacobsen F, Nerstrom B. A prospective double-blind clinically controlled multicenter trial of sodium pentosanpolysulfate in the treatment of interstitial cystitis and related painful bladder disease. J Urol. 1987;138:503–10.

59. Buffington CAT, Woodworth BE. Excretion of fluorescein in the urine of women with interstitial cystitis. J Urol. 1997;158:786–9.

59a. Chelsky MJ, Rosen SI, Knight LC, Maurer AH, Hanno PM, Ruggieri MR. Bladder permeability in interstitial cystitis is similar to that of normal volunteers: direct measurement by transvesical absorption of ^{99m}technetium-diethylenetriamine pentaacetic acid. J Urol. 1994;151:346–9.

60. Hohlbrugger G. The vesical blood–urine barrier: a relevant and dynamic interface between renal function and nervous bladder control. J Urol. 1995;154:6–14.

61. Hohlbrugger G, Lentsch P, Pfaller K, Madersbacher H. Permeability characteristics of the rat urinary bladder in experimental cystitis and after overdistension. Urol Int. 1985;40:211–6.

62. Hanno P, Levin RM, Monson FC, et al. Diagnosis of interstitial cystitis. J Urol. 1990;143:278–81.

63. Theoharides TC, Sant GR. Bladder mast cell activation in interstitial cystitis. Semin Urol. 1991;9:74–87.

64. Larsen S, Thompson SA, Hald T, et al. Mast cells in interstitial cystitis. Br J Urol. 1982;54:283–6.

65. Hofmeister MA, He F, Ratliff TL, et al. Mast cells and nerve fibers in interstitial cystitis (IC): an algorithm for histologic diagnosis via quantitative image analysis and morphometry (QIAM). Urology. 1997;49(Suppl 5A):41–7.

66. Koziol JA. Epidemiology of interstitial cystitis. Urol Clin North Am. 1994;21:7–20.

67. Koziol JA, Clark DC, Gittes RF, Tan EM. The natural history of interstitial cystitis: a survey of 374 patients. J Urol. 1993;149:465–9.

68. Hofmeister MA, He F, Ratliff TL, Becich MJ. Analysis of histochemical stains in interstitial cystitis (IC): detrusor to mucosa mast cell ratio is predictive of IC. Lab Invest. 1994;70:60A.

69. Christmas TJ, Rode J, Chapple CR, Milroy EJ, Turner-Warwick RT. Nerve fibre proliferation in interstitial cystitis. Virchow Arch A Pathol Anat Histopathol. 1990;416:447–51.

70. Lundeberg T, Liedberg H, Nordling L, Theodorsson E, Owzarski A, Ekman R. Interstitial cystitis: correlation with nerve fibers, mast cells and histamine. Br J Urol. 1993;71:427–9.

71. Nitze M. Lerbuch der Kystoscopie: Ihre Technik und Klinische Bedeuting. Berlin: JE Bergman; 1907:205–10.

72. Oravisto KJ. Epidemiology of interstitial cystitis: 1. In: Hanno PM, Staskin DR, Krane RJ, et al, eds. Interstitial cystitis. Springer-Verlag: London; 1990:25–8.

73. Held PJ, Hanno PM, Pauly MV, et al. Epidemiology of interstitial cystitis: 2. In Hanno PM, Staskin DR, Krane RJ, et al, eds. Interstitial cystitis. London: Springer-Verlag; 1990:29–48.

74. American Foundation for Urologic Diseases. Research progress and promises. Baltimore: American Foundation for Urologic Diseases; 1980.

75. Hamilton-Miller JMT. The urethral syndrome and its management. J Antimicrob Chemother. 1994;33(Suppl A):63–73.

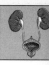
76. Oravisto KJ. Epidemiology of interstitial cystitis. Ann Chir Gynaecol Fenn. 1975;64:75–7.

77. Walsh A. Interstitial cystitis. In: Harrison JH, Gittes RF, Perlmutter AD, et al, eds. Campbell's urology, 4th edn. Philadelphia: WB Saunders; 1978.

78. Messing EM, Stamey TA. Interstitial cystitis: early diagnosis, pathology, and treatment. Urology. 1978;12:381–92.

79. Farkas A, Waisman J, Goodwin WE. Interstitial cystitis in adolescent girls. J Urol. 1977;118:837–9.

80. Bowers JE, Lattimer JK. Interstitial cystitis. Surg Gynecol Obstet. 1957;105:313–22.

81. McDonald HP, Upchirch WE, Artime M. Bladder dysfunction in children caused by interstitial cystitis. J Urol. 1958;80:354–6.

82. Lapides J. Observations on interstitial cystitis. Urology. 1975;5:610–1.

83. Parsons CL. Interstitial cystitis: clinical manifestations and diagnostic criteria in over 200 cases. Neurourol Urodyn. 1990;9:241–50.

84. Pool TL. Interstitial cystitis: clinical considerations and treatment. Clin Obstet Gynecol. 1967;10:185–91.

85. De Juana CP, Everett JC. Interstitial cystitis: experience and review of recent literature. Urology. 1977;10:325–9.

86. Hanno P, Wein A. Interstitial cystitis, Parts I and II. Baltimore: American Urological Association (Update Series, Vol. l, No 9); 1987.

87. Smith BH, Dehner LP. Chronic ulcerating interstitial cystitis (Hunner's ulcer). Arch Pathol. 1972;93:76–81.

88. Calkins B, Lilienfeld AM, Mendeloff AI, Garland C, Monk M, Garland FC. Smoking factors in ulcerative colitis and Crohn's disease in Baltimore. Am J Epidemiol. 1984;122:498–9.

89. Cope GF, Heatley RV, Kelleher J, Lee PN. Cigarette smoking and inflammatory bowel disease: a review. Hum Toxicol. 1987;6: 189–93.

90. Paulley JW. Ulcerative colitis: a study of 173 cases. Gastroenterology. 1950;16:566–76.

91. National Center for Health Statistics. Health and nutrition examination survey, cycle II, 1976–1980. Washington DC: Government Printing Office; 1985.

92. Lilienfeld AM, Lilienfeld DE. Foundations of epidemiology, 2nd edn. New York: Oxford; 1980.

93. Fall M, Johansson SL, Vahlne A. A clinicopathological and virological study of interstitial cystitis. J Urol. 1985;133:771–3.

94. Jacobo E, Stamler FW, Culp DA. Interstitial cystitis followed by total cystectomy. Urology. 1974;3:481–5.

95. Johansson SL, Fall M. Clinical features and spectrum of light microscopic changes in interstitial cystitis. J Urol. 1990;143:1118–24.

96. Burford HE, Burford CE. Hunner ulcer of the bladder: A report of 187 cases. J Urol. 1958;79:952–5.

97. Nigro DA, Wein AJ, Foy M, et al. Associations among cystoscopic and urodynamic findings for women enrolled in the Interstitial Cystitis Data Base Study. Urology. 1997;49(Suppl 5A):86–92.

98. Holm-Bentzen M, Larsen S, Hainau B, Hald T. Non-obstructive detrusor myopathy in a group of patients with chronic bacterial cystitis. Scand J Urol Nephrol. 1985;19:21–6.

99. Bumpus HC. Interstitial cystitis. Med Clin North Am. 1930;13: 1495–8.

100. Hanno PM, Buehler J, Wein AJ. Use of amitriptyline in the treatment of interstitial cystitis. J Urol. 1989;141:846–8.

101. Stewart BH, Persky L, Kiser WS. The use of dimethyl sulfoxide (DMSO) in the treatment of interstitial cystitis. J Urol. 1967;98:671–2.

102. Perez-Marrero R, Emerson LE, Feltis JT. A controlled study of dimethyl sulfoxide in interstital cystitis. J Urol. 1988;140:36–9.

103. Bohne AW, Hodson JM, Rebuck JW, Reinhard RE. An abnormal leukocyte response in interstitial cystitis. J Urol. 1962;88:387–91.

104. Simmons JL. Interstitial cystitis: an explanation for the beneficial effect of an antihistamine. J Urol. 1961;85:149–55.

105. Theoharides T. Hydroxyzine in the treatment of interstitial cystitis. Urol Clin North Am. 1994;21:113–19.

106. Badenoch AW. Chronic interstitial cystitis. Br J Urol. 1971;43: 718–21.

107. Dodson AI. Hunner's ulcer of the bladder: a report of 10 cases. Va Med Monthly. 1926;53:305–10.

108. Wishard WN, Nourse MH, Mertz JHO. Use of Clorpactin WCS90 for relief of symptoms due to interstitial cystitis. J Urol. 1957;77:420–3.

109. Smith SD, Wheeler MA, Foster HE Jr, Weiss RM. Improvement in interstitial cystitis symptom scores during treatment with oral L-arginine. J Urol. 1997;158:703–8.

110. Lose G, Frandsen B, Hojensgard JC, et al. Chronic interstitial cystitis: increased levels of eosinophil cationic protein in serum and urine and an ameliorating effect of subcutaneous heparin. Scand J Urol Nephrol. 1983;17:159–61.

111. Parsons CL, Housley T, Schmidt JD, Lebow D. Treatment of interstitial cystitis with intravesical heparin. Br J Urol. 1994;73:504–7.

112. Parsons CL, Benson G, Childs, SJ et al. A quantitatively controlled method to prospectively study interstitial cystitis and which demonstrates the efficacy of pentosanpolysulfate. J Urol. 1993;150:845–8.

113. Hanno PM. Analysis of long-term Elmiron therapy for interstitial cystitis. Urology. 1997;49(Suppl 5A):93–9.

114. Nielsen KK, Kromann-Andersen B, Steven K, Hald T. Failure of combined supratrigonal cystectomy and Mainz ileocecocystoplasty in intractable interstitial cystitis: is histology and mast cell count a reliable predictor for the outcome of surgery? J Urol. 1990;144:255–8.

115. Eigner EG, Freiha FS. The fate of the remaining bladder following supravesical diversion. J Urol. 1990;144:31–3.

116. Parsons CL, Koprowski P. Interstitial cystitis: Successful management by a pattern of increasing urinary voiding interval. Urology. 1991;37:207–12.

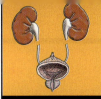

Section 6 Benign Conditions of the Lower Urinary Tract

Chapter 34

The Neuropathic Bladder

Kieran J O'Flynn

KEY POINTS

- A sound knowledge of the pathophysiology of neuropathic bladder guides clinical management.
- Preservation of renal function comes first.
- Video-urodynamics forms the cornerstone of the objective assessment of patients with neuropathic voiding dysfunction.
- Consideration of the patient's general medical and functional status and his/her expectations is vital in planning therapy.

INTRODUCTION

The term 'neuropathic bladder' includes those patients with abnormal bladder activity as a consequence of some neurologic condition. A myriad of disease processes affecting the central and peripheral nervous system may result in alterations of normal lower urinary tract function. These may range from patients with gross spinal cord injuries and congenital anomalies to those patients with less overt neurologic disturbances as seen in diabetes mellitus and following major pelvic surgery.

Numerous classifications have been proposed for neuropathic bladder disease[1]. Various neurologic diseases may result in a similar bladder response and a particular urodynamic tracing is rarely pathognomonic of a particular neurologic condition. From the clinical point of view it is probably better to accurately document the behavior of the lower urinary tract in relation to the neurologic condition under investigation. A list of diseases that may result in neurovesical dysfunction is listed in Figure 34.1.

PATHOPHYSIOLOGY

Normal lower urinary tract function

The urinary bladder has two principal functions: to act as a reservoir and to empty periodically. Urinary continence involves a complex interaction between the urethra, the internal and external sphincter, and the pelvic musculature. The bladder, unlike other visceral structures, has no integral pacemaker and its function is primarily under the control of the parasympathetic nervous system.

The spinal reflex center for micturition is situated in the conus medullaris, which contains the sacral segments of the spinal cord. The micturition reflex is integrated in the pontine micturition

Neurologic lesions resulting in lower urinary tract dysfunction		
Peripheral/lower motor neuron	Spinal	Intracranial
Spinal cord injury	Spinal cord injury	Cerebrovascular disease
Sacral agenesis	Spinal cord tumor (primary or secondary)	Brain tumor
Myelitis	Spinal cord infarction	Cerebral trauma
Herpes zoster	Multiple sclerosis	Dementia
Tabes dorsalis	Cervical spondylitis	Multiple sclerosis
Metastatic carcinoma	Spina bifida	Encephalitis
Disc disease	Myelitis	Cerebral palsy
Spinal stenosis		Parkinson's disease
Diabetes mellitus		Shy–Drager syndrome
Vitamin B_{12} deficiency		AIDS
Spina bifida		Lyme disease
Multiple sclerosis		Hereditary spastic paraplegia

Figure 34.1 Neurologic lesions resulting in lower urinary tract dysfunction.

center. Micturition is achieved by activation of the micturition reflex, which results in a co-ordinated series of events resulting in relaxation of the striated muscle of the distal sphincter, detrusor contraction, and opening of the bladder neck and urethra. For further detail see Chapter 6. Controlled co-ordinated voiding depends on an intact conus medullaris and an intact neuraxis and any lesion of the neuraxis (as in spinal cord injury), can disrupt the voiding/continence mechanism (Fig. 34.2).

The bladder, bladder neck, urethra, and striated muscles of the urethral sphincter are controlled by the following sets of peripheral nerves:

- sacral parasympathetic (pelvic nerves);
- thoracolumbar sympathetic (hypogastric and sympathetic nerves);
- sacral somatic nerves (pudendal nerves); and
- afferent pathways.

Sacral parasympathetic (pelvic nerves)

The sacral parasympathetic outflow provides the major excitatory or motor input to the urinary bladder. Motor tracts lie in the lateral corticospinal tracts and relay in the intermediolateral gray matter of the spinal cord to the anterior horn cells of the pelvic parasympathetic system or 'nervi erigentes'. The

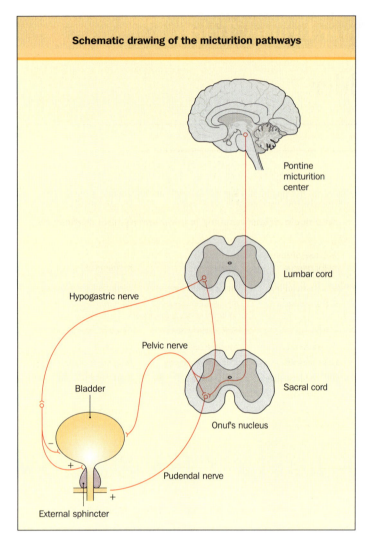

Figure 34.2 Schematic drawing of the micturition pathways.

preganglionic fibers emerge in the second, third, and fourth anterior sacral roots forming the pelvic plexus, which joins the hypogastric nerve to form the vesical plexus where they synapse with postganglionic fibers in the bladder wall. The fibers then pass to the bladder, bladder neck, and intrinsic striated smooth muscle of the distal sphincter.

Sympathetic nerves
The precise role of the sympathetic system in the neuromodulation of the detrusor is uncertain, although the anatomic pathways are well defined. Sympathetic fibers arise in the intermediolateral cell columns of the tenth thoracic to second lumbar cord segments and pass via the inferior mesenteric ganglion to the hypogastric plexus to relay in the paravesical ganglion on each side of the bladder neck. Postganglionic fibers pass to the bladder, bladder neck and distal sphincter mechanism.

Sacral somatic nerves
The striated muscle of the pelvic floor and the rhabdosphincter are supplied by the anterior horn cells of the second, third, and fourth sacral segments. These run in the internal pudendal nerves and via nerves traveling in through the pelvic plexuses. For detail see Chapter 6.

Afferent pathways
Apart from some sparse pacinian corpuscles, vesical afferent axons terminate as free nerve endings. The mechanoreceptors are activated by bladder distention, mucosal deformation, and shifts in bladder position. Afferents from the urinary tract are present in all three sets of nerves. Vesical afferents that traverse sacral nerves are silent when the bladder is empty and begin firing at small volumes. Visceral afferents accompany all three efferent pathways to the detrusor muscle and sphincter mechanism.

The visceral afferent axons synapse on interneurons and projection neurons located at the base of the posterior gray horn of the spinal cord. The interneurons participate in spinal reflexes and the axons of projection neurons form the ascending pelvic sensory vagus tract (dorsal funiculus) and the sacrobulbar tract or lateral funiculus.

Pathophysiology of neurogenic voiding dysfunction
The type of neurogenic bladder behavior seen in the clinical situation depends on both the level and extent of the lesion. Neurologic lesions above the brain stem that affect micturition generally result in involuntary bladder contractions with smooth and striated sphincter synergy. Sensation of bladder filling is usually present.

Patients with complete lesions of the spinal cord above the conus generally develop involuntary bladder contractions (termed detrusor hyperreflexia), with no sensation of bladder filling and inco-ordinated voiding due to failure of relaxation of the distal sphincter (termed sphincter dyssynergia). In patients with incomplete lesions (e.g. multiple sclerosis), some sensation may be preserved, but patients may experience urgency and urge incontinence caused by detrusor hyperreflexia and have evidence of detrusor sphincter dyssynergia.

Patients with significant trauma to the conus and cauda equina do not usually generate bladder contractions and detrusor areflexia is the commonest finding. In spinal cord injury there is no correlation between the extent of the bony injury and the neurologic damage. In lower thoracic and upper lumbar injuries it is difficult to predict the type of injury that may occur to the spinal cord. Fractures of the 11th thoracic vertebra and above cause damage to the cord above the conus, although on occasion vascular infarction of the conus may occur. Injuries to the first lumbar vertebra and below usually result in damage to the conus medullaris and cauda equina. Fractures of the 12th thoracic vertebra may result in a suprasacral or conus lesion or a combination of both.

The bladder dysfunction that occurs with injury to the peripheral reflex arc is similar to that seen in damage to the conus and cauda equina. Detrusor areflexia may occur, with a low compliant bladder and an open bladder neck. The striated sphincter may have a fixed tone.

Over time, the bladder of patients with detrusor hyperreflexia becomes trabeculated. In patients with obstructive uropathy (most commonly caused by detrusor sphincter dyssynergia), incomplete bladder emptying may occur and raised intravesical pressures are observed on urodynamic testing. The presence of large residual urines predispose to recurrent or chronic urinary tract infection, which can cause permanent damage to the smooth muscle and neural elements of the bladder wall[2]. Upper tract dilatation may result from vesicoureteric reflux, most commonly due to infection, as well as (Fig. 34.3) the altered bladder function in patients with obstructed voiding. Upper tract dilatation may be observed in the

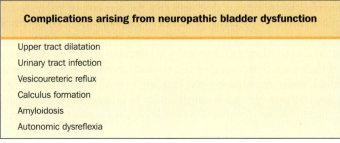

Complications arising from neuropathic bladder dysfunction
Upper tract dilatation
Urinary tract infection
Vesicoureteric reflux
Calculus formation
Amyloidosis
Autonomic dysreflexia

Figure 34.3 Complications arising from neuropathic bladder dysfunction.

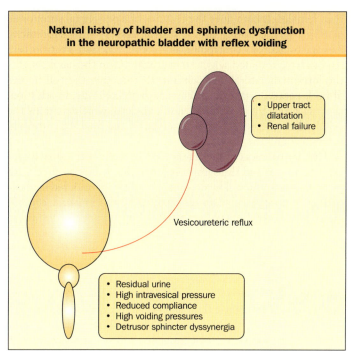

Figure 34.4 Natural history of bladder and sphincteric dysfunction in the neuropathic bladder with reflex voiding. Upper tract dilatation may occur in the absence of vesicoureteric reflux.

absence of vesicoureteric reflux, as a result of raised intravesical pressure (Fig. 34.4). For this reason, minimal degrees of upper tract dilatation detected on intravenous urogram or ultrasound should be interpreted with caution and if possible a postvoiding assessment of the upper tracts should be obtained.

The presence of infected bladder urine may lead to ascending infection, stone formation, and infection of the prostate, seminal vesicles, and epididymides. Stasis and infection predispose the patient to stone formation. Better urologic management has resulted in a reduced incidence of stone. Similarly, the incidence of renal failure that was a common cause of death in patients with congenital neuropathic bladder or spinal cord injury has declined dramatically through better understanding of the condition and continuing surveillance.

DISEASES AT OR ABOVE THE BRAINSTEM

Stroke

There are believed to be three major mechanisms responsible for urinary incontinence after stroke[3], which may be confirmed by clinical assessment and urodynamic evaluation:

- disruption of the neuromicturition pathways, resulting in detrusor hyperreflexia and urgency and urge incontinence;
- incontinence associated with cognitive, functional, or language deficits, with normal bladder function; and
- concurrent neuropathy or medication resulting in bladder areflexia and overflow incontinence.

Dementia

Dementia is a poorly understood clinical condition involving atrophy and loss of both the gray and white matter of the brain, particularly of the frontal lobes. Problems with memory and the performance of tasks that require intellectual mentation occur. The prevalence of urinary incontinence in individuals with dementia rises with the severity of the confusion and this results in increased morbidity, institutionalization, and cost. The strain on the primary carer(s) may also be significant. Urodynamic studies of patients with dementia[4] have shown that 40% had a normal bladder, 38% had detrusor instability, 16% had stress incontinence, and 5% had retention with overflow. Normal-pressure hydrocephalus may occur in dementia and is associated with incontinence due to hyperreflexia with sphincter synergia.

Treatment is complicated by the fact that bladder training is unlikely to succeed and using anticholinergic medication may increase confusion. Timed voiding may be helpful, but requires motivated carers. General measures such as the ensuring that clothing can be easily removed, regulating fluid

intake, avoiding bowel impaction and diuretics may all improve the clinical situation.

Parkinson's disease

Parkinson's disease is one of the commoner forms of neuronal degeneration in the central nervous system. It primarily affects the dopaminergic substantia-nigra–corpus-striatum pathway, resulting in a relative dopamine deficiency and cholinergic predominance in the corpus striatum. The major symptoms comprise tremor, rigidity, and akinesia. Bladder symptoms, particularly frequency, nocturia, urgency, and urge incontinence, can occur and may be exacerbated by the patient's poor mobility and cognitive function.

Urodynamic assessment of a patient with Parkinson's disease may demonstrate evidence of detrusor hyperreflexia and/or features of bladder outflow obstruction[5,6]. The urodynamic features are not disease specific and may indeed be age related. Sphincter abnormalities may also occur, e.g. sphincter bradykinesia, a delayed but co-ordinated action.

The mainstay of treatment in Parkinson's disease is an attempt to restore dopamine neurotransmitter levels in the basal ganglia with levodopa, which may improve or cause a deterioration in bladder function. Anticholinergics may be used, but can precipitate urinary retention in those patients with bladder outflow obstruction and a residual urine. Transurethral resection of the prostate (TURP) may be an appropriate treatment in those patients, with good evidence of bladder outflow obstruction on video-urodynamic assessment and a normal sphincter electromyogram (see below).

Multiple system atrophy

This condition, formerly known as Shy–Drager syndrome, typically occurs in middle age and affects males more frequently than females. It combines the features of a peripheral autonomic neuropathy (i.e. lower motor neuron lesion) with suprasacral damage to neurons controlling autonomic function. Postmortem studies have revealed selective neuronal loss in the basal ganglia, the intermediolateral cell columns that contain the cell bodies of both parasympathetic and sympathetic neurons. In addition, there is a selective lesion of Onuf's nucleus, which contains the cell bodies of the neurons innervating the anal and urethral sphincters and the pelvic floor.

Urinary frequency and urgency are frequently the first symptoms to appear and the symptoms may clearly be confused with prostatic obstruction. The diagnosis should be considered in those patients with atypical histories whose symptoms include erectile impotence and who have a postural drop in blood pressure on standing. Not infrequently, the patients have been diagnosed as having Parkinson's disease but have had a poor response to standard treatment.

The diagnosis of Shy–Drager syndrome is made on pelvic floor electromyogram (EMG)[7] (Fig. 34.5), which shows evidence of denervation of the pelvic floor and sphincters resulting from neuronal loss in Onuf's nucleus. Urodynamic evaluation shows a wide open bladder neck with phasic instability and incontinence through a deficient urethral sphincter. Decreased bladder compliance may also occur. Unfortunately, the disease is progressive and is generally associated with a poor prognosis. Currently there is no treatment available to prevent the progressive deterioration and anticholinergic medication is of little benefit. Ultimately, patients may require an indwelling catheter and surgery should be avoided.

Other diseases

Both primary and secondary brain tumors have been reported to be associated with detrusor hyperreflexia and urinary incontinence. Cerebral palsy is a permanent disorder of movement and posture caused by a defect or disease of the brain that usually appears in the first 3 years of life. The disease is not progressive, although the manifestations may alter. As there are a number of conditions that may give rise to cerebral palsy, so are there different patterns of bladder behavior, although detrusor hyperreflexia is most commonly seen. Sphincter dyssynergia may also be observed if spinal cord damage is present. Diseases of the cerebellum may give rise to poor coordination, dysarthria, and choreiform movements. Patients may also complain of urinary frequency and incontinence. Urodynamic investigation typically shows detrusor hyperreflexia with sphincter synergy.

DISEASES PRIMARILY INVOLVING THE SPINAL CORD

Spinal cord injury

Suprasacral spinal cord injury

In patients with damage to the spinal cord above the sacral cord segments, the sacral micturition center is separated from higher centers and reflex bladder activity gradually returns following the period of spinal shock. In spinal shock there is a withdrawal of the many excitatory and inhibitory influences on the alpha motor neurons, resulting in a state of hypoactivity, flaccidity, or areflexia. In humans this areflexic state may last from days to months[2].

Reflex activity first returns to the striated muscle of the pelvic floor and is heralded by the return of the bulbocavernosus and anal skin reflex. The presence of these reflexes confirms the integrity of the conus parasympathetic micturition center and has important prognostic implications for the return of bladder activity (Fig. 34.6). These reflexes may reappear shortly after spinal injury and in some instances do not disappear. In incomplete transection deep tendon reflexes may return within a few hours of injury.

Bladder activity is characterized by uninhibited reflex detrusor contractions, termed detrusor hyperreflexia. These contractions are initially unable to open the bladder neck and initiate voiding, but with time gradually increase in strength. Unlike the person with an intact neuraxis, coordinated relaxation of the distal

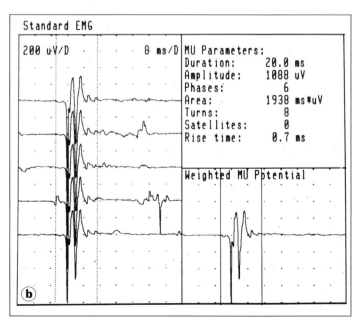

Figure 34.5 Normal and abnormal electromyograph in multiple system atrophy. (a) Normal electromyograph, duration at very upper limit of normal, 9.4msec. (b) Electromyograph in Shy–Drager syndrome with significantly prolonged duration, 28msec. Note difference in vertical and horizontal scales (μV per division, msec per division) between the two studies.

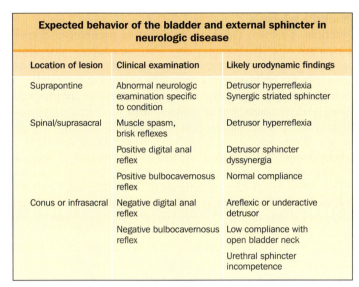

Figure 34.6 Expected behavior of the bladder and external sphincter in neurologic disease.

Location of lesion	Clinical examination	Likely urodynamic findings
Expected behavior of the bladder and external sphincter in neurologic disease		
Suprapontine	Abnormal neurologic examination specific to condition	Detrusor hyperreflexia Synergic striated sphincter
Spinal/suprasacral	Muscle spasm, brisk reflexes	Detrusor hyperreflexia
	Positive digital anal reflex	Detrusor sphincter dyssynergia
	Positive bulbocavernosus reflex	Normal compliance
Conus or infrasacral	Negative digital anal reflex	Areflexic or underactive detrusor
	Negative bulbocavernosus reflex	Low compliance with open bladder neck
		Urethral sphincter incompetence

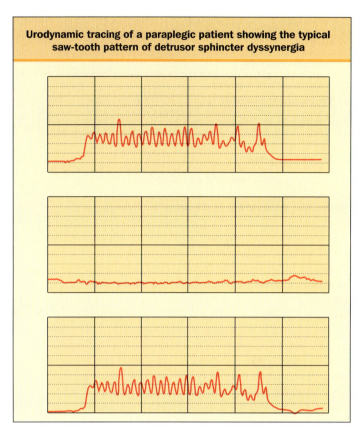

Figure 34.7 Urodynamic tracing of a paraplegic patient showing the typical saw-tooth pattern of detrusor sphincter dyssynergia.

sphincter is usually lost and spasm of the striated distal sphincter mechanism during a voiding contraction produces a functional obstruction, termed detrusor sphincter dyssynergia. In the presence of weak detrusor activity, this sphincteric imbalance may be sufficient to prevent voiding altogether. More commonly, detrusor sphincter dyssynergia results in incomplete bladder emptying and high residual urines. The functional obstruction may lead to a high-pressure voiding system and hydronephrosis.

Following spinal cord injury, return of detrusor activity is seen over the first few months and is usually established by 6 months. Once reflex voiding is established, it may be initiated or reinforced by tapping the suprapubic area. In a small number of patients return of reflex activity may take up to 2 years. Detrusor recovery following an incomplete suprasacral lesion is generally quicker than in patients with complete lesions. In a minority of patients with supraconal lesions, reflex bladder activity never returns despite the presence of conus reflexes. The reason for this is unknown, although it may be due to a second occult lesion.

Detrusor sphincter dyssynergia is characterized by contraction of the external urethral sphincter during an involuntary detrusor contraction (Fig. 34.7). Unlike neurologically intact patients, there is no prevoiding decrease in urethral pressure and external sphincter contraction occurs simultaneously with or immediately after the onset of a detrusor contraction. Detrusor sphincter dyssynergia is seen in between 70% and 100% patients with suprasacral cord lesions following spinal cord injury [8,9].

From the practical point of view, detrusor sphincter dyssynergia may result in the development of large residual urines, recurrent urinary tract infections, high voiding pressures, and hydronephrosis. In patients with lesions above T6, sphincter dyssynergia may present as recurrent episodes of autonomic dysreflexia (see below). Detrusor sphincter dyssynergia is exaggerated in conditions such as infection (urinary or pressure sores), constipation, or anal fissure.

Injury to the sacral cord segments or sacral roots

When the conus or sacral roots are irrevocably damaged, all detrusor contractions are lost and the bladder becomes an acontractile sac. This may also occur in supraconal lesions where distal vascular infarction of the cord and conus has occurred. Bladder emptying may only be achieved by abdominal straining or suprapubic compression (Credé maneuver) or catheter drainage. Often the bladder neck is incompetent at low bladder volumes or becomes incompetent at higher volumes. The bladder fills to a point where the bladder neck passively becomes incompetent and leakage occurs. By straining and increasing abdominal pressure many patients are able to void, albeit incompletely. However, patients with supraconal lesions and distal infarction of the cord cannot strain satisfactorily and need to perform suprapubic compression with a fist. With the introduction and popularization of intermittent self-catheterization [10,11] this has ceased to be a management problem.

Difficulty in straining may be due to an inability to open the bladder neck, but in males there may be a functional obstruction at the level of the distal sphincter, despite the complete paralysis of the striated muscle of the pelvic floor. An appropriate descriptive term is 'isolated distal sphincter obstruction'. This is believed to be sympathetically mediated.

Partial damage to the sacral roots may result in a mixed pattern of very weak or absent detrusor activity or low compliance, but considerable amounts of reflex activity in the pelvic floor muscles.

Congenital cord lesions

In myelomeningocele the neural grove fails to close early in intrauterine life and the neural plaque remains on the surface as a raw, reddened area, covered by a thin, transparent membrane,

Figure 34.8 Assessment of the sacral arc reflexes.

which represents the meninges. The incidence of myelomeningocele has fallen spontaneously and also as a result of antenatal screening for α-fetoprotein. In general, neurologically complete lesions occur in patients with thoracolumbar and lumbar myelomeningocele. Incomplete lesions occur with some lumbosacral and sacral lesions. Patients with a neurologic level at or below L3 usually remain ambulant, but those with higher levels usually adapt to a wheelchair existence. Thoracolumbar lesions tend to cause severe spinal deformities, which can render urologic management problematic. Sacral agenesis may occur as an isolated anomaly or be associated with imperforate anus, cloacal exstrophy, or myelomeningocele. The cord lesion is almost always incomplete. Other cord lesions include lumbosacral lipoma, diastemomyelia, intra- and extradural lipomas, dermoid cysts, and tethered cord syndrome.

Whereas obvious lesions are clearly evident in most patients, more subtle findings should be looked for in the young patient presenting with voiding dysfunction of possible neurologic etiology. These include the presence of telangiectasia, spinal dimple, a hairy patch, or an abnormal gluteal cleft (a common finding in sacral agenesis). A detailed neurologic examination should also be performed as detailed, with particular reference to the sacral reflexes (Fig. 34.8).

A urodynamic classification commonly used in patients with congenital cord lesions is that proposed by Rickwood and Mundy[12,13], which comprises:

- **Contractile bladder.** Hyperreflexic detrusor contractions occur and are the only means of voiding. The patient does *not* have sphincter weakness incontinence.
- **Acontractile bladder.** Detrusor activity is completely absent. Sphincter weakness incontinence is present to some degree so that voiding occurs either by overflow or by raising intra-abdominal pressure by straining or suprapubic compression.
- **Intermediate bladder.** There is a combination of detrusor hyperreflexia and sphincter weakness incontinence so that voiding may occur by both detrusor contractions or by straining or by suprapubic compression.

In myelomeningocele, urodynamic studies are performed on infants as part of their routine evaluation, with annual upper tract imaging, usually by ultrasound and/or renography. Urodynamics are then repeated as clinically indicated. The essential aim of management is to preserve upper tract function with a secondary aim of promoting urinary continence. Detrusor sphincter dyssynergia, decreased bladder compliance, and elevated leak-point pressures ($>40cmH_2O$) are strong risk factors for upper tract deterioration[14].

Multiple sclerosis

Multiple sclerosis (MS) is a disabling neurologic disease frequently affecting young adults. The characteristic pathologic features are zones of demyelination or plaques in the white matter of the brain or spinal cord. The etiology of the condition is unknown, but increasing evidence supports an autoimmune cause. MS is commoner in women than men (3:2 ratio) and is frequently diagnosed in patients between 20 and 50 years of age. There appears to be an uneven worldwide distribution of the disease, with a higher incidence in the northern latitudes.

The clinical course of patients with MS is variable. Approximately 80–85% of patients follow a relapsing remitting pattern, followed by a secondary progressive phase. Other patients develop primary progressive MS or have a benign course with no disability after 10 years.

Primary diagnosis of MS by a urologist is unusual, but suspicion may be raised in a patient presenting with lower urinary tract symptoms together with neurologic symptoms, or abnormalities on a neurologic examination (evidence of spasticity, extensor plantar reflexes) and an abnormal urodynamic investigation. More commonly, the diagnosis is known and the patient is referred by the neurologist for management of lower urinary tract symptoms. Over 80% of patients with MS have lower urinary tract symptoms and this increases in patients with MS for more than 10 years[15].

The clinical assessment of MS patients should include an assessment of the residual urine and a urodynamic assessment. The majority of patients will typically have irritative and obstructive symptoms and will demonstrate detrusor hyperreflexia on urodynamic evaluation[16]. This is consistent with the frequent incidence of suprasacral spinal cord demyelinating lesions. Patient may also exhibit evidence of detrusor hyperreflexia with detrusor external sphincter dyssynergia (DESD). It appears that, in contrast to spinal cord injury, the presence of DESD is usually harmless and does not predict the development of upper tract deterioration[17]. Up to 40% of patients may show evidence of hypocontractility or areflexia. Stress incontinence may also be seen in parous women.

As with the clinical condition, the demyelinating lesions responsible for voiding dysfunction in MS may change with time and it is not surprising that urodynamic patterns may differ in those patients who are retested.

DISEASE DISTAL TO THE SPINAL CORD

Disc disease and spinal stenosis

Disc protrusions most frequently compress the spinal roots at the level of L4–L5 or L5–S1 interspaces. The classic presentation is that of a cauda equina syndrome with acute back pain, saddle anesthesia, and painless urinary retention. The patient usually presents to the urologist after surgery with difficulty voiding, straining, or urinary retention. There is no evidence that laminectomy improves bladder function. Examination may reveal a distended bladder, sensory loss of the sacral dermatomes, and absent sacral reflexes. The most consistent urodynamic finding is that of a normally compliant areflexic bladder with normal or incomplete denervation of the perineal floor muscles. Occasionally, patients may show features of detrusor hyperreflexia and reduced compliance[18].

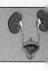

As a consequence of straining, female patients may develop stress incontinence, which may be treated with a colposuspension or sling procedure and starting the patient on intermittent self-catheterization (ISC). Male patients with symptomatic incomplete bladder emptying are best treated with ISC.

Spinal stenosis is a term applied to any narrowing of the spinal canal, nerve root canals, or intervertebral foramina. Back pain and lower extremity pain, cramp, and paresthesia related to exercise and relieved by rest are the classic symptoms of lumbar stenosis. The urodynamic abnormalities are dependent on the level of the lesion and the degree of damage to the spinal cord and/or spinal nerves.

Sequelae of pelvic surgery

Radical pelvic surgery is well recognized to be associated with bladder dysfunction. Abdominoperineal resection, low anterior resection, simple and radical hysterectomy, and vaginal surgery have all been implicated in damaging the peripheral innervation of the bladder and sphincter. Lower urinary tract dysfunction has been reported in 10–60% of patients and in 15–20% voiding dysfunction is permanent, but it should be remembered that pre-existing outflow obstruction is common in men, as is genuine stress incontinence in women in this age range. Leveckas[19] described a prospective series of 20 patients who were assessed urodynamically before and after major pelvic surgery. Before surgery only 6 patients had normal bladder function and following surgery 8 patients had developed identifiable bladder dysfunction. The bladder dysfunction is caused by damage to the pelvic and hypogastric nerves, which are located outside the pelvic fascia. In the female they pass beneath the uterine artery and are close but inferiomedial to the cervix. The pudendal nerve can be injured by either traction or perineal dissection.

Urodynamics will rarely influence the early management of patients following injury to the pelvic plexus and are best left for a least 6 weeks after the injury. Typical video-urodynamic features include a reduced sensation during bladder filling, detrusor hyporeflexia, increased compliance, and an open bladder neck. There may be evidence of stress incontinence. An EMG study of the external sphincter may show evidence of denervation with abnormal motor unit potentials.

In men with retention following major pelvic surgery, a TURP should not be performed unless there is urodynamic evidence of unequivocal obstruction and reasonable detrusor function. If detrusor function is poor or absent the patient is best managed with intermittent self-catheterization or a long-term catheter in the hope that there will be a gradual improvement in detrusor function with time. Gradually, over a period of months, spontaneous voiding will usually return. Some patients will continue to leave large postvoid residual urines and careful followup is required.

Diabetes mellitus

The pathogenesis of autonomic dysfunction in diabetes mellitus is thought to be the result of chronic hyperglycemia leading to axonal damage followed by demyelination at multiple sites in the nervous system. Diabetic cystopathy is part of a spectrum of autonomic dysfunction, including gastroesophageal atonia, hyperhydrosis, nocturnal diarrhea, postural hypotension, erectile dysfunction, and autonomic cardiac abnormalities. The

pudendal nerves appear to be relatively spared compared with autonomic peripheral nerves.

Epidemiologic studies suggest that up to 40% of patients with diabetes will have some form of voiding dysfunction although classic diabetic cystopathy is now uncommon. The clinical onset is insidious, with bladder sensation becoming impaired, with increased voiding intervals and decreased detrusor contractions leading to increased postvoid residual urines and retention, sometimes with overflow incontinence.

Urodynamic assessment may show an increased bladder capacity with reduced sensation and evidence of detrusor hyperreflexia, low voiding pressures, or areflexia. Men may have concomitant urodynamic features of bladder outflow obstruction[20]. Sphincter EMG is usually abnormal, with evoked potentials displaying increased latency with a reduced or absent bulbocavernosal reflex. As many elderly patients with diabetes mellitus will have co-existing pathology (bladder outflow obstruction, stroke, etc.), urodynamic testing is important before embarking on surgical therapy.

Herpes zoster

Herpes zoster is caused by the varicella virus. The prodromal illness with malaise and slight fever is often so slight that the rash is the first sign of the disease. Invasion of the dorsal root ganglia and posterior nerve roots with the herpes zoster virus results in a painful, vesicular dermatomal rash, which may produce a variety of urinary symptoms, including urinary retention and detrusor areflexia, detrusor hyperreflexia, or a cystitis-like syndrome with urinary frequency, dysuria, or hematuria.

Spontaneous resolution usually occurs in a month or two.

Guillain–Barré syndrome

Guillain–Barré syndrome is an inflammatory demyelinating disorder of the peripheral nervous system. It may be preceded by a mild respiratory or gastrointestinal infection. It is believed to result from an abnormal immune response directed against the peripheral nerves. The syndrome typically presents with weakness involving proximal and distal limbs as well as trunk muscles. The motor paralysis occurs first in the lower extremities and progresses proximally. Autonomic neuropathy may occur, with cardiac arrhythmias, hyper- and hypotension, and urinary retention. The patient is best managed by an indwelling catheter or intermittent catheterization during the acute phase.

ASSESSMENT OF THE NEUROPATHIC PATIENT

Clinical assessment
Disease at or above the brain stem
Patients with intracranial lesions typically present with urinary frequency and urgency with or without incontinence. Patients with intracranial lesions may have impaired cognitive function and void inappropriately. A neurologic examination is clearly important as it may help distinguish patients with dementia, stroke, Parkinson's disease, and cerebellar problems. Patients with Parkinson's disease typically have bradykinesia, cogwheel rigidity, and impaired equilibrium (see Fig. 34.6).

Disease primarily involving the spinal cord
Patients with suprasacral spinal cord lesions with preservation of the conus typically complain of urinary incontinence with little

sensation of bladder filling or the need to void. Few patients with incomplete suprasacral lesions are left with completely normal detrusor function, even if there is a remarkable degree of motor and sensory neurologic recovery. Most are left with uninhibited detrusor contractions and detrusor sphincter dyssynergia. In patients with cortical control, this may be characterized by severe frequency and urgency with incomplete bladder emptying. As the sacral arc is intact, reflex erections are usually preserved.

Physical examination of the patient will usually reveal brisk tendon reflexes and spasticity of the extremities below the level of the lesion. Rectal tone may be increased and the sacral arc reflexes are usually brisk.

Autonomic hyperreflexia. Patients with complete or incomplete lesions above the sympathetic outflow of the spinal cord (T6) may develop paroxysmal hypertension, throbbing headache, sweating, and bradycardia in response to many forms of stimulation below the level of the lesion. These include bladder distention, detrusor hyperreflexia, and detrusor sphincter dyssynergia. This sympathetic response to extreme bladder volumes occurs in normal humans as well as in patients with high cord lesions, varying only in degree of severity. Sympathetic stimulation results in sweating and increased catecholamine production[21]. To counteract the raised blood pressure, bradycardia is achieved via the baroreceptors and vagal stimulation. Prompt recognition and appropriate management of this emergency are essential, as untreated, autonomic hyperreflexia may result in a subarachnoid hemorrhage and death.

Lesions affecting the conus and peripheral nerves

In patients with lesions at or below the conus, there is usually evidence of skeletal muscle flaccidity of the lower extremities. The Achilles tendon reflex (L5–S2) and the knee jerk reflex (L2–L4) should be tested, in addition to the sacral reflexes, which provide significant information about detrusor and external sphincter (see Fig. 34.8) and may predict bladder function on urodynamic evaluation. The absence of a sacral reflex suggests a neurologic lesion of the conus, cauda equina, or a peripheral nerve. However the presence of a sacral reflex does not exclude a lesion as a patient may have an incomplete lower motor neuron lesion with an areflexic bladder. Patients with damage to the conus, cauda equina, or peripheral nerves often complain of alteration in erectile function. Reflex erections rely on the somatic function of the pudendal nerve and the autonomic function of the pelvic nerves.

Urodynamic assessment

Urodynamic assessment forms the cornerstone of the management of patients with neuropathic bladder dysfunction. Unlike conventional urodynamics, where the study is provocative, in the neuropathic patient the study should be performed under as nearly physiologic conditions as possible. Ideally a video-urodynamic study should be performed with X-ray screening, which will provide extra information about the bladder neck and distal sphincter and demonstrate vesicoureteric reflux should it occur during filling or voiding[9]. The principal indications for urodynamic assessment are listed in Figure 34.9.

Many patients with neuropathic bladder will have asymptomatic bacteriuria and should be covered with a broad-spectrum

---

Indications for urodynamic assessment in neuropathic bladder
New-onset incontinence or change in voiding pattern
Recurrent urinary tract infection
Development of upper tract dilatation
Onset of autonomic dysreflexia
Prior to reconstructive surgery

Figure 34.9 Indications for urodynamic assessment in neuropathic bladder.

Key questions in the urodynamic assessment of neuropathic bladder
Is voluntary detrusor activity present?
Is there evidence of detrusor hyperreflexia? If so, what are the pressures?
Is detrusor dyssynergia present?
Is dyssynergia related to high detrusor pressures?
Is dyssynergia related to incomplete bladder emptying?
What is the state of compliance during bladder filling?
In low compliance, does the bladder neck open during filling?
Is there evidence of vesicoureteric reflux?
Is there evidence of urethral sphincter incompetence?

Figure 34.10 Key questions in the urodynamic assessment of neuropathic bladder.

---

antibiotic (i.e. an aminoglycoside or cephalosporin) given one hour prior to the study.

Paralyzed patients who are unable to stand may be assessed in the right oblique position, with a triangular wedge of foam placed behind their backs, which allows maximum visualization of the bladder neck and urethra. Two small-diameter catheters are introduced into the bladder, piggybacked on a 14G Nelaton catheter. Once in the bladder, the Nelaton catheter is removed and the filling line and pressure recording line are correctly connected. In patients with suspected or known detrusor hyperreflexia, the residual urine should not be emptied as this may alter the pattern of reflex detrusor activity and the pattern of detrusor sphincter dyssynergia. Rapid bladder filling may also change the pattern of detrusor activity and fill rates in the range of 10–30ml/min should be used. A number of voiding sequences should be observed to establish a regular pattern of reflex voiding. A typical pattern of detruser sphincter dyssynergia is shown in Figure 34.7.

The aim of the study is to give as much objective information on detrusor and sphincteric dysfunction under as nearly physiologic conditions as possible. The key questions to be answered are listed in Figure 34.10. Low-compliance bladders and high leak-point pressures (>40cmH$_2$O) may herald the onset of vesicoureteric reflux and hydronephrosis in patients with myelomeningocele[14]. Hydronephrosis has been reported in up to 20% of patients with spinal cord injury at 15–20 years followup[8] and this is associated with low compliance, high resting pressures, detrusor sphincter dyssynergia, reflux, and calculous disease.

The ice water test

In patients with lower urinary tract symptoms, a positive ice water test is an indicator of a silent or overt neurologic disorder and may help differentiate upper and lower motor neuron lesions[22]. The ice water test is performed after standard cystometry with the patient in a supine position. A volume of 100mL of sterile water at 0°C is infused as rapidly as possible into the patient's bladder through an 8F plastic catheter (infusion time approximately 15–20s). The cold fluid is left in the bladder for 1 minute. If a sustained bladder contraction occurs during this period and the fluid is expelled the test is considered positive.

Sphincter electromyography

Sphincter electromyography (EMG) is the study of minute potentials produced by depolarization of the muscle membrane. It has been employed in conjunction with cystometry to record the electrical activity of the perineal muscles during micturition. EMG has proved to be particularly valuable in identifying patients with parkinsonism who have multiple system atrophy (see Fig. 34.5). EMG of the striated muscle of the urethral sphincter is essential in recognizing the abnormal spontaneous activity responsible for urinary retention in young women[23]. EMG is not routinely employed in the evaluation of patients with detrusor sphincter dyssynergia, as a functional assessment of the external sphincter can be made at the time of the video-urodynamic study.

MANAGEMENT

General principles
These can be simply stated as follows:
- Preservation of renal function is the principal consideration.
- An objective assessment of the patient's bladder function by urodynamics forms the cornerstone of management to re-establish continence or preserve upper tract function.
- Consideration of the patient's general medical and functional status and his/her expectations is vital prior to embarking on treatment.
- Surgical treatment should be reserved for cases where a more conservative approach has been tried and failed.
- Because of the complexity of other problems the patient may have, treatment needs to be individualized.

Medical management
Treatment options for patients with detrusor hyperreflexia range from simple behavioral measures (which may be useful in patients with dementia and cerebrovascular disease) through to highly invasive surgical procedures. Many patients are managed with antimuscarinic drugs (e.g. oxybutynin and tolterodine), but their use is limited by systemic adverse events, most notably dry mouth and constipation. Patients who have large residual urines may be treated with clean intermittent self-catheterization (CISC) and, if appropriate, an antimuscarinic drug. Intravesical instillation of oxybutynin[24] and capsaicin[25] has been reported to produce clinical and urodynamic improvement in patients with detrusor hyperreflexia, but because of manufacturing problems their use has not become widespread.

Men with detrusor hyperreflexia and incontinence can be satisfactorily managed with a condom sheath and leg bag. In women, however, detrusor hyperreflexia poses a significant clinical problem as there is no suitable incontinence appliance available. In patients managed with an indwelling catheter, it is important to use a small balloon (5mL) if possible. Asymptomatic bacteriuria

Considerations for clean intermittent self-catheterization
What is the bladder capacity?
Is the residual urine large?
Is infection or incontinence a problem?
Can the patient do CISC?
Will the patient do CISC?
How often is it necessary?
Is mobility a problem?

Figure 34.11 Considerations for clean intermittent self-catheterization. CISC, clean intermittent self-catheterization.

can usually be ignored. Long-term catheterization in women may cause urethral erosion, causing catheter expulsion, leading to the insertion of larger catheters and further problems. A suprapubic catheter with a small balloon may avoid such problems.

Clean intermittent self-catheterization
Since its introduction by Lapides in 1972, clean intermittent self-catheterization (CISC) has assumed a pivotal role in the management of patients with neuropathic bladder problems. For it to be successful, both the doctor and the patient need to be realistic about what can be expected. CISC is suitable for managing patients with incomplete bladder emptying who have a large bladder capacity (Fig. 34.11). It is rarely worthwhile starting a patient on CISC if the residual urine is less than 100mL. Many patients are wary of performing CISC and may find the procedure both embarrassing and distasteful to start with. For these reasons, the technique is best taught by a fully trained therapist who can spend time with the patient sorting out any worries. Ideally it should not be performed more than four times per day, as this may pose problems for the patient with limited mobility. It is rarely suitable for patients who leak in between catheterizations.

Clean intermittent self-catheterization does, however, have limitations. Continence may only be achieved where there is an adequate functional bladder capacity. In patients with severe hyperreflexia, CISC may need to be combined with oxybutynin or some form of cystoplasty. CISC may be impractical in patients with impaired mentation (e.g. hydrocephalus), major physical disabilities (MS, stroke, spinal deformity, obesity, hip contractures), and in some patients with well-preserved urethral sensation. Good hand function is important and poor co-ordination may preclude its use, unless the patient has a dedicated carer who is willing to undertake the procedure.

Urinary tract infection
Risk factors that predispose patients with neuropathic bladder to urinary tract infection (UTI) include outflow obstruction caused by detrusor sphincter dyssynergia, high detrusor pressures, large postvoid residual urines, vesicoureteric reflux, and stones. Indwelling catheters, CISC, and external collecting devices are all associated with bacteriuria. In general, asymptomatic bacteriuria is not associated with an adverse effect on the urinary tract or renal function and prophylactic antibiotics are not indicated. However patients with bacteriuria due to *Proteus* species or vesicoureteric reflux should be treated.

Follow-up

Irrespective of the underlying condition, followup of patients with neuropathic voiding dysfunction is usually worthwhile. Patterns of bladder behavior can change and in some patients there is a risk of upper tract deterioration. Predisposing factors for the development of upper tract complications are listed in Figure 34.12. In spinal cord injury, hydronephrosis has been reported in up to 20% of patients during a 15–20-year follow-up[8]. Patients with congenital neuropathic bladder dysfunction are also at risk of developing secondary upper tract complications and, in myelomeningocele, this may occur during puberty. Annual upper tract imaging is advisable.

In spinal cord injury an intravenous urogram or ultrasound should be performed early in the course of the patient's rehabilitation to have a baseline assessment of the urinary system. Urodynamic assessment should be undertaken once reflex voiding is established. Further upper tract imaging should be obtained if the patient's urologic condition deteriorates and also on a yearly basis. If indicated a renal scan can be done as a more accurate and sensitive assessment of renal function. By contrast, the development of hydronephrosis in MS patients is uncommon[17] and many urologists have now abandoned routine yearly upper tract imaging.

Surgical management

When appropriately chosen, surgical procedures can substantially improve the quality of life in patients with neuropathic bladder. The endoscopic approach of hydrodistention in patients with detrusor hyperreflexia or low compliance normally offers only temporary relief of symptoms. Transvesical phenol injection is more effective in MS patients with hyperreflexia although the procedure may need to be repeated and fistulae have been reported following the procedure.

Transurethral sphincterotomy

Transurethral sphincterotomy (TURS) is primarily used in male neuropathic patients with spinal cord injury or spina bifida who have severe voiding dysfunction. The main indications for TURS are persistent high voiding pressures with DESD, hydronephrosis, recurrent urinary tract infection, vesicoureteric reflux, urolithiasis, prostatoejaculatory reflux, recurrent epididymo-orchitis, and severe autonomic dysreflexia. Following the procedure the external sphincter is incompetent and the patient will need to be managed with an external condom drainage device and leg bag. TURS should not be undertaken in patients who are candidates for bladder reconstruction.

The procedure is usually performed under spinal block, which reduces the incidence of autonomic dysreflexia. The TURS incision is typically made at 12 o'clock, extending from the bladder neck, through the prostatic urethra and distal sphincter, just into the bulbar urethra, cutting through all the fibers. Some peripheral fat may be exposed.

Reconstructive surgery

This has undergone a revolution over the past decade with the widespread use of procedures to augment or totally substitute the dysfunctional bladder. Augmentation cystoplasty is used routinely in patients with neuropathic bladder. The procedure acts by both increasing the patient's bladder capacity and reducing the amplitude of phasic detrusor contractions. Where indicated a Mitrofanoff procedure may be performed at the same time. Detrusor myotomy can be used in preference to using bowel to augment the bladder.

Although modern surgical techniques have the potential to render most patients continent of urine, reconstructive surgery demands patience, tact, and a thorough knowledge of the patient's medical condition and its natural history. Prior to embarking on surgery, it is essential to have a thorough video-urodynamic assessment performed on the patient, including evaluation of the distal sphincter to see if sphincter incompetence is present. Attention should be paid to the patient's mentation, co-ordination, obesity, and mobility, as problems with any of these factors may mitigate against a successful outcome. CISC is frequently required after reconstructive surgery and it is essential that the patient is not only happy to use the technique but also committed to self-catheterization in the future. The patient should also be aware of the complication rates and revision procedures that may be required (particularly when an artificial urinary sphincter is inserted) and the need for continuing urologic surveillance.

Urinary diversion

Urinary diversion still has a place in the urologist's armamentarium, particularly in female patients with MS or high spinal lesions. In such cases, detrusor hyperreflexia results in catheter bypassing and expulsion and CISC may be difficult to perform because of poor hand function or problems in transferring (Fig. 34.13).

Causes of upper tract complications in neuropathic bladder

Low compliance

Vesicoureteric reflux

High resting detrusor pressures

Detrusor hyperreflexia

Bladder outflow obstruction

Urinary tract infection

Figure 34.12 Causes of upper tract complications in neuropathic bladder.

Therapeutic options in patients with detrusor hyperreflexia

Men	Women
Anticholinergic medication	Anticholinergic medication
Sheath and leg bag	CISC (if residual urine large)
TURS (if obstructed)	Cystodistention
CISC (if residual urine large)	Phenol or capsaicin
Capsaicin	Urinary reconstruction (depending on disease process)
Urinary reconstruction (depending on disease process)	Urinary diversion
Urinary diversion	SARS (see text)
SARS (see text)	Suprapubic indwelling catheter
Indwelling catheter	

Figure 34.13 Therapeutic options in patients with detrusor hyperreflexia. CISC, clean intermittent self-catheterization; SARS, sacral anterior root stimulation; TURS, transuretheral sphincterotomy..

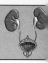
Sacral anterior root stimulation

Intradural sacral posterior rhizotomy combined with intradural sacral anterior root stimulation (SARS) using the Finetech–Brindley device is an alternative method of managing patients with complete supra conal spinal cord lesions[26]. At operation the posterior roots S2–S4 are identified and cut. Electrodes are implanted on the anterior roots and these allow transmitter-controlled stimulation via a receiver placed subcutaneously on the abdominal wall. Continence is achieved as a result of the posterior root deafferentation effectively abolishing reflex detrusor activity and increasing bladder capacity. The transmitter can then be programmed to achieve controlled low-resistance voiding and, in some patients, bowel evacuation.

REFERENCES

1. Fall M, Geirsson G, Lindstrom S. Towards a new classification of overactive bladders. Neurourol Urodyn. 1995;14:635–46.
2. Thomas DG, Lucas MG. The urinary tract following spinal cord injury. In: Chisholm GD, Fair W, eds. Scientific foundations of urology, 3rd edn. Chicago: Year Book Medical Publishers; 1990:286–99.
3. Gelber DA, Good DC, Layven LJ, Verhulst SJ. Causes of urinary incontinence after acute hemispheric stroke. Stroke. 1993;24:378–82
4. Skelly J, Flint AJ. Urinary incontinence associated with dementia. J Am Geriat Soc. 1995;43:286–94.
5. Berger Y, Blavias JG, DeLaRoche ER, Salinas JM. Urodynamic findings in Parkinson's disease. J Urol. 1987;138:836–8.
6. Fitzmaurice H, Fowler CJ, Richards D. Micturition disturbances in Parkinson's disease. Br J Urol. 1985;57:652–6.
7. Chandiramani VA, Palace J, Fowler CJ. How to recognize patients with parkinsonism who should not have urological surgery. Br J Urol. 1997;80(1):100–4.
8. Hackler RH. A 25 year prospective study mortality study in the spinal cord injured patients: comparison with the long-term living paraplegic. J Urol. 1977;117:486
9. Thomas DG, O'Flynn KJ. Spinal cord injury. In: Mundy AR, Stephenson TP, Wein AJ, eds. Urodynamics, principles, practice and application, 2nd edn. Edinburgh: Churchill Livingstone; 1994:345–58.
10. Guttman L, Frankel H. The value of intermittent catheterization in the early management of traumatic paraplegia and tetraplegia. Paraplegia. 1966;4:63.
11. Lapides J, Diokno AC, Silber SJ, et al. Clean intermittent self-catheterization in the treatment of urinary tract disease. J Urol. 1972;107:458.
12. Rickwood AMK, Thomas DG, Philp NH, Spicer RD. Assessment of congenital neuropathic bladder by combined urodynamic and radiological studies. Br J Urol. 1982;54:502–11
13. Mundy AR, Shah PJR, Borzyskowski M, Saxton HM. Sphincter behaviour in myelomeningocele. Br J Urol. 1985;57:647–651.
14. McGuire EJ, Woodside JR, Borden TA, et al. Prognostic value of urodynamic testing in myeloplastic patients. J Urol. 1981;126:205.
15. Awad SA, Gajewski JB, Sogbein SK, Murray TJ, Field CA. Relationship between neurological and urological status in patients with multiple sclerosis. J Urol. 1984;1323:499–502.
16. Hinson JL, Boone TB. Urodynamics and multiple sclerosis. Urol Clin North Am. 1996:23:475–481.
17. Koldewijn EL, Hommes OR, Lemmens WAJG, et al. Relationship between lower urinary tract abnormalities and disease-related parameters in multiple sclerosis. J Urol. 1995;154;169–73.
18. O'Flynn KJ, Murphy R, Thomas DG. Long-term follow-up of neurogenic bladder dysfunction in lumbar intervertebral disc prolapse. Br J Urol. 1992;69:38–41.
19. Leveckis I, Boucher NR, Parys BT, Reed MW, Dhorthouse AL, Anderson JB. Bladder and erectile dysfunction before and after surgery for rectal cancer. Br J Urol. 1995;76(6):752–6.
20. Nichell K, Boone TB. Peripheral neuropathy and peripheral nerve injury. Urol Clin North Am. 1996;23:491–9.
21. Trop CS, Bennett CJ. Autonomic dysreflexia and its urological implications: a review. J Urol. 1994;146;1461–9.
22. Geirsson G, Fall M, Lindstrom S. The ice-water test – a simple and valuable supplement to routine cystometry. Br J Urol. 1993;71:681–5.
23. Fowler CJ, Christmas TI, Chapple CR, Parkhouse HF, Kirby RS, Jacobs HS. Abnormal electromyographc activity of the urethral sphincter, voiding dysfunction and polycystic ovaries: a new syndrome? Br Med J. 1988;297:1436–8.
24. O'Flynn KJ, Thomas DG. Intravesical instillation of oxybutinin hydrochloride for detrusor hyper-reflexia. Br J Urol. 1993;72:566–71.
25. Fowler CJ, Jewkes D, McDonald WI, Lynn B, de Groat WC. Intavesical capsaicin for neurogenic bladder dysfunction. Lancet. 1992;339:1239.
26. Van Kerrebroeck EV, van der Aa HE, Bosch JL, Koldewijn EL, Vorsteveld JH, Debruyne-FM (Dutch Study Group on Sacral Anterior Root Stimulation) Sacral rhizotomies and electrical bladder stimulation in spinal cord injury. Part I: Clinical and urodynamic analysis. Eur Urol. 1997;31(3):263–7.

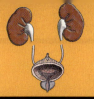

Chapter 35
The Use of Bowel in Urinary Tract Reconstruction

James Hall and John B Anderson

KEY POINTS

- Ileum and colon are most often used for urinary tract reconstruction.
- The appendix may be employed to produce a catheterizable stoma.
- Meticulous technique is as essential for entero–enteric anastomosis as it is for bowel–urinary tract anastomosis.
- Detubularization and reconfiguration maximize the capacity available from a given length of bowel.
- It is essential to understand and identify potential metabolic complications of using bowel to store urine.

INTRODUCTION

The normal physiology of a healthy urinary tract depends upon antegrade urinary drainage from the renal pelvices via the ureters and the storage of an adequate volume of urine at low pressure in a highly compliant bladder, which is then voided to completion without excessive pressure at a socially convenient time via the urethra. A wide range of disease can affect the urinary system, destroying its normal function and necessitating removal of the ureter, bladder, or urethra. Inevitably this will result in a need to divert, augment, or substitute variable amounts of the urinary tract. For this, tissue is needed and most commonly segments of the gastrointestinal tract are used. The principles by which bowel is used to restore or maintain the physiologic function of the urinary tract will be discussed in this chapter. Despite advances in technique the use of bowel under these circumstances is still subject to a wide variety of complications and these will also be reviewed.

HISTORY

Bowel has been used in urinary tract reconstruction for over a century. Its increasing use has only been made possible by advances in anesthesia and improvements in per- and postoperative patient care. An appreciation of how complications became apparent is important as it can help the modern urologist anticipate future problems. In 1852 Simon first reported the ureterosigmoidostomy to divert the flow of urine in a patient with bladder exstrophy[1], but it was many decades before the alarming malignancy rates within the sigmoid colon were appreciated[2].

The incontinent ileal loop urinary diversion was described by Bricker in 1950[3] and rapidly gained widespread popularity. It initially appeared to be the panacea for progressive deterioration of upper urinary tracts in a wide range of pathologies, but with prolonged followup it has become apparent that up to 50% of patients with a loop diversion have some degree of ongoing upper urinary tract compromise[4].

Although Mikulicz originally described bladder augmentation in 1899 it was not carried out with any frequency until the last 25 years. One of the key reasons for the more recent use of the technique, and the development of a plethora of other reconstructive urologic operations using bowel, was the successful introduction and popularization of intermittent self-catheterization (CISC) by Lapides in the early 1970s[5].

ANATOMIC CONSIDERATIONS

The segments of bowel commonly used for urinary tract reconstruction are the ileum and colon and less frequently the stomach and rectum. The appendix may be employed to produce a catheterizable stoma. Jejunum is generally avoided because of a far higher rate of metabolic complications. The most important factor in helping decide which segment of bowel to use is an adequate blood supply once the bowel is isolated, mobilized, and, if necessary, refashioned. The donor area of bowel must also have adequate perfusion to ensure viability of the segment and a safe anastomosis.

Stomach

When using the stomach for urinary tract reconstruction vascular pedicles to support the segment can be based on the greater curvature of the stomach supported by the right gastroepiploic artery. The proximal extent of such a pedicle will be determined be the quality of the right-to-left gastroepiploic arterial anastomosis, which is not always extensive[6]. The distal extent can include some antrum but should not encroach on the pylorus (Figs 35.1 & 35.2).

Small bowel

The ileum is up to 4m in length and provides extensive amounts of tissue for urinary tract reconstruction. It derives its arterial supply from multiple arcades arising from the superior mesenteric artery (Fig. 35.3). Ileal segments of varying lengths can therefore be isolated on one or more of these arcades. Identification of the small bowel vasculature is most easily achieved by transilluminating the mesentery at the time of resection. Ileum up to 10cm lateral to a straight vessel has been

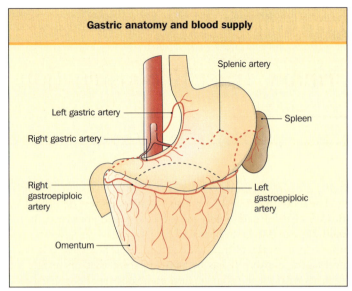

Figure 35.1 Gastric anatomy and blood supply.

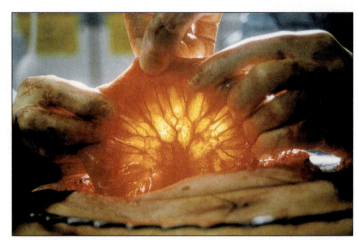

Figure 35.3 The arterial arcades supplying the distal ileum displayed by transillumination.

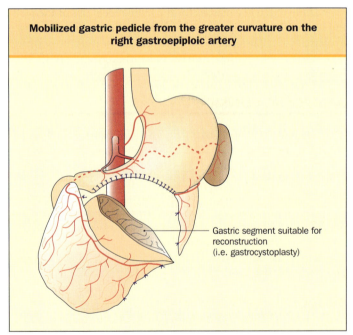

Figure 35.2 Mobilized gastric pedicle from the greater curvature on the right gastroepiploic artery.

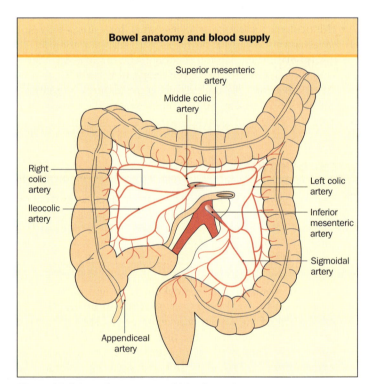

Figure 35.4 Bowel anatomy and blood supply.

shown to be viable[7], although in practice this should be kept to the minimum possible. The distal 15cm of terminal ileum is supplied by the ileocolic artery, which itself anastomoses with the terminal branch of the superior mesenteric artery. Branches from the ileocolic artery also supply the appendix, cecum, and proximal ascending colon.

Colon
The right and middle colic branches of the superior mesenteric artery supply the ascending and proximal two thirds of the transverse colon. Left colic and sigmoidal arteries arise from the inferior mesenteric artery. Hence, segments of large bowel can be isolated on one or more of the colic or sigmoidal arteries (Fig. 35.4). The anastomotic integrity can sometimes be poor between the middle and right colic arteries and between the sigmoidal and superior hemorrhoidal arteries (supplying the upper rectum). If there is any doubt about the quality of perfusion at any bowel end a further resection should be undertaken.

BOWEL SEGMENT SELECTION

The perfusion of the bowel segment and its donor site anastomosis usually dictate which parts of the bowel are suitable for reconstructive purposes. Removal of any given bowel segment from the gastrointestinal tract should cause minimal physiologic upset, and bowel previously subjected to radiotherapy or inflammatory bowel disease should be avoided.

Although the segment of bowel to be used for a particular procedure is usually constant and identified preoperatively, the urologic surgeon must be familiar with the range of possible options in case the preferred segment is not available or suitable. In the occasional difficult case, such as bladder substitution in a patient with spina bifida, where the enteric anatomy can be variable, the most suitable segment for reconstruction may only be determined intraoperatively.

BOWEL PREPARATION

Preparation of the gastrointestinal tract prior to urinary tract reconstruction requires both mechanical and antimicrobial consideration. Mechanical preparation aims to ensure that the bowel is empty at the time of surgery to facilitate access, to minimize spillage of bowel contents, and to reduce the fecal stream crossing the anastomosis in the early postoperative period. There are a variety of regimens described comprising combinations of low-residue diets, osmotic and stimulant laxatives, bowel irrigation and enemas. Mechanical bowel preparation reduces the total number of bacteria but does not reduce the bacterial concentration of the fecal fluid[8]; hence any intraoperative spillage will result in potential contamination.

Typically, mechanical bowel preparation involves a low-residue diet in the 3 days leading up to surgery. On the day prior to surgery two sachets of sodium picosulfate are given, with the addition of a third sachet if the result is poor. Mechanical bowel preparation can lead to dehydration so most patients commence an intravenous infusion to cover their preoperative night (crystalloid at 1000mL/8 hours).

The beneficial role of antibiotic preparation aiming to sterilize the bowel content is contentious. It adds to the risk of diarrhea, thrush and pseudomembranous colitis. The regimen in our own unit is metronidazole and cefuroxime at induction continued for 48 hours postoperatively, assuming there is no gross intraoperative contamination.

ANASTOMOTIC CONSIDERATIONS

While the anastomosis between the bowel and the urinary tract (either bladder or ureter) is of paramount importance, the anastomotic technique used to re-establish intestinal integrity also needs to be meticulous.

Enteroenteric anastomoses

Complications involving bowel are most commonly associated with the anastomosis and give rise to some of the commonest morbidity, and even result in mortality in the early postoperative period. To minimize these complications basic surgical principles must be observed.

- **Bowel mobilization and exposure**. Bowel mobilization is essential to avoid any tension at the anastomotic site to decrease the chance of dehiscence; for example, the whole of the left colon often needs to be mobilized to allow safe use of the sigmoid colon. Adequate exposure is important to allow careful suture placement.

- **Good blood supply**. Divided bowel ends should be pink and seen to bleed readily.
- **Avoidance of spillage**. Soft bowel clamps should be used to isolate the segments 5–10cm from the line of bowel division. The segments should be milked empty prior to application of the second clamp. A heavily soiled bowel segment should be irrigated clean with the abdominal cavity protected by packs.
- **Serosal apposition**. Since the bowel serosa contains the vast bulk of collagen and elastic tissue present in the bowel wall it must be included within the anastomotic suture to give an anastomosis optimal strength.
- **Mesentery to mesentery**. Apposition should be achieved where possible, ensuring that neither end of the bowel is twisted.

Technique of bowel anastomosis

The technique of anastomosis used is variable and, as is so often the case in surgery, the one actually employed by any surgeon is the one that is right for her/him. Our preferred technique is an interrupted extramucosal single layer anastomosis[9], using a 3/0 polydioxanone (PDS) suture (Fig. 35.5).

The use of staples for the enteric anastomosis has its proponents, who claim that it saves time. However, considering that operations often take in excess of 200 minutes, reducing around 10 minutes of handsewing time is of doubtful significance. Stapled anastomoses are also more expensive and there are concerns about possible higher anastomotic leakage rates. If nonabsorbable staples remain in contact with urine they can act as a nidus for stone formation[10,11]. Absorbable staples are now commercially available.

Complications of the bowel anastomosis are leakage, giving rise to peritonitis or fistulae, obstruction as a result of adhesions, stricture formation, and internal herniation.

Ureteroenteric anastomoses

There is considerable debate as to whether the ureterointestinal anastomosis should be created in a manner that prevents reflux of urine to the renal pelvis or not. There are reported series in

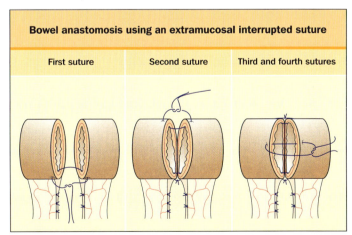

Figure 35.5 Bowel anastomosis using an extramucosal interrupted suture. (Left) First suture at mesenteric borders; (center) second suture at antimesenteric border; (right) third and fourth sutures between the first and second, dividing the anastomosis into quarters. Then interposing sutures every 4–5mm.

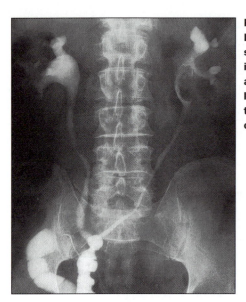

Figure 35.6 Loopogram study showing free reflux into the upper tract and demonstrating a left-side pelvic transitional cell cancer.

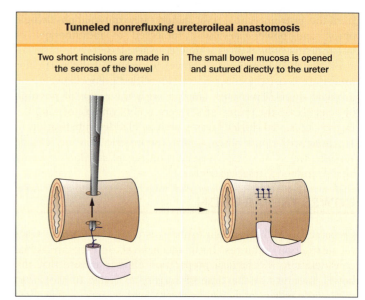

Tunneled nonrefluxing ureteroileal anastomosis	
Two short incisions are made in the serosa of the bowel	The small bowel mucosa is opened and sutured directly to the ureter

Figure 35.8 Tunneled nonrefluxing ureteroileal anastomosis. Two short incisions are made in the serosa of the bowel approximately four times the ureteric diameter apart. A submucosal tunnel is created by blunt dissection; the ureter is then drawn through this. At the distal ureteric end the small bowel mucosa is opened and sutured directly to the ureter. The serosa is then closed over this.

which up to 50% of kidneys deteriorate after conduit diversion, usually secondary to infection, stones, or obstruction. Some reports have suggested that this rate can be reduced with a non-refluxing anastomosis[12], but this is not a consistent finding[13].

With a system that allows reflux of urine, the intrarenal pressure is not significantly elevated above normal, and even with an antirefluxing anastomosis, bacterial colonization of the renal pelvis can often occur. We use a standard refluxing anastomosis, feeling it is quicker, easier, and has the added advantage that radiographic contrast can freely reflux into the upper tracts (Fig. 35.6). As the bulk of patients have had treatment for urothelial malignancy, this makes followup easier.

The principles of ureteroenteric anastomosis are similar to those of the intestinal anastomosis. Stripping of adventitia from the ureter should be minimized. Fine, absorbable, ideally non-braided sutures are used (such as 4/0 absorbable). The ureters should be adequately spatulated (opened along their length for about 2.5cm), thus increasing the circumference of the actual

anastomotic line and minimizing the risk of stricture formation. Performing the anastomosis over a fine Silastic® stent further reduces the risk of stricture formation[14]. These principles are well illustrated by the Wallace-type refluxing ureteroileal anastomosis[15], such as is used in an ileal loop urinary diversion (Fig. 35.7).

Nonrefluxing anastomoses are created either by tunneling a length of ureter through the bowel wall, as in the Leadbetter anastomosis[16] (Fig. 35.8), or the use of a split nipple technique, as popularized by Griffith (Fig. 35.9). The third option is the creation of an intestinal antireflux valve such as a Koch[17] nipple valve or an intussuscepted ileocecal valve.

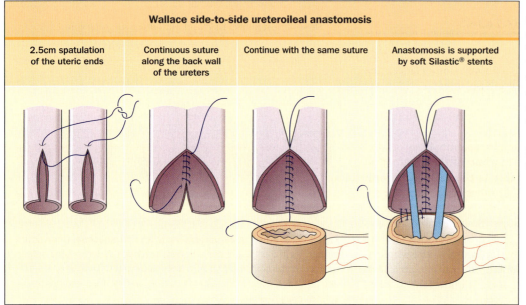

Wallace side-to-side ureteroileal anastomosis			
2.5cm spatulation of the uteric ends	Continuous suture along the back wall of the ureters	Continue with the same suture	Anastomosis is supported by soft Silastic® stents

Figure 35.7 Wallace side-to-side ureteroileal anastomosis. 2.5cm spatulation of the ureteric ends. First throw of the suture is at the apex of the spatulations, with the knot on the outside. Create a continuous suture along the back wall of the ureters, creating a 'boat' shape. Continuing with the same suture the rim of the 'boat' is anastomosed to the proximal bowel end with the anastomosis supported by soft Silastic® stents.

Complications of the ureteroenteric anastomosis include leakage giving rise to urinary fistulae and stricture formation. This often necessitates open correction, although in some cases it is amenable to either balloon dilatation or endourologic incision[18]. Pyelonephritis and the formation of upper tract stones may also occur.

DETUBULARIZATION

The ideal urinary reservoir is one that maximizes its volume with a minimal surface area (i.e. a sphere) and one that is devoid of any muscular activity within the wall, certainly during the storage phases. A low surface area is desirable as it reduces the length of bowel used and minimizes the area over which water and solute exchange can take place. Reconfiguration of the bowel to create a more spherical structure maximizes the capacity achieved for a given length of bowel.

Bowel is able to propel its luminal contents in a peristaltic fashion by coordinated contraction of the outer longitudinal and inner circular layers of muscle within its wall. These contractions cannot be abolished in the long term and will, when bowel is used to create reservoirs, result in tension in the reservoir wall. According to Laplace's law the tension in the wall is proportional to the product of the radius and the pressure; hence if the tension (i.e. the bowel wall contractions) is kept constant and the radius is increased the generated pressure falls. Thus formation of a near-spherical reservoir will reduce the pressure created.

Simple splitting of the bowel along its antimesenteric border, with reconfiguration, leads in the short term to a marked

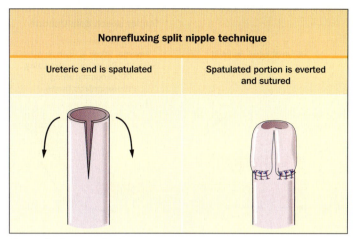

Figure 35.9 Nonrefluxing split nipple technique. The ureteric end is spatulated. The spatulated portion of ureter is everted and sutured back on to its own adventitial surface. This 'nipple' can then be implanted into a variety of bowel segments.

interruption of the coordinated muscular activity within the wall and results in reduced pressures. It has been shown, however, that over several months the muscular contractions within the bowel wall become more coordinated and, in some forms of reconstruction using detubularized right colon and ileum, pressures a year postoperatively have been recorded to be as high as that of normal large bowel (Fig. 35.10).

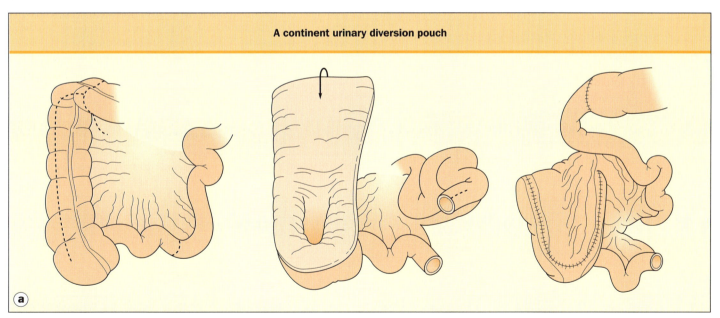

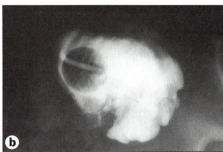

Figure 35.10 A continent urinary diversion pouch (an 'Indiana' pouch created from detubularized right colon and terminal ileum). (a) Line diagram. (b) Contrast study of pouch.

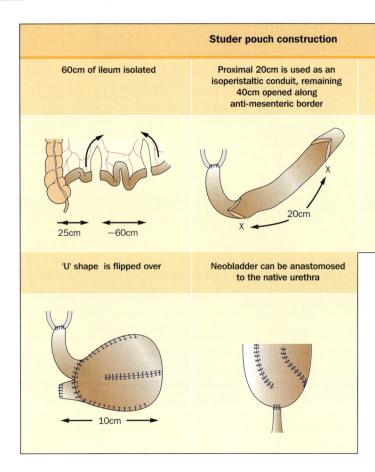

Studer pouch construction

| 60cm of ileum isolated | Proximal 20cm is used as an isoperistaltic conduit, remaining 40cm opened along anti-mesenteric border | One edge of small bowel is sutured to itself |
| 'U' shape is flipped over | Neobladder can be anastomosed to the native urethra | |

Figure 35.11 Studer pouch construction. (Top left) 60cm of ileum is isolated leaving 25cm of terminal ileum. (Top center) The proximal 20cm is used as an isoperistaltic conduit from the ureters. The remaining 40cm is opened along its antimesenteric border. (Top right) One edge of the small bowel is sutured to itself, giving a 'U' shape 20cm long (x–x). (Bottom left) This 'U' shape is then flipped over on to itself (y–y) to give a wide-diameter (approximately 8cm) cylinder about 10cm long, i.e. nearly spherical. (Bottom right) Finally, the near-spherical neobladder can then be anastomosed to the native urethra.

There are many different types of reconstructive procedure that illustrate the principles of bowel detubularization. A good example is the Studer-type bladder substitution[19] in which a crossfolded U configuration of detubularized ileum is employed (Fig. 35.11). This converts a 40cm length of ileum with a radius of 1cm and a volume of 125mL to a near-spherical shape 10cm long with a 4cm radius and a volume of around 500mL. As the radius of the reservoir created is quadrupled so the actual pressure generated for a given wall tension will be quartered (Fig. 35.12).

CATHETERIZABLE PORTS

Many patients are unable to generate adequate, sustained intravesical voiding pressures and need to perform intermittent self-catheterization to ensure complete bladder emptying. This is normally performed through the native urethra, but in some the urethra may have been removed or may be unsuitable, such as in neuropaths with urethral hypersensitivity. Under these circumstances the Mitrofanoff principle[20] allows creation of a continent extra-anatomic catheterization port. The Mitrofanoff principle is where a tubular structure, usually the appendix, is placed within a submucosal tunnel in the bladder or reservoir wall, creating a flap-valve effect. The intrareservoir pressure keeps the tube collapsed and hence continent during filling. To empty, the patient or carer passes a standard catheter (Figs 35.13 & 35.14).

Detubularization

	Length	Radius	Volume	Pressure (tension/radius)
	40cm	1cm	125	T/1
	10cm	4cm	500	T/4

Figure 35.12 Detubularization. Considering a 40cm section of ileum (radius 1cm) reconstructed into a pouch 10cm long with a radius of 4cm. By Laplace's law the tension in the wall is proportional to the product of the pressure and the radius.

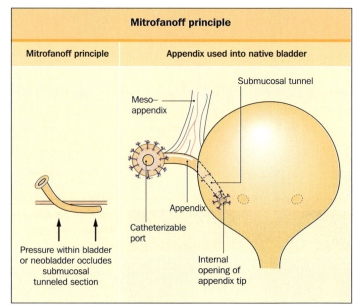

Mitrofanoff principle

Mitrofanoff principle | Appendix used into native bladder

Submucosal tunnel

Meso–appendix

Appendix

Catheterizable port

Internal opening of appendix tip

Pressure within bladder or neobladder occludes submucosal tunneled section

Figure 35.13 The Mitrofanoff principle. Pressure within the bladder or neobladder occludes the submucosal tunneled section, leading to fill phase continence. This example shows the appendix joined to the native bladder.

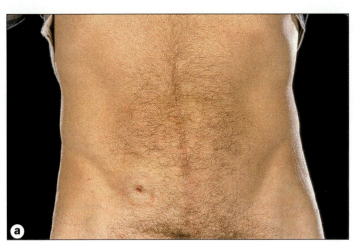
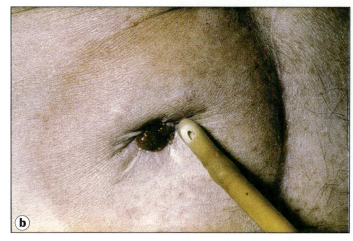

Figure 35.14 Continent catheterizable port. (a) Whole abdomen. (b) Close up.

The Monti procedure		
Isolate 2cm of ileum on mesentery	Segment opened	Tubularized over a suitable catheter

Figure 35.15 The Monti procedure.
(Left) A segment of ileum about 2cm in length is isolated on its mesentery. (Center) The segment is opened along the antimesenteric border and (right) tubularized over a suitable catheter.

The appendix may have been lost at previous appendicectomy or may be unsuitable because of scarring. In these situations other tubular structures such as ureter and fallopian tube can be used. Monti[21] described the creation of a narrow-gauge ileal tube using a short section of ileum. This technique uses a 2cm section of small bowel, which is isolated on its mesentery and then opened, usually on the antimesenteric border. This small sheet of small bowel is then retubularized over a suitable stent (approx. 12F), providing a tube of around 5–6cm in length, which can be used in a similar mechanism to those described for the appendix (Fig. 35.15). If this tube is rather short then two 'Montis' can be anastomosed together, doubling the length.

ABDOMINAL STOMAS

If an incontinent urinary diversion such as an ileal loop is performed a suitable abdominal stoma is necessary. Stomas are usually created in a protruding rosebud fashion to minimize urine contact with the skin and also reduce the rate of stomal stenosis. The stoma is created at a premarked site and should ideally traverse the rectus muscle to minimize parastomal hernia formation. The diameter of the abdominal wall defect should comfortably admit the base of an average-sized index finger.

The eversion of the bowel end is achieved by placing four absorbable sutures through skin, bowel serosa about 5cm from the cut end then all layers of the cut end in the 3, 6, 9, and

Creation of the urostomy stoma	
Four sutures inserted	Sutures tied

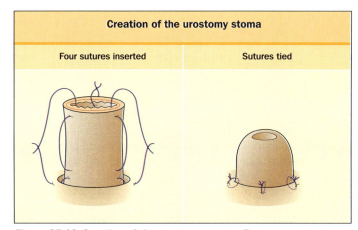

Figure 35.16 Creation of the urostomy stoma. Four sutures are inserted at 3, 6, 9, and 12 o'clock, each passing through the full thickness of the bowel end, a serosal bite about 5cm from the margin and the skin edge (only three sutures are illustrated here). The sutures are tied, leading to good eversion and the formation of a 'rosebud'.

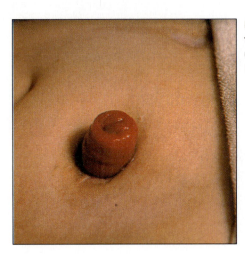

Figure 35.17 A well-fashioned rosebud urostomy. (Courtesy of Mr A T Tappe.)

12 o'clock positions. The gaps between these four sutures are closed with three or four cutaneous-to-bowel-end sutures (Figs 35.16 & 35.17).

Complications of stenosis and skin irritation can occur, as mentioned above. Other complications are stomal necrosis, obstruction, and parastomal hernias.

COMPLICATIONS OF THE USE OF BOWEL IN URINARY TRACT RECONSTRUCTION

Despite the many advances over the last three decades in the use of bowel for urinary tract reconstruction, a variety of complications are still recognized. These vary according to which segment of bowel has been used, which area of the urinary tract has been reconstructed, and the comorbidity of the patient. The patient should, where possible, be counseled preoperatively with regard to the frequency of these complications.

Renal deterioration

Reports as to the incidence of renal deterioration vary depending on the criteria used, i.e. upper tract dilatation on imaging, elevated serum creatinine, or the need for dialysis. The rates also vary depending on the original procedure. In patients with an ileal conduit urinary diversion, around 6% will ultimately die from renal failure[22] with over half showing some actual deterioration of one or both upper tracts. For many of the newer, continent diversions, long-term follow up of the incidence of renal impairment is not yet available.

Patients with already impaired renal function need very careful evaluation before long segments of intestine are used for possible continent diversions. The ability to acidify the urine after an ammonium chloride challenge, an increase in urine osmolality over 600mosmol/kg after water deprivation, and a glomerular filtration rate of over 35mL/min all suggest that the patient has enough renal reserve to prevent progressive renal deterioration[7].

The determination of renal function once urinary tract reconstruction has taken place is difficult. Urea and creatinine are reabsorbed from the urine by both ileum and colon and the serum levels will therefore not accurately reflect renal function. Water deprivation studies in these patients are also inappropriate as the 'leakiness' of bowel segment leads to dilution of the concentrated urine, hiding a true change of the urinary osmolality. Since bowel

also tends to alkalinize the urine, studies of renal acidification can be difficult to interpret[23].

Metabolic complications

In view of the morphologic makeup of the native urothelium, with its widespread tight junctions between the cells, the transfer of solvent and solutes across the bladder wall is virtually unknown. By contrast, bowel mucosa is inherently very different, allowing the diffusion of water and solutes quite readily and also transfer of different ions by active exchange. Bladder mucosa is almost flat; bowel has villi and microvilli, which lead to a vast increase in the surface area available for this exchange to occur.

A simple *aide memoire* for the junior doctor as to which metabolic complication can occur when bowel is used for urinary tract reconstruction is as follows. The stomach secretes hydrochloric acid. If the stomach is used to augment the bladder hydrochloric acid will inevitably be lost in the urine, which can result in a hypochloremic metabolic alkalosis. When small bowel or colon is used the opposite situation of a hyperchloremic metabolic acidosis may occur.

Hyperchloremic metabolic acidosis

The exact mechanism by which this occurs is not clear. Studies can be performed sampling venous blood returning from the bowel segment in patients or in animal models or by instilling radioisotope-labeled ions into the reservoir. The absorption of ammonium ions accompanied by chloride appears to be important[24]. In the liver, ammonium ions are converted to urea, releasing protons, which increases the acidic load on the body. Hydrogen ions associate with bicarbonate, forming carbon dioxide, which is excreted by the lungs in an attempted compensatory respiratory alkalosis, leading in the long term to a gross depletion of this important body buffer (Fig. 35.18).

Around 20% of patients with an ileal loop and up to 70% of patients with an ureterosigmoidostomy will develop hyperchloremic metabolic acidosis[25]. The secretion of bicarbonate by the bowel segment is greater in the latter and may account for the higher rate of this complication.

Patients in whom bowel is in contact with urine are in a continual osmotic diuresis due to the water reabsorption by their bowel segment; as the nephrons strive to maintain serum sodium levels there is an inevitable loss of potassium into the urine. Ileum tends to reabsorb potassium whereas colon does not; hence hypokalemia tends to be more of a problem where ureterocolonic diversions have been performed[26].

Symptoms of hyperchloremic metabolic acidosis are anorexia, weight loss, polydipsia, lethargy, and easy fatigability. Its correction involves systemic alkalization with sodium bicarbonate or potassium citrate. Chloride transport blockers such as chlorpromazine or nicotinic acid have also occasionally been used. It is important that, if potassium replacement is needed, it is undertaken concurrently with correction of the acidosis.

Hypochloremic metabolic alkalosis

The hypochloremic metabolic alkalosis associated with the use of stomach in urinary tract reconstruction also tends to be associated with hypokalemia but rarely gives rise to clinically significant problems unless the patient has associated renal failure. It does have some theoretic advantages in the patient

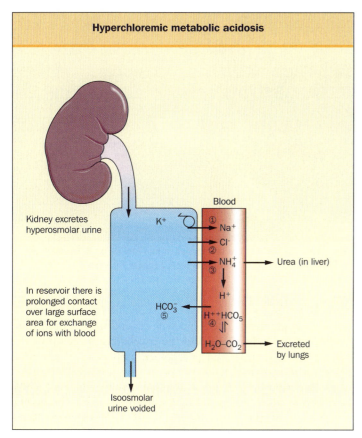

Figure 35.18 Hyperchloremic metabolic acidosis. (1) Sodium is absorbed from the hypertonic urine, some in exchange for potassium. (2) Chloride is absorbed with sodium. (3) Ammonium is absorbed, which is then converted to urea in the liver, releasing hydrogen ions. (4) Buffering of hydrogen ions with bicarbonate creates carbon dioxide, which is excreted by the lungs. (5) Bicarbonate is also excreted by the bowel wall (more so by the colon), leading to further loss of this buffer. K^+, potassium; Na^+, sodium; Cl^-, chloride; NH_4^+, ammonium; HCO_3^-, bicarbonate; CO_2, carbon dioxide; H_2O, water.

who is unable to satisfactorily acidify the urine. Some patients complain of dysuric syndrome, which is not always corrected by deacidification of their urine with agents such as proton pump blockers[27].

Jejunal conduit syndrome

Jejunum is generally avoided for urinary tract diversion[28] because of its excessive 'leakiness'. Severe hyponatremia, hypochloremia, hyperkalemia, renal failure, and acidosis can occur in up to at least a quarter of patients who have a high small bowel diversion.

Mucus

Bowel normally secretes mucus to aid lubrication and as a protective barrier for its own mucosa. Transplanted bowel will continue to do this and in fact may do this with higher rates of mucus production (diversion colitis)[29]. Mucus can lead to problems if it is not adequately cleared by the urine, predisposing to infection, catheter blockage, and stones. Ensuring adequate hydration, the use of suitably large intermittent catheterization catheters, and regular use of bladder washouts enhances mucus

clearance. Cranberry juice consumption has its proponents. Occasionally, drugs such as N-acetylcysteine can be instilled into the pouch to help break down mucus[30].

Infection

Bacteriuria is common after the insertion of bowel into the urinary tract such that around three quarters of urinary specimens from patients with ileal conduits contain organisms[31]. Many of these conduits are just colonized at the distal end and do not come to any chronic harm. It would appear that pure cultures of *Proteus* and *Pseudomonas* are more likely to be associated with deterioration of the upper tracts and significant septic episodes and an attempt should be made to sterilize the urine under these circumstances.

Stones

Persistent alkalization, frequent bacteriuria, and abnormal anatomy all contribute to a higher incidence of stones in conduits and pouches. Mucus and any foreign body such as staples will form a nidus for stone formation[32] (Fig. 35.19). Stones are generally formed of a mix of calcium, magnesium, and ammonium phosphate and are managed by standard techniques. Clearly, retrograde instrumentation of the urinary tract may be more difficult or impossible. Stones within pouches can adequately and safely be dealt with by percutaneous means, unless they are large[33].

Perforation

Transposed segments of bowel lack the normal sensory innervation of the native urinary tract. Hence, if structures such as ileal neobladders are overdistended as a result of either obstruction or patient failure to ensure adequate emptying, this can cause minimal symptoms until neobladder rupture occurs[34]. Unless diagnosed and treated appropriately by prompt laparotomy the resulting urinary peritonitis can be life-threatening. Patients need clear education on the importance of regular drainage of urine to avoid this potentially catastrophic complication.

Osteomalacia

Demineralization of the bone can occur and is probably the result of many factors, of which metabolic acidosis is probably the most important[35]. A gradual release of calcium from the bones occurs in an attempt to buffer excessive hydrogen ions; calcium is then excreted by the kidneys. In some patients correction of the acidosis itself does not result in remineralization and these patients may require supplementation with 1α–hydroxy-cholecalciferol.

Growth and development

Delay in growth has been found in children who have undergone enterocystoplasty[36]. It is unclear as to the exact cause of this: whether it is the result of bone demineralization indirectly or via hyperchloremic acidosis.

Altered sensorium

This may occur in patients for a variety of reasons, such as magnesium deficiency, drug intoxication, or abnormalities of ammonia metabolism[7]. Ammoniogenic coma can occur, particularly in those with previously altered liver function. This may be

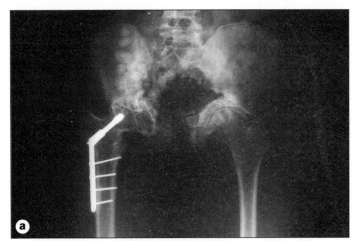

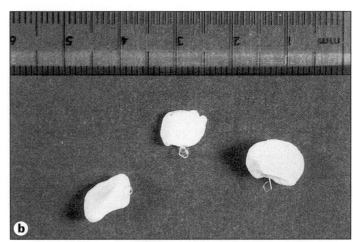

Figure 35.19 Stones within a continent diversion pouch. (a) The patient had received radiotherapy many years ago for a cervical neoplasm leading to a fibrotic bladder and the bony destruction seen in the radiograph. (b) Many of the stones had in fact formed on the staples used to create the reservoir. (Courtesy of Mr K J Hastie.)

corrected by adequate drainage of the urinary segments and the use of antibiotics such as neomycin to reduce the ammonium load in the enteric tract.

Abnormal drug metabolism

Abnormal drug absorption can occur when either the drug or the active metabolite is excreted by the kidney and then reabsorbed by the gastrointestinal segment. An example of this is methotrexate toxicity, which has been reported in patients with an ileal conduit[37]. Generally, patients with continent diversion receiving chemotherapy should have the pouch catheterized to minimize the quantity and time that either drug or its metabolite is in contact with the bowel segment.

Nutritional effects of removal of segments of the gastrointestinal tract

Loss of significant lengths of bowel can lead to a short bowel syndrome, with increase in gastrointestinal transit times. This can be exacerbated by loss of the ileocecal valve. Fatty acid absorption and bowel salt reabsorption are deranged when the terminal ileum has been sacrificed, which results in diarrhea. Diarrhea will exacerbate any problems with dehydration. The lack of fat absorption can lead to deficiencies of fat-soluble vitamins such as A and D. Correction of the diarrhea can be helped by cholestyramine to sequest the bile salts, and a low-fat diet[38].

Loss of the terminal ileum can lead to vitamin B_{12} deficiency. Monitoring and early institution of vitamin B supplementation is needed to prevent anemia and neurologic abnormalities in these patients[39].

Removal of sections of stomach is usually without problems, although it can result in a diminished appetite. Again, theoretically vitamin B_{12} absorption may be deranged because of a reduction in secretion of intrinsic factor from the stomach.

Psychologic effects

Around one quarter of patients with a stoma experience clinically significant psychologic symptoms postoperatively[40]. The psychologic effects of the use of bowel in urinary tract reconstruction are debated and will depend on the procedure performed, its indications, and the psychologic makeup of the patient. For example, the psychologic impact of a continent diversion in a patient who was previously urologically normal until the diagnosis of his/her muscle-invasive bladder cancer will be different from the impact on a spina bifida adult undergoing undiversion of the incontinent urinary loop diversion their doctors (and parents) blessed them with as a child.

Many studies have assessed whether patients undergoing continent versus incontinent urinary diversions have a better quality of life. Sexual problems, disturbed relationships with partners, emotional, and mental problems have been found to be common, occurring with the same frequency in both groups[41]. More recent studies have challenged this, showing that the number of sexual and nonsexual physical contacts was reduced for the majority of ileal conduit patients but only in the minority who had undergone bladder substitution[42]. Superior self-ratings of physical strength, mental capacity, leisure time activities, and social competence have been reported in patients undergoing continent reservoir construction[43]. None of these studies randomized the patients, so conclusions need to be treated with some caution.

Malignancy risk

Patients who had undergone ureterosigmoidostomies without diversion of fecal stream have been found after many years of followup to have an alarmingly high rate of adenocarcinoma at or near the anastomosis. In one series, patients who had a ureterosigmoidostomy for exstrophy had an excess risk 7000 times normal, with over 40% of patients developing this form of malignancy[44]. The mixture of urine and feces appears to be responsible for these malignancies, probably as a result of formation of nitroso compounds due to the action of fecal bacteria on the urinary nitrites[45].

The malignancy risks of ureterosigmoidostomy took many decades to become fully appreciated. The actual malignant potential of use of bowel elsewhere in the urinary system is not yet fully known and remains a concern to the urologic surgeon of today, particularly in the younger patient.

Neoplasms in bladder augmentations have occurred, though the numbers remain small. The bulk of these occurred in patients who were reconstructed for tuberculosis. The mean time to diagnosis was around 18 years[46]. There are very few cases of primary neoplasm in ileal conduits (two cases of adenomatous polyps)[47]. Despite primary colon adenocarcinoma being common there are only three cases of this tumor arising in colonic conduits. To date there are no established cases of adenocarcinoma in continent enteric diversions[48].

In view of the possible malignancy risks of bowel transplanted into the urinary system, patients in whom these procedures have been performed require long-term followup. How best this should be done is not yet clear but it should probably include endoscopic, cytologic, and radiographic studies.

SUMMARY

Bowel is an essential material for the reconstructive urologic surgeon. By observing basic principles a wide range of reconstructive procedures can be performed, the technical details of which will be covered in other chapters. While complications can and do occur, careful technique and patient selection can minimize their occurrence. The use of bowel in reconstructive urology is still an evolving field of surgery. The change is being driven by the need to minimize complications, the discovery with time of new complications, and the demands and needs of the patients.

REFERENCES

1. Simon J. Ectopia vesicae; operation for directing the orifices of the ureter into the rectum; temporary success; subsequent death; autopsy. Lancet. 1852;2:568.
2. Spence HM, Hoffman WW, Fosmire GP. Tumour of the colon as a late complication of ureterosigmoidostomy for extrophy of the bladder. Br J Urol. 1979;51:466–70.
3. Bricker EM. Bladder substitution after pelvic evisceration. Surg Clin North Am. 1950;30:1511–21.
4. Neal DE. Complications of ileal conduit diversion in adults with cancer followed up for at least five years. Br Med J (Clin Res Ed). 1985;290(6483):1695–7.
5. Lapides J, Diokno AC, Gould FR, et al. Further observations and self-catheterisation. J Urol. 1976;116:169.
6. Bissada SA, Bissada NK. Choice of gastroepiploic vessels for gastrocystoplasty. J Urol. 1993;150:707–9.
7. McDougal WS. Use of intestinal segments in urinary diversion. In: Walsh PC et al. (eds) Campbell's urology, vol. 3, 7th edn. Philadelphia: WB Saunders; 1997:3121–61.
8. Nichols RL, Condon RE, Gorback SL, Nyhus LM. Efficacy of preoperative antimicrobial preparation of the bowel. Ann Surg. 1972;176:227–32.
9. Carty NJ, Keating J, Campbell J, Karanjia N, Heald RJ. Prospective audit of an extramucosal technique for intestinal anastomosis. Br J Surg. 1991;78(12):1439–41.
10. Didolkar MS, Reed WP, Elias EG, et al. A prospective randomized study of sutured versus stapled bowel anastomoses in patients with cancer. Cancer. 1986;57(3):456–60.
11. Dangman BC, Lebowitz RL. Urinary tract calculi that form on surgical staples: a characteristic radiologic appearance. AJR. 1991;157(1):115–7.
12. Richie JP, Skinner DG. Urinary diversion: the physiological rationale for non-refluxing colonic conduits. Br J Urol. 1975;47(3):269–75.
13. Hill JT, Ransley PG The colonic conduit: a better method of urinary diversion? Br J Urol. 1983;55(6):629–31.
14. Regan JB, Barrett DM. Stented versus nonstented ureteroileal anastomoses: is there a difference with regard to leak and stricture? J Urol. 1985;134(6):1101–3.
15. Wallace DM. Uretero-ileostomy. Br J Urol. 1970;42:529–34.
16. Leadbetter WF, Clarke BG. Five years' experience with the ureteroenterostomy by the combined technique. J Urol. 1954;73:67–82.
17. Nieh PT. Use of bowel in urological surgery: the Kock pouch urinary reservoir. Urol Clin North Am. 1997;24(4):755–72.
18. Meretyk S, Clayman RV, Kavoussi LR, Kramolowsky EV, Picus DD. Endourological treatment of ureteroenteric anastomotic strictures: long-term followup. J Urol. 1991;145(4):723–7.
19. Studer UE, Zingg EJ. Use of bowel in urological surgery: ileal orthotopic bladder substitutes. Urol Clin North Am. 1997;24(4):781–93.
20. Mitrofanoff P. [Trans-appendicular continent cystostomy in the management of the neurogenic bladder]. Chir Pediatr. 1980;21(4):297–305.
21. Monti PR, Lara RC, Dutra MA, de Carvalho JR. New techniques for construction of efferent conduits based on the Mitrofanoff principle. Urology. 1997;49(1):112–5.
22. Richie JP. Intestinal loop urinary diversion in children. J Urol. 1974;111(5):687–9.
23. McDougal WS, Koch MO. Accurate determination of renal function in patients with intestinal urinary diversions. J Urol. 1986;135(6):1175–8.
24. Djavan B, Fakhari M, Roehrborn CG, Marberger M. Metabolic consequences of urinary diversion with intestinal segments. Tech Urol. 1998;4(4):177–81.
25. Allen TD, Roehrborn CG, Peters PC. Long term follow-up of patients after cystectomy and urinary diversion via ileal loop versus ureterosigmoidostomy. J Urol. 1989;141:350A.
26. Koch MO, Gurevitch E, Hill DE, McDougal WS. Urinary solute transport by intestinal segments: a comparative study of ileum and colon in rats. J Urol. 1990;143(6):1275–9.
27. Gosalbez R Jr, Woodard JR, Broecker BH, Warshaw B. Metabolic complications of the use of stomach for urinary reconstruction. J Urol. 1993;150(2 Pt 2):710–12.
28. Mansson W, Lindstedt E. Electrolyte disturbances after jejunal conduit urinary diversion. Scand J Urol Nephrol. 1978;12(1):17–21.
29. Edwards CM, George B, Warren B. Diversion colitis – new light through old windows. Histopathology. 1999;34(1):1–5.
30. Gillon G, Mundy AR. The dissolution of urinary mucus after cystoplasty. Br J Urol. 1989;63(4):372–4.
31. Guinan PD, Moore RH, Neter E, Murphy GP. The bacteriology of ileal conduit urine in man. Surg Gynecol Obstet. 1972; 134(1):78–82.
32. Ginsberg D, Huffman JL, Lieskovsky G, Boyd S, Skinner DG. Urinary tract stones: a complication of the Kock pouch continent urinary diversion. J Urol. 1991;145(5):956–9.
33. Woodhouse CRJ, Lennon GM. Management and aetiology of stones in intestinal urinary reservoirs. Br J Urol. 1998;81(suppl 4):47.
34. Desgrandchamps F, Cariou G, Barthelemy Y, et al. Spontaneous rupture of orthotopic detubularized ileal bladder replacement: report of 5 cases. J Urol. 1997;158(3 Pt 1):798–800.
35. Siklos P, Davie M, Jung RT, Chalmers TM. Osteomalacia in ureterosigmoidostomy: healing by correction of the acidosis. Br J Urol. 1980;52(1):61–2.

36. Woodhouse CRJ. The infective, metabolic and histological consequences of enterocystoplasty. EBU Update Series. 1994;3(2):10–5.

37. Bowyer GW, Davies TW. Methotrexate toxicity associated with an ileal conduit. Br J Urol. 1987;60(6):592.

38. Einarsson K Metabolic effects caused by exclusion of intestinal segments. Scand J Urol Nephrol Suppl. 1992;142:21–6.

39. Steiner MS, Morton RA, Marshall FF. Vitamin B_{12} deficiency in patients with ileocolic neobladders. J Urol. 1993;149(2):255–7.

40. White CA, Hunt JC. Psychological factors in postoperative adjustment to stoma surgery. Ann R Coll Surg Engl. 1997;79(1):3–7.

41. Mansson A, Johnson G, Mansson W. Quality of life after cystectomy. Comparison between patients with conduit and those with continent caecal reservoir urinary diversion. Br J Urol. 1988;62(3):240–5.

42. Bjerre BD, Johansen C, Steven K. Health-related quality of life after cystectomy: bladder substitution compared with ileal conduit diversion. A questionnaire survey. Br J Urol. 1995;75(2):200–5.

43. Gerharz EW, Weingartner K, Dopatka T, et al. Quality of life after cystectomy and urinary diversion: results of a retrospective interdisciplinary study. J Urol. 1997;158(3 Pt 1):778–85.

44. Krishnamsetty RM, Rao MK, Hines CR, et al. Adenocarcinoma in extrophy and defunctional ureterosigmoidostomy. J Ky Med Assoc. 1988;86(8):409–14.

45. Stewart M. Urinary diversion and bowel cancer. Ann R Coll Surg Engl. 1986;68(2):98–102.

46. Filmer RB, Spencer JR Malignancies in bladder augmentations and intestinal conduits. J Urol. 1990;143(4):671–8.

47. Tomera KM, Unni KK, Utz DC. Adenomatous polyp in ileal conduit. J Urol. 1982;128(5):1025–6.

48. Malone MJ, Izes JK, Hurley LJ. Carcinogenesis. The fate of intestinal segments used in urinary reconstruction. Urol Clin North Am. 1997;24(4):723–8.

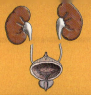
Chapter 36

Urinary Diversion and Augmentation

Christopher RJ Woodhouse

KEY POINTS

- The lower urinary tract has three components – a reservoir, a continence mechanism, and a conduit.
- If any part is congenitally absent, or irretrievably damaged, reconstruction is usually possible.
- The main justification for bladder reconstruction is the patient's quality of life.
- Some patients may accept the stoma of an ileal conduit rather than risk the complications associated with reconstruction.
- Especially in younger patients, there is overwhelming enthusiasm for anything that avoids 'a bag'.
- Many techniques for reconstruction are now available; the choice should be tailored to the individual patient and their particular needs.

INTRODUCTION

The lower urinary tract can be considered as three largely independent components – a reservoir in which the urine is stored, a continence mechanism, and a conduit to the surface. The natural bladder, its sphincters, and the urethra are better than anything that can be constructed by a surgeon and should be preserved if at all possible. If some of the natural components are congenitally absent or have to be removed, reconstruction is usually possible. If all are to be removed the urine may be diverted into a continent reservoir or to a wet stoma.

Great ingenuity has gone into devising operations for urinary diversion. Historically, three distinct phases can be seen. From the beginning of modern surgery in the second half of the 19th century, the urine was diverted into the colon and continence depended on the integrity of the anal sphincter. The ureterosigmoidostomy was the most commonly used but there were several variations designed to limit the infective complications.

The second phase began in 1950 with the introduction of the ileal conduit[1]. It is ironic that the management of the complications of ureterosigmoidostomy was just beginning to be understood at the time when its replacement was devised. The third phase, continent urinary diversion, first became practical with the adaptation of the Kock pouch for the storage of urine[2]. Since then a large number of different continent diversions have been devised. Many differ from each other only in small details.

Throughout this development, but particularly in the last 50 years, small but neurologically normal bladders have been augmented with ileum. The introduction of clean intermittent self-catheterization (CISC) by Lapides has allowed this technique to be extended to patients with a neuropathic bladder[3].

THE ILEAL CONDUIT

Indications

The ileal conduit (Fig. 36.1) waxes and wanes in popularity according to the perceived problems of the alternatives. It could, therefore, be thought of as the 'standard' diversion. In spite of all the alternatives, some patients, particularly those requiring cystectomy for cancer, may still opt for a stoma: the advantages of reconstruction are primarily cosmetic and the increased complication rate may be unacceptable.

It is difficult to appreciate just how much of an advance the ileal conduit was. The early complications were severe: in a series of 212 patients (claimed to be too small for statistical analysis) the mortality and major morbidity rate was 25%. However, nearly half the patients were undergoing cystectomy for cancer and their mortality was 30%. It is more striking to note that 27 of 39 (69%) hydronephrotic kidneys in surviving patients were improved at 3- to 6-month follow-up. The incidence of pyelitis in 156 patients discharged from hospital was only 7%. Improvement in general wellbeing and vigor were 'constant features'[4]. In another series, 29 of 30 patients managed their cutaneous appliance satisfactorily with only an occasional leakage[5]. In the spina bifida children there was an opportunity, for the first time, to control incontinence and upper tract deterioration.

In the last 40 years there have been some changes in the technique of ureteric anastomosis and in the formation of the stoma. Appliances for urine collection have improved considerably. The basic idea has stood the test of time.

The ileal conduit
Well-established operative technique
Low complication rate of about 9%
No significant metabolic complications
Requires stoma
Quality of life reduced in some physical and sexual aspects

Figure 36.1 The ileal conduit.

It is difficult to give a complication rate for ileal conduit alone as most of such operations are done in association with an exenteration for cancer. In Hendry's series of 118 survivors, there were 10 complications (8.5%) related to the conduit[6].

It would, therefore, seem reasonable to accept that the ileal conduit is the simplest form of definitive diversion. In the longer term, the results are much less good, but it should not be assumed that any of the newer forms of continent diversion will be any better (Fig. 36.2).

Long-term aspects

All external urinary diversions impose a severe burden on the child and adolescent. The more philosophical view of the older adult may allow an easier acceptance of such a change in body image. It must be remembered that many children, especially with exstrophy, have grown up to be well-adjusted and normal adults in spite of the bag. In considering 58 young adults for operations to remove the bag in one way or another, I have found 6 who claimed to be happy as they were.

There have been several large reviews of the long-term results of ileal conduits. All testify to the high complication and reoperation rates. For example, in a series with 75 children who could be reviewed between 10 and 16 years after diversion, only 12 had not had at least one complication[7]. With such poor surgical results it would be difficult to identify psychosocial problems specifically related to the bag. Dunn found a 27% incidence of psychologic problems in 55 children followed for a mean of 10 years. The children attended special schools for the handicapped. They had educational problems through lack of contact with teachers and normal children. Older children restricted their social lives and suffered sexual problems[8].

Psychologic problems have been found in adults with ileal conduits. In a group largely of cancer patients it was commented that many of the problems could be avoided by good preoperative counseling and surgical techniques that gave an easily managed stoma. Of 29 working patients, 20 returned to their previous jobs but nearly two thirds of all the patients restricted their social lives because of the stoma[6].

It has been presumed that a continent diversion gives a better quality of life (QOL) than a conduit. However, the first survey that attempted to look at this issue found that there was little to choose between the ileal conduit and the Kock pouch. Patients with each type of diversion felt happy in their social surroundings and there was no difference in the rate of return to work or the performance of daily tasks. Ileal conduit patients had lower expectations, poor self-image, and less physical contact. Some 22% of ileal conduit patients were sexually active compared to 48% of Kock pouch patients[9]. Although this survey was done largely on cancer patients, it does have some important lessons for other groups. More recent reviews have shown an advantage in QOL for continent reconstructions (see below).

Renal aspects

The short-term follow-up of patients with ileal conduits was very encouraging. Although it was recognized that some normal kidneys were damaged by the diversion, the commoner situation was improvement of grossly distended kidneys or stabilization of moderately distended ones. For example 83% of 62 children undergoing ileal conduit diversion because of renal deterioration were improved or stable according to the first postoperative urogram. Even at 10- to 16-year follow-up Shapiro found that 70% of previously normal kidneys remained so[7]. With longer followup the rate of renal deterioration is high. Three types of renal damage are seen: dilated kidneys, small scarred kidneys, and stones. Early renal damage is symptomless but can be detected by careful followup. Advanced renal damage is a tragedy that could have been avoided.

Dilatation is usually due to obstruction. The commonest site is the stoma and the distal conduit, secondly the ureteroileal junction, and thirdly where the left ureter passes behind the root of the intestinal mesentery to reach the conduit lying on the other side.

Stomal stenosis is reported in 5–75% of patients (Fig. 36.3). It is important to put a finger in the stoma at routine follow-up to search for this complication as the obstruction is commonly at fascial level. The stoma itself may look normal. Stomal prolapse may occur if the conduit is too long (Fig. 36.4).

The residual urine on catheterization of the conduit should be small: 3–15mL has been quoted[7]. However, it is difficult to make a big fuss of a single high residual, especially if the urine is sterile on culture. A repeatedly high residual of infected urine, especially if the bacteriuria is not cleared by appropriate antibiotic therapy, suggests outlet obstruction and is also an indication for upper tract imaging.

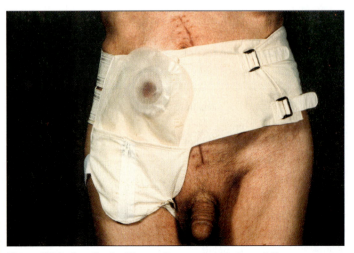

Figure 36.2 A patient with a well-managed ileal conduit.

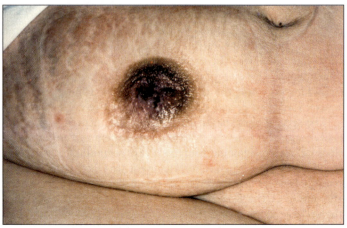

Figure 36.3 An ileal stoma that is flush with the skin and stenosed.

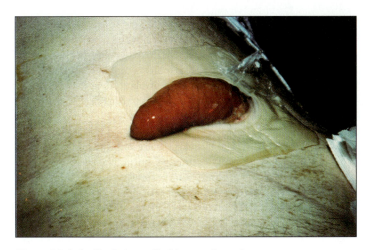

Figure 36.4 An ileal stoma that has prolapsed.

The stenosis may also provoke vigorous peristaltic waves that are of high amplitude and are associated with raised resting pressure. Kidneys draining into conduits with this activity are almost invariably dilated. True anatomic or functional obstruction of the stoma appears to be the cause and the dilatation will be improved by stomal revision[10].

Ureteroileal stenosis may occur at any time. It is much less common than stomal stenosis, being reported in 5–10% of patients. It may be the cause of up to 25% of episodes of renal dilatation[7]. If the Wallace system of anastomosing the ureters side to side and then joining them to the ileum is used, it is likely that both will stenose together.

Small, scarred kidneys are caused by infection with or without obstruction. An ileal conduit should not be infected. The urine in the bag and swabs of the stoma are invariably positive on culture. Urine collected from the depths of the conduit by catheter should not be. Ideally, specimens should be collected with a catheter passed down the lumen of an outer catheter to avoid contamination. In practice a pure culture of a typical organism in a catheter specimen is acceptable.

A statistically significant association has been shown between the urographic finding of small kidneys and the antibody titer of *Escherichia coli* or *Proteus mirabilis*. In 26 patients with raised antibodies only four had normal kidneys, whereas 89% of patients with normal urograms had normal titers[11]. Although this does not prove cause and effect, others have noted the association between bacteriuria, urinary tract dilatation, and renal damage. It would certainly support the clinical observation.

Stones are seen in 5–30% of patients. They most often occur in the kidneys but have been seen in the ureters and even, occasionally, in the conduit. In patients who are not stone-formers before diversion, 90% of stones are associated with *Proteus* infection. Other precipitating factors are ureteral dilatation, recurrent pyelonephritis, conduit residuals above 10mL, and minor degrees of hyperchloremic acidosis (HCA)[12].

Metabolic problems

In practice, the metabolic consequences of forming an ileal conduit are negligible. Experiments have usually been done on relatively fresh conduits that still maintain their normal villi. There can be difficulty in diabetics, who may not have glycosuria with a high blood sugar. Well-established conduits with the villous atrophy that occurs within a year or so of their formation have little metabolic function.

A problem may arise in patients with bladder cancer who are given methotrexate. Elevated blood levels of this drug were found in 8 of 11 patients 2 days after administration of 250mg/m^2. Patients with conduits less than 2 years old or that were unusually long were particularly at risk[13]. This may require dose reduction or delay in therapy, problems that were found in 84% of patients in one series[14].

COLON CONDUITS

The colon conduit is newer than the ileal conduit and large, long-term series are lacking. Its stoma is unlikely to be different in its psychologic effects from that of the ileum. In follow-up to 21 years colon conduits have been shown to have similar complication rates to ileal conduits. There has been some suggestion that the antireflux mechanism, when successful (about 50% of anastomoses) protects the kidneys from parenchymal scarring[15].

CUTANEOUS URETEROSTOMY

The cutaneous ureterostomy is seldom used as a permanent form of diversion. It is difficult to make a satisfactory stoma. In a group of children followed for at least 6 years, 8 of 16 survivors had to have an intestinal conduit formed for stomal complications. Although stomal stenosis can largely be avoided by suturing a triangular flap of skin into the spatulated end of the ureter, this modification only improved the revision rate to 30%[16].

In patients who are dying of cancer and who require a diversion, usually for intractable incontinence, the procedure is useful. It is easiest if there is at least one dilated ureter, although I have used it successfully in patients with two normal ureters. It is more convenient to transfer one ureter across and anastomose it to the other as a transureteroureterostomy than to make two stomas. The dilated ureter will make a satisfactory stoma with a skin flap and a small spout. In one series, all 8 patients had an acceptable outcome with maximum survival of 1 year[17].

URETEROSIGMOIDOSTOMY AND VARIATIONS

The ureterosigmoidostomy (Fig. 36.5) has had a minor resurgence since 1990 as the shortcomings of the other diversions are realized. Furthermore, lessons can be learnt from the long-term follow-up of the ureterosigmoidostomy that are relevant to the newer forms of diversion and reconstruction.

It is surprising that the main mechanical drawback to the ureterosigmoidostomy was not recognized earlier. The need for a low-pressure reservoir has been known for at least 25 years and yet no one attempted to reduce the intrarectal pressure, which has been known to be up to 200cmH$_2$O since Coffey's work in 1911[18]. High storage pressure leads to recurrent pyelonephritis and incontinence. The newer versions with reduced rectal pressures have a lower rate of complications.

In the Mansoura system, the rectum is opened longitudinally and augmented with an opened segment of ileum. The ureters are implanted into the rectum. The sigmoid colon is intussuscepted to prevent reflux of urine into the rest of the colon (Fig. 36.6)[19].

A simpler system, called the Mainz 2, avoids the use of an augment or a nipple. The rectosigmoid is opened longitudinally over about 20cm and the ureters are implanted. It is then closed transversely to create a low-pressure reservoir (Fig. 36.7)[20].

Indications

As with all diversions, the indications are relative and it is easier to consider the contraindications. Continence depends on a competent anus. Therefore, no patient with a neuropathy should have a ureterosigmoidostomy of any type. Women who have had several pregnancies and elderly patients may have a weak anus: it is helpful to ask to what extent they can control diarrhea or flatus. The anus can be tested by filling the rectum with 500mL of a slurry made from water and a cereal (porridge

---

The modified ureterosigmoidostomy

Old technique improved by the formation of a low-pressure reservoir

Anal continence in 95% of patients

Offensive-smelling slurry

50% incidence of hyperchloremic acidosis

Complicated by anastomotic tumors in 20% of patients after 20 years

Suitable for patients requiring urethrectomy for cancer

Figure 36.5 The modified ureterosigmoidostomy.

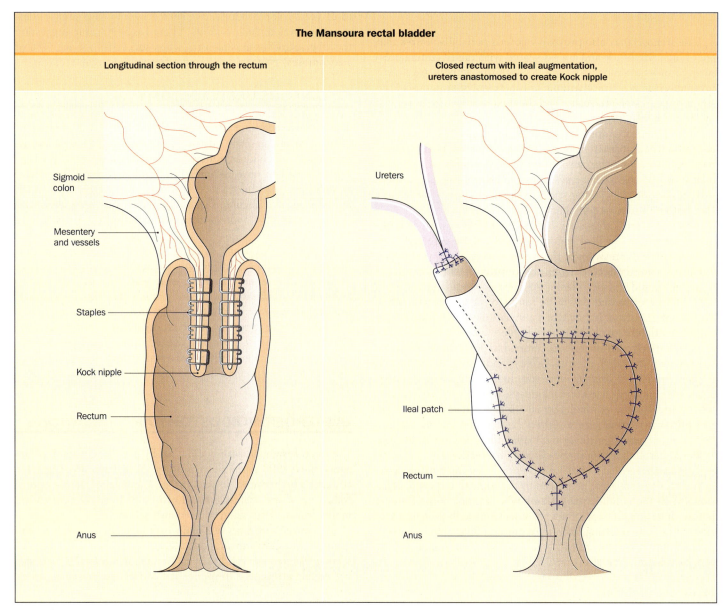

Figure 36.6 The Mansoura rectal bladder. (Left) Longitudinal section through the rectum. The sigmoid colon has been intussuscepted as a Kock nipple; (right) the rectum is closed with an ileal augmentation. The ureters have been anastomosed to a Kock nipple in the ileum. (Reproduced with permission from Mundy AR, et al. Urodynamics: principles, practice and application, 2nd edn. Edinburgh: Churchill Livingstone; 1994.)

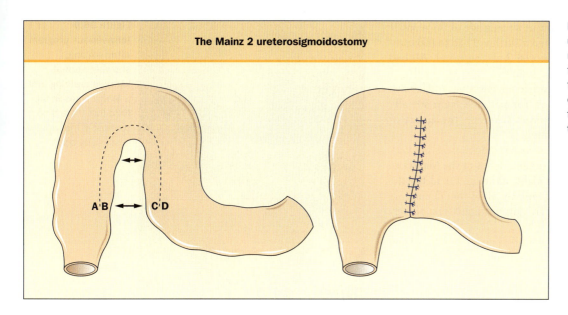

The Mainz 2 ureterosigmoidostomy

Figure 36.7 The Mainz 2 ureterosigmoidostomy. The rectum and sigmoid are laid in a 'U' formation and incised over 20cm from AB to CD. After implantation of the ureters, the reservoir is formed by closing the bowel transversely, A to D and B to C.

test); the mixture should be held easily for at least an hour. Anorectal manometry and electromyelography have also been recommended[20]. Patients who have had pelvic radiotherapy or who have extensive diverticular disease also should not be considered for this diversion.

Modified ureterosigmoidostomy is probably less satisfactory as a diversion than an orthotopic bladder reconstruction. There are a few patients for whom the risk of incontinence or the possibility of requiring CISC with an orthotopic reconstruction are unacceptable, and who would prefer a modified ureterosigmoidostomy.

In patients with bladder cancer who have to lose the urethra as well as the bladder, I believe that the modified ureterosigmoidostomy is preferable to the suprapubic continent diversions. The complication rate is lower and the ability to 'void' rather than to use a catheter is welcome. Conversely, gay men require careful and sensitive counseling before recommending a ureterosigmoidostomy.

The modified ureterosigmoidostomy is particularly useful in poorer countries. The simplicity of construction, low complication rate and freedom from expensive catheters and bags all contribute. Even the main complication, HCA, is relatively cheap to treat.

Short-term complications

The surgical complications of the modified ureterosigmoidostomies appear to be uncommon. It is difficult to give figures as the modifications are new and experience is limited. Reports of large series of the original operation are so old as to be irrelevant: infection and fistulae were common. Now, bowel preparation, antibiotics, and better suture materials have considerably reduced such problems. In the published work on the modified operations, the surgical complication rate is about 5%.

Subsequent radiologic testing of the antireflux mechanism has proved difficult: even when watery contrast is put into the rectum it does not reflux. The presence of gas in the ureter and in the renal pelvis is the best indication that reflux is occurring and this is seldom seen in the modified ureterosigmoidostomies (Fig. 36.8).

Long-term results
Continence

Patients who have had a conventional ureterosigmoidostomy since early childhood are satisfied with their lot. I have never encountered one who wanted to change the diversion. Even in 6 patients operated on for neoplasm of the ureteric anastomosis, all wished to have a new ureterosigmoid anastomosis rather than a safer diversion. In my own series of 28 patients followed since childhood for a mean of 20 years, 5 had minor leakage. Late onset of incontinence has only been seen once[21].

This group, however, is highly selected – those who had an unsatisfactory result during childhood had the diversion changed. In patients operated as adults, the results were poor and illustrate why the procedure fell from favor. In 22 patients diverted to a

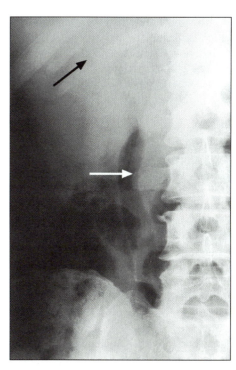

Figure 36.8 Plain abdominal X-ray showing gas in the right ureter and in a calyx (arrowed).

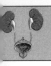

conventional ureterosigmoidostomy at a mean age of 66 years, it was found that 2 were incontinent but a further 9 had to take precautions against leakage (6 at night and 3 all the time). All had urgency and a best dry interval of 2 hours[22].

The effluent of mixed urine and feces has a very offensive smell. It is not a suitable diversion for patients from socially deprived families with shared lavatories. Likewise, the misery of incontinence is worsened by the smell.

The results of the modified ureterosigmoidostomies are very much better. All 65 patients in the original series of the Mansoura operation were continent day and night, although 6 had to take imipramine to stay dry at night[19]. Similarly, all of the 33 patients with Mainz II diversions were dry by day, with only one elderly lady wet at night[20].

The accumulated results of the modified diversions have been reviewed. There were 243 adults and 18 children available from seven publications. All of the children were completely dry. One adult was wet by day, 8 (all in one series) by night[23].

Renal consequences

Although the metabolic problems are better understood and antibiotics have lessened the consequences of infection, the long-term effect on the kidneys are still worrying.

In children, it must be remembered that many renal units were already damaged at the time a ureterosigmoidostomy was made. At a minimum follow-up of 18 years, about 50% of kidneys were damaged to some extent, 30% sufficiently to warrant a change of diversion, usually to an ileal conduit[24]. Late renal dilatation was usually due to a ureterocolic malignancy.

In adults, the early renal complication rate was less than 10% and no different from that of other diversions. Many of the patients had stones, infection, or benign strictures within the first few years. Few adults, most of whom were diverted for cancer, lived long enough to develop late renal damage.

The very early results that are available for the modified operations give an overall incidence of upper tract complications of 5%. On the other hand, most renal units that were dilated preoperatively improved after diversion. In my experience, gas is not seen in the renal pelvis, suggesting that there is no reflux. This, combined with the low storage pressure, may reduce the incidence of pyelonephritis and late renal damage (Fig. 36.9).

Ureterosigmoid cancer

The first case of carcinoma of a ureterosigmoidostomy was reported in 1929[25]. Only 18 further cases were reported in the literature up to 1970, presumably because few patients lived long enough to develop one.

The tumor arises at the anastomosis or very close to it in 90% of cases. It should, therefore, be regarded as an anastomotic tumor and not just a consequence of mixing urine and feces in bowel. In patients diverted for benign disease, 95% are adenomatous (adenomas or adenocarcinomas)[26]. The most important etiologic factor, both experimentally and clinically, is the mixture of feces and urine at the anastomosis.

At least in humans, a malignant transformation is initiated early and it is not reversed by subsequent exclusion of urine unless the anastomosis is excised as well. The shortest period of exposure to risk (that is the period with a ureterosigmoidostomy before conversion to an ileal conduit) is 9 months[27]. The mean

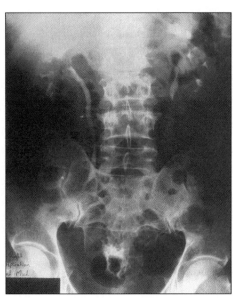

Figure 36.9 Intravenous urogram after voiding, showing normal kidneys draining into a Mainz 2 reservoir. Note that there is no contrast in the descending colon.

time from exposure to the development of a benign tumor is 18 years and a malignant one is 23 years. Mean age at presentation is 35 years[26].

In the absence of a mixture of urine and feces neoplasms are very rare and do not necessarily occur at the anastomosis (Fig. 36.10). Only 3 carcinomas have been reported in colonic conduits[28]. No neoplasms were found in a 37-year follow-up of diversion into the isolated rectum (Mauclaire or Boyce–Vest operation)[29].

The increased risk of neoplasia in patients with ureterosigmoidostomy (Fig. 36.11) has been variously estimated at 100–7000 times that in the normal population[30]. In an adult exstrophy population, Strachan estimated the increased risk at 1726 times normal by comparing those who had ever had a ureterosigmoidostomy with those who had never had one[31].

The carcinogenic agent may be an *N*-nitroso compound, although it is unproved. These potent carcinogens are present in ureterosigmoid effluent in a concentration 10 times greater than in normal bladder urine. The concentration found in isolated intestinal conduits and reservoirs is variable between patients and in individuals at different times of day: the only consistent finding is low concentrations when the diverted urine is sterile[32,33].

Hyperchloremic acidosis

The only clinically important biochemical abnormality is hyperchloremic acidosis, in which there is an excess of chloride, diminished bicarbonate, and, sometimes, potassium deficiency. The mechanisms involved in the development of this condition are discussed in Chapter 30.

Persistent HCA is common: the incidence ranges from 50% to 100%. This wide range is due, in part, to the definition used. Some authors define it as a raised chloride and low bicarbonate on a venous blood sample. Others consider a base excess below a certain figure to be critical. Arterial blood gas analysis is impractical to use in routine management. In its chronic form, HCA is symptomless.

Bone demineralization and osteomalacia have been recognized consequences of HCA for many years. All of the small number of cases reported in the literature have occurred in patients with

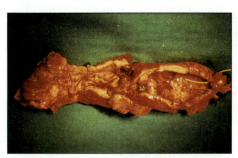

Figure 36.10 A resected ileal conduit opened longitudinally. There is a carcinoma in the mid portion, remote from the ureteric anastomoses, which have been marked with a red and a yellow tube.

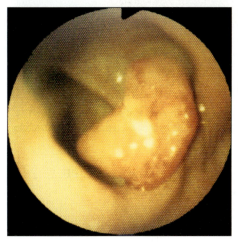

Figure 36.11 View through a flexible sigmoidoscope of a carcinoma of the ureterosigmoid junction.

Tissues that may be used in the construction of continent urinary diversions		
Reservoir	Conduit	Control mechanism
Bladder	Urethra	Urethral sphincters
Stomach	Appendix	Mitrofanoff
Ileum	Ileum (tubed)	Kock
Cecum	Ileum (natural)	Ileocecal valve
Colon	Ureter	Anal sphincter
Rectum	Skin tube	Artificial sphincter

Figure 36.12 Tissues that may be used in the construction of continent urinary diversions.

severe and uncorrected acidosis. Patients present with bone pains, tenderness, and weakness but the demineralization must be far advanced before radiologic changes are seen. Bone biopsies in fit adults with normal renal function show an increase in trabecular bone and a decreased apposition rate, which may delay healing (Davidsson, personal communication, 1995). In growing rats we have found decreased trabecular bone density and expansion of marrow cavity independent of HCA[41]. Subclinical demineralization of the spine has been found in Kock pouch patients by dual-energy X-ray absorptiometry[34].

Acute hyperchloremic acidosis is rare except when there is a severe intercurrent illness and impairment of renal function. Presentation is, therefore, usually with that illness. The symptoms of acute HCA are, most strikingly, extreme thirst in spite of nausea and vomiting and a salty taste in the mouth. Other symptoms include fatigue, weakness, weight loss, susceptibility to cold, anorexia, polyuria, rectal urgency, and diarrhea[35]. The accompanying hyperammonemia causes coma and encephalopathy.

Treatment consists of drainage of the rectum with a large catheter and slow correction of the acidosis with bicarbonate. The dehydration should not be corrected with sodium chloride, of which the patient already has an excess.

By far the most important aspect is prophylaxis. The plasma bicarbonate and chloride should be measured at least annually. On the assumption that potassium deficiency is not a problem, I prescribe sodium bicarbonate tablets. Most patients require 90–150mmol/day.

CONTINENT INTERNAL DIVERSION

There have been many attempts over the last 50 years to create a continent urinary reservoir. They have generally failed because it was not appreciated that there were two essential components: a low-pressure reservoir and a passive continence mechanism. Even having created such a continent system, evacuation depended on self-catheterization, which was only popularized by Lapides et al. in 1972[3].

Several different systems of continent internal diversion have been described. It is not necessary to know the precise details of every system. It is necessary to know the basic principles so that the most appropriate system can be used for each patient.

Continent internal diversion implies that the bladder, the urethra, and its sphincters are unusable. It is, therefore, necessary to build a low-pressure reservoir from intestine, a conduit to the surface, and a continence mechanism. The components that have been used are shown in Figure 36.12.

Choice of reservoir

The urinary reservoir can be made from one or more of the items in the first column of Figure 36.12. The stomach may be useful in children with renal failure because of the acid that is secreted but its reported use so far has been confined to bladder augmentations[36]. Jejunum is not suitable as it is too metabolically active.

There is no generally agreed ideal segment of bowel for a urinary reservoir. Sometimes circumstances dictate a choice. For example, if a patient already has a conduit that is to be converted to a continent system, it is usual to find that it is long enough to form at least half the reservoir. On the other hand, in a patient who has had radiotherapy for pelvic malignancy, much of the ileum, the ileocecal valve, the cecum, and the appendix may be damaged; transverse colon may then be the best choice.

Reservoir construction

The distinction between bladder augmentation and bladder substitution is rather artificial. If the bladder has a disease only of the muscle, e.g. a neuropathy, it is usually unnecessary to remove any tissue. The requirement is to reduce the intraluminal pressure and to bring the capacity up to normal.

If the bladder disease affects epithelium and muscle, e.g. in cancer, some or all of the bladder will have to be removed. A new reservoir can be formed and anastomosed to the sphincter mechanism or it may be drained by a continent suprapubic channel for self-catheterization.

Benign Conditions of the Lower Urinary Tract

There is therefore a spectrum from adding a small segment of bowel to a reasonable bladder (augmentation or clam cystoplasty) to a complete bladder replacement (substitution cystoplasty or pouch construction). In all cases the consequences of intestinal urine storage and voiding abnormalities will occur. In general, the bowel segment should be kept as small as possible.

To replace the bladder completely, 40cm of ileum or 20cm of large bowel or a combination of both is needed. The intrinsic peristaltic contractions of the bowel must be reduced if there is to be an acceptably low pressure within the reservoir. If an extrapolation can be made from the neuropathic bladder, a maximum storage pressure of $40cmH_2O$ should prevent upper tract damage[37]. Most authors believe that a passive reservoir is best achieved by longitudinal incision of the bowel to divide the circular muscle. The bowel is then reconfigured to form a reservoir that is as nearly spherical as possible[38].

Gonzalez used intact bowel segments to augment the bladder; 50% of the reservoirs had unacceptably high pressures and required anticholinergic drugs[39]. Alternatively, a very long bowel segment may be used so that the stored volume of urine is never large enough to stimulate peristaltic contractions[40]. Urodynamic studies have shown that the lowest intrinsic pressures are found in colon reservoirs augmented with ileum[41]. However, no system can completely guarantee a passive reservoir. The effect of detubularization is to delay the onset of contractions to a higher volume and to reduce their amplitude.

In a very small number of cases a chronically dilated ureter may be available to use as a clam. The kidney is removed if it is not functioning or a transureteroureterostomy made to preserve it. In pigs, tissue expanders have been used to create urothelium-lined cavities of 15–1000mL for this purpose[42]. In the laboratory it is possible to grow sheets of urothelium and to use them to create small pouches in sheep[43]. It remains to be seen whether these techniques can be translated into practice.

The choice of conduit

The choice of conduit cannot be entirely divorced from the choice of continence mechanism. A tube is needed with an adequate blood supply. It must be long enough to include a continence mechanism and must be easily catheterizable. Wide tubes must be intussuscepted to make a flutter valve, as originally described by Kock for continent ileostomies[2]. Narrow tubes must be buried in the reservoir wall to make a tunnel (Mitrofanoff)[44]. Combinations of these two principles can be used. For example, a wide tube such as ileum may be imbricated to make a narrow tube suitable for burying. In the Indiana system, continence depends on the ileocecal valve with some reinforcement, so the conduit must be made from ileum. In the original Mainz I pouch, the ileum is intussuscepted through the ileocecal valve and fixed as a Kock nipple so, again, the conduit must be made from ileum.

Of the narrow tubes, the appendix seems to be the most resilient. A 12F catheter will normally pass easily and it can usually be dilated to 16F[45]. It can be lengthened by inclusion of a cuff of cecum (Fig. 36.13) or by a skin tube (or both). Unfortunately, the appendix, even when present, is unusable in 31% of cases[46].

A dilated ureter is satisfactory, especially for the conversion of a conduit to a continent system[47]. Neither a ureter of normal caliber nor the fallopian tube has proved durable in the long run.

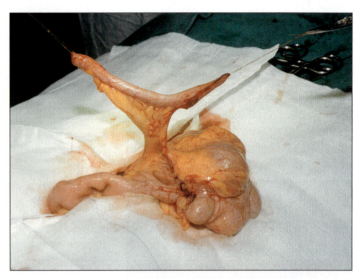

Figure 36.13 Appendix mobilized in preparation for implantation as a Mitrofanoff. The tip (to the left) has been resected. A cuff of cecum (to the right), is used to give extra length.

Orthotopic reconstruction
Allows urethral voiding
Diurnal incontinence rate in up to 7% of patients
Nocturnal incontinence in up to 43% of patients
Self-catheterization needed in up to 30% of patients after 5 years
Probably the best choice after cystectomy if the urethra can be retained

Figure 36.14 Orthotopic reconstruction.

A constant and reliable source of narrow tubes is ileum after reconfiguration. Originally a 7–8cm length was narrowed down longitudinally, usually with staples[47]. However, the system originally described by Yang and investigated by Monti has proved to be more useful[48,49]. In clinical practice good results have been reported in 14 of 16 patients, with 2 incontinent. A unique complication of this system is the development of an internal fistula between the conduit and the reservoir; it is essential to prepare the tunnel with care, ensuring that the reservoir epithelium is not breached[50]

Continence systems
Natural urethral sphincters
Use of the natural sphincters is highly desirable as the only means of re-establishing normal voiding. The question is, to what extent do they provide reliable continence and allow voiding to completion with an intestinal bladder (Fig. 36.14)?

In patients who are neurologically normal and in whom both sphincters are preserved, continence is likely to be normal. Those having a clam cystoplasty for idiopathic detrusor instability or a substitution for chronic interstitial cystitis are generally dry. Even when there is incontinence, the cause may be previously unrecognized sphincter weakness, especially in parous women. Voiding to completion may be more difficult and, even when achieved initially, may not be maintained in the long term. In a series of

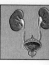

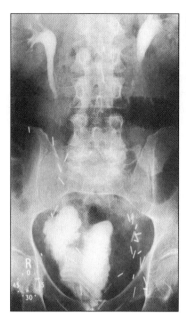

Figure 36.15 Intravenous urogram of a patient after an orthotopic substitution cystoplasty. The bladder had been removed for invasive bladder cancer.

51 women with a clam cystoplasty for detrusor instability, 82% were continent but 39% eventually needed CISC for chronic retention. Only 53% of the patients were happy with the result of their surgery[51].

After radical cystectomy and orthotopic reconstruction for cancer (Fig. 36.15), the reported continence rates vary widely. Recent papers give a nocturnal incontinence rate of 14% and 43% and a rate of incontinence by day of 0% and 7% respectively[52,53]. Nocturnal incontinence may be due to sphincter weakness (65% of cases), to chronic retention and overflow (24%), or to a combination of both (11%)[52]. Preservation of the neurovascular bundles reduces the risk of incontinence, both day and night: daytime continence was 96% with one or both nerves preserved compared to 86% with neither preserved, and continence by night was 95% and 77% respectively[53].

There has been some doubt about the advisability of radical cystectomy and orthotopic reconstruction in women. It now appears that women can be continent and void providing a small ring of bladder neck can be preserved for the anastomosis of the neobladder. It is important to limit the dissection around the urethra and to preserve the anterior vaginal wall adjacent to the urethra.

Passive sphincters

Without the urethral sphincters, there are three basic principles that may be applied to create continence and all depend on CISC for reservoir emptying.

A flutter valve is made by the intussusception of a wide-bore tube (e.g. the Kock nipple); a flap valve by the tunneling of a narrow tube into the wall of the reservoir (e.g. the Mitrofanoff principle) or by using the ileocecal valve (e.g. the Indiana). There are several variations on these themes, in some cases amounting to completely new designs[54]. The formation of continent diversions using these systems has become less common in the last decade as enthusiasm for orthotopic reconstruction after cystectomy has increased. They are primarily indicated in those with congenital anomalies or with no usable urethra.

Flutter valves

The Kock nipple, originally used to make a continent ileostomy after total colectomy, has been modified several times. To make it reliably continent it is essential to pay attention to every detail (Fig. 36.16). It is the most commonly used continence system by virtue of the large number reported from Skinner's unit. In his first 245 patients the incontinence rate was 23%; in the most recent 85 (of a total of 546) it was only 11%.

In the Benchekroun system, a length of ileum is intussuscepted, with the serosal surface turned inwards to form the catheterizable tract, unlike the Kock where the mucosal surface forms the tract[55]. Such a valve has been called the 'ink well'. Although the system seems relatively uncomplicated and Benchekroun himself reported 75% continence rate initially, rising to 93% after revisions, the technique has not been generally accepted.

The Mitrofanoff principle

Mitrofanoff first described the use of the appendix as a continent vesicostomy for children with neuropathic bladder[44]. His name is now given to the principle of burying a narrow tube within the wall of any reservoir (Figs 36.17 & 36.18). Unlike the Kock pouch, the Mitrofanoff only describes a continence mechanism rather than a complete reconstruction.

The technique is familiar to all urologists who are accustomed to reimplanting ureters. In most reported series the continence rate is more than 90% and it does seem to be a system that can easily be learned from a small number of cases[56].

Pressure studies (including our own unpublished data) have shown that the resting pressure generated within a Mitrofanoff conduit is two to three times the highest pressure generated by the reservoir[45]. Furthermore, our own studies have shown that the conduit responds to pouch pressure rises with a considerable pressure rise of its own. The difference between the conduit and pouch pressures is large, so that continence is reliably maintained. In the Kock nipples the difference between conduit and pouch pressures is small and the response to pouch pressure rises is limited so that continence is tenuous.

It is generally held that narrow tubes such as the appendix must be made continent by burying in a tunnel. Some experimental and clinical work has suggested that the tunnel is not needed[57,58]. However, until more definite proof is available, it would be foolish to abandon the use of the tunnel.

The ileocecal valve

The Indiana system is based on the competence of the ileocecal valve with a detubularized reservoir[59]. There have been important modifications to improve the competence of the valve. The valve itself is reinforced with nonabsorbable plicating sutures[60]. The terminal ileum, which forms the conduit, is tailored and may even be buried in the pouch wall, which makes the whole design very similar to a Mitrofanoff.

In the Mainz I pouch a length of terminal ileum is intussuscepted through the ileocecal valve as a Kock nipple (Fig. 36.19)[61]. It is impossible to say whether the nipple or the valve (or both) produce the continence which is reported in 96% of patients.

Artificial sphincter

As a last resort, the artifical urinary sphincter (AUS) may be considered to give continence to a reconstructed outlet. The cuff

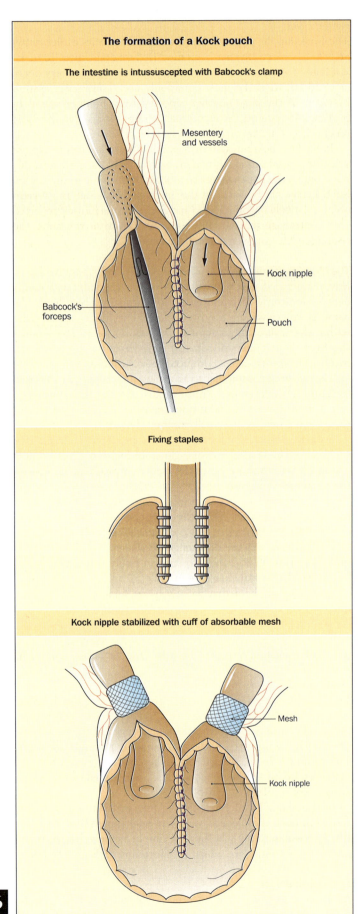

The formation of a Kock pouch

The intestine is intussuscepted with Babcock's clamp

Mesentery and vessels

Kock nipple

Babcock's forceps

Pouch

Fixing staples

Kock nipple stabilized with cuff of absorbable mesh

Mesh

Kock nipple

Figure 36.16 The formation of a Kock pouch. A total of 72cm of ileum is needed. The nipple is formed from 16cm at each end and the central 40cm is reconfigured as a reservoir. (Top) About 6–7cm is cleared of mesentery. The intestine is intussuscepted with a Babcock's clamp. (Center) The nipple is fixed to itself with three rows of staples and to the reservoir wall with a further row of staples. (Bottom) The nipple is stabilized with a cuff of absorbable mesh. The pouch is then closed. (Reproduced with permission from Mundy AR, et al. Urodynamics: principles, practice and application, 2nd edn. Edinburgh: Churchill Livingstone; 1994.)

Continent urinary diversion

Complex surgery

20% late complication rate

Good quality of life, especially for physical and sexual activities

Preferred by patients who have had previous experience of an ileal conduit

Stones occur in about 20% of patients

Figure 36.17 Continent urinary diversion.

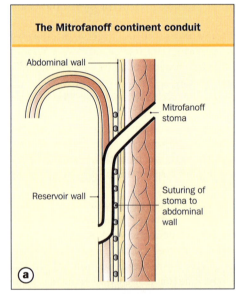

The Mitrofanoff continent conduit

Abdominal wall

Mitrofanoff stoma

Reservoir wall

Suturing of stoma to abdominal wall

(a)

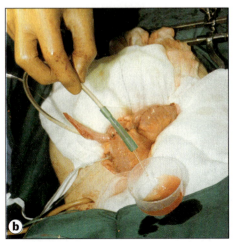

(b)

Figure 36.18 The Mitrofanoff continent conduit. (a) The principle of the formation of the conduit. (b) Operative photograph showing a reservoir with the appendix tunneled in and being drained by a catheter.

of an AUS is designed to encircle the normal urethra or bladder neck. Experimental evidence suggests that AUS cuffs can be placed safely around intestine providing the pressure is low. An AUS with a cuff pressure of 71–80cmH$_2$O has been used successfully around large bowel in three of four children with follow-up to 11 years[62].

Formation of the cutaneous stoma

The long-term success of continent diversion depends on this part of the operation more than any other. If the conduit cannot be catheterized, the whole system is useless.

The site for the stoma should be selected before surgery. The ideal site is probably the umbilicus, which provides an excellent passage way through the abdominal wall no matter how fat the patient. The stoma thus formed is not noticeable and is easy for the patient to find.

Otherwise, the site should be chosen to suit the physical and cosmetic requirements of the patient. In those who are normally mobile it should be as low as possible. In patients who are wheelchair-bound, any site below the umbilicus is likely to be inaccessible. I try to get the opening as high as possible, if necessary to a point just below the xiphisternum.

The conduit is tunneled through the abdominal wall obliquely to make the track as straight as possible. The cutaneous end is spatulated and a long triangular skin flap (2–3cm) is sutured into the spatulation. This allows the minimum of mucosa to be visible, forms a neat funnel for catheterization, and may contribute to the prevention of stenosis (Fig. 36.20).

A very neat stoma can be made by covering the spatulated skin/conduit anastomosis with a further fold of skin, the so-called VQZ stoma[63].

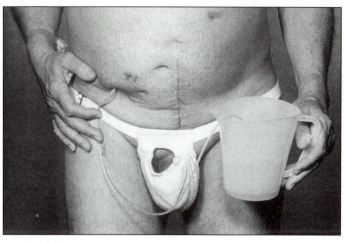

Figure 36.20 A patient catheterizing his Mitrofanoff stoma.

GENERAL CONSEQUENCES OF CONTINENT DIVERSION

Storage and emptying

In the short term, continent diversions can store urine and can be emptied, usually by CISC. There is a tendency, in the long term, for the reservoirs to enlarge. Although there has been no formal study of this phenomenon, it is likely to contribute to large residual urine volumes, recurrent infection and stones. In patients who are voiding through the urethral sphincters, emptying efficiency deteriorates with time in about 30% of patients: all patients should be warned of this risk and the practicalities of CISC considered.

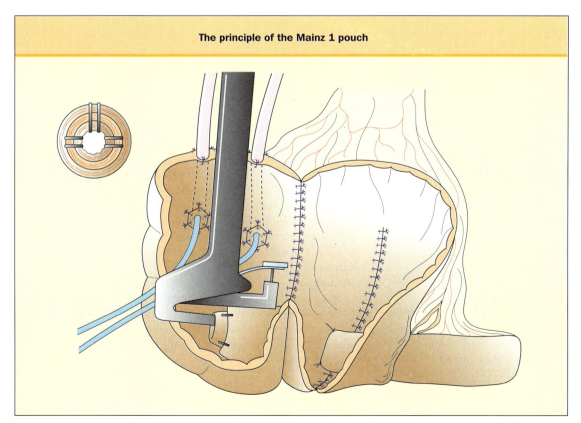

The principle of the Mainz 1 pouch

Figure 36.19 The principle of the Mainz 1 pouch. The cecum and ascending colon have been opened. The ileum has been intussuscepted through the ileocecal valve and is being fixed with staples. The inset shows a cross-section of the valve thus formed, fixed with three rows of staples.

Figure 36.21 Consequences of storage of urine in intestine.

It is already apparent that there is a constant need for review and surgical revision, especially of catheterizable diversions. My own figures suggest that patients require a mean of one surgical procedure every 10 years (unpublished data). In general, once continent, they remain continent. The problem lies more in difficulties with catheterization, particularly stenoses and false passages (Fig. 36.21).

Reservoir rupture
The incidence of spontaneous rupture varies between different units. It remains the most dangerous complication. Mansson et al. have surveyed Scandinavian centers and calculated an incidence of 1.5% in 1720 patients. Perforations occurred between 3 and 60 months postoperatively[64].

The diagnosis is often delayed, although the history of sudden abdominal pain and diminished or absent urine on catheterization should make it obvious. The patient rapidly becomes very ill with generalized peritonitis. 'Pouchogram' is commonly normal. Diagnosis is best made by peritoneocentesis of fluid collections identified on ultrasound.

If diagnosed early, catheterization and broad-spectrum antibiotics may lead to recovery. If the patient fails to respond within a few hours on this regime, or if there has been a delay in diagnosis, laparotomy should be performed at once. In a series of 23 cases of perforation in 18 patients the highest risk was with reservoirs using sigmoid colon (14.5% of 264 children having a perforation) and the lowest in ileal reservoirs (1.6%). There was one death[65].

Pregnancy
When reconstructing young females, it is essential to have a future pregnancy in mind. The position of the reservoir in relation to the uterus should be noted. The bowel pedicles should be fixed on one side of the abdomen to allow enlargement of the uterus on the other. Pregnancies may be complicated, but the urologic situation usually reverts to normal after delivery. An indwelling catheter may be needed for the last trimester. Joint urologic and obstetric care is essential[66].

Metabolic changes
Metabolic changes are common when urine is stored in intestinal reservoirs and must be carefully monitored. They are considered in more detail in Chapter 30. Much the most common is hyperchloremic acidosis. In 183 patients of all ages with any form of enterocystoplasty, we found HCA in 14% and borderline HCA in another 22%. The incidence was lower in reservoirs made solely with ileum compared to those formed with any colon (9% v. 16%)[67].

Long follow-up has shown low levels of vitamin B_{12} in 14% of children and 18.7% of adults. In the adults the mean vitamin B_{12} level was significantly lower when the ileocecal segment as opposed to ileum alone was used (257ng/mL compared to 413ng/mL)[68,69]. It is usually symptomless. In order to avoid serious neurologic complications, annual monitoring of vitamin B_{12} levels is essential from the fourth year onwards.

The terminal ileum is also the most important site for the reabsorption of bile acids. The loss of 40cm of terminal ileum trebles bile acid synthesis. This predisposes to gallstone formation and to diarrhea and steatorrhea[70].

Even with an ileal conduit 17.5% of patients may have a change in bowel habit persisting beyond the first year postoperatively (but with minimal impact on quality of life). Interestingly, in the same series 54% (of 28 patients) having a clam cystoplasty for idiopathic detrusor instability had new disturbance of bowel motility and function postoperatively. The effect on all aspects of quality of life was most marked in this group. This suggests that an intrinsic abnormality of smooth muscle or its innervation may affect both bladder and bowel; the bowel disturbance may be precipitated by the alterations in bile acid metabolism and increased transit time. It seems unlikely that the ileum needed for a clam cystoplasty would be significantly longer than that for a conduit. New bowel symptoms are commoner in patients having a clam for neuropathic disease than for non-neuropathic disease (26% against 14%) but with little effect on the quality of life.

Disturbance of bowel habit does not mean diarrhea alone. It also includes urgency, leakage, and nocturnal bowel actions, all of which may seriously undermine quality of life[71].

Renal function
In the follow-up so far available, undiversion or continent diversion do not seem to have affected renal function. In the longer term, it seems likely that the rate of renal damage will be the same as that for conduits (29% at 5–11 years). The common causes are stones, obstruction, and reflux[72]. In some patients renal function has improved after reconstruction, but probably as a result of the elimination of obstruction or high bladder storage pressures.

Infection and stones
Stones are a particular problem in the Kock pouch, where the nipple is fixed with metal staples. In Skinner's large series the incidence was 17%. In those who had formed a stone, the recurrence rate was 22%[73]. Otherwise, stones are associated with infection and retained mucus (Fig. 36.22).

In our patients 28% have troublesome infections and a further 20% have occasional infections[67]. Renal stones are uncommon (1.6%). The incidence of reservoir stones ranges from 12% to an extraordinary 52.5% at 4 years[74]. Nearly all are triple phosphate on analysis[75].

In my own practice, the incidence of stones appears to have fallen since greater attention has been paid to avoiding these known predisposing factors. Stones are seldom seen in patients who are catheterizing (or voiding) through the urethra as opposed to a suprapubic stoma[76].

Growth
The most worrying consequence of enterocystoplasty in children has been delayed growth in height. The problem appears in

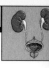

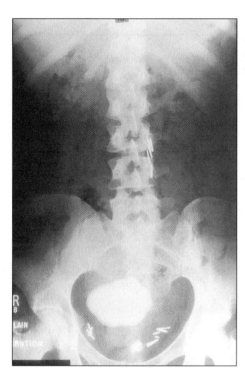

Figure 36.22 Plain abdominal X-ray showing a stone in an intestinal reservoir.

20% of children, affecting height but not weight. It is not associated with any metabolic or surgical complications[77]. Late follow-up suggests that most patients eventually catch up (unpublished data).

In rat models with ureterosigmoidostomy, uncorrected HCA delays growth unless prophylactic antibiotics are given[78,79]. In models with ileocystoplasty there is cortical and cancellous bone loss, only slightly reduced by continuous antibiotics[80].

Cancer

In patients with colonic and ileal cystoplasties high levels of nitrosamines, comparable to those in ureterosigmoidostomy slurry, have been found in the urine of most patients[32,33]. Biopsies of ileal and colonic segments show changes similar to those seen in conduits and ureterosigmoidostomies, but more severe changes correlate with higher nitrosamine levels and heavy mixed bacterial growth on culture[33].

Recently, the *MUC5AC* gene has been identified in urothelium adjacent to enteric anastomoses. This gene is not normally present in urothelium and is associated with villous adenoma of the rectum[81].

The stage is certainly set for the development of neoplasia in enterocystoplasties. Single cases of pouch neoplasia have been reported and a literature review identified 14 cases[28]. Nine were

adjacent to the bowel/urothelium anastomosis. However, special features could be found in nearly all cases. For example, 10 patients had tuberculous bladders; 4 tumors were not adenocarcinomas; 1 patient had a pre-existing adenocarcinoma of the colon; 6 patients were over 50 years old. These are not the characteristics of the ureterosigmoid cancer.

It has not been proved that nitrosamines are the cause of ureterosigmoid carcinoma and it could be presumed that, whatever the cause, the isolated pouch would be less at risk than the ureterosigmoidostomy. Nonetheless, a watch must be kept for pouch neoplasia. Their early identification will be difficult and may have to rely on the advanced technology of three-dimensional reconstruction of computed tomography and virtual reality endoscopy[81].

QUALITY OF LIFE

The main justification for performing bladder reconstruction or continent diversion is to improve an individual's quality of life. The more research that is done in this area, the more difficult it turns out to be. In young patients who have experienced both a cutaneous and a continent diversion, there is overwhelming enthusiasm for anything that avoids a bag[9].

In patients with cancer, and especially in those with idiopathic detrusor instability, reconstruction is not always the best option. There is a high level of dissatisfaction among patients, who realize that they have only changed one lot of symptoms for another[71,82].

It is also interesting to note that a wide range of complications of cystoplasty are considered to be 'acceptable' by surgeons although an ordinary urologic clinic would be full of patients trying to get rid of such symptoms: mild incontinence (50%), nocturia (37%), bladder stones (12%), infections (9%), and hydronephrosis (5%). Nonetheless, their QOL is judged to be good because 70% experienced no adverse effect on their normal daily lives[82].

With a specifically designed instrument it is possible to show that continent diversion is superior to an ileal conduit in all items related to a stoma. Continent patients have better physical and mental strength and are better adjusted socially. There is no difference in levels of satisfaction with professional, financial, family, and sexual activities[83].

Few patients who have a working continent diversion will ask for a bag. Patients with bags will usually wish to be rid of them if possible. For new patients, very careful counseling is essential. It may be that considerable physical and mental strength are needed to cope with continent diversion and its complications.

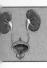

REFERENCES

1. Bricker EM, Eiseman B. Bladder reconstruction from cecum and ascending colon following resection of pelvic viscera. Ann Surg. 1950;132:77.

2. Kock NG. Ileostomy without external appliances: a survey of 25 patients provided with intra-abdominal reservoir. Ann Surg. 1971;173:545.

3. Lapides J, Diockno AC, Silber SJ, Lowe BS. Clean intermittent self catheterisation in the treatment of urinary tract disease. J Urol. 1972;107:458.

4. Wells CA. The use of intestine in urology. Br J Urol. 1956;28:335.

5. Annis D. The use of the isolated ileal segment in urology. Br J Urol. 1956;28:362.

6. Jones MA, Breckman B, Hendry WF. Life with an ileal conduit: results of questionnaire surveys of patients and urological surgeons. Br J Urol. 1980;52:21.

7. Shapiro SR, Lebovitz R, Colodny AH. The fate of 90 children with an ileal conduit urinary diversion 10 years later. J Urol. 1975;114:289.

8. Dunn M, Roberts JBM, Smith PJB, Slade N. The long term results of ileal conduit diversion in children. Br J Urol. 1979;51:458.

9. Boyd SD, Feinberg SM, Skinner DG. Quality of life survey of urinary diversion patients. J Urol. 1987;138:1386.

10. Neal DE. Urodynamic investigation of the ileal conduit: upper tract dilatation and the effects of revision of the conduit. J Urol. 1999;142:97.

11. Bergman B, Kaijser B, Nilson AE. Urinary diversion and urinary tract infection. Scand J Urol Nephrol. 1979;13:65.

12. Dretler SP. The pathogenesis of urinary tract calculi occurring after ileal conduit diversion. J Urol. 1973;109:204.

13. Fossa SD, Heilo A, Bormer O. Unexpectedly high methotrexate levels in cystectomized bladder cancer patients with an ileal conduit treated with intermediate doses of the drug. J Urol. 1990;143:498.

14. Srinivas S, Mahalati K, Freiha FS. Methotrexate tolerance in patients with ileal conduits and continent diversions. Cancer. 1998;82:1134.

15. Hill JT, Ransley PG. The colonic conduit: a better method of urinary diversion? Br J Urol. 1985;55:629.

16. Eckstein HB, Kapila L. Cutaneous ureterostomy. Br J Urol. 1970;42:629.

17. Thrasher JB, Wettlaufer JN. Transureteroureterostomy and terminal loop ureterostomy in advanced pelvic malignancies. J Urol. 1991;146:977.

18. Coffey RC. Physiologic implantation of the severed ureter or bile duct into the intestine. JAMA. 1911;56:397.

19. Ghoneim MA, Ashamallah AK, Mahran MA, Kock NG. Further experience with the modified rectal bladder (augmented and valved rectum). J Urol. 1992;147:1252.

20. Fisch M, Wammack R, Muller SC, Hohenfellner R. The Mainz pouch 2 (sigma-rectum pouch). J Urol. 1993;149:258.

21. Silverman SH, Woodhouse CRJ, Strachan JR, Cumming J, Keighley MRB. Long term management of patients who have had urinary diversions into colon. Br J Urol. 1986;58:634.

22. McConnell JB, Murison J, Stewart WK. The role of the colon in the pathogenesis of hyperchloraemic acidosis in ureterosigmoid anastomosis. Clin Sci. 1979;57:305.

23. Woodhouse CRJ, Christofides M. Modified ureterosigmoidostomy (Mainz II); technique and early results. Br J Urol. 1998;81:247.

24. Woodhouse CRJ, Ransley PG, Williams DI. The patient with exstrophy in adult life. Br J Urol. 1983;55:632.

25. Hammer E. Cancer du colon sigmoide dix ans apres implantation des uretères d'une vessie exstrophiée. J Urol (Paris). 1929;28:260.

26. Stewart M. Urinary diversion and bowel cancer. Ann R Coll Surg Engl. 1986;68:98.

27. Spence HM, Hoffman WW, Fosmire GP. Tumour of the colon as a late complication of ureterosigmoidostomy for exstrophy of the bladder. Br J Urol. 1979;51:466.

28. Filmer RB, Bruce JR. Malignancies in bladder augmentations and intestinal conduits. J Urol. 1990;143:671.

29. Kroovand RL, Boyce HH. Isolated vesicorectal internal diversion: a 37 year review of the Boyce–Vest procedure. J Urol. 1988;140:572.

30. Stewart M, Williams CB. Neoplasia and ureterosigmoidostomy: a colonoscopic review. Br J Surg. 1982;69:414.

31. Strachan JR, Woodhouse CRJ. Malignancy following uretero-sigmoidostomy in patients with exstrophy. Br J Surg. 1991;78:1216.

32. Groschel J, Riedasch G, Kalble T, Tricker AR. Nitrosamine excretion in patients with continent ileal reservoirs for urinary diversion. J Urol. 1992;147:1013.

33. Nurse DE, Mundy AR. Assessment of the malignant potential of cystoplasty. Br J Urol. 1989;64:489.

34. Poulsen AL, Overgaard K, Christiansen C, Thode J, Steven K. Bone mineral status following urinary diversion with the Kock ileal reservoir. Scand J Urol Nephrol. 1992;142:136(abstract).

35. Jacobs A, Barr-Stirling W. The late results of ureterocolic anastomosis. Br J Urol. 1952;24:259.

36. Adams MC, Mitchell ME, Rink RC. Gastrocystoplasty: an alternative solution to the problem of reconstruction in the severely compromised patient. J Urol. 1988;140:1152.

37. Wang SC, McGuire EG, Bloom DA. A bladder pressure management system for myelodysplasia: clinical outcome. J Urol. 1988;140:1499.

38. Hinman F. Selection of intestinal segments for bladder substitution: physical and physiological characteristics. J Urol. 1988;139:519.

39. Gonzalez R, Sidi AA, Zhang G. Urinary undiversion: indications, technique and results in 50 cases. J Urol. 1986;136:13.

40. Mundy AR. Cystoplasty. In: Mundy AR, ed. Current operative surgery – urology. London: Baillière Tindall; 1988:140.

41. Gerharz EW, Gasser J, Moniz C, et al. Skeletal growth and long term bone turnover after enterocystoplasty in the rat model. Br J Urol. 1998;81:28.

42. Ikeguchi EF, Stifelman MD, Hensle TW. Ureteral tissue expansion for bladder augmentation. J Urol. 1998;159:1665.

43. Schaefer BM, Lorenz C, Back W. Urothelial cell culture for transplantation. J Urol. 1998;159:284.

44. Mitrofanoff P. Cystostomie continente trans-appendiculaire dans le traitement de vessies neurologiques. Chir Paediatr. 1980;621:297.

45. Riedmiller H, Burger R, Muller SC, Thuroff J, Hohenfellner R. Continent appendix stoma: a modification of the Mainz pouch technique. J Urol. 1990;143:1115.

46. Leibovitch I, Avigad I, Nativ O, Goldwasser B. The frequency of histopathological abnormalities in incidental appendectomy in urological patients: the implications for incorporation of the appendix in urinary tract reconstructions. J Urol. 1992;148:41.

47. Woodhouse CRJ, Reilly JM, Strachan JR, Malone PR. The Mitrofanoff principle for continent urinary diversion. Br J Urol. 1989;63:53.

48. Monti PR, Lara RC, Dutra MA, Rezende de Carvalho R. New techniques for construction of efferent conduits based on the Mitrofanoff principle. Urology. 1997;49:112.

49. Yang WH. Yang needle tunneling technique in creating antireflux and continence mechanisms. J Urol. 1993;150:830.

50. Gerharz EW, Woodhouse CRJ. The transverse ileal tube as second line modification of the Mitrofanoff principle. World J Urol. 1998;16:231.

51. Awad SA, Al-Zahrani HM, Gajewski JB, Bourque-Kehoe AA. Long term results and complications of augmentation ileo cystoplasty for idiopathic urge incontinence in women. Br J Urol. 1998;81:569.

52. Park JM, Montie JE. Mechanisms of incontinence and retention after orthotopic neobladder diversion. Urology. 1998;51:601.

53. Turner WH, Danuser H, Moehrle K, Studer UE. The effect of nerve sparing cystectomy technique on postoperative continence after orthotopic bladder substitution. J Urol. 1997;158:2118.

54. Gleeson MJ, Griffith DP. Urinary diversion. Br J Urol. 1990;66:113.

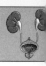

55. Benchekroun A, Essakali N, Faik M. Continent urostomy with hydraulic ileal valve in 136 patients: 13 years of experience. J Urol. 1989;142:46.

56. Woodhouse CRJ, Pope AJ. Alternatives to a cutaneous urinary diversion: results in 100 cases. Br J Urol. 1993;72:580.

57. Simforoosh N, Razzaghi MR, Danesh AK. Continent ileo caecal diversion with an unaltered appendix conduit. J Urol. 1998; 159:1176.

58. Celayir S, Dervisoglu S, Buyukunal SNC. A modified Mitrofanoff procedure using rectus abdominis muscle flap technique: a preliminary report in a rabbit model. Br J Urol. 1998;81:83.

59. Rowland RG, Mitchell ME, Bihrle R, Kahnoski PJ, Iser JE. Indiana continent urinary reservoir. J Urol. 1987;137:1136.

60. Ahlering TE, Weinberg AC, Razor B. Modified Indiana pouch. J Urol. 1991;145:1156.

61. Thuroff J, Alken P, Reidmiller H, Jakobi GH, Hohenfellner R. 100 cases of Mainz pouch: continuing experience and evolution. J Urol. 1988;140:283.

62. Light KK. Long term clinical results using the artificial sphincter around bowel. Br J Urol. 1989;64:56.

63. Mor Y, Quinn FMJ, Carr B, et al. Combined Mitrofanoff and antegrade continence enema procedures for urinary and faecal incontinence. J Urol. 1997;158:192.

64. Mansson W, Bakke A, Bergman B. Perforation of continent urinary reservoirs. Scand J Urol Nephrol. 1997;31:529.

65. Rink RC, Hollensbe DW, Adams MC, Keating MA. Is sigmoid enterocystoplasty at greatest risk for perforation? Observations and etiology in 23 bladder perforations in 264 patients. Scand J Urol Nephrol. 1992;142:179.

66. Hill DE, Kramer SA. Pregnancy after augmentation cystoplasty. J Urol. 1989;144:457.

67. Wagstaff KE, Woodhouse CRJ, Rose GA, Duffy PG, Ransley PG. Blood and urine analysis in patients with intestinal bladders. Br J Urol. 1991;68:311.

68. Kalloo NB, Jeffs RD, Gearhart JP. Long term nutritional consequences of bowel segment use for lower urinary tract reconstruction in pediatric patients. Urology. 1997;50:967.

69. Racioppi M, D'Addessi A, Fanasca E. Vitamin B_{12} and folic acid plasma levels after ileo-caecal and ileal neobladder reconstruction. Urology. 1997;50:888.

70. Einarsson K. Metabolic effects caused by exclusion of intestinal segments. Scand J Urol Nephrol. 1992;142:21.

71. N'Dow J, Leung HY, Marshall C, Neal DE. Bowel dysfunction after bladder reconstruction. J Urol. 1998;159:1470.

72. Akerlund S, Delin K, Kock NG. Renal function and upper urinary tract configuration following urinary diversion to a continent ileal reservoir (Kock pouch). J Urol. 1989;142:964.

73. Ginsberg D, Huffman JL, Lieskovsky G, Boyd SD, Skinner DG. Urinary tract stones: a complication of the Kock pouch urinary diversion. J Urol. 1991;145:956.

74. Palmer LS, Franco I, Kogan S, et al. Urolithiasis in children following augmentation cystoplasty. J Urol. 1993;150:726.

75. Blyth B, Ewalt DH, Duckett JW. Lithogenic properties of enterocystoplasty. J Urol. 1992;148:575.

76. Woodhouse CRJ, Lennon GM. Management and aetiology of stones in intestinal urinary reservoirs. Br J Urol. 1998;81:47.

77. Wagstaff KE, Woodhouse CRJ, Duffy PG, Ransley PG. Delayed linear growth in children after enterocystoplasty. Br J Urol. 1992;69:314.

78. Imler M, Schlienger JL, Batzenschlager A. Hyperammonemia following ureterocolostomy in the rat. Surg Gynecol Obstet. 1979;149:183.

79. McDougal WS, Koch MO, Shands C, Price RR. Bony demineralization following urinary intestinal diversion. J Urol. 1988;140:853.

80. N'Dow, J. M. O. Mucus production and mucin gene expression in normal bladder and in intestinal segments transposed into the urinary tract. University of Newcastle Thesis. 1999:174–206.

81. Stenzl A, Frank R, Eder R. 3-dimensional computerized tomography and virtual reality endoscopy of the reconstructed lower urinary tract. J Urol. 1998;159:741.

82. Sullivan LD, Chow VDW, Ko DSC, Wright JE, McLoughlin MG. An evaluation of quality of life in patients with continent urinary diversions after cystectomy. Br J Urol. 1998;81:699.

83. Gerharz EW, Weingartner K, Dopatke T. Quality of life after cystectomy and urinary diversion: results of a retrospective interdisciplinary study. J Urol. 1998;158:778.

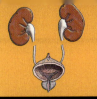

Chapter 37

Urinary Fistulae

Noel W Clarke

KEY POINTS

- Fistulae may be simple or complex.
- Diagnosis may require a combination of contrast and cross-sectional imaging, dye studies and endoscopy.
- Decisions on treatment must consider fistula location/anatomy, patient's condition and the underlying disease process.
- Closure principles include use of vascularized, healthy, tension-free anastomoses, avoidance of overlapping suture lines, use of interposition flaps, catheter and pelvic drainage, and drainage and control of sepsis.
- Complex fistulae may require a period of proximal defunction, distal drainage and patient rehabilitation before definitive surgery.

INTRODUCTION

Descriptions of urinary fistulae and their management have been recorded in numerous written records dating from the early Greek civilization to the current day[1]. The earliest report of successful surgical closure dates from the 17th century and involved the use of sharpened goose quills covered with waxed silk to oppose the cut edges of the fistula[2]. For the most part, however, such treatments were unsuccessful until the 19th-century pioneers developed the basic techniques, many of which hold true in modern practice. The leading exponent of these techniques was the gynecologist James Marion Sims. Although he was not the first to use transvaginal surgical techniques successfully, he popularized and developed this approach, expounding the virtues of the 'knee/elbows' position and the surgical principles of excision of diseased tissue, preparation of fresh tissue edges, tension free closure without overlying suture lines, and postoperative catheter drainage of the bladder[3]. Technical advances have continued thereafter with the description of the Martius flap[4] and the popularization of the transabdominal approach by the urologist O'Connor in the mid-20th century[5,6]. Today a variety of techniques and surgical approaches are available to the pelvic surgeon to enable successful fistula treatment with a good functional outcome for a condition that was previously untreatable and that can cause major morbidity and profound distress to the affected individual.

CLASSIFICATION

Urinary fistulae can be classified broadly as 'congenital' and 'acquired', and the latter may be further subdivided into 'simple' and 'complex', according to their etiology, location, and complexity. This chapter will deal specifically with the management of the acquired type.

Simple fistulae

These involve a simple communication between the urinary tract and the genital/gastrointestinal tract or external body wall without gross tissue loss or damage. They are usually amenable to repair using the basic principles of fistula tract disconnection, closure/reconstruction avoiding opposing suture lines, and postoperative drainage/stenting. Most are caused by trauma of obstetric origin in underdeveloped countries[7,8] or are of iatrogenic origin in the developed world[9,10].

Complex fistulae

These are often multiple and are usually associated with major tissue damage from repeated surgical procedures, radiation therapy, chronic inflammation/infection, or tissue loss for other reasons (e.g. necrotizing infection, trauma). These etiologic factors can occur either alone or in combination. Treatment will often require preliminary procedures as a prelude to definitive surgery and operations will often involve a complex excisional and reconstructive approach (Fig. 37.1).

Etiology

In the developing world the commonest type of urinary fistula is vesicovaginal, arising as a result of obstetric trauma[11]. This occurs mainly because of pressure necrosis of the anterior vaginal wall caused by obstructed labor (84%), although surgical cutting (Gishiri cutting) of the anterior vaginal wall to alleviate the obstruction accounts for approximately 13% of cases[12]. In the developed world, fistulae of this type are uncommon, representing less than 6% of all reported cases[13,14].

The most frequent cause of urinary fistulation in the developed world is iatrogenic trauma. Up to 74% are the result of gynecologic surgery, particularly abdominal hysterectomy[15,16], although they are seen following other procedures such as vaginal hysterectomy and anterior colporrhaphy[17]. The incidence of vesicovaginal fistulation after standard hysterectomy is less than 1%[18] and that of ureteric injury 0.5–1.5%[19,20]. Injury arises as a consequence of the close proximity of the ureter and vesicoureteric junction to the vaginal vault (Fig. 37.2). Suturing or

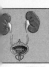

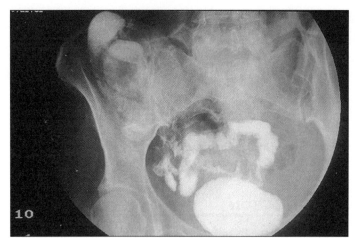

Figure 37.1 Complex enterourinary fistula arising as a consequence of curative radiotherapy for cervical cancer. Radiocontrast from the cystogram enters the pelvic small bowel and emerges from a defunctioning loop ileostomy. At laparotomy a complex entero-urinary-vaginal fistula was repaired by fistula disconnection, small bowel resection, and vaginal fistula closure with an omental interposition flap. The bladder was small and poorly compliant because of the radiotherapy; this was therefore augmented using an anteroposterior 'clam' small bowel segment.

clamp application in this area can result in ischemia of the tissues[21], while devascularization can occur during surgical dissection of the distal ureter. This risk is greatest in Wertheim's hysterectomy, particularly where there has been concomitant radiotherapy. The reported incidence of damage in this circumstance is as high as 10%[22]. Abdominal/bowel surgery can also result in urinary tract damage leading to fistulation. In severe cases this can precipitate the formation of complex enterourinary fistulae with concomitant intra-abdominal sepsis, which, in its severest form, may be life threatening (Fig. 37.3).

Radiation therapy is another factor in the etiology of fistula. This complication occurs most commonly after radiation treatment for cervical cancer, affecting 1–2% of women[23] (Figs 37.1 & 37.4); this rate can be much higher when the radiotherapy is administered after previous surgery has been undertaken. Ureteric fistulation is much less common but in susceptible individuals the pelvis can be markedly affected, leading to the development of complex radiation-related fistulae that, in the most severe cases, can communicate with bowel, vagina, and the urinary tract in combination (Figs 37.1 & 37.4). It is noteworthy that radiation fistulae can present many years after the initial course of curative treatment[23]. Radiotherapy to the prostate can also induce fistulation, predominantly prostatorectal. Fortunately, this is an uncommon complication, occurring in 0.4% of patients treated with external beam therapy. However, the incidence increases to 2.2% in men treated with brachytherapy[24]. Interestingly, the incidence of prostatorectal/urethrorectal fistulae after radical prostatic surgery is similar to that for external beam treatment[25] although perineal prostatectomy seems to confer a greater risk.

Other causes of urinary fistula formation include trauma, infectious/inflammatory conditions such as Crohn's and diverticulitis, and more commonly, direct invasion of the urinary tract in the late stages of cervical and colorectal cancer (Figs 37.5 & 37.6).

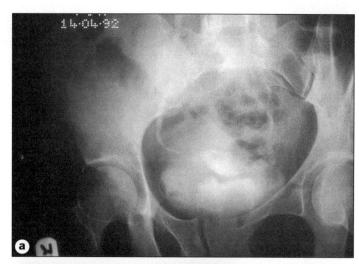

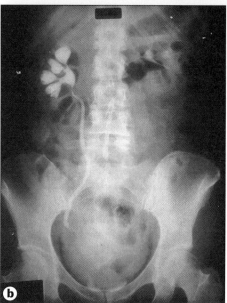

Figure 37.2 Urinary fistula arising as a consequence of gynecologic surgery. (a) Intravenous urogram showing radio contrast in the bladder and vagina 3 weeks following abdominal hysterectomy. The patient had been dry at hospital discharge but had subsequently developed urinary leakage. Repair was by psoas hitch and reimplantation. (b) Intravenous urogram showing a dilated right ureter that has been divided during laparoscopic dissection. The patient had persistent abdominal pain and pyrexia postoperatively. The ureter was repaired as in case (a).

PRESENTING FEATURES

The simple postoperative urinary fistula will usually present with partial or complete loss of urinary control. This most commonly occurs in the early days following surgery and will often be associated with a slow postoperative course complicated by prolonged ileus and abdominal pain if there is intraperitoneal leakage (see Fig. 37.26). In cases of ischemic necrosis, the signs may not be seen for 2 or more weeks postoperatively[26] (Fig. 37.2a). Typically, the patient will complain of the development of incontinence following discharge home, having previously been continent[27] (Fig. 37.2a). In some cases, patients develop signs of sepsis and, in the worst-case scenario, the patient can be acutely ill, with severe manifestations of endotoxemia. This can be a particular problem in patients with postoperative enterourinary fistulation (Figs 37.3 & 37.7).

Chronically developing fistulae will often manifest initially with irritative lower urinary tract symptoms such as urinary

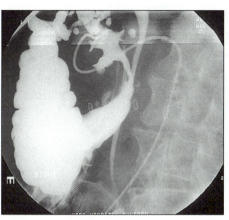

Figure 37.3 Complex enterourinary fistula. This fistula arose as a consequence of failure to recognize a right-side duplex system at cystectomy for node-positive disease. The intravenous urogram demonstrates fistulation between the divided duplex moiety and the anastomotic site of the ileal loop. Clinically, mixed urine and enteric content could be seen emerging from the abdominal wound, through the ileal loop, and via the rectum through a further defect in the anterior rectal wall. Because of the metastatic disease, life expectancy was limited. Repair was therefore undertaken by removal of the right upper urinary tract, diversion of the left upper urinary tract using an intubated cutaneous ureterostomy and defunctioning the small bowel proximally by exteriorization of the ileum after taking the previous enteric anastomosis apart.

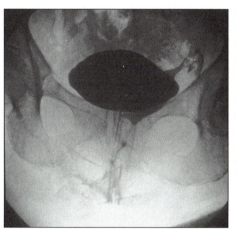

Figure 37.4 Cystogram showing a vesicouterine fistula arising following radiotherapy for cervical cancer. The fallopian tube is clearly delineated on the left. Repair was by fistula disconnection and closure with an omental pedicle flap.

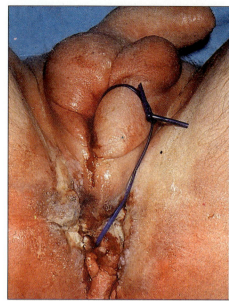

Figure 37.5 Advanced recurrent colorectal cancer infiltrating the prostate and urethra producing a urethral fistula involving the urinary sphincters. Fistulae of this type are not amenable to closure and should be treated by the simplest form of urinary diversion possible. Blue tape, fistula track.

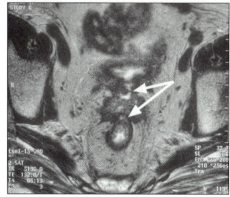

Figure 37.6 T2-weighted magnetic resonance image of the pelvis showing an anteriorly placed rectal cancer infiltrating the prostate and bladder base (arrows). The fluid (showing as white) can be seen clearly tracking back from the bladder base into the rectum. This patient was successfully treated by pelvic exenteration.

frequency/urgency, often with recurrent or refractory urinary infection. In radiation cases bladder pain is often encountered[23] with infection occurring in up to 40% of cases[28] (Fig. 37.8).

EVALUATION AND DIAGNOSIS

Simple fistulae

Diagnosis in simple fistulation is usually straightforward, although location of the exact site of the fistula can be difficult. The basis of diagnosis is biochemical analysis, contrast imaging, dye testing, and endoscopy. In the presence of involuntary loss of urine or prolonged fluid discharge from an operation site or through an abdominal drain, it is important to establish whether or not the fluid emerging is urine and, if it is, whether this is coming through a fistulous connection or is arising as a result of urethral incontinence or discharge for other reasons. Biochemical analysis of draining fluid will quickly establish if it is urine.

Intravenous urography should be performed in all patients. The characteristic features in ureteric damage are dilatation and/or extravasation. Radiocontrast may be seen in the vagina, peritoneal cavity, and other abdominal organs in both ureteral

and vesicovaginal fistulae (Figs 37.1–37.4). In some cases of simple fistula it may be necessary to supplement the IVU with antegrade or retrograde studies. It should be remembered that vesicovaginal fistulae are present in association with ureteral fistulae in 12% of cases[16].

Dye testing may be invaluable in locating the site of a fistula[17] and the most commonly used is the three-pad test[29]. The principles of the test are shown in Figure 37.9. While this test may be particularly helpful in some circumstances, it is often less valuable than direct vaginoscopy following dye instillation. This technique can enable direct visualization of the vaginal component of the fistula (Fig. 37.10). Although useful, the test has the disadvantage that it may yield false results in the presence of vesicoureteric reflux. Dye studies may need supplementation with retrograde pyelography for delineation. However, in many cases, edema and inflammation of the bladder base preclude these because of the difficulty of locating and intubating the ureter. In difficult cases it is sometimes necessary to resort to intraoperative dye/contrast studies by cannulating the pelvic ureter directly under vision with synchronous X-ray screening and/or cystoscopy and vaginoscopy.

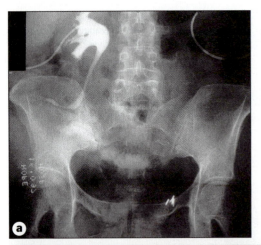

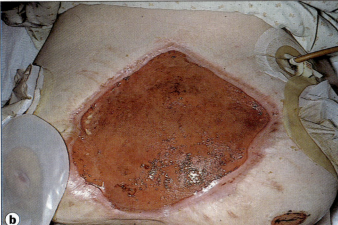

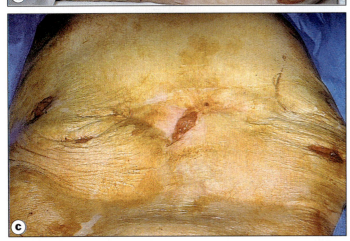

Figure 37.7 Defunction of urinary and gastrointestinal tracts and a laparostomy in a patient with severe intraabdominal sepsis following strangulation and necrosis of an ileal loop urinary diversion. (a) The ureter on the right communicates with the mid-ileum and enteric content and urine discharges through the laparostomy (b). Proximal urinary defunction is by a right nephrostomy and a left intubated ureterostomy. The bowel has been defunctioned by a gastrostomy, jejunostomy, and mucous fistulation of the distal small bowel and colon. (c) The sepsis has settled, the laparostomy has healed, and the patient has been maintained on total parenteral nutrition. Repair used a Bricker-type ileal loop with restoration of the continuity of the bowel to the colon.

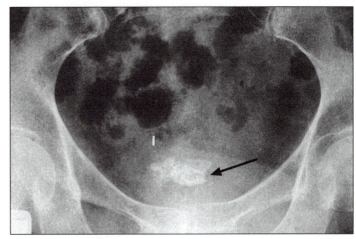

Figure 37.8 Patient presenting with postradiotherapy bladder pain as a prelude to fistulation. The X-ray shows a pelvic treatment marker and encrustation in an ulcer in the trigonal region of the bladder (arrow). This eventually fistulized. The bladder capacity was small and the base badly diseased. However, the urethra was spared and in good condition. Repair therefore used an orthotopic substitution with a Mainz-type pouch.

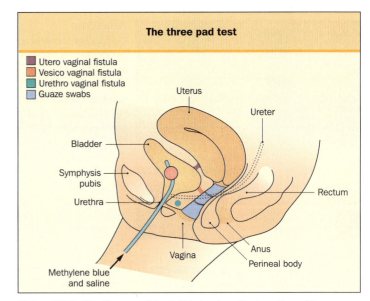

Figure 37.9 The three pad test. This involves the insertion of three small gauze swabs into the vagina followed by instillation of aqueous methylene blue to the bladder. Dye staining of the inner or middle pad is indicative of a fistulous connection. Various authors have suggested that differential staining of the pads and use of different dyes intravesically and intravenously facilitates anatomic location of the fistula site[45]. In practice, this technique is very inaccurate because of the potential for vesicoureteric reflux, the presence of multiple fistulae, and, in some cases, poor renal function. The test should be supplemented by cystoscopy, vaginoscopy, and where necessary antegrade or retrograde pyelography. In difficult cases it may be necessary to inject dye directly into the pelvic ureter intraoperatively to locate the origin of a low ureteric fistula.

Complex fistulae

Evaluation of the complex fistula requires additional imaging of the abdominopelvic cavity and, in particular, the gastrointestinal tract. The mainstay of diagnosis is cross-sectional imaging with contrast computed tomography (CT) scanning supplemented

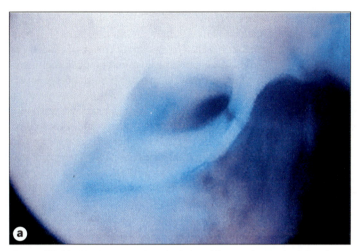

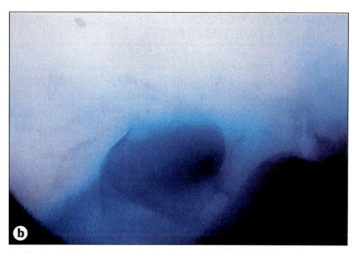

Figure 37.10 Vaginoscopy in a patient with a vesicovaginal fistula following hysterectomy. Methylene blue has been instilled into the bladder and this can clearly be seen emerging from the vaginal aspect of the fistula (a), followed by a flood of dye after further instillation (b). (a) Methylene blue begins to emerge, (b) proximity view with the endoscope confirms vesico–vaginal fistulation.

by ante- and retrograde pyelography, bowel contrast studies and where necessary, magnetic resonance imaging (MRI)[30,31] (Fig. 37.6). The patients should also undergo examination under anesthetic and endoscopy of the pelvic organs, preferably by a multidisciplinary team comprising urologists, gynecologist, and colorectal surgeons. It is important to determine the complexity of the fistula and the extent of its communication, in addition to obtaining information about anatomy and function of the bowel, bladder, and kidneys. The reason for this is that patients with fistulae of this type often have damage to more than one organ system. In patients affected by pelvic radiation disease, for example, 15–30% have injury to multiple organs[32] (Figs 37.1 & 37.4). Thus it is vital to establish whether the bladder and urethra will function if the fistula is closed, that precarious renal function will not be compromised further by metabolic problems as a consequence of inappropriate reconstructive techniques and that there is a sufficient length of healthy bowel with good sphincteric control to enable functional restoration of the gastrointestinal tract. It is also important to evaluate the patient generally, assessing nutritional status, looking for chronic sepsis and septic foci, and paying particular attention to the condition of the abdominal skin if there is an enterourinary fistula discharging on to the abdominal wall (Fig. 37.11). In situations where malignancy is suspected, examination under anesthetic, endoscopy, and biopsy are essential. The presence of primary or secondary malignancy may have an important bearing on decisions to reconstruct, exenterate, or simply to divert the urinary and/or fecal stream. Some authors suggest that in the presence of carcinoma at a urinary fistula site, omental patching is reliable[33]. However, this strategy is very risky and will usually fail. It is far safer to accept the doctrine that 'the imagination and the versatility of the most skilful surgeon cannot close all fistulae'[34] and consider exenteration or palliative diversion[9]. This may be of particular benefit in patients with incurable cancer, especially if the patient's long-term prognosis is for survival in excess of 6 months, as is often the case in cervical and rectal cancers invading the lower urinary tract (Figs 37.5 & 37.6).

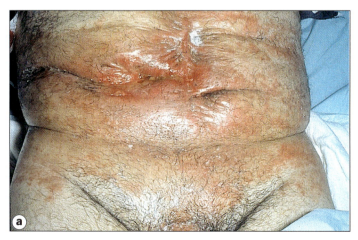

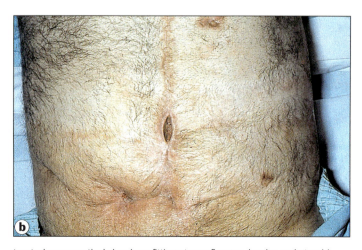

Figure 37.11 Enterourinary fistula in a male following self-mutilation of an existing ileal conduit. (a) The effect of the enteric and urinary content on the skin has produced a severe dermatitis. (b) This has been treated preoperatively by close-fitting stoma flanges, barrier and steroid creams, and low-pressure suction to keep the mixed urine and enteric fluid off the skin prior to definitive surgery.

MANAGEMENT OF SIMPLE FISTULAE – CONSERVATIVE TREATMENT

Small fistulae may heal spontaneously with prolonged catheter drainage[35] or with JJ stenting if a stent can be manipulated past a small ureteric defect. Fulguration of small fistulae followed by catheter drainage can work for defects of 3mm or less[36], as can a number of other adjunctive measures[17]. However, these procedures are reportedly effective only in the smallest fistulae; the majority will require a definitive surgical repair.

Surgical repair: general principles

Adherence to basic surgical principles is the key to a successful outcome. It is also important to remember that the best chance of success is the first attempt at repair. The principles include comprehensive preoperative evaluation and control of infection, wide exposure of the fistula and surrounding area, excision of fibrosed and damaged tissue, tension-free apposition of well vascularized edges with a dry, uninfected suture line and interposition of a vascularized tissue flap where there is the least suspicion of tissue compromise or a tenuous repair[9,17,21,37].

Timing of repair

There is considerable controversy relating to the safety and efficacy of early or delayed repair. The traditional and somewhat dogmatic approach is that there should be a delay of 3–6 months before any attempt at closure is made[17]. This doctrinaire view has been questioned in relation to cases of clean iatrogenic injury[16,38] and large series have shown that early repair of ureteral and vesicovaginal fistulae can be safely and successfully undertaken, although it should be noted that such repairs entail the use of an extensive abdominal approach and reconstruction with pedicle flaps[38]. Wise counsel would suggest that it is impossible to generalize in all cases and that final decisions on early versus delayed treatment should be taken on an individual basis in the light of the clinical condition and the bacteriologic, radiologic, and endoscopic information available. This is especially true of complex radiation and enterourinary fistula.

Surgical approach

Abdominal, vaginal, and combined approaches are all described for fistula repair. The final decision depends on various factors, including the type and anatomy of the fistula, its etiology, co-existing pathology, and the experience and preference of the individual surgeon.

The vaginal approach has the advantage of avoiding an abdominal incision and cystotomy, it has minimal blood loss, and there is a shorter postoperative recovery period[39]. For straightforward fistulae it has a high success rate, over 90% of fistulae being closed successfully using this method[14,40,41]. However, for more complex fistulae, especially those close to or involving the ureter and those with disease affecting other organ systems, the abdominal approach is preferred, this giving better exposure of the fistula, better access to other organs, and the facility to fashion an interposition flap using omentum or peritoneum. The ideal strategy is to have the facility and expertise available to deal with the problem using either technique or a combination of the two when necessary[42,43].

Vaginal techniques

The patient is ideally placed supine with the legs in Lloyd-Davies-type stirrups or boots. This facilitates optimal placement and enables modification of the patient's position intraoperatively if it becomes clear that a combined abdominoperineal approach is required. The exaggerated lithotomy position usually provides best exposure of the anterior vaginal wall with the patient tipped 15° head down and the hips abducted. Good retraction and exposure is provided by either a ring retractor or a weighted Auvard retractor in the vaginal fourchette in combination with a self-retaining retractor pulling the labia laterally. Suturing of the labia to the perineal skin will aid exposure in most patients. When the introitus is narrow, e.g. in the older patient, a posterolateral releasing incision will facilitate access[44] (Fig. 37.12). The patient is then cystoscoped and, if the fistula is in close relation to the ureteric orifices, they should be catheterized.

The fistula is then clearly visualized through the vagina and held with a tissue forceps or suture. An alternative method is to place a balloon catheter through the fistula and use the inflated balloon to retract the fistula down towards the introitus (Fig. 37.13 top left panel). The fistula is then circumcised, the track is dissected free and the vaginal wall and surrounding tissues are separated from the bladder wall (Fig. 37.13 top right panel). Having done this, some authors advocate excision of the scarred marginal edge of the fistula[45] while others maintain that this maneuver makes the fistula larger and decreases the strength of its wall on the bladder side, making the repair more difficult[46]. Once isolated, the bladder defect is closed with an absorbable 3/0 braided or monofilament suture (Fig. 37.13 bottom left panel). If the perivesical tissue or bladder wall is of good quality it is possible to suture these over the fistula suture line, adopting the principles used in the 'keel-type' repair of an incisional hernia. The vaginal skin is then closed over the defect, avoiding opposed

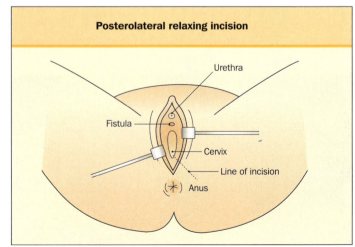

Figure 37.12 Posterolateral relaxing incision. The incision is carried out in the manner of an episiotomy to facilitate access when the introitus is narrow. This may be a particular problem following radiotherapy and in the elderly. Before carrying this out it is important to consider whether a Martius flap is required and from which side this is to be harvested, as the releasing incision may compromise the blood supply at the posterior limb of the flap.

Simple transvaginal fistula repair using balloon traction

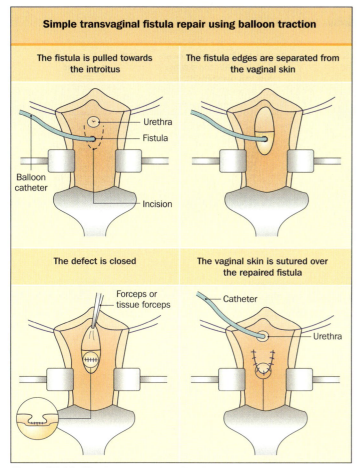

The fistula is pulled towards the introitus	The fistula edges are separated from the vaginal skin

Urethra
Fistula
Balloon catheter
Incision

The defect is closed	The vaginal skin is sutured over the repaired fistula

Forceps or tissue forceps
Catheter
Urethra

Figure 37.13 Simple transvaginal fistula repair using balloon traction. (Top left) The fistula is catheterized and gentle downward traction is applied to pull it towards the introitus. (Top right) The fistula margin is then circumcised. The fistula edges are separated from the vaginal skin; they may be left or excised according to condition. A vaginal advancement flap can be developed by incising the vaginal skin anteriorly on either side lateral to the urethra. (Bottom left) The defect is closed with 3/0 absorbable braided or monofilament suture. The paravesical tissue can then be used to oversew the defect in 'keel' fashion. (Bottom right) The vaginal skin is sutured over the repaired fistula as a 'U'.

sutures lines if possible. This can be achieved by using advancement techniques based on a 'U' incision (Fig. 37.13 bottom right panel), by a lateralization technique using a releasing incision in the lateral vaginal wall, or by excising a disc of vaginal skin laterally and suturing this, thereby pulling the suture line overlying the fistula to one side or the other. Either technique can be supplemented by the use of a Martius flap (Fig. 37.14).

In more difficult cases where the vaginal skin is scarred by surgery or damaged by radiotherapy, the technique of colpocleisis can be used[47] (Fig. 37.15). This involves incising an ellipse of vaginal skin around the fistula and lifting a flap based on a strip of that skin. This is then folded forwards and sutured to the remaining ellipse of vaginal skin, thereby closing the fistula defect without actually entering the bladder itself .

When the fistula affects the urethra, similar techniques are used as with the vesicovaginal defects. The main difference is with the initial incision; it is better in this circumstance to use an inverted 'U' configuration (Fig. 37.14). Prior infiltration with

1:250,000 epinephrine may help to maintain hemostasis and a clear field. An interposition Martius flap should be used once the defect is closed (Fig. 37.14).

Postoperatively the bladder should be drained by suprapubic and urethral catheters for a 10-day period, paying close attention to antisepsis. Bladder spasm may require anticholinergic/antispasmodic treatment. A cystogram is carried out prior to catheter removal to ensure that the repair is sealed. Thereafter, patients should be given basic advice about avoiding sexual activity for a 2-month period to allow complete healing.

Vaginal interposition flaps

When the vaginal skin is in poor condition, the defect is large, or there is concern regarding the vascularity of the tissues, an interposition flap should be used. This improves the successful closure rate in a more difficult fistula, although the exact mechanism of its action is unproven. A flap of this nature certainly provides a separation of the suture lines and it is possible that it also provides added vascularity and improved lymphatic drainage. There are three basic types, although a large number of modifications have been reported. They are:

- The Martius flap[4] (Fig. 37.14);
- The labial rotation flap[48] or Lehoczky island flap[49] (Fig. 37.16); and
- The gracilis myofascial/myocutaneous flap.

The basic technique for the Martius flap is shown in Figure 37.14. This flap is the one most frequently used as an adjunct to vaginal repair. The other types of flap repair are usually reserved for situations where the perineal damage is most severe, e.g. after radiotherapy.

Abdominal techniques
Simple fistulae

This popular method of repair has the advantage that it provides excellent exposure and can be used with other adjunctive surgical maneuvers such as omental or peritoneal interposition flaps. The principles of repair are identical to those used in the vaginal techniques.

Preoperatively, prophylactic antibiotics are administered and specific antimicrobial pathogens are eradicated. Routine precautions are taken to minimize thromboembolic complications. The patient is positioned in Lloyd-Davies with a 15° head-down tilt before opening the abdomen using a midline incision. This approach allows greater versatility in mobilizing other structures in the event that the fistula repair is more difficult than was anticipated postoperatively. If a Pfannenstiel incision has been made recently, it may need conversion to a midline type. An extraperitoneal approach can be used for the simplest fistulae but in general the transperitoneal route is preferred. The technique of repair is shown in Figure 37.17. The bladder is opened in the sagittal plane in the midline and 'bivalved' down to the fistula edge. The bladder edges are held back by stay sutures secured over an abdominal or ring retractor. The ureteric orifices are then cannulated under direct vision and the fistula is circumcised. It is important then to separate the distal bladder margin from the vaginal wall, cutting away dead and diseased tissues to well vascularized edges, which can be moved together without tension. In some cases a combined abdominal and perineal approach is required to achieve this, separating the anterior vaginal wall from

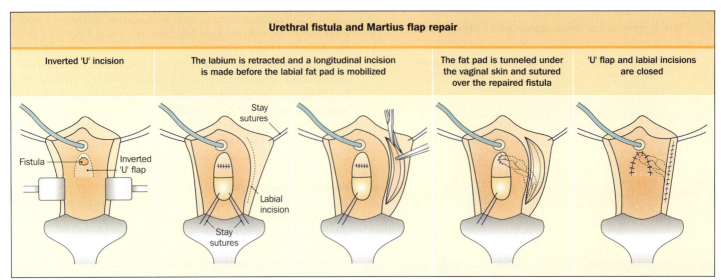

Figure 37.14 Urethral fistula and Martius flap repair. The urethra is catheterized and an inverted 'U' incision is fashioned in the overlying vaginal skin. The labium is retracted and a longitudinal incision is made before the labial fat pad is mobilized. This can be done from the anterior or posterior aspect, preserving the blood supply from one end. For fistulae lower in the vagina the anterior mobilization is preferred. The mobilized fat pad is tunneled under the vaginal skin and sutured in place over the repaired fistula using absorbable sutures. The vaginal skin 'U' flap and labial incisions are closed and the urethral catheter is left *in situ*.

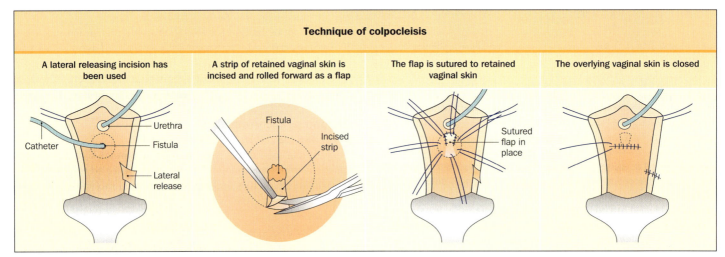

Figure 37.15 Technique of colpocleisis. For colpocleisis the fistula is excised more widely. A lateral releasing incision has been used to facilitate access. A strip of the retained vaginal skin is incised and then raised and rolled forwards as a flap. The inverted flap is sutured to the residual retained vaginal skin margin, closing the defect. The overlying vaginal skin is closed. A Martius flap may be interposed at this juncture.

below and meeting the abdominal dissection from above, thus facilitating the subsequent interposition of a long omental or peritoneal flap (Figs 37.17 bottom right, 37.18, & 37.19). If the tissues are very rigid, e.g. after radiotherapy, additional surgical procedures may be required to enable a vascularized tension-free closure and/or augmentation of the bladder capacity. This may entail the use of an enteric patch brought down on its mesenteric blood supply, usually from the small bowel, a technique that can also be used in rectovaginal fistula[50].

Once isolated, the fistula is closed with absorbable 3/0 braided or monofilament sutures to both the bladder and vagina, and the interposition flap is stitched in place (Figs 37.17–37.19). The bladder is drained via a suprapubic and urethral catheter and, if there is concern about periureteric edema, separate ureteric catheters can be brought out through the abdominal wall via a cystotomy. The pelvis is drained with a simple tube drain. Postoperatively, antispasmodics and antimicrobial therapy are usually required. The abdominal drains are left until urine output is minimal and the catheters are left in for approximately 10 days. A cystogram should be undertaken to ensure the repair is watertight before these are removed. Using this technique, most fistulae of this type are amenable to repair, with a success rate in excess of 90%[37,51].

Abdominal interposition grafts/flaps
An interposition graft or flap separates overlying suture lines and in the case of omental or myofascial flaps may also add vascular supply and lymphatic drainage. Their use is essential in

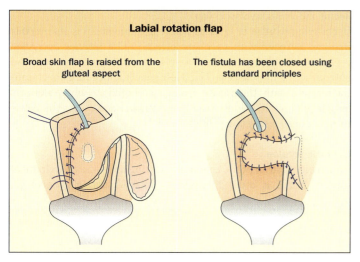

Labial rotation flap

Broad skin flap is raised from the gluteal aspect	The fistula has been closed using standard principles

Figure 37.16 Labial rotation flap. If the vaginal skin is damaged and scarred (e.g. following radiotherapy) a rotation flap using labial/perineal skin can be used. A broad skin flap is raised with its base arising from the gluteal aspect. The fistula has been closed using standard principles. The mobilized labial skin and fat are rotated across the defect and sutured in place with interrupted absorbable braided or monofilament 3/0 sutures. If the labial skin is in poor condition, a similar closure can be achieved using a tunneled gracilis myofascial or myocutaneous flap.

successful fistula closure, especially in the radiation or complex fistula case. The simplest type is a free graft of rectus sheath, peritoneum, or bladder mucosa. These have the disadvantage that they are not vascularized but, in cases where there is no easily available alternative, e.g. previously removed omentum, irradiated, or scarred pelvic peritoneum, and inability to use a rectus flap because of abdominal scarring or abdominal stomas, this alternative may be invaluable. For the most part, however, it is best to use a vascularized pedicle flap, of which there are three major types:

Peritoneal rotation advancement flap

This was originally described in 1900[52] and has subsequently been revisited[53]. The principles are described in Figure 37.18. This is a particularly useful technique and avoids the necessity of bringing an omental flap across the peritoneal cavity. In using this technique it is important to consider early in the procedure where the flap is to be mobilized from, in order to preserve the peritoneal reflection on to the pelvic side wall. Modifications of this approach include mobilizing the peritoneum off the bladder itself to give extra flap length or, alternatively, mobilizing the peritoneum off the posterior wall of the vagina and/or the anterior rectal surface and using this as an advancement flap (Fig. 37.18).

Simple fistula repair using the transabdominal approach

Bladder bivalved to fistula	Ureters cannulated, fistula circumcised	Abdominal and perineal approach may be used

- Fistula
- Uterus

Vaginal defect closed	Interposition flap sutured and bladder closed	Suprapubic and/or urethral drainage

Omental or peritoneal flap

Omental or peritoneal flap

Figure 37.17 Simple fistula repair using the transabdominal approach.
(Top left) The bladder is exposed and 'bivalved' down to the fistula. (Top center) The ureters are then cannulated and the fistula is circumcised, removing diseased tissue. (Top right) The healthy bladder edges are separated from the fistula. This can usually be undertaken abdominally but may need a combined abdominoperineal approach. (Bottom left) The free edges of the bladder and vaginal defects must be well vascularized and must come together without tension. The vaginal defect is then closed with a 3/0 braided or monofilament suture. (Bottom center) An interposition flap is sutured in place so that it completely overlies the vaginal defect. The bladder defect is then closed with a continuous 3/0 braided or monofilament suture and suprapubic and/or urethral catheters are left in situ. (Bottom right) A tube drain is left in the pelvis and, if there is any concern about the proximity or drainage of the ureters, ureteric cannulas are left *in situ* and brought out through a separate cystotomy.

Omental pedicle flap

This was first reported in 1935 and is a most valuable adjunct to fistula repair. The omentum not only provides the necessary interpositional bulk, it also adds a good blood and lymphatic supply. In radiation cases it has the advantage that it has usually been outside the radiation field during radiotherapy. The principles of its mobilization are shown in Figure 37.19. There is some controversy as to whether the flap should be raised on the left gastroepiploic pedicle[54] or the right gastroepiploic pedicle[55]. In practical terms, either can be used with good results and the choice of right or left should be individualized according to the patient's anatomy to obtain the best outcome.

Rectus abdominis myofascial flap

In complex fistulae or in cases where the omentum is absent, this flap can be used with excellent effect[56]. The inferior epigastric vessels enter the rectus abdominis muscle from the top and bottom of the muscle (Fig. 37.20 left panel). Once mobilized from the rectus sheath, the muscle can be transected anywhere along its length (Fig. 37.20 middle panel) and turned down into the pelvis to be secured with absorbable sutures.

Ureteric fistulae

The ureter is susceptible to damage during any type of abdominal surgery but it is most commonly damaged during gynecologic

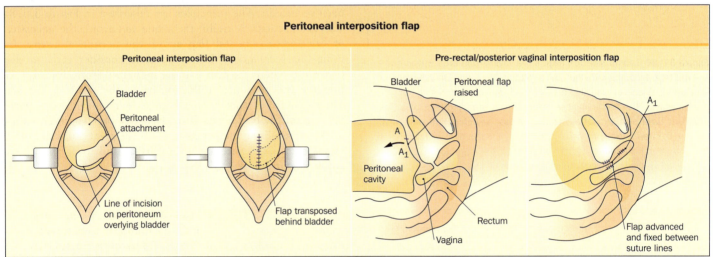

Figure 37.18 Peritoneal interposition flap. The peritoneum is raised on the lateral aspect from right or left (left, center left) or from the posterior vagina and anterior rectal surface (center right, right). It is important to make the decision about mobilization early in the operation. The flap is then interposed between the closure lines and sutured in place.

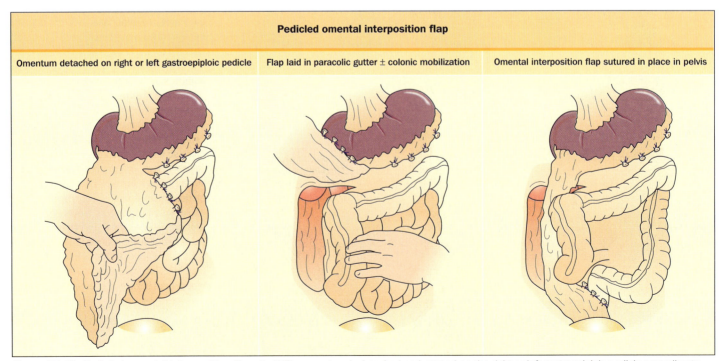

Figure 37.19 Pedicled omental interposition flap. (Left) The omentum is detached and rotated on the right or left gastroepiploic pedicle according to the patient's anatomy. (Center) The graft is laid in the paracolic gutter and, if necessary, (right) can be sutured right down on the perineal floor itself.

Rectus abdominis myofascial interposition flap

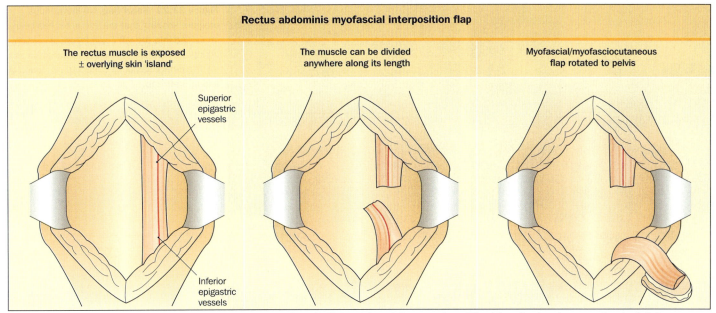

| The rectus muscle is exposed ± overlying skin 'island' | The muscle can be divided anywhere along its length | Myofascial/myofasciocutaneous flap rotated to pelvis |

Superior epigastric vessels

Inferior epigastric vessels

Figure 37.20 Rectus abdominis myofascial interposition flap. (Left) The left or right rectus is mobilized from its sheath, preserving the inferior epigastric vessels entering on the inferior and lateral aspect. (Center) The muscle is then transected, rotated into the pelvis and sutured in place. If a bowel stoma is to be used, the rectus from the opposite side should be used. The flap can be taken with or without the overlying skin (right).

procedures[57]. Injuries can also occur when an unsuspected duplex system is missed during the course of an operation (Fig. 37.3).

Surgical management depends on the type and level of the injury as well as the time to presentation, involvement of other organ systems, and the general condition of the patient. Simple 'side hole' fistulae, or those with minimal damage, e.g. as a consequence of ureteroscopy, may be managed successfully by ureteric stenting and/or nephrostomy drainage[58]. However, those with complete transection of the ureter will require surgical repair. The ureteric fistula recognized soon after the initial injury may be managed safely by early repair[38] although it may be necessary to control sepsis by proximal nephrostomy and antimicrobial therapy in the first instance. In situations where there is gross edema, sepsis, and complex fistulation making the situation hazardous it is best to delay definitive treatment (Figs 37.3, 37.7, 37.11; see Complex enterourinary fistulae, below).

If there is appropriate ureteric length and vascularity, the transected ureter can be repaired by a simple spatulated end-to-end anastomosis over a ureteric stent. The stent should be left in situ for at least 3 weeks postoperatively. In most cases, fistulae of this type are best managed using a psoas hitch (Fig. 37.21) or Boari flap if the defect is long (Fig. 37.22). This avoids the potential danger of distal avascular necrosis and anastomotic stricturing. In the well selected case success rates using this method approach 100%[59].

Postoperatively it is important to remember that ureteric stricturing can occur and renographic assessment is recommended at 3 and 6 months following the repair to enable early detection of developing obstruction.

In situations where renal function on the side of the fistula is poor or where the patient has a poor prognosis, e.g. from end-stage malignancy, ablation of the kidney may be considered. This can be carried out by renal embolization[60], nephrectomy, or ligation of the ureter proximal to the leak.

Complex fistulae

Fistulae of this type may arise from various conditions (Fig. 37.23). Straightforward vesicoenteric fistulae without multiple fistulous communications and/or concomitant intra-abdominal inflammation and sepsis are dealt with by simple disconnection and fistula closure using standard techniques. Bowel re-anastomosis may be primary or may be carried out secondarily following a period of external defunctioning. Cancers of the rectum and cervix fistulating into the lower urinary tract are best managed by exenteration if there is potential for cure, or diversion if there is not (Figs 37.5 & 37.6). Exenteration may also be considered for palliation in some cases, particularly if the patient has a relatively long life expectancy. Otherwise, the best alternative in this situation is to consider urinary and/or fecal diversion.

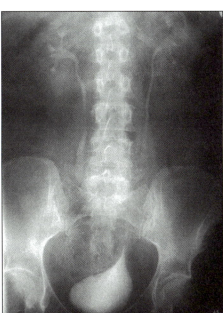

Figure 37.21 Psoas hitch. Intravenous urogram showing the typical appearance of a bladder following psoas hitch reimplantation.

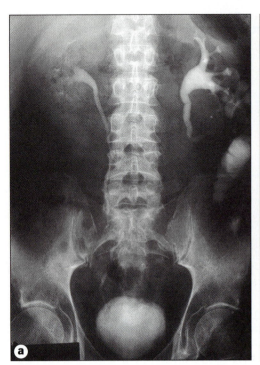
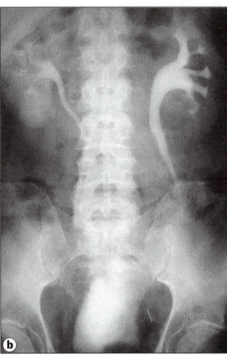

Figure 37.22 Boari flap. (a) Intravenous urogram showing that the left ureter has been implanted into the left colon following division during a laparotomy for a diverticular abscess. (b) The defect has been corrected by means of a long Boari flap.

Causes of complex fistulae

Inflammation/infection
Diverticulitis
Crohn's
Tuberculosis

Trauma
Foreign body/pessary
Obstetric
Traumatic injury
Surgery

Tumor
Primary erosion/invasion
Secondary spread
Radiotherapy-induced

Figure 37.23 Causes of complex fistulae.

Complex enterourinary fistulae are a problem of much greater magnitude. They often involve the urinary/genital and gastrointestinal tracts in combination and fistulous discharge can occur through several sites synchronously (Figs 37.1, 37.3, 37.7, & 37.11). Such cases may be particularly challenging and are best dealt with by a multidisciplinary surgical team with specific expertise that includes expert nurses, physiotherapists, and nutritionists. The techniques used for repair are the same as those for all fistulae but the essential key to success lies in the ability of the surgical team to recognize and correct the initial septic and metabolic complications before evaluating all aspects of the patient, including the nature of the fistula, the patient's general condition, and his/her overall surgical prognosis. It should be emphasized that not all fistulae can be closed (e.g. radiation fistulae affecting the bladder neck/sphincter area, extensive malignant fistulae from pelvic tumors not amenable to exenterative procedures) and that in incurable malignancy the simplest form of urinary diversion will provide the best palliation. In other circumstances, especially pelvic radiation disease, excision of

The York–Mason approach

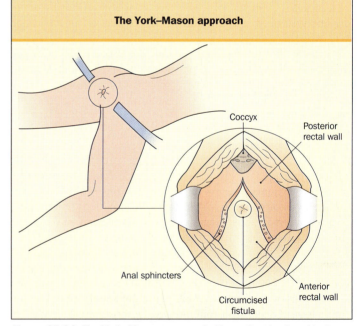

Figure 37.24 The York–Mason approach. The patient is placed in the 'prone jack-knife' position and the buttocks are taped out widely. The skin is incised from the sacrococcygeal articulation and carried down through the posterior rectal wall and anal sphincters. The fistula track is then seen and excised under vision. Healthy tissues are approximated closing first the urethra and then the anterior rectal wall. The posterior wall and sphincteric bundles can then be closed precisely by approximation with absorbable sutures. The presacral space is then drained (after Stephenson and Middleton[67]).

diseased organs and reconstruction where possible, using bowel segments, may be the only option available to achieve a good functional result[23,61].

Patients with complex enterourinary fistulae arising from postoperative and/or radiotherapy complications can present acutely and these patients may be profoundly septic. The management of these individuals can broadly be categorized into three stages:

1. Sepsis management. This involves cardiovascular stabilization and resuscitation followed by contrast imaging, usually with a CT scanner. The urinary and gastrointestinal systems are then defunctioned proximally and drained distally. This commonly involves nephrostomy insertion or cutaneous ureterostomy formation if the ureters have been transected intra-abdominally. The bladder or urostomy is drained distally. The bowel is defunctioned proximally by enterostomy above the fistula and where necessary mucous fistulation and drainage above and below the level of leakage. Septic foci should be drained, necrotic tissue excised, and if the wound/abdominal wall is compromised, the peritoneum and abdominal wound should be left open as a laparostomy (Fig. 37.7). Antimicrobial and, where necessary, antifungal therapy should be administered parenterally.

2. Recovery/rehabilitation. This stage involves controlled elimination of persistent sepsis using antimicrobials and, where necessary, further drainage procedures. Throughout this time the patient should receive total parenteral nutrition to supplement nutritional shortfall, renal replacement therapy where necessary, and intensive nursing and medical support, paying particular attention to the condition of the abdominal and perineal skin (Fig. 37.11). When the patient is sufficiently well, further anatomic delineation is undertaken to enable planning of subsequent reconstruction when the patient is rehabilitated, nutritionally restored, and the intra-abdominal sepsis has settled.

3. Reconstruction. This is usually delayed for several weeks but in some cases the delay can be for months before safe intervention can be contemplated. Reconstruction should be undertaken by a multidisciplinary team of urologists and colorectal surgeons with expertise in the field of fistula management and reconstruction.

Using the above regimen a successful outcome can be achieved in most patients provided there is adequate recovery of residual renal function following the initial septic and metabolic insult[62].

Treatment of rectoprostatic/rectourethral fistulae

Fistulae of this type may be associated with infection in the urinary tract or testis; this should be treated initially. The diagnosis should be established by cystoscopy and sigmoidoscopy with biopsy if the underlying diagnosis is in any doubt. This is particularly important in distinguishing inflammatory conditions from neoplastic ones. MRI using T2-weighted sequences may be particularly useful in identifying a connecting fistulous track in this situation when the diagnosis may be very difficult (Fig. 37.6). Some malignant and postradiotherapy fistulae are not amenable to closure (Fig. 37.5) but the majority of postsurgical ones are. In complex cases this requires an abdominal or combined abdominoperineal approach but in the majority a perineal, transanal, or transrectal approach can be used. The transanal approach, first described by Vose[63] and modified by Parks[64] has the disadvantage that access to the fistula is limited. Similar problems are encountered using the perineal approach, although it is possible to use a gracilis flap in these circumstances[65].

The direct posterior approach has now become the most popular technique for closure of fistulae of this type. This was originally described using the Kraske approach[66] but more recently the modified York–Mason technique has been employed with excellent functional results without the need for a defunctioning colostomy[67]. The technique is shown in Figure 37.24.

In circumstances where the fistula communicates with a defunctioned rectal stump, e.g. in inflammatory bowel disease, the best treatment is to remove the rectum and where necessary to lay in an omental or myofascial flap (Fig. 37.25).

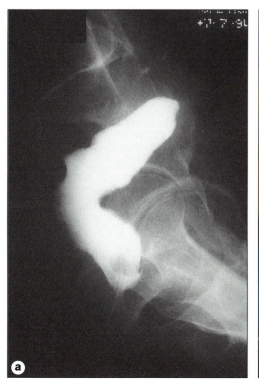

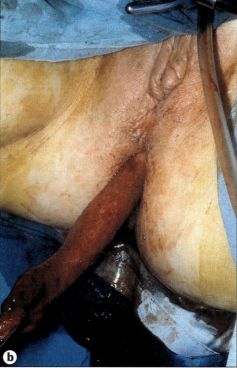

Figure 37.25 Fistula involving defunctioned rectal stump in a patient with Crohn's disease. (a) Contrast study. Urinary leakage persisted through the rectal stump and vagina despite previous attempts at closure. Definitive treatment was effected by removal of the rectal stump (b) and fashioning of a rectus abdominis myofascial flap to interpose between the bladder and vagina to enable closure of the vaginal defect. The omentum had been removed during previous surgery and the peritoneum was too scarred to use for flap closure.

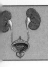
REFERENCES

1. Zacharin RE. Obstetric fistula. New York: Springer-Verlag; 1988.
2. Zacharin RF. Grafting as a principle in the surgical management of vesico-vaginal and recto-vaginal fistulas. Aust NZ J Obstet Gynaecol. 1980;20:10–17.
3. Simms JM. On the treatment of vesical fistula. Am J Med Sci. 1852; 23:59–62.
4. Martius H. Die operative Wiederherstellung der vollkommen fehlenden Harnrohre und des Schiessmuskels derselben. Zentralbl. Gynak. 1928;480:52–57.
5. O'Conor VJ Jr, Sokol JK, Bowkley GJ, et al. Suprapubic closure of vesico-vaginal fistula. J Urol. 1973;109:51–4.
6. O'Conor VJ, Sokol JK. Vesico-vaginal fistula from the standpoint of the urologist. J Urol. 1951;66:579–81.
7. Hamlin RHJ and Nicholson EC. Reconstruction of urethra totally destroyed in labour. Br Med J. 1969;1:147–50.
8. Ashworth FL. Urinary vaginal fistulas: a series of 152 patients treated in a small hospital in Ghana. West Afr Med J. 1973;22:39–43.
9. Wein AJ, Malloy TR, Carpiniello VO, et al. Repair of vesico-vaginal fistula by suprapubic transvesical approach. Surg Gynecol Obstet. 1980;150:57–60.
10. Herbert DB. Vesicovaginal fistula: a therapeutic challenge. Infect Urol. 1988;1:63–5.
11. Tahzib AU. Epidemiological determinants of vesicovaginal fistulas. Br J Obstet Gynaecol. 1983;90:389–91.
12. Davits RJ, Miranda SI. Conservative treatment of vesicovaginal fistulas by bladder drainage alone. Br J Urol. 1991;68:155–6.
13. Symmonds RE. Incontinence: vesical and urethral fistulas. Obstet Gynecol. 1984;27:499–514.
14. Massie JS. Management of urinary vaginal fistula: ten years survey. JAMA. 1964;190:902–6.
15. Lee AL, Symmonds RE, Williams TJ. Current status of genito-urinary fistula. Obstet Gynecol. 1988;72:313–19.
16. Goodwin WE, Scardino PT. Vesico-vaginal and uretero-vaginal fistulas: a summary of 25 years of experience. J Urol. 1980;123:370–4.
17. Gerber GS, Shoenberg HW. Female urinary tract fistulas. J Urol. 1993;149:229–36.
18. Little NA, Juma S, Raz S. Vesico-vaginal fistulas. Semin Urol. 1979;7:78–82.
19. Mann WJ, Arato M, Patsner B, et al. Ureteral injuries in an obstetrics and gynecology training programme: etiology and management. Obstet Gynecol. 1988;72:82–5.
20. Daly JW, Higgins KA. Injury to the ureter during gynecological surgical procedures. Surg Gynecol Obstet. 1988;167:19–22.
21. Zimmern PE, Ganabathi, Leach GE. Vesico-vaginal fistula repair. Atlas Urol Clin North Am. 1994;2:87–99.
22. Selvaggi FP, Battaglia M, Cormio L. Ureteral complications of pelvic surgery. In: Jewett MAS, ed. Urological complications of pelvic surgery and radiotherapy. Oxford: Isis Medical Media; 1995.
23. Lupton EW. Radiation urinary tract disease. In: Schofield PF, Lupton EW, eds. The causation and clinical mangement of pelvic radiation disease. London: Springer Verlag; 1989.
24. Solsona E, Iborra-Juan I, Ricos-Torrent J, et al. Urological complications of pelvic radiotherapy. In: Jewett MAS, ed. Urological complications of pelvic surgery and radiotherapy. Oxford: Isis Medical Media; 1995:51.
25. Williams RD. Urological complications of pelvic surgery. In: Jewett MAS, ed. Urological complications of pelvic surgery and radiotherapy. Oxford: Isis Medical Media; 1995:1.
26. Kirsh ED, Morse RM, Reznick MI, et al. Prevention and development of a vesico-vaginal fistula. Surg Gynecol Obstet. 1998;166:409–11
27. Keettel WC, Sehring FG, DeProsse CA, et al. Surgical management of urethro-vaginal and vesico-vaginal fistulas. Amer J Obstet Gynecol. 1978;131:425–31.
28. Graham JB. Painful syndrome of post-radiation urinary vaginal fistula. Surg Gynecol Obstet. 1966;124:1260–2.
29. Moir JC. Vesico-vaginal fistulas as seen in Britain. J Obst Gynecol Br Commonw. 1973;80:598–602.
30. Taylor PM, Johnson RJ, Eddlestone B, et al. Radiological changes in the gastro-intestinal and genito-urinary tract following radiotherapy for carcinoma of the cervix. Clin Radiol. 1990;41:165–9.
31. Johnson RJ, Carrington BM. Pelvic radiation disease. Clin Radiol. 1992;45:4–12.
32. Kimose HH, Fischer L, Spjeldnaes N, et al. Late radiation injury of the colon and rectum. Surgical management and outcome. Dis Col Rect. 1989;32:684–9.
33. Turner-Warwick R. Urinary fistulas in the female. In: Walsh PC, Gittes RF, et al, eds. Campbell's urology, 5th edn. Philadelphia, PA: WB Saunders; 1986:2718.
34. Marshall VF. Editorial comment. J Urol. 1980;123:369.
35. Zimmern PE, Leach GE. Vesico-vaginal fistula repair. Probl Urol. 1991;5:171–4.
36. Falk HC, Orkin LA. Non-surgical closure of vesico-vaginal fistulas. Obst. Gynecol. 1957;9:538–40.
37. O'Conor VJ Jr. Editorial comment. J Urol. 1980;123:374.
38. Blandy JP, Badenoch DF, Fowler CG, et al. Early repair of iatrogenic injury to the ureter or bladder after gynecological surgery. J Urol. 1991;146:761–5.
39. Wang Y, Hadley R. Non-delayed trans-vaginal repair of high lying vesico-vaginal fistula. J Urol. 1990;144:34–6.
40. Raz S, Little NA, Juma S. Female urology. In: Walsh PC, Retik AB, Stamey TA, Vaughan ED, eds. Campbell's urology, 6th edn. Philadelphia, PA:WB Saunders; 1992:2782.
41. Tancer ML. Observations on prevention and management of vesico-vaginal fistula after total hysterectomy. Surg Gynecol Obstet. 1992;175:501–6.
42. Weyrauch HM, Rous SN. Trans-vaginal trans-vesical approach for surgical repair of vesico-vaginal fistula. Surg Gynecol Obstet. 1966;123:121–5.
43. Roen PR. Combined vaginal and trans-vesical approach in successful repair of vesico-vaginal fistula. Arch Surg. 1960;80:628–30.
44. Graham JB. Vaginal fistulas following radiotherapy. Surg Gynecol Obstet. 1965;120:1019–21.
45. McVey KT, Marshall FF. Urinary fistulas. In: Gillenwater JY, Grayhack JT, Howards S, Duckett JW, eds. Adult and pediatric urology, 3rd edn. St Louis, MO: Mosby; 1996.
46. Leach GE, Trockman BA. Surgery for vesico-vaginal and urethro-vaginal fistula and urethral diverticulum. In: Walsh PC, Retik AB, Vaughan ED, Wein AJ, eds. Campbell's urology, 7th edn. Philadelphia, PA: WB Saunders; 1997.
47. Latzko W. Post-operative vesico-vaginal fistulas: genesis and therapy. Am J Surg. 1942;58:211–14.
48. Hendren WH. Construction of female urethra from vaginal wall and a perineal flap. J Urol. 1980;123:657–64.
49. Kelemen Z, Lehoczky G. Closure of severe vesico-vaginal-rectal fistulas using Lehoczky's island flap. Br J Urol. 1987;59:153–5.
50. Mraz JP, Sutory M. An alternative in surgical treatment of post-irradiation vesico-vaginal and recto-vaginal fistulas: the sero-muscular intestinal graft (patch). J Urol. 1994;151:357–9.
51. Blaivas JG, Heritz DM, Romanzi LJ. Early versus late repair of vesico-vaginal fistulas: vaginal and abdominal approach. J Urol. 1995;153:1110–12.
52. Bardescu N. Ein neues Verfahren fur die Operation der tiefen Blasen-Uterus-Scheidenfisteln. Centralbl Gynak. 1900;24:170–4.
53. Eisen M, Jurkovic K, Altwein JE, et al. Management of vesico-vaginal fistulas with peritoneal flap interposition. J Urol. 1974;112:195–8.
54. Kiricuta I, Goldstein AMB. Epiplooplastia vezicla metoda de tratament curativ al fistulelor vezico-vaginale. Obstet Ginecol Bucuresti. 1956;2:163–7.
55. Turner-Warwick RT, Wynne EJC, Handley, Ashken M. The use of the omental pedicle graft in repair and reconstruction of the urinary tract. Br J Surg. 1967;54:849–53.

56. Robertson CN, Riefklhl R, Webster GN. Use of the rectus abdominis muscle in urological reconstructive procedures. J Urol. 1986;135:963–5.

57. Lee AL, Symmonds RE. Uretero-vaginal fistula. Am J Obstet Gynecol. 1971;109:1032–5.

58. Dowling RA, Corriere JN, Sandler CM. Iatrogenic ureteral injury. J Urol. 1986;135:912–15.

59. Onuora VC, Al-Mohahal S, Yousseff A, et al. Iatrogenic urogenital fistulas. Br J Urol. 1993;71:176–8.

60. Long MA, McIvor J. Renal artery embolisation with ethanol and gelfoam for the treatment of ureteric fistulas with one year follow-up. Clin Radiol. 1992;46:270–2.

61. Chapple CR, Turner-Warwick RT. Surgical salvage of the post-irradiation frozen pelvis. In: Jewett MAS, ed. Urological complications of pelvic surgery and radiotherapy. Oxford: Isis Medical Media; 1995:89–108.

62. Shackley DC, Brew C, Bryden AAG, et al. Management of complex entero-urinary fistulas. Br J Urol. 2000 (in press) .

63. Vose SN. A technique for the repair of recto-urethral fistula. J Urol.1949; 61:790–4.

64. Tiptaft RC, Parkes M. Fistulas involving rectum and urethra: the place of Parkes' operation. Br J Urol. 1983;55:711–15.

65. Ryan JA, Beebe HG, Gibbons RP. Grascilis muscle flap for closure of recto-urethral fistula. J Urol. 1979;122:124–5.

66. Kilpatrick FR, Thompson HR. Post-operative recto-prostatic fistula and closure by Kraske's approach. Br J Urol. 1962;34:470–2.

67. Stephenson RA, Middleton RG. Repair of recto-urinary fistulas using a posterior sagittal transrectal (modified York–Mason) approach: an update. J Urol. 1996;155:1989–91.

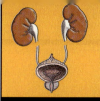

Section 6 Benign Conditions of the Lower Urinary Tract

Chapter 38

Urethral Stricture Disease

Leonard Zinman

KEY POINTS

- Common etiology of strictures is endoscopic trauma and instrumentation. Inflammatory strictures result most frequently from balanitis xerotica obliterans.
- The diagnosis requires dynamic fluoroscopic ascending urethrogram, voiding cystourethrogram, and meticulous urethroscopy to completely identify stricture and non-obstructive spongiofibrosis.
- Location, length of the stricture and coexisting genital pathology governs the selection of final management options for repair of a urethral stricture.
- The methods for stricture management involve regenerative (dilation/urethrotomy), anastomotic, and substitution techniques.
- Regenerative procedures are best performed in anterior strictures less than 2cm in length.
- Anastomotic repair is exclusively limited to post-traumatic, bulbar, and prostatomembranous strictures.
- Circumferential tube grafts and flaps frequently fail and should be avoided.

INTRODUCTION

Strictures have plagued humankind since the beginning of time as a sequel to inflammatory urethritis, but times have changed and gonorrhea, the historical basis of strictures, has been replaced by urethral instrumentation and external trauma as the common cause of the disease[1]. Strictures are scars of various depths, densities, and lengths, replacing portions of the corpora spongiosa with loss of urothelium and subsequent circular contracture of the lumen. They are most often located in the proximal portion of the urethra but vary in length and location, depending upon etiology and the extent of prior endoscopic surgery and instrumentation[2]. Inflammatory strictures continue to appear with a decreased incidence but of greater length than those seen after gonorrheal urethritis. The most common cause of inflammatory strictures at present may be balanitis xerotica obliterans (BXO), which often involves the submeatal and pendulous segments of the urethra but may first present as a panurethral stricture[3,4] and appears to be a much more common and more extensive disease than previously reported. This disease classically involves the glans and prepuce but may vary in its extent to include the entire genital skin along with coexistent scrotal edema[4].

A significant number of strictures have been designated as of unknown origin but are presumed to follow infection, with a history clouded by the prior effects of repeat instrumentation.

SURGICAL ANATOMY

Urethra and corpus spongiosa

The location and length of a stricture ultimately dictates the appropriate reparative surgical procedure selected. The urethra is best thought of in terms of five separate divisions rather than the traditional concept of an anterior and a posterior segment. The prostatic and membranous portions are considered as one unit, since they are both difficult to access and harbor a sphincter active area below and proximal to the pubic arch. The anterior urethra includes the bulbar and bulbomembranous segments, the pendulous portion, and a submeatal portion. Anastomotic and substitution procedures have specific limitations on the basis of this anatomy. The bulbar and membranous segments need to be considered together, since the repair of these two locations requires similar exposure and tissue transfer techniques, but the membranous component can be difficult to distinguish from the bulbous component by standard retrograde imaging assessment. The urethra itself is central in location as it passes through the pendulous portion of the corpus spongiosa but changes to a more dorsal, eccentric location in the proximal bulbar site. This anatomic feature permits a relatively avascular proximal dorsal urethrotomy if the corpus spongiosum is first mobilized circumferentially[5].

The blood supply to the male genitalia arises from both the internal and external pudendal systems. The penile skin circulation comes from the external pudendal vasculature, both deep and superficial. This vascular tree arborizes with the scrotal blood supply coming from the scrotal and perineal branches of the internal pudendal artery[6]. This biaxial system feeds the skin of the penis and scrotum through perforators in a fasciocutaneous complex that permits safe retrieval of skin islands in both penis and scrotum for the entire anterior urethra. The blood supply to the corpus spongiosum arises entirely from the common penile division of the terminal portion of the internal pudendal artery but divides into a bipedal system. The proximal system consists of the bulbar arteries, which communicate with the distal system coming from the dorsal artery of the penis in a retrograde manner to the glans and spongiosa. These two circulations maintain the viability of some of the most fibrotic bulbous urethras after transection, partial excision, and a roof-strip anastomosis, if properly mobilized. A unique anatomic aspect of the penile skin is the subdermal supply, which maintains viability of all remaining donor

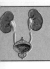

site skin after a cutaneous island has been retrieved with the entire dartos fascial envelope and its axial pedicles.

ASSESSMENT OF ANTERIOR URETHRAL STRICTURE DISEASE

Strictures present with a variety of clinical patterns. The most common ones are gradual decrease in caliber and force of urinary stream, insidious onset of irritative and obstructive voiding symptoms, which have been tolerated for years, acute urinary retention, spontaneous meatal bleeding, or recurrent responsive urinary tract infections. The physical examination reveals a firm, almost nodular, palpable urethra in a quarter of patients at the time of presentation. A palpable urethra portends a severe stricture that will not respond to regenerative procedures such as dilation or urethrotomy. The presence of a palpable nodular urethra, a septic spontaneous fistula or sinus, or recurrent periurethral abscesses should immediately lower the threshold for the suspicion of a urethral cancer. Careful examination of the penile and glans skin may reveal various degrees of balanitis xerotica obliterans, which will alter the choice of skin substitute used in repair and forewarn the surgeon of the presence of a more extensive stricture. The anatomy and character of the stricture will ultimately dictate its future course and management. Failure to recognize the extent of proximal and distal wide-caliber spongiofibrosis is the major cause of recurrent stricture. It is best defined by careful scrutiny of retrograde urethrogram studies along with endoscopic examination using both adult and pediatric instruments. Retrograde balloon catheter bougienage has been an invaluable tool during intraoperative evaluation of a stricture when the surgeon is trying to pinpoint the proximal margin of disease. This is best performed by introducing a no. 5 Fogarty catheter, as you would a filiform, filling the balloon with 1mL (26F) and withdrawing the balloon until an obstructive point is identified. Wide-caliber spongiofibrosis is subtle and difficult to assess, but a carefully performed endoscopy will reveal the abnormal, pale, rigid urethra, which appears radiologically equivocal. The extent of wide-caliber fibrous replacement of the spongiosal wall is best noted during the surgical urethrotomy when the diseased urethra can be compared to the normal vascular bed. The cryptic extension of a stricture from the bulbar urethra across into the trans-sphincteric membranous segment can be elusive on routine retrograde urethrography. A micturating study may be an additional aid along with intraoperative endoscopy through the open urethrotomy. Recognizing this entity changes the surgical repair dramatically but should not compromise the surgeon's ability to include this segment in reconstruction.

OVERVIEW AND GENERAL PRINCIPLES OF URETHRAL STRICTURE MANAGEMENT

Urethral reconstruction falls into the general category of either regenerative conservative management or open urethroplasty, which includes an increasingly complex repertoire of tissue transfer methods that include the general use of either substitution or anastomotic techniques. Regenerative procedures include urethral dilation, direct vision cold knife urethrotomy, intermittent self-dilation, the placement of an intraluminal

stainless steel stent, and the use of chronic dilatation by tissue expansion. Open surgical approaches to urethral stricture[3] are the integral components of a reconstructive triangle, including anastomotic technique, graft onlays and the retrieval of genital cutaneous island flaps[7]. Surgical reconstruction should be seriously entertained early in the course of all refractory strictures that do not respond to one adequate urethrotomy and a 3-month course of intermittent self-dilation. Panurethral strictures, posthypospadias strictures, complex bulbomembranous pathology, and segmental loss of urethra are best managed initially by an appropriate open reconstructive procedure. Urethral dilatation continues to be the mainstay of management of strictures in older or poor-risk individuals who require infrequent bougienage, men with postprostatectomy trans-sphincteric strictures when continence is an issue[8], and those patients in whom formidable open urethroplasty has failed and who wish to be treated conservatively. Recent data suggests that appropriate gentle urethral dilation is as effective as incisional endoscopic urethrotomy and that this approach is most effective in superficial strictures less than 2cm in length[9].

A patient being selected for a formal open urethral reconstruction is carefully and exhaustibly informed about the potential complications of the procedure, a realistic expectation of the voiding pattern and the subsequent need for 5–10 years of surveillance[10]. Surgical exposure and other adjunctive measures have a significant impact on the outcome of urethral reconstruction. The use of contemporary protective stirrups for the surgical repair of a proximal or panurethral stricture is crucial to prevent pressure-induced peripheral nerve injuries or compartment space syndromes[11]. One should avoid extreme exaggerated flexion of the thighs and employ a more moderate lower dorsolithotomy position. The addition of the so-called direct OR supporting stirrups with pneumatic compression boots has been a major advance for surgery on patients in the lithotomy position. Instruments that permit proper exposure and gentle movement of tissue include a perineal, self-retaining ring retractor, a posterior long-blade nasal speculum retractor, bipolar cautery, fine Bishop–Harman forceps, short and medium length tenotomy scissors, a halogen headlight, and the exclusive use of fine absorbable sutures.

Some of the changing concepts in surgical technique that have clearly improved the long-term cure rate of stricture repair include an aggressive stricturotomy with an extension into normal urethra for at least 2–3cm proximally and distally, partial excision of very fibrotic spongiosa with a pinpoint lumen and a roof-strip anastomosis combined with an onlay patch, the use of the dorsal urethrotomy after an extensive proximal bulbar urethral mobilization and the shift to buccal grafts. The compulsive use of appropriate urinary diversion and urethral stents along with early and delayed monitoring and surveillance are measures integral to achieving a patent urethral lumen. Wide spongiosal mobilization is required in the presence of a fibrotic urethra to avoid the serious sequela of ventral chordee. The urethral onlay augments used in a roof-strip anastomosis or in traditional urethral reconstruction should be placed over a 28–30F catheter template when a graft is used and over a 22–24F catheter when a flap is used. A 14F Silastic intraurethral stent is left in place for 7–10 days, and all patients undergo diversion by suprapubic cystotomy for a minimum of 3 weeks. The urethral lumen is monitored at 3 weeks by a voiding cystourethrogram to identify extravasation before removing the cystotomy tube, and retrograde urethrograms are obtained with flow studies at 3 months, 8 months, and annually if a change in voiding pattern, urinary tract infection, or decreased flow rate develops.

An important form of stricture management continues to be urethral dilation in its classic form, a procedure that is rarely curative but can selectively maintain an acceptable voiding pattern in patients with stable fibrotic walls that are not burdened by the complexity of fistulae, radiation, or full-length spongiofibrosis. For a sustaining effect, gentle graduated introduction of bougies at 4–7-day intervals followed by the use of an indwelling catheter at the onset of a dilation course until a lumen of 24F is achieved. The introduction of filiforms with the use of a flexible urethroscope will avoid the sequelae of false passages and troublesome bleeding.

The perception that direct vision endoscopic urethrotomy is more effective than dilation has been questioned by many reports of lower cure rates for urethrotomy than had previously been noted[12]. A report by Steenkamp and colleagues[9] demonstrates optical urethrotomy to be no more effective than standard dilation in a prospective study of 210 men randomized to undergo filiform dilation (106) or direct vision urethrotomy (104) on an outpatient basis. Recurrence at 12 months was significantly lower in patients with strictures shorter than 2cm (40%) as opposed to dilation or urethrotomy for strictures longer than 4cm (80%). The length of the stricture, as defined radiologically, was the only feature of this large series of prospectively studied strictures to predict recurrence. They concluded that strictures less than 2cm should be managed by a dilation protocol and that direct vision urethrotomy should be exclusively limited to the non-negotiable lumen that cannot be dilated and those strictures located in the bulbous urethra where a deep cleft is possible. The logic behind urethrotomy is that a focal, nontraumatic, well-placed incision will create a deep enough cleft in the spongiosa, which can then develop an epithelial cover to prevent cross-adherent contracture. The ideal location for endoscopic urethrotomy is the proximal urethra where there is a thick, relatively normal spongiosa. A deep incision is created at the 6 o'clock position to avoid injury to the corpus cavernosum circulation, using a no. 5 vascular balloon catheter as a guide to the distal margins of the stricture. When urethrotomy is performed in the pendulous portion of the urethra, two incisions may be made at the 3 o'clock and the 9 o'clock locations to prevent an increase in periurethral fibrosis and subsequent ventral chordee. An indwelling silicone-coated catheter should routinely be used for any urethrotomy to prevent the noxious wound effects of urinary extravasation on an open urethral incision. This is best maintained for a minimum of 7–10 days. The value of a subsequent 2–3-month posturethrotomy intermittent self-catheterization dilation program is controversial and not clearly proved to enhance the development of a durable patent lumen[12,13].

The more recent development of an indwelling endoprosthetic stent to prevent recurrent stricture after urethrotomy appears to show some promise, but followup is less than 5 years with a low incidence of complications noted at this early date. The present stent is a nonmagnetic alloy of steel that is woven into a tubular mesh with a self-expansile property that produces a 42F internal lumen diameter[14]. It is currently recommended for use in short strictures located in the bulbar segment of the urethra and has been used successfully in trans-sphincteric and postradical

prostatectomy vesical neck contractures when combined with an artificial AMS-800 urinary sphincter. Recurrent stricture will inevitably develop in patients with a long, post-traumatic, or complete disruption stricture with significant intraluminal tissue growth and should not be used in this group of patients.

This stent fares poorly after failed substitution urethroplasty, with recurrent obstructing tissue developing at the proximal or distal margin. The tissue growing through the fenestrations of the stent is usually a hypertrophic scar mixed with hyperplastic glandular histology. The addition of a second stent either in tandem or placed inside a first stent does decrease the incidence of recurrent scar infiltration[15]. Stent migration may occur early, but no instance of erosion, infection, encrustation, or erectile dysfunction has been recorded. Recurrent strictures in the presence of a Urolume stent requires a segmental resection of urethra and stent, since the prosthesis cannot be removed without formal resection of the remainder of the urethra. This is a challenging, complex problem that requires a roof-strip anastomosis combined with either a penile or scrotal island flap augment. The results of bulbar anastomotic urethroplasty of short post-traumatic strictures are so good in this location that they are best managed surgically rather than inviting the potential risks of a prosthesis in someone with decades of life to live. The short-term results of this technique have been satisfactory and it will undoubtedly have an important place in the future management of strictures.

OPEN SURGICAL REPAIR OF URETHRAL STRICTURES

Definitive resolution of stricture disease is obtained by the appropriate selection of an open reconstructive surgical procedure that either excises the lesion or corrects the obstructed lumen with an extensive stricturotomy and repair. The repertoire of techniques that has been introduced during the past two decades continues to evolve and will undoubtedly follow the tissue transfer innovations emerging from the investigation of wound care and problems with tissue remodeling noted in other organ systems. Patients with strictures in whom conservative maneuvers have failed may undergo reliable repair with a 5–10-year sustaining success of a stricture-free lumen in 85–90% of cases using one of the five contemporary modified, newly developed reconstructive concepts[16]. These include circumferential excision with end-to-end anastomosis, penile island flaps, scrotal nonhirsute island flaps, free grafts of buccal mucosa or skin with and without muscle buttress support, and the multi-stage mesh graft technique. The exact role of each of these operations and management of varied strictures has yet to be clearly defined and continues to remain a reflection of the surgeon's bias and experience. The emerging algorithm in stricture care depends, again, primarily on location, length, extension into the trans-sphincteric segment, and the availability of healthy penile and scrotal skin.

CIRCUMFERENTIAL EXCISION AND PRIMARY END-TO-END ANASTOMOTIC URETHRAL REPAIR

Primary anastomotic urethroplasty is the ideal method of reconstruction and the gold standard for the spectrum of urethral stricture surgery because urethra is clearly the best substitute for urethra. This operation should be limited exclusively to the proximal bulbar and bulbomembranous segments of urethra for post-traumatic strictures less than 2cm in length because the elasticity of the pendulous urethra is inadequate to prevent ventral chordee. A tension-free, watertight, spatulated, end-to-end anastomosis is dependent on adequate mobilization of the corpus spongiosum and division of the enveloping Buck's fascia to permit an average extension of 4cm of elastic lengthening of a proximal urethra. In patients in whom potency is not an issue, 3–4cm of a well-defined, post-traumatic stricture can be excised and subsequently repaired by this technique without the concern that a ventral erectile deformity will develop.

Strictures that occur secondary to instrumentation or urethritis are rarely suitable for this technique, because they either are longer or may have significant spongiofibrosis that interferes with the normal intrinsic elastic lengthening required for a tension-free connection.

Technique

This procedure is performed with patients in the low lithotomy position, counseling them beforehand that an alternative procedure might be required if a more extensive, wide-caliber stricture is encountered unexpectedly. A midline bifurcated perineal incision is made and carried deep to Colles fascia, which is retracted, exposing the bulbocavernosus muscle (Fig. 38.1). This is divided and reflected laterally without injuring the scrotal circulation or the corpus spongiosal surface. A self-retaining ring retractor (Turner-Warwick) is used to maintain exposure, and a 5F vascular balloon is introduced into the urethra like a filiform, distended with 1mL of saline solution and partially withdrawn to identify the proximal margin of the stricture (Fig. 38.1 right panel). A 24F bougie is then inserted in a retrograde fashion to define the distal limit of the stricture and establish that it is suitable for an anastomotic approach by measuring the distance between these two bougies. This judgment can also be aided by transperineal

ultrasonography where the urethrographic length is measured to be 2.5–3cm[17]. This study is followed by careful but complete mobilization of the bulbospongiosus from the intercrural membrane and membranous urethra to the suspensory ligament to achieve a 3–5cm increase in length. This length is obtained by virtue of releasing the intrinsic elasticity of a bulbar component of the spongiosa (Fig. 38.2 left panel). The proximal and distal spongiosal blood flow is controlled with vascular clamps or an occlusive drain tourniquet with the bougie and Fogarty catheter in place (Fig. 38.2 right panel). A distal ventral urethrotomy is made to open the urethra in its normal portion against the bougie and extending the urethrotomy proximally to the mid portion of the stricture (Fig. 38.3 left panel).

To gain vision and excise the precise margin of the fibrotic urethral wall, the stricture is transected at midpoint and suture tags are placed on both ends (Fig. 38.3 center panel). The proximal urethra is incised on its dorsal side, spatulating the lumen well into normal tissue (Fig. 38.3 right panel). The fibrotic wall can be distinguished readily and excised without much question of its extent, and the two free ends of the urethra are easily brought together without tension if the bulbospongiosus has been mobilized adequately. If tension exists, the distal end can be mobilized further up to the penile mid-shaft with the potential for some ventral chordee. The course of the urethra can be shortened further by separating the proximal corpora cavernosa and incising the intercrural membrane. A 2cm spatulation should be made of both ends, which may, at times, include some fibrotic wall at that point. A 20F suprapubic cystotomy Silastic Foley catheter is placed by introducing a fenestrated Van Buren sound with an exaggerated curve to execute a pull-in technique through an incision over the palpable tip, withdrawing the catheter into the bladder and out of the urethra before releasing the sound from the end of the Silastic catheter.

The inner aspects of the proximal and distal spatulated lumen are first approximated with three sutures of 4-0 absorbable at the

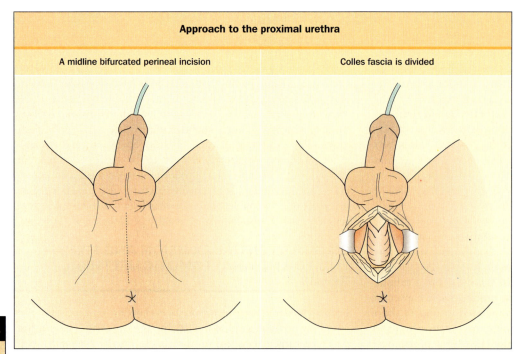

Approach to the proximal urethra	
A midline bifurcated perineal incision	Colles fascia is divided

Figure 38.1 Approach to the proximal urethra. (Left) A midline bifurcated perineal incision offers good exposure for proximal bulbospongiosal mobilization. (Right) Colles fascia is divided and reflected laterally without injuring the scrotal or penile circulation.

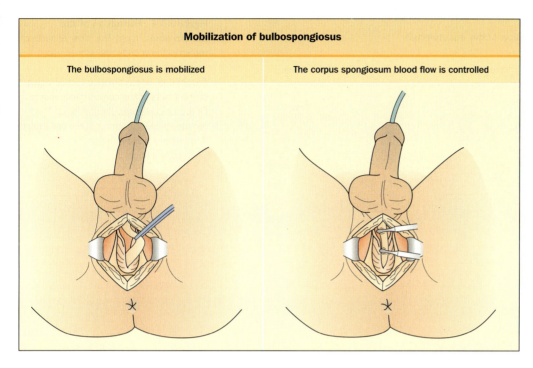

Mobilization of bulbospongiosus

The bulbospongiosus is mobilized	The corpus spongiosum blood flow is controlled

Figure 38.2 Mobilization of bulbospongiosus. (Left) The bulbospongiosus is mobilized from the membranous urethra to the suspensory ligament to release its intrinsic elasticity. (Right) The corpus spongiosum blood flow is controlled with vascular clamps or an occlusive drain tourniquet.

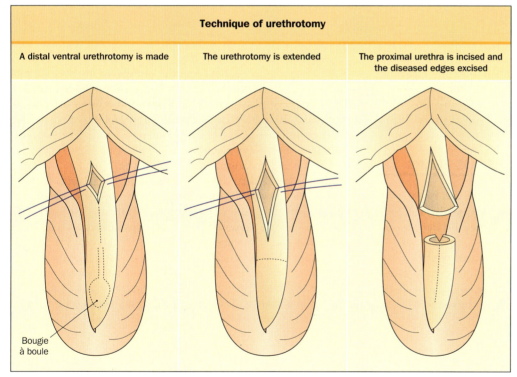

Technique of urethrotomy

A distal ventral urethrotomy is made	The urethrotomy is extended	The proximal urethra is incised and the diseased edges excised

Bougie
à boule

Figure 38.3 Technique of urethrotomy. (Left) A distal ventral urethrotomy is initially made into 2cm of normal urethra. (Center) The urethrotomy is extended proximally to a midpoint of the stricture where it is transected. The palpable balloon bougie identifies the proximal margin of the disease. (Right) The proximal urethra is incised on its dorsal surface, spatulating the lumen into normal nonfibrotic wall. The diseased edges are excised.

12 o'clock position with the knots on the outside of the lumen (Fig. 38.4 left panel). The remaining anastomotic sutures are initially placed before finally securing the knots, which are located in an external position (Fig. 38.4 center panel). A no. 16 Silastic stent is placed intraluminally at the completion of the anastomosis and is sutured to the meatal margin. The bulbocavernosus muscle is approximated with interrupted sutures of 4-0 absorbable (Fig. 38.4 right panel). Colles fascia is closed with 4-0 absorbable and the skin incision is closed completely with interrupted, closely placed 5-0 absorbable.

The urethral catheter is removed in 7–10 days and the suprapubic cystotomy tube is left for 3 weeks, removing it after voiding cystourethrography confirms an intact, sealed anastomotic suture line without extravasation. A urine culture is obtained, and the patient is treated with 5 days of antibiotics. Our experience with 66 patients obstructed by a short bulbar and bulbomembranous stricture measuring 1–4cm in length and managed by excision and primary anastomosis resulted in a stricture-free lumen in 64 patients. The two failures occurred within 3 months in patients with a 2–3cm stricture and a segment of urethra with

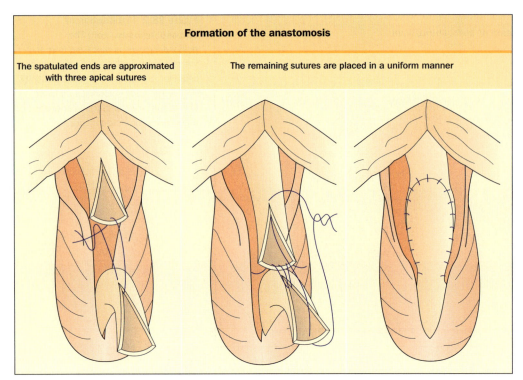

Formation of the anastomosis

| The spatulated ends are approximated with three apical sutures | The remaining sutures are placed in a uniform manner |

Figure 38.4 Formation of the anastomosis. (Left) The inner aspects of the spatulated ends are approximated with three apical sutures of 4-0 absorbable, which are also tacked down to the fascia of the corpus cavernosa to fix the anastomosis. (Center, right) The remaining anastomotic sutures are placed in a uniform manner before finally securing the knots.

a fibrotic wall, which was incorporated as part of the anastomosis. Of these patients, 14 had prior unsuccessful internal urethrotomy that did not alter a final success, but 2 patients experienced sustained erectile dysfunction. One was successfully treated by an arterial bypass revascularization procedure using an inferior epigastric artery to dorsal penile artery end-to-end anastomosis.

PENILE ISLAND FASCIOCUTANEOUS FLAPS

Penile skin flaps have become the workhorse and mainstay of anterior urethral reconstruction. The use of penile skin as an island one-stage procedure has been validated by the observations of long-term success achieved in hypospadias surgery through the decades. These skin islands adapt well to a wet milieu, are nonhirsute, and are well vascularized by a robust biaxial circulation that permits wide flap mobility. The onlay patch is the most successful design of this technique with the potential for use in every portion of the urethra, depending on the distensibility of the penile skin, its ventral location, a history of prior circumcision, the presence of balanitis xerotica obliterans, and the absence of prior penile surgery.

Orandi[18] first introduced the technique of a penile island flap, which was conceived as a random ventral longitudinal skin strip harvested on a short pedicle adjacent to the penile urethral stricture to be repaired. In reality, however, the penile island is a fasciocutaneous flap with an axial circulation, which supplies well-defined skin territories irrespective of the specific penile location or design.

The penile skin blood supply has been shown by Quartey[19] and Salmon[20] to arise from a group of dorsolateral and ventrolateral branches of the external pudendal artery and arborize with dependable cross-connections from the scrotal branches of the internal pudendal artery. This vascular pedicle is carried in the

dartos fascia, which, in essence, is the vehicle for penile skin islands. The anatomy of this flap is characterized by two distinct surgical planes, one just deep to the dermis, where a subdermal plexus exists, and one below the dartos's shiny fascial surface. The superficial plane permits a dissection between the pedicle containing the dartos fascia during flap development. Residual penile skin that is left after extensive mobilization of this dartos pedicle survives by virtue of a unique rich, supportive subdermal circulation and prevents a penile deformity.

Various penile flap designs can be used for anterior urethral repair depending on location of the stricture and surgeon preference. Ventral longitudinal penile islands (Orandi) and transverse dorsal or ventral preputial flaps[21] are particularly suited to the pendulous and submeatal segments. The transverse ventral flap is ideal for fossa navicularis and submeatal strictures but is usually affected by balanitis xerotica obliterans, which is the common etiology of the fossa navicularis and meatal lesions[22]. Circular preputial[23] and ventral bipedicle island penile flaps (BIPIPS) were developed for panurethral and more proximal bulbomembranous disease[24,25]. The ventral longitudinal island of skin combined with a circular distal penile extension is a very reliable substitution procedure for panurethral strictures and bulbomembranous lesions when the skin of these areas are healthy and intact.

PENILE FLAP RECONSTRUCTION FOR PENDULOUS AND SUBMEATAL STRICTURES

Short, midshaft, pendulous strictures can readily be repaired by the Orandi ventral linear flap, but this is an uncommon stricture event. Most complex pendulous, meatal and submeatal strictures that require repair are associated with balanitis xerotica obliterans of the ventral preputial and penile skin and a stricture that extends proximally beyond the penoscrotal junction. Because the dorsal surface of the penis is commonly free of this atrophic, troublesome skin disease, a transverse dorsal preputial flap combined with a lateral or ventral penile skin island resolves most distal urethral disease.

The supine position is usually adequate for exposure of the pendulous, penoscrotal, and distal bulbar strictures and prevents the lower extremity potential nerve injury that might occur with a prolonged lithotomy position. In the event that the proximal extent has been misjudged, the patient can readily be placed in the lithotomy position after the distal urethral pathology has been repaired. This maneuver is facilitated by the use of the Direct OR stirrups, which permit lower extremity mobility without changing the exposure and drapes.

A Fogarty vascular balloon catheter is inserted into the proximal bulbous urethra and drawn out with the distended balloon to help identify the proximal extent of the stricture. The presence of hair on the proximal penile skin is carefully marked, and an incision is started in the ventral shaft of the penis just lateral to the midline, exposing initially the spongiosa (Fig. 38.5 left panel). The deep surface of dartos fascia is reflected off the ventral surface of the spongiosa, where it is readily identified and dissected to the contralateral side, where a flap will be developed. A urethrotomy begins distally and is extended proximally well beyond the distended balloon bougie into 2–3 cm of normal urethra (Fig. 38.5 right panel). Bleeding is controlled with a running lock suture of 4-0 plain catgut, and a bridge of submeatal skin is preserved to maintain the integrity of the meatal contour. Some of the preputial and shaft skin can be excised if the patient is disabled by the pain or pruritus of balanitis xerotica obliterans. The urethra is dissected subcutaneously distally to the edge of the meatus, which is enlarged by lateral extension of the meatal incision (Fig. 38.5 right panel). The proximal extent of the urethrotomy should be well into normal spongiosa.

The flap construction is dependent on the length of the urethral defect and the width based on the measurement obtained using a 22–24F catheter template placed against the intact roof-strip. The skin incision for the flap begins on the ventral surface after an outline is made with a skin marker. It continues laterally 1 cm proximal to the frenulum and coronal groove into a circumferential extension, depending upon the length of flap needed. Combining a ventral strip and a distal complete circular extension is referred to as a Q-flap and is the longest penile island available (Fig. 38.6). Skin flap and subcutaneous dartos vascular bundle are dissected laterally, developing a plane underneath the dartos fascial surface all the way to the contralateral corpus cavernosa (Fig. 38.6 center panel).

A second parallel incision is made lateral to the first, achieving a width of 1.7–2.3 cm, depending upon the urethral measurements. The incision is deepened into the superficial layer of the subcutaneous tissue and the flap is created by dissecting on the cleavage plane between the dartos pedicle and the subdermal plexus of vessels. Great care is required to prevent injury to the subdermal circulation by keeping the dissection closer to the dartos, avoiding trauma to the deep dermis. The penile skin is reflected off the vascular pedicle down to the base of the penis, and the dartos pedicle is incised laterally to create a mobile flap. The flap is sutured in place, fitting the distal margin of the transverse dorsal circular component under the meatal bridge and suturing first the inner margin with continuous 5-0 absorbable reinforced with interrupted 5-0 absorbable (Fig. 38.6 right panel).

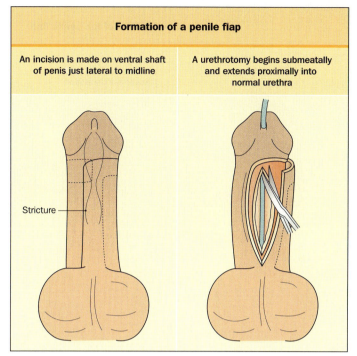

Formation of a penile flap

| An incision is made on ventral shaft of penis just lateral to midline | A urethrotomy begins submeatally and extends proximally into normal urethra |

Stricture

Figure 38.5 Formation of a penile flap. (Left) When the proximal extent of the pendulous stricture has been identified, an incision is made just lateral to midline, preserving the submeatal shaft skin in preparation for a penile fasciocutaneous flap. An appropriate penile flap is outlined with the penile skin maximally stretched, based on the length and width of the prior preparatory urethrotomy measurements. The distal hockey-stick extension is added to the ventral island, creating a penile flap with additional length. (Right) The dartos fascia is reflected off the ventral surface of the spongiosa and dissected to the contralateral side in anticipation of a longitudinal ventral or lateral penile island flap. A urethrotomy begins submeatally and extend proximally into normal urethra.

A no. 14 Silastic stent is fixed to the meatal sutures, and the outer side of the patch is sutured in place with running 5-0 absorbable from distal to proximal apex, reinforcing the absorbable with interrupted sutures of 5-0 absorbable, widely spaced (Fig. 38.7). This outer suture line is covered with either some redundant dartos fascia or a separate flap of tunica vaginalis. Any obvious devascularized ischemic skin should be excised and viable skin approximated with a compression dressing that maintains the penis in an elevated position for 5 days. The stent is removed in 7–10 days, and micturating cystourethrography is performed in 3 weeks at the time of removal of the suprapubic cystotomy tube. Recurrent stricture is uncommon in pendulous urethral reconstruction because an accurate mucocutaneous anastomosis is always performed in this location, and the skin flap is rarely ischemic if properly retrieved.

BIAXIAL PENILE FLAP FOR BULBAR AND BULBOMEMBRANOUS STRICTURES

The proximal bulbar and bulbomembranous parts of the urethra are the most common locations for strictures and the most challenging sites to treat. The proximity to the distal sphincter and the inaccessible nature of this site in the deep perineum make this urethroplasty a technically more demanding procedure.

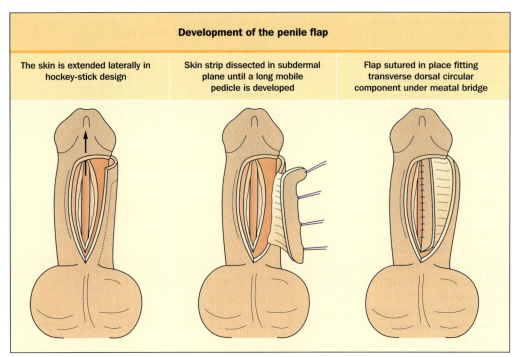

Development of the penile flap

The skin is extended laterally in hockey-stick design	Skin strip dissected in subdermal plane until a long mobile pedicle is developed	Flap sutured in place fitting transverse dorsal circular component under meatal bridge

Figure 38.6 Development of the penile flap. (Left) The skin is extended laterally in a hockey-stick design with the aim of placing the distal flap subcutaneously under the submeatal bridge. The length of the lateral circumferential incision can be extended around the entire distal penile shaft, depending on the length of the skin flap required. (Center) The skin flap and subcutaneous dartos bundle is separated laterally on tunica albuginea of the corpora cavernosa all the way to the contralateral corpora. The skin strip is then created and dissected in the subdermal plane until a long, mobile pedicle is developed. (Right) Flap is sutured in place fitting distal margin of transverse dorsal circular component under meatal bridge.

Suturing the penile flap

The suture line is covered	The skin is closed

Figure 38.7 Suturing the penile flap. (Left) The medial completed suture line is covered by tacking the subcutaneous vascular tissue over it to the fascia of the corpus cavernosum. (Right) The skin is closed and a dorsal relaxing incision may be used if tension is found in the closure.

The most reliable flap and first choice of urethral reconstruction for this location would be the BIPIP ventral penile island with or without a hockey-stick extension designed and established by Turner-Warwick and Chapple[26]. It is an extremely reliable repair when the length of the stricture does not permit a primary anastomotic procedure. This flap is a natural outgrowth of the Quartey preputial flap and was originally designed to permit the use of penile skin in circumcised patients without the need for total penile subcutaneous dartos mobilization required for the circular flap. It incorporates two robust blood supplies, is non-hirsute and has the potential of a circular extension to increase its length and mobility so that it can be transferred comfortably to the trans-sphincteric and prostate urethra without tension. The hairless distal edge of this flap can readily be used to reach even the bladder neck and to replace simultaneously the bulbar and pendulous urethra. In uncircumcised patients, flap lengths of 17–21cm have been retrieved with a combination of a ventral and distal circular component combined with a scrotal component when a nonhirsute segment exists. Penile strips of skin can also be used as a double composite with scrotal island pedicle flaps or buccal grafts when panurethral strictures are too long and burdened by the complexities of fistulae, sinuses, and prior penile surgery. The BIPIP concept decreased the ischemic loss of residual penile skin left behind after pedicle mobilization, because a dorsal segment of dartos fascia remains intact after the flap is transferred. The technique of a biaxial penile island pedicle flap combined with a urethral resection and roof-strip anastomosis is the standard of care in bulbar and bulbomembranous strictures that are complex and have failed prior treatment. We excise a 2–4cm segment of bulbar urethra after an extensive urethrotomy and do a roof-strip anastomosis to prevent a complete circumferential replacement (Figs 38.8 & 38.9). A patient with a proximal stricture may initially be placed in the supine or the lithotomy position depending upon whether the plan is to retrieve the penile skin substitute at the start of the procedure without actually measuring the urethrotomy defect. This limits the time spent in the lithotomy position and, therefore, prevents peripheral nerve injury. A modified low lithotomy position is adequate with a wedge or Gel-pack support under the sacrum and upper buttocks.

The urethra is exposed through a midline, bifurcating incision as for an anastomotic repair. The spongiosa is fully mobilized from the suspensory ligament to the intercrural membrane by separating it from the corpora cavernosa, and the urethrotomy is

The bipedicle island penile strip

Fascial layers of penis	The dorsolateral portion of the subcutaneous tissue carries the blood supply	The skin island can be divided from its lateral attachments

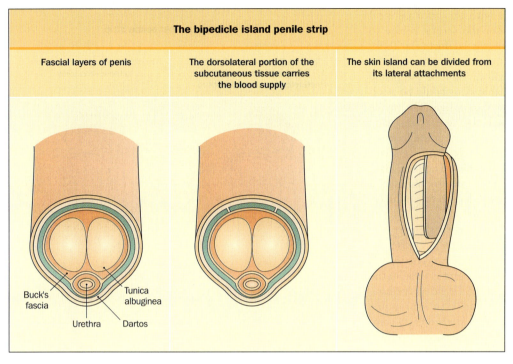

Buck's fascia

Tunica albuginea

Urethra   Dartos

Figure 38.8 The bipedicle island penile strip. (Left) The dartos fascia is dissected laterally around the penile circumference, avoiding damage to the underlying vascular pedicle and the subdermal plexus. (Center) The dorsolateral portion of the subcutaneous tissue carries the blood supply to the ventral and distal penile skin from the external pudendal vessels. Preserving a dorsal strip of subcutaneous tissue helps maintain residual penile skin viability. (Right) The ventral penile skin island with subcutaneous tissue pedicle can now be divided from its lateral attachments.

The bipedicle island penile strip

The penile flap and dartos fascia can be lifted off	A wide subscrotal tunnel is developed, a segment of urethra is resected and dorsal edges approximated

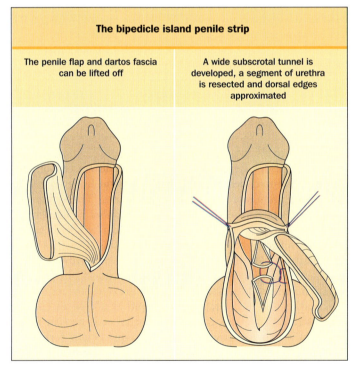

Figure 38.9 The bipedicle island penile strip. (Left) The penile flap and dartos fascia can be lifted off the spongiosa and corpora cavernosa. (Right) A wide subscrotal tunnel is developed to reach the proximal bulbous urethra. The narrowest fibrotic segment of urethra is resected. The dorsal edges are approximated in a roof-strip (or floor-strip) anastomosis with interrupted sutures of 4-0 absorbable.

aggressively extended well into normal, patent, distal, and proximal urethra over the intraluminal vascular balloon stent. This urethrotomy can be directed on to the dorsal surface when the

ventral spongiosal wall is thick and presents the potential for severe bleeding. The narrow segment of urethra is obliquely excised, and the stomal lumens are spatulated on their dorsal sides. These ventral ends are then sutured together in a tension-free anastomosis with interrupted sutures of 4-0 absorbable, creating a wider dorsal half of the urethral circumference in preparation for a penile flap to augment and close the urethral defect (Fig. 38.9). The defect length and width are measured over a no. 24 Foley catheter template, and suprapubic cystotomy diversion is established by a pull-in technique.

The patient is placed temporarily in the supine position, maintaining perineal wound sterility and cover. A glans suture is placed vertically for traction, and the urethrotomy measurements are used to outline the appropriate penile flap (Fig. 38.9). The width of this flap varies between 1.7cm and 2.2cm. This is accomplished with penile skin maximally stretched using calipers and a skin marking pen. The ventral and distal extent of the penile flap is incised just to the dermis into the superficial subdermal plane around the penile circumference, establishing a 240° circumferential dissection (Fig. 38.9 left panel). This dissection is carried on to the proximal scrotum to include the tunica-dartos pedicle and preserve the cross connections of the internal and external pudendal vessels. The distal transverse incision behind the coronal margin is deepened into the dartos fascia superficial to the spongiosa and the dorsal neurovascular bundle of the penis, elevating the penile skin island and its pedicle (Fig. 38.8 left and middle panels). The plane is easily established and extends proximally, incising the lateral border as the dissection progresses and avoiding any major vessels, thus procuring a 240° circumferential flap and subcutaneous tissue composite, being raised on dartos fascia as the vehicle. The dorsal penile skin and the contralateral shaft skin are maintained in continuity with the glans, thus supporting the subdermal circulation of the remaining skin (Fig. 38.8 right panel).

A space is created to communicate with the prior perineal dissection, and a tunnel is formed under the scrotal bridge to reach the previously prepared proximal urethral defect (Fig. 38.9). Any tension at this point may require further development of the scrotal portion of the pedicle and lateral division of the penile component of the pedicle. Adequate viable skin should be available for coverage of the penis using this flap design. The penile flap and pedicle are transferred through the connecting wide tunnel to the perineum and approximated to the urethral mucosal defect with continuous sutures of 5-0 absorbable reinforced with interrupted 5-0 absorbable (Fig. 38.10 left panel). The redundant skin is excised, if excessive, but the urethrotomy should be extended if it is a matter of 1–2cm of extra length to produce a more uniform lumen (Fig. 38.10 right panel).

The bulbocavernosus muscle is over-closed to support this repair and prevent sacculation. This step helps decrease the amount of postvoiding bulbar urethral residual urine. The wound does not need a drain; a 16F Silastic catheter stent is fixed at the meatus. The penile dressing is applied as in the Orandi procedure, and the patient is kept at bedrest for 5 days on suprapubic drainage. Biaxial penile island, nonhirsute flap urethroplasty combined with the adjuncts of aggressive use of extended urethrotomies, partial proximal bulbar urethral excision, and the use of continuous, fine absorbable sutures has resulted in a successful, long-term, stricture-free lumen.

GRAFTS

The mainstay and standard of care for urethral reconstruction in the mid-1970s was the full-thickness penile skin graft as popularized by Devine and colleagues[26]. Our early expectations of the free full-thickness patches and tube grafts have not been achieved, but the relative simplicity and the numerous potential donor sites are hard to overlook. Grafts are easy to apply, are versatile, have multiple hairless donor sources and result in a conduit that most clearly resembles a normally functioning urethra with rare diverticulum formation. Failure to accomplish this, however, is multifactorial and is associated with the use of an extrapenile donor site, tube graft design and improper harvesting. The most important negative factor is selection of a patient with a fibrotic or impaired recipient bed in which neovascularity for graft take is unlikely to develop. The best contemporary reported results in graft onlay repairs reveal a recurrent stricture rate of 14–30%[2,27].

The four major advances in enhancing graft take and rekindling the interest in this technique are the introduction of a buccal mucosal graft, the use of muscle-assisted full-thickness skin graft urethroplasty, a proximal dorsal urethrotomy graft placement[28], and the selected application of multistage mesh graft repair for complex and panurethral strictures.

BUCCAL MUCOSAL GRAFT FOR URETHRAL RECONSTRUCTION

The use of a buccal mucosal patch onlay is a relatively new and promising technique for both pendulous and bulbar strictures. It does not fare well in tubular form or when placed in a trans-sphincteric portion of the urethra, where graft take is less dependable. Complex hypospadias repairs have been the

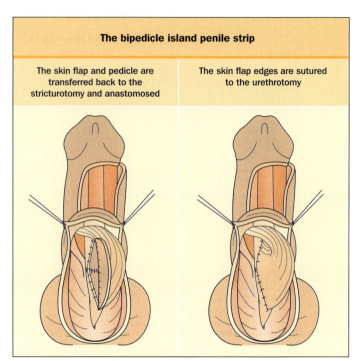

The bipedicle island penile strip

The skin flap and pedicle are transferred back to the stricturotomy and anastomosed	The skin flap edges are sutured to the urethrotomy

Figure 38.10 The bipedicle island penile strip. (Left) The skin flap and pedicle are transferred back to the stricturotomy and the roof-strip anastomosis performed. If there is tension on the pedicle, more length can be achieved by dissecting the pedicle into the proximal scrotum. (Right) The skin flap edges are sutured to the urethrotomy with continuous 5-0 absorbable reinforced with widely placed, interrupted 5-0 absorbable, and the bulbocavernosus muscle is closed over this to support the repair.

impetus for the use of buccal mucosa in urethral replacement[29], but further reports by El-Kasaby and colleagues[30] and Morey and McAninch[31] show superior graft take in stricture reconstruction with short-term followup.

This quality of improved graft take and decreased contracture over full-thickness skin patches is thought to be related to the unique anatomic aspects of oral mucosa. These features include a thick epithelium with a large number of basal cells, thin lamina propria with rich vascularity, and a firm body to the graft, permitting greater ease of handling. This tissue has rapid regenerative ability, obvious adaptation to a wet environment, is less likely to have scar formation and has a natural inherent barrier to the threat of local sepsis. Experimental studies comparing skin epithelium with oral mucosal epithelial cells in culture demonstrate that cheek mucosal epithelial cells possess faster proliferative growth curves and a more rapid colony formation than skin epithelium[32,33]. These inherent growth features of buccal mucosa may be the basis for the success of this tissue transfer technique. Grafts, in general, are most often used in shorter bulbar strictures with good results, but the buccal mucosal repair has extended the use of free graft material to a longer stricture with a significant early record of success[34].

TECHNIQUE OF A BUCCAL MUCOSAL ONLAY GRAFT

Buccal mucosal onlay graft can be used in both pendulous and bulbar strictures with a potential length of 9–12cm, but

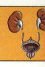

instances of successful repair of strictures up to 17cm have been reported[31]. Pendulous or penile shaft disease is probably best managed through a degloving maneuver after a circumferential, subcoronal incision has been made and the dartos fascial surface well preserved. The more proximal bulbar stricture can be approached by either a ventral or dorsal urethrotomy[28], depending on the extent of spongiofibrosis. The graft is fixed on to the urethrotomy defect after an appropriate roof-strip excision and anastomosis is completed. The proximal spongiosal urethra is generally mobilized to the suspensory ligament, and the stricturotomy performed well into normal spatulated urethra, starting distally and continuing proximally to the margin identified by the vascular balloon bougie. Trans-sphincteric extension of the stricture is probably a contraindication to any free graft technique, and a buccal mucosal segment should be abandoned in that circumstance for a penile or scrotal flap if it is available.

The length and width of the defect should be measured over a no. 28 catheter template using calipers for accurate estimates. The patient is taken out of the lithotomy position temporarily, and the graft is harvested. It can be retrieved from either the inner cheek or lower lip, depending upon the length required. Our technique for harvesting buccal mucosa is to hyperextend the head with some cervical spine support and clean the face, neck, and perioral skin surface. The face and jaw are draped and a side bit retractor or a small Weitlaner is placed in the mouth with an endotracheal tube toward the side and a moist sponge mouth gag to prevent any collection of blood or saliva from reaching the pharynx. This retractor can be replaced by a small Weitlaner with a protective guard. Two short right angle retractors are placed under the lips at the angle of the mouth or cheek of the graft donor site being exposed. A rectangle of buccal mucosa measuring $2.5 \times 6–9$ cm is outlined with a skin marker after excluding and marking the opening to Stensen's duct below the second or third molar (Fig. 38.11 left panel). The incision is carried just within the cheek margin, and a 5-0 absorbable tagging suture is placed at each corner of the distal graft edge. The plane between the graft lamina propria and the buccinator is developed, taking great care not to injure the muscle or its neurovascular supply.

Segments of buccal mucosa are placed in a saline soaked sponge, and the donor site defect is closed with a running 4-0 chromic catgut suture. The lower lip defects are often left open to prevent a contraction deformity. The graft is carefully cleaned and defatted after fixing it to a sterile Silastic block (Fig. 38.11 right panel). The graft is placed in the urethral defect with a stabilizing apical suture of 5-0 absorbable at each end.

A 3-0 silk traction suture is placed in the glans. The lumen of the urethra is cannulated with a no. 5 Fogarty catheter, and a grooved erector is inserted. A ventral midline incision is made to a depth that includes the urethrotomy over the trough of the grooved director, using a 6-0 chromic running lock suture to control bleeding from the spongiosal edge (Fig. 38.12). The graft is then placed in the urethral defect with stabilizing apical sutures of 5-0 absorbable. If several strips of oral mucosa are needed, these are sutured together before the onlay patch is applied. Edges of the graft are sutured to the urethrotomy margins with running 5-0 absorbable (Fig. 38.12). The skin margins are approximated after the graft surface is firmly covered by quilting sutures between the dartos fascia and the lamina propria of the graft (Fig. 38.12). If an avascular fibrotic subcutaneous tissue is noted, a tunica vaginalis flap is raised and transferred over the pendulous and submeatal urethral reconstruction. An 18F Silastic stenting catheter is inserted and fixed to the meatus with a plan to maintain the stent for 12 days.

Proximal bulbar strictures are the most favorable location for grafts, because the bulbocavernosus and Buck's fascia deep to the wound provide a more favorable recipient bed for an inosculation. Poor graft take with contracture is less likely to produce a ventral chordee in this perineal location.

The bulb is exposed and mobilized through a wide perineal and scrotal inverted Y incision. The urethrotomy is performed on the dorsal surface to increase compression of the graft and prevent excessive blood loss (Fig. 38.13 left panel). Bulbar strictures lend themselves to a roof-strip or floor-strip excision of irregular narrow segments that aid in creating a more uniform wide lumen (Fig. 38.13 right panel). The buccal mucosal onlay patch can then be applied to the dorsal urethrotomy and fixed to the urethral edges (Fig. 38.14).

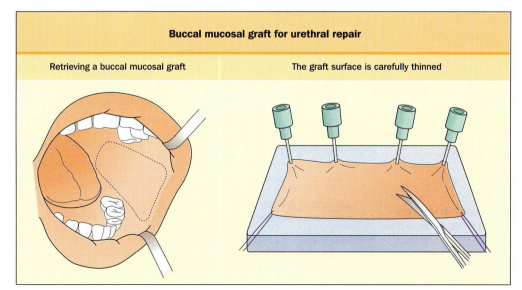

Buccal mucosal graft for urethral repair

| Retrieving a buccal mucosal graft | The graft surface is carefully thinned |

Figure 38.11 Buccal mucosal graft for urethral repair. (Left) Retrieving a buccal mucosal graft from one or both cheeks. The opening to Stensen's duct is opposite the second molar and should be preserved. A 9×2.5 cm graft can be harvested from each side if the dissection is carried to the proximal edge of the gum line. (Right) The graft surface is carefully thinned by placing it on the forefinger, followed by repeat removal of any fat or fascia on a Silastic board.

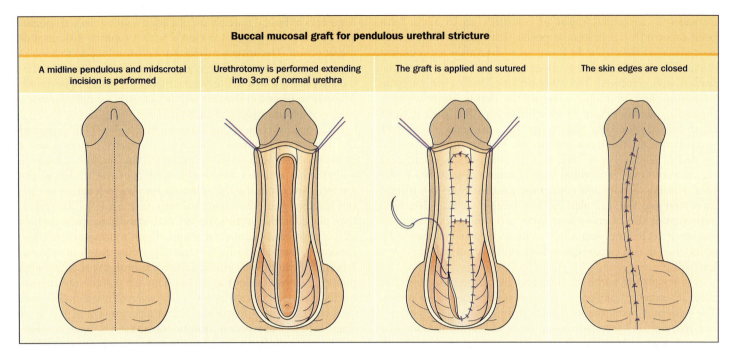

Buccal mucosal graft for pendulous urethral stricture

| A midline pendulous and midscrotal incision is performed | Urethrotomy is performed extending into 3cm of normal urethra | The graft is applied and sutured | The skin edges are closed |

Figure 38.12 Buccal mucosal graft for pendulous urethral stricture. (Left) A midline pendulous and midscrotal incision is performed over a grooved director probe. (Center left) The urethrotomy is made on either the ventral or dorsal side with aggressive extension into 3cm of normal urethra. The segments of oral mucosa from both cheeks are needed for strictures longer than 7–9cm. These are first sutured together before developing the onlay. (Center right) The graft is applied to the urethrotomy defect and sutured to the margins with 5-0 absorbable. (Right) The skin edges are closed with a two-layer 5-0 absorbable suture, securing the dartos against the graft surface and compressing the penile surface in a foam dressing with an 18F Silastic catheter for 12 days.

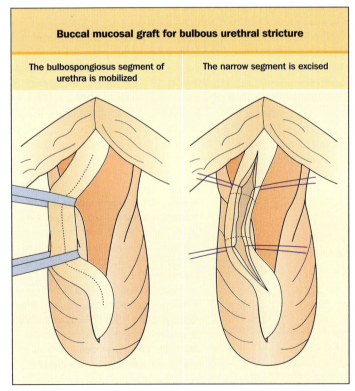

Buccal mucosal graft for bulbous urethral stricture

| The bulbospongiosus segment of urethra is mobilized | The narrow segment is excised |

Figure 38.13 Buccal mucosal graft for bulbous urethral stricture.
(Left) The bulbospongiosus segment of urethra is mobilized widely to place the urethrotomy on the dorsal surface. (Right) Bulbous urethral strictures lend themselves to an excision of the narrow segment after the urethrotomy.

The graft is compressed by the tension of the stretched spongiosa against the midline fascia between the corpora cavernosa (Fig. 38.14). The bulbocavernosus is closed with sutures of 4-0 absorbable and the skin with 5-0 absorbable. An 18F Silastic stent is fixed to the meatus. A 20F Silastic pubic cystotomy diversion is established. A compression dressing is used in all graft reconstructions, including the graft onlay placed in a dorsal urethrotomy position. The stent is maintained for a longer period than that required for flaps, and a voiding cystourethrogram is studied for extravasation at 3 weeks before removing the suprapubic tube to insure that the graft has healed securely.

Our experience with 21 buccal graft repairs included 14 patients with onlay patches that varied from 5–17cm in length, and 7 patients in whom a patch was combined with flap. This latter group had shorter segments varying from 3–5cm. Eight pendulous and 13 bulbar strictures were repaired with the use of this graft, and patients were observed at 3–38 months. Recurrent stricture developed in 2 patients, and a fistula with loss of a graft in association with a complicating infected hematoma developed in 1 patient. The characteristics of buccal mucosal grafts in the onlay technique, including vascular characteristics, ease of handling, and ease of retrieval, along with the characteristic of a wet epithelial surface, have contributed to the enthusiasm for this tissue transfer technique, which seems to be well founded.

MESH GRAFT URETHROPLASTY

Mesh graft multistage urethral reconstruction was introduced in 1989 by Schreiter and Noll to treat the cohort of patients with complex failed hypospadias, panurethral strictures, or long

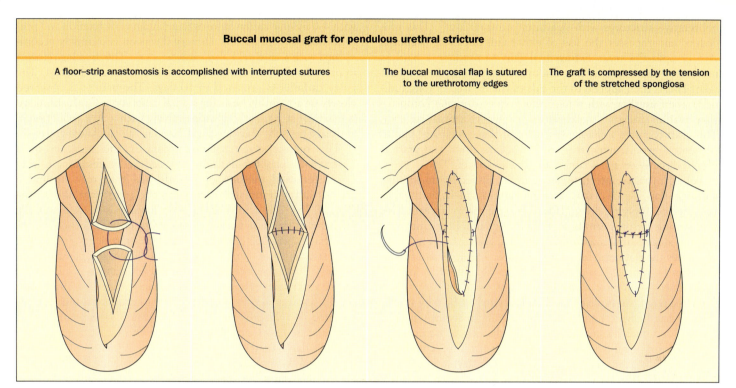

Buccal mucosal graft for pendulous urethral stricture

A floor–strip anastomosis is accomplished with interrupted sutures	The buccal mucosal flap is sutured to the urethrotomy edges	The graft is compressed by the tension of the stretched spongiosa

Figure 38.14 Buccal mucosal graft for bulbous urethral stricture. (Left, center left) A floor-strip anastomosis is accomplished with interrupted sutures of 4-0 absorbable. The urethrotomy can be extended if the graft or flap is longer. (Center right) The buccal mucosal patch is sutured to the urethrotomy edges with running suture of 5-0 absorbable. (Right) The graft is compressed against the dorsal midline fascia by the tension of the stretched spongiosa.

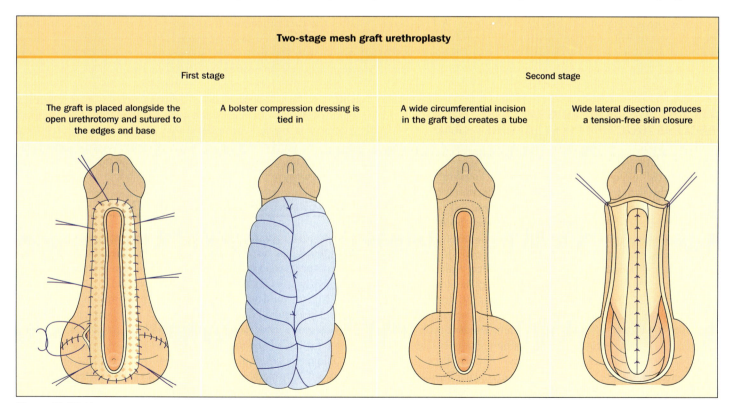

Two-stage mesh graft urethroplasty

First stage		Second stage	
The graft is placed alongside the open urethrotomy and sutured to the edges and base	A bolster compression dressing is tied in	A wide circumferential incision in the graft bed creates a tube	Wide lateral disection produces a tension-free skin closure

Figure 38.15 Two-stage mesh graft urethroplasty. (Left) A full-length urethrotomy is used to define normal distal and proximal urethra. The scrotum is sutured laterally to cover the testes and decrease wound surface. The completed graft is placed alongside the open urethrotomy; sutures of 5-0 absorbable are used to fix the graft to both the edges and base. A 16F Foley catheter is inserted through both stomas. (Center left) A bolster compression dressing is tied in with suture ties from the margin of the skin to immobilize the graft and secure it to the bed. (Center right) Second-stage reconstruction requires a wide circumferential incision in the graft bed to create a tube around a 26F catheter template. The strip is tapered with Babcock clamps and closed with running extraepithelial inverting suture of 5-0 absorbable reinforced at intervals with sutures of 5-0 absorbable. (Right) Skin closure is accomplished after a wide lateral dissection to produce a tension-free closure. If the outer skin is compromised, a tunica vaginalis is used as a buttress over the urethral suture line.

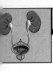

obliterative strictures with significant urethral loss[35]. This procedure encompasses the use of either full-thickness preputial skin or split-thickness extragenital skin to produce a hairless urethra by first meshing the skin to a 1:1.5 ratio to insure graft take. This is then applied to the side of the excised or longitudinally open urethra with a meticulous stent dressing compression, waiting for graft stabilization and secure stomal patency. This graft requires a pliable, vascularized tissue recipient bed to prevent a hypertrophic scar, which occurs when the graft is placed directly on a raw tunica albuginea surface.

A healthy tissue interface can be accomplished by transposing a muscle flap, penile dartos fascia or tunica vaginalis on the corpora before applying the graft in adverse circumstances[36]. This intervening tissue permits a greater graft mobility, improves second stage tubularization, decreases graft shrinkage, and decreases the potential for penile chordee. This mesh graft concept can be replaced by a split-thickness (15/1,000) skin graft using multiple piecrust incisions with less resultant contracture if the recipient bed is pliable, well vascularized, or healthy gracilis muscle has been applied. The mesh graft onlay, when fully mature, becomes a smooth, supple, and hairless structure with waterproofing qualities and a sufficient surface for a uniform, wide-lumen urethra with a low risk for the development of a pseudodiverticulum.

A second-stage procedure is scheduled for 9–15 months later, when a stable, mature skin surface has been achieved and a time-proven, patent proximal and distal stoma is present. The longer the interval before the second-stage tubularization procedure the better is the quality of urethral skin substitute. A long-term, durable, successful outcome depends on careful interim management. Osteal stenosis can be managed successfully by careful calibration with a bougie à boule to insure a 26–30F caliber proximally and a 24–26 caliber distally.

TECHNIQUE OF MESH GRAFT URETHRAL RECONSTRUCTION FOR PANURETHRAL STRICTURE

The surgical exposure for this difficult urethral pathology requires the lithotomy position. The penile and scrotal skin is incised in the midline, splitting the scrotum and suturing the scrotum laterally. An aggressive, full-length urethrotomy is used for the panurethral stricture to open and define normal distal and proximal urethra (Fig. 38.12 center left panel).

The split skin graft can be retrieved from the inner portion of the posterior thigh, buttocks, or lateral lower groin area. A Padgett dermatome procures a medium-thickness graft (0.4mm), averaging 5–8cm in width and 15–18cm in length, depending on the length of the defect. This depth eliminates any hair follicles, but the accuracy of the setting in the dermatome should be confirmed by measuring the blade interval with a no. 15 Bard–Parker scalpel blade edge. The donor site should be covered with DuoDerm and a firm compression dressing. The graft can be meshed with the commonly used Zimmer mesher using a 1:1.5 ratio sheet. It is then sutured to the edge of the urethrotomy with running 5-0 absorbable and fixed to the recipient bed with interrupted 5-0 absorbable placed evenly to aid the bolster dressing. Fibrin glue can also be used (Fig. 38.15 left panel). A compression stent dressing bolster is placed over a graft cover of Zerofom gauze and sutured

with 4-0 nylon fixation sutures to maintain graft fixation and prevent motion (Fig. 38.15). Urinary diversion is routinely accomplished with a urethral Foley catheter stent. The dressing remains in place for 5–7 days while keeping the patient at bedrest. The Foley catheter is removed in 10 days. The patient is observed closely on a monthly basis for stomal calibration. Graft shrinkage is maximal at 3 months postoperatively with a 50% reduction in graft size for split-thickness and 20% for full-thickness grafts.

The second stage reconstruction is the creation of a Thiersch–Duplay tubularization procedure by designing a wide circumferential incision of a graft bed that rolls around a 26F catheter template, narrowing the strip near the stoma (Fig. 38.15). The width of the strip initially is in excess of the diameter of the catheter and is tapered by either Babcock clamps or a straight vascular clamp to proper measurements. It is closed with two or three running extraepithelial inverting sutures of 5-0 absorbable, reinforced at intervals with interrupted sutures of 5-0 absorbable (Fig. 38.15 right panel). Penile skin and transected scrotum are dissected laterally to produce a tension-free covering skin closure (Fig. 38.12 right panel). If the outer skin is compromised with any skin disease or fibrotic surface, a tunica vaginalis flap is used to cover the skin tube suture line. The penile and scrotal skin is widely mobilized, and the penile skin is brought around the ventral surface after incising the glans for a subcoronal meatoplasty. The urethral closure is stented with a 16F Silastic catheter and drained by a suprapubic cystotomy for 3–4 weeks. The urethral catheter is removed in 7–10 days, and a followup micturating cystourethrogram is obtained at 3 weeks. Graft take after the first procedure is consistently high, with no more than a 5% loss observed in any patient. During the interval of observation after the first stage, 30% of some patients require some form of osteal revision in the form of a side Y–V plasty.

Mesh graft urethroplasty is technically a challenging procedure with an unprecedented success rate in patients with complex hypospadias, an unresolved stricture and numerous prior surgical attempts at repair with a deficiency of useful penile or scrotal skin. It cannot be overemphasized that patients should be counseled that the operation may be a multistage rather than a two-stage procedure[37].

POSTERIOR URETHRAL STRICTURES

The posterior prostatomembranous urethral stricture or distraction defect has historically been the most formidable challenge of stricture surgery. It is an uncommon lesion and occurs most frequently as a consequence of pelvic fracture or straddle injury and is associated with serious urethral disruption and separation. The injury is often complicated by inappropriate initial management using substitution skin flap techniques with the development of recurrent stenosis, irreversible impotence, and occasional incontinence. Management by endoscopic techniques plays a role in patients with short strictures or after prostatectomy but is rarely helpful in resolving the complex obliterated urethra with a significant defect[2,38,39]. The management of this post-traumatic posterior urethral distraction defect and other posterior urethral pathology has dramatically improved over the past two decades, despite an inaccessible subpubic location involving exposed sphincter-active and erectile neurovascular anatomy. A contemporary perineal, one-stage bulboprostatic anastomotic operation as popularized by Turner-Warwick[40] with selective scar excision is a versatile procedure with a high patent lumen success. The anastomotic urethroplasty has a sustained patent urethral lumen success rate approaching 100% versus those who have undergone urethral skin flap or patch repair, where the re-stricture rate in 5 and 10 years increases two- to threefold[41]. A patent urethra, after anastomotic urethroplasty at 6 months, is free from further recurrent stricture, and it gives credence to Mr Turner-Warwick's admonition that 'urethra is the best substitute for urethra'.

Other etiologies of complex posterior urethral strictures are those following endoscopic trans-sphincteric injury, postoperative vesicourethral stricture following radical prostatectomy and radiation bulbomembranous strictures following radiation for prostatic carcinoma. These nontraumatic posterior urethral strictures offer an entirely different set of issues with more serious potential for incontinence and its resolution. They do not lend themselves to anastomotic repair but require management by some regenerative or substitution technique. The marked increase in the number of patients undergoing radical prostatectomy over the past decade accounts for an emergence of the still unresolved entity of vesicourethral anastomotic stricture. This complication has been reported to occur in 0.5–11% of patients undergoing both a retropubic and perineal approaches[42]. Keetch et al.[43] reported in 1994 an experience of 42 of 810 patients (5%) in whom an anastomotic stricture developed. The incidence in the latter 310 patients reported by Keetch et al, however, had a dramatic decrease to 0.6% when the bladder neck lumen was increased from 18F to 24F size using a traditional mucosa-to-mucosa watertight anastomosis with bladder mucosal eversion. The major risk factors in the development of this stricture were identified by Igel et al.[44] and Surya et al.[45] as a prior transurethral prostatectomy, a tight anastomosis, a vest suture technique, excessive intraoperative blood loss, or prolonged leakage of urine.

Two types of stricture have been encountered in patients who have had radical prostatectomy. One is an anastomotic disruption with separation of the urethra and bladder neck resulting in a distraction defect, and the second is an early or delayed stricture with a vesicourethral anastomosis that is still in continuity. In both situations, patients may have retained an intact continence mechanism, which will alter the management approach. The algorithm for management depends very much on whether the patients have undergone prior radiation therapy for margin-positive disease, the severity of the stricture, continence, a history of prior endoscopic surgery, and the length of the gap. Intermittent, gentle, filiform-guided urethral dilatation after careful urethroscopic examination followed by intermittent, gentle balloon dilatation is the initial approach to the nonobliterated stricture[42]. If this therapy fails, then a sustained balloon dilatation of the area on a regular basis for anywhere from 20 minutes to 2 hours should be performed. Holmium laser stricturotomy with steroid infiltration is another possible option. The incontinent patient with an anastomotic stricture is a candidate for a more aggressive, deep but careful transurethral resection or urethrotomy at the 3 o'clock and the 9 o'clock position, avoiding any incisions at the 6 o'clock position where a rectal fistula can readily follow endoscopic trauma and an inadvertent rectal injury. Virulent recurrent strictures, prior radiation therapy, and failed attempts at open reconstruction can be managed by a

urethrotomy at the 3 o'clock and 9 o'clock position, placement of a 2cm Wallstent (American Medical Systems, Minitonka, MN) and subsequent placement of an AMS-800 artificial urinary sphincter after the patency of a lumen has been established.

The vesicourethral anastomotic disruption obliteration defect is, fortunately, a rare lesion that can only be resolved by open surgical reconstruction with or without a subsequent AMS-800 artificial urinary sphincter, depending upon the preservation of continence. This procedure can be performed by an exclusively abdominal retropubic route or a combined abdominoperineal approach when the membranous urethra has retracted to a low infrapubic position. The primary perineal technique we have used has resulted in total incontinence in 2 patients. The retropubic approach with partial pubectomy and the use of an anterior bladder tube has been employed successfully in 4 patients, 3 of whom have remained continent and 1 of whom has required a subsequent artificial sphincter. Schlossberg et al.[46] successfully managed 2 patients with a combined approach using an anterior perineal dissection to complete the anastomosis after repairing a bladder tube from the retropubic route. Two of our patients with an anastomotic stricture and radiation injury to the bladder with a bladder contracture and urinary incontinence underwent continent urinary diversion.

Strictures of the membranous urethra that follow transurethral resection of the prostate are a particularly difficult group since the bladder neck continence mechanism has been destroyed and only a distal intrinsic or external sphincter mechanism exists. This is an uncommon problem and one that may be seen with both obstruction and incontinence. In the absence of a complicating factor, such as chronic retention, obstructive nephropathy, or recurrent urinary tract infection, this stricture is best untreated but carefully monitored if the patient is continent[47]. Treatment that is least likely to cause further sphincter damage is gentle urethral dilatation with twice-weekly catheter self-dilatation. Urethrotomy or perineal anastomotic urethroplasty will leave this group of patients totally incontinent. Bladder neck reconstruction in the patient after prostatectomy has a poor record, with a significant incidence of failure to achieve continence. Edwards et al.[48] reported cure of a postprostatectomy trans-sphincteric stricture using a multistage scrotal flap technique and a conservative trans-sphincteric stricturotomy at the 6 o'clock position. In a more contemporary study of 25 patients with trans-sphincteric strictures, reported by Mundy[7,47] in 1989, urethral dilatation controlled the stricture in 14 patients, 6 of whom continued with occasional dilatation or soft catheterization to maintain control; 11 patients have persistent recurrent strictures requiring perineal anastomotic urethroplasty and artificial sphincter. The incidence of erosion in the urethra in this group of patients was significant. Urethral mobilization required for bulboprostatic anastomotic urethroplasty and the division of the proximal blood supply leaves the urethra completely dependent on a retrograde spongiosal blood flow, which can be compromised by the artificial sphincter cuff, resulting in ischemia and erosion. Any urethral reconstruction in this patient population should keep the spongiosa in continuity and be managed by a scrotal or penile flap technique requiring an artificial sphincter at a subsequent operation and at a more distal site.

In a group of 28 patients with troublesome trans-sphincteric strictures after transurethral surgery referred to our institution,

11 patients underwent two-stage scrotal posterior flap urethroplasty without the development of incontinence. They were selected by subjecting them to vigorous dilatation, excluding patients who became incontinent after a dilatation procedure. None of the 11 patients had preoperative urinary incontinence, and 5 were subsequently closed by a second-stage procedure 11–18 months after the scrotal inlay. A total of 17 patients were managed by interval dilatation, including 8 who maintained patency by intermittent self-catheterization over a 6-month/6-year interval. Three patients have had transurethral resection of the stricture and insertion of a wall stent followed by subsequent successful placement of an artificial sphincter.

POSTERIOR URETHRAL DISRUPTION INJURY

Early management of the posterior urethral separation injury that follows either a pelvic fracture or straddle fall-astride trauma continues to be controversial. The specific extent of a blunt posterior urethral injury must be defined to include the proximal anterior urethra, the bladder neck, and bladder base as well as the prostatic and membranous urethra, since involvement of this entire anatomy will alter the therapeutic approach. The classification by Colapinto and McCallum[49], modified by Goldman et al.[50], is comprehensive and anatomic and includes all the post-traumatic lesions commonly seen in clinical practice. Type 1 injury involves a stretched urethra caused by rupture of the puboprostatic ligaments with an intact urethra, and type 2 describes a partial or complete disruption of the membranous urethra above the perineal membrane. These two patterns of injury occur 30% of the time, and the remainder of the postpelvic fracture disruptions are predominantly type 3, which is an injury with membranous urethral disruption extending through the urogenital diaphragm to involve the proximal bulbous urethra. Because the potential sequelae of bladder neck injury are so important, Goldman et al.[50] included a type 4 and type 4A classification that includes the bladder neck and/or extraperitoneal bladder injuries, which should be distinguished because they demand early intervention. These are best identified by using retrograde urethrography under fluoroscopic control. The type 4 injury is seen more often when there is an associated pubic symphysis separation or a severe straddle fracture. Goldman et al.[14] also added a type 5 injury, which represented a partial or complete pure anterior urethral injury, because it is not uncommon to confuse proximal bulbar injuries with a type 3 membranous injury, since both show contrast extravasation below the urogenital diaphragm.

After the diagnosis of membranous urethral rupture has been established and hemodynamic stability and serious nonurologic trauma has been resolved or excluded, several methods of repair are available, each with a convincing enthusiast based on a relatively small number of cases. It is clear that exploration and immediate suturing of the urethral ends results in an unacceptable 40–50% incidence of impotence and a 20% incidence of incontinence and should be abandoned as a management option[51]. Primary realignment should be limited to patients with a long separation defect, an injured bladder, an injured bladder neck or rectum, and patients undergoing open reduction and internal fixation by the orthopedic surgeon for pelvic girdle stabilization. Primary open realignment should probably not be considered an option in younger patients who are sexually active until the complication rate of erectile dysfunction is resolved or the endoscopic techniques reported to manage the acute phase injury are substantiated to achieve effective urethral continuity and to be free of significant morbidity. Potency is reported to be impaired in 3–60% of patients after pelvic fracture and urethral distraction injury. The most likely cause is disruption of the cavernosal nerves posterolateral to the prostatomembranous urethra behind the symphysis pubis as a result of the trauma and, uncommonly, as a result of surgical repair. Preoperative risk factors that correlated with the development of impotence included patient's age, a longer urethral defect, bilateral pubic rami fractures, and pelvic fractures following fall-astride trauma[52,53].

DELAYED RECONSTRUCTION OF POST-TRAUMATIC URETHRAL DISRUPTION INJURIES

The ultimate expectation of a long-term patent posterior urethra in a continent and potent patient after pelvic fracture is most often seen after a primary anastomotic urethroplasty in experienced hands. This uncommon injury occurs in 5–10% of pelvic fractures following auto accidents, occupational crush trauma, or fall-astride trauma from varying heights (17%). Minor short obliteration defects that occur in less than 5% of patients may be managed by endoscopic means, but there is rarely any long-term success.

A predictable cure of this urethral defect requires a bulboprostatic anastomosis, an approach that has been one of the significant advances in reconstructive urologic surgery over the past two decades. Turner-Warwick[40] and Carr & Webster popularized and extended the concept of end-to-end transperineal[54] one-stage bulboprostatic anastomosis for this lesion and revolutionized repair of these previously unresolved strictures with minimal morbidity. Primary anastomotic repair by the infrapubic perineal approach will resolve urethral defects up to 7cm in length and result in outcomes approaching 95–98% patency. Mundy[41] reported 5- and 10-year followup data comparing anastomotic and substitution procedures in patients with posterior urethral disruption defects not burdened by a history of prior stricture, spongiofibrosis, hypospadias, or prior anterior urethra injury. He firmly demonstrated that the anastomotic procedure has a significant advantage and a higher success rate than substitution skin procedures. A circumferential, spatulated, overlapping anastomotic urethroplasty with a mucosa-to-mucosa, tension-free urethral repair is now the golden standard of urethral reconstruction, but it is clearly limited to strictures of the bulb and bulbomembranous urethra with post-traumatic or congenital causes.

It is a rare occasion when a membranous urethral distraction injury cannot be reconstructed by a perineal approach. The abdominal perineal transpubic route is reserved for the uncommon orthopedic injury that limits proper positioning, a post-traumatic, 6–9cm urethral defect, or the patient with an obviously badly injured bladder neck that requires an attempted repair. The most common cause of severe re-stricture is ischemic necrosis of the proximal corpora spongiosa secondary to compromised retrograde blood flow from the glans and dorsal penile arteries. Generally, the reported success rate associated with this operation approaches 98% when managed by delayed reconstruction.

Our experience with 87 patients undergoing primary anastomotic repair revealed a sustained, unobstructed urethra in 79 patients. Two of these patients underwent continent augmentation cystoplasty with closure of the bladder neck since they were incontinent following an extensive bladder neck injury. Recurrent stricture developed in 8 patients. Three of these were managed successfully by endoscopic urethrotomy. A total of 82 cases were managed by the perineal route, while 5 underwent an abdominal perineal approach. Bladder neck reconstruction was repaired in 3 patients 4–8 months following the urethral repair. Two were continent and one underwent insertion of an AMS-800 artificial urinary sphincter[55].

REFERENCES

1. Attwater HL. The history of urethral stricture. Br J Urol. 1943;15:39.
2. Roehrborn CG, McConnell JD. Analysis of factors contributing to success or failure of one-stage urethroplasty for stricture disease. J Urol. 1994;151:869.
3. Jordan GH, Schellhammer PF. Urethral surgery and stricture disease. In: Droller MJ, ed. Surgical management of urologic disease: an anatomic approach. St Louis: Mosby Yearbook 1992:1218–37.
4. Venn SN, Mundy AR. Urethroplasty for balanitis xerotica obliterans. Br J Urol. 1998; 81:735–7.
5. Barbagli G, Selli V, decello Mottola A. A one-stage dorsal free-graft urethroplasty for bulbarurethral strictures. Br J Urol. 1996;78:929.
6. Grossman JA, Caldamone A, Khouri R, Kenna DM. Cutaneous blood supply of the penis. Plast Reconstr Surg. 1989;83:213;83:213.
7. Mathes S, Nahai F. The reconstructive triangle. In: Reconstructive surgery. New York: Churchill Livingstone; 1997:9–36.
8. Mundy AR. The treatment of sphincter strictures. Br J Urol. 1990;64:626.
9. Steenkamp JW, Heyn GF, DeKock ML. Internal urethrotomy versus dilation as treatment for male urethral strictures: a prospective randomized comparison. J Urol. 1997;157:98.
10. Mundy AR. The long-term results of skin inlay urethroplasty. Br J Urol. 1995;75:59.
11. Angermeier KW, Jordan GH. Complications of the exaggerated lithotomy position. A review of 177 cases. J Urol. 1994;151:866.
12. Stormont TJ, Suman VJ, Oesterling JE. Newly diagnosed bulbar urethral strictures: etiology and outcome of various treatments. J Urol. 1993;150:1725.
13. Roosen JU. Self-catheterization after urethrotomy: prevention of urethral stricture recurrence using clean intermittent self-catheterization. Urol Int. 1993;50:90.
14. Milroy EJ. Treatment of sphincter strictures using permanent uroLume stents. J Urol. 1993;150:1729.
15. Pansadoro J, Scarpone P, Emiliozzi P. Treatment of a recurrent penobulbar urethral stricture after wall stent implantation with a second inner wall stent. Urology. 1994;43:248.
16. Zinman L. Surgical management of anterior urethral strictures. In: Ehrlich R, Alter G. Reconstructive and plastic surgery of the external genitalia. Philadelphia: WB Saunders; 1999:369–84.
17. Morey AF, McAninch JW. Role of intraoperative sonourethrography in bulbar urethral reconstruction (Abstract 848). J Urol. 1997; 157(Suppl):217.
18. Orandi A. One-stage urethroplasty: 4 year follow-up. J Urol. 1972; 107:977.
19. Quartey JK. One-stage penile/preputial cutaneous island flap urethroplasty for urethral stricture: a preliminary report. J Urol. 1983;129:284.
20. Salmon M. Artères de la peau. Paris: Masson, 1936; English translation Taylor GI, Tempest MN, ed. Arteries of the skin. Edinburgh: Churchill Livingstone; 1988.
21. Mundy AR, Stephanson TP. Pedicled preputial patch urethroplasty. Br J Urol. 1988;61:48.
22. Jordan GH. Management of anterior urethral stricture disease. In: Webster GD, ed. Reconstructive urology, vol 2. Boston: Blackwell Scientific Publications; 1993:703–22.
23. McAninch JW. Reconstruction of extensive anterior urethral strictures: circular fasciocutaneous penile flaps. J Urol. 1993;149:488.
24. Turner-Warwick RT, Chapple CR. The bilaterally pedicled island skin (BIPIPS) urethral substitution procedure: 10 year follow-up. Presented at Annual Meeting of the British Association of Urologic Surgeons, London, June 1990.
25. Zinman L, Vereb MJ, Gaertner R, et al. Bipedicle ventral penile island flap urethroplasty (BIPIP) (Abstract 763). J Urol. 1996;155 (Suppl.):501A.
26. Devine PC, Sakati LA, Poutasse EF, Devine CJ. One-stage urethroplasty: repair of strictures with free full thickness patch of skin. J Urol. 1968;99:191.
27. Wessels H, McAninch JW. Use of free grafts in urethral stricture reconstruction. J Urol. 1996;155:1912.
28. Barbagli G, Selli C, Tosto A. Reoperative surgery for recurrent stricture of the penile and bulbous urethra. J Urol. 1996;156:76.
29. Duckett JW, Coplen D, Ewalt D, Baskin LS. Buccal mucosal urethral replacement. J Urol. 1995;153:1660.
30. El-Kasaby AW, Fath-Alla M, Noweir AM, et al. The use of buccal mucosa patch graft in the management of anterior urethral strictures. J Urol. 1993;149:276.
31. Morey AF, McAninch JW. When and how to use buccal mucosal grafts in adult bulbar urethroplasty. Urology. 1996;48:194.
32. Hata K, Hideaki K, Minoru U, et al. The characteristics of cultured mucosal cell sheet as a material for grafting: comparison with cultured epidermal cell sheet. Ann Plast Surg. 1995;34:530.
33. Thompson AM, Scholma J, Blaauw EH, et al. Improved in vitro generation of epithelial grafts with oral mucosa. Transplantation. 1994;58:1282.
34. Fichtner J, Fisch M, D'Elia G, et al. Buccal mucosa onlay graft for urethral reconstruction. the first 100 cases (Abstract 966). J Urol. 1997;157 (Suppl.):247.
35. Schreiter F, Noll F. Mesh graft urethroplasty using split thickness skin graft or foreskin. J Urol. 1989;142:1223.
36. Ehrlich R, Alter G. Split thickness skin graft urethroplasty and tunica vaginalis flaps for failed hypospadias repairs. J Urol. 1996;155:131.
37. Schreiter F. The two-stage mesh graft urethroplasty using split thickness skin. Urol Clin North Am. 1997;5:75
38. Koraitim MM. Pelvic fracture urethral injuries: evaluation of various methods of management. J Urol. 1996;156:1288–91.
39. Zinman L. Editorial: the management of traumatic posterior urethral distraction defects. J Urol. 1997;157:511–2.
40. Turner-Warwick R. Complex traumatic posterior urethral strictures. J Urol. 1977;118:564.
41. Mundy AR. Urethroplasty for posterior urethral strictures. Br J Urol. 1996;78:243–7.
42. Mark S, Perez LM, Webster GD. Synchronous management of anastomotic contracture and stress urinary incontinence following radical prostatectomy. J Urol. 1994;151:1202–4.
43. Keetch DW, Andriole GL, Catalona WJ. Complications of radical retropubic prostatectomy. AUA Update Ser. 1994;13:46–51.
44. Igel TC, Barrett DM, Sequra JW, Benson RC Jr, Rife CC. Perioperative and postoperative complications from bilateral pelvic lymphadenectomy and radical retropubic prostatectomy. J Urol. 1987;137:1189.

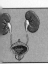

45. Surya BV, Provet J, Johanson KE, Brown J. Anastomotic strictures following radical prostatectomy: risk factors and management. J Urol. 1990;143:755.

46. Schlossberg S, Jordan G, Schellhammer P. Repair of obliterative vesicourethral stricture after radical prostatectomy: a technique for preservation of continence. Urology. 1995;45:510–3.

47. Mundy AR. Treatment of sphincter strictures. Br J Urol. 1989; 64:626–8.

48. Edwards L, Singh M, Notley R, Blandy J. Continence after scrotal flap urethroplasty. Br J Urol. 1972;44:23–30.

49. Colapinto V, McCallum RM. Injury to the male posterior urethra in fractured pelvis: a new classification. J Urol. 1977;118:575–9.

50. Goldman SM, Sandleer CM, Corriere JN, McGuire EJ. Blunt urethral trauma: a unified anatomical mechanical classification. J Urol. 1997;157:85–9.

51. Mundy AR. The role of delayed primary repair in the acute management of pelvic fracture injuries of the urethra. Br J Urol. 1991;68:273.

52. Mark SD, Keane TE, Vandemark RM, Webster GD. Impotence following pelvic fracture urethral injury: incidence, etiology and management. Br J Urol. 1995;75:62–4.

53. Kotkin L, Koch MO. Impotence and incontinence after immediate realignment of posterior urethral trauma: result of injury or management? J Urol. 1996;155:1600.

54. Carr LK, Webster GD. Posterior urethral reconstruction. Ann Urol Clin North Am. 1997;5:125–37.

55. Iselin CE, Webster GD. Significance of the open bladder neck associated with pelvic fracture urethral distraction defects. J Urol. 1999;162:347–51.

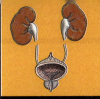

Section 7 Andrology

Chapter 39

Male Infertility

Roy A Brandell and Peter N Schlegel

KEY POINTS

- Male infertility may be primary or secondary.
- A male factor alone may be responsible for 20% of cases.
- 30% are secondary to combined male and female factors.
- Advances in assisted reproductive technology have dramatically changed clinical practice.
- Procreation is now theoretically possible for any man for whom a single viable sperm can be isolated.

INTRODUCTION

Traditionally, *infertility* has been defined as the inability to achieve conception after 1 year of unprotected intercourse. As more couples delay parenthood until later in life, however, it may be appropriate to initiate evaluation of both partners earlier. Female fertility declines with advancing age, especially beyond 35 years.

Male infertility is classified as either *primary* or *secondary* (Fig. 39.1). A male factor alone is responsible for 20% of infertility cases and an additional 30% are secondary to combined male and female factors (Fig. 39.2). These statistics emphasize the importance of thoroughly evaluating the male and female partners concurrently.

Over the past several years, advances in assisted reproductive technology (ART) have dramatically changed male infertility practice. Men who would have been labeled sterile just a few years ago are now capable of fathering their own biologic offspring. Intracytoplasmic sperm injection (ICSI), reported as successful in humans for the first time in 1994[1], is performed by injecting a solitary spermatozoon into the cytoplasm of a mature ovum (Fig. 39.3). Thus, procreation is now theoretically possible for any man for whom a single viable sperm can be isolated.

An unfortunate consequence of the success and widespread availability of ART is the tendency to bypass thorough evaluation and treatment of the male partner while proceeding directly to *in vitro* fertilization (IVF) with ICSI. This practice may be unwise for a number of important reasons. First, it subjects the female partner to medical and procedural interventions for what may be an entirely correctable male factor problem. Second, potentially life-threatening conditions in the male such as testicular cancer or hormonal abnormalities could be missed[2]. Third, genetic abnormalities (discussed later) are associated with male factor infertility and could be transmitted to offspring. Finally, recent reports have shown convincingly that appropriate evaluation of the male partner and specific, diagnosis-focused treatment is more cost-effective and may yield higher success rates than proceeding directly to ART[3].

INVESTIGATION

History

The important components of a complete history are listed in Figure 39.4. Each of these areas needs to be addressed since any one could affect the patient's fertility status. A detailed sexual

Definitions of male infertility	
Primary infertility	The infertile or subfertile patient who has never achieved conception in his lifetime.
Secondary infertility	The infertile or subfertile patient who has successfully achieved conception previously.

Figure 39.1 Definitions of male infertility.

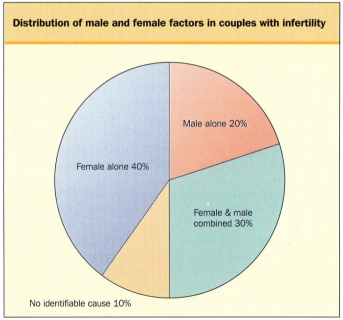

Figure 39.2 Distribution of male and female factors in couples with infertility.

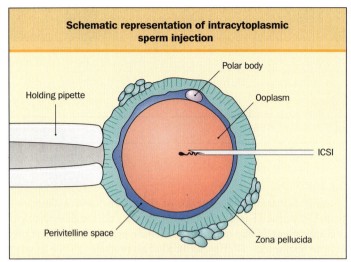

Schematic representation of intracytoplasmic sperm injection

Holding pipette

Polar body

Ooplasm

ICSI

Perivitelline space

Zona pellucida

Figure 39.3 Schematic representation of intracytoplasmic sperm injection (ICSI).

Important history components for evaluation of male infertility

History of infertility	Gonadotoxins
Duration	Chemicals (pesticides)
Prior pregnancies – present partner – another partner	Drugs (prescription, over-the-counter, recreational)
Previous evaluation and treatment	Thermal (hot tubs, saunas)
Evaluation and treatment of wife	Radiation
	Smoking
Sexual history	**Family history**
Potency	Cystic fibrosis
Lubricants	Infertility
Frequency and timing of coitus	
Childhood and development	**Review of symptoms**
Cryptorchidism, orchidopexy	Respiratory infections
Herniorrhaphy	Anosmia
Testicular torsion	Libido
Onset of puberty	Gynecomastia or galactorrhea
	Impaired visual fields
	Headaches
Medical history	**Infection**
Systemic illness (e.g. diabetes, multiple sclerosis)	Viral, febrile
	Mumps orchitis
Previous or current treatment	Epididymitis
	STD
	TB (rare)
	Urinary tract infection
Surgical history	
Orchiectomy (torsion, cancer)	
Retroperitoneal surgery	
Pelvic, inguinal, or scrotal surgery/injury	
Y–V plasty, TURP	
Spinal cord injury	

Figure 39.4 Important history components for evaluation of male infertility. STD, sexually transmitted disease; TB, tuberculosis; TURP, transurethral resection of the prostate.

history includes duration of the problem, previous pregnancies (together or with other partners), frequency and timing of intercourse, potency and ejaculatory function, prior methods of birth control, and the use of vaginal lubricants. Unless absolutely necessary for successful intercourse, lubricants should be avoided as most have been shown to inhibit sperm motility.

The couple need to have a basic understanding of the ovulatory cycle to maximize their chances of natural conception. Sperm are known to survive in the cervical mucus for up to 48 hours. The oocyte can be fertilized within the fallopian tube for 12–24 hours or more after ovulation. Thus, engaging in intercourse too frequently can result in inadequate numbers of sperm being deposited in the vaginal vault, whereas intercourse performed too infrequently may result in the ovulatory period being missed. The time of ovulation can be determined by monitoring basal body temperature or by daily measurements of urinary luteinizing hormone (LH) levels. A less precise approach is to simply have intercourse every 2 days during the middle of the menstrual cycle.

A thorough past medical history should be obtained, since virtually any disease process can potentially affect fertility. Unfortunately, the treatments rendered for some conditions can make the fertility problem even worse. For example, testicular cancer is known to cause impaired spermatogenesis and infertility even prior to any form of treatment. All the available therapeutic modalities such as surgery, radiation, and chemotherapy can result in further deterioration of semen parameters either temporarily or permanently.

Cryptorchidism causes oligospermia (defined in Fig. 39.5) in 30% and 50% of men with unilateral and bilateral abnormalities respectively[4,5]. The higher the location of the testis during descent, the worse the testicular dysfunction. The treatment of choice is orchidopexy prior to puberty and preferably within the first 2 years of life. However, the procedure itself can cause infertility if the vasculature of the testis is compromised or if the vas deferens is traumatized. Fortunately, the vast majority of orchidopexy procedures are entirely successful, and boys undergoing the procedure prior to puberty have fertility rates approaching normal[6].

It seems that any abnormality or trauma affecting the testis on one side can have deleterious effects on the contralateral, 'normal' testis as well. In addition to testicular cancer and cryptorchidism, this phenomenon has been observed with varicoceles and torsion. All procedures performed in the inguinal region, scrotum, pelvis, or retroperitoneum can potentially result in infertility. Patients may not recall procedures performed during infancy or early childhood and any unexplained surgical scars observed during physical examination should lead to further questioning.

It takes just under 3 months for a spermatogonium to appear in the ejaculate as a mature spermatozoon. Therefore special attention should be paid to any illness occurring in this time period. High fevers or other systemic ailments can cause substantial, albeit temporary, declines in sperm quantity and quality.

Commonly used terms for description of semen analysis results	
Term	**Definition**
Normospermia	Semen specimen meets normal WHO criteria
Azoospermia	Complete absence of sperm in the ejaculate (even after centrifugation)
Cryptozoospermia	Rare sperm found after centrifugation ('virtual azoospermia')
Oligospermia	Sperm density $<20 \times 10^6$/mL
Asthenospermia	<50% of sperm have good quality movement (grade 3–4)
Teratospermia	<30% normal sperm forms by WHO criteria
OAT	Oligoasthenoteratozoospermia (abnormalities of all three parameters)
Pyospermia	$>1 \times 10^6$WBC/mL
Necrospermia	Satisfactory density but viability stain shows no living sperm
Hematospermia	Presence of gross or microscopic blood in the ejaculate
Aspermia	Absence of any ejaculate

Figure 39.5 Commonly used terms for description of semen analysis results. WBC, white blood cells.

A history of urinary tract infection, prostatitis, or sexually transmitted disease should be noted. Postpubertal mumps orchitis has historically been a cause of infertility, but the development of effective vaccines has made the condition quite rare. Patients should be questioned about the onset and progression of puberty as abnormalities in this area may suggest an endocrinopathy. Finally, exposure to potential gonadotoxins should be identified (Fig. 39.6).

PHYSICAL EXAMINATION

A complete physical examination should be performed, with special attention to the genitalia. The patient's general appearance, including body habitus, limb length, and degree of virilization (e.g. gynecomastia, body hair) should be noted. Head, neck, chest, abdomen, extremities, and nervous system are each meticulously evaluated. Although relatively rare, there are several recognized syndromes, summarized in Figure 39.7, that should be kept in mind while performing the systemic review and physical examination.

The genital examination begins with inspection of the penis for lesions, urethral discharge, and position of the urethral meatus. More severe cases of hypospadias can impair the patient's ability

Potential gonadotoxins
Heat
Radiation
Commonly used substances
Alcohol
Cigarettes
Caffeine
Marijuana
Cocaine
Medications
Diethylstilbestrol
Testosterone
Ketoconazole
Nitrofurantoin
Cimetidine
Sulfa drugs
Calcium channel blockers
Chemotherapy
Pesticides
DDT
Organophosphates
Heavy metals
Lead
Manganese
Solvents
Carbon disulfide
Toluene
Ethylene glycol

Figure 39.6 Potential gonadotoxins. DDT, dichlorodiphenyltrichlorethane.

to deposit an ejaculate deep in his partner's vagina near the cervix. The scrotal contents are examined in both the supine and standing positions. A warm room facilitates palpation of important structures. The testicles are examined for masses, tenderness, size, and consistency. Testicular size can be quantified using calipers or an orchidometer. A normal testis is over 4cm in length with a volume greater than 16mL. The spermatogenic region of the testis, the seminiferous tubules, occupies 80% of its volume. Therefore, abnormally small testicles suggest impaired spermatogenesis. Very firm testes indicate fibrosis and testicular failure whereas abnormally soft testes are frequently encountered in

Clinical syndromes to remember when evaluating infertile men			
Syndrome	**Genetics**	**Cause**	**Features**
Kartagener's	Autosomal recessive	Ciliary axoneme defect	Immotile sperm, respiratory infections, situs inversus
Kallman's	Sporadic or familial	Defective GnRH release	Delayed puberty, anosmia, somatic midline defects, long limbs
Klinefelter's	De novo event	Meiotic non-disjunction (47XXY)	Elevated gonadotrophins, gynecomastia, small and firm testicles

Figure 39.7 Clinical syndromes to remember when evaluating infertile men. GnRH, gonadotrophin-releasing hormone.

men with hormonal abnormalities. A completely normal testis in a man with azoospermia is suggestive of reproductive tract obstruction.

The finding of swelling, tenderness, or scarring of the epididymis is consistent with current or previous infection. The epididymis may also become indurated secondary to obstruction. The vas deferens is usually easy to palpate through the scrotal skin. Congenital absence or atresia of the vas is not uncommon and may occur unilaterally or bilaterally. Some but not all of these patients will also have seminal vesicle and/or renal anomalies.

Varicoceles are dilated tortuous veins in the pampiniform plexus of the testis and have been reported in up to 40% of men presenting with subfertility[7]. With the patient in the standing position, the size of the varicocele is graded I–III using the system shown in Figure 39.8. The varicocele should essentially disappear when the patient assumes a recumbent position. If it does not, obstruction of the internal spermatic vein by a retroperitoneal mass (e.g. kidney tumor, sarcoma, lymphoma) may be present and further radiographic imaging is warranted.

Because of venous anatomy, varicoceles are more common on the left side. The left internal spermatic vein is 8–10cm longer than the right, which may result in an increased hydrostatic pressure[8]. Compression of the left renal vein between the aorta and superior mesenteric artery ('nutcracker effect') may also contribute to higher internal spermatic vein pressure[9]. Bilateral varicoceles are frequently detected with careful examination but isolated right varicoceles are relatively rare.

The exact pathophysiologic mechanism whereby varicoceles cause impaired testicular function remains poorly understood. Theories include abnormally high scrotal temperature, hypoxia due to venous stasis, dilution of intratesticular substrates (e.g. testosterone), hormonal imbalances, and reflux of renal and/or adrenal metabolites down the spermatic vein. Data exist to both support and refute each of these possibilities. Most probably, the etiology is multifactorial[10].

Lastly, a digital rectal examination should be performed, noting the size and consistency of the prostate gland. A tender or 'boggy' gland is indicative of inflammation or infection (prostatitis). Asymmetry, induration, or discrete nodules are all, of course, suggestive of carcinoma. The seminal vesicles may be subtly palpable. Easily palpated, dilated seminal vesicles are abnormal and require further evaluation with transrectal ultrasound.

Female evaluation

Although the female evaluation is generally carried out by a gynecologist, it is imperative that urologists caring for infertile men have a good understanding of the etiologies, evaluation, and treatment of female infertility. The most common causes of female infertility are uterine or fallopian tube abnormalities (e.g. uterine leiomyomas, adhesions, endometriosis) and ovulatory dysfunction.

LABORATORY EVALUATION

Semen analysis

Although the semen analysis remains a critical component of the evaluation of infertile men, it is not, strictly speaking, a measure of fertility. Substantial overlap exists between the semen parameters of fertile and infertile men. Also, significant fluctuations in seminal quality can occur in any one individual. Therefore, at least three separate specimens, each with a consistent 48–72 hour abstinence period, should be obtained over several months.

The physical characteristics of the specimen are assessed first, including color, volume, viscosity, pH, and liquefaction. Freshly ejaculated semen is a white–gray coagulum that gradually liquefies over 10–20 minutes. Substances in the seminal vesicles (SV) are responsible for coagulation while proteinase enzymes from the prostate gland cause liquefaction. SV fluid has a relatively basic pH whereas prostatic secretions are acidic (pH6.0–6.5). The two fluids combine to form an ejaculate in the high physiologic pH range (7.4–8.0). Roughly 60% of the ejaculate volume comes from the SV. The prostate is responsible for about 30% and the remaining 10% is produced by the epididymis, ampulla of the vas, and periurethral glands. The SV produce high concentrations of fructose through an androgen-dependent process and are the only significant source of this sugar in the reproductive tract. Therefore, patients with obstruction or congenital absence of the SV will typically have a fructose-negative, low-volume, low pH ejaculate that does not coagulate.

A microscopic evaluation of the semen specimen is performed quantifying three general parameters: sperm density, motility, and morphology. It is clear that *average* semen parameters for normal, fertile men far exceed what is actually *necessary* for conception. Therefore, it is more appropriate to discuss the 'limits of adequacy' or perhaps the 'low end of normal' rather than average values (Fig. 39.9). This highlights an important difference between *subfertility* and *sterility*. As semen quality declines below 'normal', the chances of pregnancy statistically decrease. They do

Varicocele grading system

Grade	Definition
I	Palpable only with Valsalva
II	Palpable in standing position
III	Visible through scrotal skin

Figure 39.8 Varicocele grading system.

Normal values for semen analysis

Variable	Normal
Volume	1.5–5.0mL
pH	7.2–8.0
Density	>20 × 10^{6}sperm/mL
Motility	>50%
Forward progression	>2 (scale 0–4)
Morphology	>30% normal forms
Leukocytes	<1 × 10^{6}WBC/mL
Fructose	>13μmol/ejaculate
Plus: absence of significant agglutination and hyperviscosity	

Figure 39.9 Normal values for semen analysis (1992 World Health Organization guidelines). The 'limits of adequacy' are indicated. WBC, white blood cells.

not reach zero, however, until a total absence of motile sperm is demonstrated. Some of the terms commonly used to describe semen analysis results are outlined in Figure 39.5.

If no sperm are found on routine semen analysis, the specimen is centrifuged and the pellet is resuspended in a microliter volume for inspection. It is not uncommon to find rare sperm, which would effectively rule out complete obstruction of the reproductive tract (cryptozoospermia). Absence of sperm in the pellet makes a definitive diagnosis of azoospermia.

Sperm motility is expressed both as the percentage of sperm moving and the general quality of motion (Fig. 39.10). If motility is low (<50%) a viability stain must be performed. ICSI can be successfully performed with viable immotile sperm but not with dead sperm.

Morphology is the most subjective semen parameter. A normal spermatozoon is represented schematically in Figure 39.11. It should have an oval head with a clearly distinguishable acrosome. Immature sperm have larger, rounded heads and the midpiece may contain retained cytoplasmic droplets. Normal specimens should contain more than 30% normal forms with fewer than 3% immature forms, using World Health Organization (WHO) criteria for analysis of morphology[11]. More strict criteria have been described by Kruger and associates[12]. They found that semen specimens with less than 14% normal forms by their strict criteria yielded substantially decreased success rates with conventional IVF.

When assessing morphology, 'round cells' are commonly encountered that could represent either immature germ cells or leukocytes. Differentiating between the two is important as the presence of numerous white blood cells suggests infection, which may be amenable to antibiotic therapy. Traditionally, peroxidase staining has been used but immunohistochemical techniques are also available for consistent and accurate differentiation of round cells[13]. Pyospermia should be further evaluated with aerobic and anaerobic cultures including analysis for *Mycoplasma*, *Ureaplasma*, *Chlamydia*, and gonorrhea.

Hormonal studies

Normal sperm production, maturation, and transport requires the presence of certain hormones in appropriate amounts (Fig. 39.12). The cascade of hormonal production begins at the level of the hypothalamus with pulsatile release of gonadotrophin-releasing hormone (GnRH). This stimulates the release of luteinizing hormone (LH) and follicle-stimulating hormone (FSH) from the anterior pituitary. FSH acts on Sertoli cells in the testis to quantitatively maintain spermatogenesis. Sertoli cells release activin and inhibin, which feed back to the pituitary

to modulate FSH release. LH stimulates testicular Leydig cells to synthesize and release testosterone. High levels of testosterone in the seminiferous epithelium are required for initiation and maintenance of normal spermatogenesis. Testosterone is converted in most androgen-sensitive organs into a more potent form, dihydrotestosterone, by the enzyme 5α-reductase. Estradiol is required in small amounts for normal testicular function but may impair spermatogenesis when excess levels are present.

Patients with primary testicular failure may have significantly elevated gonadotrophins, especially FSH, caused by the absence of negative feedback. Abnormally low gonadotrophin levels are secondary to hypothalamic or pituitary dysfunction. Prolactin (PRL), another hormone made in the pituitary, can affect fertility when present in excess. High PRL levels cause decreased LH release and may impair libido. Hyperprolactinemia can be idiopathic or caused by macroadenomas of the pituitary. In addition to diminished sex drive, men with macroadenomas may complain of headaches or impaired visual fields.

Only about 3% of male infertility cases are due to a primary hormonal problem. Such abnormalities are especially rare in men with a sperm density greater than $5-10 \times 10^6$/mL. What constitutes an appropriate endocrine evaluation depends upon the clinical situation and the nature of one's practice. Some practitioners obtain a complete profile on virtually all patients but others have argued for a more limited initial evaluation consisting only of FSH and testosterone[14].

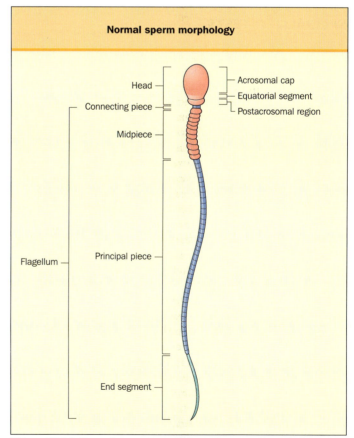

Normal sperm morphology

Figure 39.11 Normal sperm morphology. Note smooth, oval shape; acrosome comprising 40–70% of head; no neck, midpiece, or tail anomalies; no cytoplasmic droplets.

Grade	Definition
0	No motility
1	Sluggish, nonprogressive
2	Slow, meandering progression
3	Straight motion, moderate speed
4	Straight motion, high speed

Quality of sperm motility

Figure 39.10 Quality of sperm motility (forward progression).

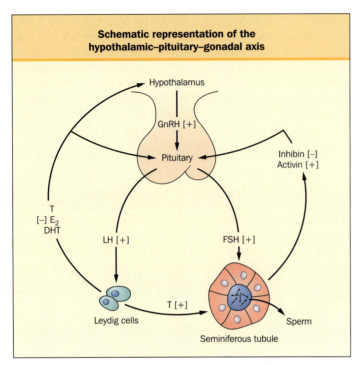

Schematic representation of the hypothalamic–pituitary–gonadal axis

Figure 39.12 Schematic representation of the hypothalamic–pituitary–gonadal axis. E₂, estradiol; DHT, dihydrotestosterone; FSH, follicle-stimulating hormone; GnRH, gonadotrophin-releasing hormone; LH, lunteinizing hormone; T, testosterone.

SPECIALIZED TESTS

The history, physical, and initial laboratory work usually suggest a short list of potential diagnoses that may be extended, if necessary, with additional, more sophisticated testing.

Antisperm antibodies

Tight junctions between cells are largely responsible for creating a blood–testis and blood–epididymis barrier that prevents exposure of sperm to the immune system. When these barriers are disrupted, sperm are recognized as 'foreign' by the man's immune system, resulting in antibody production. Conditions that may trigger antisperm antibody formation include ductal obstruction (e.g. vasectomy), infection, torsion, cryptorchidism, trauma, and varicoceles[15]. Antisperm antibodies are occasionally found in normal, fertile men but high titers are much more common in infertile men[16]. Various studies have shown that only antibodies on the surface of the spermatozoon are clinically significant. Antibodies to internal sperm antigens and those found only in serum probably have little or no impact on fertility[17]. Patients who should be considered for testing are those with any of the previously mentioned risk factors, abnormal sperm agglutination (clumping), impaired motility, an abnormal postcoital test, or unexplained infertility.

Postcoital test

The postcoital test (PCT) evaluates the interaction between a man's sperm and the cervical mucus environment in his partner. Important information is obtained, since sperm must travel through the cervical mucus en route to the uterus and fallopian

Potential reasons for an abnormal postcoital test

Inappropriate timing of test (most common)
Abnormal semen (volume, viscosity, count, etc.)
Antisperm antibodies (in semen or cervical mucus)
Anatomic abnormalities (e.g. hypospadias)
Inappropriately performed coitus (e.g. lubricants)
Poor-quality mucus (ferning, *Spinnbarkeit*)

Figure 39.13 Potential reasons for an abnormal postcoital test.

tubes for fertilization. Cervical mucus is obtained just prior to ovulation but several hours after intercourse. A normal specimen will show more than 10 sperm per high power field (400 ×) with the majority having progressive motility. A PCT is indicated in cases of hyperviscous semen, low- or high-volume ejaculates with good sperm density, abnormal penile anatomy (e.g. hypospadias), or unexplained infertility. It is also used to obtain information about semen quality from men who are unable to provide a specimen by other means for religious reasons. A patient with an abnormal semen analysis does not require a PCT, since results are invariably also poor. Some of the causes of an abnormal PCT are listed in Figure 39.13.

Sperm function tests
Sperm penetration assay
Species-specific fertilization is regulated by the zona pellucida, a layer of glycoproteins surrounding the ovum. When this layer is removed, interspecies sperm–oocyte interaction is possible. The sperm penetration assay (SPA) is an *in vitro* test of human sperm interaction with hamster oocytes. A positive (normal) SPA requires that sperm be capable of several important functions: capacitation, the acrosome reaction, fusion with the oolema, and incorporation into the ooplasm. The total number of hamster ova penetrated and the number of penetrations per ovum is determined. Normal results vary between laboratories but, in general, 10% of eggs penetrated and more than 5 penetrations per egg is desirable.

Because the SPA is a nonstandardized bioassay, it is difficult to compare results from different laboratories. It has been reported that patients with a positive SPA have a 95% chance of fertilizing human ova in vitro while those testing negative have a 50% chance[18]. Thus, the test may be used in some cases of unexplained infertility when the couple is considering assisted reproduction. A normal SPA suggests a good chance of success with conventional IVF whereas a negative result is a strong indication for ICSI. When other clear indications for ICSI are already present, the SPA is unnecessary.

Hypo-osmotic swelling test
Exposing viable sperm to hypo-osmotic solutions causes sperm swelling that results in a typical tail-coiling pattern identifiable under a light microscope. Up to 80% of sperm from normal fertile donors develop this swelling pattern[19]. The hypo-osmotic swelling (HOS) test is probably the only test of sperm function that has been increasingly used since the advent of ICSI. It functionally evaluates sperm membrane integrity and individual

sperm viability without lethal toxicity. Therefore, it may be used to pick out viable sperm for ICSI from an immotile population of cells.

Other tests

The hemizona assay measures the ability of sperm to interact with the zona pellucida, a prerequisite to natural fertilization. It requires the use of human oocytes. Sperm must also undergo capacitation and the acrosome reaction for natural fertilization to take place. Using specific stains and light or transmission electron microscopy, it is possible to detect abnormalities of these processes (ultrastructural abnormalities). While still useful in the research setting, these tests are seldom performed for clinical evaluation of the infertile male.

Genetic testing

Advances in molecular biology have allowed the detection of genetic abnormalities in a significant proportion of infertile men, particularly those with azoospermia or severe oligospermia. The advent of ICSI has made it possible for men with genetic abnormalities that would have rendered them sterile in the past to now successfully father children. Since many genetic defects can be transmitted to offspring or affect the chances of fertility treatment success, it is important to provide appropriate counseling to couples when testing reveals an abnormality.

Karyotype analysis

Widely available, karyotype testing is used to detect abnormalities of chromosomal number and/or structure. Patients with Kleinfelter's syndrome (47 XXY) or XX male syndrome can be identified in this manner. Large terminal deletions and certain translocations may also be detected. Karyotype analysis should be performed on men with azoospermia or severe oligospermia (<10 million sperm per mL).

Y chromosome microdeletion analysis

Approximately 7% of men presenting for infertility evaluation will prove to have a deletion of the Y chromosome that is too small to be detected by routine karyotype analysis[20]. These 'submicroscopic' deletions are associated with severe spermatogenic defects and may be detected by polymerase chain reaction. Y chromosome microdeletion screening is only available at a few centers but should be considered for men with azoospermia or severe oligospermia.

Cystic fibrosis gene mutation analysis

Over 95% of men with cystic fibrosis (CF) have abnormalities of wolffian duct derivatives (vas deferens, seminal vesicles, ejaculatory ducts)[21]. Interestingly, it has recently been observed that anywhere from 50% to 80% of healthy men with bilateral congenital absence of the vas (BCAVD) have mutations of the CF gene[22]. Thus it appears that some cases of vasal agenesis may represent mild forms or reproductive-tract-specific forms of cystic fibrosis. All men with unilateral or BCAVD who are considering assisted reproduction should be screened for CF gene mutations. Their partners should also be screened as approximately 4% of the Caucasian population in North America are silent carriers. Vasal agenesis (especially when unilateral) is also frequently found in combination with renal agenesis but this

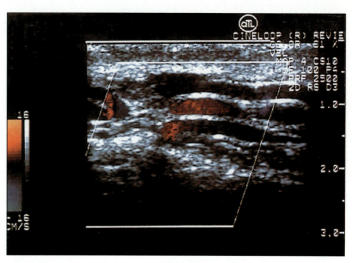

Figure 39.14 Scrotal sonogram showing a large varicocele.

appears to be a distinct clinical entity not associated with CF gene mutations.

Radiologic studies

Scrotal ultrasonography

As discussed previously, varicoceles represent the most common correctable cause of male infertility. Using ultrasonography, the diameter of dilated veins in the pampiniform plexus can be measured and retrograde flow confirmed using color Doppler flow imaging (Fig. 39.14). This technology is so sensitive that 'subclinical' varicoceles can be diagnosed that are too subtle to be appreciated on physical examination. Typically, subclinical varicoceles have a venous diameter less than 2.7mm. Most experts agree that little, if any, benefit is gained by diagnosing and treating these lesions. In general, scrotal ultrasound is most useful for *confirming* pathology already suspected on physical examination.

Scrotal masses such as testicular tumors, hydroceles, and spermatoceles can be well visualized by ultrasonography. Very accurate estimates of testicular size may also be obtained. In addition, color flow analysis has proved to be quite helpful in ruling out testicular torsion in equivocal cases.

Abdominal ultrasonography

Varicoceles should markedly diminish in turgidity when patients move from the standing to supine positions. If they do not, it suggests the presence of a retroperitoneal process (e.g. tumor) causing obstruction of the venous outflow. Ultrasonography is an excellent screening tool for evaluation of the retroperitoneum, including the kidneys. Abnormalities should be further confirmed and delineated with a computed axial tomography scan or magnetic resonance imaging (MRI).

Renal ultrasonography is indicated for men with vasal anomalies. Unilateral congenital absence of the vas deferens is associated with agenesis of the ipsilateral kidney in up to 90% of cases, whereas men with bilateral vasal agenesis have a 10–15% prevalence of unilateral renal anomalies.

Transrectal ultrasound

Transrectal ultrasound (TRUS) has gained widespread use in urology, mainly in evaluating men for prostate cancer. It also has

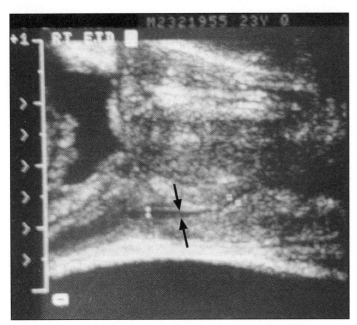

Figure 39.15 Transrectal ultrasound showing dilatation of the ejaculatory duct in a man with ejaculatory duct obstruction. The seminal vesicles are not visualized in this longitudinal image.

applications in male infertility, primarily to assess the seminal vesicles and ejaculatory ducts. Dilatation of these structures suggests obstruction (Fig. 39.15). Absence or atresia of the seminal vesicles is found in most, but not all, patients with congenital absence of the vas deferens. On rare occasions, the retroperitoneal portion of the vas can be detected when the scrotal vas is absent. TRUS may also be used to guide needle aspiration of the seminal vesicles[23]. This technique has been used to obtain sperm for assisted reproduction and to confirm the diagnosis of ejaculatory duct obstruction. Under normal conditions, very few sperm reside in the seminal vesicles within the first 5 days after ejaculation but, in the presence of obstruction or prolonged abstinence, substantial numbers of sperm may be observed.

Vasography

Used to identify sites of obstruction on the vas deferens, vasography should only be performed at the time of planned reconstruction, not at the time of diagnostic testis biopsy. A classic vasogram is performed by cannulating the vas deferens near the junction of its straight and convoluted portions. Contrast is injected while applying gentle traction on a Foley catheter to occlude the bladder neck. Visualization of contrast media in the urethra on a plain radiograph of the pelvis rules out obstruction (Fig. 39.16). Retrograde injection toward the testicle is never attempted because of the potential for epididymal rupture and injury to the testicle.

Testicular biopsy

To definitely distinguish obstructive from nonobstructive azoospermia, a testis biopsy is required. Often, the biopsy simply confirms what was already suspected clinically. For men with small testes (<10cm) and an elevated FSH in the absence of epididymal fullness, the diagnosis of nonobstructive azoospermia does not require a biopsy. For men with BCAVD, normal testicular volume, and normal FSH, a biopsy is also unnecessary to confirm the presence of adequate sperm production for retrieval. In equivocal cases, histologic material should be obtained. Bilateral biopsies should be performed whenever two testicles are present. Testicular biopsy is generally not indicated in cases of oligospermia since results will rarely alter therapy. Histologic findings are rarely pathognomonic and do not, by themselves, provide a clinical diagnosis.

Prior to the advent of ICSI, testicular biopsies were performed strictly for diagnostic purposes. Therapeutic biopsy for sperm retrieval may now be performed in a procedure called testicular sperm extraction (TESE). This technique is appropriate to retrieve sperm for ICSI from men with nonobstructive azoospermia. For men with obstructive azoospermia, percutaneous biopsies are less invasive and equally effective. However, some patients with nonreconstructable, obstructive azoospermia may be better served by procuring sperm from the epididymis using a procedure called microscopic epididymal sperm aspiration (MESA). Sperm from the epididymis are usually more plentiful and mature than those in the testis (Fig. 39.17).

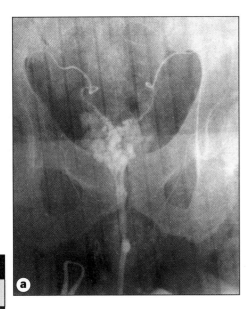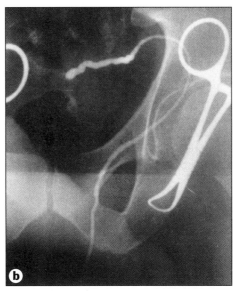

Figure 39.16 Retroperitoneal obstruction.
(a) Normal vasogram (courtesy of M Goldstein).
(b) Vasogram showing retroperitoneal obstruction.

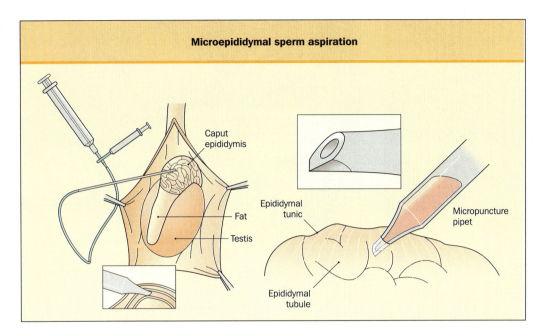

Microepididymal sperm aspiration

Caput epididymis

Fat

Testis

Epididymal tunic

Micropuncture pipet

Epididymal tubule

Figure 39.17 Microepididymal sperm aspiration. A specially designed glass micropet is inserted into an epididymal tubule for retrieval of sperm. (Adapted with permission from Schlegel PN, Berkeley AS, Goldstein M, et al. Epididymal micropuncture with *in vitro* fertilization and oocyte micro-manipulation for the treatment of unreconstructable obstructive azoospermia. Fertil Steril. 1994; 61: 895–901.)

Microscopic evaluation of diagnostic biopsy specimens should initially be quantified by calculating the average number of elongated spermatids per round seminiferous tubule. A diagnosis of obstruction can safely be made if more than 15–20 mature spermatids are seen per tubule. Histologic findings generally fall into one of five categories: normal, hypospermatogenesis, maturation arrest, Sertoli-cell-only pattern (germinal aplasia), and sclerosis. Examples of these histologic patterns, along with brief descriptions of important histologic features, are shown in Figures 39.18–39.22. It is important to realize that different spermatogenic patterns may be present within the same testis. For men with nonobstructive azoospermia, we have found that it is the most advanced pattern of spermatogenesis seen, not the most abundant pattern, that best predicts the chances of retrieving sperm with TESE (Fig. 39.23)[24].

MANAGEMENT

When discussing the various causes and treatments of infertility, it is useful to group patients into one of four categories based upon their initial semen analysis results: (1) all parameters normal, (2) azoospermia, (3) diffuse abnormalities in all parameters, or (4) isolated problems restricted to one parameter. This approach provides an opportunity to consider further evaluation and/or treatment in the clinical setting.

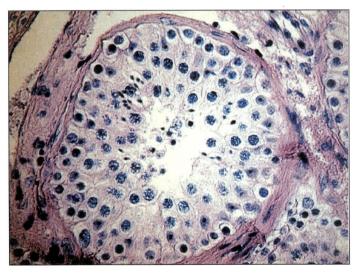

Figure 39.18 Normal testis biopsy histology. Seminiferous tubules are separated by a thin interstitium containing acidophilic Leydig cells, blood vessels, lymphatics, and connective tissue. The basement membrane of the tubules is lined by Sertoli cells and spermatogonia. Germ cells are visible in all stages of spermatogenesis.

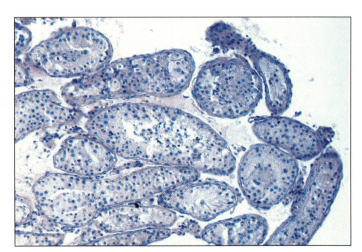

Figure 39.19 Hypospermatogenesis. Seminiferous tubules contain reduced numbers of all germinal elements. Disorganization of the germinal epithelium may be present in places with immature germ cells in the lumen. Some of the tubules in this micrograph show maturation arrest at the spermatocytic level.

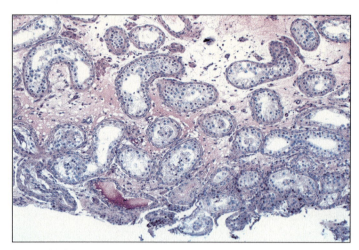

Figure 39.20 Maturation arrest. May occur early (at primary or secondary spermatocyte stage) or late (at spermatid stage). This example shows arrest at the spermatocytic level.

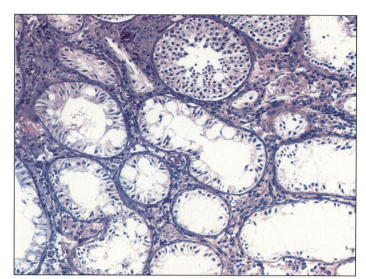

Figure 39.22 Mixed pattern. Note the general pattern of Sertoli cell only (germinal aplasia) with one seminiferous tubule displaying a 'pocket' of spermatogenesis.

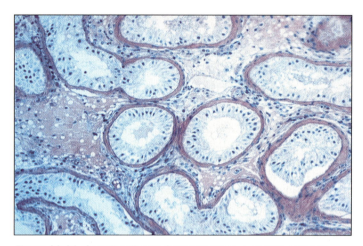

Figure 39.21 Sertoli cell only. Complete absence of germ cells with reduced seminiferous tubule diameter. Sertoli cells are identified by their basal location in the seminiferous tubules and the single, prominent nucleolus in the nucleus of each cell. Leydig cell hyperplasia may be present.

Sperm retrieval rates after testicular sperm extraction	
Histologic findings	Sperm retrieval rate (%)
Hypospermatogenesis	79
Maturation arrest	47
Sertoli cell only	24

Figure 39.23 Sperm retrieval rates after testicular sperm extraction, based on the testis histology from open diagnostic biopsy. The most advanced stage of spermatogenesis seen on biopsy is predictive of testicular sperm extraction results.

Normal

If all semen parameters are normal on repeated analyses, a thorough evaluation of the female partner by a gynecologist experienced in female infertility should be completed. If her work-up proves normal, or if pregnancy does not result following adequate treatment of identified problems, then a postcoital test and antisperm antibody studies should be performed. A sperm penetration assay may also be helpful for directing treatment of these couples with 'unexplained infertility'. Couples with a normal SPA may elect to pursue intrauterine insemination (IUI) or conventional IVF whereas those with few egg penetrations should probably proceed directly to ICSI.

Azoospermia

Men with azoospermia either have impaired spermatogenesis or ductal obstruction (or both). Causes for impaired spermatogenesis include varicoceles, genetic abnormalities, endocrinopathies,

gonadotoxins, and idiopathic causes. Obstruction can be structural or functional. As discussed previously, if the initial semen analysis shows no sperm, the specimen should be centrifuged and the pellet re-examined. The presence of rare sperm in the pellet rules out complete obstruction as an etiology. Azoospermia may also occasionally occur as a result of retrograde ejaculation. This condition is ruled out by performance of a postejaculate urine analysis.

Endocrinopathies

A complete hormonal evaluation should be performed on all azoospermic men, including those for whom an apparent diagnosis is already present (e.g. CBAVD). Elevated serum FSH levels *result from* impaired testicular function; they do not *cause* testicular dysfunction. It appears that FSH levels are reflective of the number of germ cells present in the seminiferous tubules of the testis[25]. Therefore, a man with normal spermatogenesis in a solitary testis will have an elevated FSH but a man with maturation arrest in both testes may have a normal FSH despite the complete absence of mature sperm in the testes. Although significantly elevated FSH levels have traditionally been a poor prognostic sign, they do not appear to reflect the chances of sperm recovery with TESE. A man with a diffuse Sertoli-cell-only pattern but isolated pockets of spermatogenesis will typically have an elevated FSH level but retain an excellent chance of sperm retrieval, whereas with maturation arrest (and frequently normal FSH), no mature sperm may be found despite intensive efforts at TESE because of the uniform, complete blockade of spermatogenic development throughout the testis.

If the serum FSH is extremely high (two to three times normal), traditional teaching has been that taking a biopsy is unnecessary because some degree of testicular failure is clearly present and the chances of finding obstruction are very low. These patients have 'hypergonadotrophic hypogonadism'. However, testicular biopsy may still be useful in these men to confirm the diagnosis, evaluate the prognosis for sperm retrieval, and rule out the presence of intratubular germ cell neoplasia (testicular carcinoma-in-situ).

A low FSH and LH combined with a reduced serum testosterone level is indicative of 'hypogonadotrophic hypogonadism'. The condition may be congenital (e.g. Kallman's syndrome), acquired (e.g. pituitary tumor), or idiopathic. These patients should undergo a complete endocrine evaluation including MRI of the sella turcica to rule out a pituitary tumor.

Elevated serum prolactin levels have been associated with both infertility and impotence. Hyperprolactinemia may be idiopathic or secondary to a macroadenoma of the pituitary ('prolactinoma'). High circulating PRL levels cause decreased gonadotrophin release and depressed testosterone levels. A direct detrimental effect on the testis has also been postulated. Mild elevations in PRL require no treatment if asymptomatic, but significant hyperprolactinemia should be managed with bromocriptine. Surgery and radiation are reserved for those patients unresponsive to bromocriptine. Hypogonadotrophic hypogonadism in the absence of hyperprolactinemia is managed with gonadotrophin replacement.

Isolated deficiencies of LH or FSH are extremely rare. They typically cause azoospermia or oligospermia and are treated by replacing the appropriate hormone. Conditions that cause androgen excess (e.g. congenital adrenal hyperplasia), estrogen excess (hepatic dysfunction), or cortisol excess (e.g. Cushing's disease) may also result in infertility but the vast majority of these patients present with other symptoms first. A summary of endocrine etiologies and the expected results of hormonal analysis is provided in Figure 39.24.

Genetic abnormalities

All men with suspected nonobstructive azoospermia should undergo karyotyping and Y chromosome microdeletion screening. Most men with Klinefelter's syndrome will be azoospermic but mosaics may have some sperm in the ejaculate. Patients with Klinefelter's syndrome have a hormonal profile similar to that of other patients with testicular failure. Men with the XYY syndrome are occasionally fertile but XX males are uniformly azoospermic. Submicroscopic deletions of the Y chromosome result in either azoospermia or severe oligospermia depending on the size and location of the deletion. Patients with these genetic abnormalities can now father children by combining TESE with ICSI. The risks of passing on genetic defects to offspring

Typical results of hormonal testing for various etiologies				
Diagnosis	FSH	LH	T	PRL
Eugonadotropism	nl	nl	nl	nl
Hypogonadotrophic hypogonadism	↓	↓	↓	nl
Primary testicular failure	↑	↑	nl/↓	nl
Germ cell aplasia	↑	nl	nl	nl
Exogenous androgens	↓	↓	↑	nl
Hyperprolactinemia	nl	nl	nl	↑

Figure 39.24 Typical results of hormonal testing for various etiologies. FSH, follicle-stimulating hormone; LH, luteinizing hormone; nl, normal levels; PRL, prolactin; T, testosterone.

necessitates testing and counseling prior to treatment. In some cases, preimplantation genetic diagnosis may also be performed during IVF to further minimize the risks of transmission of genetic anomalies.

Varicoceles

While many men with varicoceles causing infertility display abnormal motility and decreased sperm concentration on semen analysis, some patients with varicoceles will be azoospermic. Up to 55% of azoospermic men with varicoceles will have sperm return to their ejaculate following varicocelectomy and some will even regain sufficient spermatogenesis to achieve unassisted pregnancies[26].

Gonadotoxins

Although the list of potential gonadotoxins is long (Fig. 39.5), there are relatively few exposures that consistently induce azoospermia. All commonly used chemotherapeutic agents have an adverse affect on spermatogenesis but alkylating agents and procarbazine seem to result in the greatest testicular damage. The specific combination of drugs used, the dose administered, and the age of the patient during treatment are all factors that impact the level of gonadotoxicity. Cisplatin-based chemotherapy regimens (PEB, PVB) at the doses commonly used to treat testicular germ cell tumors will cause azoospermia in nearly all patients, with most displaying a rise is FSH levels. The majority of patients will have recovery of spermatogenesis and normalization of FSH levels 2–4 years after the regimen is completed[27].

Like chemotherapy, the effects of radiation on testicular function are dose-dependent. Irreversible azoospermia commonly occurs when the testicular dose exceeds 6–8Gy, with fractionated schedules causing more damage than a single large dose. In one study, men receiving 1Gy had a 100% chance of recovering spermatogenesis whereas those receiving 2Gy had a 60% chance[28]. Testosterone levels usually remain normal after radiation exposure.

Despite their significant health risks, anabolic steroids remain quite popular among certain groups of athletes. The androgenic component of these steroids may induce hypogonadotrophic hypogonadism. As discussed earlier, high intratesticular levels of testosterone are required for maintenance of normal spermatogenesis. When testosterone is administered systemically, negative feedback at the pituitary ultimately leads to diminished

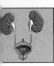

intratesticular testosterone levels and azoospermia. In fact, exogenous testosterone has even been advocated as a contraceptive agent[29].

Ductal obstruction

Azoospermic men with normal hormone parameters and normal-volume testicles on physical examination should be suspected of having ductal obstruction. This suspicion may be supported by the finding of a full or indurated epididymis on physical examination. Acquired and congenital obstructions can occur anywhere along the reproductive tract. Men with ejaculatory duct obstruction or congenital absence of the seminal vesicles will typically have a low-volume, low-pH, fructose-negative ejaculate in addition to azoospermia. These patients should be further evaluated with TRUS. Ejaculatory duct obstruction may be treated by transurethral resection or dilation of the ejaculatory ducts, whereas congenital absence of the vas and seminal vesicles requires sperm retrieval with assisted reproduction. As mentioned previously, all men with vasal agenesis and their partners must undergo testing for CF gene mutations prior to proceeding with sperm procurement and ICSI. In addition, men with idiopathic epididymal obstruction are at risk for CF gene mutations as well.

Men with low-volume ejaculates or those who are aspermic should be evaluated for retrograde ejaculation. This condition usually has an obvious cause such as diabetes, prior retroperitoneal surgery, or transurethral resection of the prostate (TURP), but occasionally idiopathic cases will present. A finding of more than 10 sperm per high powered field (400 ×) from the postejaculatory urine is diagnostic. Initial treatment is with sympathomimetic agents (e.g. ephedrine), which help to close the bladder neck prior to emission and ejaculation. If this is unsuccessful, sperm can be retrieved from the urine by centrifugation and used for IUI or IVF. In general, men with azoospermia and a normal-volume antegrade ejaculate will not prove to have sperm in the postejaculate urine.

Occasionally, aspermia can also occur from failure of seminal emission. For these men, semen does not enter the urethra or bladder following climax due to failure of the ejaculatory mechanism. Some cases are idiopathic or psychogenic but most are secondary to a neurologic insult (e.g. spinal cord injury, retroperitoneal surgery). Therapeutic options include psychotherapy, sympathomimetics, penile vibratory stimulation, or electroejaculation.

Azoospermic men with normal testicles, normal FSH, palpable vasa, and no evidence of ejaculatory duct obstruction should undergo a diagnostic testis biopsy. If quantitatively limited spermatogenesis is found (<5 spermatids/tubule), a diagnosis of nonobstructive azoospermia is made and management options include TESE–ICSI, adoption, or donor insemination. If biopsy results are normal, scrotal exploration to determine the site of obstruction is warranted (a site is often suspected on the basis of the history). Vasography should be performed as previously described. Patency of the testicular end of the vas is confirmed by the finding of sperm in the vasal fluid. When no sperm are found in the vasal fluid, a diagnosis of epididymal obstruction is likely. Points of focal obstruction can be repaired with the microsurgical techniques of vasoepididymostomy or vasovasostomy. Another therapeutic option, especially if the obstruction is beyond repair,

is retrieval of spermatozoa by MESA for subsequent IVF and ICSI. This is also the procedure of choice for patients with congenital absence of the vas. To avoid the need for subsequent sperm retrieval procedures in the event of microsurgical reconstruction failure, sperm retrieval and cryopreservation should be considered during the reconstructive procedure.

Diffuse semen abnormalities

Many patients present with abnormalities involving all semen parameters (density, motility, and morphology), a condition called oligoasthenoteratozoospermia (OAT). Repeated specimens are needed since transient stresses like fever can cause a temporary decline in overall semen quality. Most cases of OAT are associated with varicoceles or are idiopathic. A small percentage of patients may have other factors involved, such as infection, antisperm antibodies, partial obstruction, or exposure to a gonadotoxin.

Varicoceles

Clinically significant varicoceles are diagnosed by physical examination with ultrasonographic confirmation reserved for equivocal cases. Current literature does not support the diagnosis and treatment of subclinical varicoceles. A variety of approaches for correcting varicoceles exist, including open surgery, laparoscopy, and percutaneous methods. Improved semen parameters are seen in 60–70% of patients postoperatively with pregnancy rates in the 30–40% range. It should be noted that not all varicoceles cause infertility and that treatment should only be performed for a clear indication. Varicocele ligation purely for the relief of pain may be reasonable in some situations but symptomatic improvement is by no means guaranteed.

Idiopathic

Up to 25% of men with diffuse semen analysis abnormalities will not have an identifiable etiology. Empiric treatment of men with idiopathic subfertility is controversial. Some of the agents that have been used are summarized in Figure 39.25. The largest experience has been with the antiestrogen clomiphene citrate. Early trials seemed to show significant improvements in semen analysis results and pregnancy rates but more strictly controlled, randomized studies have failed to confirm this benefit.

Patients with idiopathic infertility frequently require assisted reproduction with IUI or IVF–ICSI to achieve a pregnancy. Generally, IUI is best suited for men with more than 10 million motile sperm per ejaculate but IUI with ovarian stimulation of the female partner has been successful in men with much lower counts (500,000 motile sperm/ejaculate).

Other causes

Many of the conditions causing azoospermia may also result in OAT when present in a milder form. Partial obstructions of the epididymis, vas, and ejaculatory ducts probably do occur but are very difficult to diagnose. They are treated in a similar fashion to complete obstruction. Some Y chromosome deletions will result in OAT rather than azoospermia as well. Likewise, hormonal abnormalities and less severe gonadotoxins (e.g. some prescription medications) can also cause OAT. If treatment of the underlying cause proves unsuccessful, assisted reproduction is necessary.

Empiric treatment of idiopathic subfertility	
Therapy	Comment
Testosterone-rebound therapy	No longer recommended. Rarely effective and may result in permanent azoospermia.
Gonadotrophin-releasing hormone	Requires subcutaneous administration every 90–120 minutes to simulate normal, pulsatile release.
Human chorionic gonadotrophin	Requires intramuscular injections 3 times per week for 3–4 months.
Clomiphene citrate	Estrogen antagonist. Results in improved testosterone levels but may also result in elevated estradiol levels.
Testolactone	Aromatase inhibitor. Results in an improved testosterone:estradiol ratio.
Mesterolone	Synthetic androgen. Widely used in Europe.

Figure 39.25 Empiric treatment of idiopathic subfertility. No large, prospective, placebo-controlled, randomized studies have either proved or disproved the effectiveness of these regimens.

Single parameter abnormalities

Low sperm motility with poor forward progression (asthenospermia) is the most common isolated semen parameter abnormality. This problem is frequently due to antisperm antibodies and evidence of sperm agglutination may be present in the semen specimen. A definitive diagnosis is ultimately made using the direct assays previously described. Treatment of immunologic infertility with corticosteroids is controversial. Results have been inconsistent and the devastating complication of aseptic necrosis of the femoral head is worrying. Semen processing followed by IUI or IVF–ICSI is the most commonly pursued therapeutic option.

Other potential causes of asthenospermia are genital tract infection, spermatozoal structural defects, prolonged abstinence periods, partial ductal obstruction, and idiopathic causes. Although a causal relationship between infection and subfertility has never been firmly established, the presence of white blood cells in semen appears to be detrimental to sperm function[30]. Documented infections should be treated, bearing in mind that some antibiotics impair spermatogenesis (e.g. nitrofurantoin, sulfa). The immotile cilia syndrome (also called primary ciliary dyskinesia) is an autosomal recessive disorder that results in asthenospermia due to defective dynein arms or radial spokes in the microtubules of the sperm tail. The same ciliary defect is present in the respiratory tract of these patients, resulting in chronic pulmonary infections. Some 50% of patients with the immotile cilia syndrome will also have situs inversus, a condition known as Kartagener's syndrome. Many cases of asthenospermia are associated with high reactive oxygen species (ROS) levels in semen. The role of antioxidants to decrease ROS production is controversial, although 100mg/day of vitamin E may increase the antioxidant capacity of semen.

Most cases of isolated morphologic abnormalities (teratospermia) are idiopathic. However, many of the previously discussed diagnoses such as varicocele can result in defects that are primarily morphologic in nature. Electron microscopy may be used to detect ultrastructural abnormalities in sperm such as acrosomal absence. Spermatozoa with abnormal morphology perform poorly with conventional IVF and these patients may be better served by proceeding straight to ICSI.

Physical seminal abnormalities such as an abnormally high volume or viscosity should only be treated if the postcoital test is abnormal. Mechanical concentration of sperm by centrifugation or the use of a split ejaculate can be used to treat high volume. Hyperviscosity may be managed with vitamin C (250mg/day), mucolytics (guaifenesin), or sperm processing followed by IUI.

SUMMARY

The development of new diagnostic tests and treatment alternatives over the past few years has revolutionized the management of infertility and brought hope to many couples struggling with this emotionally charged problem. There is still much we do not know, however, especially in the area of impaired spermatogenesis. Too many patients remain without a clear diagnosis, falling into the 'catch-all' category of idiopathic infertility. If we hope to continue making significant strides in the areas of reproductive medicine and andrology, it is imperative that the male partner be thoroughly evaluated and provided with treatments that are diagnosis specific.

REFERENCES

1. Palermo GD, Joris H, Devroey P, VanSteirteghem A. Pregnancies after intracytoplasmic sperm injection of a single spermatozoan into an oocyte. Lancet. 1994;340:17–8.

2. Jarrow JP. Life threatening conditions associated with male infertility. Urol Clin North Am. 1994;21:409–15.

3. Pavlovich CP, Schlegel PN. Cost-effectiveness of treatments for male infertility: A review. Assisted Reprod Rev. 1997;8:40–6.

4. Lipshultz LI, Caminos-Torres R, Greenspan CS, Snyder PJ. Testicular function after orchidopexy for unilaterally undescended testis. N Engl J Med. 1976;295:15–8.

5. Okuyama A, Nonomura N, Nakamura M, et al. Surgical management of undescended testis: retrospective study of potential fertility in 274 cases. J Urol. 1989;142:749–51.

6. Puri P, O'Donnell B. Semen analysis of patients who had orchiopexy at or after seven years of age. Lancet. 1988;2:1051–2.

7. Cockett ATK, Takihara H, Cosentino MJ. The varicocele. Fertil Steril. 1984;41:5–11.

8. Shafik A, Bedeir GA. Venous tension patterns in cord veins. 1. In normal and varicocele individuals. J Urol. 1980;123:383–5.

9. Coosaet BL. The varicocele syndrome: venography determining the optimal level for surgical management. J Urol. 1980;124:833–9.

10. Turek PJ, Lipshultz LI. The varicocele controversies I. Etiology and pathophysiology. AUA Update Series. 1995; vol XIV: lesson 13.

11. World Health Organization. WHO laboratory manual for the examination of human semen and semen–cervical mucus interaction, 3rd edn. Cambridge: Cambridge University Press; 1992.

12. Kruger TF, Menkveld R, Stander FS, et al. Sperm morphologic features as a prognostic factor in in vitro fertilization. Fertil Steril. 1986;46(6):1118–23.

13. Homyk M, Anderson DJ, Wolff H. Differential diagnosis of immature germ cells in semen utilizing monoclonal antibodies MHS-10. Fertil Steril. 1990; 53:323–30.

14. Sigman M, Jarow JP. Endocrine evaluation of infertile men. Urology. 1997;50:659–64.

15. Jarow JP, Sanzone JJ. Risk factors for male partner antisperm antibodies. J Urol. 1992;148:1805–7.

16. Rumke P, VanAmstel N, Messer EN, Bezemar PD. Prognosis of fertility of men with sperm agglutinins in the serum. Fertil Steril. 1974;25:393–8.

17. Hellstrom WJ, Overstreet JW, Samuels SJ, Lewis EL. The relationship of circulating antisperm antibodies to sperm surface antibodies in infertile men. J Urol. 1988;140:1039–44.

18. Smith RG, Johnson A, Lamb D, Lipshultz LI. Functional tests of spermatozoa: sperm penetration assay. Urol Clin North Am. 1987;14:451–8.

19. Jeyendran RS, Van der Van HH, Perez-Pelaez M, et al. Development of an assay to assess the functional integrity of the human sperm membrane and its relationship to other semen characteristics. J Reprod Fertil. 1984;70:219–28.

20. Pryor JL, Kent-First M, Muallem A, et al. Microdeletions in the Y chromosome of infertile men. N Engl J Med. 1997;336:534–9.

21. Taussig LM, Lobeck CC, di Sant'Agnese PA, et al. Fertility in males with cystic fibrosis. New Engl J Med. 1972;287:586–9.

22. Mak V, Jarvi KA. The genetics of male infertility. J Urol. 1996;156:1245–57.

23. Jarow JP. Transrectal ultrasonography in the diagnosis and management of ejaculatory duct obstruction. J Androl. 1996;17:467–72.

24. Su LM, Palermo GD, Pavlovich CP, et al. Testicular sperm extraction with intracytoplasmic sperm injection for nonobstructive azoospermia: testicular histology can predict success of sperm retrieval. J Urol. 1998;159 (5 suppl.):Abst 809, p 210.

25. Kim ED, Gilbaugh JH, Patel VR, et al. Testis biopsies frequently demonstrate sperm in men with azoospermia and significantly elevated follicle stimulating hormone levels. J Urol. 1997;157:144–6.

26. Matthews GJ, Matthews ED, Goldstein M. Induction of spermatogenesis and achievement of pregnancy after microsurgical varicocelectomy in men with azoospermia and severe oligoasthenospermia. Fertil Steril. 1998;70:71–5.

27. Petersen PM, Giwercman A, Skakkebaek NE, Rorth M. Gonadal function in men with testicular cancer. Semin Oncol. 1998;25:224–34.

28. Hansen PV, Trykker H, Svennekjaer IL, et al. Long-term recovery of spermatogenesis after radiotherapy in patients with testicular cancer. Radiother Oncol. 1990;18:117–25.

29. WHO Task force on methods for regulation of male fertility. Contraceptive efficacy of testosterone-induced azoospermia in normal men. Lancet. 1990;336:955–9.

30. Wolff H, Politch JA, Martinez A, et al. Leukocytospermia is associated with poor semen quality. Fertil Steril. 1990;53: 528–536.

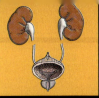

Chapter 40 Erectile Dysfunction

Tom F Lue and Ahmed I El-Sakka

KEY POINTS

This chapter discusses the following aspects of erectile dysfunction:
- Physiology;
- Pathophysiology;
- Evaluation of the patient with erectile dysfunction; and
- Medical and surgical treatment.

INTRODUCTION

The ultimate goal of treating a man with erectile dysfunction (ED) is to enable the sexually crippled patient and his frustrated partner to resume satisfactory sexual intercourse. The therapeutic strategy is to correct the underlying cause of ED or, if it is not feasible, to bypass the cause and offer a nonspecific but personally and socially accepted treatment. The physician should also consider the patient's age and general health, as well as patient and partner's expectations and treatment goals. In this chapter we will discuss the anatomy and physiology of erection and the evaluation and management of erectile dysfunction.

ANATOMY AND PHYSIOLOGY OF THE PENIS

Arterial supply

The main source of blood supply to the penis is usually via the internal pudendal artery, a branch of the internal iliac artery. In many instances, however, accessory arteries exist, arising from the external iliac, obturator, vesical, and femoral arteries, and may occasionally become the dominant or only arterial supply to the corpus cavernosum[1]. Damage to these accessory arteries during radical prostatectomy or cystectomy may result in vasculogenic ED after surgery[2,3]. The internal pudendal artery becomes the common penile artery after giving off a branch to the perineum. The three branches of the penile artery are the dorsal, the bulbourethral, and the cavernous arteries. The cavernous artery is responsible for tumescence of the corpus cavernosum and the dorsal artery for engorgement of the glans penis during erection. The bulbourethral artery supplies the bulb and corpus spongiosum (Fig. 40.1).

Venous drainage

The venous drainage from the three corpora originates in tiny venules leading from the peripheral sinusoids immediately

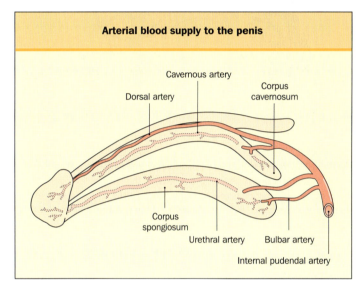

Figure 40.1 Arterial blood supply to the penis. The figure shows the common penile artery and the three branches: dorsal, cavernous, and bulbourethral arteries. (With permission from Lue[4].)

beneath the tunica albuginea. These venules travel in the trabeculae between the tunica and the peripheral sinusoids to form the subtunical venular plexus before exiting as the emissary veins. Outside the tunica albuginea, the venous drainage is as follows:

- *The pendulous portion of the penis*: The emissary veins from the corpus cavernosum and spongiosum drain dorsally to the deep dorsal, laterally to the circumflex, and ventrally to the periurethral veins. Beginning at the coronal sulcus, the prominent deep dorsal vein is the main venous drainage of the glans penis and distal two-thirds of the corpora cavernosa and corpus spongiosum. Usually a single vein, but sometimes more than one deep dorsal vein, runs upwards behind the symphysis pubis to join the periprostatic venous plexus.
- *The infrapubic penis*: Emissary veins draining the proximal corpora cavernosa join to form cavernous and crural veins. These veins join the periurethral veins from the urethral bulb to form the internal pudendal veins (Fig. 40.2).

In addition, multiple superficial veins run subcutaneously and unite near the root of the penis to form a single (or paired) superficial dorsal vein, which in turn drains into the saphenous veins. Occasionally the superficial dorsal vein may also drain a portion of the corpora cavernosa[4].

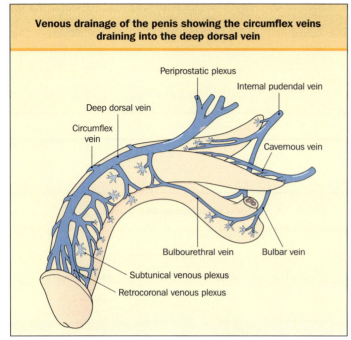

Venous drainage of the penis showing the circumflex veins draining into the deep dorsal vein

Periprostatic plexus

Internal pudendal vein

Deep dorsal vein

Circumflex vein

Cavernous vein

Bulbourethral vein

Bulbar vein

Subtunical venous plexus

Retrocoronal venous plexus

Figure 40.2 Venous drainage of the penis showing the circumflex veins draining into the deep dorsal vein. At the base of the penis, the deep dorsal vein continues as the periprostatic plexus. The deeper veins such as the cavernous and crural veins drain the proximal portion of the penis and empty into internal pudendal veins. (With permission from Lue[4].)

Innervation

The penis is richly innervated by autonomic (sympathetic, parasympathetic) and somatic (sensory and motor) nerves.

The sympathetic pathway originates from the 11th thoracic to the second lumbar spinal segments and passes via the white rami to the sympathetic chain ganglia (Fig. 40.3). Some fibers then travel via the lumbar splanchnic nerves to the inferior mesenteric and superior hypogastric plexuses, from which fibers travel in the hypogastric nerves to the pelvic plexus. In man, the T10–T12 segments are most often the origin of the sympathetic fibers, and the chain ganglia cells projecting to the penis are located in the sacral and caudal ganglia[5].

The parasympathetic pathway arises from neurons in the intermediolateral cell columns of the second, third, and fourth sacral spinal cord segments. The preganglionic fibers pass in the pelvic nerves to the pelvic plexus, where they are joined by the sympathetic nerves from the superior hypogastric plexus.

The cavernous nerves are branches of the pelvic plexus that innervate the penis. Other branches of the pelvic plexus innervate the rectum, bladder, prostate, and sphincters. The cavernous nerves are easily damaged during radical excision of the rectum, bladder, and prostate. A clear understanding of the course of these nerves is essential to the prevention of iatrogenic erectile dysfunction[6].

The somatosensory pathway originates at the sensory receptors in the penile skin, glans, urethra, and within the corpus cavernosum. In the human glans penis, there are numerous afferent terminations: free nerve endings and corpuscular receptors. The nerve fibers from the receptors converge to form bundles of the dorsal nerve of the penis, which joins other nerves to become the pudendal nerve. Activation of these sensory receptors sends messages of pain, temperature, and touch via the dorsal and pudendal nerves, spinal cord, and spinothalamic tract to the thalamus and sensory cortex for sensory perception.

Onuf's nucleus in the second to fourth sacral spinal segments is the center of somatomotor penile innervation. These nerves travel in the sacral nerves to the pudendal nerve to innervate the ischiocavernosus and bulbocavernosus muscles (Fig. 40.4). Contraction of the ischiocavernosus muscles produces the rigid erection phase. Rhythmic contraction of the bulbocavernosus muscle is necessary for external ejaculation.

The tunica albuginea

The covering of the corpora cavernosa is a bilayered structure with multiple sublayers. Inner-layer bundles support and contain

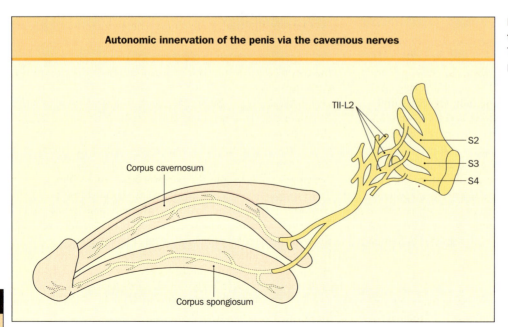

Autonomic innervation of the penis via the cavernous nerves

TII-L2

S2

S3

S4

Corpus cavernosum

Corpus spongiosum

Figure 40.3 Autonomic innervation of the penis via the cavernous nerves. These contain both sympathetic and parasympathetic neurotransmissions.

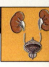
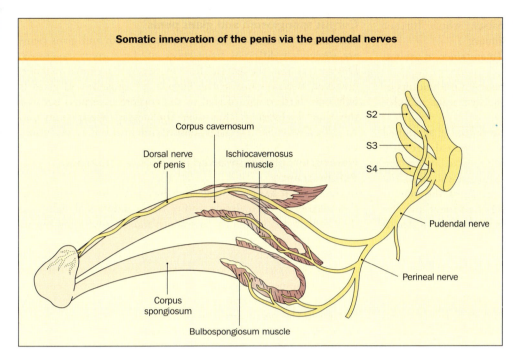

Somatic innervation of the penis via the pudendal nerves

Figure 40.4 Somatic innervation of the penis via the pudendal nerves. The pudendal receives sensory input from the penile skin and glans while its motor component innervates the bulbocavernous and ischiocavernous muscles.

the cavernous tissue, and are oriented circularly. Radiating from this inner layer are intracavernosal pillars (ICPs) acting as struts, augmenting the septum that provides support to the erectile tissue. Outer-layer bundles are oriented longitudinally, extending from the glans penis to the proximal crura; they insert into the inferior pubic ramus but are absent between the 5 and 7 o'clock positions. In contrast, the corpus spongiosum lacks an outer layer or intracorporeal struts, assuring a low-pressure structure during erection[4] (Fig. 40.5).

The tunica albuginea is composed of elastic fibers that form an irregular, latticed network on which the collagen fibers rest (Fig. 40.6). Emissary veins run between the inner and outer layers for a short distance, often piercing the outer bundles in an oblique manner. Branches of the dorsal artery, however, take a more directly perpendicular route and are surrounded by a periarterial fibrous sheath.

Mechanism and phases of erection involving the corpus cavernosum

Sexual stimulation triggers release of neurotransmitters from the cavernous nerve terminals. This results in relaxation of the smooth muscles and the following events:
1. dilation of the arterioles and arteries and increased inflow;
2. trapping of the incoming blood by the expanding sinusoids;
3. compression of the subtunical venular plexuses between the tunica albuginea and the peripheral sinusoids, reducing the outflow;

The tunica albuginea of the corpus cavernosum and corpus spongiosum

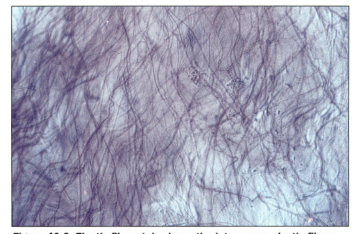

Figure 40.6 Elastic fiber stain shows the interwoven elastic fibers and the collagen fibers. This unique structure provides the elasticity for stretching and recoiling of the tunica albuginea during erection and detumescence.

Figure 40.5 The tunica albuginea of the corpus cavernosum and corpus spongiosum. Note the intracavernosal pillars and the septum.

4. stretching of the tunica to its capacity, which further decreases the venous outflow to a minimum;
5. an increase in intracavernous pressure (maintained at around 100mmHg) – the full erection phase);
6. a further pressure increase (to several hundred millimeters of mercury) with contraction of the ischiocavernosus muscles (rigid erection phase)[3] (Fig. 40.7).

Three phases of detumescence have been reported in an animal study[7]. The first entails a transient intracorporeal pressure increase, indicating the beginning of smooth muscle contraction against a closed venous system. The second phase shows a slow pressure decrease, suggesting a slow reopening of the venous channels with resumption of the basal level of arterial flow. The third phase shows a fast pressure decrease with fully restored venous outflow capacity.

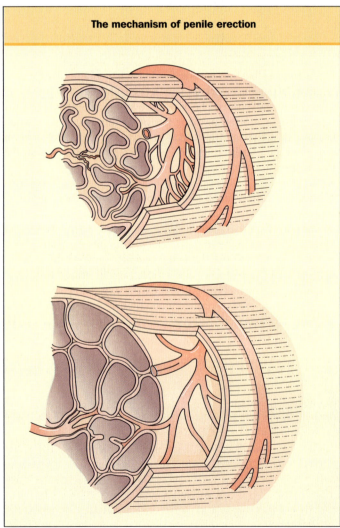

The mechanism of penile erection

Figure 40.7 The mechanism of penile erection. In the flaccid state, contraction of the smooth muscles in the trabeculae and the arterioles allows little inflow into the sinusoids and the venous channels remain open. Relaxation of the smooth muscles during erection maximally dilates the arterioles and drops the resistance to a minimum. The inflow expands the entire sinusoidal system and compresses the subtunical venules against the tunica albuginea. This stretches the tunica albuginea to its limit and gives rigidity to the penis. (With permission from Lue[4].)

Corpus spongiosum and glans penis

The hemodynamics of the corpus spongiosum and glans penis are somewhat different from those of the corpora cavernosa. During erection, the arterial flow increases in a similar manner; however, the pressure in the corpus spongiosum and glans is only one third to half of that in the corpora cavernosa because the tunical covering (thin over the corpus spongiosum and virtually absent over the glans) ensures minimal venous occlusion.

Neurotransmitters involved in penile erection and detumescence

In the penis, it has been suggested that acetylcholine stimulates the release of nitric oxide (NO) from endothelial cells and thus contributes indirectly to smooth muscle relaxation during erection.

Nitric oxide was first described in 1979 as a potent relaxant of peripheral vascular smooth muscle, with an action mediated by cyclic guanidine monophosphate (cGMP)[8]. Nitric oxide is synthesized from endogenous L-arginine by NO synthase (NOS) located in the nerve terminal or vascular endothelium[9]. Nitric oxide can also be synthesized and released as a neurotransmitter by nonadrenergic noncholinergic (NANC) neurotransmission after their excitation by either electrical or chemical stimulation. Many studies have indicated that NO is the principal neurotransmitter for penile erection[10,11].

Cyclic guanidine monophosphate is mainly degraded by a type V phosphodiesterase, PDE-5. Sildenafil is a PDE-5 inhibitor that increases cGMP and has been used to enhance smooth muscle relaxation and penile erection.

Other investigators believe that vasoactive intestinal polypeptide (VIP) may be one of the neurotransmitters responsible for erection. Kim et al.[12] suggest that NO generation is involved in VIP-stimulated smooth muscle relaxation. Other potential candidates include calcitonin-gene-related peptide (CGRP)[13], peptide histidine methionine[14], pituitary adenylate cyclase activating polypeptide[15], and prostaglandins[16]. These agents may act through increased production of cyclic adenosine monophosphate (cAMP) (Fig. 40.8).

The maintenance of intracorporeal smooth muscle in a semi-contracted state may result from three factors: intrinsic myogenic activity, adrenergic neurotransmission, and endothelium-derived contracting factors.

By acting on postjunctional α-adrenoceptors, norepinephrine constricts the arteries and contracts the trabecular smooth muscle. Although its role in maintaining penile flaccidity has not been definitively characterized, most researchers agree that norepinephrine is involved in the return of the penis to the flaccid state after ejaculation.

Several endothelium-derived contracting factors may contribute to flaccidity. A study of rabbit erectile tissue suggests that resting smooth muscle tone may be mediated by prostaglandins E_2 or $F_{2\alpha}$ or both. The endothelins, on the other hand, may augment the contractile responses of other vasomodulators (e.g. the contractile responses to sympathetic activity). In addition, angiotensin may also play a role in modulating cavernous smooth muscle tone.

PATHOPHYSIOLOGY OF ERECTILE DYSFUNCTION

Penile erection is a neurovascular event modulated by psychological input and hormonal levels. Therefore, we prefer to

Intracellular mechanism of penile erection

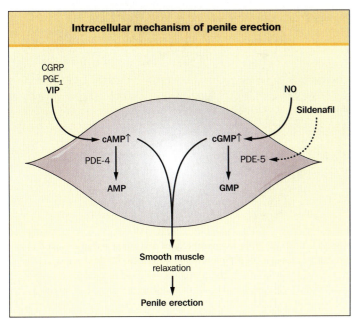

Figure 40.8 Intracellular mechanism of penile erection. The principal neurotransmitter for penile erection is the nitric oxide (NO) released from nerve endings and the endothelium. AMP, adenosine monophosphate; cAMP, cyclic adenosine monophosphate; cGMP, cyclic guanidine monophosphate; CGRP, calcitonin-gene-related peptide; PDE-4, type 4 phosphodiesterase; PDE-5, type 5 phosphodiesterase; PGE_1, prostaglandin E_1; VIP, vasoactive intestinal polypeptide.

classify ED as psychogenic, neurogenic, hormonal, arterial, and cavernosal[17] (Fig. 40.9).

Psychogenic

Previously, psychogenic ED was believed to be the most common, accounting for 90% of cases. This belief has given way to the realization that, in most men, ED has both a physical and a psychological component.

Two mechanisms might be involved in psychogenic ED:
- Exaggeration of the normal suprasacral inhibition of the spinal erection center; and
- Inadequate release of erectile neurotransmitters.

Neurogenic

Pathologic processes in the brain, spinal cord, and peripheral nerves may disrupt nerve conduction and cause ED. Examples are Parkinson's and Alzheimer's diseases, stroke, head trauma, spinal cord injury, diabetes, and radical prostatectomy.

Hormonal

Androgen deficiency is known to suppress nocturnal erection and decrease sexual drive. Hyperprolactinemia, whether from a pituitary adenoma or drugs, results in both reproductive and sexual dysfunction owing to the inhibition of prolactin on central dopaminergic activity and gonadotrophin-releasing hormone. Symptoms may include loss of libido, erectile dysfunction, galactorrhea, gynecomastia, and infertility.

Arterial

Atherosclerotic or traumatic arterial occlusive disease of the pudendal–cavernous–helicine arterial tree can decrease the perfusion pressure and arterial flow to the sinusoidal spaces, thus

Classification of erectile dysfunction according to the organ systems involved in the pathogenesis of erectile dysfunction

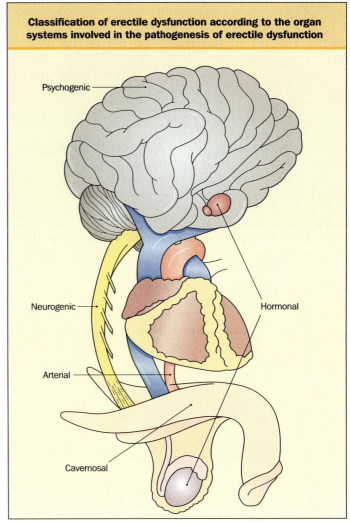

Figure 40.9 Classification of erectile dysfunction according to the organ systems involved in the pathogenesis of erectile dysfunction.

increasing the time to maximal erection and decreasing the rigidity of the erect penis. Common risk factors include hypertension, hyperlipidemia, cigarette smoking, diabetes mellitus, and pelvic injury.

Cavernosal (venogenic)

Veno-occlusive dysfunction may result from one or more of the following pathologic processes:
- large venous channels draining the corpora cavernosa (as often seen in patients with primary ED);
- degenerative changes (Peyronie's disease, old age, diabetes) or traumatic injury to the tunica albuginea (penile fracture);
- structural alterations of the cavernous smooth muscle and endothelium;
- insufficient trabecular smooth muscle relaxation (seen in anxious patients with excessive adrenergic tone or in patients with inadequate neurotransmitter release); and
- acquired shunts – the result of operative correction of priapism.

Since smooth muscle relaxation is the final pathway of penile erection, normal smooth muscles with intact innervation and

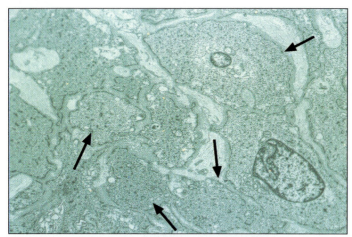

Figure 40.10 Electron micrography of normal intracavernosal tissue.
This slide shows the healthy smooth muscle cells (arrows) with abundant myofilaments and gap junctions.

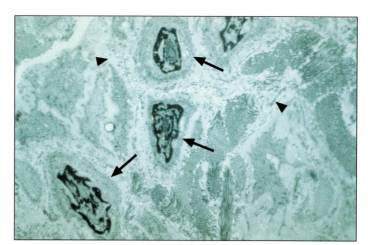

Figure 40.12 Electron micrography of abnormal erectile tissue of a man with diabetes and hypercholesterolemia. Atrophy of the smooth muscle cells (arrows) with loss of myofilament and gap junctions is seen. In addition, large amount of collagen fibers (arrowheads) can be noted.

Smooth muscle content in the corpora cavernosa	
Patient category	% smooth muscle (corpora cavernosa)
Potent (age)	
2–20	46.1
21–40	46.2
41–60	40.6
61–73	35.3
Old impotent	
with venous leakage	19–36
with arterial insufficiency	10–25

Figure 40.11 Smooth muscle content in the corpora cavernosa.
(Data from Wespes et al.[18,19])

adequate intercellular communication via gap junctions are essential in penile erection (Fig. 40.10). Wespes et al.[18,19] have determined the smooth muscle content in potent and impotent young and old men (Fig. 40.11).

In men with long-term diabetes and atherosclerosis, atrophy of penile smooth muscle, loss of myofilaments, decrease in cell size, increase in collagen fibers, and loss of gap junctions can result in incomplete relaxation of the muscle and venous leakage (Fig. 40.12).

Drug-induced

Many therapeutic agents have been reported to cause ED, although the mechanism of action is largely unknown and there are few well-controlled studies on the sexual effects of a particular drug. In general, drugs that interfere with central neuroendocrine or local neurovascular control of penile smooth muscle have the potential to cause erectile dysfunction. Central neurotransmitter pathways, including 5-hydroxytryptaminergic, noradrenergic, and dopaminergic pathways involved in sexual function, may be disturbed by antipsychotics, antidepressants, and centrally acting antihypertensive drugs.

Cigarette smoking may induce vasoconstriction and penile venous leakage because of its contractile effect on the cavernous

smooth muscle. Alcohol in small amounts improves erection and sexual drive because of its vasodilatory effect and the suppression of anxiety; however, large amounts can cause central sedation, decreased libido, and transient erectile dysfunction. Chronic alcoholism may result in liver dysfunction, decreased testosterone and increased estrogen levels, and alcoholic polyneuropathy, which may also affect penile nerves. Cimetidine, a histamine-H_2 receptor antagonist, has been reported to suppress the libido and produce erectile failure. It is thought to act as an antiandrogen and to increase prolactin levels.

Other drugs known to cause erectile dysfunction are estrogens and drugs with antiandrogenic action, such as ketoconazole and cyproterone acetate.

Aging and systemic diseases

A number of studies have indicated a progressive decline in sexual function in 'healthy' aging men. About 50% of patients with chronic diabetes mellitus reportedly have ED. In addition to the disease's effect on small vessels, it may also affect the cavernous nerve terminals and endothelial cells, resulting in deficiency of neurotransmitters.

Patients with severe pulmonary disease often fear aggravating dyspnea during sexual intercourse. Patients with angina, heart failure, or myocardial infarction can become impotent from anxiety, depression, or concomitant penile arterial insufficiency. Other systemic diseases, such as cirrhosis of the liver, scleroderma (involving the erectile tissue), chronic debilitation, and cachexia, are also known to cause ED.

DIAGNOSIS OF ERECTILE DYSFUNCTION

We prefer a patient's goal-directed approach to the diagnosis and treatment of erectile dysfunction[20] (Fig. 40.13). We believe that the following should be obtained in every patient:
- a detailed medical and psycho-sexual history;
- a thorough physical examination; and
- appropriate laboratory tests (complete blood count, urinalysis, fasting glucose, lipid profile, testosterone, and others if indicated)[21].

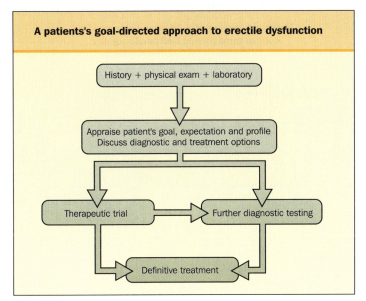

A patients's goal-directed approach to erectile dysfunction

History + physical exam + laboratory

Appraise patient's goal, expectation and profile
Discuss diagnostic and treatment options

Therapeutic trial → Further diagnostic testing

Definitive treatment

Figure 40.13 A patient's goal-directed approach to erectile dysfunction.

Diagnostic tests for chosen treatment options	
Treatment options	**Diagnostic tests**
Oral medication or vacuum constriction device	None (CIS or duplex ultrasound optional)
Intracavernous injection	CIS (duplex ultrasound optional)
Penile prosthesis	NPT with Rigiscan® or CIS or duplex ultrasound
Venous surgery	CIS + duplex ultrasound + cavernosonography (or DICC); NPT
Arterial surgery	CIS + duplex ultrasound (or DICC) + arteriography (NPT optional)

Figure 40.14 Diagnostic tests for chosen treatment options. CIS, combined intracavernous injection and stimulation test; DICC, dynamic infusion cavernosometry and cavernosography; NPT, nocturnal penile tumescence. (With permission from Lue and Broderick[25].)

Differentiation between psychogenic and organic erectile dysfunction		
Characteristic	**Organic**	**Psychogenic**
Onset	Gradual	Acute
Circumstances	Global	Situational
Course	Constant	Varying
Non-coital erection	Poor	Rigid
Psychosexual problem	Secondary	Long history
Partner problem	Secondary	At onset
Anxiety and fear	Secondary	Primary

Figure 40.15 Differentiation between psychogenic and organic erectile dysfunction. Testing to be undertaken after complete history, physical examination and laboratory testing. (With permission from Lue and Broderick[25].)

The patient is given a pamphlet explaining the physiology of erection, diagnostic tests, and treatment options including advantages, disadvantages, and cost. After the patient has finished reading the pamphlet, the physician will answer any questions he may have and ascertain his (and his partner's, if available) expectations and treatment goals.

The physician then evaluates the patient's overall profile and works with him to decide the next step (diagnostic or therapeutic). If additional workup is necessary, it is tailored according to the patient's age, general heath, and treatment goal. Figure 40.14 lists the diagnostic tests we perform for patients' chosen treatment options.

History and physical examination

Obtaining a detailed medical and psychosexual history is the most important part of the diagnostic evaluation. It should include the quality of erection, the duration of ED, the level of libido, and a complete inventory of sexual partners. Although exceptions are not uncommon, an assessment of the onset of dysfunction, the presence of morning erection, and any psychological conflict may help determine whether the dysfunction is mostly psychogenic or organic (Fig. 40.15). Often the sexual history provides the most helpful information in directing further evaluation and treatment.

A psychologic disorder may occasionally be the primary cause of erectile dysfunction. Early recognition not only allows the physician to avoid further costly workup, but saves the patient from unnecessary, sometime invasive diagnostic tests as well. As erectile dysfunction is known to be associated with many common medical conditions and medications, careful questioning may yield insights. Clinically, an older patient with a long history of diabetes and vascular disease is likely to have ED secondary to vascular and neuropathic disease. On the other hand, a young patient with psychiatric illness is more likely to have psychogenic ED or possibly ED secondary to psychotropic medications.

Currently, the most commonly used ED drug is sildenafil; the patient's cardiovascular status, exercise tolerance, and use of nitrate or any medications that might increase or decrease the blood level of sildenafil should therefore also be assessed.

Physical examination should include the following:
- breast, hair distribution, testis, thyroid (to detect an endocrine abnormality);
- femoral and pedal pulses (for vascular insufficiency);
- genital and perineal sensation (neurologic deficit); and
- penile abnormalities.

If no correctable cause of ED is found (e.g. hypogonadism), we will instruct the patient in the correct use of the first-line therapy (usually sildenafil or a vacuum device) and begin ED therapy.

Advanced investigations

Some patients may benefit from more sophisticated testing. For example, a nocturnal penile tumescence test may help to differentiate psychogenic causes from vascular insufficiency in a young man with primary ED. Advanced vascular testing is also helpful in selecting patients with localized arterial or venous insufficiency for vascular surgery.

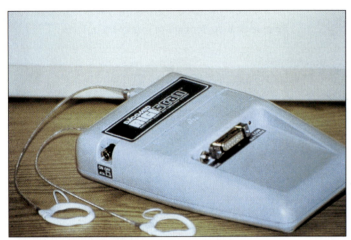

Figure 40.16 The Rigiscan® device. (Courtesy of Timm Medical Inc.)

Nocturnal penile tumescence testing

Nocturnal penile tumescence (NPT) or sleep-related erection is a recurring cycle of penile erections associated with REM sleep in virtually all potent men. This test is helpful in differentiating psychogenic from organic erectile dysfunction (Fig. 40.16)[22,23]. For example, the demonstration of normal penile erections during NPT in a man complaining of inability to achieve and maintain erection for sexual intercourse confirms the psychogenic nature of his ED. The introduction of an ambulatory monitoring device, Rigiscan, has simplified the study. The patient is instructed to take this computerized device home and place the two loops around the penis, one at the base and the other just proximal to the glans. The device automatically records the total sleep time, the frequency and duration of the erectile events, the circumference, and rigidity changes. Figure 40.17 shows a normal tracing with normal tumescence and penile rigidity. In Figure 40.18, the abnormal tracing indicates that the cause of erectile dysfunction in this man is most probably neurologic deficit or vascular insufficiency. It is to be noted that anxiety, depression, and sleep disturbances such as sleep apnea and motor agitation can at times influence the content of the dream state, negatively affecting spontaneous nocturnal erections. When in doubt, a formal sleep lab NPT or psychologic consultation may be needed to reach the correct diagnosis.

Combined intracavernous injection and stimulation test

Intracavernous injection (ICI) of papaverine or alprostadil is a useful diagnostic tool. Our technique involves injecting 10µg of alprostadil through a 28G 16mm needle into the corpus cavernosum. The erectile response is periodically evaluated for both rigidity and duration. Normally, a full erection is achieved within 15min (i.e. an erection of more than 90° that is firm to palpation) and lasts longer than 15min.

A normal finding rules out venous leakage (although about 20% of patients with arterial insufficiency may achieve a rigid erection). An abnormal pharmacologic test suggests penile vascular disease (arterial or cavernosal) and further evaluation may be indicated. The patient's fear of injection may produce a heightened sympathetic response and a false-positive result. To obtain a better result, patients are also instructed to perform self-stimulation (or view X-rated material) if a rigid erection does

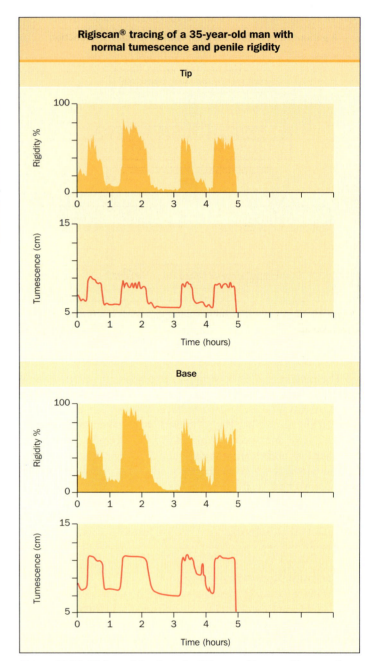

Figure 40.17 Rigiscan® tracing of a 35-year-old man with normal tumescence and penile rigidity. If this man complains of erectile dysfunction, it is most probably psychogenic in origin.

not occur within 15min. This technique is known as the combined intracavernous injection and stimulation (CIS) test.

Duplex ultrasound

Duplex sonography employs high-resolution sonography and pulsed Doppler blood flow analysis to investigate penile vascular function[24]. The color-coded Doppler device provides an additional advantage of easier detection of blood flow and communication vessels among the cavernous, dorsal, and spongiosal arteries, which are crucial in penile vascular and reconstructive surgeries (Figs 40.19 & 40.20). The study is performed before and after intracavernous injection of a vasodilator (10µg of

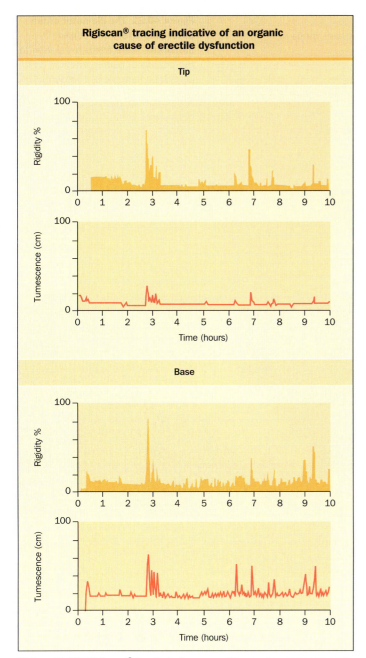

Figure 40.18 Rigiscan® tracing of a man with poor tumescence and penile rigidity indicative of an organic cause of erectile dysfunction.

Rigiscan® tracing indicative of an organic cause of erectile dysfunction

Tip

Base

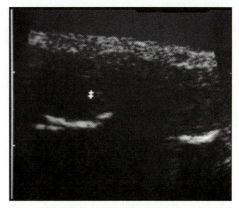

Figure 40.19 Cross-section of the penis. High-resolution ultrasound shows the paired corpora cavernosa and corpus spongiosum. The cursor shows the inner diameter of the cavernous artery in the flaccid state.

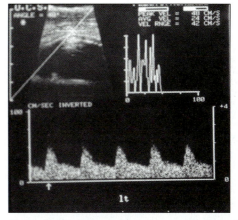

Figure 40.20 Duplex ultrasound examination of the penis after intracavernous injection of 10μg of alprostadil. The trace shows the flow velocity of the systolic and diastolic phases. This is a normal response of the cavernous artery in the first few minutes after intracavernous injection of a vasodilator. However, if the diastolic component persists after 15–20min, or after self-stimulation, the study should be repeated on another day to rule out psychologic inhibition before making a diagnosis of venous leakage.

alprostadil is our drug of choice) so that the functional capacity of the cavernous arteries can be assessed. The normal Doppler response is a peak systolic flow velocity of more than 30cm/s in both cavernous arteries and a strong phasic pulsation of the cavernous arteries. An adequate veno-occlusive mechanism is characterized by a sustained rigid erection and absence of end-diastolic flow after 15–20min.

One should be familiar with the changes of diameter and wave form of the cavernous artery during different phases of erection so that misdiagnosis can be avoided (Fig. 40.21)[25].

Pharmacologic arteriography

Penile arteriography was introduced by the pioneering work of Michal and Pospichal (1978)[26]. Arteriography is most useful in

providing anatomic rather than functional information. Owing to the relatively high cost and invasive nature of the study, only a small percentage of ED patients are appropriate candidates (those who are candidates for arterial revascularization). Perhaps the strongest indication is in the young man with ED secondary to a traumatic arterial disruption or in the rare patient with pelvic steal syndrome. In these selected cases, a detailed roadmap of the arterial anatomy provided by arteriography is essential to surgical reconstruction (Fig. 40.22). The objectives of the arteriography are to localize the site of obstruction and assess the condition of the donor and recipient arteries[25].

Pharmacologic cavernosometry and cavernosography

Pharmacologic cavernosometry involves simultaneous saline infusion and intracavernous pressure monitoring after intracavernous injection of vasodilators such as papaverine + phentolamine, alprostadil or a combination of the three drugs. The saline infusion rate required to maintain erection and the

The diameter of the cavernous artery and duplex ultrasound wave forms in relation to the phases of penile erection

Flaccid	Latent	Tumescent	Full	Rigid	Detumescent

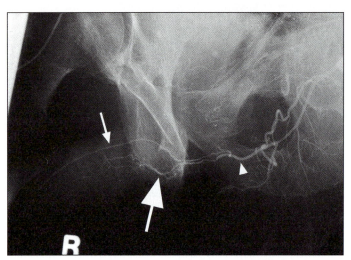

Figure 40.21 The diameter of the cavernous artery and duplex ultrasound wave forms in relation to the phases of penile erection. (With permission from Lue and Broderick[25].)

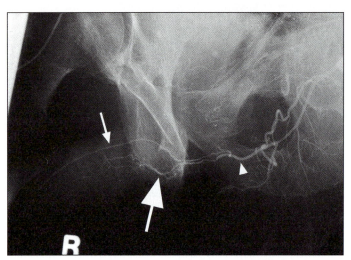

Figure 40.22 Pharmacologic arteriography visualization of the internal pudendal (arrowhead), dorsal (small arrow) and cavernous arteries. Penile arteriography without intracavernous injection of a vasodilator will not obtain optimal visualization of the cavernous artery (large arrow) and can be misleading.

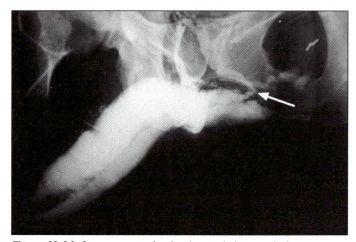

Figure 40.24 Cavernosography. An abnormal pharmacologic cavernosogram shows venous leakage through the cavernous (arrow) and dorsal veins in a man with primary erectile dysfunction. His erectile dysfunction was cured after bilateral cavernous vein and crural ligation.

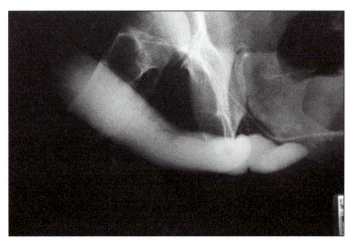

Figure 40.23 Cavernosography. A normal cavernosogram after intracavernous injection of a solution containing papaverine and phentolamine shows opacification of both corpora cavernosa without evidence of venous leakage.

intracorporeal pressure drop 30s after cessation of infusion are the parameters of venous leakage most often used. The normal maintenance rate in patients with complete smooth muscle relaxation is reported to be less than 5mL/min with a pressure decrease from 150mmHg to less than 45mmHg in 30s.

Cavernosography during visual sexual stimulation was first used to detect venous leakage by Wagner[27]. Cavernosography involves the infusion of diluted contrast solution into the corpora cavernosa during a pharmacologically induced erection to visualize the site of venous leakage (Figs 40.23 & 40.24). These two tests should always be performed after activation of the veno-occlusive mechanism by intracavernous injection of vasodilators. In the majority of patients, more than one venous leakage sites can be visualized by cavernosography[28]. It is to be noted that, because these studies are done in a nonsexual setting with little privacy, patient anxiety may lead to a false-positive result. When in doubt, repeated injections of vasodilators should be given to achieve complete smooth muscle relaxation[29].

Treatment options for erectile dysfunction: costs, advantages and disadvantages			
Treatment	Cost ($)	Advantages	Disadvantages/ side effects
Psychosexual therapy	75–200/ session	Noninvasive, resolves conflict	Moderately successful; high recurrence rate
Sildenafil	10/dose	Noninvasive	Systemic side effects
Vacuum constriction device	150–550/ device	Low cost; noninvasive	Unnatural erection/ petechiae, pain
Transurethral therapy	25/dose	Minimally invasive	Low success rate/penile pain
Intracavernous injection	5–25/dose	Natural erection; highly successful	More invasive/ priapism, fibrosis, pain
Prosthesis	6,000–15,000	Highly successful	Requires surgery, anesthesia/ infection, fibrosis
Vascular surgery	8,000–15,000	Restores natural erection	Moderate success rate/requires surgery, anesthesia

Figure 40.25 Treatment options for erectile dysfunction: costs, advantages and disadvantages. (With permission from Lue and Broderick[25].)

Advanced hormonal, neurologic, and psychosexual evaluation

We refer patients with suspected pituitary, thyroid, or adrenal diseases to an endocrinologist for further evaluation and treatment. When a spinal or central nervous system lesion is suspected, consultation with a neurologist should be requested. If a patient is likely to be suffering from deep-seated psychological, relationship, or psychiatric problems, involvement of a mental health professional is highly recommended.

TREATMENT OF ED

A summary of costs, advantages and side effects of the various treatment options for ED is shown in Figure 40.25.

Oral medications

Phosphodiesterase inhibitor

Sildenafil (Viagra®) is a selective inhibitor of the cGMP-specific, cGMP-binding phosphodiesterase type 5 (PDE-5). Since its release in 1998, it has become the drug of choice for most men with ED. When sexual stimulation releases NO into the penile smooth muscle, inhibition of PDE-5 by sildenafil causes a higher cGMP level in the glans penis, corpus cavernosum, and corpus spongiosum, resulting in enhanced smooth muscle relaxation, better rigidity, and a more sustained erection. It is to be noted that sildenafil has little effect on the penis in the absence of sexual stimulation, when NO and cGMP are at low basal levels (Fig. 40.8).

In clinical studies, sildenafil has been evaluated at doses of 25mg, 50mg, and 100mg in 21 randomized, double-blind, placebo-controlled trials of up to 6 months in over 3,000 patients with mixed etiologies (organic 58%, psychogenic 17%, mixed 24%). The percentage of patients reporting improved erection is as follows: placebo 24%, 25mg 63%, 50mg 74%, and 100mg 82%. When the patients' and partners' diaries were analyzed, weekly

Recommendations for sildenafil and the cardiac patient
1. Sildenafil is absolutely contraindicated in patients taking long-acting or short-acting nitrate drugs.
2. If the patient has stable coronary disease and does not need nitrates on a consistent basis, the risks of sildenafil should be carefully discussed with him.
3. Patients must be warned of the danger of taking sildenafil in the 24-hour period before or after taking a nitrate preparation.
4. Pre-sildenafil treadmill test may be indicated in some cardiac patients to assess the risk of cardiac ischemia during sexual intercourse.
5. Initial monitoring of hypotensive effect after taking sildenafil may be indicated in: (a) patients with congestive heart failure who have borderline low blood pressure and low volume status; (b) patients following a complicated, multidrug, antihypertensive therapy regimen.

Figure 40.26 Recommendations for sildenafil and the cardiac patient. (Data from Cheitlin et al.[32])

successful intercourse rates averaged 1.3 on 50–100mg of sildenafil versus 0.4 on placebo. The main effect of sildenafil is the improvement in rigidity and duration of erection; it has little effect on sexual drive.

The major adverse reactions are headache (16%), flushing (10%), dyspepsia (7%), and abnormal vision (3%)[30]. Abnormal vision includes mild and transient blue color tinge and increased sensitivity to light or blurred vision. This is due to the effect of sildenafil on PDE-6, an enzyme found in the retina. (Sildenafil is about 10 times as potent for PDE-5 as for PDE-6.)

Adverse cardiovascular events were mild and transient in the majority of cases. The rates of serious cardiovascular events were 4.1 and 5.7 and of myocardial infarction 1.7 and 1.4 events (per 100 man-years of treatment) for the sildenafil and placebo groups respectively[31]. However, because studies excluded patients using nitrates and those with significant concomitant medical conditions, the incidence of serious cardiovascular events could be expected to be higher in the general population. From late March to mid-November 1998, more than 6 million outpatient prescriptions were dispensed (about 50 million tablets) to more than 3 million patients. During the same period, 130 deaths in the USA were reported to the Food and Drug Administration (FDA). In response to the concern of physicians, the American Heart Association has published a guideline for sildenafil therapy (Fig. 40.26)[32]. In addition, patients should be warned to contact their physician if an erection lasts for more than 4 hours, as more than 25 cases of prolonged erection or priapism have occurred.

Sildenafil is eliminated predominantly by the liver. The terminal half-life is about 4 hours. Taken in the fasted state, the maximal plasma concentrations are reached within 30–120min (mean 60min). The recommended dose is 50mg taken 1 hour before sexual activity. On the basis of effectiveness and toleration, the dose may be increased to 100mg or decreased to 25mg. The maximal recommended frequency is once per day. Some researchers speculated that sildenafil might improve sexual function in women; however, a pilot study of a small number of postmenopausal women did not show much improvement in overall sexual satisfaction[33]. Thus, its use in women should not be encouraged until placebo-controlled, double-blind trials prove its effectiveness and identify its indications.

Adrenoceptor antagonists

Yohimbine is an α_2-adrenergic receptor antagonist produced from the bark of the yohim tree. It acts at the adrenergic receptors in the hypothalamic centers associated with libido and penile erection. In a recent meta-analysis of seven randomized, placebo-controlled studies of yohimbine therapy[34], it was reported to be superior to placebo. In several other controlled randomized studies of patients with organic ED, no significant difference from placebo was found[35]. The most frequently reported side effects include palpitation, fine tremor, elevation of blood pressure, and anxiety. As its effect is marginal, yohimbine is not recommended in patients with organic ED.

Oral *phentolamine* (Vasomax®) has been reported to improve erectile function[36,37]: in a clinical trail in patients with mild to moderate ED, the response rates (improved erections) were 37% to 40mg, 45% to 80mg, and 16% to placebo. Side effects include headache, facial flushing, and nasal congestion. Oral phentolamine has not been approved by the FDA.

Dopaminergic agonist

Apomorphine acts on central dopaminergic (D_1/D_2) receptors. When injected subcutaneously, it induced erections in rats and humans[38], but the side effects, notably nausea, seriously limited its clinical usefulness. A sublingual formulation (Uprima®) is now in clinical trials. In one study, in patients with psychogenic or mild organic ED taking a 4mg dose, 52% attained erection compared with 35% in the placebo group. Further, sexual intercourse was achieved in 43% of the treated group compared with 27% of the placebo group. However, nausea was reported in 17% of patients, with 4% requiring antiemetics[38]. Sublingual apomorphine has not received FDA approval.

Serotonergic drugs

Trazodone is a serotonin antagonist and reuptake inhibitor used as a sedative and antidepressant, with a rare incidence of priapism. Its effect on erection is thought to be the result of serotonergic and α-adrenolytic activity. Although trazodone alone or in combination with yohimbine has been reported to improve erectile function in some men[39–41], its beneficial effects could not be substantiated in a double-blind, placebo-controlled, multicenter trial with a dosage of 150mg/day[41]. Therefore, its use in patients with ED is not recommended.

Hormonal therapy

Although endocrinopathy can certainly contribute to ED, its role may result from its effects on central mechanisms (libido) rather than on the penile tissue itself. In a young hypogonadal man, testosterone replacement is clearly the treatment of choice. However, the risks may outweigh the benefits in older patients, in whom testosterone may speed up the growth of an enlarged prostate or occult prostate cancer. The effectiveness of hormonal replacement in ED has been rather disappointing. Morales and associates[42] reported only a 9% response rate for patients treated with oral androgen replacement. The majority of older patients are more likely to suffer from concomitant neurovascular insufficiency than from androgen deficiency alone. If the aim of androgen replacement therapy is to restore erectile function, testosterone is a relatively poor choice when compared with others. A list of androgen preparations is shown in Figure 40.27. Because of their potential hepatotoxicity, oral preparations are the least desirable.

Vacuum constriction device

The vacuum constriction device (Fig. 40.28) has become popular in the last decade as an effective and safe treatment for ED. It consists of a plastic cylinder connected directly or by tubing to a vacuum-generating source (manual or battery-operated pump). After the penis is engorged by the negative pressure, a constricting ring is applied to the base to maintain the erection. To avoid injury, the ring should not be left in place for longer than 30min. The treatment is effective in over 70% of patients with erectile dysfunction.

The erection produced by a vacuum device is different from a physiologic erection or one produced by intracavernous injection. The blood oxygen level in the corpus cavernosum is less and the portion of the penis proximal to the ring is not rigid,

Androgen preparations for patient with hypogonadism			
Preparation	Dose (mg)	Route	Schedule
17-alkylated androgens			
Methyltestosterone (Android®, Metandren®, Oreton®)	25–50	Sublingual	Daily
Fluoxymesterone (Halotestin®)	5–10	Oral	Daily
Methandrostenolone	5–10	Oral	Daily
Transdermal			
Testoderm®	4–6	Scrotal skin	Daily
Androderm®	5	Skin	Daily
Esterified testosterone			
Propionate	50	IM	3×/week
Cypionate (depo-testosterone)	200	IM	Every 2–3 weeks
Enanthate (Delatestryl®)	200	IM	Every 2–3 weeks

Figure. 40.27 Androgen preparations for patients with hypogonadism. (With permission from Lue and Broderick[25].)

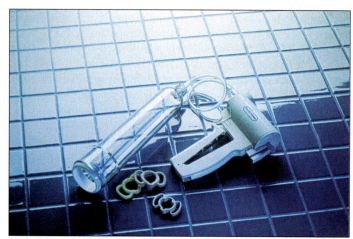

Figure 40.28 A vacuum constriction device. This consists of a negative pressure pump, a plastic cylinder, and a rubber or Silastic® constriction ring. (Courtesy of Timm Medical Inc.)

which may produce a pivoting effect. The device is more acceptable to older men in a steady relationship than to young single men in search of a partner. It is safe when used properly and is one of the least costly treatment options available. Although it can be used by any patient with erectile dysfunction, we still recommend that a reasonable workup be conducted so that some easily correctable cause of the dysfunction is not overlooked. Side effects include: numbness of the penis, hinged erection, trapped ejaculation, pain and pulling of scrotal tissue into the cylinder. The device also can be used to prevent penile shortening after explantation of a penile prosthesis.

Transurethral therapy

Transurethral administration of alprostadil (prostaglandin E1) (Fig. 40.29) was approved by the FDA in the USA in 1996. In a double-blind, placebo-controlled study of 1,511 men with organic ED[43], 996 men (65.9%) had erections sufficient for intercourse when tested in the clinic. Of these men, when they tried the drug at home 64.9% had intercourse successfully at least once. To improve efficacy, a constricting device (Actis®) placed at the base of the penis is recommended and the combination gives a success rate of about 50–60%. The most common side effects are penile pain and urethral bleeding.

Intracavernous injection therapy

In 1982, Virag[44] reported the incidental finding of erection induced by intracavernous injection of papaverine. Subsequently, Zorgniotti and Lefleur[45] reported their experience of instructing patients in the technique of autoinjection of a mixture of papaverine and phentolamine for home use. In the last decade, intracavernous injection therapy has gradually gained worldwide acceptance. A list of drugs that have been used clinically is presented in Figure 40.30, and the drugs used to prevent or treat priapism are shown in Figure 40.31. The most often reported side effects are penile fibrosis, ecchymosis, and occasional priapism. A high dropout rate of up to 70% has also been reported by several investigators. In clinical practice,

we usually begin with a test dose of 5–10μg of alprostadil in the office. This initial testing helps determine the dose required for home injection therapy. The patient or the partner is instructed in the injection technique and drug dosage during the next visit before home injection is started. Regular followup visits every 3–6 months for dose adjustment or medication change as well as examination for penile fibrosis are recommended as long as the patient is on the therapy. Although intracavernous injection therapy has lost its predominance it remains one of the most effective and reliable second line therapies for ED.

Vascular surgery

Because of the multiple risk factors, the overlapping causes of ED, and the diffuse nature of the arterial lesions, the majority of older patients with arteriogenic ED are not candidates for arterial revascularization.

However, a small subset of patients with arteriogenic ED can benefit from penile arterial revascularization. This group consists mostly of young patients with discrete arterial lesions secondary to traumatic pelvic or perineal injuries. In these patients, duplex sonography and cavernosometry and cavernosography should be performed to assess both arterial and veno-occlusive function. In addition, a pharmacologic pudendal arteriogram to locate the site of occlusion and the condition of the donor vessel (most commonly the inferior epigastric artery) and the recipient vessel (the dorsal artery) should also be performed. The most successful surgical approach is the epigastric to dorsal artery bypass (Fig. 40.32) or epigastric artery to dorsal vein anastomosis.

Common intracavernous agents			
Drug	Dose range	Advantages	Disadvantages/side effects
Papaverine	7.5–60mg	Low cost; stable at room temperature	Fibrosis, priapism Elevation of liver enzymes
Papaverine + phentolamine	0.1–1mL	More potent than papaverine alone	Fibrosis, priapism
Alprostadil	1–60μg	Metabolized in penis; priapism rare	Painful erection Requires refrigeration Relatively expensive
Moxisylyte	10–30mg	Priapism rare	Less potent
Papaverine + phentolamine + alprostadil	0.1–1mL	Most potent	Requires refrigeration

Figure 40.30 Common intracavernous agents. (With permission from Lue and Broderick[25].)

α-adrenergic agents for the treatment of priapism	
Drug	Usual dose
Epinephrine (adrenaline)	10–20μg
Phenylephrine	250–500μg

Figure 40.31 α-adrenergic agents for the treatment of priapism. Intracavernous injection every 5min until detumescence after aspiration of 10–20mL of blood. (With permission from Lue and Broderick[25].)

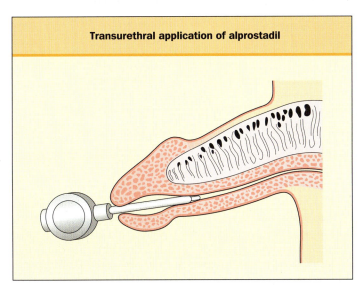

Transurethral application of alprostadil

Figure 40.29 Transurethral application of alprostadil through an applicator. (Courtesy of Vivus Inc.)

Epigastric artery to dorsal artery bypass

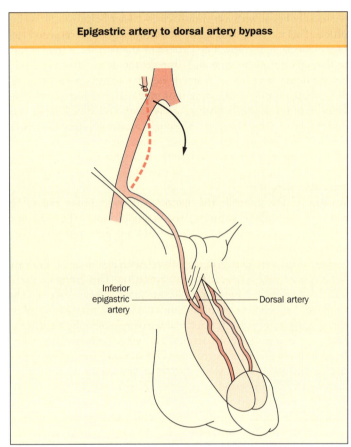

Inferior
epigastric
artery
— Dorsal artery

Figure 40.32 An epigastric artery to dorsal artery bypass in a young patient with obstruction of the internal pudendal artery from pelvic trauma.

Penile venous surgery

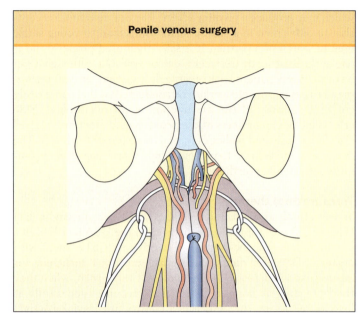

Figure 40.33 Penile venous surgery showing resection of the deep dorsal vein and ligation of both crura in a patient with primary erectile dysfunction.

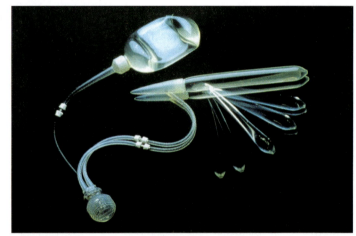

Figure 40.34 A three-piece inflatable penile prosthesis. (Courtesy of Mentor Corporation.)

Despite the promising early results of penile venous surgery, longer-term results have been disappointing. Although several authors have reported short-term success rates of up to 70% in selected patients, longer-term followups show a significant decline. Development of venous collaterals and persistent venous leakage appear to be contributing factors in many patients who fail to improve following venous surgery. However, in patients under 40 years old, with congenital or traumatic venous leakage, we have noted a success rate after venous surgery of more than 75%. The most common pathology in patients with primary ED is maldeveloped crura with crural and cavernous venous leakage. The surgical approach consists of resection of deep dorsal vein and ligation of the crura, as shown in Figure 40.33.

Prosthetic surgery
Penile prostheses are divided into three general types: malleable (semirigid), mechanical and inflatable. The malleable devices are made of silicone rubber and several models contain a central intertwined metallic core. The mechanical device is also made of silicone rubber but contains polytetrafluorethylene-coated interlocking polysulfone rings in a rod column, which provides rigidity when the rings are lined up in a straight line and flaccidity when the penis is bent. Inflatable (hydraulic) prostheses are further divided into one-piece, two-piece, and three-piece devices. The one-piece device consists of a pair of hydraulic cylinders implanted within the corpora cavernosa. A pump at the distal end cycles fluid from a rear tip reservoir into a central chamber to produce penile rigidity. Two-piece inflatable prostheses consist of a pair of cylinders attached to a scrotal pump or pump-reservoir. Three piece inflatable penile prostheses consist of paired penile cylinders, a scrotal pump, and a suprapubic fluid reservoir, as shown in Figure 40.34.

In general, the malleable devices last longer than the inflatable ones. Patients should be informed that a 5–15% failure rate is expected in the first 5 years and the majority of devices will fail in 10–15 years and need to be replaced. Potential complications include mechanical failures, cylinder leaks, tubing leaks, infection, perforation, persistent pain, and self-inflation. The past decade has seen a marked improvement in the reliability and durability of the prostheses. In addition, the introduction of a salvage procedure to reimplant the prosthesis after thorough irrigation with several antiseptics and antibiotics in cases of infection and erosion has also improved the outcome tremendously.

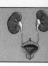
PERSPECTIVES

The past two decades have witnessed a phenomenal advance in the understanding of penile physiology and several revolutionary new treatments for patients with erectile dysfunction. With the progress of molecular biology technique and its introduction into the field, instead of symptomatic treatment, we may see cure of various types of erectile dysfunction in the near future.

REFERENCES

1. Breza J, Aboseif SR, Orvis BR, Lue TF, Tanagho EA. Detailed anatomy of penile neurovascular structures: surgical significance. J Urol. 1989;141:437.

2. Aboseif S, Shinohara K, Breza J, Benard F, Narayna P. Role of penile vascular injury in erectile dysfunction after radical prostatectomy. Br J Urol. 1994;73:75.

3. Kim ED, Blackburn D, McVary KT. Post-radical prostatectomy penile blood flow: assessment with color flow Doppler ultrasound. J Urol. 1994;152:2276.

4. Lue TF. Physiology of penile erection and pathophysiology of impotence and priapism. In: Walsh PC, Retik AB, Vaughan ED Jr, Wein A, eds. Campbell's urology, 7th edn. Philadelphia: WB Saunders; 1997:1157.

5. DeGroat WC, Booth AM. Neural control of penile erection. In: Maggi CA, ed. The autonomic nervous system. Nervous control of the urogenital system. London: Harwood; 1993: ch 13:465.

6. Walsh PC, Brendler CB, Chang T, et al. Preservation of sexual function in men during radical pelvic surgery. M Med J. 1990;39:389.

7. Lue TF, Takamura T, Schmidt RA, Palubinskas AJ, Tanagho EA. Hemodynamics of erection in the monkey. J Urol. 1983;130:1237.

8. Gruetter CA, Barry BK, McNamara DB, Gruetter DY, Kadowitz PJ, Ignarro LJ. Relaxation of bovine coronary artery and activation of coronary arterial guanylate cyclase by nitric oxide, nitroprusside and a carcinogenic nitrosoamine. J Cyclic Nucleotide Res. 1979;5:211.

9. Palmer RMJ, Ashton DS, Moncada S. Vascular endothelial cells synthesize nitric oxide from L-arginine. Nature. 1988;333:664.

10. Ignarro LJ, Bush PA, Buga GM, Wood KS, Fukuto JM, Rajfer J. Nitric oxide and cyclic GMP formation upon electrical field stimulation cause relaxation of corpus cavernosum smooth muscle. Biochem Biophys Res Comm. 1990;170:843.

11. Kim N, Azadzoi KM, Goldstein I, Saenz de Tejada I. A nitric oxide-like factor mediates nonadrenergic-noncholinergic neurogenic relaxation of penile corpus cavernosum smooth muscle. J Clin Invest. 1991;88:112.

12. Kim YC, Kim JH, Davies MG, Hagen PO, Carson CC. Modulation of vasoactive intestinal polypeptide (VIP)-mediated relaxation by nitric oxide and prostanoids in the rabbit corpus cavernosum. J Urol. 1995;153:807.

13. Stief CG, Benard F, Bosch RJ, Aboseif SR, Lue TF, Tanagho EA. A possible role of calcitonin-gene-related peptide in the regulation of the smooth muscle tone of the bladder and penis. J Urol. 1990;143:392.

14. Kirkeby HJ, Fahrenkrug J, Holmquist F, Ottesen B. Vasoactive intestinal polypeptide (VIP) and peptide histidine methionine (PHM) in human penile corpus cavernosum tissue and circumflex veins: localization and in vitro effects. Eur J Clin Invest. 1992;22:24.

15. Hedlund P, Alm P, Hedlund H, Larsson B, Andersson KE. Localization and effects of pituitary adenylate cyclase-activating polypeptide (PACAP) in human penile erectile tissue. Acta Physiol Scand. 1994;150:103.

16. Adaikan PG, Ratnam SS. Pharmacology of penile erection in humans. Cardiovasc Intervent Radiol. 1988;11:191.

17. Carrier S, Brock G, Kour NW, Lue TF. Pathophysiology of erectile dysfunction. Urology. 1993;42:468.

18. Wespes E, Goes PM, Schiffmann S, Depierreux M, Vanderhaeghen JJ, Schulman CC. Computerized analysis of smooth muscle fibers in potent and impotent patients. J Urol. 1991;146:1015.

19. Wespes E, Moreira de Goes P, Schulman CC: Age-related changes in the quantification of the intracavernous smooth muscles in potent men. J Urol. 1998;159:99.

20. Lue TF. Impotence: a patient's goal-directed approach to treatment. World J Urol. 1990;8:67.

21. El-Sakka AI, Lue TF. A rational approach to investigation of the sexually dysfunctional man. In: Morales, A, ed. Erectile dysfunction: issues in current pharmacotherapy. London: Martin Dunitz; 1998:49.

22. Morales A, Condra M, Heaton JP, Johnston B, Fenemore J. Diurnal penile tumescence recording in the etiological diagnosis of erectile dysfunction. J Urol. 1994;152:1111.

23. Kessler WO. Nocturnal penile tumescence. Urol Clin North Am. 1988;15:81.

24. Lue TF, Hricak H, Marich KW, Tanagho EA. Vasculogenic impotence evaluated by high-resolution ultrasonography and pulsed Doppler spectrum analysis. Radiology. 1985;155:777.

25. Lue TF, Broderick G. Evaluation and nonsurgical management of erectile dysfunction and priapism. In: Walsh PC, Retik AB, Vaughan ED Jr, Wein A, eds. Campbell's urology, 7th edn. Philadelphia: WB Saunders; 1997:1181–214.

26. Michal V, Pospichal, J. Phalloarteriography in the diagnosis of erectile impotence. World J Surgery. 1978;2:239.

27. Wagner G. Methods of differential diagnosis of psychogenic and organic erectile failure. In: Wagner G, Green R, eds. Impotence. New York: Plenum Press; 1981:89.

28. Shabsigh R, Fishman IJ, Toombs RD, Skolkin M. Venous leaks: anatomical and physiological observations. J Urol. 1991;146:1260.

29. Hatzichristou DG, Saenz de Tejada I, Kupferman S, et al. In vivo assessment of trabecular smooth muscle tone, its application in pharmaco-cavernosometry and analysis of intracavernous pressure determinants. J Urol. 1995; 153:1126.

30. Goldstein I, Lue TF, Padma-Nathan H, Rosen RC, Steers WD, Wicker PA. Oral sildenafil in the treatment of erectile dysfunction. Sildenafil Study Group. N Engl J Med. 1998;338:1397.

31. Morales A, Gingell C, Collins M, Wicker PA, Osterloh IH. Clinical safety of oral sildenafil citrate (VIAGRA) in the treatment of erectile dysfunction. Int J Impotence Res. 1998;10:69–73.

32. Cheitlin MD, Hutter AM Jr, Brindis RG, et al. Use of sildenafil (Viagra) in patients with cardiovascular disease. Technology and Practice Executive Committee. Circulation. 1999;99:168–77.

33. Kaplan SA, Reis RB, Kohn IJ, et al. Safety and efficacy of sildenafil in postmenopausal women with sexual dysfunction. Urology. 1999;53:481–6.

34. Ernst E, Pittler MH. Yohimbine for erectile dysfunction: a systematic review and meta-analysis of randomized clinical trials. J Urol. 1998;159:433–6.

35. Morales A, Surridge DH, Marshall PG, Fenemore J. Nonhormonal pharmacological treatment of organic impotence. J Urol. 1982;128:45–7.

36. Gwinup G. Oral phentolamine in nonspecific erectile insufficiency. Ann Intern Med. 1988;109:162–3.

37. Zorgniotti AW. Experience with buccal phentolamine mesylate for impotence. Int J Impotence Res. 1994;6:37–41.

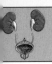
38. Heaton JP, Morales A, Adams MA, Johnston B, el-Rashidy R. Recovery of erectile function by the oral administration of apomorphine. Urology. 1995;45:200–6.

39. Lance R, Albo M, Costabile RA, Steers WD. Oral trazodone as empirical therapy for erectile dysfunction: a retrospective review. Urology. 1995;46:117–20.

40. Montorsi F, Strambi LF, Guazzoni G, et al. Effect of yohimbine-trazodone on psychogenic impotence: a randomized, double-blind, placebo-controlled study. Urology. 1994;44:732–6.

41. Meinhardt W, Schmitz PI, Kropman RF, de la Fuente RB, Lycklama à Nijeholt AA, Zwartendijk J. Trazodone, a double blind trial for treatment of erectile dysfunction. Int J Impotence Res. 1997;9:163–5.

42. Morales A, Johnston B, Heaton JW, Clark A. Oral androgens in the treatment of hypogonadal impotent men. J Urol. 1994;152:1115.

43. Padma-Nathan H, Hellstrom WJG, Kaiser FE, et al. Treatment of men with erectile dysfunction with transurethral alprostadil. N Engl J Med. 1997;336:1.

44. Virag R: Intracavernous injection of papaverine for erectile failure (letter). Lancet. 1982;2:938.

45. Zorgniotti AW, Lefleur RS. Auto-injection of the corpus cavernosum with a vasoactive drug combination for vasculogenic impotence. J Urol. 1985;133:39.

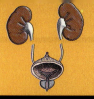

Chapter
41

Benign and Malignant Disorders of the Penis

John P Pryor and David J Ralph

KEY POINTS

- Most congenital disorders of the penis present in childhood.
- Careful technique for circumcision is essential to avoid complications, some of which can be devastating.
- Surgery for Peyronie's disease should be delayed until the disease has stabilized – usually about 1 year.
- Priapism can be low-flow, high-flow or recurrent (stuttering); treatment should be tailored to the underlying pathophysiology..
- The prognosis of cancer of the penis is directly related to stage at diagnosis.

CONGENITAL DISORDERS IN ADULT LIFE

Most congenital disorders of the penis present during childhood and this is particularly so when they are visible or interfere with urinary tract function. Some abnormalities do not present until the boy becomes sexually active; these are shown in Figures 41.1–41.3. It should be noted that minor abnormalities may have a profound effect on the psychologic makeup of the sexually inexperienced man. For this reason it is often necessary to correct minor congenital erectile deformities, 15–30°, whereas the average deformity of men undergoing the Nesbit procedure for Peyronie's disease was 70°[3].

CIRCUMCISION

Routine circumcision of all infants is unnecessary. The prepuce may be adherent to the glans at birth but it separates over the next 5 years. Neonatal circumcision may reduce the incidence of a urinary tract infection during the first year of life but 195 circumcisions would need to be performed to prevent one hospital admission for urinary tract infection in the first year of life[4].

Circumcision should be performed for a tight phimosis with ballooning of the foreskin on micturition or in adult life when it is causing difficulties. Diabetes should always be excluded in an acquired phimosis and the possibility of a hidden penile carcinoma should be suspected if there is phimosis and bleeding.

Circumcision may be performed for religious reasons and it is desirable that the operation should be performed skillfully to avoid the complications listed in Figure 41.4.

There are many techniques for circumcision and plastic devices are useful for neonates. The preferred surgical technique is to use double circumferential incisions and dissection. Careful hemostasis is essential and care should be taken to align the median raphe with the frenulum.

Congenital penile disorders in adult life		
Condition	**Problem**	**Solution**
Hypospadias	Residual chordee	Nesbit or complete reconstruction
Epispadias	Curvature/shortness	Reconstruction ± counseling
Tight frenulum (Fig. 41.2)	Pain/bleeding	Transverse incision and suture longitudinally
Phimosis	Pain on erection	Dorsal slit, preputial plasty[1], circumcision
Paraphimosis	Pain and swelling after erection	Reduce (Fig. 41.3) Elective circumcision
Penoscrotal web	Cosmesis/pain	Divide and suture longitudinally
Congenital short urethra	Ventral erectile deformity	Nesbit procedure (see above)
Chordee without hypospadias	Ventral erectile curvature with chordee	Nesbit procedure
Corporal disproportion	Erectile deformities, palpation normal	Nesbit procedure
Deficient suspensory ligament	Unstable penis	Fixation to symphysis pubis[2]
Micropenis	Sexual difficulty/anxiety	See text

Fig. 41.1 Congenital penile disorders in adult life.

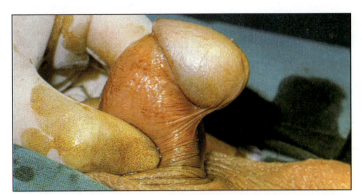

Fig. 41.2 Tight frenulum. It should be noted that a tight frenulum does not cause an erectile deformity. In some men it is necessary to divide the frenulum as a first procedure in order to convince them of this.

THE SMALL PENIS

The penis increases in length at puberty and the stretched penile length of the flaccid adult penis is about 12.5 ± 1.5cm. The penis is classified as small when it is less than 2 standard deviations from the normal length – i.e. less than 9.5cm. There are many causes for a small penis (Fig. 41.5) and it is necessary to investigate the patient further looking for etiologic factors[5]. A small penis associated with hypospadias is called *microphallus*, in contrast to a *micropenis* where there are no associated abnormalities. The sexual function of men with a small penis is surprisingly good[6,7]; however, vaginal penetration would seem to be impossible when the stretched penile length is less than 7cm. In these circumstances a penile lengthening procedure[8], whereby the suspensory ligament is divided and the corpora cavernosa are mobilized off the symphysis may give an apparent increase in length of 2–3cm (Fig. 41.6) with a dramatic impact on the patient's sexual performance and wellbeing.

An increasing number of men with a normal-sized penis are presenting for surgical lengthening procedures. These men do not have a problem with sexual function but may be severely handicapped by their perception of the problem. The psychologic effect ranges from shyness in the locker room to such a fear of needing to expose the penis in the public urinal that they will avoid all travel and new circumstances. These men are rarely helped by psychologic or surgical means. Surgical procedures do not increase the length of the erectile tissue and, although there may be apparent lengthening of the flaccid penis, the man's dissatisfaction often persists.

Penile lengthening is often combined with the introduction of fat or a dermal graft and is known as an enhancement phalloplasty[9]. The long-term results remain to be validated and the tendency is to combine the lengthening procedure with the use of weights to stretch the penis. It may be that the latter will have persistent value and replace surgery.

INFECTIONS AND BENIGN SKIN DISORDERS

These are summarized in Figure 41.7 and an accurate diagnosis should always be made. If there is any doubt the man should be referred to a genitourinary physician.

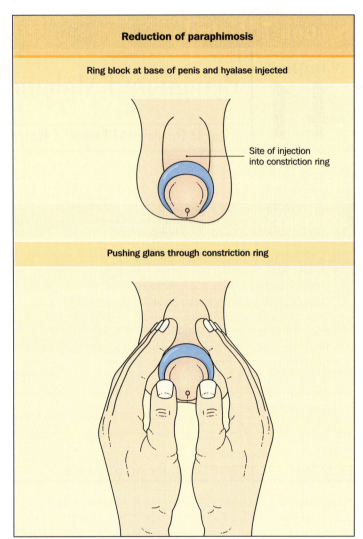

Fig. 41.3 Reduction of paraphimosis. (Top) Swollen edematous foreskin with a tight constriction ring more proximal. Ring block at base of penis and hyalase injected into this area. Some of the edema fluid may be squeezed out of the foreskin before reduction is attempted. (Bottom) Reduction is performed by holding the penis with the index and third fingers of both hands and gently pushing the glans penis, with the thumbs, through the constriction ring. Should reduction not be possible then in early instances circumcision may be performed but, if there has been a late presentation, it is wiser to divide the constricting band, reduce the paraphimosis, and perform the circumcision 2 weeks later.

Complications of circumcision
Bleeding
Bruising
Minor sepsis
Meatal stenosis
Buried penis
Death from hemorrhage
Amputation of glans
Loss of penis from infection/thrombosis
Urethral fistula

Fig. 41.4 Complications of circumcision.

Causes of a small penis	
Category	**Example**
Chromosome disorders	e.g. Klinefelter's syndrome
Intersex	Impaired Leydig cell function
	Androgen insensitivity
	Incomplete differentiation of testes
Hormone disorders	Hypogonadotrophic hypogonadism
	Hypergonadotrophic hypogonadism
Idiopathic	
Acquired cavernous fibrosis	Hypospadias cripple
	Postradiotherapy in childhood

Fig. 41.5 Causes of a small penis.

LYMPHEDEMA OF THE PENIS

The enlarged penis with lymphedema (elephantiasis) is easily recognized. In many instances the disease is localized to the penis whereas in other patients the scrotum and/or lower limbs may be involved. The first objective is to diagnose and treat the underlying cause of the problem (Fig. 41.8) and this requires full blood counts and urine analysis, and may involve lymphography, computed tomography and/or magnetic resonance imaging of the pelvis, and biopsy for culture and histology.

Penile lymphedema often requires little treatment although recurrent bouts of streptococcal infection are common. These require urgent antibiotic treatment with penicillin-like antibiotics and in some instances this needs to be for a relatively long period of time. Surgical treatment is only required when the size of the swelling is such as to interfere with function. Local excision of an affected area may be possible and the wounds heal

surprisingly well, although prophylactic antibiotics should always be given. More extensive disease may require skin grafting to cover the defect[11].

PEYRONIE'S DISEASE

This is a benign disorder of the penis that predominantly affects middle-aged men. They usually complain of pain and deformity on erection and some may have noticed a lump in the flaccid penis. The incidence increases from 4.3/100,000 men aged 20–29 years to 66/100,000 men aged 50–59 years[12]. The age range of 408 men presenting with Peyronie's disease[13] is shown in Figure 41.9.

Pathology
The early stages of Peyronie's disease are painful and characterized by the appearance of an inflammatory infiltrate consisting of T cells, macrophages, and plasma cells in the loose connective tissue between the tunica albuginea and the corpus cavernosus. Fibroblast proliferation leads to the deposition of collagen, which may be absorbed or mature into fibrous tissue. Calcification and ossification sometimes occur (Fig. 41.10).

Etiologic factors
The precise etiology remains obscure but recognizable etiologic factors may be found in Figure 41.11. It is likely that the origin is multifactorial and the problem is triggered by minor trauma in a patient with decreased perfusion of the penis and susceptible genetic predisposition.

Metabolic changes following trauma elsewhere in the body may play a role in some patients and the early histologic appearances suggest that an immunologic mechanism may be involved[14], although the mechanism for this is unknown. Similarly, it is possible that metabolic changes following trauma elsewhere in the body may play a role in some patients.

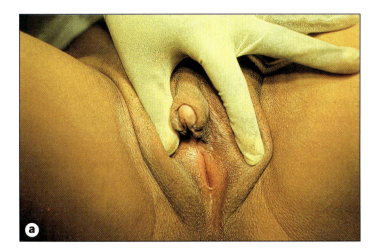
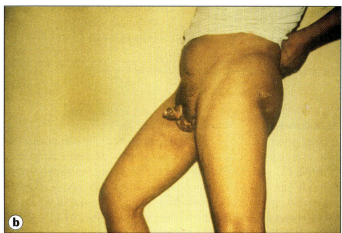

Fig. 41.6 Penile lengthening may improve the quality of life. (a) Small penis associated with perineal hypospadias of a 26-year-old male pseudohermaphrodite schoolteacher who was suicidal. (b) Postoperative photograph 3 months after two-stage penile lengthening, hypospadias repair, and bilateral orchidopexy. He subsequently married and has had no further psychological troubles.

Infections and benign skin disorders

Condition	Treatment
Acute urethritis	Appropriate antibiotics
Balanoposthisis, *Candida* infection	Antibiotics, hygiene, circumcision, antifungal agents
Balanitis simplex	Hygiene, corticosteroids, circumcision
Balanitis plasmacelluris (Zoon's)	Hygiene, corticosteroids, circumcision
Lichen planus (balanitis xerotica obliterans)	Hygiene, corticosteroids, circumcision
Herpes genitalis	Aciclovir
Condylomata acuminata (human papilloma virus)	Podophylline
Syphilis – primary/secondary	Penicillin
Chancroid	Erythromycin
Lymphogranuloma venereum	Doxycycline
Necrotizing fasciitis (Fournier's gangrene)	Antibiotics/debridement*

Fig. 41.7 Infections and benign skin disorders. * The etiology of Fournier's gangrene remains obscure[10] and may be the result of many different organisms. These include anaerobic streptococci but also other anaerobes from the bowel. Urgent treatment is indicated as the superficial tissues rapidly become gangrenous. Large doses of broad-spectrum antibiotics and debridement are necessary. The role of hyperbaric oxygen is uncertain. The previous high mortality rates have been reduced except in debilitated men.

Classification of lymphedema of the penis

Congenital (Milroy's)	
Traumatic	Postpenile surgery
	Constricting devices
	Inguinal node dissection
Chronic infection	Filariasis, tuberculosis, syphilis
Crohn's disease	
Neoplastic	Carcinoma of the prostate
	Pelvic node disease
	Postradiotherapy

Fig. 41.8 Classification of lymphedema of the penis.

Assessment

A good history and clinical examination is usually sufficient. The man is usually able to simulate the degree of penile deformity (Fig. 41.12) with a bent finger but a Polaroid photograph is also helpful. The deformity may be demonstrated by giving an intracavernous injection of alprostadil, which is also a useful adjunct if there is any associated erectile impairment (Fig. 41.13). Color Doppler examination is an invaluable investigation in distinguishing the different causes of erectile failure[15–19]. Cavernosometry and cavernosography (Fig. 41.14) are now rarely performed[20,21], nor is it necessary to assess the plaque by X-ray, ultrasound[22] or magnetic resonance imaging[23].

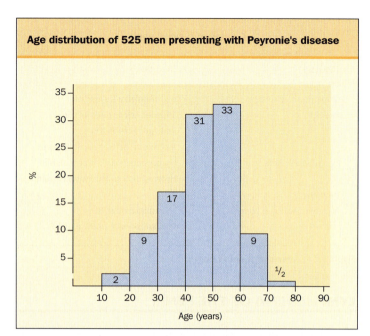

Age distribution of 525 men presenting with Peyronie's disease

Fig. 41.9 Age distribution of 525 men presenting with Peyronie's disease.

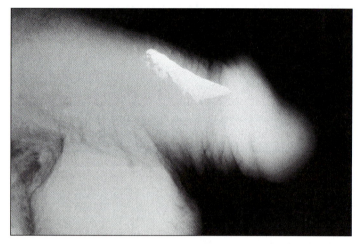

Fig. 41.10 Calcification in a plaque of Peyronie's disease.

Management

Early disease

Peyronie's disease is a benign condition and many men require no treatment once they are reassured that the lump is not a malignant tumor. In men with early Peyronie's disease, characterized by pain on erection, it is worthwhile commencing treatment with twice-daily tamoxifen, 20mg for 6 weeks[24]. This may be continued for 6 months when there is evidence of a response. Attempts to interfere with fibroblast activity with colchicine or verapamil have met with mixed success.

In those men with persistent pain it is worthwhile using vitamin E, 200mg thrice daily, as it is easy to take and well tolerated. Potassium paraaminobenzoate (Potaba) is unpleasant to take and has more side effects, but also has the merit that it should be taken for 12 months. Patients should not be operated upon until

Etiologic factors in 408 men with Peyronie's disease (%)	
Genetic	17
Trauma	22
Infection	4
Atherosclerosis/hypertensive	30
Miscellaneous	6
Idiopathic	33

Fig. 41.11 Etiologic factors in 408 men with Peyronie's disease.

Erectile dysfunction in men with Peyronie's disease	
Problem	Effect/causation
Deformity	Prevents erection
	Causes performance anxiety
Flail penis	Segment of erectile tissue fails to 'erect' normally
Distal flaccidity	Anxiety or impaired hemodynamics
Erectile deficit	Arterial input diminished
	Myogenic
	Veno-occlusive dysfunction

Fig. 41.13 Erectile dysfunction in men with Peyronie's disease.

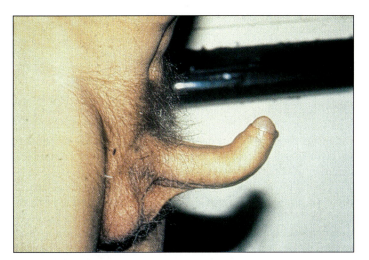

Fig. 41.12 Erectile deformity in Peyronie's disease.

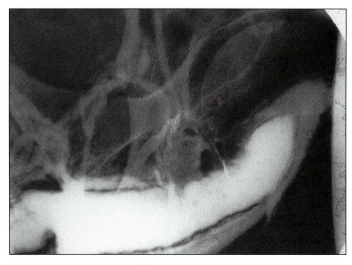

Fig. 41.14 Cavernosogram in Peyronie's disease showing dorsal plaque.

the disease has stabilized and this usually takes 1 year to occur. There have been numerous reports of treatment with steroids but there is little evidence that it is better than the natural history of the condition, which usually leads to an improvement in pain over the course of 3–4 months. The deformity itself may improve either through resolution of the disease or through progression to balance up the effects of the plaque. Progression of the Peyronie's disease is associated with shrinkage in size of the penis.

Stable Peyronie's disease
This is characterized by the absence of pain on erection and the deformity having been constant for 3–6 months. This usually occurs 9–12 months after the onset of the disease and surgery should not be considered before this time. Men who are able to have sexual intercourse without any difficulty do not usually require surgery. The choice of surgery depends upon the quality of the erection and the size of the penis (Fig. 41.15).

Correction of penile deformity
The operation of plaque excision and dermal grafting[25,26] often gives a poor result and is best avoided. In a recent series of 418 men[27] it was found that 20% had a significant postoperative impairment of erection and 17% required further surgery to correct the erectile deformity. In contrast, the Nesbit procedure was found to give good results in 82% of 359 men operated upon between 1977 and 1992[3].

In the Nesbit operation an ellipse of tunica albuginea is removed from the convex side of the bend, and it is 1mm wide for each 10° of deformity. It is important to close the tunica albuginea with a nonabsorbable or poorly absorbed suture such as polyglycolic acid sutures with the knots buried on the inside. Some authors favor a plication technique or a corporoplasty without excision of the ellipse. Such procedures are simpler but the long-term results are less favorable.

Peyronie's disease is associated with penile shortening and this may be increased by the Nesbit procedure. Penile shortening of more than 2cm was found in 17 (4.7%) of 359 men following the Nesbit procedure but intercourse was possible in 15 of these men[3].

During the past 5 years attempts have been made to lengthen the penis by incising the fibrous plaque and covering the defect with a vascular graft that does not contract. Dorsal penile or saphenous vein[28,29] may be used to fill the defect following division of the fibrous plaque. The vein patch operation has given promising results in a group of 112 patients, with 96% reporting the penis to be straight. Shortening was less than 2.5cm in 15% of patients and less than 2.5–5cm in 2% of patients. Only 2 patients felt that the shortened penile length negatively affected their sexual activity. In men who have not been circumcised,

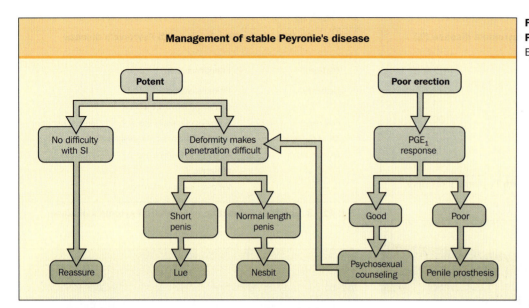

Management of stable Peyronie's disease

Fig. 41.15 **Management of stable Peyronie's disease.** PGE$_1$, prostaglandin E$_1$; SI, sexual intercourse.

a pedicled dermal graft from the foreskin is an alternative procedure[30].

In those men with Peyronie's disease and an erectile deficit it is sensible to implant a penile prosthesis. A malleable prosthesis is sufficient to correct any deformity but with a hydraulic prosthesis it may be necessary to perform a straightening procedure. Penile modeling may be sufficient[31] but otherwise it is necessary to incise the plaque. Patching is not usually necessary.

PRIAPISM

A priapism is a prolonged and painful penile erection that is not accompanied by sexual desire. Our understanding of the pathophysiology of the condition owes much to the concept of high- and low-flow priapism[32], the introduction of intracavernous pharmacotherapy for the treatment of erectile dysfunction[33,34], and the need to reverse prolonged erections that were induced[35]. The management of priapism is an emergency and in the past they were considered to require operation but nowadays the treatment is pharmacologic[36].

Clinical presentation

There are three main types of priapism, which are known as low-flow or anoxic priapism, high-flow or arteriogenic priapism, and recurrent or stuttering priapism. A high-flow or recurrent priapism may convert to an anoxic priapism and the relationship between these three types is not always clearcut[36].

Clinical features

These are summarized in Figure 41.16. The anoxic priapism is usually present on waking but it may follow sexual intercourse or an intracavernous injection for the treatment of erectile dysfunction. The incidence varies with different drugs used but in general terms alprostadil is the favored treatment at the present time and when this drug was used priapism occurred 5 times in 683 men in the clinical trial who received a total of 13,762 injections[37]. Certain drugs (Fig. 41.17) are thought to have an etiologic role in some patients with priapism and other factors are

shown in Figure 41.18. Priapism is not uncommon in patients with sickle-cell disease but also seems to have an increased incidence in men with sickle-cell trait and thalassemia.

A low-flow priapism is characterized by increasing anoxia of the cavernous smooth muscle. The longer the erection persists, the greater the degree of ischemia and after 3–4 hours the erection becomes painful. After 12 hours there is interstitial edema with damage to the sinusoidal endothelium. Smooth muscle necrosis occurs after 24–48 hours and this is often patchy – more severe in the penile shaft than the crura. Untreated, detumescence occurs slowly over 2–4 weeks and the necrotic corporal muscle is replaced by fibrous tissue. The man is then unable to obtain a full erection.

High-flow priapism was first noted after arterial reconstructive surgery for erectile dysfunction but now occurs mainly after perineal trauma. High-flow priapism occurs in young men (in a group of 11 the mean age was 27 with a range of 9–54 years) and the onset of priapism may be delayed for up to 4 days (mean onset was 19 hours in the 11 men). The trauma need not be

Clinical features of priapism		
	Low flow	**High flow**
Onset	During sleep	Following trauma
Pain	Little at first becomes severe	Little to moderate
Penis	Rigid	Turgid
Cavernous blood	Black	Red
P_{O_2}[18]	<30mmHg	>50mmHg
P_{CO_2}[18]	>80mmHg	<50mmHg
pH[18]	<7.25	>7.5
Color Doppler	No flow	Present, fistula
Arteriography	Vessels intact	Arteriovenous malformation

Fig. 41.16 **Clinical features of priapism.**

Drugs that may cause priapism
Anticoagulants
Antihypertensives
Antidepressants
Phenothiazides
Recreational drugs
Intracavernous drugs

Fig. 41.17 Drugs that may cause priapism.

Etiologic factors in 116 men with priapism	
Etiology	No. of patients
Idiopathic	36
Sickle cell disease	29
Other hematologic problems	5
Chronic renal failure/dialysis	4
Oral medications	6
Intracavernous injection	20
Perineal trauma	11
Neoplastic infiltration	2
Miscellaneous	3

Fig. 41.18 Etiologic factors in 116 men with priapism.

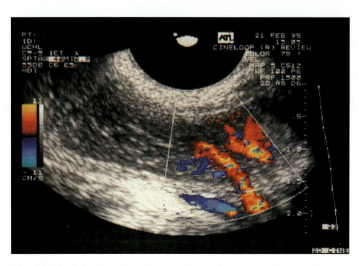

Fig. 41.19 Color Doppler ultrasound examination of the penis in high-flow priapism caused by a fistula.

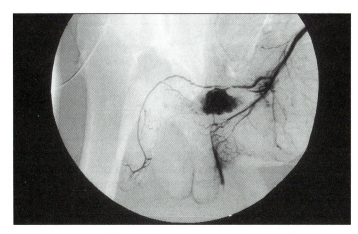

Fig. 41.20 Selective arteriogram of patient with a high-flow priapism caused by a fistula.

severe (fall astride 4, football injury 3, kick 1, skateboard 1, sat on tow bar 1, tourniquet 1). The diagnosis should be made from the clinical presentation and confirmed by color Doppler ultrasound examination (Fig. 41.19) and arteriography (Fig. 41.20). The management is by embolization rather than surgical[38]. The outlook in a high-flow priapism is very good even when the priapism persists for months. The return of normal erectile function is almost inevitable.

Management

The importance of the history and clinical examination must be stressed but it may be useful to arrange for the initial investigations and first aid measures to be instituted immediately – particularly if there is any delay before the man can be seen. Exercise may divert blood to the gluteal muscles and cause detumescence and the same effect may be obtained with ice packs placed around the penis to increase reflex sympathetic nervous activity.

It is convenient to insert a 19 gauge butterfly needle and aspirate 10–20mL of blood. Bright red blood signifies a high-flow priapism (see above) but dark blood indicates a low-flow situation. The penis often immediately becomes less painful and rigid when the priapism is of recent origin and this may be all the treatment that is required. When the cavernous muscle has been anoxic for some time it does not contract and it is necessary to maintain sufficient flaccidity to enable the muscle to recover. This may take 60–90 minutes. The use of α-adrenoagonists is often required[39] but care should be taken to prevent undue hypertension. The blood pressure should be monitored and phenylephrine[40] is preferred to metaraminol or epinephrine. Detumescence usually occurs when the patient feels nauseous and develops a reflex bradycardia.

Failure to control a low-flow priapism of long duration is caused by muscle necrosis and there is now little role for surgical interference – glans shunt, spongiocavernous anastomosis, or long saphenous cavernosus shunts – as these too will fail because the anoxic muscle is unable to contract. When there is a failure to control the priapism it is sensible to biopsy the muscle for medicolegal reasons and possibly insert a penile prosthesis. The recovery of erectile function following a priapism is variable and related to the duration of ischemia (Fig. 41.21).

Recurrent or stuttering priapism

This condition is not uncommon in men with sickle-cell disease but also occurs in Caucasians. The precise mechanism is unknown and some patients have abnormal patterns of nocturnal penile tumescence, which suggests a neurologic origin. It has also occurred following a low-flow anoxic priapism[41]. The management of this condition is difficult and procyclidine (10mg at night and/or 5mg three times daily) may be used, although the

Relationship between the incidence of postpriapism impotence and its duration			
Duration (hours)	No.	Potent (%)	Impotent (%)
<24	32	18 (57)	14 (43)
>24	38	4 (10)	34 (90)

Fig. 41.21 Relationship between the incidence of postpriapism impotence and its duration.

atropine-like side-effects may prove troublesome. Concordin, protriptyline, and clonazepam[42] have been tried, as has phenyl-propanolamine[41]. The recurrent prolonged erections in sickle-cell disease have been controlled by stilboestrol[43] or gonadotrophin releasing hormone analogues[44] but long-term use causes testicular atrophy. Priapism occurring in a patient with sickle-cell disease requires general management with good oxygenation and possible exchange blood transfusion.

PENILE TUMORS

Benign tumors are uncommon and are usually a hemangioma or neurofibroma. Malignant melanoma occurs rarely and the majority of tumors are squamous carcinoma. Premalignant lesions occur and present either as a whitish patch (leukoplakia) or as a reddish area usually without ulceration. The distinction between erythroplasia of Queyrat, Bowen's disease, and Paget's disease is difficult even after histologic examination. These are intraepithelial tumors or carcinoma in situ and may be treated with topical chemotherapy with 5% 5-fluorouracil cream, local excision, or laser surgery. Bowen's disease is sometimes associated with carcinoma of the bladder.

CARCINOMA OF THE PENIS

Etiologic factors

Lack of penile hygiene is the major risk factor for this rare (in Western societies) tumor[45]. The protective effect of circumcision is well known and its effectiveness decreases with increasing age at the time of circumcision.

Infection with human papillomavirus type 16 is a recognized etiologic factor but the role of other genital infections and smoking are more difficult to quantify. The premalignant lesions already mentioned may develop into invasive tumors and, in addition, the Buschke–Lowenstein tumor may be locally invasive but rarely metastasizes.

Clinical features

The tumor usually starts as an ulcerative lesion in the coronal sulcus. It causes bleeding and discharge and is often hidden behind a phimosis (Fig. 41.22). Through fear or embarrassment the man may present late with a large fungating mass and/or inguinal lymph nodes. The TNM (tumor, nodes, and metastasis) classification of penile tumors is given in Figure 41.23.

Management of the primary tumor

Biopsy is essential and this often requires a dorsal slit or circumcision in order to expose the tumor. Occasionally an unsuspected tumor is removed at the time of circumcision and, if the removal was complete, no further treatment may be necessary. Antibiotics are given at the time of surgery to help bring about resolution of infection. Radiation is the treatment of choice in a sexually active man as it preserves penile function. Should it fail to control the disease then surgical salvage still permits cure. The choice between mold therapy, interstitial therapy, or beam therapy depends upon the experience of the radiotherapist[46–48]. Gross sepsis or a short penis in a fat patient may make radiotherapy more difficult unless interstitial implants are used.

Surgical treatment aims to remove the tumor completely and is successful unless the tumor involves the corpora. Surgery is particularly useful in older men who are no longer sexually active and when there is gross sepsis. Sexual function is satisfactory when the penile stump is more than 7cm in length[49]. Partial amputation gives good results when the tumor is confined to the superficial tissues but radical amputation rarely gives good results because of spread into the vascular spaces.

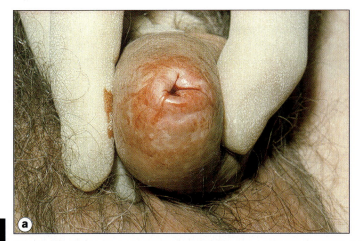

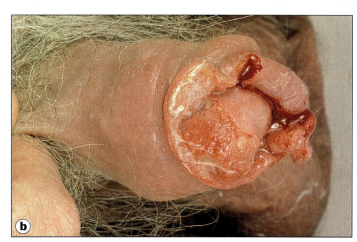

Fig. 41.22 Phimosis and carcinoma of the penis. (a) Bloody discharge and phimosis. (b) Carcinoma revealed after a dorsal slit procedure.

TNM clinical classification	
Stage	**Description**
Primary tumor (T)	
TX	Primary tumor cannot be assessed
T0	No evidence of primary tumor
Tis	Carcinoma in situ
Ta	Noninvasive verrucous carcinoma
T1	Tumor invades subepithelial connective tissue
T2	Tumor invades corpus spongiosus or cavernosus
T3	Tumor invades urethra or prostate
T4	Tumor invades adjacent structures
Regional lymph nodes (N)	
NX	Regional lymph nodes cannot be assessed
N0	No regional lymph node metastasis
N1	Metastasis in a single superficial inguinal lymph node
N2	Metastasis in multiple or bilateral superficial inguinal lymph nodes
N3	Metastasis in deep inguinal or pelvic lymph node(s), unilateral or bilateral
Distant metastases	
MX	Presence of distant metastases cannot be assessed
M0	No distant metastasis
M10	Distant metastasis

Fig. 41.23 TNM (tumor, nodes, and metastasis) clinical classification.

Management of regional nodes and metastatic disease

Enlargement of the inguinal nodes is common at the time of presentation but is usually caused by infection. Most urologists treat with antibiotics until the penile lesion is controlled and then perform a lymphadenectomy if the nodes remain palpable. Approximately 50% of patients with palpable nodes will be free of tumor.

Impalpable nodes will be found to contain tumor in 20% of patients and there may be an advantage in performing a prophylactic node dissection[50,51]. Inguinal node dissection is not without complications. Wound infection and skin necrosis are common and it is desirable to transfer the gracilis muscle to cover the femoral vessels. This lessens morbidity and permits earlier skin grafting. Seroma formation and lymphedema are frequent and resolve slowly.

Prophylactic radiotherapy is of no value for inguinal node metastases but may be used to treat fixed nodes for palliation[50-52].

Combination chemotherapy may have some benefit but there is no universal agreement as to which agents should be used.

Prognosis

Localized disease of the penis is associated with a good prognosis and a 70–95% 5-year survival free of disease. This falls to 50% when the nodes are microscopically involved[47] and survival is rare when there is macroscopic node involvement or spread to soft tissues.

REFERENCES

1. Cuckow PM, Rix G, Mourignand PDE. Preputial plasty: a good alternative to circumcision. J Pediatr Surg. 1994;29:561–3.

2. Pryor JP, Hill JT. Abnormalities of the suspensory ligament of the penis as a cause for erectile dysfunction. Br J Urol. 1979;51:402–3.

3. Ralph DJ, Al-Akraa M, Pryor JP. The Nesbit operation for Peyronie's disease: 16-year experience. J Urol. 1995;154:1362–3.

4. To T, Agha M, Dick PT, Felman W. Cohort study on circumcision of newborn boys and subsequent risk of urinary tract infection. Lancet. 1998;352:1813–6.

5. Aaronson IA. Micropenis: medical and surgical implications. J Urol. 1994;152:4–14.

6. Reilly JM, Woodhouse CRJ. Small penis and male sexual role. J Urol. 1989;142:569–71.

7. Miller MAW, Grant DB. Severe hypospadias with genital ambiguity: adult outcome after staged hypospadias repair. Br J Urol. 1997;80:485–8.

8. Johnston JH. Lengthening of the congenital or acquired short penis. Br J Urol. 1973;46:685–7.

9. Burman SO, Kelly TP. Enhancement phalloplasty with girth augmentation by autologous fat transfer: a further report of 700 cases. In: Porst H, ed. Penile disorders. Berlin: Springer-Verlag; 1997:251–76.

10. Clayton MD, Fowler JE, Sharifi R, Pearl RK. Causes, presentation and survival of 57 patients with necrotising fasciitis of the male genitalia. Surg Gynecol Obstet. 1990;170:49–55.

11. Morey AF, Meng MV, McAninch JW. Skin graft reconstruction of chronic genital lymphedema. Urology. 1997;50:423–6.

12. Lindsay MB, Schain DM, Grambsch P, et al. The incidence of Peyronie's Disease in Rochester, Minnesota, 1950 through 1984. J Urol. 1991;146:1007–9.

13. Chilton CP, Castle WM, Westwood CA, Pryor JP. Factors associated in the aetiology of Peyronie's Disease. Br J Urol. 1982;54:748–50.

14. Ralph DJ, Mirakian R, Pryor JP, Bottazzo GF. The immunological features of Peyronie's disease. J Urol 1996;155:159–62.

15. Ralph DJ, Hughes T, Lees WR, Pryor JP. Pre-operative assessment of Peyronie's disease using colour Doppler sonography. Br J Urol. 1992;69:629–32.

16. Amin Z, Patel U, Friedman EP, et al. Colour Doppler and duplex ultrasound assessment of Peyronie's Disease in impotent men. Br J Radiol. 1993;66:398–402.

17. Lopez JA, Jarow JP. Penile vascular evaluation of men with Peyronie's Disease. J Urol. 1993;149:53–55.

18. Montorsi F, Guazzoni G, Bergamaschi F, et al. Vascular abnormalities in Peyronie's Disease: The role of colour Doppler sonography. J Urol. 1994;151:373–5.

19. Levine LA, Coogan CL. Penile vascular assessment using color duplex sonography in men with Peyronie's disease. J Urol. 1996;155:1270–3.

20. Jordan GH, Angermeier KW. Preoperative evaluation of erectile function with dynamic infusion cavernosometry/cavernosography in patients undergoing surgery for Peyronie's disease: correlation with postoperative results. J Urol. 1993;150:1138–42.

21. Gasior BL, Levine FJ, Howannesian A, et al. Plaque-associated corporal veno-occlusive dysfunction in idiopathic Peyronie's Disease: a pharmacocavernosometric and pharmacocavernosographic study. World J Urol. 1990;8:90–6.

22. Hamm B, Friedrich M, Kelami A. Ultrasound imaging in Peyronie's Disease. Urology. 1986;6:540–5.

23. Helweg G, Judmaier W, Buchberger W, et al. Peyronie's disease: MR findings in 28 patients. AJR. 1992;158:1261–4.

24. Ralph DJ, Brooks MD, Bottazzo GF, Pryor JP. The treatment of Peyronie's Disease with tamoxifen. Br J Urol. 1992;70:648–51.

25. Devine CJ, Horton CE. Surgical treatment of Peyronie's disease with a dermal graft. J Urol. 1974;111:44.

26. Bystrom J, Johansson B, Edsmyr F, et al. Induratio penis plastica (Peyronie's disease): the results of the various forms of treatment. Scand J Urol Nephrol. 1972;6:1–5.

27. Austoni E, Colombo F, Mantovani F, et al. Chirurgia radicale e conservazione dell'erezione nella malattia di La Peyronie. Arch It Urol. 1995;67:359–64.

28. Brock G, Kadioglu A, Lue TF. Peyronie's disease: a modified treatment. Urology. 1993;42:300–4.

29. Al-Sakka AI, Lue TF. Venous grafting for the correction of penile curvature in Peyronie's disease. Curr Opin Urol. 1998;8:541–6.

30. Krishnamurti S. Penile dermal flap for defect reconstruction in Peyronie's disease: operative technique and four years' experience in 17 patients. Int J Impotence Res. 1995;7:195–208.

31. Wilson SK, Delk JR. A new treatment for Peyronie's disease: modeling the penis over an inflatable prosthesis. J Urol. 1994;152:1121–3.

32. Hauri D, Spycher MA, Brühlmann W. Erection and priapism: a new physiopathological concept. Urol Int. 1983;153:138–45.

33. Virag R. Intracavernosal injection of papaverine for erectile failure. Lancet. 1982;2:938

34. Brindley GS. Cavernosal alpha blockade: a new technique for investigating and treating erectile impotence. Br J Psychiat. 1988;149:210–5.

35. Brindley GS. New treatments for priapism. Lancet. 1984;2:220–1.

36. Lue TF, Hellstrom WJG, McAninch JW, Tanagho EA. Priapism: a refined approach to diagnosis and treatment. J Urol. 1986;136:104–8.

37. Linet OI, Ogrinc FG. Efficacy and safety of intracavernosal alprostadil in men with erectile dysfunction. N Engl J Med. 1996;334:873–7.

38. Wear IJ, Crummy AB, Munson BO. A new approach to the treatment of priapism. J Urol. 1993;117:252–4.

39. Pryor JP. Conservative management of priapism. Int J Androl. 1984;7:449–50.

40. Lee M, Cannon B, Sharifi R. Chart for preparation of dilutions of alpha adrenergic agent for intracavernosal use investigation of priapism. J Urol. 1995;153:1182–3.

41. Levine JF, Saenz de Tejada I, Payton TR, Goldstein I. Recurrent prolonged erections and priapism as a sequela of priapism. J Urol. 1991;145:764–7.

42. Pryor JP, Hehir M. The management of priapism. Br J Urol. 1982;54:751–4.

43. Serjeant GR, de Cenlaer K, Maude GH. Stilboestrol and stuttering priapism in homozygous sickle cell disease. Lancet. 1985;2:1274–6.

44. Levine LA, Guss SP. Gonadotrophin-releasing hormone analogues in the treatment of sickle cell anaemia-associated priapism. J Urol. 1993;150:475–7.

45. Maden C, Sherman KJ, Beckmann AM et al. History of circumcision, medical conditions and sexual activity and risk of penile cancer. J Nat Cancer Inst. 1993;85:19–24.

46. Gerbaulet A, Lambin P. Radiotherapy of cancer of the penis. Indications, advantages, pitfalls. Urol Clin North Am. 1992;19:325–32.

47. Ravi R, Chaturvedi HK, Sastry DVLN. Role of radiation therapy in the treatment of carcinoma of the penis. Br J Urol. 1994;74:646–51.

48. Neave F, Neal AJ, Hoskin PJ, Hope-Stone HF. Carcinoma of the penis: a retrospective review of treatment with iridium mould and external beam irradiation. Clin Oncol. (R Coll Radiol.) 1993;5:207–10.

49. Opjordsmoen S, Fossa SD. Quality of life in patients treated for penile cancer. A follow-up study. Br J Urol. 1994;74:652–7.

50. McDougal WS, Kirchner FK Jr, Edwards RH, Killion LT. Treatment of carcinoma of the penis: the case for primary lymphadenectomy. J Urol. 1986;136:38–41.

51. Ornellas AA, Seixas ALC, Marota A et al. Surgical treatment of invasive squamous cell carcinoma of the penis: retrospective analysis of 350 cases. J Urol. 1994;151:1244–9.

52. Kulkarini JN, Kamat MR. Prophylactic bilateral groin dissection versus prophylactic radiotherapy and surveillance in patients with N0 and N1–2A carcinoma of the penis. Eur Urol. 1994;26:123–8.

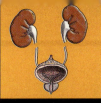

Section 8 Miscellaneous

Chapter 42

Extracorporeal Shock-wave Lithotripsy

Jeffrey A Moody, Andrew P Evans, and James E Lingeman

KEY POINTS

- Lithotripsy is effective for 80–85% of stone patients.
- The long-term effects of shock wave lithotripsy on renal function remain unknown.
- Effective lithotripsy requires some form of analgesia or sedation.
- Complex stone problems usually demand percutaneous nephrolithotomy.
- Endourologic skills are the critical factor in positive outcomes for stone patients.

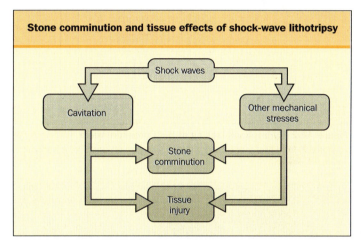

Figure 42.1 Stone comminution and tissue effects of shock wave lithotripsy.

INTRODUCTION

Extracorporeal shock-wave lithotripsy (ESWL or SWL) has revolutionized the treatment of urolithiasis. SWL is now the most common urologic procedure performed for symptomatic renal lithiasis, because of its noninvasive nature, efficacy for selected stones and wide availability of lithotriptors (either fixed or mobile)[1]. The physics and material science behind lithotripsy and stone fragmentation remain to be fully characterized, but shock wave generation, fragmentation theory, and the tissue effects are beginning to be understood. SWL acts via transmission of energy to a stone through tissue until the stone has been pulverized to a sufficiently small size that the fragments will pass spontaneously from the urinary tract. SWL has effects on tissue and can cause short-term and possibly long-term injury. Since the first clinically used lithotriptor, the Dornier HM3, an evolution of shock wave generators, type of anesthesia, and clinical efficacy has occurred, for better or worse. The efficient use of lithotripsy as a treatment modality relies upon a thorough understanding of its indications, contraindications, and limitations. SWL has, like any surgical procedure, risks and potential complications.

At the end of this chapter, the reader should be able to complete the following objectives:
- Understand the basic principles of shock-wave generation and stone fragmentation.
- Learn about the various types of lithotriptors, mechanisms of action, capabilities, and limitations.
- Understand the indications, contraindications, clinical algorithm for use of SWL, and techniques to enhance efficacy.
- Understand the complications of SWL and their subsequent management.

LITHOTRIPSY PRINCIPLES

Shock-wave lithotripsy acts via a number of mechanical and dynamic forces on stones, resulting in fragmentation. The most important force is thought to be cavitation[2-5]. Other forces are shear and spalling[6-8] (Fig. 42.1). Cavitation occurs when dissolved gases (which are essentially microscopic bubbles from sizes 1–30μm) in solution in and around stones and tissue are first compressed, then expanded up to 500μm in fluid by the positive and negative pressure of a passing hydrodynamic wave. Figure 42.2 illustrates the hydrophonic waveform of a passing shock wave. The passage of the wave form occurs in a relatively short time period (8–10μs). Subsequently, a large and unstable bubble (Fig. 42.3a) is transiently created, in a period from 0–1400μs before collapse. Because of impurities inherent in biologic systems, these bubbles can collapse asymmetrically, producing a destructive microjet (Fig. 42.3b) that causes pitting and, ultimately, fragmentation of stones but may also cause trauma to tissue, especially thin-walled vessels in the kidney[9,10]. Hemorrhage, release of cytokines/inflammatory cellular mediators, and infiltration of tissue by inflammatory response cells occur acutely. These lead to formation of scar and possible loss of renal function chronically[11].

Shear and spalling are dynamic mechanical forces that describe the interaction between shock waves and the stone material itself, acting to 'pull' the stone apart, typically along weak points or fracture planes[6]. Fragmentation of urinary stones is related to the separation of layers of crystals in stones that are laminated

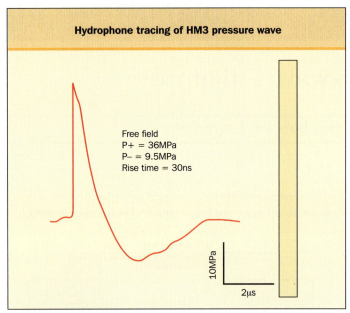

Hydrophone tracing of HM3 pressure wave

Free field
P+ = 36MPa
P– = 9.5MPa
Rise time = 30ns

10MPa

2μs

Figure 42.2 Hydrophone tracing of HM3 pressure wave. (With permission from McAteer et al.[15] ©1998 Acoustical Society of America.)

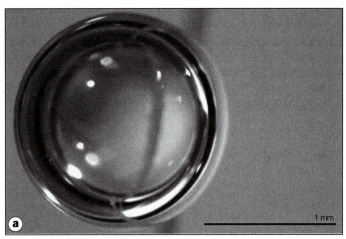

a

1 mm

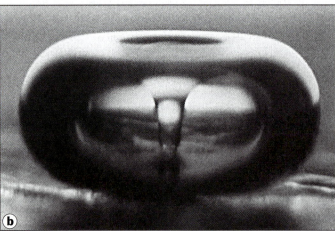

b

Figure 42.3 Cavitation bubble. (a) Cavitation bubble – size 800μm. (Courtesy George Kapodistrias, Department of Graduate Engineering, University of Washington.) (b) Microjet from collapsing bubble impacting adjacent surface. (Courtesy Lawrence Crum, Acoustic Physics Laboratory, University of Washington.)

during formation (calcium oxalate, uric acid) and fracture of the crystals themselves in amorphous stones (struvite)[12].

There are several different ways in which shock waves can be generated – electrohydraulic (EHL), electromagnetic (EMG) and piezoelectric (PZE) – and they will be described in detail in the section of this chapter covering the different types of lithotriptor.

TISSUE EFFECTS OF SHOCK-WAVE LITHOTRIPSY

The dichotomy of clinically effective SWL is the balance between delivery of adequate power to the stone for fragmentation and the tissue effects of this energy (Fig. 42.1). The biologic effects of SWL are related to the manner in which the shock waves and subsequent effects (cavitation, shear, etc.) interact with tissue. Risk factors for increased renal tissue damage after SWL are reduced renal mass, either in pediatric or elderly populations, bleeding diatheses, pre-existing hypertension or hypertension during therapy (Fig. 42.4).

In vitro studies[2,13] have proved the damaging effects of cavitation on inert materials as well as on cell suspensions[14]. Further work has shown that the tissue-damaging effects of SWL attributed to cavitation may be eradicated by varying ambient pressure during application of shock waves to both inert materials and cell suspensions[15]. Figure 42.5 illustrates the effects of increasing ambient pressure on damage to aluminum foils and LLC-PK1 cells. At modest degrees of overpressurization (3–5 atmospheres), cellular damage is reduced by more than 50%, while cavitation-induced foil pitting paradoxically increases. Foil damage is reduced almost completely as pressure continues to increase to over 60 atmospheres. Cellular damage also decreases as

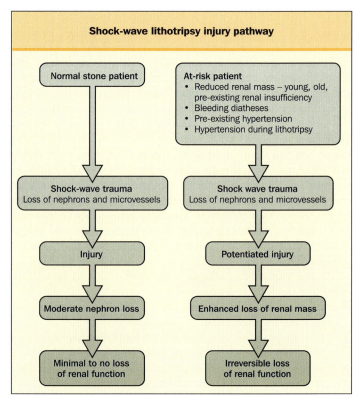

Shock-wave lithotripsy injury pathway

Normal stone patient

At-risk patient
• Reduced renal mass – young, old, pre-existing renal insufficiency
• Bleeding diatheses
• Pre-existing hypertension
• Hypertension during lithotripsy

Shock-wave trauma
Loss of nephrons and microvessels

Shock wave trauma
Loss of nephrons and microvessels

Injury

Potentiated injury

Moderate nephron loss

Enhanced loss of renal mass

Minimal to no loss of renal function

Irreversible loss of renal function

Figure 42.4 Shock-wave lithotripsy injury pathway.

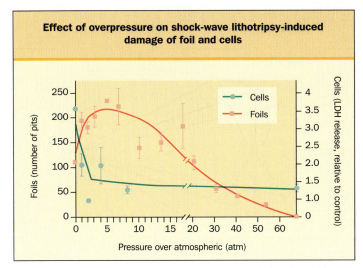

Figure 42.5 **Effect of overpressure on shock-wave lithotripsy-induced damage of foil and cells.** (With permission from McAteer et al[15] ©1998 Acoustical Society of America.)

Possible renal effects of shock-wave lithotripsy

Acute
  Hematoma – subcapsular or perirenal
  Increased occurrence of hematoma in patients with hypertension
  Low signal intensity changes in perinephric fat on MRI
  Loss of corticomedullary demarcation on MRI
  Perirenal or capsular fluid on MRI
  Delayed to complete loss of contrast excretion with or without ureteral obstruction
  Hematuria
  Enlargement of kidneys (excretory urogram)
  Decrease in effective plasma flow in treated kidneys
  Marked congestion of kidney with mild tubular degeneration
  Rupture and congestion of perirenal capillaries
  Disruption and edema of urothelium
  Increased N-acetylglucosaminidase
  Increased β-galactosidase
Chronic
  New onset of hypertension
  Perirenal fibrosis
  Patchy fibrosis of ureter
  Loss of renal function

Figure 42.6 **Possible renal effects of shock wave lithotripsy.** MRI, magnetic resonance imaging.

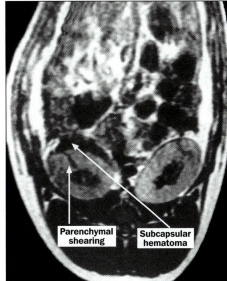

Figure 42.7 **Renal effects of shock waves.** Frontal magnetic resonance image of juvenile porcine kidneys after 2000 shock, 24kV treatment, with disruption of parenchyma, extravasation of blood, and subcapsular hematoma around right kidney.

Parenchymal shearing | Subcapsular hematoma

atmospheric pressure increases, but is not eliminated completely, even at 60 atmospheres, possibly indicating the effect of other SW-induced stress (i.e. shear, spall) on cells.

The effects of SWL in vivo depend upon the tissue impacted, medicines given to ameliorate injury and the shock wave regimen. Hemorrhage and hematoma can be seen in lung, kidney, liver, and bowel[16–19]. Chemical pancreatitis may develop after SWL treatment[20]. New cortical bone formation with minimal marrow alterations can be seen in long bone treated with SWL[21]. There are preliminary data on protective effects of some compounds (nifedipine, allopurinol) on renal injury indicators when given before SWL[22]. Further, the timing and dosing of SWL may affect renal function, with data in an animal model indicating that large solitary doses of shock waves induce a greater degree of periglomerular and intratubular fibrosis than either lower or high, divided doses of lithotripsy[23].

The mechanism of injury after SWL is a combination of injury and an exuberant injury response. Figure 42.6 lists the possible renal injuries after SWL. The degree of effect SWL has on patients' renal function and possibility of inducing hypertension depends on the risk factors for injury (age >60, pediatric, pre-existing hypertension, pre-existing renal disease). Evidence that risk factors are important in determining outcome after lithotripsy was reported by Janetschek et al., who found that intrarenal resistive indices increased in patients over age 60 after SWL. New-onset hypertension was also seen in 45% of this group of patients with increased resistive indices and hypertension being highly correlated. (See also Figure 42.26)

The pathophysiology of SWL injury is a two-armed process in the kidney. First, shock waves lead to vascular and tissue shearing, extravasation of blood, ischemia, and renal vasoconstriction, which stimulates an acute injury response, with local recruitment of inflammatory mediators (prostaglandin[24], thromboxane[25], endothelin[26]) and injury response cells[27], which release cellular chemotactic mediators [interleukin-1 (IL-1), interleukin-2 (IL-2), (TGF-β)]. Figures 42.7 and 42.8 illustrate the radiologic and histologic correlates of tissue and vascular shear in the same porcine kidney after SWL. In the kidney, these mediators promote

fibrosis and healing. The fibrosis may encompass as much as 1% of the renal mass[27]. Second, tubular function (glomerular filtration rate (GFR)) and renal plasma flow (RPF) are severely compromised for 24 hours after SWL[28]. In a mini-pig model, SWL significantly reduced GFR and RPF in those kidneys at 1 and 4 hours after ESWL[28]. Gross renal function returned to normal after 1 week in young adult animal models and humans[29].

Inflammatory mediators are also possibly recruited in response to tubular injury. Patients have been found to have transient enzymuria with glycosaminoglycans (GAGs) after SWL, indicating urothelial and/or tubular injury[30]. Further, morphologic analysis of tubules shows a dose-dependent cellular injury

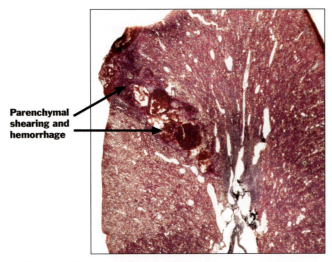

Figure 42.8 Renal effects of shock waves. Light microscopy of kidney from Figure 42.7, showing parenchymal disruption, extravasation of blood, and perirenal hematoma.

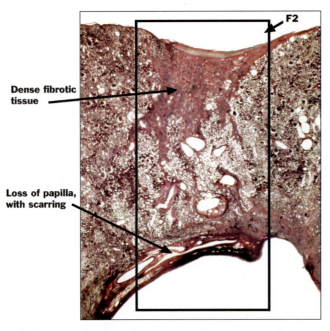

Figure 42.9 Renal effects of shock waves. Light microscopy of renal parenchyma, juvenile porcine kidney, 2000 shocks at 24kV, 3 months after SWL. Note extensive transparenchymal scarring, with loss of papilla in collecting system. F2, focus of shockwave.

response to SWL[31]. Tubular injury and response also lead to interstitial fibrosis and loss of functional nephrons (Fig. 42.9). Both vascular and tubular injury play important roles in the renal response to SWL, and may lead to decreased renal function or renal failure after SWL, termed 'lithotripsy nephritis'[11].

While clinical experience has shown that the vast majority of patients undergo SWL without any apparent short-term or long-term sequelae, what is not known is whether repeated treatments with SWL in normal patients or solitary treatments in patients with risk factors as defined above ultimately induce 'lithotripsy nephritis'. Clearly, the long-term biologic sequelae of SWL are still to be determined.

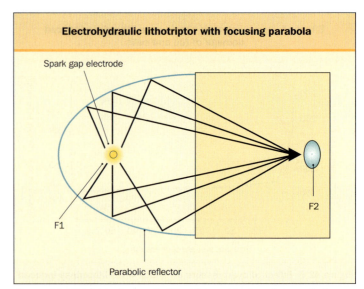

Figure 42.10 Electrohydraulic lithotriptor with focusing parabola.

LITHOTRIPTORS

The first lithotriptors developed used the principle of electrohydraulic (EHL) generation of shock waves. An underwater spark discharge generates a hydrodynamic pressure wave, which is released at the focal point of a parabolic reflector, or F1. The parabolic reflector refocuses the shock wave at a definable point (F2), as demonstrated in Figure 42.10. F2 is the point at which the stone is localized by fluoroscopy or ultrasound to achieve fragmentation. The Dornier HM (Human Model) series is based on this principle, with the HM3 most widely used of the so-called first-generation lithotriptors. As a model of the first generation of lithotriptors, the characteristics of the HM3 are as follows: an EHL generator, use of water bath for shock wave transmission, a fixed position, no endourologic capabilities, cost of approximately $100,000 (used), and no longer manufactured.

Lithotriptor manufacturers sought other methods to generate shock waves, hoping to reduce general anesthesia requirements and the need for electrode replacement. This led to the development of electromagnetic (EMG) and piezoelectric (PZE) shock-wave generators. The principle of EMG lithotripsy is that charge differences between two plates will cause motion and generation of a shock wave, which can be focused by an acoustic lens or parabolic reflector (Fig. 42.11). The Siemens Lithostar is a representative EMG lithotriptor. Its characteristics are as follows: EMG generator, a water cushion for shock wave transmission, fixed position, endourology capability and cost of $300,000 (used). Finally PZE generators were developed, based on the principle that an array of piezocrystals arranged in a semicircular fashion, focused at the center of its sphere, generate peak pressures at F2 sufficient for stone fragmentation, with lower peak pressures at skin level, leading to less pain and lower anesthesia requirements (Fig. 42.12). EMG and PZE generators, along with modified, non-water-bath EHL machines, were the next generation of lithotriptors.

Other factors were incorporated into lithotriptors as indications and demand grew. Variations included ultrasound and/or fluoroscopic localization, use for nonurologic applications (salivary,

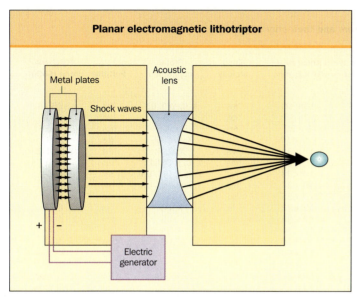

Figure 42.11 Planar electromagnetic lithotriptor.

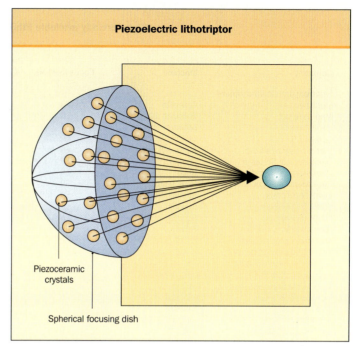

Figure 42.12 Piezoelectric lithotriptor.

biliary, and pancreatic lithotripsy, orthopedic tissue applications), addition of a multifunctional table for combined endoscopic use, and modularity with portability, which have subsequently been termed by manufacturers the third generation of lithotriptors. Two examples are the Medirex Tripter X-1, which uses an EHL generator, is modular and portable, and has endourologic capacity, and the Karl Storz Modulith SLX with an EMG generator, which adds ultrasound localization for concomitant use for biliary tract stones.

For all lithotriptors, individual or stone center treatment needs dictate which machine best serves the needs of its users. Considerations in choosing a lithotriptor include patient population to be treated, desire to incorporate endourologic or percutaneous capability, costs (including reusable/disposable items, generator life span, additional service contract) and need for multifunctionality (salivary/biliary, orthopedic, or radiologic use). The evolution of the lithotriptor will continue as indications, technology, and patient care issues change and expand. Currently available lithotriptors are detailed in Figure 42.13.

ANESTHESIA AND LITHOTRIPSY

Anesthesia and lithotripsy have always been a balance between the shock wave system, and the type of anesthetic techniques available at that time, which, taken together, demonstrate the efficacy of a lithotriptor (Fig. 42.14). Both have evolved considerably since the HM3 was introduced in 1984. Early lithotriptors (HM3) had large focal volumes and higher pressures at the skin level. Shock wave energy levels at the skin have been found to cause cavitation in subcutaneous tissue and may be the reason for pain during lithotripsy[32]. There have been general trends in lithotripsy towards alternate and less powerful shock wave generation, as it became apparent that most urinary stones will fragment at lower power levels than that provided by the unmodified HM3[33–35]. Subsequent generations of lithotriptors and modifications of the original HM3 progressed towards lower energy levels at the skin–shock-wave-medium interface, leading to decreased anesthesia requirements[36]. Trends towards

outpatient lithotripsy and the realization that there were few obvious deleterious side effects of SWL led to lower-power lithotripsy, but often to higher retreatment rates as well.

Anesthesia techniques have advanced equally over the past 15 years along with advances in the technology of SWL. Figure 42.15 depicts the different types of anesthetic agents that have been developed, and their use. Local application of anesthetic cream (EMLA) to the skin in an effort to decrease pain perceived at skin level have been effective in reducing perceived pain. However, double-blinded placebo-controlled studies did not note a decrease in additional anesthetic agents or shortened recovery time after SWL[37,38]. If used, it is important to apply the cream over a sufficiently large area at least 45 minutes prior to the procedure. Some lithotriptors use topical agents exclusively without need for subsequent anesthesia[39], although the use of additional agents may be needed[40]. Local infiltration of the skin with lidocaine has also been effective in reducing the pain of lithotripsy[41,42].

Intravenous sedation, or sedoanalgesia, has allowed SWL to be conducted on all lithotriptors at standard treatment energy levels. The short-acting duration of these agents allows rapid relief of pain, titration of analgesia to increasing pain, and rapid recovery after the procedure. Intravenous anesthesia has also been shown to be more time-efficient, with equal pain-control efficacy when compared to epidural anesthesia[43]. An extension of decreasing anesthetic techniques is the use of oral premedication to provide most, if not all, of the anesthesia required for SWL. In a large study, oral premedication prior to SWL with an EMG lithotriptor was the only anesthetic required in 83% of patients[44].

The trend towards decreasing anesthetic techniques must always be balanced with the lithotripsy needs of the stone and the patient. Stone that classically require higher energy level (brushite, cystine) or large stone burdens will most probably not be treated with adequate energy under minimal anesthetic

Commercially available lithotriptors and their characteristics

Company	Machine	Focus method	Pressure at F2 (MPa)	Focal zone (W × L, mm)	Endo urology	Stone localization	Portable	Purchase Price ($000)
Electrohydraulic lithotripters								
Medispec Ltd	Econolith	ER	72.6	13 × 60	Yes	X, C, OPT. US	Yes	350
Medispec Ltd	Econolith 2000	ER	120	13 × 60	Yes	X, C	Yes	390
Healthtronics	Lithotron	ER	53	8 × 38	Yes	X, C	Yes	595
Comair AB	Lithocut C-3000S**	ER	120	3.5 × 12	No	X, OPT. US	Yes	250
Medirex Systems Corp.	Tripter X-1 Compact	ER	110	10 × 34	Yes	X, C, F	Yes	395–445
Direx Medical Systems	Compact**	ER	110	10 × 34	Yes	X, C, F, OPT. US	Yes	350
Direx Medical Systems	Nova**	ER	110	10 × 34	Yes	X, C, F, OPT. US	Yes	600
Direx Medical Systems	Nova Ultima**	ER	110	10 × 34	Yes	X, C, F, OPT. US	Yes	600
EDAP Technomed	Sonolith 3000	ER	78*	15 × 55	No	US	Yes	N/A
EDAP Technomed	Sonolith 4000	ER	130	12 × 23	No	X, US	Yes	800
EDAP Technomed	Sonolith Praktis**	ER	130	12 × 23	No	X, US	Yes	500
Medstone International	STS	ER	120	13 × 50	No	X, US	No	500
Medstone International	STS-T	ER	120	13 × 50	No	X, US	Yes	N/A
Dornier Medical Systems	HM-3	ER	50*	15 × 90	No	X	No	100 used
Dornier Medical Systems	HM-4	ER	130	15 × 90	No	X	No	N/A
Dornier Medical Systems	MPL 9000	ER	130	3 × 20	No	CO-AX US, X	No	250 used
Dornier Medical Systems	MFL 5000	ER	100	10 × 40	Yes	X	No	750 used
PCK Co., Ltd	Stonelith**	ER	120	7.7 × 30	Yes	X, OPT. US	Yes	80–130
PCK Co., Ltd	Stonelith Smart**	ER	120	7.7 × 30	Yes	X, OPT. US	Yes	80–130
ELMED	Multimed 2001**	ER	120	7.5 × 22	Yes	X, US	Yes	125
ELMED Lithotripsy Sys.	Complit	ER	120	7.5 × 22	Yes	X, OPT. US	Yes	175
Electromagnetic lithotripters								
Siemens Medical Systems	Lithostar-standard	AL	44*	11 × 90	Yes	X	No	300 used
Siemens Medical Systems	Lithostar-Shock Tube C	AL	50	7 × 70	Yes	X	No	500 used
Siemens Medical Systems	Lithostar Multiline	AL	80	5 × 80	Yes	CO-AX US, X	No	N/A
Siemens Medical Systems	Lithostar Modularis	AL	50	7 × 70	Yes	X	Yes	600
Karl Storz Lithotripsy	Modulith SL20	PR	105.6	3 × 37	Yes	CO-AX US, X	No	295 used
Karl Storz Lithotripsy	Modulith SLX	PR	105.6	3 × 37	Yes	CO-AX US, X	No	695
Karl Storz Lithotripsy	Modulith SLX-T	PR	105.6	3 × 37	Yes	C, X	Yes	525
Dornier Medical Systems	Compact-S	AL	46	6.4 × 70	Limited	X	Yes	495
Dornier Medical Systems	DoLi/50	AL	46	6.4 × 70	Yes	X	No	795
Piezoelectric lithotripters								
EDAP Technomed	LT.01	SD	105*	5 × 23	No	CO-AX US	No	N/A
EDAP Technomed	LT.02	SD	140	1.8 × 29	No	CO-AX US, X	No	600
Richard Wolf	Piezolith 2300	SD	114*	3 × 11	No	CO-AX US	Yes	995
Richard Wolf	Piezolith 2500**	SD	150	3 × 11	No	CO-AX US, X	Yes	N/A
Richard Wolf	Piezolith 2501**	SD	150	3 × 11	No	CO-AX US, X	Yes	N/A

Figure 42.13 Commercially available lithotriptors and their characteristics. * Measured MPa by polyvinylidene difluorine (PVdF) hydrophone; remainder of values converted from bar data from manufacturers. ** Not Food and Drug Administration approved. Al, acoustic lens; C, C-arm; CO-AX, co-axial ultrasound; ER, ellipsoid reflector; F, fluoroscopy; OPT.US, optical ultasound; PR, parabolic reflector; X, X-ray; US, ultrasound.

Lithotriptor efficacy

Power = Volume of F_2 × peak pressure

Pain = relates to energy density at point of skin entry

Figure 42.14 Lithotriptor efficacy.

Recent anesthetic agents used for shock-wave lithotripsy

Local – Eutectic mixture of local anesthetics)

Intravenous sedation – midazolam, propofol, alfentanil

Figure 42.15 Recent anesthetic agents used for shock-wave lithotripsy.

---

conditions (Fig. 42.16). Pediatric patients and patients requiring lithotripsy in uncomfortable positions will require general anesthesia. Additionally, reduced anesthesia techniques and technology have increased treatment times[36], retreatment rates and reduced efficacy[45].

In conclusion, advances in anesthetic techniques have allowed nearly any lithotriptor to be used efficiently, with a minimum of both lithotriptor and anesthetic complications.

TREATMENT OUTCOMES AND EFFICACY OF SHOCK-WAVE LITHOTRIPSY

In analyzing results from clinical trials of lithotripsy, it is critical for the urologist or urologist-in-training to discern the type and generation of lithotriptor, whether the trial was randomized, controlled and prospective, and what were the criteria for success or failure of SWL[46]. Significant differences exist across the

Figure 42.16 Lingeman's law of lithotripsy and anesthesia. IV, intravenous.

spectrum of lithotriptors with respect to stone free rates, and little comparative clinical data exists[47]. Randomized studies have been performed only rarely. Assessing success for lithotripsy can mean widely varying definitions, from complete fragmentation to stone-free rates, which can be determined by KUB, ultrasound, renal tomograms, noncontrast computed tomography (CT) scan, or secondary nephroscopy, in order of increasing sensitivity. Plain abdominal radiographs and renal tomograms have been shown to underestimate stone-free rates by 35% and 17% respectively when compared to nephroscopy[48].

The power of a lithotriptor and, ultimately, stone fragmentation, are dependent on two factors: peak pressure (measured in pascals $\times 10^6$, or MPa) and the focal volume or size of F2 (Fig. 42.14). Not coincidentally, the clinical efficacy is directly related to the product of these two factors. For example, the peak pressure of the Dornier HM3 is 38.6MPa[49] and its focal volume is 15×90mm, delivering the largest amount of energy per shock wave of any lithotriptor. The clinical efficacy of the HM3 is the baseline for efficacy against which other lithotriptors are compared, and nears 67–90% for long-term stone-free rates for a wide range of stones[50,51]. In contrast, the PZE generators, like the EDAP Technomed LT.02 or the Wolf Piezolith 2501 generate much higher peak pressures, in the 140–150 MPa range, but with a much smaller focal volume (1.8×29mm and 3×11mm, respectively). The total joules of energy delivered to the stone per shock wave (SW) is therefore only a fraction of that produced by the HM3, but the pain generated at the skin level and anesthesia requirements are also greatly reduced. Clinical efficacy is lower (50–60% stone-free rates) and retreatment rates are higher than with the HM3[47]. In general, no lithotriptor has exceeded the ability of the HM3 to effectively fragment stones to passable size with a minimum rate of retreatment.

Clinical fragmentation of stones in the urinary system is dependent on three factors:
- correct localization of stone (either by fluoroscopy or ultrasound);
- application of appropriate energy to the stone for fragmentation; and
- spontaneous passage of fragments of sufficiently small size to cause minimal symptoms.

Although localization of renal and ureteral calculi can be accomplished by two methods, fluoroscopy and ultrasound, fluoroscopy is generally preferred for urologic lithotripsy applications. Fluoroscopic localization is adequate for radio-opaque renal stones and is essential for ureteral stones. It can be used for in situ SWL, during retrograde stone manipulation or catheter placement, or while performing simultaneous ureteroscopic or percutaneous stone extraction. Fluoroscopy may also be used for radiolucent stones when combined with injected contrast. Fluoroscopy is readily available on most lithotriptors or can be added as a C-arm

in modular systems, and most urologists are familiar with the characteristics of stones displayed on fluoroscopy.

Ultrasound can localize most stones of all radio-densities in the kidney and upper ureter, provides real-time, continuous monitoring of stone fragmentation, and does not expose patients to radiation. However, stones that are further from the skin (e.g. renal pelvis, upper ureter) can be difficult or impossible to image well with ultrasound, especially in obese patients. Further, most mid and many pelvic ureteral stones are not possible to localize with ultrasound. Ultrasound should be considered optional on all lithotriptors, particularly since urologists may not be as familiar with the imaging of stones via ultrasound. Clinical experience has demonstrated that fluoroscopy and lithotripsy are sufficient for virtually all types of stone.

Directing adequate fragmentation energy to the stone depends on patient body habitus, intervening organs, or bony structures, patient position and lithotriptor limitations. Obesity may make SWL impossible through inability to localize F2 on the stone. Organomegaly (hepatosplenomegaly, cardiomegaly, chronic obstructive pulmonary disease) or any other disease state that potentially interposes organs between the shock waves and the stone under treatment may cause injury to these organs and make directing clinically useful energy to the stone dangerous or impossible. Mid-ureteral stones overlying the bony pelvis or ureteral stones overlying transverse vertebral processes or aortic aneurysms may be impossible or dangerous to fragment in the supine position. Prone lithotripsy may be necessary for distal and mid-ureteral stones. Finally, lithotriptor-specific limitations (focal length, power) may preclude SWL in certain situations.

The last criterion for successful lithotripsy is clearance of stone fragments of sufficient size to cause minimal symptoms and complications for the patient. For this reason, complex or abnormal renal or ureteral anatomy often makes SWL a poor choice because of the lower clearance rate[52–55]. Stones greater than 2cm have poorer clearance rates and higher incidence of obstruction and steinstrasse than smaller stones and are more effectively removed via percutaneous methods[56].

CLINICAL INDICATIONS AND CONTRAINDICATIONS FOR SHOCK-WAVE LITHOTRIPSY IN UROLOGY

After initial enthusiasm in the use of SWL for all types of stones, irrespective of size, composition, or location, clinical outcomes have delineated what are the most useful and efficacious applications for SWL[57,58] (Fig. 42.17).

After adhering to the indications and contraindications for SWL, many clinical situations remain in which the most efficacious method of stone treatment may not be clear. We present here the 'laws' and clinical algorithms proved for use of ESWL in the most practical and efficient manner (Figs 42.18–42.20).

'Simple' stone situations have been shown to respond well to lithotripsy. Complex stone situations have been shown historically to respond poorly to SWL. The first complex stone situation is stone burden greater than 2cm. Stone clearance after SWL is dramatically reduced when stone size exceeds 2cm, falling from near 90% for stones less than 1cm to 62% for stones greater than 2cm in a large series[59]. Retreatment also increased to 32% in the same >2cm patient group. Patients also suffered more renal colic,

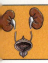

Indications and contraindications for shock-wave lithotripsy	
Indications	**Contraindications**
Renal stones <2cm	Morbid obesity
Ureteral stones	Coagulopathy (uncorrected)
	Urinary tract obstruction
	Sepsis or active urinary tract infection
	Pregnancy
	Renal artery or aortic aneurysm
	Cystine or brushite stones (relative)

Figure 42.17 Indications and contraindications for shock wave lithotripsy.

Lingeman's law for management of renal lithiasis
'If the stone problem is simple, do shock-wave lithotripsy.
If the stone problem is complex, do percutaneous nephrolithotomy.'

Figure 42.18 Lingeman's law for management of renal lithiasis.

The simple situation
Stones <2cm
Normal renal anatomy

Figure 42.19 The simple situation.

The complex situation
Stone burden >2cm
Staghorn calculi
Abnormal renal anatomy
Dilated calyces
Ureteropelvic junction obstruction
Horseshoe kidney
Calyceal diverticulum
Lower pole stones
Cystine/brushite stones

Figure 42.20 The complex situation.

obstruction, and need for cystoscopic stone manipulation. Percutaneous nephrolithotomy (PCNL) is the preferred method for treatment of large (>2cm) renal calculi. Staghorn renal calculi are an even more extreme example of large, complex renal stones that benefit most from PCNL, with fewer post-SWL fragment-related complications[60].

Abnormal renal anatomy will preclude passage of even the most adequately fragmented stones, leading to stone recurrence, retreatment, and morbidity. Several classifications of abnormal renal anatomy are detailed below.

Dilated calyces or hydronephrosis imply a previous long-standing obstruction or loss of renal parenchyma. Hydronephrosis may be associated with poorer renal function, decreased GFR and urinary stasis, leading to decreased clearance of fragments and formation of new stone on residual fragments.

Ureteropelvic junction (UPJ) obstruction may be a cause of nephrolithiasis secondary to stasis, as well as a hindrance to effective passage of stone fragments after SWL. Evaluation with excretory urography, diuretic renograms, or more invasive pressure-flow studies preoperatively will define whether a true UPJ obstruction is present. If a true UPJ obstruction is present, concomitant PCNL and incision of the UPJ obstruction (endopyelotomy) with stenting are more appropriate than SWL alone. If there is no UPJ obstruction, but ureteral narrowing and hydronephrosis are present, the patient should be counseled that SWL alone may not be successful.

Horseshoe kidneys pose an interesting and sometimes difficult anatomic obstacle, as a large renal pelvis combined with high insertion of the ureter will hinder passage of fragments after SWL. Clearance of 55% with SWL alone has been accomplished in a small series[61], but adjunctive procedures, including stent placement, ureteroscopy, and PCNL, are necessary in up to 65% of patients. PCNL is a highly effective treatment option for stones in horseshoe kidney[62].

Calyceal diverticula are an uncommon, troublesome entity that can be very symptomatic for patients and traditionally

responds poorly to SWL, with stone clearance rates of 4–20%[63,64]. However, symptomatic improvement in a highly selected population without complete stone clearance may be as high as 58%[65]. Percutaneous removal of stones in diverticulas is more efficient with 80–90% stone-free rates[63,66]. Ureteroscopy or laparoscopy can also be performed for stone removal[67,68].

Lower pole renal anatomy is a hindrance to efficient passage of fragments after SWL. Acute infundibulopelvic angle, long infundibular length, and narrow infundibular width are factors that negatively impact stone clearance[69]. For stones less than 1cm, SWL may successfully treat up to 80%[70], but stone clearance rapidly falls as stone size increases, to 44% for stones 1–2cm[2,71]. PCNL has higher stone-free rates, from 70–100%, is not affected by stone size, and is more cost effective for stones greater than 1cm[72,73]. However, PCNL has longer hospital stays, and potential for increased morbidity[71,72].

Poor stone fragility excludes SWL as a viable treatment option for patients with brushite or cystine stones, unless known to fragment from prior experience with a specific patient[74].

Adherence to the 'laws' for treatment of urolithiasis form the basis for the most efficient clearance of urinary tract stones with the least total morbidity and cost for the patient. Below are clinical situations that illustrate the treatment algorithms.

The guidelines in Figure 42.21 apply to 'noncomplex' cases (Figs 42.18–42.20). Abnormal anatomy, obstruction or stones known to be resistant to SWL require direct fragmentation by the most direct and least morbid access (either percutaneous or ureteroscopic) for the patient.

SHOCK-WAVE LITHOTRIPSY: TECHNIQUE AND 'PEARLS'

Shock-wave lithotripsy for ureteral stones can be accomplished either in situ or using the 'push-smash' or retrograde stone manipulation technique, which enhances stone fragmentation and subsequent stone-free rates[75,76]. Clinical studies confirm

Figure 42.21 Treatment algorithm for urolithiasis and shock-wave lithotripsy. PCNL, percutaneous nephrolithotomy; SWL, shock-wave lithotripsy.

earlier in vitro work regarding the importance of fluid surrounding the stone and subsequent stone fragmentation[77].

If stones are too radiolucent to be easily seen with fluoroscopy alone, a ureteral catheter can be placed at an appropriate location below the stone to allow injection of contrast to illuminate the filling defect. Use of dilute contrast will allow visualization of the stone without obscuring the subsequent view of success of SWL.

Bilateral SWL at the same sitting can be safely undertaken in the patient with small bilateral stones and normal renal function.

Stent use in SWL should have a rational basis. Studies have documented the morbidity of stents[78], and lack of efficacy in preventing complications with smaller stones[79–81]. Stent use for large stones (>25mm) undergoing lithotripsy has been shown to decrease symptomatic steinstrasse and the need for auxiliary procedures[82]. In general, stent use should be reserved for patients with solitary kidneys, with a large stone burden, or undergoing concomitant ureteral manipulation.

COMPLICATIONS OF SHOCK-WAVE LITHOTRIPSY AND MANAGEMENT

A thorough understanding of the principles that underlie shock-wave lithotripsy is important, not only for mechanism of action but also for the possible ways in which lithotripsy can cause injury and subsequent complications. The complications of SWL can be divided into immediate or short-term complications (fragment-related complications, infection, hemorrhage/hematoma, adjacent organ injury) and delayed or long-term complications (effects on renal function, blood pressure and stone recurrence; Fig. 42.22).

Immediate complications

Fragment-related complications can be divided into retained residual fragments and steinstrasse. Recall that stone size, composition, and intrarenal anatomy are important factors that affect whether or not a fragment is retained. The fate of residual fragments after SWL has been debated since lithotripsy began 15 years ago. Referring to the 'Lingeman laws of lithotripsy', fragments of a noninfection stone in an unobstructed system

Complications after shock-wave lithotripsy	
Immediate	**Delayed**
Fragment-related	Renal function
Infection	Hypertension
Hemorrhage/hematoma	Stone recurrence
Adjacent organ injury	
Arrhythmia	

Figure 42.22 Complications after shock-wave lithotripsy.

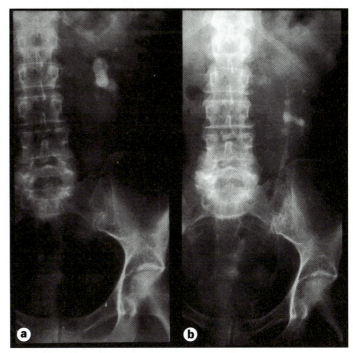

Figure 42.23 Steinstrasse. (a) Pre- and (b) postlithotripsy plain radiographs on patient who developed steinstrasse with obstruction. Stent was placed to relieve obstruction.

with favorable drainage characteristics[69] may be expected to pass with a high degree of certainty. However, even fragments 4mm or less are associated with an increase in stone burden (18% of patients) and retreatment (43% of patients) in a 5-year study[83]. Complete treatment of calculi to clinically and radiographically insignificant size (<4mm) as assessed by renal tomograms is therefore important. SWL should be selectively used in 'simple' situations only, as defined above.

Steinstrasse, literally 'stone street', is defined as complicated when more than 5cm of ureter is filled with fragments or a concomitant urinary tract infection is present, or simple, when less than 5cm of ureter is occupied with fragments (Fig. 42.23). Steinstrasse occurs in 1–4% of patients undergoing SWL overall,[84,85] in up to 5–10% of patients with large stone burdens (>200mm²)[79] and can occur in up to 40% of patients with partial or complete staghorn nephrolithiasis treated with SWL[60]. Patients may not have significant symptoms but are usually obstructed and may have concurrent infection. Sepsis is rare but demands prompt attention. Treatment of steinstrasse consists of relieving the obstruction, treatment of any infection, and endoscopic removal of the stone burden. Aggressive treatment can prevent irreversible renal damage and ureteral stricture disease[86]. Patients with complex steinstrasse are best managed with percutaneous nephrostomy, with subsequent percutaneous or ureteroscopic stone removal. A simple steinstrasse can be treated with ureteral stenting and ureteroscopic removal of stone. Prevention of steinstrasse is most important when considering treatment options for large stone burdens. Stent use has been shown to reduce subsequent complications of steinstrasse in patients with large (>25mm) stone burden[82].

Steinstrassen and their complications are rare now for several reasons: urologists have learned the limitations of SWL for large stone burdens, stents are used more frequently for large stone burdens undergoing SWL, and PCNL has been employed more frequently for large stone burdens.

Infection post-SWL is more common in patients with struvite stones, multiple or complex stones, or patients who undergo periprocedural stone or urologic manipulation[87]. Fortunately, preoperative urine culture and appropriate prophylactic antibiotics can prevent infectious complications after SWL. If urosepsis should ensue, appropriate drainage of the affected renal unit, aggressive fluid resuscitation, hemodynamic support with vasoactive agents, and invasive monitoring in an intensive care setting ameliorate further deterioration and speed recovery.

Some bleeding probably occurs in and around the kidney with nearly every SWL treatment. If examined for by CT or magnetic resonance imaging (MRI), the incidence of renal hematoma following SWL may be as high as 25%, but typically resolves without sequelae. Symptomatic renal hemorrhage or hematoma has been reported in approximately 0.66% of patients undergoing SWL[88] (Fig. 42.24). While this incidence is low, several factors increase the risk of perirenal hematoma. Anticoagulation, either by pharmacologic (aspirin, warfarin, anti-inflammatory medicines, etc.) or pathologic means (liver failure, spherocystosis, von Willebrand disease), without recognition and treatment prior to SWL increases the risk of hematoma and hemorrhage. However, appropriate preoperative therapy directed at the specific disease can allow SWL safely[89]. An uncorrected bleeding diathesis remains a contraindication to SWL. Pre-existing hypertension or untreated hypertension at the time of treatment are also risk factors for renal hematoma and hemorrhage, increasing the risk four- to fivefold[88]. Others have reported atherosclerosis as a risk factor for post-SWL hematoma or hemorrhage[90]. Patients with significant perirenal bleeding present with flank pain and falling hematocrit (Fig. 42.25). The consequences of renal hemorrhage can be severe, and life-threatening if unrecognized. Aggressive monitoring and transfusion as necessary with conservative operative management are generally successful. The rare patient with a large renal hematoma may develop a 'Page' kidney, with subsequent severe hypertension caused by renal ischemia from compression of parenchyma[90]. Such patients may warrant operative decompression.

Adjacent organ injury can rarely occur with lithotripsy, as organs in the blast path are subjected to the focused shock wave. The injuries are organ-specific. Pancreatic injury is a rare but possible result of lithotripsy for left-sided renal stones[20]. Conservative measures until clinical pancreatitis resolves are often the only treatment necessary. Splenic hematoma, rupture, and abscess

Risk of perinephric hematoma			
	Rx	Hematomas	%
Study patients	3,260	21	0.666
Pre-existing hypertension	479	12	2.5*
Pre-Rx diastolic blood pressure >90	265	10	3.8*
* p<0.001			

Figure 42.24 Risk of perinephric hematoma. Incidence of perirenal hematomas after shock wave lithotripsy. (Data from Knapp et al.[88])

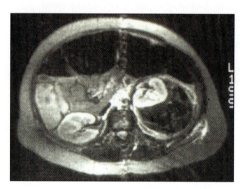

Figure 42.25 Unilateral hematoma in patient after shock-wave lithotripsy.

have been reported as possible complications after lithotripsy[91–93]. Surgical removal of the spleen may be necessary, depending on the patient's clinical situation. Hepatic hematoma is also possible after SWL[18]. Pulmonary, duodenal, and colonic contusions are also possible but can be managed expectantly[94].

Arrythmias caused by stimulation and proximity of the heart to SWs are possible with all types of lithotriptor, the incidence ranging from 11–59%[95–97]. The incidence is reduced with gating of the SW to the electrocardiogram pulse[94]. Ungated SWL can be performed but the incidence of arrhythmia is increased[96,98]. However, the incidence of morbid cardiac events in the presence of arrhythmia is not increased[95]. Ungated SWL can safely be performed with cardiac monitoring during and after therapy.

Patients with pacemakers can also safely undergo SWL with appropriate monitoring and adjustment of pacemaker[99]. Single-chamber ventricular pacemakers can safely undergo SWL without modification. Dual-chamber atrially paced patients should have the pacemaker set to the VVI mode. Patients with piezoelectric sensing rate-responsive single-chamber pacemakers should have this feature programmed off. Abdominal placement of a piezoelectric pacemaker is a contraindication to SWL[100]. Life-threatening arrhythmia is managed with aggressive, cardiac algorithm-based treatment and termination of the procedure.

Delayed complications

There is no doubt that SWL has short-term deleterious effects on RBF, GFR, and urine output[11]. However, the long-term effects of SWL on renal function are unknown. Renography performed on a series of patients undergoing SWL showed increased parenchymal transit time of tracer with decreased renal function 2–3 days post-ESWL on the treated side, which returned to the pretreatment level by 3 weeks post-ESWL. Patients who received more than 1,000 shocks as compared with those who received fewer than 1,000 shocks had significantly greater increases in parenchymal transit time of nuclear tracer[101]. A functional study of scars left after PNCL and SWL revealed that scarring was similar but generally solitary when associated with the percutaneous access site for PCNL. Scarring could be multifocal after SWL. Therefore, PCNL was preferred if multiple sessions of SWL were anticipated[102]. Comparison of various methods of treatment of stones and their effects on renal function yielded no differences in an animal model, although the percentage of renal parenchymal scarring was significantly increased with percutaneous nephrostolithotomy[103]. Elevated creatinine was noted in 50% of patients with initial creatinine above 1.5mg/dl who underwent bilateral SWL, with significant rises in creatinine if multiple stones were treated[104]. The long-term effect of SWL on renal function in patients without pre-existing renal impairment appears to be minimal.

The incidence of hypertension (new-onset) after lithotripsy was initially reported to be 8%[105,106]. Further studies, however, consistently reported the incidence of new-onset hypertension in patients after lithotripsy not to be increased over that of the general population[107-110]. While systolic hypertension per se has not been shown to be increased after SWL, diastolic hypertension has been found in multiple studies[108,109,111]. Diastolic hypertension may be a dose-related phenomenon, with increasing number of shock waves correlating with more severe diastolic hypertension[108], although the renal pathophysiologic significance of diastolic hypertension is unclear. For all patients who undergo SWL, untreated hypertension, even small elevations, can have serious sequelae and should receive appropriate therapy[112].

Most of the preceding studies analyzing hypertension post-SWL did not stratify patients into at-risk groups or excluded patients with pre-existing hypertension, renal disease, or other risk factors for potentiated renal injury after SWL. These are the patients in whom the risk for hypertension after SWL may be the highest. In a recent study, patients over age 60 (who may have reduced renal mass or pre-existing hypertension) were found to develop hypertension at a higher rate than the control population, and this hypertension could be predicted by increased intrarenal resistive indices[113] (Figs 42.26 & 42.27). Therefore, it is reasonable to closely monitor at-risk patients for development of hypertension after SWL, and follow any post-SWL patient with developing diastolic hypertension for deterioration of renal function.

Stone recurrence after SWL is related to patient factors and lithotripsy factors. A large, longitudinal human study showed that significant increases in stone recurrence after SWL were correlated with previous history of stones, and number of stones. The 10-year stone recurrence rate was 41%[114]. However, a lithotripsy-specific causal relationship to increased stone recurrence has not been

Resistive index: increased risk of hypertension aged over 60				
Age	n	Pre-SWL	Post-SWL	p
<40	16	0.590 ± 0.041	0.597 ± 0.047	NS
40–59	21	0.650 ± 0.053	0.633 ± 0.052	NS
>60	20	0.644 ± 0.038	0.740 ± 0.050	<0.0001

Figure 42.26 Resistive index: increased risk of hypertension aged over 60. (Data from Janetschek et al.[113])

Hypertension in the elderly
9/20 patients aged >60 became hypertensive. Strong correlation between resistive index and diastolic blood pressure ($R^2 = 0.903$).

Figure 42.27 Hypertension in the elderly. (Data from Janetschek et al.[113])

Shock-wave lithotripsy in 2000
Lithotriptors less efficient but still effective for 80–85% of stones. Types of lithotriptor **not** important as long as endourologic skills adequate to manage cases not well treated with shock-wave lithotripsy.

Figure 42.28 Shock-wave lithotripsy in 2000.

identified. An animal model of SWL injury demonstrated rabbits that had undergone lithotripsy and then had hyperoxaluria induced showed crystal deposition in intercellular and intratubular regions of the kidney versus none in control animals[115]. This data poses the interesting question of whether SWL-induced trauma to the kidney predisposes that same kidney to increased crystal deposition with subsequent increased stone-formation in the future. Clinically, patients who are recurrent stone formers may simply have underlying metabolic or anatomic abnormalities which predispose them to further stone formation.

CONCLUSIONS

Over the past 15 years, lithotripsy has undergone revolutions in technology, anesthetic techniques, and indications. As indicated in Figure 42.28, SWL in 2000 reflects the decrease in efficacy of newer lithotriptors but the continuing ability to treat patients effectively by combining endourology and SWL for complete stone removal.

REFERENCES

1. Dyer RB, Zagoria RJ, Auringer ST, et al. Radiologic contribution to the management of patients undergoing extracorporeal shock-wave lithotripsy. Crit Rev Diag Imag. 1988;28:295–330.

2. Lifshitz DA, Williams JC Jr, Sturtevant B, et al. Quantitation of shock wave cavitation damage in vitro. Ultrasound Med Biol. 1997;23:461–71.

3. Crum LA. Cavitation microjets as a contributory mechanism for renal calculi disintegration in ESWL. J Urol. 1988;140:1587–90.

4. Delacretaz G, Rink K, Pittomvils G, et al. Importance of the implosion of ESWL-induced cavitation bubbles. Ultrasound Med Biol. 1995;21:97–103.

5. Zhong P, Cocks FH, Cioanta I, et al. Controlled, forced collapse of cavitation bubbles for improved stone fragmentation during shock-wave lithotripsy. J Urol. 1997;158:2323–8.

6. Howard D, Sturtevant B. In vitro study of the mechanical effects of shock-wave lithotripsy. Ultrasound Med Biol. 1997;23:1107–22.

7. Dahake G, Gracewski SM. Finite difference predictions of P-SV wave propagation inside submerged solids. II. Effect of geometry. J Acoust Soc Am. 1997;102:2138–45.

8. Dahake G, Gracewski SM. Finite difference predictions of P-SV wave propagation inside submerged solids. I. Liquid–solid interface conditions. J Acoust Soc Am. 1997;102:2125–37.

9. Newman R, Hackett R, Senior D, et al. Pathologic effects of ESWL on canine renal tissue. Urology. 1987;29:194–200.

10. Evan AP, McAteer JA Q-effects of shock-wave lithotripsy. In: Coe FL, Favus MJ, Pak CYC, Parks JH, Preminger GM, eds. Kidney stones: medical and surgical management. Philadelphia: Lippincott-Raven; 1996:549–70.

11. Evan AP, Willis LR, Lingeman JE, et al. Renal trauma and the risk of long-term complications in shock-wave lithotripsy. Nephron. 1998;78:1–8.

12. Khan SR, Hackett RL, Finlayson B. Morphology of urinary stone particles resulting from ESWL treatment. J Urol. 1986;136:1367–72.

13. Coleman AJ, Saunders JE, Crum LA, et al. Acoustic cavitation generated by an extracorporeal shockwave lithotripter. Ultrasound Med Biol. 1987;13:69–76.

14. Brummer F, Brenner J, Brauner T, et al. Effect of shock waves on suspended and immobilized L1210 cells. Ultrasound Med Biol. 1989;15:229–39.

15. McAteer JA, Stonehill MA, Colmenares K, et al. SWL cavitation damage in vitro: pressurization unmasks a differential response of foil targets and isolated cells. Seattle: American Institute of Physics; 1998;vol 4:2497–8.

16. Amouretti M, Perissat J, Collet D, et al. Effets tissulaires de la lithotritie extracorporelle sur un modele de lithiase biliaire experimentale du chien. Gastroenterol Clin Biol. 1989;13:489–94.

17. Donahue LA, Linke CA, Rowe JM. Renal loss following extracorporeal shock-wave lithotripsy. J Urol. 1989;142:809–11.

18. Meyer JJ, Cass AS. Subcapsular hematoma of the liver after renal extracorporeal shock-wave lithotripsy. J Urol. 1995;154:516–7.

19. Abrahams C, Lipson S, Ross L. Pathologic changes in the kidneys and other organs of dogs undergoing extracorporeal shock-wave lithotripsy with a tubeless lithotripter. J Urol. 1988;140:391–4.

20. Mullen KD, Hoofnagle JH, Jones EA. Shock wave-induced pancreatic trauma. Am J Gastroenterol. 1991;86:630–2.

21. Delius M, Draenert K, Al Diek Y, et al. Biological effects of shock waves: in vivo effect of high energy pulses on rabbit bone. Ultrasound Med Biol. 1995;21:1219–25.

22. Li B, Zhou W, Li P. Protective effects of nifedipine and allopurinol on high energy shock wave induced acute changes of renal function. J Urol. 1995;153:596–8.

23. Morris JS, Husmann DA, Wilson WT, et al. Temporal effects of shock-wave lithotripsy. J Urol. 1991;145:881–3.

24. Hasanoglu E, Buyan N, Bozkirli I, et al. The role of prostanoids in the complications of extracorporeal shock-wave lithotripsy (ESWL) in children. Prostagl Leukot Essent Fatty Acids. 1994;51:381–4.

25. Horgan PG, Hanley D, Burke J, et al. Extracorporeal shock-wave lithotripsy induces the release of prostaglandins which increase ureteric peristalsis. Br J Urol. 1993;71:648–52.

26. Masui N, Kobayashi S, Kurokawa J, et al. [Endothelin levels after extracorporeal shock waves, effects of renal function and blood pressure in rats]. Nippon Hinyokika Gakkai Zasshi – Jpn J Urol. 1996;87 1018–25.

27. Begun, FP, Lawson RK, Kearns CM, et al. Electrohydraulic shock wave induced renal injury. J Urol. 1989;142:155–9.

28. Willis LR, Evan AP, Connors BA, et al. Effects of extracorporeal shock-wave lithotripsy to one kidney on bilateral glomerular filtration rate and PAH clearance in minipigs. J Urol. 1996;156:1502–6.

29. Strohmaier WL, Carl AM, Wilbert DM, et al. Effects of extracorporeal shock-wave lithotripsy on plasma concentrations of endothelin and renin in humans. J Urol. 1996;155:48–51.

30. Winter P, Ganter K, Leppin U, et al. Glycosaminoglycans in urine and extracorporeal shock-wave lithotripsy. Urol Res. 1995; 23:401–5.

31. Weichert-Jacobsen K, Scheidt M, Kulkens C, et al. Morphological correlates of urinary enzyme loss after extracorporeal lithotripsy. Urol Res. 1997;25:257–62.

32. Heidenreich A, Bonfig R, Wilbert DM, et al. Painless ESWL by cutaneous application of vaseline. Scand J Urol Nephrol. 1995;29:155–60.

33. Pettersson B, Tiselius HG, Andersson A, et al. Evaluation of extracorporeal shock-wave lithotripsy without anesthesia using a Dornier HM3 lithotriptor without technical modifications. J Urol. 1989;142:1189–92.

34. Tiselius HG. Treatment of large staghorn stones and ureteral stones without anesthesia. Scand J Urol Nephrol Suppl. 1989;122:25–8.

35. Tiselius HG. Anesthesia-free in situ extracorporeal shock-wave lithotripsy of ureteral stones. J Urol. 1991;146:8–12.

36. Allman DB, Richlin DM, Ruttenberg M, et al. Analgesia in anesthesia-free extracorporeal shock-wave lithotripsy: a standardized protocol. J Urol. 1991;146:718–20.

37. Ganapathy S, Razvi H, Moote C, et al. Eutectic mixture of local anaesthetics is not effective for extracorporeal shock-wave lithotripsy. Can J Anaesth. 1996;43:1030–4.

38. Monk TG, Ding Y, White PF, et al. Effect of topical eutectic mixture of local anesthetics on pain response and analgesic requirement during lithotripsy procedures. Anesth Analg. 1994;79:506–11.

39. Barcena M, Rodriguez J, Gude F, et al. EMLA cream for renal extracorporeal shock-wave lithotripsy in ambulatory patients. Eur J Anaesthesiol. 1996;13:373–6.

40. Bierkens AF, Maes RM, Hendrikx JM, et al. The use of local anesthesia in second generation extracorporeal shock-wave lithotripsy: eutectic mixture of local anesthetics. J Urol. 1991;146:287–9.

41. Knudsen F, Jorgensen S, Bonde J, et al. Anesthesia and complications of extracorporeal shock-wave lithotripsy of urinary calculi. J Urol. 1992;148:1030–3.

42. Loening S, Kramolowsky EV, Willoughby B. Use of local anesthesia for extracorporeal shock-wave lithotripsy. J Urol. 1987;137:626–8.

43. Monk TG, Boure B, White PF, et al. Comparison of intravenous sedative-analgesic techniques for outpatient immersion lithotripsy [published erratum appears in Anesth Analg 1992;74(2):324]. Anesth Analg. 1991;72:616–21.

44. Vandeursen H, Pittomvils G, Matura E, et al. Anesthetic requirements during electromagnetic extracorporeal shock-wave lithotripsy. Urol Int. 1991;47:77–80.

45. Rassweiler J, Schmidt A, Gumpinger R, et al. ESWL for ureteral calculi. Using the Dornier HM 3, HM 3+ and Wolf Piezolith 2,200. J Urol (Paris). 1990;96:149–53.

46. Grenabo L, Lindqvist K, Adami HO, et al. Extracorporeal shock-wave lithotripsy for the treatment of renal stones. Treatment policy is as important for success as type of lithotriptor and patient selection. Arch Surg. 1997;132:20–6.

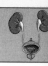
47. Bierkens AF, Hendrikx AJ, de Kort VJ, et al. Efficacy of second generation lithotriptors: a multicenter comparative study of 2,206 extracorporeal shock-wave lithotripsy treatments with the Siemens Lithostar, Dornier HM4, Wolf Piezolith 2300, Direx Tripter X-1 and Breakstone lithotriptors. J Urol. 1992;148:1052–6.

48. Denstedt JD, Clayman RV, Picus DD. Comparison of endoscopic and radiological residual fragment rate following percutaneous nephrolithotripsy. J Urol. 1991;145:703–5.

49. Coleman AJ, Saunders JE, Preston RC, et al. Pressure waveforms generated by a Dornier extra-corporeal shock-wave lithotripter. Ultrasound Med Biol. 1987;13:651–7.

50. Drach GW, Dretler S, Fair W, et al. Report of the United States cooperative study of extracorporeal shock-wave lithotripsy. J Urol. 1986;135:1127–33.

51. Lingeman JE, Coury TA, Newman DM, et al. Comparison of results and morbidity of percutaneous nephrostolithotomy and extracorporeal shock-wave lithotripsy. J Urol. 1987;138:485–90.

52. Kirkali Z, Esen AA, Mungan MU. Effectiveness of extracorporeal shockwave lithotripsy in the management of stone-bearing horseshoe kidneys. J Endourol. 1996;10:13–5.

53. Esuvaranathan K, Tan EC, Tung KH, et al. Stones in horseshoe kidneys: results of treatment by extracorporeal shock-wave lithotripsy and endourology. J Urol. 1991;146:1213–5.

54. Chen WC, Lee YH, Huang JK, et al. Experience using extracorporeal shock-wave lithotripsy to treat urinary calculi in problem kidneys. Urol Int. 1993;51:32–8.

55. Baltaci S, Sarica K, Ozdiler E, et al. Extracorporeal shockwave lithotripsy in anomalous kidneys. J Endourol. 1994;8:179–81.

56. Ackermann D, Claus R, Zehntner C, et al. Extracorporeal shock-wave lithotripsy for large renal stones. To what size is extracorporeal shock-wave lithotripsy alone feasible? Eur Urol.1988;15:5–8.

57. A consensus conference. Prevention and treatment of kidney stones. JAMA. 1988;260:977–81.

58. Segura, JW, Preminger GM, Assimos DG, et al. Ureteral Stones Clinical Guidelines Panel summary report on the management of ureteral calculi. J Urol. 1997;158:1915–21.

59. Lingeman JE, Newman D, Mertz JH, et al. Extracorporeal shock-wave lithotripsy: the Methodist Hospital of Indiana experience. J Urol. 1986;135:1134–7.

60. Wirth MP, Theiss M, Frohmuller HG. Primary extracorporeal shock-wave lithotripsy of staghorn renal calculi. Urol Int. 1992;48:71–5.

61. Locke DR, Newman RC, Steinbock GS, et al. Extracorporeal shock-wave lithotripsy in horseshoe kidneys. Urology. 1990;35:407–11.

62. Saw KC, Lingeman JE Percutaneous operative procedures in horseshoe kidneys. New York: Slack; 1998:17–1.

63. Jones JA, Lingeman JE, Steidle CP. The roles of extracorporeal shock-wave lithotripsy and percutaneous nephrolithotomy in the management of pyelocaliceal diverticula. J Urol. 1991;146:724–7.

64. Psihramis KE, Dretler SP. Extracorporeal shock-wave lithotripsy of caliceal diverticula calculi. J Urol. 1987;138:707–11.

65. Streem SB, Yost A. Treatment of caliceal diverticular calculi with extracorporeal shock-wave lithotripsy: patient selection and extended followup. J Urol. 1992;148:1043–6.

66. Bell BB, Lingeman JE Absence of metabolic activity following percutaneous treatment of calyceal diverticular calculi. Dallas: Slack; 1999.

67. Ruckle HC, Segura JW. Laparoscopic treatment of a stone-filled, caliceal diverticulum: a definitive, minimally invasive therapeutic option. J Urol. 1994;151:122–4.

68. Baldwin DD, Beaghler MA, Ruckle HC, et al. Ureteroscopic treatment of symptomatic caliceal diverticular calculi. Tech Urol. 1998;4:92–8.

69. Elbahnasy AM, Shalhav AL, Hoenig DM, et al. Lower caliceal stone clearance after shock-wave lithotripsy or ureteroscopy: the impact of lower pole radiographic anatomy. J Urol. 1998;159:676–82.

70. Ilker Y, Tarcan T, Akdas A. When should one perform shockwave lithotripsy for lower caliceal stones? J Endourol. 1995;9:439–41.

71. Havel D, Saussine C, Fath C, et al. Single stones of the lower pole of the kidney. Comparative results of extracorporeal shock-wave lithotripsy and percutaneous nephrolithotomy. Eur Urol. 1998;33:396–400.

72. Lingeman JE, Siegel YI, Steele B, et al. Management of lower pole nephrolithiasis: a critical analysis. J Urol. 1994;151:663–7.

73. May DJ, Chandhoke PS. Efficacy and cost-effectiveness of extracorporeal shock-wave lithotripsy for solitary lower pole renal calculi. J Urol. 1998;159:24–7.

74. Newman DM, Lingeman JE, Mertz JH, et al. Extracorporeal shock-wave lithotripsy. Urol Clin North Am. 1987;14:63–71.

75. Lingeman JE, Shirrell WL, Newman DM, et al. Management of upper ureteral calculi with extracorporeal shock-wave lithotripsy. J Urol. 1987;138:720–3.

76. Carini M, Selli C, Fiorelli C. Elective treatment of ureteral stones with extracorporeal shock-wave lithotripsy. Eur Urol. 1987;13:289–92.

77. Holmer NG, Almquist LO, Hertz TG, et al. On the mechanism of kidney stone disintegration by acoustic shock waves. Ultrasound Med Biol. 1991;17:479–89.

78. Bregg K, Riehle RA Jr. Morbidity associated with indwelling internal ureteral stents after shock-wave lithotripsy. J Urol. 1989;141:510–2.

79. Bierkens AF, Hendrikx AJ, Lemmens WA, et al. Extracorporeal shock-wave lithotripsy for large renal calculi: the role of ureteral stents. A randomized trial. J Urol. 1991;145:699–702.

80. Kirkali Z, Esen AA, Akan G. Place of double-J stents in extracorporeal shock-wave lithotripsy. Eur Urol. 1993;23:460–2.

81. Preminger GM, Kettelhut MC, Elkins SL, et al. Ureteral stenting during extracorporeal shock-wave lithotripsy: help or hindrance? J Urol. 1989;142:32–6.

82. Libby JM, Meacham RB, Griffith DP. The role of silicone ureteral stents in extracorporeal shock-wave lithotripsy of large renal calculi. J Urol. 1988;139:15–7.

83. Streem SB, Yost A, Mascha E. Clinical implications of clinically insignificant store fragments after extracorporeal shock-wave lithotripsy. J Urol. 1996;155:1186–90.

84. Kim SC, Moon YT, Kim KD. Extracorporeal shock-wave lithotripsy monotherapy: experience with piezoelectric second generation lithotriptor in 642 patients. J Urol. 1989;142:674–8.

85. Elhilali MM, Stoller ML, McNamara TC, et al. Effectiveness and safety of the Dornier compact lithotriptor: an evaluative multicenter study. J Urol. 1996;155:834–8.

86. Grasso M, Loisides P, Beaghler M, et al. The case for primary endoscopic management of upper urinary tract calculi: I. A critical review of 121 extracorporeal shock-wave lithotripsy failures. Urology. 1995;45:363–71.

87. Cochran JS, Robinson SN, Crane VS, et al. Extracorporeal shock-wave lithotripsy. Use of antibiotics to avoid postprocedural infection. Postgrad Med. 1988;83:199–204.

88. Knapp PM, Kulb TB, Lingeman JE, et al. Extracorporeal shock-wave lithotripsy-induced perirenal hematomas. J Urol. 1988;139:700–3.

89. Streem SB, Yost A. Extracorporeal shock-wave lithotripsy in patients with bleeding diatheses. J Urol. 1990;144:1347–8.

90. Dominguez Molinero JF, Arrabal Martin M, Mijan Ortiz JL, et al. Hematomas renales secundarios a litotricia extracorporea por ondas de choque. Arch Esp Urol. 1997;50:767–71.

91. Chen CS, Lai MK, Hsieh ML, et al. Subcapsular hematoma of spleen – a complication following extracorporeal shock-wave lithotripsy for ureteral calculus. Chang Keng i Hsueh – Chang Gung Med J. 1992;15:215–9.

92. Marcuzzi D, Gray R, Wesley-James T. Symptomatic splenic rupture following extracorporeal shock-wave lithotripsy. J Urol. 1991;145:547–8.

93. Fugita OE, Trigo-Rocha F, Mitre AI, et al. Splenic rupture and abscess after extracorporeal shock-wave lithotripsy. Urology. 1998;52:322–3.

94. Fuchs GJ, David RD, Fuchs AM. Complicaciones de la litotricia extracorporea por ondas de choque. Arch Esp Urol. 1989;42 (Suppl. 1):83–9.

95. Lingeman JE, Newman DM, Siegel YI, et al. shock-wave lithotripsy with the Dornier MFL 5000 lithotriptor using an external fixed rate signal. J Urol. 1995;154:951–4.

96. Kataoka H. [Cardiac dysrhythmias related to extracorporeal shock-wave lithotripsy using a piezoelectric lithotriptor in patients with kidney stones]. J Cardiol. 1995;26:185–91.

97. Elabbady A, Mathes G, Morehouse DD, et al. Safety and effectiveness of Lithostar shock tube C in the treatment of urinary calculi. J Endourol. 1995;9:225–31.

98. Winters JC, Macaluso JN Jr. Ungated Medstone outpatient lithotripsy. J Urol. 1995;153:593–5.

99. Drach GW, Weber C, Donovan JM. Treatment of pacemaker patients with extracorporeal shock-wave lithotripsy: experience from 2 continents. J Urol. 1990;143:895–6.

100. Cooper D, Wilkoff B, Masterson M, et al. Effects of extracorporeal shock-wave lithotripsy on cardiac pacemakers and its safety in patients with implanted cardiac pacemakers. Pacing Clin Electrophysiol. 1988;11:1607–16.

101. Bomanji J, Boddy SA, Britton KE, et al. Radionuclide evaluation pre- and postextracorporeal shock-wave lithotripsy for renal calculi. J Nucl Med. 1987;28:1284–9.

102. Lechevallier E, Siles S, Ortega JC, et al. Comparison by SPECT of renal scars after extracorporeal shock-wave lithotripsy and percutaneous nephrolithotomy. J Endourol. 1993;7:465–7.

103. Wilson WT, Husmann DA, Morris JS, et al. A comparison of the bioeffects of four different modes of stone therapy on renal function and morphology. J Urol. 1993;150:1267–70.

104. Cass AS. Renal function after bilateral extracorporeal shockwave lithotripsy. J Endourol. 1994;8:395–9.

105. Lingeman JE, Kulb TB. Hypertension following extracorporeal shock-wave lithotripsy. J Urol. 1987;137:142A.

106. Williams CM, Kaude JV, Newman RC, et al. Extracorporeal shock-wave lithotripsy: long-term complications. AJR. 1988;150:311–5.

107. Zanetti G, Montanari E, Trinchieri A, et al. Long-term follow-up of blood pressure after extracorporeal shock-wave lithotripsy. J Endourol. 1992;6:195–7.

108. Yokoyama M, Shoji F, Yanagizawa R, et al. Blood pressure changes following extracorporeal shock-wave lithotripsy for urolithiasis. J Urol. 1992;147:553–7.

109. Lingeman JE, Woods JR, Toth PD. Blood pressure changes following extracorporeal shock-wave lithotripsy and other forms of treatment for nephrolithiasis. JAMA. 1990;263:1789–94.

110. Dannenberg AL, Garrison RJ, Kannel WB. Incidence of hypertension in the Framingham study. Am J Pub Health. 1988;78:676.

111. Claro JdA, Lima ML, Ferreira U, et al. Blood pressure changes after extracorporeal shock-wave lithotripsy in normotensive patients. J Urol. 1993;150:1765–7.

112. Prevention of stroke by antihypertensive drug treatment in older persons with isolated systolic hypertension. Final results of the Systolic Hypertension in the Elderly Program (SHEP). SHEP Cooperative Research Group [see comments]. JAMA. 1991;265 3255–64.

113. Janetschek G, Frauscher F, Knapp R, et al. New onset hypertension after extracorporeal shock-wave lithotripsy: age related incidence and prediction by intrarenal resistive index. J Urol. 1997;158:346–51.

114. Kato S, Tanda H, Ohnishi S, et al. [Recurrence of stones after extracorporeal shock-wave lithotripsy]. Hinyokika Kiyo – Acta Urol Jpn. 1996;42:717–22.

115. Sarica K, Soygur T, Yaman O, et al. Stone recurrence after shockwave lithotripsy: possible enhanced crystal deposition in traumatized tissue in rabbit model. J Endourol. 1996;10:513–7.

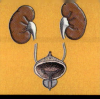

Section 8 Miscellaneous

Chapter 43

Genitourinary Trauma

Jack W McAninch and Michael H Safir

KEY POINTS

- Most blunt renal trauma can be managed conservatively. Indications for exploration include intraoperative identification of an expanding perirenal hematoma, persistent renal derived hemorrhage, and injury to major renal vasculature.
- Although low grade penetrating renal injuries, in a stable patient, can be managed conservatively, higher grade injuries, because of the risk of delayed hemorrhage, should be explored.
- Almost all extraperitoneal bladder injuries can be managed nonoperatively, usually with a Foley catheter. In contrast, intraperitoneal bladder injuries almost always mandate surgical repair.
- Controversy exists as to whether to treat acute urethral injury with a suprapubic cystostomy and delayed reconstruction, or with primary repair.
- If at all feasible, penile amputation is treated with replantation.

INTRODUCTION

As surgeons who are trained to diagnose and treat victims of trauma, we also inherit an obligation to educate about trauma, both intentional and accidental. As an example, physicians have taken a leadership role in seat belt safety and have spearheaded efforts both to improve seat belt design (use of shoulder harness versus lap belt[1]) and to promote widespread routine usage[2]. Despite this effort, health care providers have quite variable compliance toward this educational effort[3]. While the direct implications of seatbelt use on genitourinary injury is the subject of some debate[4], widespread use has been supported by all major medical societies, including the American College of Surgeons and the American Medical Association.

As urologists, we need to take a leadership position in the development of guidelines for genitourinary trauma or we may be relegated to following guidelines instead of creating them. As clinicians, we are frequently called on to evaluate a variety of injuries, some innocuous and some lethal, and are asked to contribute to developing a diagnostic and treatment plan for the individual patient. Often, these injuries are uncommon, either uncommon in the specialty of urologic trauma or, more appropriately, uncommon within our own practice. Although it is helpful to refer to

algorithms related to trauma, it is more important to understand the rationale underlying these algorithms. Initial decision-making for urologic trauma, and indeed for any organ injury, may be thought of as an evolving process: Detection, Diagnosis, and Disposition. Within this chapter, we hope to illustrate some important concepts in acute genitourinary trauma and help the individual reader develop a working understanding about care of the injured patient.

ACUTE ASSESSMENT

By the time the urologist has been consulted to evaluate the acutely injured patient, the patient has usually been seen by the emergency department physician and, often, by the trauma surgeon. Since it is unusual that trauma within the urologic domain represents the sole life-threatening injury, initial trauma evaluation and intervention is appropriately relegated to support of the patient's airway and provision of volume resuscitation. Following standard resuscitation in the field, triage for trauma patients is focused on identifying patients who are likely to have sustained major trauma and will require the participation of a designated trauma center. These criteria have been developed to reflect the severity of physiologic, anatomic, and mechanical alterations (Fig. 43.1) present in significant trauma[5].

Following establishment of a stable airway and assurance of ventilation, circulatory function must be assessed. It is important to note that, in young patients, hypotension is an unreliable indicator of shock, since compensatory mechanisms of vasoconstriction and tachycardia may be surprisingly effective. Young patients may sustain as much as 30% loss in circulatory volume without an appreciable decrease in blood pressure, although careful and directed examination early on may reveal a narrowed pulse pressure. In unusual cases, despite an apparently adequate circulatory reserve, hypovolemic shock is irretrievable in some 'well-resuscitated' young patients[6], a phenomenon that most probably results from inotropic decompensation accompanying myocardial depression.

Since the primary survey of the trauma patient investigates immediate life-threatening injuries, it is during the 'secondary survey', after resuscitation, that physical examination may reveal direct genitourinary (GU) trauma (e.g. genital skin loss) or may reveal the potential for GU trauma (e.g. flank ecchymosis). During this appraisal, all trauma patients should be questioned regarding their medical and surgical history, recent medication and illicit drugs use, medicinal allergies, and time of last meal. As we will discuss, it is during this stage of evaluation that we begin to undertake diagnostic studies to answer important clinical questions.

Criteria for transfer of patient to Level I trauma facility	
Criteria type	Specific criteria
Physiologic	Systolic blood pressure <90
	Glasgow Coma Score <13
	Respiratory rate <10 or >30
	By a prehospital trauma index, e.g. revised trauma score, circulation, respiration, abdomen, motor, and speech, etc.
Anatomic	All penetrating injuries to head/neck, thorax, and abdomen
	Flail chest
	Pelvic fractures
	Para- or quadriplegic
	Two or more proximal long bone fractures
	Proximal amputations
Mechanism of injury	Ejection or roll-over motor vehicle crash
	Other death in same passenger compartment
	Fall from a height (>6m)
	Pedestrian struck
	Motorcycle crash with separation of rider and bike

Figure 43.1 Criteria for transfer of patient to Level I trauma facility. (With permission from Mackersie and Gillon[5].)

RENAL TRAUMA

Renal injuries are the most common type of urinary trauma and are believed to occur in approximately 10% of patients sustaining abdominal trauma. To appropriately treat renal trauma, we must accurately diagnose it. To accurately diagnose renal trauma, we must first be able to discover it by entertaining the diagnosis of renal injury in appropriate patients. Clinically, it may be suggested in some patients:

- those demonstrating significant flank ecchymosis;
- those presenting with lower (T8–12) rib fractures;
- those sustaining major deceleration injuries, either falls or motor vehicle injuries; and
- those sustaining a penetrating abdominal or flank injury.

Despite the attractiveness of such guidelines, in actuality they are all quite poor when used to predict the significance of renal injury. Since it is economically impractical and clinically inappropriate to subject all patients to radiographic and, perhaps, surgical exploration, certain 'tools' such as hematuria may be applied to assist clinical decision-making.

Hematuria and the need for imaging studies

The presence or absence of hematuria is the single most important factor available to help gauge the presence or severity of renal injury. Does the presence of microscopic hematuria mandate radiographic imaging in all instances? Not necessarily. Ideally, imaging studies should only be obtained when they are likely to demonstrate significant injury. At San Francisco General Hospital, our group has elected to selectively manage blunt renal trauma, based upon retrospective and prospective review of patients entered into a trauma database over the last 22 years[7,8]. These data provided many valuable insights; the most prominent are as follows.

- The management of blunt and penetrating injuries must be separately considered.
- Adult blunt renal trauma patients presenting with microhematuria but without shock (BP_{sys} <90mmHg.) virtually never are identified to have significant renal injury. Radiographic staging is seldom necessary in these patients.
- A special case exists for blunt trauma coincident with microhematuria and shock, since major renal vascular injury cannot be excluded. Radiographic imaging in these patients is indicated.

Sometimes we are unable to obtain the imaging studies that we want. The stabilized 30-year-old unrestrained automobile passenger who presents with gross hematuria should be evaluated with upper urinary tract imaging [computed tomography (CT or intravenous urography (IVU)] and cystography. However, in the unstable patient, we may be unable to complete the secondary survey and may simply be provided with a 'one-shot' intravenous pyelogram prior to meeting the patient in the operating room. Since trauma care requires a team approach, our recommended studies should be synchronized with studies mandated by other surgical services to avoid confusion and repetition and to avert any potentially harmful delays.

Choice of radiographic imaging

Computed axial tomography (CAT) has risen to the forefront of available technologies for evaluation of blunt trauma because of its availability, its resolution of parenchymal detail, and its suitability for evaluation of other abdominal and retroperitoneal injuries. The advent of the helical CT technique has potentially provided a valuable new tool for the evaluation of real trauma[9]. This value is apparent both in the speed of image acquisition for the kidney and other imaged organs and in the propriety for multidimensional reconstruction. Despite the obvious benefit of a 'faster' study, it is important to remember that initial images may represent only corticomedullary filling, and may miss important diagnoses such as urinary extravasation, unless delayed (5 minute) images demonstrating the collecting system are obtained.

Although it is too early to predict whether it will be of value for evaluating the acutely injured patient, three-dimensional CT reconstruction of the injured kidney is an enticing possibility of helical imaging. Specifically, its greatest benefit may be in the evaluation of blunt renal trauma, when the surgeon is considering conservative management via observation. Rendered images may more accurately mimic what we find at renal exploration and may provide a unique 'window' into the surgical anatomy of the patient. We believe that this form of imaging may indeed be suitable to evaluate the patient who is being managed conservatively and shows promise as a noninvasive means of renal angiography, since the technique can demonstrate subtle arterial injuries of both the main artery and its branches.

Unfortunately, recent accounts of magnetic resonance imaging (MRI) have failed to demonstrate any advantage of the more costly and time-consuming MRI over a conventional CT scan, particularly with regard to injury staging[10]. However, MRI may be a worthwhile consideration for the patient with renal insufficiency or contrast allergy. In the future, magnetic resonance angiography (MRA) may have a role as a safe alternative to conventional contrast angiography for the evaluation of the stable patient suspected of segmental arteriolar injury.

Staging of injury

To simplify and standardize the evaluation and treatment of such patients, urologists have applied a system of staging paradigms and treatment algorithms, analogous to systems successfully used in the less chaotic arena of, for example, urologic oncology. To address this need, accurate, safe, and cost-conscious 'staging' algorithms have been devised, which use available information from clinical, radiographic and surgical findings (Fig. 43.2).

Management of renal trauma

For the management of blunt trauma, absolute indications for exploration include intraoperative identification of a pulsatile expanding perirenal hematoma, persistent hemorrhage believed to stem from renal injury, and known injury to the major renal vasculature (grade 5 injury; Fig. 43.3). Relative indications for renal exploration include (1) obvious urinary extravasation (Fig. 43.4), (2) shattered kidney with bulky, nonviable tissue, or (3) inability to convincingly stage the patient's injury. Most injuries are potential candidates for observational treatment (Fig. 43.5).

In contrast with the infrequent need for renal exploration for blunt trauma, urologic surgeons usually have historically a reduced threshold for exploring the patient who has sustained penetrating renal trauma. Since associated abdominal injury often mandates renal exploration, urologists are frequently consulted during the course of laparotomy regarding the need to proceed with renal exploration. Velmahos and colleagues at the University of Southern California retrospectively investigated 52 patients sustaining renal gunshot wounds[11] and avoided renal exploration in 20 patients (38%), concluding that many patients may unnecessarily be subjected to renal exploration. In the series, stable patients with low-grade injuries and without coincident surgical abdominal injuries avoided laparotomy. For patients undergoing laparotomy for nonrenal injury, the renal hematoma was explored only if bleeding was active or the hematoma was large. Overall, however, 92% (48/52) patients underwent laparotomy for renal and nonrenal indications. Exploration was carefully considered,

since 53% of patients explored required nephrectomy for severe (grade IV and V) injuries. The necessity of nephrectomy at exploration has been reported less frequently[12] in other series (14%) and may be avoided by liberal application of partial nephrectomy and renorrhaphy techniques.

To evaluate selective management of stab wounds, Tavioglu in Istanbul retrospectively investigated 387 patients sustaining abdominal stab wounds over a 3-year period[13], finding a 1.3% risk of renal injury requiring renal surgery. Our own retrospective investigation of significant penetrating renal trauma (grade 2–4 injuries) focused on 120 patients managed either with observation or renal exploration[14]. The group treated with observation were (1) significantly more likely to have sustained a stab wound rather than a gunshot, (2) less likely to have coincident abdominal injury

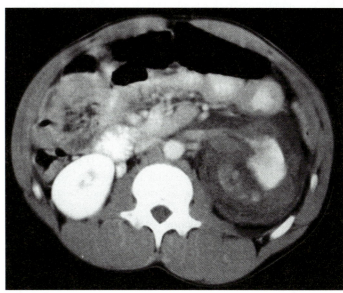

Figure 43.3 Grade 5 injury. The left kidney has been completely disrupted and is not in complete continuity.

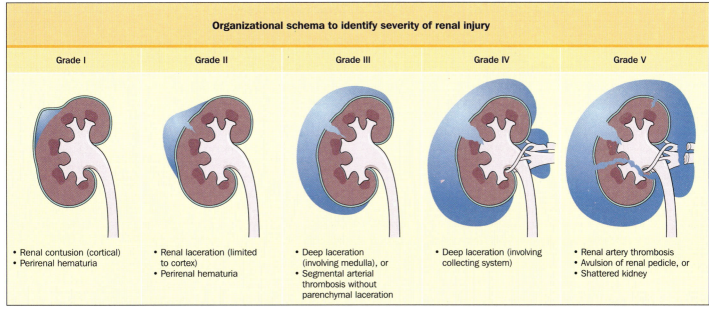

Figure 43.2 Organizational schema to identify severity of renal injury.

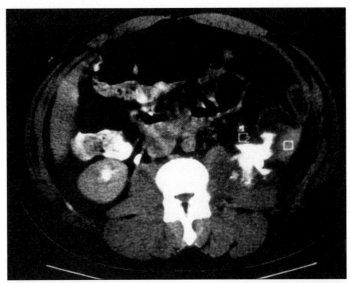

Figure 43.4 Blunt trauma resulting from motor vehicle injury. Contrast adjacent to the left psoas muscle represents urinary extravasation (Grade 4).

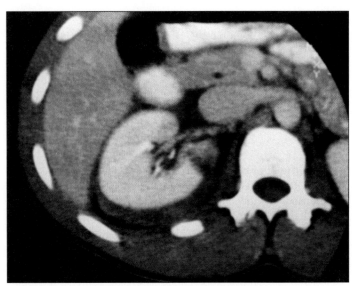

Figure 43.5 Deceleration injury resulting in Grade 3 parenchymal injury in the posteromedial aspect of the right kidney. A small perirenal hematoma is easily apparent.

requiring surgery, and (3) less likely to require transfusion ($p<0.0001$). Specifically among stab wound victims, patients were more likely to require surgery if (1) they presented in shock, (2) had associated intra-abdominal injury, or (3) required transfusion. We were particularly troubled by the significant risk of delayed bleeding among patients with grade 3 and 4 injuries in the observation group (23%) (Fig. 43.4).

Overall, as a general guideline regarding penetrating trauma, surgical decision-making should focus on signs of clinical stability, grade of injury and presence of associated injuries. All unstable intra-abdominal injuries should be explored. Stable patients with grade 1 or 2 renal injuries may be managed with observation. Because of the strong association of delayed bleeding with higher grade injuries (grades 3 or 4), severe renal trauma should mandate synchronous renal exploration for patients undergoing laparotomy for nonrenal injuries (Fig. 43.5).

There are a few recent reports regarding the management and sequelae of renal arterial injuries[15] (Fig. 43.6). Overall, these injuries are quite rare[16] and seldom result in successful outcomes. Haas and coworkers at Case Western reviewed hospital records on 12 patients sustaining renal arterial occlusion following blunt trauma[17]. Their salvage rate was poor: of 5 patients undergoing attempt at surgical revascularization, 1 patient required nephrectomy, 3 patients' kidneys demonstrated no function and 1 patient demonstrated 9% function on postoperative renal scan.

Less invasive means of renal reconstruction have evolved, most prominently endovascular repair using vascular stents; however, these attempts are mostly reflected in individual case reports. Goodman and colleagues presented recent successful treatment of an occlusive injury to the main renal artery from an intimal flap, which is the most common form of vascular injury following blunt renal trauma[18] (Fig. 43.7). After identification of the injury, a Palmaz stent was placed under angiographic guidance, after which the patient underwent a 2-month interval of anticoagulation. Follow-up nuclear renal scintigraphy identified normal renal function. We have been disappointed with our rates of renal salvage via open surgery (15–20%) and consider this pilot angiographic procedure a reasonable alternative to retrieve ischemic injury.

Operative approach to the injured kidney

Suspected renal trauma should be explored via a midline transperitoneal incision. Since renal bleeding is the predominant issue forcing nephrectomy in the trauma setting, we obtain vascular control of the kidney prior to renal exploration. Incision of the parietal peritoneum over the aorta allows access to the renal arteries and veins prior to retroperitoneal exploration (Fig. 43.8 left panel). This maneuver provides rapid vascular access to contend with uncontrolled renal hemorrhage. After looping the vessels, the right or left colon, as appropriate, is reflected medially and the white line of Toldt is incised, providing access to Gerota's fascia. Incision into the fascia releases tamponade of the perirenal hematoma and, again, should be performed only if vascular control is established (Fig. 43.8 right panel). The kidney is then mobilized within Gerota's fascia to enable complete surface inspection of the four items: kidney, renal vessels, renal pelvis, and ureter. If grossly devitalized renal parenchyma is encountered, it is conservatively debrided until healthy bleeding tissue is encountered.

The surgical assistant provides the essential hemostatic maneuver of manually compressing the kidney, to allow more definitive and directed hemostasis using 4-0 figure-of-eight chromic sutures (Fig. 43.9). By focusing on local hemostatic control, it is unusual that bleeding necessitates clamping of the main renal artery or surface renal hypothermia. After control of bleeding is established, any violations of urothelium are repaired with 4-0 chromic sutures. Occult collecting system injuries may be made more conspicuous by instilling 3ml methylene blue into the renal pelvis while compressing the ureter.

Three types of parenchymal injury may be described:
- Superficial parenchymal injury without tissue loss. Principles of repair include meticulous hemostasis and repair or replacement of renal capsule, usually with perinephric fat or omentum (Fig. 43.10).

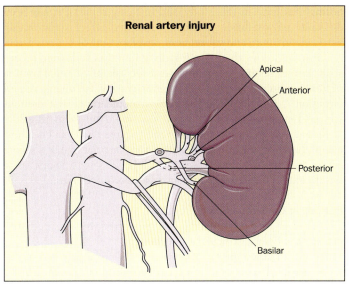

Figure 43.6 Renal artery injury. Arterial injury may manifest within the main renal artery, the posterior branch, or any of four main divisions of the anterior branch.

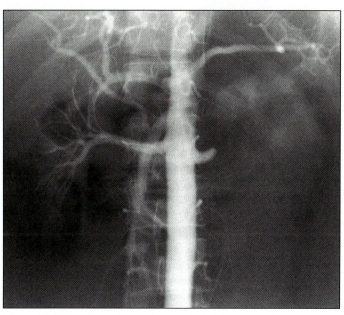

Figure 43.7 Arteriography performed for non-visualization of the left kidney following blunt trauma. This image demonstrates abrupt contrast cessation within the proximal renal artery.

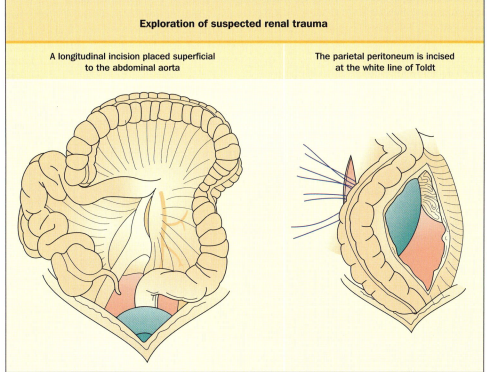

Figure 43.8 Exploration of suspected renal trauma. (Left) A longitudinal incision is placed directly superficial to the abdominal aorta. If the size of the hematoma precludes facile identification of the aorta, the incision is placed medial to the inferior mesenteric vein. (Right) Following vascular control, the parietal peritoneum is incised at the white line of Toldt. Release of tamponade without prior vascular control may result in significant hemorrhage.

Exploration of suspected renal trauma

A longitudinal incision placed superficial to the abdominal aorta

The parietal peritoneum is incised at the white line of Toldt

- Polar injury with tissue loss. Partial nephrectomy is appropriate for debridement of devitalized tissue caused by severe polar trauma (Fig. 43.10).
- Mid-organ injury with tissue loss. Renorrhaphy may include suture closure over Gelfoam for hemostasis, use of omentum for coverage, or placement of a mesh bag to prevent hemorrhage (Fig. 43.10).

Nephrectomy should be performed only for shattered kidneys that cannot be reconstructed or in the rare setting that attention to life-threatening coincident intra-abdominal injury prevents time necessary for renorrhaphy. Penrose or Jackson–Pratt drains are important adjuncts to renorrhaphy, since short-term drain complications are preferable to urinoma or infection. Peripheral collecting system injuries do not mandate double-J

43

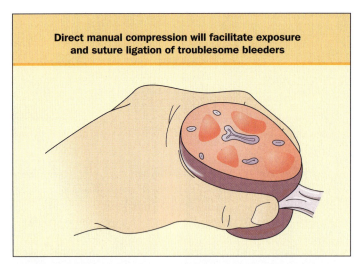

Direct manual compression will facilitate exposure and suture ligation of troublesome bleeders

Figure 43.9 Direct manual compression will facilitate exposure and suture ligation of troublesome bleeders.

stenting, although stenting is recommended for injuries to the renal pelvis or ureteropelvic junction.

Sequelae of renal injury

Two outcomes of renal trauma that have received ongoing attention are (1) development of renovascular hypertension following occult renal injury and (2) quantitative assessment of renal function following post-traumatic reconstruction. To address the former issue, Montgomery and colleagues reviewed a trauma database and identified 7 patients who were pre-traumatically normotensive, in whom hypertension developed between 2 weeks and 8 months following 'occult' trauma[19]. However, no patient was actually diagnosed with a renal injury; indeed, 6 patients underwent contrast urography (3 CT, 3 IVU) with

normal findings. In this study, and in many reports, it has been difficult to establish a clear cause-and-effect relationship between an injury and subsequent development of hypertension.

How well does the injured kidney function following reconstruction? A recent report reviewed records of 52 renal trauma patients who underwent renal scintigraphy following reconstruction[20]. At follow-up, the reconstructed renal unit demonstrated a mean of 39.3% of overall function. Approximately 20% of reconstructed kidneys were found to have less than one third overall function. As univariate issues, renovascular injuries, severe coincident injuries, and extensive blood loss with shock were significant factors related to poor function outcomes.

Pediatric considerations

The special case of renal trauma sustained by the pediatric patient has been distinguished because:

- a child's kidney may be more vulnerable to injury because of physical differences such as proportionally increased size and a relatively poor perinephric 'cushion'[21];
- indicators of clinical 'shock' may be veiled, as hypotension is not a reliable sign among the young; and
- accurate paradigms for evaluation and treatment are not as well defined as in the adult population.

Brown and coworkers[22] investigated whether children are more at risk for major renal injury caused by blunt trauma. Comparison between a small consecutive cohort of adults (35 patients) and children (34) identified major injury (grade 4 or 5) more commonly in the pediatric sample ($p<0.04$). A conclusion that children are more at risk for severe injury may require a larger cohort investigation, but it is clear that children are at least at commensurate risk with adults.

Recent data has explored whether application of adult criteria mandating radiographic imaging is appropriate for the pediatric population and if our diagnostic testing can be accurately applied

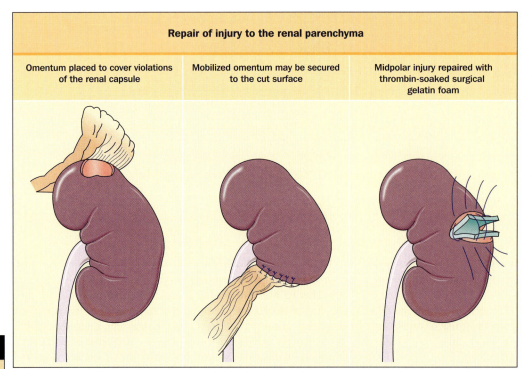

Repair of injury to the renal parenchyma

| Omentum placed to cover violations of the renal capsule | Mobilized omentum may be secured to the cut surface | Midpolar injury repaired with thrombin-soaked surgical gelatin foam |

Figure 43.10 Repair of injury to the renal parenchyma. (Left) Available omentum may be placed to cover significant violations of the renal capsule. (Center) Following polar nephrectomy for severe direct and blast injury, the mobilized omentum may be circumferentially secured to the cut surface. This maneuver will aid hemostasis and may reduce the risk of urinary leak. (Right) Midpolar injury with or without parenchymal loss may be repaired with a wedge of thrombin-soaked surgical gelatin foam, secured in place with imbricating capsular sutures.

in clinical decision-making[23]. Within a group of 180 patients 16 years or younger, decision to perform radiographic imaging was retrospectively analyzed according to degree of hematuria at presentation. Only one child with microscopic hematuria (0.7% of the subpopulation) had sustained significant (grade 2 or higher) injury. This contrasts with gross hematuria, a finding with which 27% of children were identified as having significant renal injury. We are convinced that selective imaging is appropriate for the management of stable pediatric renal injury, and support use of (>50RBC/high-power field) as a benchmark, on the basis of the findings of the above study.

URETERAL INJURY

Since the ureter travels from the upper flank to the base of the pelvic diaphragm, it is potentially exposed to external trauma directed anywhere between the ribs and the base of the bony pelvis. Despite this potential, it is injured very rarely (<1% of urinary trauma), owing both to its protected location in the retroperitoneum and to its small cross-sectional area. Because of the comparatively small volume of clinical experience with ureteral injuries, compared with, say, renal trauma, heuristics for diagnosis and treatment are not well established. Additionally, we are forced to use imaging studies (IVU, CT) that have documented benefit for evaluation of renal injuries but unproven efficacy for the diagnosis of ureteral injury.

As opposed to renal and bladder injuries, penetrating injuries are most common, gunshot wounds more frequently causing injury than stab wounds. If present, direct injury from blunt trauma may take the form of ureteral contusion, which is most commonly seen from impaction of the ureter against vertebral bodies.

At present, the most commonly used methods for preoperative evaluation of suspected ureteral trauma are IVU or CT of the retroperitoneum with intravenous contrast. Injuries, when present, may be manifest as extravasation of contrast at the level of injury, often with lateral deviation of the ureter from hematoma or urinoma. Unfortunately, injuries may escape recognition since hematuria, excluding those with coincident renal or bladder trauma, may be present in as few as 53% of patients[24]. Of equal concern is the fact that as few as 40% of imaging studies (CT, IVU) may display any radiographic features of injury.

Since penetrating injuries to the ureter are virtually always associated with synchronous intraperitoneal injury (small bowel most common, followed by colon and stomach), recognition of injury is frequently performed at laparotomy. Reflection of the ascending or descending colon, as appropriate, will provide access to the ureter, at which point the ureter may be inspected for injury. Intravenous injection of indigocarmine (5mL) will reveal the site of injury within 10 minutes in the well-resuscitated patient. Infrequently, retrograde pyelography can be used for diagnosis if laparotomy is not otherwise mandated. After diagnosis, the type of ureteral repair should be tailored to the site of injury and to the viable length of the remaining proximal segment (Fig. 43.11).

Complete disruptions of the ureteropelvic junction are quite rare. Injuries are believed to occur more commonly among children as a result of a hyperextensible vertebral column.

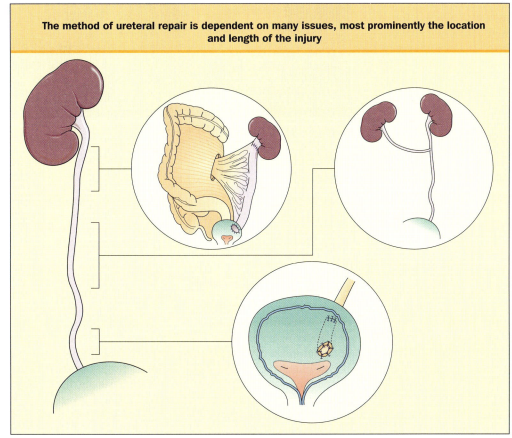

The method of ureteral repair is dependent on many issues, most prominently the location and length of the injury

Figure 43.11 The method of ureteral repair is dependent on many issues, most prominently the location and length of the injury. As examples, distal ureteral injuries (bottom) are usually repaired with simple reimplantation, using psoas hitch or Boari flap when necessary if tissue loss is more extensive. Midureteral injuries (center) are virtually always treated with ipsilateral ureteroureterotomy (IUU), or rarely by crosstransfer of the ureter, transureteroureterotomy (TUU). Severe tissue loss in the proximal ureter (top) frequently makes IUU or TUU impossible, leading to transposition of ileum to replace the ureter (ileal ureter).

Because of a paucity of clinical stigmata specific for the diagnosis of ureteropelvic junction injury, the diagnosis is made radiographically[25]. A tetrad of radiologic signs at urography have previously been described[26]:

- unremarkable renal excretion of intravenous contrast;
- intact calyceal system;
- extravasation of contrast in the region of the ureteropelvic junction (UPJ); and
- nonfilling of the affected ureter.

Surgical management of ureteropelvic avulsion focuses on re-establishing continuity by watertight anastomosis and provision of reliable drainage (Penrose or Jackson–Pratt).

BLADDER INJURY

Since the urinary bladder is a pliable organ and may occupy both the abdomen and the pelvis, it is vulnerable to the myriad injuries that may occur in either anatomic location. For instance, fixation of the bladder within the pelvis by endopelvic fascia and neurovascular pedicles, as well as proximity of the organ to adjacent pelvic bones, makes bladder injuries opportune to blunt injuries to the pelvis. Bladder rupture, in fact, is associated with pelvic fracture in approximately 90% of cases. Although seemingly protected from trauma by the bony pelvis, the bladder is vulnerable to penetrating trauma as well, through displacement to an intra-abdominal position following physiologic distention.

Triage of suspected bladder injury

The possibility of bladder injury should be considered in virtually all patients seen for traumatic hematuria. Indeed, similar caveats mandating upper and lower urinary tract evaluation for hematuria and suspected malignancy are true for evaluation of traumatic hematuria. Patients in whom hematuria demands bladder imaging include those sustaining blunt lower abdominal trauma, those with pelvic trauma and those sustaining penetrating imaging to the abdomen or pelvis. As a single sign, gross hematuria is present in 95% of bladder ruptures occurring from blunt trauma, although even microscopic hematuria may be absent[27] despite significant injury. To best understand the diagnosis and treatment of bladder injuries, it is helpful to distinguish injuries according to mechanism and type of injury:

- extraperitoneal bladder rupture resulting from blunt trauma, usually in association with pelvic fracture (Fig. 43.12);
- intraperitoneal bladder rupture resulting from blunt trauma, usually in association with a full bladder and deceleration injury (Fig. 43.13); or
- penetrating bladder injury.

A retrograde cystogram is essential to provide a diagnosis of bladder injury. The bladder is filled under gravity to a volume of 300mL using iodinated contrast material. Anteroposterior radiographic images are most commonly performed to assess for urinary extravasation, although many centers include oblique images to facilitate identification of posterior bladder injuries. It is essential to obtain images following evacuation of the bladder, since overlying contrast from bladder filling may mask subtle extravasation.

- Intraperitoneal injuries result in contrast outlining of the peritoneal contents (especially small bowel) and contrast may characteristically settle into the paracolic gutters.

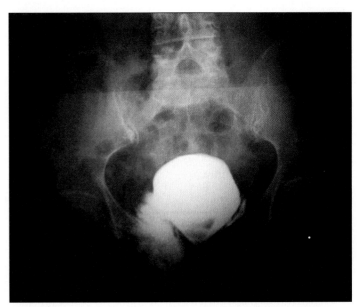

Figure 43.12 Extravasation of urine from the bladder following pelvic trauma. This may appear as a radio-opaque flare or 'flame' adjacent to the organ, without evidence of contrast within the peritoneum.

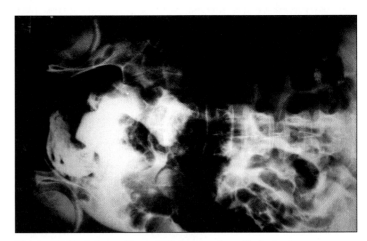

Figure 43.13 Intraperitoneal bladder rupture. Cystogram demonstrating partial opacification of the bladder with contrast outlining the bowel and dependent collection of urine in the left paracolic gutter.

- Extraperitoneal injuries may be revealed when contrast extravasates but remains confined within the space of Retzius.

The CT cystogram is equivalent to conventional cystography, provided the bladder is sufficiently filled under gravity. False-negative studies may result if the bladder is simply allowed to physiologically fill with urine while the catheter is clamped, since distention may be necessary to detect if a blood clot or portion of omentum occludes a tear in the bladder. Signs and symptoms of bladder injury are fairly nonspecific and may manifest as pain and tenderness in the suprapubic region, although accompanying pelvic fracture may make it difficult to discern bladder injury distinctly on the basis of these findings. Unusually, fluid placed into the abdomen during diagnostic peritoneal lavage may be recovered from the Foley catheter collection bag, a finding that is diagnostic of intraperitoneal bladder injury.

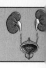

Injuries to the bladder include minor injuries such as bladder contusion (no disruption) and interstitial rupture (partial-thickness breach of bladder wall). Major injuries (bladder rupture) may simply be referred to as either extraperitoneal or intraperitoneal injuries.

Extraperitoneal bladder rupture

Because of tight ligamentous fixation of the bladder within the bony pelvis by the endopelvic fascia and pelvic diaphragm, inertia associated with deceleration injury may cause shearing of the bladder, especially when points of fixation are moving in different directions (e.g. pelvic fracture). Indeed, it is these shearing forces that are believed to most commonly cause bladder injury, rather than direct laceration of the bladder by bony spicules[28]. These forces generally result in injuries at the bladder base and are beneath the peritoneum that rests upon the dome.

Because as many as 93% of extraperitoneal bladder injuries occur synchronous with pelvic fracture[29], some orthopedic knowledge is requisite. Injuries to the pelvic ring may occur in discrete vectors, either singly or in combination[30]:

- Lateral compression injury, the most common type of pelvic ring disruption, results in 'closed book injury', such that the pubic symphysis may be overlapped as the pelvis is crushed inward. This injury is frequently seen in association with rami fractures.
- Anteroposterior injury results in external rotation of the hemipelvis ('open book injury') and may be associated with rami fractures, symphysis diastasis, and sacroiliac disruption. Because of disruption of tethering ligaments to the bladder base (i.e. condensations of endopelvic fascia), bladder injuries are quite common.
- Vertical shear injuries, as may occur following a fall, result in unpredictable but often devastating injuries both to the bony pelvis and to neurovascular structures of the lower urinary tract.

Despite this description of injury mechanism, it is impossible to predict presence or severity of injury in the individual patient based solely on fracture. We therefore recommend lower urinary tract contrast imaging for all patients in whom gross hematuria occurs together with pelvic fracture. Additionally, since 10–29% of male patients may have sustained urethral injury coincident with bladder injury, an aroused level of suspicion for this injury in this setting is appropriate and retrograde urethrography should be liberally performed if the usual clinical variables suggest it.

Virtually all extraperitoneal injuries can be managed nonoperatively, usually with a Foley catheter for 10 days. The catheter can be removed at that time if a contrast cystogram is normal; otherwise, contrast cystography can be performed weekly until disappearance of extravasation. The unusual decision to explore the patient who otherwise does not require laparotomy may be caused by presence of intravesical bony fragments, concerns regarding continence if injury includes the bladder neck, or synchronous injury to the anterior vaginal wall. If the patient's care requires abdominal exploration for associated injury, it is reasonable to perform bladder repair. For patients undergoing laparotomy for other reasons, repair of bladder injuries should be strongly considered.

Intraperitoneal bladder injuries

In contrast to conservative measures applied to extraperitoneal injuries, intraperitoneal injuries almost always mandate surgical repair. Undetected intraperitoneal injuries are associated with serious complications such as peritonitis and sepsis. Intraperitoneal bladder injuries related to trauma are of two types:

- 'Blowout' injuries to the bladder as a consequence of direct blunt trauma. The dome of the bladder, which is sheathed in peritoneum, represents the weakest part when the bladder is distended.
- Penetrating injuries including, most prominently, gunshot and stab wounds to the abdomen, buttocks, and genitalia.

Blowout injuries of the bladder occur when a sharp increase in intra-abdominal pressure exceeds the compliance of the body wall. A model of the intoxicated unrestrained driver with a full bladder incurring deceleration injury is instructive as an illustration. The bladder injury that results is usually approximately 3–5cm and is located on the dome, where the bladder is thinnest and most poorly supported. Treatment is via open repair of the laceration, usually in two layers with absorbable sutures.

Isolated penetrating injuries to the bladder are uncommon, so urologists most often explore injured patients in tandem with general trauma surgeons. When addressing penetrating injury to the bladder certain questions arise to gauge the extent of injury:

- Is the obvious injury the only one?
- What is the status of the ureteral orifices?
- Does any coincident injury (e.g. rectum) complicate management?

With these questions in mind, exploration for intraperitoneal injury should begin with a transperitoneal anterior cystotomy that is suitably large to allow visual inspection of the entire bladder urothelium. It is a mistake to see a hole and to extravesically repair it, since both gunshot and stab wounds may typically cause both entrance and exit injuries. Indigocarmine may be given intravenously to confirm ureteral patency and ureteral stents may be advisable if the injury is proximal to the ureteral orifice or if a high-velocity injury raises the question of blast damage. The bladder incision and the injuries may be closed in two layers with 2-0 or 3-0 absorbable suture. A Penrose or Jackson–Pratt drain and a formal suprapubic cystostomy secured with purse-string sutures are essential adjuncts.

A special case may be made for synchronous rectal and bladder injury. Any injury to the trigone or bladder base of a male patient should provoke question about the integrity of the rectum, since the trigone directly overlies the rectum. Conversely, known penetrating trauma to the rectum endangers the lower urinary tract. In approximately 200 cases of penetrating rectal trauma over a 13-year period, Franco et al. identified 17 concomitant GU tract injuries (13 bladder, 3 urethral, and 1 ureteral injury). Complications were significant and consisted of pelvic, suprapubic, or subphrenic abscesses in 3 of 17 cases (18%), rectovesical or rectourethral fistulae in 24%, chronic urinary tract infections in 18%, bladder stones in 12%, and the development of urethral strictures in 12%[31]. Although knowledge of a rectal injury does not alter the technique of bladder repair per se, this extremely complex subpopulation of injuries clearly distinguish themselves from 'simple' bladder injuries, the repair of which is seldom associated with major complications.

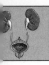

URETHRAL INJURY

Virtually all (90%) injuries to the urethra are sustained as a result of blunt trauma. Anterior urethral injuries usually result from perineal straddle injuries, but uncommonly may arise from penetrating trauma or in association with sexual corporal rupture. Injuries to the posterior urethra are almost always stereotypical distraction injuries and are seen accompanying approximately 5% of pelvic fractures, especially anterior pelvic ring fractures from a pelvic crush injury.

The mainstay of diagnosis of urethral injury is the properly performed retrograde urethrogram. Retrograde urethrography is relatively simple, fast, inexpensive, and safe and may identify important injuries that contraindicate urethral catheter placement. The retrograde urethrogram is properly performed by:

- oblique positioning of the patient toward the physician using a wedge;
- stretch of the penis to avoid redundant contrast; and
- urethral injection of contrast using a Brodney clamp or partially inflated 14F Foley catheter.

Particular clinical findings raise suspicion for urethral injury. Blood seen at the urethral meatus is an absolute indication for retrograde urethrography. A high-riding prostate, while intellectually conceivable, is a flawed assessment, since pelvic hematoma is often difficult to distinguish from prostate and the significantly distracted prostate may not feel so dramatically displaced on examination. Extravasation of contrast confirms urethral injury. If no extravasation is seen, a urethral catheter may be placed. If extravasation is seen, a suprapubic tube should be placed instead. Following successful placement of a urethral or suprapubic catheter a contrast cystogram should be performed to exclude concomitant bladder injury.

Blunt injuries to the anterior urethra causing extravasation should be treated with suprapubic urinary diversion and delayed urethroplasty, since immediate exploration may not reveal the extent of injury. Most penetrating injuries to the urethra occur anteriorly, mainly because of the sequestered position of the posterior urethra within the penis. As a general rule, an ideal method of handling low-velocity gunshot wounds to the penile and bulbar urethra includes debridement of superficial wounds and meticulous repair of any cavernosal injuries. Although primary repair may be appropriate for injuries not associated with tissue loss (e.g. clean stab wounds), delayed repair and suprapubic cystostomy is generally best, especially in the setting of significant tissue loss or devitalization from higher-velocity injuries[32].

Prostatomembranous urethral injuries are a horrific complication of pelvic fracture and pelvic ring disruptions. They result from distraction forces that occur as shear forces at the level of the membranous urethra and separate the prostate, which is relatively immobilized by endopelvic fascial condensations, from the more mobile membranous urethra (Fig. 43.14). Pelvic magnetic resonance imaging is the single best test to document the span of the disruption, as the prostate may retreat as much as 5–6cm as a result of posterosuperior displacement.

Should repairs be attempted in the acute setting or should initial treatment consist of a suprapubic cystostomy and delayed urethral reconstruction? This remains an area of substantial controversy. Clearly, the issues of contention have focused upon three major issues, namely the ability to provide successful and

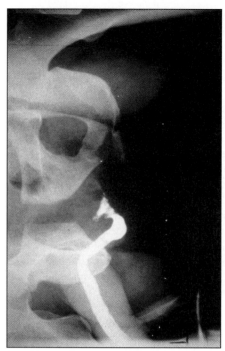

Figure 43.14
Prostatomembranous urethral injury. Retrograde urethrogram demonstrating a normal anterior urethra, although contrast extravasates at the prostatomembranous urethral junction. No contrast is seen to enter the bladder.

durable establishment of a patent anastomosis, preservation of continence, and preservation of sexual potency.

Acceleration of the debate regarding early versus delayed management occurred in 1972, when Morehouse questioned the advisability of early repair, voicing concerns regarding excessively high impotence and incontinence rates in a group of patients referred to him following failed attempts at immediate repair of these injuries[33]. Proponents of early repair maintain that it has the advantage of managing the problem immediately, thereby avoiding the need for prolonged suprapubic catheterization while awaiting secondary repair. However, others argue that operating through a pelvic hematoma threatens infection of the hematoma, prolongs pelvic bleeding by releasing the tamponade, and delays interventions such as angiographic embolization, which may be essential to control pelvic hemorrhage.

Immediate reconstruction may be accomplished by digital passage of a catheter by palpation, use of linked catheters[34], magnetically attracted catheters, and via endoscopic realignment. We are unaware of any studies comparing various means of acute repair with identification of distinct technical idiosyncrasies, so it is inappropriate to consider these methods collectively. At Vanderbilt, suture-linked catheters have successfully been implemented for immediate realignment to achieve 90% continence, 80% potency, while 15% of patients ultimately required open urethroplasty for stricture and 20% required dilation or endoscopic incision. Immediate realignment was aborted in 17% of patients[35].

At San Francisco General Hospital, our group reviewed our experience with 82 patients who underwent delayed repair following suprapubic tube placement[36]. With median follow-up of more than 1 year, continence was achieved in 95% of patients, impotence decreased from 54% prior to reconstruction to 38% postoperatively while 15% needed urethrotomy to achieve an overall success rate of 97%. Preoperative potency should always be recorded, both to monitor progress and to provide sufficient medicolegal documentation of existing pathology. Impotence is a devastating outcome following posterior urethral disruption and

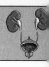

is believed to result from disruption of the cavernosal nerves lateral to the prostatomembranous urethra behind the symphysis pubis[37]. As an unusual category of patient, Ahmed et al. reviewed the results of their delayed repair of posterior urethral disruptions in boys 3–12 years old, identifying no postoperative strictures, 67% total continence and no loss of any preoperatively confirmed erections[38].

Immediate realignment, when indicated, is achieved via a lower abdominal midline incision. In one technique, the prostate is carefully palpated in a superolateral distortion from its orthotopic position. Care must be taken when exploring through the retropubic pelvic hematoma, both to avoid injury to the surgeon from jutting bony fracture spicules and to avoid unexpected release of hematoma tamponade. Two catheters are used at the outset: one is placed via the urethral meatus into the hematoma, while the other is placed via the anteriorly incised bladder through the bladder neck into the hematoma. The catheters are joined via sutures through the eyeholes to allow delivery of the urethral catheter. After closure of the bladder, the site of urethral injury is not reapproximated, either with suture or with traction. A retropubic drain is placed along with a suprapubic catheter. The urethral catheter is used for at least 4 weeks, after which a voiding cystourethrogram (VCUG) is performed. Persistent extravasation is managed with extended Foley catheter use. Most other means of primary repair, either endoscopic or open, adhere to the basic principles of this description.

Although most high-velocity injuries to the anterior urethra are best managed with suprapubic drainage alone, selected injuries without tissue loss or significant devitalization may be repaired primarily with a spatulated end-to-end anastomosis with 6-0 monofilament absorbable suture. A urethral catheter is left indwelling for at least 4 weeks, after which it may be removed if a voiding cystourethrogram shows no extravasation.

The female urethra is rarely injured as a consequence of blunt trauma. A retrospective chart review identified urethral injury to accompany pelvic fracture in approximately 5% of female patients[39]. Since only 50% of such injuries were diagnosed upon erectile dysfunction (ED) presentation, careful observation of blood at the urethral meatus (80% of urethral injuries) and thorough vaginal exam is important to arrive at the diagnosis. Primary urethral repair is recommended and cautious follow-up is essential in order to avert deep periurethral infection or urethrovaginal fistula.

INJURY TO GENITALIA

Scrotal injuries

Minor scrotal injuries are common because of the physically vulnerable position of the male genitalia. Injuries requiring urologic attention usually distinguish themselves by involving scrotal skin loss or by having potential for major testicular injury (breach of tunica albuginea). Although the presence of a gaping skin defect may be obvious, the diagnosis of 'major' testicular injury may be difficult to achieve by clinical means alone. Classically, patients sustaining testicular rupture usually report acute, severe pain associated with dramatic scrotal swelling (hematocele). Physical examination, if possible, may reveal ecchymosis, tenderness, and scrotal swelling. Frequently, however, these factors may render physical examination impossible. As a general guideline, scrotal ultrasound is essential for evaluation of any testicle that, by virtue of hematoma, edema, or pain, cannot reliably be examined.

The primary goal of testis ultrasound is to establish whether the tunica albuginea of the testis (usually able to withstand 50kg of blunt trauma[40]) has been ruptured and whether the underlying parenchyma has sustained injury. Sonographically, the most sensitive feature is hypoechogenicity of the parenchyma subtending the region of injury, and is supported by focal disruption of the echogenic tunic[41]. Although ultrasound examination remains the best adjunctive test to compliment physical examination of blunt trauma, accuracy may be as low as 56%, owing to significant false positives (hematocele without rupture) and false negatives (inability to distinguish the region of disruption)[42].

Recall that the bulbar urethra is vulnerable to many forms of trauma that cause scrotal injuries. In particular, straddle injuries to the scrotum and penetrating scrotal trauma are worrisome mechanisms. Because missed urethral injuries can be disastrous, it is our practice to liberally perform retrograde urethrography on these types of injury and whenever clinical suspicion is raised by proximity of injury.

Why explore suspected testicular trauma? The goal of scrotal exploration for testis injury is to preserve endocrine parenchyma, since germ cells are more sensitive to injury and may sustain both direct sperm cell line injury and injury to transport mechanism (efferent ductules and epididymis). In order to provide access to both testes, scrotal exploration should be performed via a midline raphe incision. Since hematoma and edema may obfuscate clean layers of dissection, the initial goal of exploration is to visualize the remaining glistening surface of the visceral tunica vaginalis. Since intraparenchymal edema and hematoma may hamper attempt at primary closure, excision of ischemic tubules is often necessary to allow tension-free closure of the tunica albuginea.

As a general rule, all penetrating injuries to the scrotum should be explored in the operating room. If any question is raised about bilateral involvement, both scrotal compartments may be explored through a common midline raphe incision. While testicular salvage is generally possible, high-velocity missile injuries have been associated with testicular salvage in only half of cases[43].

Injury to the spermatic cord usually requires little more than meticulous hemostasis. If, indeed, testicular viability is questioned, a small incision can be made in the albuginea, as active bleeding from testicular parenchyma is reassuring. Only in very rare cases is injury so complete as to necessitate orchidectomy. Vasal injuries should not be primarily repaired for fertility since the extent of tissue ischemia and blast injury may not be demarcated at the time of exploration. Silk sutures may be employed at the cut ends to provide easy identification if infertility mandates repair.

Scrotal skin, by virtue of reliable blood supply and extensibility, can usually be closed primarily, even when 50% or more of skin is lost. Closure, however, must be meticulous and should involve two-layer approximation of the skin and dartos fascia for hemostasis. The scrotum should be elevated postoperatively using fluffs and an athletic supporter. A Penrose drain, if placed, may be removed after 24 hours.

Certain injuries such as burns and extensive avulsions mandate employing various forms of tissue transfer, most commonly a split-thickness skin graft. Debridement and placement of testicles into thigh pouches is the easiest means of providing coverage of the testis, but used as monotherapy provides no coverage for

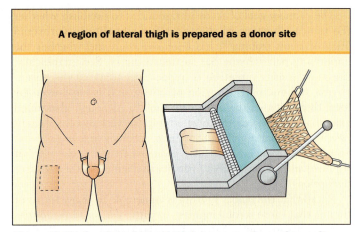

Figure 43.15 A region of lateral thigh is prepared as a donor site. Following harvest of the graft at appropriate thickness, the graft is 'meshed' at 2:1 for application to the scrotum.

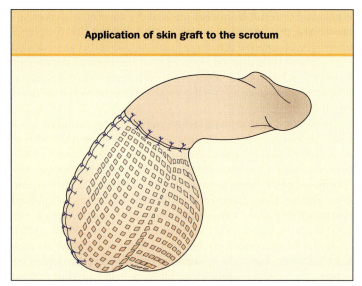

Figure 43.16 Application of skin graft to the scrotum. The testes are sutured together and the graft is placed as a 'clamshell' and sutured in place.

missing skin. Meshed split-thickness skin grafts (2:1 and 0.015" thick) harvested from the anterior thigh (Fig. 43.15) provide an excellent cosmetic result while allowing exudative runoff through the interstices during early graft survival (Fig. 43.16).

Penile injuries

Penile amputation is primarily seen in two settings: self-mutilation and intentional assault by a secondary individual. As might be expected, psychotic illness is endemic to self-mutilation (65% of patients), and frank schizophrenia is identified in 29%[44]. In all cases, penile replantation should be attempted if medically feasible, since remorse following acute psychiatric disease is the rule. To protect and preserve the severed portion, it should be packed in ice but insulated from 'freeze injury' by placing the specimen within an isolated bag. Despite the unlikely possibility that the 'free flap' will survive warm ischemia longer than 18–24 hours, replantation should be attempted unless the 'free flap' is necrotic or grossly contaminated.

Principles of repair (Fig. 43.17) include[45]:

- initial closure of urethra over Foley catheter to provide stabilization for more delicate portions of the repair (two-layer anastomosis);
- minimal dissection along neurovascular bundle only as necessary to exhume severed vessels and nerves;
- re-approximation of cavernosal artery if technically feasible using 11-0 nylon suture;
- closure of tunica albuginea with 4-0 polyglycolic suture;
- anastomosis of dorsal arteries with 11-0 nylon;
- dorsal vein repair with 9-0 nylon; and
- re-approximation of epineurium with 10-0 nylon.

Penetrating trauma to the penis primarily involves gunshot wounds, although human and animal bites are sometimes seen. A common pattern of gunshot wounds to the genitalia is a triad of injury to the penis, scrotum, and thigh, not infrequently causing vascular injury to the lower limb. In part because of the use of semi-automatic and automatic weapons, associated injuries are quite common (83%) and, in addition to lower extremity vascular injuries, may include trauma to the fingers, buttocks, and sigmoid

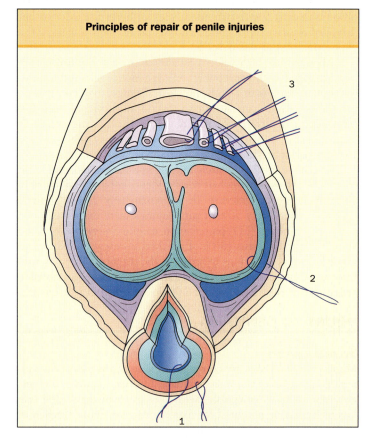

Figure 43.17 Principles of repair of penile injuries. The urethra is re-approximated in two layers with 5-0 and 6-0 monofilament absorbable suture (1) and is stented with a Foley catheter to provide stability for more delicate stages of repair. The corporal bodies are repaired in a single layer with 4–0 absorbable suture (2), taking care to 'bury the knots' on the dorsal aspect such that the limbs of the knots will not interfere with microvascular repair (3) of the dorsally based neurovascular bundle.

colon, often curiously sparing the urinary tract[46].

Dog bite injuries to the phallus are uncommon and morbidity is directly related to the severity of the initial wound. Irrigation and debridement are the cornerstones of management of any penetrating genital trauma, along with broad-spectrum anti-microbial agents. Dog bite lacerations can be sutured closed safely if there is no infection. Skin avulsion from the penis may require extensive debridement and skin grafts or flaps[47]. Victims of human bites to the penis often do not seek timely medical attention and dangerous progression of infection may ensue[48].

Injuries to the female genitalia

Because anatomic concealment may protect the female external genitalia from injury, isolated genital injuries are uncommon, except in the setting of sexual assault. To specifically address injuries seen in the setting of felonious assault, most emergency departments have in place both acute counseling and supportive care, as well as routine procedures for evidence collection.

Most superficial injuries to the external female genitalia may be closed primarily using fine absorbable sutures. Vaginal injuries may be associated with significant blood loss, especially if pelvic injury has disrupted pudendal vessels[49]. Except for closure of small lacerations that may tolerably be performed in the emergency department, most significant injuries are best addressed in the operating room, where anesthesia allows thorough painless speculum examination. Lacerations may be closed using running, locked chromic gut for hemostasis. A vaginal pack is left for 24 hours.

Although vaginal laceration has been identified as occurring in association with pelvic fracture from blunt trauma, blunt trauma is rarely the cause of injury to the labia or vaginal introitus. As for female urethral injuries, vaginal examination is essential to provide the diagnosis, since as many as 30% of vaginal injuries may have an associated urethral injury[50].

CONCLUSIONS

Trauma care is significantly different from elective patient care. As thoughtful cancer surgeons, we are esteemed for our careful patient evaluation and for a well-rehearsed operative plan. As trauma surgeons, we lose all luxuries of anticipatory planning and are called on at odd hours to employ scattered information to cure a life-threatening disease in a patient we have never met before. The best way to wrestle the dichotomy is to think and rehearse the principles of trauma care in our minds, so that some of the surprise is lost by the time we are actually called to see the patient.

REFERENCES

1   Grace DM, Fenton JA, Duncanson ME. Devastating lap-belt injury: a plea for effective rear-seat restraints. Can Med Assoc J. 1994;151:331–3

2.   Hazinski MF, Eddy VA, Morris JA Jr. Children's traffic safety program: influence of early elementary school safety on family seat belt use. J Trauma. 1995;39:1063–8.

3.   Hunt DK, Lowenstein SR, Badgett RG, Steiner JF. Safety belt nonuse by internal medicine patients: a missed opportunity in clinical preventative medicine. Am J Med. 1995;98:343–8.

4.   Siegel JH, Mason-Gonzalez S, Dischinger P, et al. Safety belt restraint and compartment intrusions in frontal and lateral motor vehicle crashes: mechanisms of injuries, complications, and acute care. J Trauma. 1993;34:736–58.

5.   Mackersie RC, Gillon JW. Initial resuscitation of the trauma patient. In: McAninch JW, Carroll PR, eds. Problems in urology: genitourinary trauma. Philadelphia: JB Lippincott; 1994.

6.   Abou-Khali B, Scalea TM, Trooskin SZ, Henry SM, Hitchcock R. Hemodynamic responses to shock in young trauma patients: need for invasive monitoring. Crit Care Med. 1994;22: 633–9.

7.   Nicolaisen GS, McAninch JW, Marshall GA. Renal trauma: reevaluation of the indications for radiographic assessment. J Urol. 1985;133: 183–7.

8.   Mee SL, McAninch JW, Robinson AK. Radiographic assessment of renal trauma: a 10-year retrospective study of patient selection. J Urol. 1989;141:1095–100.

9.   Goldman SM, Sandler CM. Upper urinary tract trauma – current concepts. World J Urol. 1998;16:62–8.

10. Marcos HB, Noone TC, Semelka RC. MRI evaluation of acute renal trauma. JMRI. 1998;July/August:989–90.

11. Velmahos GC, Demetriades D, Cornwell EE, et al. Selective management of renal gunshot wounds. Br J Surg. 1998;85: 1121–4.

12. Nash PA, Bruce JE, McAninch JW. Nephrectomy for traumatic renal injuries. J Urol. 1995;153: 609–11.

13. Taviloglu K, Kayihan K, Erekin C, Calis A, Turel O. Abdominal stab wounds: the role of selective management. Eur J Surg. 1998;164: 17–21.

14. Wessells H, McAninch JW, Meyer A, Bruce JE. Criteria for nonoperative treatment of significant penetrating renal injuries. J Urol. 1997;157:24–27.

15. Carroll PR, McAninch JW, Wong A, Wolf JS Jr, Newton C. Outcome after temporary vascular occlusion for the management of renal trauma. J Urol. 1994;151(5):1171–3.

16. Carroll PR. In: McAninch JW, ed. Traumatic and reconstructive urology. Philadelphia: WB Saunders; 1996:113–25.

17. Haas CA, Dinchman KH, Nasrallah PF, Spirnack JP. Traumatic renal artery occlusion: a 15-year review. J Trauma. 1998;45: 557–61.

18. Goodman DNF, Saibil EA, Kodama RT. Traumatic intimal tear of the renal artery treated by insertion of a Palmaz stent. Cardiol Intervent Radiol. 1998;21:69–72.

19. Montgomery RC, Richardson JD, Harty JI. Posttraumatic renovascular hypertension after occult renal injury. J Trauma. 1998;45: 106–110.

20. Wessels H, Deirmenjian J, McAninch JW. Preservation of renal function after reconstruction for trauma: quantitative assessment with radionuclide scintigraphy. J Urol. 1997;157:1583–6.

21. Elshihabi I, Elshihabi S, Arar M. An overview of renal trauma. Curr Opin Pediatr. 1998;10:162–6.

22. Brown SL, Elder JS, Spirnak JP. Are pediatric patients more susceptible to major renal injury from blunt trauma? J Urol. 1998;160: 138–40.

23. Morey AF, Bruce JE, McAninch JW. Efficacy of radiographic imaging in pediatric blunt trauma. J Urol. 1996;156: 2014–8.

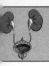

24. Medina D, Lavery R, Ross SE, Livingston DH. Ureteral trauma: preoperative studies neither predict nor prevent missed injuries. J Am Coll Surg. 1998;186: 641–4.

25. Kenney PJ, Panicek D, Witanowski LS. Computed tomography of ureteral disruption. J Comput Asst Tomogr. 1987;11:480–4.

26. Kawashima AK, Sandler CM, Corriere JN, Rodgers BM, Goldman SM. Ureteropelvic junction injuries secondary to blunt abdominal trauma. Radiology. 1997;205:487–92.

27. Cass AS. Diagnostic studies in bladder rupture: indications and techniques. Urol Clin North Am. 1989;16:267.

28. Corriere JN Jr, Sandler CM. Management of the ruptured bladder: seven years of experience with 111 cases. J Trauma. 1986;26:830–3.

29. Cass AS. The multiply injured patient with bladder trauma. J Trauma. 1984;23:731–7.

30. Molligan HJ. Pelvic ring disruptions. In: McAninch JW, ed. Traumatic and reconstructive urology. Philadelphia: WB Saunders; 1996:357.

31. Franco ER, Ivatury RR, Schwalb DM. Combined penetrating rectal and genitourinary injuries: a challenge in management. J Trauma. 1993;34(3):347–53.

32. Hall SJ, Wagner JR, Edelstein RA, Carpinito GA. Management of gunshot injuries to the penis and anterior urethra. J Trauma. 1995;38(3):439–43.

33. Morehouse DD, Belitsky P, MacKinnon K. Rupture of the posterior urethra. J Urol. 1972;107: 255.

34. Herschorn S, Thijssen A, Radomski SB. The value of immediate or early catheterization of the traumatized posterior urethra. J Urol. 1992;148:1428.

35. Follis HW, Koch MO, McDougal WS. Immediate management of prostatomembranous urethral disruptions. J Urol. 1992;147(5):1259–62.

36. Morey AF, McAninch JW. Reconstruction of posterior urethral disruption injuries: outcome analysis in 82 patients. J Urol. 1997;157:506–10.

37. Mark SD, Keane TE, Vandermark RM, Webster GD. Impotence following pelvic fracture urethral injury: incidence, etiology and management. Br J Urol. 1995;75(1):62–4.

38. Kardar AH, Sundin T, Ahmed S. Delayed management of posterior urethral disruption in children. Br J Urol. 1995;75(4):543–7.

39. Perry MO, Husman DA. Urethral injuries in female subjects following pelvic fractures. J Urol. 1992;147(1):139–43.

40. Wesson MB. Traumatism of the testicle: report of a case of a rupture of a solitary testicle. Urol Cutaneous Rev. 1946;50:16–19.

41. Fournier GR, McAninch JW. Sonography in the staging of testicular trauma. In: McAninch JW, ed. Traumatic and reconstructive urology. Philadelphia: WB Saunders; 1996.

42. Corrales JG, Corbel L, Cipolla B, et al. Accuracy of ultrasound diagnosis after blunt testicular trauma. J Urol. 1993;150(6):1834–6.

43. Brandes SB, Buckman RF, Chelsky MJ, Hanno PM. External genitalia gunshot wounds: a ten-year experience with fifty-six cases. J Trauma. 1995;39(2):266–71, discussion 271–2.

44. Aboseif S, Gomez RG, McAninch JW. Genital self-mutilation. J Urol. 1993;150(4):1143–6.

45. Jordan GH. Initial management of male genital amputation injuries. In: McAninch JW, ed. Traumatic and reconstructive urology. Philadelphia: WB Saunders; 1996:673–681.

46. Gomez RG, Castanheira AC, McAninch JW. Gunshot wounds to the male external genitalia. J Urol. 1993;150(4):1147–9.

47. Wolf JS Jr, Turzan C, Cattolica EV, McAninch JW. Dog bites to the male genitalia: characteristics, management and comparison with human bites. J Urol. 1993;149(2):286–9.

48. Wolf JS Jr, Gomez R, McAninch JW. Human bites to the penis. J Urol. 1992;147(5):1265–7.

49. Knudson MM, Crombleholme WR. Female genital trauma and sexual assault. In: Blaisdell FW, Trunkey DD, eds. Abdominal trauma. New York: Thieme Medical Publishers; 1993: 311.

50. Goldman HB, Idom CB, Dmochowski RR. Traumatic injuries to the female external genitalia and their association with urological injuries. J Urol. 1998;159:956–959.

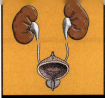

Chapter 44   Lasers in Urology

Graham M Watson

LASER PHYSICS

A laser beam is light energy of a single wavelength with almost no divergence of the beam and with a very high intensity. The essential components of a laser are a lasing medium surrounded by two mirrors, one of which is partly transmissive and the other partly reflective.

The laser process is generated by stimulated emission. This occurs when an electron of a specific element can exist in an outer or inner shell (Fig. 44.1). When the electron falls from an outer to an inner shell a photon is emitted. This photon will have a wavelength that is dictated by the energy shift of the electron, and this is constant for that particular element. If a photon collides with an electron in an outer shell then the electron will be stimulated to emit a second photon, which is in phase and in a similar direction to the stimulating photon. Throughout the process of stimulated emission an external energy source is applied to the laser medium to return the electrons to an excited state. Any photons that are emitted in the optical axis of the laser (Fig. 44.2) will continue to propagate backwards and forwards, increasing in power with each pass. The word laser is an acronym for **l**ight **a**mplification by **s**timulated **e**mission of **r**adiation. The laser process will therefore always produce a beam of intense light with a nearly parallel beam of light of a single wavelength.

The different types of laser describe the laser medium and therefore the wavelength at which that laser emits. This wavelength determines most of the interactions that the laser beam will have with tissue. Lasers have been developed that span most of the electromagnetic spectrum of light (Fig. 44.3). Those lasers that emit at a wavelength at which tissue absorbs intensely have

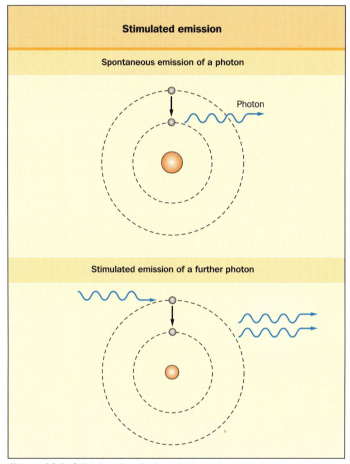

Figure 44.1 Stimulated emission. A photon is emitted when an electron falls from a high-energy to a low-energy state. When a photon collides with an electron at a high-energy level, then a second photon is emitted in phase with the first photon.

a very short path length through tissue and therefore tend to vaporize the tissue surface. Examples of this are the excimer, carbon dioxide, and holmium lasers. Those lasers emitting with a wavelength that is absorbed poorly by tissue will have a long path length and will tend to coagulate. Examples of this are the neodymium:YAG and semiconductor diode lasers.

Tissue may contain a number of different pigments (chromophores) and some wavelengths may be absorbed unevenly according to the distribution of the chromophores. This can be taken advantage of when using the selective effects of a laser. The best example of this is the selective destruction of portwine

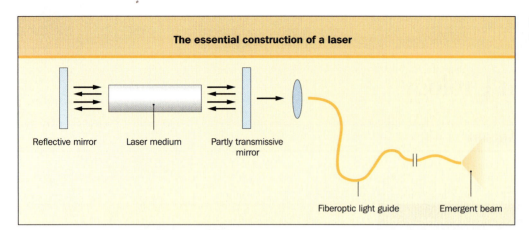

Figure 44.2 The essential construction of a laser.

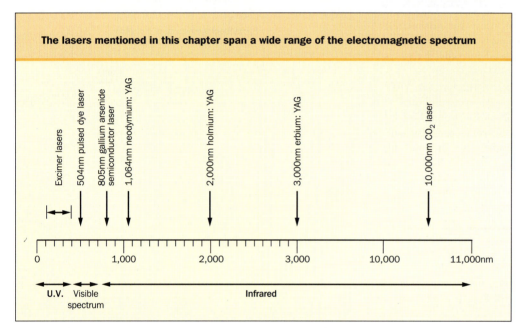

Figure 44.3 The lasers mentioned in this chapter span a wide range of the electromagnetic spectrum.

stains, where the laser wavelength is absorbed by the blood vessels and to a minimal extent by surrounding tissue. The pulsed dye laser, when used for fragmentation of urinary calculi, also makes use of the greater absorption of green light by stones rather than the ureter.

Photodynamic therapy is an interesting variation on this in that an agent is given to the patient prior to therapy. The drug is retained in malignant tissue for longer than in normal tissue. Laser irradiation is given at a power that does not affect the tissue but does activate the agent to produce a cytotoxic effect. The laser and the agent on their own have no effect but in combination do destroy the tumor. Lasers can also be delivered as a continuous beam of energy or can be pulsed. Short pulses cause vaporization when in the millisecond range and can even cause fragmentation when in the nano- to microsecond range. By pulsing a laser emission a very small amount of energy can cause such a high power density that an ionization bubble results, with a consequent acoustic effect.

Lasers are inherently complex and inefficient machines. It is rare to find an action that cannot be replicated by simpler and cheaper technology. It is therefore very important to have a considered approach to any specific application. The expense of

purchasing a laser makes it necessary for that expense to be justified. It is therefore not a level playing field and the laser must be seen to be superior to cheaper technologies if it is to be justified. The two main arenas for laser applications at present are fragmentation of stone and prostatectomy. The holmium laser can be used for both of these applications and indeed for all laser applications in urology apart from photodynamic therapy. This chapter will therefore address how different lasers compare with alternative cheaper technologies.

A summary of the properties of lasers
- A laser is an intense beam of light energy.
- There is wide diversity in the wavelengths of different lasers.
- The wavelength defines the penetration depth of the light through tissue.
- The penetration depth defines the action of the laser on the tissue.
- Thus different lasers have widely different effects on tissue.
- Selective effects are possible if the target has a specific chromophore.
- Pulsing the laser modifies the action allowing fragmentation or cutting.

LASER APPLICATIONS

Stone fragmentation

When considering a modality for fragmenting calculi the modality must be considered alongside the ureteroscopes required for accessing the calculi. The history of the development of the first laser systems for lithotripsy was linked to the development of ureteroscopes to access the stones. Thus if one uses a pneumatic kinetic device one has to use a rigid ureteroscope with an offset eyepiece. If one uses a holmium or pulsed dye laser one can use a flexible ureteroscope and thus access stones anywhere in the urinary tract. The complications are predominantly those of the ureteroscopy. Therefore a discussion on laser lithotripsy has to include at least in part a reference to the ureteroscopes it can be used with.

The first attempt to fragment a calculus was made by Mulvaney in 1968[1] when he placed calculi in the path of a ruby laser beam. He described using energies of 50–300J on various stones. He was able to fragment struvite stones but not calcium oxalate. The precise pulse durations of the ruby laser were not mentioned but were presumably 100–1000ms. In 1978, Fair[2] described the use of an optomechanical coupler that converted a laser beam into a shock wave that fragmented a calculus. He used a Q-switched Nd:YAG laser aimed at a thin layer of aluminum confined between glass and brass. It was possible to fragment calculi if they were enclosed within the brass chamber but the glass was fragmented more readily than the stone. Trains of Q-switched laser pulses of lower pulse energies produced an effect rather like extracorporeal shock-wave lithotripsy (ESWL), with the elimination of tiny fragments, but it was very difficult to transmit these down fibers[3].

The first clinical system to be developed was the pulsed dye laser developed by Watson et al.[4] The optimum parameters were a pulse duration of 1ms because this could be transmitted down a fiber with the fiber in contact with the stone. The optimum wavelength was green light at 504nm because the differential absorption between stone and ureter was greatest at this point (Fig. 44.4) and because the laser performed efficiently at this wavelength. The fiber size chosen was 200–320μm. The repetition rate was up to 20Hz. Although these were designed to be the optimum parameters it was always recognized that there were many possible laser systems for stone fragmentation.

The differential absorption between stone and ureter results in a degree of selectivity of the laser. When the laser pulse is directed at a stone there is an obvious impulse felt in the fiber but when the laser is directed at the ureter there is no impulse and no action for the first few pulses until purpura changes the absorption properties.

The mechanism of action of the pulsed dye laser has been shown by Teng et al.[5] to be by formation of a plasma. This is an ionization bubble that forms at the stone surface. Fragmentation occurs with the water jets that rush in as the bubble collapses. The pulsed dye laser can induce a plasma because the peak power density at the tip of the fiber exceeds 100×10^6W/cm^2 as a result of the short pulse duration. The holmium laser has a pulse duration that is 300 times longer and uses pulse energies 10 times those of the pulsed dye laser; consequently the holmium laser has a peak power density of less than 5×10^6W/cm^2, which is insufficient to form a plasma. Teng et al. showed that one could record

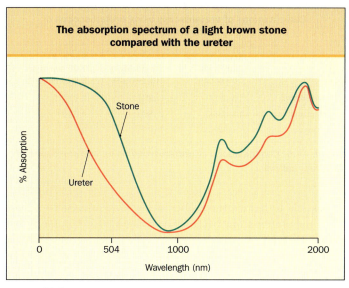

Figure 44.4 The absorption spectrum of a light brown stone compared with the ureter.

the plasma signal back down the very fiber that delivered the laser energy. Only stones gave this signal: tissue, guidewires, and catheters would not[6]. There was therefore a potential for using this plasma feedback to diagnose that one was in contact with stone rather than ureter.

Engelhardt et al.[7] studied the spectroscopy pattern of light remitted from the stone surface during the first 10% of the laser pulse from a pulsed dye laser emitting at 590nm. They then went on to develop a system that diagnosed whether or not it was stone at the tip of the fiber. Only if there was stone would the laser deliver sufficient energy to cause a plasma and therefore fragment the stone. This system was commercialized as the Lithognost® device.

Animal experiments have been performed that give some insights into the need for feedback devices with lasers for stone fragmentation. Watson et al. used a pulsed dye laser at 504nm in the pig ureter under endoscopic control[8]. There was no significant injury at the site of laser fragmentation of a urinary calculus. By contrast, Muschter et al.[9] found that pulsed dye laser energy delivered to rabbit bladder that had been opened surgically caused purpura and healed with fibrosis. Watson et al. had impacted urinary calculi in the upper ureters of pigs and compared the action of the laser with that of the electrohydraulic probe. Electrohydraulic probe fragmentation was significantly more aggressive to the ureter. However by far the most important factor was the diameter of the ureteroscope used to reach the stone. The distal ureter bore the brunt of this injury. Clinical experience after many thousands of ureteroscopic treatments with the pulsed dye laser corroborates this view.

Initially the laser was used via the then standard sized 11.5F ureteroscopes. The laser had to be passed through a ureteric catheter in order to stabilize it in the 5F working channel. The rod lens ureteroscopes were reduced in caliber down to 10.5, 9.5, and even 8.5F. There were difficulties with bending of these narrow rod lens instruments causing half-moon distortion to the view. The development of a purpose-built ureteroscope for use with the laser using a fiberoptic image bundle in a semirigid sheath made

Complications of ureteroscopy using ureteroscopes of different calibers			
	Series 1 11.5F rigid 100 patients	Series 2 8.5–11.5F 100 patients	Series 3 7.2F semirigid 2,000 patients
Perforations	10 (10%)	3 (3%)	2 (0.1%)
Nephrostomy	12 (12%)	6 (6%)	4 (0.2%)
Stricture	3 (3%)	2 (2%)	0

Figure 44.5 Complications of ureteroscopy using ureteroscopes of different calibers.

it possible to reduce the caliber of the ureteroscope to a mere 7.2F and ureteroscopy became much easier[10]. Ureteroscopy also became safer.

We have compared our results in our first 100 patients using predominantly an 11.5F ureteroscope, our second 100 patients using predominantly 8.5–11.5F ureteroscopes, and the next 2000 patients treated with the 7.2F MiniScope[11]. The success rate increased as we progressed through these series in spite of treating an increasing proportion of upper-third stones. Most important of all was the reduced complication rate shown in Figure 44.5. Harman et al.[12] from the Mayo clinic have reported an increasing success rate and have noted a reduction in complications related to ureteroscopy when comparing audits of 1982 to 1985 with a second audit of 1992 (Fig. 44.6). In both series the improved results were due to the reduced trauma from the smaller caliber ureteroscope. The laser was therefore just the means by which miniaturization was made possible.

Nevertheless the pulsed dye laser performed well as a safe modality for fragmenting calculi. There have been no reported cases of the laser injuring the ureteric wall. Fragmentation of cysteine calculi was inefficient but was made possible by introducing rifampicin 2% solution as the irrigant to coat the calculi and improve absorption[13]. The alexandrite laser was also developed for stone fragmentation though with less impact commercially. It also had limited efficacy on cysteine stones, but this could be remedied by irrigating with a 0.01% solution of cardiogreen.

The holmium laser has already been mentioned as a tool for stone fragmentation. The holmium laser has a higher pulse energy but lower peak power than the pulsed dye laser. It does however have the advantage of excellent absorption at the stone surface whatever the stone composition. The peak powers are insufficient to produce a plasma but it does cause local vaporization of the stone, causing a crater and eventually cracking of the stone. The temperatures required to vaporize the stone are in excess of 4,000°C. It is possible to fragment a stone safely because the laser is pulsed and therefore there is a sudden jump and fall in temperature right at the tip of the fiber and the surrounding

ureter is protected by the heat sink of the water. However, if the fiber is deployed too close to the ureteric wall significant trauma can occur.

The advantage of the holmium laser over the pulsed dye laser is that it will vaporize and eventually fragment any stone no matter how hard or how pale. Watson and Smith[14] showed that the pulsed dye laser at 65mJ was equivalent to the holmium laser at 1J per pulse. The percentage of fragments less than 0.5mm was greater with the holmium laser. Teichmann et al.[15] reported on a clinical series comparing the holmium laser and electrohydraulic probe. The holmium laser produced the smaller fragments. The differences between the two laser systems is shown in Figure 44.7.

There have been a number of reports into the effectiveness of the holmium laser on ureteric calculi. There have not been cases that could not be fragmented by the laser and the success rates were really just evaluating the success rates of the ureteroscopy and the ability to remove all the fragments. Shroff et al. achieved an 86.8% rate of complete clearance of calculi in one session[16]. Grasso cleared 33 of 34 stones in one session[17]. Of interest is that the mean size of stones in his series was 13.2mm, one stone being 6cm in diameter. With the holmium laser one has the assurance that any stone in the ureter can be fragmented. With the pulsed dye laser one knows it can be used safely in a very impacted stone where the visibility is impaired. The holmium laser has proved to be very useful for intrarenal lithotripsy[18]. One can either fragment a calculus in its peripheral position or else grasp it and withdraw it into the pelvis before fragmenting it and clearing it from there. The increasing use of active flexible ureteroscopes has made this a very important application. Finally, the holmium laser can be used for bladder stones. McIver et al. have described using the holmium laser via a 550µm fiber and a 23F cystoscope. The laser was used at 15–30W to fragment the stones, which were an average of 36×43mm with an average

A comparison of the pulsed dye and holmium lasers		
	Pulsed dye laser	Holmium laser
Typical pulse energy	80mJ	800mJ
Typical peak power	80kW	2.5kW
Action on stone	Fragmentation	Drilling
Mechanism	Plasma formation	Local heat formation
Tissue damage	Minimal	Potentially great
Propulsion	Slight	Minimal
Consistency of action	Less efficient with cysteine/white stones	Consistent effect on all stones

Figure 44.7 A comparison of the pulsed dye and holmium lasers.

Figure 44.6 Improved results and reduced complications in Harman's series.

Improved results and reduced complications in Harman's series						
	Overall success (%)	Stone success (%)	Distal (%)	Above iliacs (%)	Complications (%)	Significant complications (%)
1982–85	86	89	95	72	20	6.6
1992	96	95	97	77	12	1.5

anesthesia time of 50min. One of the cases had failed a previous attempt using electrohydraulic lithotripsy. In the bladder one can take the power right up to 80W if necessary, in contrast to the ureter, where the maximum suggested power is 10W.

The main impact of the pulsed dye and holmium lasers has been the effect on the size of the ureteroscopes used to access the stones. Other fragmentation modalities have also been reduced in size and can therefore be used via similarly small ureteroscopes. These modalities are often a fraction of the cost of a laser system. Figure 44.8 compares the cost and main features of these competing devices.

It is only sensible to consider purchasing a laser for stone fragmentation if the cost can be justified either on the basis of the numbers of patients likely to be treated or because of the site of the stones. The pneumatokinetic devices, including the electromagnetic device, are the most cost-effective but are limited in that they cannot be used via flexible ureteroscopes. There is an increasing use of the laser to fragment stones in peripheral calyces via flexible ureteroscopes because of the high rate of rendering the patient completely stone-free in contrast to ESWL.

Lasers and the prostate

The first attempt to use a laser to treat benign prostatic outflow obstruction was made by Johnson et al. using a sidefiring reflector on a quartz fiber to deliver neodymium:YAG laser energy to the prostate[20]. They delivered 60W for 60s at four different points of the dog prostate. By 6 weeks there was a large central cavity in the prostate. This work launched a series of phase I trials and then randomized trials comparing sidefire Nd:YAG laser with transurethral resection of the prostate[21,22]. There was initially a great deal of enthusiasm for this approach because the laser procedure was bloodless except on very rare occasions. The patients emerged from the procedure with minimal trauma looking as though they had just had a cystoscopy apart from the presence of an indwelling catheter. On the negative side they required approximately 10 days of catheterization; approximately 40% of them had prolonged dysuria and perineal pain lasting for over 6 weeks, and finally it took 6 weeks before any disobstruction occurred. With 5 years followup[23] there was a higher retreatment rate than with conventional transurethral resection of the prostate (TURP).

Interstitial laser therapy partly gets around the problem of postoperative dysuria because of the sparing of the urethra but it does not get around the time required for the coagulated tissue to be removed. Coagulative necrosis can also be induced by microwave therapy without the need for anesthesia and therefore one wonders what advantage there might be in interstitial laser therapy. Meanwhile, sidefiring laser therapy has fallen out of fashion as a general treatment for the obstructive prostate. It might be considered for the occasional young man with obstruction from adenoma rather than bladder neck who is intent on keeping the capacity for ejaculation.

The holmium laser has been developed for the treatment of benign prostatic outflow obstruction. The technique that has been developed by Gilling and Fraundorfer[24] is to use the holmium laser at 80W to cut the prostate using a bare fiber close to the tissue. Radial incisions are made from the veru to the trigone to separate the middle lobe from the lateral lobes and again from the anterior lobe. These incisions are made down to the capsule and dividing the bladder neck. They are then widened into trenches. One then works from the veru to the bladder sweeping the prostatic tissue off from the capsule until the tissue is freed into the bladder.

Prior to the development of the morcellator for removal of these lobes it was necessary to interrupt the freeing of the lobes and to then divide the lobes into segments to facilitate extraction[25]. The morcellator, however, has allowed the procedure to be performed without having to divide the lobes prior to freeing them from the capsule. The result is a prostatic fossa which resembles that from a TURP but with preservation of an almost bloodless field. Gilling et al. have performed a randomized controlled trial comparing holmium laser resection with TURP[26]. The results are shown in Figure 44.9.

Our group has performed a small study comparing holmium enucleation with TURP. The hemoglobin drop was from 13.8 to 12.3 in the TURP group and was 13.9 pre- and postoperatively in the holmium group. The sodium fell from 140 to 129 in the TURP group and remained unchanged at 139 in the holmium group. The degree of debulking of the prostate was assessed by measuring the PSA and transrectal ultrasound volume. The results are shown in Figure 44.10.

Finally the patients were asked to score their postoperative pain on an analogue scale. Six out of 13 patients felt that there was some pain following TURP versus 1 of 18 patients in the

A comparison of different modalities for fragmentation				
Modality	Price (£; approx.)	Flexibility	Potential trauma to ureter	Propulsion
Pulsed dye laser	100,000	+++	–	+
Holmium laser	60,000+	+++	++	–
Ultrasound	10,000	–	+/–	+
Electrohydraulic	10,000	++	++	++
Pneumatokinetic	15,000	–	–	+++

Figure 44.8 A comparison of different modalities for fragmentation.

Holmium laser enucleation versus conventional TURP		
	Holmium laser	TURP
No. of patients	61	59
Preoperative AUA score	21.9	23.0
Postoperative AUA score (6 months)	3.9	5.1
Preoperative $\dot{Q}_{max}$	8.9	9.1
Postoperative $\dot{Q}_{max}$	23.9	22.4
Reoperation rate	1.6%	3.4%
Strictures	3.3%	8.5%
Blood transfusion	None	6.8%
Duration of surgery	41.5min	25.3min
Length of stay	26.2h	47.5h
Nursing time	36.1min	105.6min

Figure 44.9 Holmium laser enucleation versus conventional transurethral resection of the prostate (TURP) (Adapted from Gilling et al.[26]).

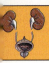

Degree of debulking of the prostate				
	Holmium laser		TURP	
	Pre	Post	Pre	Post
TRUS volume	46	24	41	23
PSA	5.4	4.9	4.8	3.9

Figure 44.10 Degree of debulking of the prostate. PSA, prostate-specific antigen; TRUS, transrectal ultrasound; TURP, transurethral resection of the prostate.

holmium laser group. There was no difference in dysuria between the two groups.

Holmium laser enucleation of the prostate does therefore seem to have some advantages over conventional TURP in that bleeding is less with no risk of hyponatremia and with a reduced hospital stay and intensity of nursing care. On the negative side one has to consider the learning curve of mastering a new technique and the cost of hiring or purchasing the laser plus the increased operating time. Other technologies can be used to perform the enucleation technique without recourse to laser technology. What we do not know is whether these alternative technologies can produce the same hemostasis. We also need to know that the technique of holmium laser enucleation can be taken on and used widely. Certainly the technique is extremely promising and perhaps it is superior to TURP.

Other applications

A recurring theme in this chapter is that laser energy is light energy and that it produces a unique effect only when it uses some aspect of the property of light. Otherwise its effect can be replicated by other, cheaper modalities. We have already heard about how the fiber delivering laser energy to a stone can be used to transmit energy back giving information about the stone. Information can also be obtained from tissue.

Kriegmair et al.[27] have investigated the use of 5-aminolevulinic acid (5-ALA) in the bladder. This agent can be given intravenously or, more interestingly, intravesically and taken up by the transitional epithelium. Here it is metabolized to protoporphyrin IX and its level is very much greater in malignant or dysplastic tissue than in normal tissue a few hours after administration. These sites fluoresce bright red when illuminated with blue light. The sensitivity of the system is close to 100% but the specificity is as low as 60% in some series.

Jichlinski et al.[28] administered 5-ALA into the bladder 6 hours prior to cystoscopy. They then used a white light to view the bladder and a blue light of 380–450nm to excite the agent. The protoporphyrin accumulating in the tissue has an emission peak at 635nm, which is red light. A long-pass filter filtering out all light of wavelength longer than 490nm is placed over the optics and areas high in protoporphyrin fluoresce red, with normal urothelium looking green and blood vessels appearing as darker tracks. Jichlinski et al. viewed the bladder first under normal light in order to select normal sites for biopsy. Prior to biopsy they then viewed with the long-pass filter to see if the area fluoresced.

In 31 patients studied they took a total of 132 biopsies of which 51 fluoresced and 81 did not fluoresce. Of the 51 biopsies that were positive for fluorescence, 17 had normal histology, i.e.

33% false positives; 7 out of the 81 that were negative for fluorescence had an abnormal histology, i.e. 8.7% false negatives. There were 47 'tumors' in 22 patients that were invisible under white light but which fluoresced; 6 were papillary tumors, 27 were grade 1–2 dysplasia, 3 were grade 3 dysplasia and 11 were carcinoma in situ. Fluorescence detected additional atypia in 85% of patients with multiple tumors and 41% of patients with a single tumor.

This agent does therefore enhance the optical feedback available to the urologist using just light. An extra dimension to the application of 5-ALA is that it can be activated by intense light at one of its excitation peaks to produce singlet oxygen in sufficient quantities to produce cell death within that cell. It can therefore be used selectively to destroy malignant cells in which the protoporphyrin IX has accumulated. The intensity of light at these specific wavelengths generally requires the use of a laser.

Anidjar et al.[29] have investigated the potential for using low-energy laser light to fluoresce the bladder epithelium without the use of drugs to enhance fluorescence. The fluorescence is caused by the increased levels of endogenous molecules in dysplastic or malignant tissue such as tryptophan, collagen, NADH, riboflavins, and porphyrins. Using an optical multichannel analyzer they recorded the autofluorescence spectrum from the bladder prior to resection for biopsy. The tissue was first stimulated with light from a xenium chloride laser at 308nm, a nitrogen laser at 337nm and a coumarin dye laser at 480nm. The nitrogen laser caused a band of excitation centered on 440nm with normal bladder giving the highest levels; visible tumor gave levels 2.5 times lower in intensity and carcinoma in situ gave levels 100 times lower. There was an excitation band centered on 360nm which was proportionally higher in malignant tissue. The authors felt that an ultraviolet light combined with alternating narrow pass filters and a charge coupled device camera would allow accurate mapping of carcinoma in situ. Koenig et al[30] studied the autofluorescence spectra from bladders using a nitrogen laser. They compared the fluorescence signals emitted at 385nm and 455nm. They were able to differentiate malignant from non-malignant areas with a sensitivity of 97%, a specificity of 98%, a positive predictive value of 93%, and a negative predictive value of 99%. They thought that the emission bands were detecting differences of collagen at 385nm and of NADH at 455nm.

The realm of diagnosis using fluorescence and autofluorescence spectra is a fascinating offshoot of laser applications. The potential has been grasped by the leading endoscopy companies, who have developed filter systems for use with the 5-ALA spectra.

CONCLUSIONS

Laser energy is light energy. Lasers tend to be expensive and when they compete with other technologies they have to outperform the alternative technologies in order to justify the extra expense. In their short history laser techniques in urology have arisen and caused an impact in an area only to be caught up by alternative technologies. Laser lithotripsy achieved some prominence because the fiber was smaller and more flexible than any alternative and also because the pulsed dye laser was safer than the electrohydraulic probe. Laser lithotripsy is currently under threat from pneumatokinetic and electromagnetokinetic devices, which are extremely efficient at fragmentation and extremely safe. However the potential to use the holmium laser in the kidney via flexible ureteroscopes has caused an enormous increase in the interest in laser lithotripsy. This is because the laser is flexible and can reduce the stone to such minute fragments. In the field of holmium laser resection of the prostate it is uncertain whether other modalities could replace the holmium laser. Certainly electrical techniques can be used to enucleate the gland, but are they as hemostatic?

Where lasers are unassailable is where some aspect of their use of light energy is exploited. In dermatology lasers have a very important role in treating portwine stains and other vascular lesions because the specific wavelength employed is preferentially absorbed by the blood and not by surrounding tissue. The result is a *smart laser* with inbuilt selectivity. In urology we can use specific wavelengths of light to fluoresce agents that are themselves selectively absorbed by tumor. The same principle is used to activate these same agents for an antitumor effect. We can also use lasers for in vivo autofluorescence emission spectroscopy as a way of detecting chemical differences in tissue and discriminating between benign and malignant tissue.

Lasers can be used for the very important actions discussed in this chapter of fragmentation and hemostatic cutting. The development of the laser was a potent factor in the miniaturization of ureteroscopes. Now alternative modalities can be used via similarsized semirigid ureteroscopes. The laser is now one of the instruments of choice for use with flexible ureteroscopes in the kidney. It competes with the electrohydraulic probe. The use of the holmium laser in the prostate has shown that the laser can reduce the morbidity and hospital stay compared to TURP. The gauntlet has been thrown down in that other studies must be done to see if other units can replicate the observations of Gilling et al. and, if so, conventional resection should be abandoned or improved.

REFERENCES

1. Mulvaney WP, Beck CW. The laser beam in urology. J Urol. 1968; 99,112–5.
2. Fair HD. In vitro destruction of urinary calculi by laser-induced stress waves. Med Instrument. 1978;12:100–5.
3. Watson GM. Principles of laser stone destruction. In: Smith JA, Stein BS, Benson RC, eds. Lasers in urologic surgery. St Louis: CV Mosby; 1994:183–9.
4. Watson GM, Dretler S, Parrish JA. The pulsed dye laser for fragmenting urinary calculi. J Urol. 1987; 138:195–8.
5. Teng P, Nishioka NS, Anderson RR. Optical studies of pulsed laser fragmentation of biliary calculi. Appl Phys B. 1987;42:73–8.
6. Shah T, Watson GM, Xiang ZX, King TA. Non-visual laser lithotripsy aided by plasma spectral analysis: viability study and clinical application. J Urol. 1993;149:1431–6.
7. Engelhardt R, Meyer W, Hering P. Spectroscopy during laser induced shock wave lithotripsy. In: Optical fibers in medicine 111. Proc SPIE. 1988;906:200–3.
8. Watson GM, Murray S, Dretler SP, Parrish JA. An assessment of the pulsed dye laser in the pig ureter. J Urol. 1987;138:199–203.
9. Muschter R, Knipper A, Maghraby H. Laser lithotripsy – experience with different laser systems in the treatment of urinary calculi. In: Katzir A, Anderson RR, eds. Laser surgery: advanced characterisation, therapeutics and systems. Proc SPIE. 1990;1200:118–21.
10. Watson GM, Wickham JEA. The development of a laser and miniaturised ureteroscope system for ureteric stone management. World J Urol. 1989;7:147–50.
11. Watson GM, Landers B, Nauth-Misir B, Wickham JEA. Developments in the ureteroscopes, techniques and accessories associated with laser lithotripsy. World J Urol. 1993;11:1–5.
12. Harmon, WJ, Sershon PD, Blute ML, Patterson DE, Segura JW. Ureteroscopy: current practice and long term complications. J Urol. 1997;157:28–32.
13. Cechetti W, Tasca A, Guazzieri S, Zattoni F, Villi G, Pagano F. Optical coupling method to improve laser lithotripsy. J Endourol. 1992;6:229–31.
14. Watson GM, Smith N. A comparison of the pulsed dye and holmium lasers for stone fragmentation: in vitro studies and clinical experiences. Proc Lasers Urol Gynecol Gen Surg SPIE. 1993;1879:139–42.
15. Teichman JMH, Rao RD, Rogenes VJ, Harris JM. Ureteroscopic management of ureteral calculi: electrohydraulic versus holmium:YAG lithotripsy. J Urol. 1997 158:1357–61.
16. Shroff S, Watson GM, Parickh A, Thomas R, Soonawalla PF, Pope A. The holmium YAG laser for ureteric stones. Br J Urol. 1996;78:836–9.
17. Grasso M. Experience with the holmium laser as an endoscopic lithotrite. Urology. 1996;48:199–206.
18. Bagley D, Erhard M. Use of the holmium laser in the upper urinary tract. Tech Urol. 1995;1:25–30.
19. McIver BD, Griffin KP, Harris JM, Teichman JMH. Cystoscopic holmium lithotripsy of large bladder calculi. Tech Urol.1996;2:65–7.
20. Johnson DE, Proce RE, Cromeens DM. Pathological changes occurring in the prostate following transurethral laser prostatectomy. Lasers Surg Med. 1992;12:254–63.
21. Cowles RS, Kabalin JN, Childs S, et al. A prospective randomized comparison of transurethral resection to visual laser ablation of the prostate for the treatment of benign prostatic hyperplasia. Urology. 1995;46:155–60.
22. Anson K, Nawrocki J, Buckley J, et al. A multicentre, randomised, prospective study of endoscopic laser ablation versus transurethral resection of the prostate. Urology. 1995;46:305–10.
23. McAllister WJ, Absalom MJ, Mir K, et al. Does endoscopic laser ablation of the prostate stand the test of time? 5 year results from a multi-centre randomised controlled study of endoscopic laser ablation versus transurethral resection of the prostate. BJU Int. 2000;85:437–9.
24. Gilling PJ, Cass CB, Creswell MD, Fraundorfer MR. Holmium laser resection of the prostate: preliminary results of a new method for the treatment of benign prostatic hyperplasia. Urology. 1996;47:48–50.
25. Fraundorfer MR, Gilling PJ. Holmium laser enucleation of the larger prostate combined with mechanical morcellation. J. Endourol. 1997;11(suppl. 1):S159.
26. Gilling PJ, Mackey M, Creswell M, Fraundorfer MR. The perioperative care of patients undergoing holmium laser resection of the prostate compared with transurethral resection of the prostate. Proc Lasers Urol Gynecol Gen Surg SPIE. 1998;3245:75–9.
27. Kriegmair M, Baumgartner R, Knuechel R, Steinbach P, Ehsan A, Lumper W. Fluorescence photodetection of neoplastic urothelial lesions following intravesical instillation of 5-aminolaevulinic acid. Urol. 1994;44:836–9.
28. Jichlinski P, Forrer M, Mizeret J, Braichotte D, Wagnieres G, Zimmer G. Fluorescence photodetection of urothelial neoplastic foci in superficial bladder cancer. In: Lasers in surgery: advanced characterisation, therapeutics and systems VII. SPIE. 1997;2970:470–4.
29. Anidjar M, Ettori D, Cussenot O, Meria P, Desgrandchamps F, Cortesse A. Laser induced autofluorescence diagnosis of bladder tumors: dependence on the excitation wavelength. J. Urol 1996;156:1590–6.
30. Koenig F, McGovern FJ, Althausen AF, Deutsch TF, Schomacker KT. Laser induced autofluorescence diagnosis of bladder cancer. J Urol. 1996;156:1597–601.

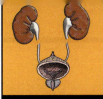

Chapter 45

Radiation Therapy in Urology

Richard A Cowan

- Placing a radioactive source close to a tumor produces a regression that may lead to a cure.
- In bladder cancer, radiotherapy may offer an alternative to radical surgery.
- In prostate cancer, radiotherapy offers treatment for early disease, locally advanced disease, and metastatic disease.
- Radiotherapy has a significant role in palliative therapy in malignant disease.

HISTORICAL PERSPECTIVE

The therapeutic potential of ionizing radiation as a treatment of cancer was recognized soon after its discovery over 100 years ago.[1,2]

In the early half of last century doctors learned that placing a radium source in close proximity to a tumor produced significant tumor regression, which could lead to cure. In the second half of the century machines were developed capable of generating beams of high energy X-rays, electrons, neutrons, and latterly protons. During this time we have harnessed advances in radiobiology and radiation technology to enhance tumor eradication while keeping damage to surrounding normal tissue to a minimum.

PRINCIPLES OF RADIOTHERAPY

When a beam of X-rays penetrates the body it deposits energy along its path. The higher the energy the deeper the penetration of the beam (Fig. 45.1).

The major characteristics of X-rays, electrons, and protons are illustrated in Figure 45.2.

On entering the cell the ionizing radiation interacts with the cellular constituents, producing highly reactive free radicals, which are responsible for damaging the cell. The DNA molecule is the most sensitive structure within the cell to free radical damage. As a consequence of impaired DNA function radiation damage manifests when the cell comes to divide. Radiation damage is therefore seen early in most malignant tumors with a high cell turnover and in normal tissues of high proliferative activity. In contrast, organs with low rates of cell division (lung and kidney) show radiation damage as a late phenomenon 6–18 months postradiotherapy (Fig. 45.3).

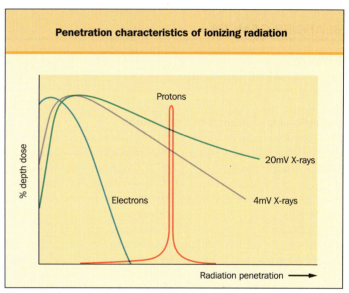

Figure 45.1 Penetration characteristics of ionizing radiation.

Characteristics of ionizing radiation	
Ionizing radiation	**Characteristics**
X-rays	Energy falls off gradually along its path
Electrons	Energy deposition close to the surface – less penetration
Protons	All energy is deposited at a specific distance from the surface – deep penetration

Figure 45.2 Characteristics of ionizing radiation.

An increase in radiation dose leads to an increased cure rate and a similar relationship exists between radiation dose and the chance of normal tissue damage (Fig. 45.4, top panel).

The aim of radiation therapy is to maximize the therapeutic ratio by separating the two curves illustrated in Figure 45.4 (center & bottom panels).

The selectivity of radiation therapy is caused by normal cells having a better capacity to repair radiation damage. The phenomenon is exploited by administering radiotherapy in a series of small exposures usually 24 hours apart, a process termed *fractionated radiotherapy* (Fig. 45.5). The gap between exposures is designed to permit maximum normal tissue DNA repair while allowing insufficient time for the malignant cell to repair the DNA damage.

Early and late responding tissues	
Early response to radiotherapy (weeks)	**Late response to radiotherapy (6–18 months)**
Most cancers	Slow growing tumors (rarely)
Bone marrow	Kidney
Gastrointestinal tract	Liver
Skin	Lung
	Brain/spinal cord

Figure 45.3 Early and late responding tissues.

BLADDER CANCER

Radiotherapy in transitional cell carcinoma of the bladder offers the potential for cure with preservation of a satisfactorily functioning bladder.

Superficial transitional cell carcinoma

The role of radiotherapy in superficial bladder cancer is not well defined[3]. Radiotherapy may be considered when the disease progresses beyond endoscopic control. Conventionally, intravesical therapy represents the initial treatment of recurrent tumors but the place of early radiation therapy to prevent recurrence and progression is being evaluated in ongoing trials including a study in the UK run by the Medical Research Council (MRC). For uncontrolled superficial disease refractory to intravesical therapy radiotherapy to the bladder offers an alternative to cystectomy (Fig. 45.6).

In summary, it would be appropriate to offer radiotherapy to patients with uncontrollable superficial disease as an alternative to cystectomy if they have good bladder function and are eager to avoid surgery. However, patients should be made aware that the treatment may delay cystectomy rather than prevent it.

Muscle-invasive transitional cell carcinoma
Background

Both radiotherapy and cystectomy offer curative potential in this disease and no satisfactory randomized comparisons have been published to indicate the relative roles of the two options. Currently there is considerable geographic variation in clinical practice. In the USA cystectomy continues to predominate while primary radiotherapy is more commonly employed in parts of Europe and particularly in the UK (BA06/3089 trial)[4].

Comparison of published results between cystectomy and radiotherapy may be misleading (Fig. 45.7).

Primary radiotherapy with salvage cystectomy if required

Who should be considered for primary radiotherapy (Fig. 45.8)?

With good pretreatment staging [magnetic resonance imaging (MRI) ± laparoscopic lymph node sampling] and modern techniques involving conformal radiotherapy ± chemoradiation, the results of primary radiotherapy treatment in the group of patients listed in Figure 45.8 may be comparable with equivalent surgical series, with the advantage of offering the patient a well-functioning bladder. Over 50% of these patients should be cured[5] (Fig. 45.9).

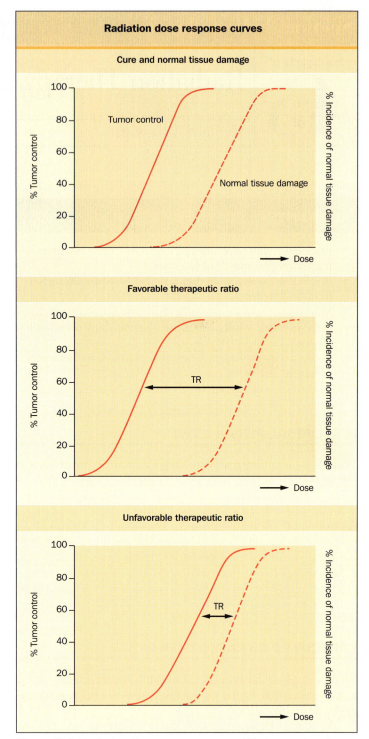

Figure 45.4 Radiation dose response curves. TR, therapeutic ratio.

The results of primary radiotherapy in the group of patients with the features listed in Figure 45.10 are less good, with approximately 30% of patients surviving 5 years[6–8]. Radiotherapy may be considered in this group of patients in cases where there is poor surgical risk or the patient has a clear preference for organ preservation (Fig. 45.11).

Representation of fractionated radiotherapy

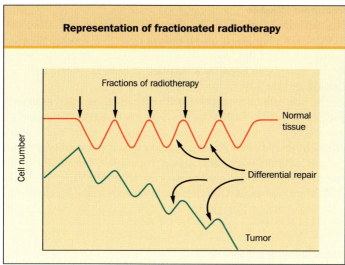

Figure 45.5 Representation of fractionated radiotherapy.

Radiotherapy in superficial transitional cell carcinoma of the bladder

Relative indications for radiotherapy	Contraindications to radiotherapy
Good bladder function	Poor bladder capacity/function
Poor surgical risk	Widespread CIS with unhealthy urothelium
Patient preference	Previous pelvic radiotherapy
Healthy unaffected urothelium	

Figure 45.6 Radiotherapy in superficial transitional cell carcinoma of the bladder. CIS, carcinoma in situ.

Flaws in nonrandomized comparisons between cystectomy and radiotherapy

Patient selection favoring fitter patients for surgery

Radiotherapy patients tend to be understaged clinically compared with pathologic staging at cystectomy

Cystectomy series usually report treatment received rather than 'intention to treat' and as a consequence patients whose cystectomy was abandoned because of advanced disease are excluded from the results

Radical radiotherapy series include patients who have received radiotherapy as a 'palliative' procedure whose disease was deemed incurable by surgery

There are very few recently published radiotherapy results and therefore current surgical series are compared with old radiotherapy results where staging was inaccurate and outmoded radiotherapy techniques were used

Figure 45.7 Flaws in nonrandomized comparisons between cystectomy and radiotherapy.

Features favoring a good prognosis following radiotherapy

Good performance status

Single muscle-invasive tumor

Healthy remaining urothelium

Good bladder function (and capacity)

Aggressive TURT to leave minimal residual disease

No extravesical infiltration or nodal metastatic disease

Figure 45.8 Features favoring a good prognosis following radiotherapy. TURT, transurethral resection of tumor.

Overall survival following radiotherapy combined with concomitant cisplatin in muscle invasive transitional cell carcinoma of the bladder

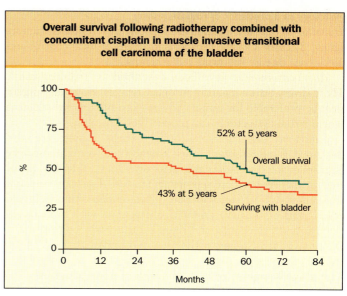

Figure 45.9 Overall survival following radiotherapy combined with concomitant cisplatin in muscle invasive transitional cell carcinoma of the bladder[5].

Features suggesting an intermediate prognosis following radiotherapy

Multiple tumors

Residual disease post-TURT

Extravesical infiltration

Hydronephrosis

Heavy hematuria

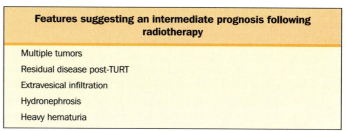

Figure 45.10 Features suggesting an intermediate prognosis following radiotherapy. TURT, transurethral resection of tumor.

Overall survival, cancer-specific survival, and relapse-free survival for an unselected group of patients receiving radiotherapy in the 1970s

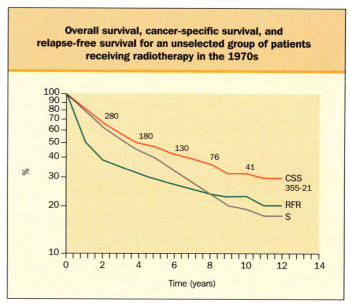

Figure 45.11 Overall survival (S), cancer-specific survival (CSS), and relapse-free survival (RFR) for an unselected group of patients receiving radiotherapy in the 1970[8].

Histology as a predictor of radiosensitivity

Transitional cell carcinoma (TCC): Poorly differentiated tumors (grade 3) carry a worse prognosis in terms of local control and metastatic disease following radiotherapy.

Adenocarcinomas have been described as 'radioresistant'. There is very little supporting evidence for this. However, surgery may be preferable for tumors arising from the urachal remnant when partial cystectomy can produce good results.

Squamous cell carcinoma(SCC): These tumors are also described as radioresistant. Their prognosis, however, is also very poor following cystectomy and, in locally advanced disease, radiotherapy may offer a more appropriate method of palliative therapy.

In summary, patients with poorly differentiated tumors (grade 3TCC and SCC) have an inferior prognosis with both radiotherapy and cystectomy and there is little evidence to support the premise that surgery is the preferred option.

The place of palliative radiotherapy in poor prognosis bladder cancer

When the disease is deemed incurable the question arises: Will palliative radiotherapy help the patient?

In the presence of metastases or extensive local disease causing a rapid deterioration in the patient's general condition local radiotherapy will not prolong life.

Pelvic radiotherapy may be administered in this setting to relieve symptoms. However, not all bladder symptoms are amenable to relief by radiotherapy (Fig. 45.12).

The patient's life expectancy has to be sufficient to allow enough time for the radiotherapy to be administered and the inevitable delay of a few weeks before the therapeutic benefits are experienced. In general, the life expectancy needs to be in excess of 3 months for the patient to experience significant benefit from a course of palliative pelvic radiotherapy.

The radiotherapy procedure

Definition of field of treatment (treatment volume)

The radiotherapy field must encompass the entire bladder and immediate extra vesical tissues plus or minus the pelvic lymph nodes (Fig. 45.13).

Visualizing the treatment volume

A computed tomography (CT) scan (or MRI) of the pelvis is used to plan the radiotherapy treatment volume (Fig. 45.14).

Treatment schedule

The standard schedule involves an administered dose of 6,000–7,000cGy given on weekdays over 6–7 weeks. Shorter treatment schedules, e.g. 5,500cGy in 20 daily fractions over 4 weeks, have been used by a number of centers, particularly in Canada and the UK.

The side effects from this treatment can be regarded as *immediate* or *late* (Fig. 45.15). In less than 5% of patients postradiation bladder symptoms persist for many months and are of sufficient severity to warrant cystectomy. This eventuality is more likely in patients with poor bladder function, diminished capacity, and severe bladder symptoms prior to radiotherapy. Although cystectomy for irradiation damage is very undesirable, the long-term outcome in this group of patients is superior to that in patients undergoing cystectomy for tumor recurrence.

Postradiotherapy follow-up

Treatment failure necessitates salvage cystectomy. Careful cystoscopic followup is therefore mandatory, as a delay in diagnosis of recurrence may lead to tumor progression beyond salvage cystectomy. The optimum time for postradiotherapy cystoscopic assessment is conventionally considered to be between 3 and 6 months following completion of radiotherapy. This allows adequate time for tumor regression and healing of

Inclusion of pelvic lymph nodes in the radiation field	
Advantages	**Disadvantages**
Potentially prevent subsequent pelvic nodal relapse	Unselective
Reduces the need for accurate pretreatment staging of lymph nodes	Increases the treatment volume and thereby the toxicity
	May lead to a reduction in administered dose of radiotherapy
	Potentially makes salvage cystectomy a more difficult procedure

Figure 45.13 Inclusion of pelvic lymph nodes in the radiation field.

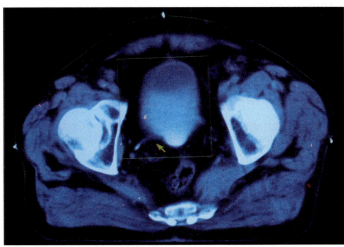

Figure 45.14 Computed tomography scan visualizing the bladder and demonstrating the radiotherapy treatment volume (arrow).

The role of palliative pelvic radiotherapy	
Symptoms relieved by radiotherapy	**Symptoms not helped by radiotherapy**
Hematuria	Fatigue
Pain, particularly bone metastases or lymph node metastases	Anorexia
	Dysuria
	Frequency
	Incontinence

Figure 45.12 The role of palliative pelvic radiotherapy.

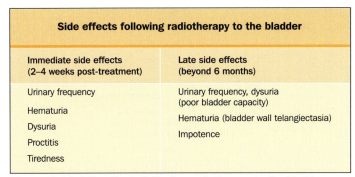

Figure 45.15 Side effects following radiotherapy to the bladder.

Immediate side effects (2–4 weeks post-treatment)	Late side effects (beyond 6 months)
Urinary frequency	Urinary frequency, dysuria (poor bladder capacity)
Hematuria	Hematuria (bladder wall telangiectasia)
Dysuria	Impotence
Proctitis	
Tiredness	

the acute radiation-induced mucosal inflammation. The key features for postradiotherapy cystoscopic assessment are:
• No residual tumor – cystoscopic followup initially 4-monthly progressing to 6-monthly and annually
• Residual tumor – confirmed histologically → to cystectomy
When superficial tumor occurs at the site of the initial muscle invasive cancer, immediate cystectomy should be recommended, although some patients can do well with resection alone.

Cystectomy following radiotherapy
There has been concern that cystectomy following radiation treatment is technically more difficult but this has not been borne out in experienced hands. However, neobladder reconstruction represents a more demanding procedure in the postradiation pelvis.

Advances in radiotherapy for bladder cancer
Conformal radiotherapy
Modern linear accelerators are now capable of producing a beam of any desired shape. This permits the beam to accurately follow the contour of the tumor and reduces the volume of normal tissue unnecessarily irradiated. Conformal radiotherapy offers the potential to:
• reduce the acute and long term toxicity of conventional dose of radiotherapy; and
• increase the dose to the tumor while maintaining the same incidence of radiation side effects.
The incorporation of conformal radiotherapy in the treatment of bladder cancer has been accompanied by improved imaging techniques (e.g. MRI) enabling more accurate tumor visualization and staging.

Chemoradiation
The concurrent administration of chemotherapy and radiation has recently been shown to improve the response rate for bladder cancer[9,10]. The most commonly used chemotherapy agent has been cis-platinum but 5FU and methotrexate have also been shown to enhance the radiation effect. A typical treatment scheme incorporating chemoradiation is shown in Figure 45.16.

In vitro testing of radiosensitivity
It is recognized that approximately 50% of muscle-invasive bladder tumors are not eradicated by conventional radiotherapy. This has prompted interest in identifying predictors of radiosensitivity. A number of in vitro assays have been developed and

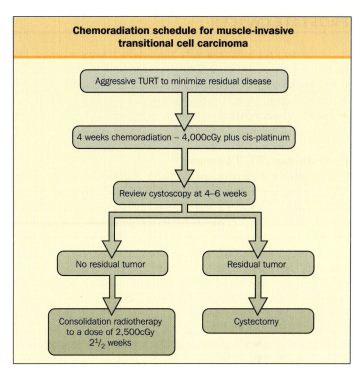

Figure 45.16 Chemoradiation schedule for muscle-invasive transitional cell carcinoma. TURT, transurethral resection of tumor.

some have shown a close correlation with tumor control[11]. It is hoped that as these develop it may be possible to use results from radiosensitivity assays in the selection process between cystectomy and radiotherapy.

Radiosensitizers and radioprotectors
A number of agents have been identified that sensitize tumors to the effects of radiation and trials are ongoing that evaluate their efficacy in bladder cancer. Conversely, radioprotectors are chemicals that bestow a degree of radio-resistance to irradiated tissue. Targeting these agents appropriately to surrounding normal tissue offers the potential to significantly improve the therapeutic ratio of radiation therapy.

Gene therapy
Recent studies have shown that gene expression can be modified by ionizing radiation. Models being developed involve the insertion of radiation-activated genes into tumors. These offer the promise of manipulating tumor sensitivity for both radiation and chemotherapy.

Summary
In the management of muscle-invasive bladder cancer, the prospect for the future is that we will be able to identify a group of patients who can be successfully treated by modern conformal radiotherapy plus or minus chemotherapy. Following treatment, these patients should enjoy a good quality of life with a well-functioning bladder.
    In addition, patients showing a poor response to chemoradiation will undergo early cystectomy with the potential that the preoperative chemoradiation will improve outcome compared with surgery alone.

PROSTATE CANCER

Radiotherapy represents a very important treatment modality in the management of prostate cancer and its role may be considered under the following headings;
- early disease;
- locally advanced disease; and
- metastatic disease.

Early disease (T1, T2 tumors)

The prognosis of early prostate cancer is determined by T-stage serum prostate-specific antigen (PSA) and Gleason score. Patients with T1 and T2 well-differentiated tumors and a PSA below 20 have an excellent prognosis with radical prostatectomy or radiotherapy[12,13]. Indeed, some of these patients may be better served by observation alone. As the Gleason score increases, however, active treatment becomes the most appropriate option[14] and the question remains: Surgery or radiotherapy? There are no published large randomized trials comparing the outcome of these treatment approaches. In the UK an attempt by the Medical Research Council to compare watchful waiting with radiotherapy or surgery failed because of poor accrual (MRC PRO6 1994). It is clear that men are not happy to have three very different treatments offered on a random basis and they prefer to come to their own decision[15]. If survival is the endpoint, we know that the results of such randomized studies will take many years to become available.

As a consequence, in current practice it is deemed appropriate to offer the patient a full explanation of the treatment options with a broad reassurance that there is no proven superiority of one option over the others. The patient should then be free to make his own decision on the basis of the current evidence. A study performed in Manchester examining the reasons why men chose not to be randomized revealed two major factors influencing the patient's decision:
- Patients who opt for surgery are happier with the idea of having the entire tumor removed.
- Patients preferring radiotherapy are keen to avoid a surgical procedure.

For patients who express no particular preference the decision may be determined by comparison of the side effect profiles of the two options (Fig. 45.17).

The results of external beam radiotherapy in early prostate cancer

What end points should we consider in assessing the results for external beam radiotherapy?

The potential endpoints are:
- overall survival;
- local recurrence;
- the development of metastatic disease; and
- PSA failure.

The problems with overall survival as an endpoint for radiotherapy in prostate cancer are:
- The expected long survival of men following radiotherapy means that many years will elapse before the treatment can be evaluated.
- Intercurrent deaths – in an elderly population, deaths from other causes are to be expected and will have a significant impact on survival.

Figure 45.17 Side effects following radiotherapy and prostatectomy.

Side effects following radiotherapy and prostatectomy	
Surgery	Radiotherapy
Urinary incontinence	Proctitis
Impotence	Urinary frequency and dysuria
Postoperative complications	Impotence

Figure 45.18 Problems with local recurrence as an endpoint for radiotherapy in prostate cancer. MR, magnetic resonance.

Problems with local recurrence as an endpoint for radiotherapy in prostate cancer	
	Problem
Digital rectal examination	Difficult to evaluate postradiotherapy and therefore low sensitivity and low specificity
Transrectal ultrasound	Difficult interpretation of postradiotherapy prostate
Trans rectal biopsy	Invasive Difficulties in histologic interpretation Sampling error
MR staging	Low sensitivity/specificity postradiotherapy Expensive

The problems with local recurrence as a measure of treatment success are illustrated in Figure 45.18.

The incidence of local failure and the time to local failure will be influenced by which parameter is used to evaluate local recurrence and the frequency with which these tests are done. In most published series local failure has not been a reliable endpoint. The recommended measurement for local failure is transrectal biopsy at a fixed timepoint, e.g. 18 months–2 years following radiotherapy.

Development of metastatic disease

The development of metastases does not represent a logical endpoint to assess the success of a local treatment. However there is a recognized correlation between local failure and metastatic spread.

Development of metastatic disease is usually identified as bone metastases visualized on a bone scan or lymph node metastases on CT/MRI. The incidence of metastases and the time to the development of metastatic spread are dependent on the frequency with which these investigations are performed. Therefore the time to asymptomatic metastatic disease does not represent a reliable parameter for evaluating the efficacy of radiotherapy and the time to symptomatic metastatic disease is rather more meaningful.

PSA failure

The use of PSA failures as an endpoint for evaluating radiotherapy treatment has the following advantages:
- early identification of treatment failure;
- cheap and noninvasive; and
- reliable surrogate of local failure metastatic disease and cancer death.

However, in contrast to patients undergoing prostatectomy, the PSA postirradiation does not fall to undetectable levels as the residual prostate gland is capable of producing small amounts of PSA. The American Society for Therapeutic Radiology and Oncology (ASTRO) has produced criteria for the definition of PSA failure following radiation treatment[16]:

- three consecutive rises in PSA following a nadir value post-radiotherapy; and
- the time to PSA failure taken as the time from the end of radiotherapy to the first rise in PSA.

PSA failure represents the most appropriate endpoint for evaluating the success of local radiotherapy in early prostate cancer.

The results of external beam radiotherapy in favorable disease

Favorable disease is defined as tumor stage T1/T2 and PSA less than 20.

Worldwide, radiotherapy for the prostate is administered over 6–7 weeks although within the UK accelerated treatment schedules are used over 3–4 weeks with broadly similar outcomes[17].

With standard dose radiotherapy (64–74Gy), approximately 65% of patients will be in biochemical complete remission 5 years after treatment[12] (Fig. 45.19).

In recent years we have seen the use of conformal radiotherapy in early prostate cancer. This technique allows the beam of radiation to be individually shaped to conform to the outline of the prostate, thereby reducing the volume of surrounding normal tissue within the radiation field. Conformal radiotherapy has allowed us to increase the radiation dose to over 80Gy[20].

The results from the high-dose treatments are encouraging but longer followup will be required in order to allow a meaningful comparison with conventional dose radiotherapy.

Toxicity from prostate radiotherapy

Acute side effects are experienced by all patients. They include:

- proctitis;
- urinary frequency;
- dysuria;
- urinary retention (rarely); and
- fatigue.

Acute side effects develop in the latter half of the course of treatment and continue for 3–4 weeks following completion of therapy.

Late side effects include:

- impotence; and
- persistent proctitis.

Prolonged bladder or bowel symptoms as a late complication of radiotherapy may be mild in up to 10% of patients and are severe in less than 5% of men. These figures are continuing to improve with the more widespread use of conformal radiotherapy[21].

Reliable data on impotence levels following radiotherapy are scarce. Evaluation of postradiation potency is hindered by varying levels of potency pretreatment and the increasing use of neoadjuvant hormone therapy. However, in general approximately one third of men are largely unaffected, one third show a partial fall in potency and one third are rendered completely impotent. A proportion of these men will be helped by impotence therapy.

The results of external beam radiotherapy in locally advanced disease

Locally advanced disease is defined as tumor stage T3 and PSA more than 20.

It is recognized that the prognosis following prostatectomy is significantly worse once the tumor has penetrated the capsule and the PSA has risen above 20. Similar results have been reported following external beam radiotherapy[12].

The reduced chance of cure has made radical prostatectomy more difficult to justify and the mainstay of therapy for this group of patients is conformal external beam radiation. Results of radiotherapy series in this group of patients are illustrated in Figure 45.20[18].

Adjuvant hormonal manipulation

In view of these disappointing results the question has been asked as to whether the addition of hormone manipulation to radiotherapy would improve the results A randomized study published by the European Organization for Research and Treatment of Cancer (EORTC)[22] shows a significant improvement in survival in

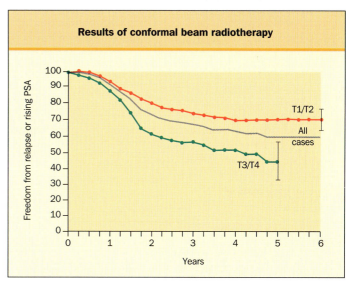

Figure 45.20 Results of conformal beam radiotherapy comparing early (T1/T2) with locally-advanced (T3/T4) disease. PSA, prostate-specific antigen. (From Zagars et al.[18] with permission from Elsevier Science.)

Results of external beam radiotherapy on favorable early prostate cancer				
Reference	Date	No. of patients	Median followup (months)	Biochemically relapse-free (%)
Zietman et al.[12]	1995	504	49	60
Zagars et al.[18]	1995	461	31	65
Kubin et al.[19]	1995	384	78	65

Figure 45.19 Results of external beam radiotherapy on favorable early prostate cancer.

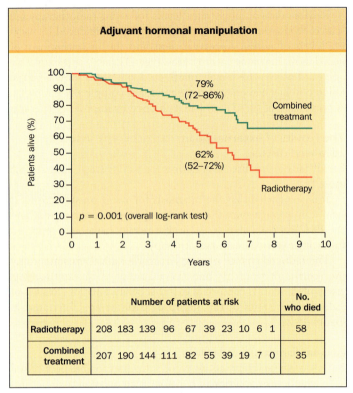

Figure 45.21 **Adjuvant hormonal manipulation.** Overall survival in patients treated with a combination of hormone therapy and radiotherapy compared with radiotherapy alone. (From Bolla et al.[22] © 1997 Massachusetts Medical Society. All rights reserved.)

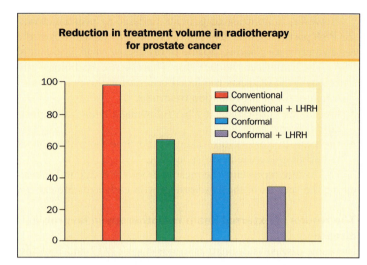

Figure 45.22 **Reduction in treatment volume in radiotherapy for prostate cancer.** LHRH, luteinizing hormone-releasing hormone. (Adapted from Dearnaley[24].)

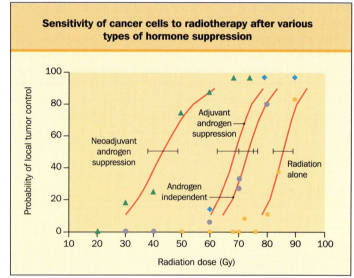

Figure 45.23 **Sensitivity of cancer cells to radiotherapy after various types of hormone suppression.** (From Zeitman et al.[25])

patients receiving radiotherapy in addition to 3 years of hormone therapy compared with radiotherapy alone (Fig. 45.21).

The Radiation Therapy Oncology Group (RTOG) randomized 977 patients to receive radiotherapy and 2 years adjuvant hormone therapy or radiotherapy alone followed by hormone therapy on relapse[23]. This study showed an improvement in local control and freedom from progression in the adjuvant hormone arm but, with a median followup of 4.5 years, there has not been a significant impact on overall survival.

Hormonal downstaging

There are theoretical advantages whereby the results of radiotherapy could be improved by pretreating patients with 3–6 months of hormone therapy.

The rationale for this approach is:
- Hormone therapy may eradicate occult metastatic disease.
- Reducing the volume of the prostate by hormone therapy permits a smaller volume of tissue to be included within the radiation field. This may reduce the normal tissue side effect and permit dose escalation.
- The hormone therapy may render the tumor more radiosensitive.
- The hormone therapy reduces the number of viable malignant cells to be killed by the radiation treatment.

Studies have shown a significant reduction in radiotherapy volume following hormone therapy[24] (Fig. 45.22).

Zietman et al.[25] showed in animal studies evidence that prostate cancer cells may be more sensitive to radiotherapy after hormone deprivation (Fig. 45.23).

The evidence to suggest that hormone therapy removes occult metastatic disease is less compelling. Experience in patients with proven metastatic disease implies a temporary remission rather than cure with hormone manipulation. In addition, the use of neoadjuvant hormone therapy prior to surgery has not satisfactorily reduced the risk of subsequent metastatic disease[26].

The clinical evidence to support the approach of hormonal downstaging prior to radiotherapy is still accruing. Laverdiere and colleagues have published preliminary results on 118 patients[27] and these are summarized in Figure 45.24.

The RTOG 86-10 randomized study compared 226 patients receiving hormone therapy 2 months prior to and during radiotherapy with 230 patients receiving radiotherapy alone. The results at a median followup of 5.9 years are illustrated in Figure 45.25[28].

Effect of hormonal downstaging in combination with radiotherapy for prostate cancer						
Time postradiotherapy (months)	PSA value (ng/mL)			Residual tumor in prostate biopsy (%)		
	Group 1	Group 2	Group 3	Group 1	Group 2	Group 3
12	1.56	0.60	0.20	62	30	4
24	1.20	0.65	0.50	65	28	5

Figure 45.24 Effect of hormonal downstaging in combination with radiotherapy for prostate cancer. Results in terms of post-treatment prostate-specific antigen (PSA) and biopsy. Group 1, radiotherapy alone; Group 2, neoadjuvant hormones plus radiotherapy; Group 3, neoadjuvant hormones and radiotherapy followed by adjuvant hormones. (Adapted from Laverdiere et al.[27])

Effect of adjuvant hormone therapy on success rate of radiotherapy for prostate cancer			
Therapy regimen	No. of patients	Local failure at 5 years (%)	PSA failure at 5 years (%)
Hormones and radiotherapy	226	25	61
Radiotherapy alone	230	36	80

Figure 45.25 Effect of adjuvant hormone therapy on success rate of radiotherapy for prostate cancer. (From ref[28] © by the Lancet Ltd 1999.)

In summary

Current recommended practice for T3 tumors with a PSA of greater than 20 is 3–4 months of hormone downstaging followed by external beam conformal radiotherapy. The question remains as to whether hormone therapy should be continued for 3 years as described in the EORTC study[22] and an ongoing EORTC trial is addressing this question comparing 3 years of hormone therapy with a reduced period of 6 months.

Are there any disadvantages with hormone downstaging?

Inevitably these patients are subjected to the expected side effects of testosterone deprivation. This should, however, resolve on discontinuing the treatment, although preliminary evidence is emerging that impotence rates following radiotherapy may be higher in men receiving neoadjuvant hormone therapy than in those treated with radiotherapy alone.

Technical aspects of radiotherapy for localized prostate cancer

The radiotherapy treatment volume should encompass the entire prostate gland, with the immediate periprostatic tissue. The treatment volume is usually outlined on a series of CT sections through the pelvis.

Should the seminal vesicles be routinely included in the radiation treatment volume?

Data accumulated from large prostatectomy series have indicated the likelihood of seminal vesicle involvement taking into account clinical stage, PSA, and Gleason grade. Indications for inclusion of seminal vesicle in the radiotherapy treatment volume are:
- Evidence of seminal vesicle involvement:
  - biopsy;
  - transrectal ultrasound or MR scanning;
- PSA greater than 20;
- T3 tumors; and
- Gleason score greater than 7.

Should pelvic lymph nodes be included within the radiation treatment volume?

There is a low likelihood of nodal disease in patients with T1/T2 tumors, favorable Gleason score, and a PSA below 20ng/ml[29]. In this setting, pelvic lymph nodes would not be routinely included in the radiation field.

The results of external beam radiotherapy in poor-risk locally advanced prostate cancer

This is defined as tumor stage T3 and PSA greater than 50.

Despite there being no evidence of bone or lymph node metastases on standard imaging, these patients remain at high risk of occult metastatic disease. Therefore hormone manipulation would appear the most appropriate initial management on the current data[30]. The issue that has not been resolved is whether local radiotherapy should be added to the hormone manipulation. An MRC study[31] compared hormone therapy versus radiotherapy versus combined radiotherapy and hormone therapy in 227 patients and found no significant survival advantage. This issue is being addressed by a study set up by the National Cancer Institute of Canada (NCIC), which now has multinational participation. The treatment scheme is illustrated in Figure 45.26. The results of this study will not be known for a number of years.

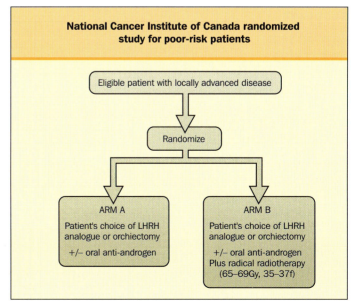

Figure 45.26 National Cancer Institute of Canada randomized study for poor-risk patients. LHRH, luteinizing hormone-releasing hormone.

Radiotherapy following prostatectomy

The place of postoperative radiotherapy has not been clearly defined. It has been suggested that radiotherapy to the prostatic bed may be of value in patients who have histologically positive resection margins but this has not been proved.

Data is accumulating for the use of radiotherapy in patients with a rising PSA following prostatectomy. The evidence would suggest that postoperative prostatic bed radiotherapy is most effective when the PSA is still below 3[32].

Brachytherapy

Brachytherapy or interstitial therapy refers to the delivery of very localized radiation treatment within the prostate by inserting radioactive seeds (iodine-125 or palladium-103). Initial studies evaluating this approach were performed at the Memorial Sloan–Kettering Hospital in New York in the 1970s. However, it has only been in the last 10 years that the procedures has been incorporated into standard clinical practice.

Indications for brachytherapy
- T1, T2 tumors;
- no previous transurethral resection of the prostate; and
- minimal benign prostatic hypertrophy (prostate volume <50cm^2).

Practical details

The volume of the prostate gland is accurately estimated using transrectal ultrasound scanning, usually under general anesthesia. Calculations are then made of the precise positioning and the appropriate number of radioactive seeds to be inserted into the gland. Under general anesthetic the seeds are inserted via transperineal needles using a template (Fig. 45.27).

The seeds remain in situ and the radiation treatment is essentially delivered over several weeks (iodine-125 half-life, 60 days;

palladium-103 half-life 17 days). Usually this treatment can be administered as an outpatient procedure. The major side effect is urethritis, which may last for up to 3 months.

Results

In early favorable prognosis disease (T1/T2 PSA <20) the results are comparable with surgery and conformal radio-therapy[33]. Inevitably, this data is less mature and longer followup is required to adequately assess the outcome.

The advantages of brachytherapy (Fig. 45.28) are:
- localized therapy treats less normal tissue, potentially giving rise to less side effects in terms of less proctitis and less impotence;
- it is delivered as an outpatient procedure.

Palliative radiotherapy in metastatic cancer of the prostate
Bone metastases

External beam radiotherapy is highly effective at relieving pain from bone metastases and may enhance bone healing.

Radiotherapy is not routinely recommended for asymptomatic bone metastases visualized on bone scan or plain radiology. The indications for radiotherapy for bone metastases are:
- pain;
- prevention/treatment of pathologic fracture; and
- prevention/treatment of spinal cord compression.

In the majority of cases adequate analgesia can be achieved by administering between one and 10 daily fractions of radiation to the affected bone, with pain relief expected 10–14 days following treatment.

Spinal cord compression requires emergency intervention. The therapeutic options include surgical decompression or radiotherapy and the relative indications are shown in Figure 45.29.

Figure 45.27 Technique of brachytherapy.

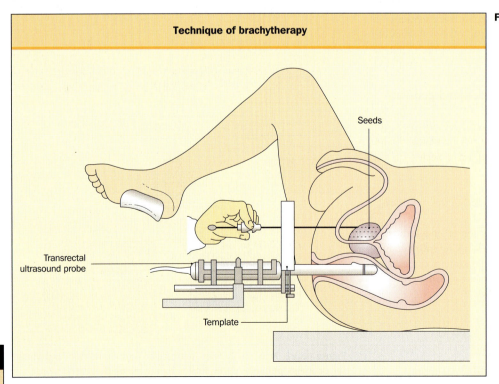

Technique of brachytherapy

Seeds

Transrectal ultrasound probe

Template

Comparison of surgery, external beam radiotherapy, and brachytherapy for prostate cancer

	Surgery	External beam radiotherapy	Brachytherapy
Ease of therapy	–	–	+
Proctitis	–	+	–
Urethral symptoms	+	–	+
Impotence	+	+	*
*Data emerging for impotence following brachytherapy is conflicting			

Figure 45.28 Comparison of surgery, external beam radiotherapy, and brachytherapy for prostate cancer.

Surgery versus radiotherapy for spinal cord compression

Factors favoring surgery	Factors favoring radiotherapy
A need for a tissue diagnosis	Patient unfit for surgical intervention and/or a short life expectancy
A need for spinal stabilization procedure	Multiple lesions
	A need for pain relief

Figure 45.29 Surgery versus radiotherapy for spinal cord compression

The likelihood of neurologic recovery from the emergency radiotherapy is dependent upon the presence of favorable features:

- minor neurologic deficit pre treatment;
- neurologic deficit of less than 24 hours duration; and
- good neurologic response to dexamethasone.

Isotope therapy – strontium/sumarium

Strontium and sumarium are both bone-seeking radionuclides that, when injected intravenously, will target radiation to the bony skeleton. Comparative studies have shown the equivalence in pain relief compared with conventional radiotherapy[34]. Isotope therapy offers the advantage of simultaneous treatment to multiple areas of bone metastases and is relatively easy to administer. It remains, however, a rather costly treatment.

Interest has been expressed in the potential of these therapies in a prophylactic setting in patients with asymptomatic bone metastases in an attempt to prevent or delay symptomatic disease progression. This issue is a subject of ongoing studies.

Radiotherapy for nodal metastases

Patients with symptomatic nodal progression refractory to hormone therapy may be helped by radiation treatment. The more common situations are pelvic nodal disease causing pain and/or lower limb swelling. Retroperitoneal nodal metastases may lead to pain or inferior venacaval obstruction. A degree of symptomatic improvement is seen in the majority of appropriately selected patients receiving radiotherapy to these nodal areas (Fig. 45.30).

Local radiotherapy in metastatic disease

Occasionally, men with documented metastatic disease experience distressing local symptoms from progression within the prostate gland unresponsive to hormone manipulation. In this

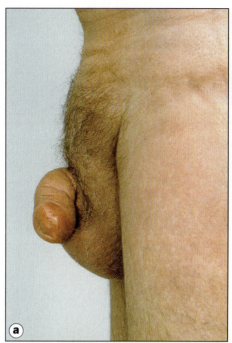

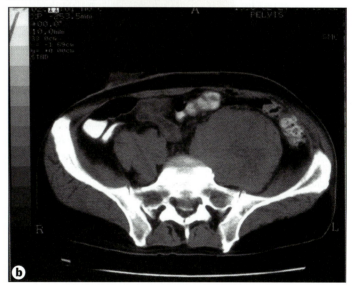

Figure 45.30 Radiotherapy for nodal metastases. (a) Lower limb and penile edema due to inferior vena caval compression. (b) Computed tomography scan showing substantial metastatic nodal enlargement

setting local radiotherapy to the prostate may provide relief of local symptoms for the remainder of the patient's life.

CARCINOMA OF THE PENIS

The management of this disease has been discussed in Chapter 41. Radiotherapy offers an opportunity of preserving the full penis, reserving amputation as a salvage procedure. Radiotherapy is appropriate for men with early disease (Jackson stage 1) with no evidence of nodal metastases.

A purpose built immobilization device is made to encompass the penis during treatment (Fig. 45.31a, b). The treatment is delivered as shown in Figure 45.32.

Side effects include:

- acute skin reaction lasting several weeks post radiotherapy; and
- late effects – telangiectasia, urethral stricture.

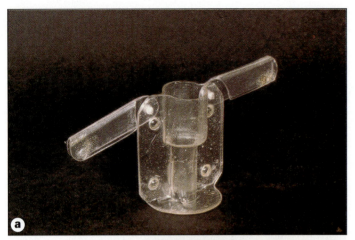

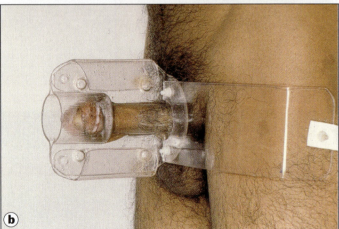

Figure 45.31 Immobilization device used in radiotherapy for carcinoma of the penis. The immobilization device (a) is secured using the pelvic wings and a PVC strap and wax is used to compensate for the cylindric shape (b).

The place of prophylactic nodal irradiation is unclear. Patients receiving radiotherapy to the penis alone require close followup. Most treatment failures (local and nodal) develop within the first 2 years. Local or nodal failure, if discovered early, should be amenable to surgical salvage.

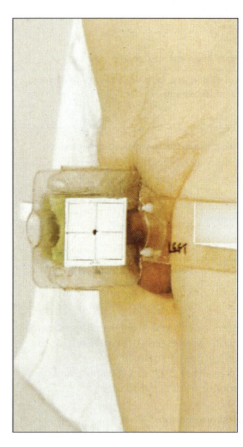

Figure 45.32 Administration of radiotherapy for carcinoma of the penis.

REFERENCES

1. Roentgen WC. On a new kind of rays (preliminary communication). Translation of the Paper read on 28 December 1895. Br J Radiol. 1931;4:32.

2. Curie P, Curie Mme P, Bemont G. Sur une nouvelle substance fortement radioactive contenue dans la pechblende. Compt Rend Acad Sci (Paris). 1898;127:1215–7.

3. Sawchuk IS, Olsson CA, deVere White R. The limited usefulness of external beam radiotherapy in the control of superficial bladder cancer. Br J Urol. 1988;61:330–2.

4. International collaboration of trialists on behalf of the Medical Research Council Advanced Bladder Cancer Working Party, et al. Neoadjuvant cisplatin, methotrexate and vinblastine chemotherapy for muscle-invasive bladder cancer: a randomised controlled trial (BA06/3089 trial).

5. Kachnic LA, Kaufman DS, Griffin PP, et al. Bladder preservation by combined modality therapy for invasive bladder cancer. J Clin Oncol. 1997;15:1022–9.

6. Duncan W, Quilty PM. The results of a series of 963 patients with transitional cell carcinoma of the urinary bladder primarily treated by radical megavoltage X-ray therapy. Radiother Oncol. 1986;7:299–310.

7. Pollack A, Gunar K, Zagars GK, Swanson DA. Muscle-invasive bladder cancer treated with external beam radiotherapy: prognostic factors. Int J Radiat Oncol Biol Phys. 1994;30:267–77.

8. Gospadorowicz MK, Rider WD, Keen CW, et al. Bladder cancer: long-term follow-up results of patients treated with radical radiation. Clin Oncol. 1991;3:155–61.

9. Kaufman DS, Shipley WU, Griffin PP, et al. Selective bladder preservation by combination treatment of invasive bladder cancer. N Engl J Med. 1993;329:1377–82.

10. Dunst J, Sauer R, Schrott KM, Reinhold K, Wittekind C, Altendorf-Hofmann A. Organ-sparing treatment of advanced bladder cancer: a 10-year experience. Int J Radiat Oncol Biol Phys. 1994;30:261–6.

11. West CML, Davidson SE, Elyan SAG, et al. The intrinsic radiosensitivity of normal and tumour cells. Int J Radiat Biol. 1998;73:409–13.

12. Zietman AL, Coen JJ, Dallow KC, Shipley WU. The treatment of prostate cancer by conventional radiation therapy: An analysis of long-term outcome. Int J Radiat Oncol Biol Phys. 1995;32:287–92.

13. Keyser D, Kupelian PA, Zippe CD, Levin HS, Klein EA. Stage T1–2 prostate cancer with pretreatment prostate-specific antigen level 10ng/ml: radiation therapy or surgery? Int J Radiat Oncol Biol Phys. 1997;38:723–9.

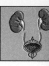

14. Chodak, GW, Thistad, RA, Gerber, GS. et al. Results of conservative management of clinically localized prostate cancer. N Engl J Med 1994;330:242–8.

15. Livsey JE, Cowan RA, Brown SEW, et al. Trial of randomisation between radical prostatectomy and radiotherapy in early prostate cancer. Clin Onc. 2000;12:63.

16. American Society for Therapeutic Radiology and Oncology Consensus Panel. Consensus statement: guidelines for PSA following radiation therapy. Int J Radiat Oncol Biol Phys. 1997;37:1035–41.

17. Read G, Pointon RCS. Retrospective study of radiotherapy in early carcinoma of the prostate. Br J Urol. 1989;63:191–5.

18. Zagars GK, Pollack A, Kavadi VS, von Eschenback AC. Prostate-specific antigen and radiation therapy for clinically localized prostate cancer. Int J Radiat Oncol Biol Phys. 1995;32:293–306.

19. Kuban DA, el-Mahdi AM, Schellhammer PF. Prostate-specific antigen for pre-treatment prediction and post-treatment evaluation of outcome after definitive irradiation for prostate cancer. Int J Radiat Oncol Biol Phys. 1995;32:307–16.

20. Zelefsky MJ, Leibel SA, Gaudin PB, et al. Dose escalation with three-dimensional conformal radiation therapy affects the outcome in prostate cancer. Int J Radiat Oncol Biol Phys. 1998;41:491–500.

21. Dearnaley DP, Khoo VS, Norman AR, et al. The comparison of radiation side-effects of conformal and conventional radiotherapy in prostate cancer: a randomised trial. Lancet. 1999;353:267–72.

22. Bolla M, Gonzalez D, Warde P, et al. Improved survival in patients with locally advanced prostate cancer treated with radiotherapy and goserelin. N Engl J Med. 1997;337:295–300.

23. Pilepich MV, Caplan R, Byhardt RW, et al. Phase III study of androgen suppression using goserelin in unfavourable prognosis carcinoma of the prostate treated with definitive radiotherapy. (Report of RTOG Protocol 85-31.) J Clin Oncol. 1997;15): 1013–21.

24. Dearnaley DP, Nahum A, Lee M, et al. Radiotherapy of prostate cancer. Reducing the treated volume. Conformal therapy, hormone cytoreduction and protons. Br J Cancer. 1994;70(suppl. 22):16.

25. Zietman AL, Prince EA, Nakfoor BM, Park JJ. Androgen deprivation and radiation therapy: Sequencing studies using the Shionogi *In VIVO* Tumor System. Int J Radiat Oncol Biol Phys. 1997;38:1067–70.

26. Goldenberg SL, Klotz LH, Srigley J, et al. Randomized, prospective, controlled study comparing radical prostatectomy alone and neoadjuvant androgen withdrawal in the treatment of localized prostate cancer. Canadian Urological Oncology Group. J Urol. 1996;156:873–7.

27. Laverdiere J, Gomez JL, Cusan L, et al. Beneficial effect of combination hormonal therapy administered prior and following external beam radiation therapy in localized prostate cancer. Int J Radiat Oncol Biol Phys. 1997;37:247–52.

28. International collaboration of trialists on behalf of the Medical Research Council Advanced Bladder Cancer Working Party, EORTC Genito-Urinary Group, Australian Bladder Cancer Study Group, National Cancer Institute of Canada Clinical Trials Group, Finnbladder, Norwegian Bladder Cancer Study Group, and Club Urologico Espanol de Tratamiento Oncologico (CUETO) Group. Neoadjuvant cisplatin, methotrexate, and vinblastine chemotherapy for muscle-invasive bladder cancer: a randomised controlled trial. Lancet. 1999;354:533–40.

29. Partin AW, Yoo J, Carter HB, et al. The use of prostate-specific antigen, clinical stage and Gleason score to predict pathological stage in men with localised prostate cancer. J Urol. 1993;150:110–4.

30. Medical Research Council Prostate Cancer Working Party Investigators Group. Immediate versus deferred treatment for advanced prostatic cancer: initial research results of the Medical Research Council Trial. Br J Urol. 1997;79:235–46.

31. Fellows GJ, Clark PB, Beynon LL, et al. Treatment of advanced localised prostatic cancer by orchidectomy, radiotherapy or combined treatment. A Medical Research Council Study. Br J Urol. 1992;70:304–9.

32. Wu JJ, King SC, Montana GS, McKinstry CA, Ancher MS. The efficacy of postprostatectomy radiotherapy in patients with an isolated elevation of serum prostate-specific antigen. Int J Radiat Oncol Biol Phys. 1995;32:317–23.

33. Blasko JC, Wallner K, Grimm PD, et al. Prostate-specific antigen based disease control following ultrasound guided I 125 implantation for stage T1/T2 prostatic carcinoma. J Urol. 1995;154:1096–9.

34. Porter et al. Results of a randomized phase III trial to evaluate the efficacy of strontium-89 (^{89}Sr) adjacent to local field external beam irradiation in the management of endocrine resistant prostate cancer. Int J Radiat Oncol Biol Phys. 1993;25:805–13.

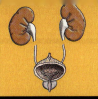

Chapter 46

Chemotherapy in Urology

CHEMOTHERAPY IN UROLOGY: TESTIS CANCER

R Tim D Oliver

KEY POINTS

- Cure rate of testicular germ cell cancer is now in excess of 95% for all cases and 85% for patients with metastatic disease.
- The standard chemotherapy for metastatic disease is bleomycin, etoposide and cisplatin.
- There is ongoing debate as to whether surveillance, adjuvant treatment for all or adjuvant treatment for patients at high risk of relapse is optimum management for patients with stage 1 disease.
- Despite the high cure, both patient and physician related delay remains a major factor in the extent of tumor spread and chance of failing primary treatment and education about this risk should continue to be encouraged.

Since the success from use of chemotherapy to treat choriocarcinoma in women in late 1950s, patients with metastatic nonseminomatous testicular germ cell cancers have been a test bed that has made a significant contribution to the development of chemotherapy for adult cancers. Today, compared to other cancers there is an almost embarrassing excess of choice for first-, second- and third-line treatment and in excess of 85% of metastatic disease patients achieve durable primary long-term disease-free survival[1,2,3] and in excess of 95% of all cases survive[4,5].

Much of the work on chemotherapy in testis cancer has been in patients with metastatic nonseminoma. However with evidence that nonseminomas arise by clonal evolution from seminomas[5], the chapter will also review the observations that have been noted from chemotherapy of seminoma.

CHEMOTHERAPY IN THE PRIMARY MANAGEMENT OF GERM CELL CANCERS

Delay in diagnosis and treatment

Before the advent of cisplatin, early diagnosis and immediate orchidectomy were paramount. Today less attention is paid to this issue and there has been a tendency to treat these patients as less of an emergency. There is some evidence to support this attitude as today the overall results are so good, with more than 95% alive[4], that it is difficult to see any gain from reduction in delay in terms of overall survival[1]. However when delay is correlated with stage, which directly correlates with the amount of treatment needed, it is clear that there is still a direct relation between delay and extent of disease (Figs 46.1 & 46.2). A further demonstration of the significance of delay comes from analysis of extent of delay in those needing salvage chemotherapy and those cured by primary chemotherapy. With the average delay in those needing bone marrow transplant (6.2 months) being nearly double that of those cured by primary

Influences of changes in preorchidectomy delay on cure of testis germ cell cancer 1978–1984						
	1978–1983 (*n* =113)		1984–1988 (*n* =155)		1989–1994 (*n* =185)	
Delay	Proportion in cohort (%)	% currently nem (*n*)	Proportion in cohort (%)	% currently nem (*n*)	Proportion in cohort (%)	% currently nem (*n*)
<1 month	17	89 (19)	23	94 (36)	31	100 (57)
2–3 months	30	79 (34)	36	93 (56)	28	98 (52)
4–11 months	33	81 (37)	24	89 (37)	32	100 (59)
>12 months	20	57 (23)	17	89 (26)	9	94 (17)
All cases						
Median delay/ currently nem (%)	4 months/77		3 months/92		3 months/98	
Median tumor size (cm)	4.8		4.5		4.0	

Figure 46.1 Influences of changes in preorchidectomy delay on cure of testis germ cell cancer 1978–1984. nem, no evidence of malignancy.

Delay and proportion of true stage 1 testis cancer

Months delay	No. cases	Stage 1 (%)	Relapse on surveillance (%)	True stage 1 (%)
>1	40	80	18	66
1–2	70	60	26	44
2–3	143	46	29	33
<3	200	45	38	28

Figure 46.2 Delay and proportion of true stage 1 testis cancer.

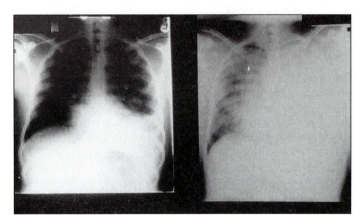

Figure 46.3 Acute respiratory failure occurring 2 weeks after orchidectomy.

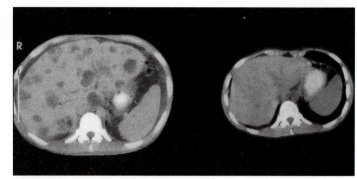

Figure 46.4 Vena cava tumor invasion. (Left) Budd–Chiari syndrome from vena cava tumor invasion causing hepatorenal failure and (right) resolving after chemotherapy.

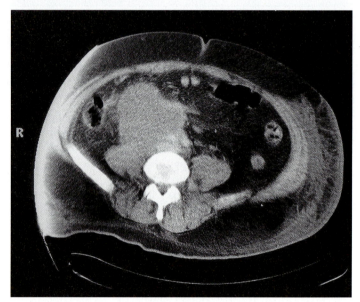

Figure 46.5 Vena cava tumor invasion. Mass of lymph nodes invading vena cava leading to death from renal failure and gangrene of both legs 14 days after first consultation.

chemotherapy (3.4 months), it is clear that avoidance of delay in diagnosis is still of primary importance in management of this disease.

A further factor justifying attention to delay is the rare occurrence (1–2% of metastatic cases) of hurricane growth of these tumors after orchidectomy as illustrated in Figure 46.3, where a patient developed acute respiratory failure within 2 weeks of orchidectomy, Figure 46.4, where a patient developed Budd–Chiari hepatorenal shutdown from para-aortic lymph node metastasis invasion of vena cava, hepatic, and renal veins within 2 weeks of initial histologic diagnosis; and Figure 46.5, where the patient developed lower limb venous infarction from a low para-aortic lymph node mass invading the bifurcation of the vena cava but also spreading up the vena cava, causing hepatorenal failure, and died within 2 weeks of presentation without being able to have any chemotherapy.

The lesson from the analysis of effect of delay and extent of spread and the anecdotes on hurricane growth is that it is vital that all clinicians involved in diagnosis of this disease must be aware of these possibilities and prepared to organize for the patients to be treated as an emergency. In such a circumstance it may be necessary to make the diagnosis on the basis of the clinical situation and tumor markers that can be performed as an emergency, using the urinary pregnancy test with or without a fine needle biopsy depending on the circumstance.

Fertility

A further factor that has made it of considerable importance to consider medical management before orchidectomy is the issue of fertility. There is now evidence that 10% of patients presenting

with a primary testis tumor have no sperm production from the contralateral testis and orchidectomy of patient with a small tumor in a testis with a normally functioning rim of germ cells can lead to induction of infertility in these patients and a 50% reduction of sperm count in half of the other patients[6], demonstrating the importance of not doing orchidectomy unnecessarily in patients who are going to have to proceed to chemotherapy. It is important in such cases that at least some thought is given to preserving sperm before any treatment, i.e. chemotherapy or orchidectomy, is undertaken.

PRACTICAL ISSUES WITH USE OF CHEMOTHERAPY FOR TREATING GERM CELL CANCERS

While there is little doubt that prescribing the standard regimen of bleomycin, etoposide, and cisplatin (BEP) is not particularly difficult, it is the actual decisions taken during the period of treatment that is crucial to the success of the therapy. This is why it is of paramount importance that these patients are treated in major centers treating adequate numbers of patients to gain sufficient experience in the minutiae of treatment. All major centers have demonstrated improvement in results as a result of the experience of using the regimen[2,4,7]. This experience relates to management issues such as the need to ensure that the treatment is done on time according to the 21-day schedule, the need to ensure that treatment-related death is avoided by intensive treatment of neutropenic sepsis and, in particularly at-risk patients, using antibiotic prophylaxis over the neutropenic phase, avoiding aminoglycoside use or having extremely careful dosage control if this is the only antibiotic that can be used, as this agent is synergistic with cisplatin and in the past has led to patients having to be put on to hemodialysis. A recently identified risk has been use of intravenous contrast in the week after cisplatin. Monitoring for cisplatin-induced magnesium leak in sick patients and adjusting bleomycin dosage in the event of any cisplatin-induced reduction of renal function to avoid bleomycin lung are other critical aspects of management. Finally, once cured, as well as monitoring for relapse on follow up, it is also important to assess testicular function and organize testosterone replacement for any patients with Leydig cell failure. This occurs in the majority of patients in the first 6 months after chemotherapy, and for some of these patients a short period of monthly intramuscular testosterone replacement helps. Only a small minority require continuous replacement.

SELECTION OF PATIENTS FOR CHEMOTHERAPY

In the late 1970s, when cisplatin-based curative treatment first became available, treatment was restricted to patients with blood-borne metastatic M+ disease or those who had failed conventional local treatment with surgery or radiation for node-positive patients. These were initially mainly nonseminomas, as whole-lung radiation could cure a proportion of seminomas with lung metastases. As confidence grew in the durability of cures and it became apparent that previously irradiated patients had higher risks of neutropenic deaths, nodal disease N+ patients in centers using radiotherapy began receiving chemotherapy first. With increasing recognition of the value of postchemotherapy surgery for establishing when it was safe to stop chemotherapy, this began to be increasingly used in these centers and it is now the practice in our center to use chemotherapy for all patients with metastatic nonseminoma with early surgery for localized disease if there is marker response but no obvious shrinkage by d21[8]. If the markers fail to respond, salvage chemotherapy is usually the treatment of choice, although in patients with alpha-fetoprotein-positive disease there is a subgroup who become long-term cured following surgery alone despite persistent viable malignancy.

CHOICE OF CHEMOTHERAPY FOR NONSEMINOMA

It was the demonstration that etoposide cisplatin produced 37% continuous disease-free survival after failure of cisplatin, vinblastine, and bleomycin (PVB) that led to etoposide being substituted for vinblastine and proved to be significantly better as first-line therapy in both good and poor risk patients[9]. Subsequently, three salvage strategies of BEP failures (Fig. 46.6)

Salvage studies in germ cell cancer			
	No. cases	Relapse-free (%)	Currently nem (%)
EP/BEP	30	37	37
VIP	135	24	32
M-BOP	65	45	60
High dose	283	30	30
High dose × 2	25	52	52

Figure 46.6 Salvage studies in germ cell cancer. EP, etopside, cisplatin; BEP, bleomycin, etopside, and cisplatin; M-BOP, methotrexate-bleomycin, oncovin, and cisplatin; nem, no evidence of malignancy; VIP, velbe, ifosfamide, and cisplatin.

have been explored in reasonable numbers[10]. Vinblastine, ifosfamide, and cisplatin (VIP) was the first and, although it salvaged 24% of BEP failures, it failed to improve survival over BEP when used in a randomized trial for previously untreated patients.

Two strategies of dose intensification have been explored in salvage setting (Fig. 46.6). The first used 'horizontal' dose intensification with weekly bleomycin, oncovin, and cisplatin (BOP). This uses doses similar to those standard regimens. When used as first-line salvage it does not show cross-resistance with the other standard salvage regimen (VIP) and 47% achieve primary salvage and 60% are salvaged overall after third-line regimens[11].

However when BOP was combined with VIP as a first-line regimen (BOP/VIP) it failed to demonstrate any superiority over BEP in poor-risk patients.

Currently most research on salvage treatment internationally is being made on the effects of 'vertical' dose intensification using 1–4 high-dose treatments with chemotherapy and peripheral blood stem cell rescue[12]. Although this approach is currently being investigated in a randomized trial against VIP without high dose, to date there is no evidence that it is better than BEP, which remains the universal standard at the present time.

Several drugs both old and new (methotrexate, paclitaxel, and gemcitabine) are working after failed high dose and hold promise that there will be even further progress in the future.

In addition to new chemotherapy regimens there is increasing recognition that surgery can salvage patients with chemotherapy-resistant disease[13]. Most centers report in excess of 50% durable relapse-free survival after retroperitoneal lymph node dissection (RPLND) of patients with persistent tumor marker elevation after chemotherapy. However reports of accelerated tumor recurrence after surgery, if done in totally unresponsive patients[14], emphasizes the importance of case selection for such surgery.

TRIALS IN NONSEMINOMA: GOOD AND POOR RISK PATIENTS

Today using level of α-fetoprotein, β-human chorionic gonadotrophin and lactic dehydrogenase with extent of disease it is possible to define three prognostic groups for outcome after chemotherapy[2,3].

Three principal questions have been addressed in the good risk patients (Fig. 46.7): a) dropping bleomycin because of the risk of mortality from bleomycin lung; b) changing cisplatin to carboplatin because of oto- and nephrotoxicity; and c) reducing

Overview of trials in good-risk patients			
Trial	Number of trials	Number of cases	Progression free (%)
Platinum combination			
+ bleomycin	4	434	86
– bleomycin	4	425	77
Combination plus			
cisplatin	3	256	91
carboplatin	3	240	79
Number of courses			
BEP × 4	1	96	92
BEP × 3	1	88	92

Figure 46.7 Overview of trials in good risk patients. BEP, bleomycin, etoposide, and cisplatin.

Comparison of BEPq21 and phase II studies of accelerated cisplatin (q<14) regimens verses high dose regimens as first-line therapy in 'poor risk' nonseminoma			
Study	No. of cases	Progression- free (%)	Toxic deaths (%)
BEP[33]	81	77	4
BOP[34,35]	58	83	NA
BOP/VIP[36]	91	63	2
C-BOP/BEP[37,38]	91	82	7
MD Anderson[39]	22	82	Nil
HD VIP × 4[16]	141	68	8
VIP + HD[40]	30	50	NA
VIP v.	145	64	3
PEB[15]	141	60	4
BOP-VIP v.	185	53	8
BEP[41]	185	60	3

Figure 46.8 Comparison of BEPq21 and phase II studies of accelerated cisplatin (q<14) regimens verses high dose regimens as first line therapy in 'poor risk' nonseminoma. BEP, bleomycin, etopside, and cisplatin; BOP, bleomycin, oncovin, and cisplatin.

treatment from four courses to three. Only the last of these has been proved to be free from risk of reduced cure[10].

Despite several phase II studies suggesting that there are regimens better than BEP in poor risk patients (Fig. 46.8), for no regimen tested in poor risk patients to date has there been significant progression-free survival advantage over BEP and all have to a greater or lesser extent increased toxicity problems[15], including treatment-related mortality[16].

LATE EVENTS

Apart from the treatment-related mortalities discussed in the previous section, the most serious treatment-related event seen in these patients has been etoposide-associated leukemia. Although this has been predominantly in patients who have accumulated a high dose over a long period of treatment, it has occurred in patients with low doses[17]. Interestingly, the ultra high doses used with stem cell rescue do not seem to be associated with any increased risk over conventional doses. With radiation-induced secondary cancers it is known that most of the risk is associated with low dose prolonged treatment. So far followup after etoposide is too short to exclude any risk in terms of late solid cancers. As has been seen after radiation, the risk of solid tumors does not develop until 10–20 years have passed[18]. This issue is of some importance when one contemplates using etoposide in an adjuvant setting (see below).

Gonadal toxicity is one other area where there is increasing information. It is now becoming clear that the majority (circa 80%) of patients treated with bleomycin, etoposide and cisplatin recover spermatogenesis, though in about 1 in 3 it is delayed beyond the conventionally stated time of 2 years and can return as late as 5 years[19]. It is of interest that about 20% of patients with absolute azoospermia prior to chemotherapy can recover normospermic counts while some with normal sperm counts never recover. It is thought that in the majority of the former, human chorionic gonadotrophin (hCG) is suppressing spermatogenesis, although some effect of chemotherapy on pre-existing in-situ carcinoma has not been excluded as yet. In keeping with the poorer cure of metastases by regimens using carboplatin, spermatogenesis recovery is generally 6–12 months quicker after carboplatin than cisplatin[19].

ROLE OF CHEMOTHERAPY IN STAGE 1 AND 2 NONSEMINOMA

Chemotherapy for stage 2 disease

In the USA two courses of chemotherapy are used as an adjunct to surgery in the management of early stage 2a/b tumors (for review see Bajorin et al.[3]). In the UK chemotherapy has been primary management for small-volume stage 2 cases, with salvage surgery for patients left with residual disease after achieving marker remission with similar results to those achieved by surgery[4]. In the UK there has been a tendency to leave residual masses after chemotherapy rather than doing post-treatment surgical staging and this has been identified as one factor that may reduce cure[20]. It would seem that, given the fact that more than 50% of tumor bulk can disappear after one course of chemotherapy[8] and the observation that ejaculatory nerve damage is more frequent when removing large masses while chemotherapy-induced loss of spermatogenesis is also increased the longer treatment is continued[19], one course of chemotherapy followed by d21 scanning should be the standard strategy for stage 2 cases. Treatment should then be based on response, with those showing less than 50% response prepared for surgery early after two to three courses unless a delayed response is seen, while the rest are allowed to complete three courses of chemotherapy. It is of course incumbent on any center that uses the medical approach to stage 2 disease not to treat on the basis of a small para-aortic mass on computed tomography (CT) alone unless it is enlarging or there are rising tumor markers, as it is known from surgical series that 10% of patients staged as stage 2 on CT scan have enlarged nodes due to reactive hyperplasia[21].

Chemotherapy for stage 1 disease

In the course of the last 40 years the relapse rate for stage 1 nonseminoma after radiotherapy fell from 55% to 15% because of the advent of improvements in staging from lymphangiogram,

CT scan, and tumor markers[22]. Until recently in the UK it was conventional to define stage 1 disease as any patient with less than 2cm lesion visible on CT scan. With the increasing accuracy of spiral CT scans it is possible to define many smaller lesions. Although the chances of malignancy are known to increase with increasing size, use of a full lymph node dissection to prove this is increasingly accepted as 'overkill', as the risk of relapse remains 10% after surgery[23]. However, laparoscopic RPLND, positron emission tomography (PET) scanning, and new approaches to immunohistochemistry of the primary tumor are improving the prediction of relapse. The critical issue is whether enough precision in diagnosis of early metastatic risk has been achieved to justify adjuvant chemotherapy (Fig. 46.9). As the risk of relapse after adjuvant therapy is very low and salvage of such relapse is good, this is increasingly used as the standard approach. Despite this, standard treatment is still unresolved. Reduced hair loss after BOP regimens is one factor in increasing interest in this combination instead of BEP. The 100% relapse-free results after RPLND plus single-agent actinomycin D or mithramycin in historic studies suggest that there would be justification for single-agent chemotherapy regimens in good risk situations.

Testis conservation with chemotherapy

Despite the overall cure of testes cancer being so high it was thought until recently that the risks of second cancers from carcinoma-in-situ precluded the use of chemotherapy for testes conservation. With suggestions that 75% of patients with germ cell cancer are subfertile, evidence that atrophy is a major risk factor for testis cancer development[24], and a report that 1 in 10 patients with sperm in ejaculate pre-orchidectomy actually became azoospermic after orchidectomy[25], more attention is being paid to this issue[1,26,27].

In one study[26] 14 of 42 with metastases and 3 of 10 with stage 1 tumor were salvaged by chemotherapy, although there were two recurrences salvaged by orchidectomy. So far there has been one pregnancy and 2 others have recovered spermatogenesis.

CHEMOTHERAPY FOR SEMINOMA

It is now more than 50 years since the classic paper by Friedman[28] demonstrated that patients with metastatic seminoma had more lasting complete remissions with lower doses of radiation than malignant teratoma/nonseminoma. This led to adjuvant radiation becoming the standard treatment for stage 1 seminoma. This occurred in the late 1950s and early 1960s, with the cure increasing from 90–95% in most recently treated cohorts of patients[29]. Because relapse has occurred in patients as late as 9 years after orchidectomy alone and patients have presented with signs and symptoms of spinal cord compression as first manifestation of relapse, the need for use of adjuvant treatment has been accepted by most physicians involved in treatment of these patients. Because of the high success rates with radiation, this has remained the standard treatment for stage 1 seminoma[29].

As mentioned earlier, when cisplatin chemotherapy first begun to be used in metastatic nonseminoma because of the exquisite radiosensitivity of seminoma, chemotherapy was being used even more as a last resort treatment in seminoma than in nonseminoma. This was illustrated by the use of whole-lung radiation for seminoma lung metastases, as this cured over 50% of patients with lung metastases. As a consequence, some of the early reports suggested that outcome of metastatic seminoma after cisplatin-based chemotherapy was worse than in nonseminoma. It has only been in the last few years that data has clearly emerged demonstrating that, when using single-agent platinum or BEP as first line and VIP or BOP as second treatment, the results from cisplatin-based chemotherapy treatment of seminoma are substantially better than that from treatment of nonseminoma and this is most pronounced when single-agent cisplatin is used (Fig. 46.10). The importance of pure seminoma histology as an independent good risk factor for response to cisplatin-based therapy has only recently been incontrovertibly confirmed[5,6].

The UK Medical Research Council (MRC) trial TE12 was set up to compare single-agent versus combination therapy in seminoma. This was terminated because of poor results when carboplatin was used in nonseminoma and a nonsignificant excess of relapses that developed in the carboplatin arm. Subsequent analysis showed no significant difference in relapse rate[30]. Recent in vitro studies suggest that oxaliplatin, a new platinum analog, is better than either cisplatin or carboplatin. Given increasing anxiety about etoposide-related leukemia and questions about cancers

Adjuvant studies for stage 1 nonseminoma			
Study	No. of cases	Relapse-free (%)	Survival (%)
RPLND	263 (unselected)	89	97
Radiotherapy[42]	73 (unselected)	85	97
+ RPLND neo adj actinomycin[43]	42 (unselected)	95	100
RPLND + mithramycin[44]	21 (unselected)	100	100
Rad/vinblastine/bleo[45]	16 (poor risk)	87	94
BEP × 2[46–49]	216 (poor risk)	97	99
BEP × 1[49]	44 (poor risk)	93	100
BOP q14[50]	115 (poor risk)	98	99
BOP q10[49]	33 (poor risk)	100	100

Figure 46.9 Adjuvant studies for stage 1 nonseminoma. BEP, bleomycin, etopside, and cisplatin; BOP, bleomycin, oncovin, and cisplatin; RPLND, retroperitoneal lymph node dissection.

Differential chemosensitivity of seminoma and nonseminoma		
	Seminoma (%)	Nonseminoma (%)
Cisplatin as first line	90	10
Carboplatin as first line	78	NA
BEP as first line	95	85
VIP as salvage	67	24
BOP as salvage	85	47

Figure 46.10 Differential chemosensitivity of seminoma and nonseminoma. BEP, bleomycin, etopside, and cisplatin; BOP, bleomycin, oncovin, and cisplatin; VIP, vinblastine, isosfamide, and cisplatin.

after radiation, there is clearly a case for further investigation of single-agent platinum analogues in seminoma. This needs to be both in metastatic disease and in stage 1 disease[31], where one course of carboplatin has been given to 134 patients and there has only been one relapse. Given this apparently lower relapse rate than radiation and its potential to be less toxic, this is being assessed in the latest MRC trial (TE20). Currently, more than 400 patients have been recruited but it will be some time before we get any indication as to the comparative impact on relapse-free survival and even longer in respect of late events.

CLINICAL SIGNIFICANCE OF EXCESSIVE CHEMOSENSITIVITY OF SEMINOMA OVER NONSEMINOMA

With increasing evidence that nonseminoma can develop by clonal evolution from seminoma[5] and with evidence that a p53-related mechanism could be involved in the greater chemosensitivity of germ cell cancers[32], there is clearly more to be learnt from further study of the molecular basis of germ cell cancer chemosensitivity. As well as helping to design molecular approaches to treatment of common solid cancers, it might also help to develop ideas to counteract the continuing anxiety over the declining sperm count that has become increasingly associated with the rising incidence of testis cancer[24].

CONCLUSION

Bleomycin 30mg d2, 9, 19, etoposide 165mg/m² d1–3 or 100mg/m² d1–5, cisplatin 50mg/m² d1–2 or 20mg/m² d1–5 has been established as the standard regimen for all cases of metastatic nonseminoma with in excess of 85% durable relapse-free survival. There are at least three established salvage regimens, VIP, weekly BOP, and high dose chemotherapy, that have

salvaged patients who fail first-line treatment. Despite increasingly strict criteria for definition of poor risk as well as evidence that patients are being diagnosed earlier with less advanced disease, no regimen has done better than BEP when used as first-line therapy. With paclitaxel and gemcitabine showing activity, there may be newer regimens in the near future.

So far, apart from a possible excess of acute myeloid leukemias after high cumulative doses of etoposide, there have been no serious late events. However more detailed and more prolonged followup is required to exclude late solid cancer and vascular problems.

Chemotherapy with salvage surgery or surgery with adjuvant/salvage chemotherapy produces equivalent survival for patients with early stage 2 disease. The recent introduction of a policy of d21 CT assessment of response provides the most cost-effective approach to reduce exposure to chemotherapy in these patients.

Low-toxicity chemotherapy regimens are also becoming established as adjuvants for high-risk stage 1 patients because of their low risks of relapse (less than 4%). Encouraged by these results and the increasing recognition of the need to conserve germinal epithelium in patients, 75% of who will have subfertile levels of sperm count there is increasing interest in the use of chemotherapy for testis conservation.

Multivariate analysis and phase 2 studies in first-line and salvage patients has demonstrated that pure seminoma is a predictor of a more favorable response to both single-agent and combination chemotherapy. A further demonstration of this exquisite chemosensitivity of seminoma comes from data on use of one course of carboplatin as adjuvant in 134 patients, with a solitary relapse comparing favorably with the 4% relapse in the contemporarily treated series receiving radiation. Further confirmation from randomized comparison with radiation is now in progress.

CHEMOTHERAPY IN UROLOGY: BLADDER CANCER

Stephen J Harland

KEY POINTS

- For patients with primary disease, the benefit of adjuvant therapy remains relatively marginal at the present time.
- For patients with recurrent disease, temporary responses are frequently seen with combination chemotherapy.

INTRODUCTION

Muscle-invasive bladder cancer is aggressive, with only the minority of patients surviving more than 5 years in prospective studies. Significant numbers of patients return with recurrent

disease following their primary radical treatment (surgery or radiotherapy). These patients are going to request palliation of their symptoms and prolongation of their life. From the surgeon's point of view, however, the desire to improve the primary treatment of patients with invasive disease is considerable.

PALLIATION OF SYMPTOMS

General

Some of the symptoms associated with metastatic or locally recurrent bladder cancer – for example, the pain from bone or pelvic lymph node metastases – may respond satisfactorily to radiotherapy given to the site of recurrence if this is not within the previous field of irradiation. The advantages of this treatment are its brevity and lack of systemic toxicity. The problems with this type of palliation are shown in Figure 46.11.

Chemotherapy is an alternative method of palliating symptoms. The improvement in wellbeing in those responding to chemotherapy is familiar to those who treat metastatic bladder cancer. There is a trade-off, however, since in multicenter studies at least as many patients fail chemotherapy as respond and these patients will have to tolerate the burden of chemotherapy toxicity as well as that of their disease.

Palliation of metastatic bladder cancer with initial radiotherapy – the disadvantages
The time until the development of further symptoms is often short.
Although local symptoms are well controlled it is rare to see improvement in systemic symptoms.
Radiotherapy to marrow-bearing areas can impair a patient's tolerance of any subsequent chemotherapy.

Figure 46.11 Palliation of metastatic bladder cancer with initial radiotherapy – the disadvantages.

Assessing suitability for chemotherapy
Factors reducing the likelihood of durable benefit:
Poor performance status
Hematogenous (as opposed to lymphatic) spread
Recurrence within a recently irradiated field
Factors associated with an increased risk of toxicity:
Poor performance status
Significant prior irradiation of bone marrow
Renal or hepatic impairment for drugs cleared by these organs

Figure 46.12 Assessing suitability for chemotherapy.

How should patients with recurrent bladder cancer be chosen for chemotherapy? One 'computes' the likelihood of severe toxicity and the likelihood of durable benefit of course (Fig. 46.12) but there are few rules. There is no clinical pointer or in vitro test which reliably predicts tumor sensitivity.

Single-agent chemotherapy

Agents with activity in bladder cancer were reviewed in 1987[51]. Essentially, such a review comprises a compilation of patient-series where single agents have been used. Cisplatin and methotrexate appeared to be the most potent in terms of response rates. The value of these series is limited, since the response rate for any agent varies so much. A common observation is that single-center studies have higher response rates than multicenter studies. The reason for this is not certain, although most accept that the difference is a function of performance status: patients who attend tertiary referral centers, because of the distance traveled, are likely to be fitter than those in secondary care.

Drug combinations

Combination chemotherapy including methotrexate and cisplatin in the early 1980s produced impressive response rates[51–54]. For some years the M-VAC combination (methotrexate, vinblastine, Adriamycin, and cisplatin) has been considered by many to be the most potent treatment for metastatic bladder cancer. Initially response rates of 70% were reported[52]. These have not consistently been seen at other institutions[56] but when it has been compared in randomized fashion with other regimes, M-VAC has been shown to be superior to them (Fig. 46.13). The M-VAC regimen is not without toxicity, which includes neutropenia, sepsis, renal damage, mucositis, nausea, and vomiting. It is the author's experience that only about a half of patients with metastatic bladder cancer in a general hospital setting are suitable for this type of chemotherapy.

CHEMOTHERAPY AS A RADICAL TREATMENT

The frequent failure of radical therapies in muscle-invasive bladder cancer has led to the exploration of the use of chemotherapy in this area. Substantial responses in primary bladder cancer are frequently seen following combination chemotherapy. Assessment of response of primary bladder tumor masses is notoriously difficult but complete responses of masses not completely removed by transurethral resection (TUR) are reported in 10–20% of cases[60–62]. If this could be achieved with palpable masses, could not microscopic metastatic disease – in many cases the presumed cause of subsequent failure – be sterilized by such treatment? Would not primary disease already in remission at the time of radiotherapy be much less likely to produce local recurrence?

Adjuvant therapy had in the past consisted of single-agent chemotherapy and had been completely unsuccessful (Fig. 46.14). But the superiority of combination chemotherapy over single-agent treatment and its activity – at least in the short term against primary tumors – encouraged the setting up of further studies (Fig. 46.15). Although at the time of writing a survival benefit for the

Randomized trials involving methotrexate–platinum combinations in metastatic or locally recurrent bladder cancer

Reference	Study arms	Patients	Response rate (%)	Median survival (months)
Saxman et al. 1997[57]	Regime 1: M-VAC: methotrexate, vinblastine, adriamycin, cisplatin	133	33	12.5
	vs			
	Regime 2: Cisplatin	122	9 ($p<0.001$)	8.2
Logothetis et al. 1990[58]	Regime 1: M-VAC: as above	55	65	19
	vs			
	Regime 2: CisCA: cisplatin, cyclophosphamide, doxorubicin	55	46 ($p<0.05$)	9.3 ($p=0.0003$)
Mead et al. 1998[59]	Regime 1: CMV: cisplatin, methotrexate, vinblastine	108	46	7
	vs			
	Regime 2: MV: methotrexate, vinblastine	106	19	4.5 ($p=0.0065$)

Figure 46.13 Randomized trials involving methotrexate–platinum combinations in metastatic or locally recurrent bladder cancer.

Adjuvant studies in muscle-invasive bladder cancer using single-agent chemotherapy

1. Chemotherapy used 2. Definitive radical treatment 3. Reference		Chemotherapy arm	Control arm
1. Methotrexate	No. of patients	188	188
2. Radiotherapy or radiotherapy + cystectomy	Median survival (months)	20	23 (NS)
3. Shearer et al. 1988[63]			
1. Cisplatin	No. of patients	83	76 (W. Midlands, UK)
2. Radiotherapy		42	54 (Australia)
3. Wallace et al. 1991[64]	Median survival (months)	24	24 (W. Midlands, UK)
		15	22 (Australia) (NS on meta-analysis)
1. Cisplatin (concurrent)	No. of patients	51	48
2. Radiotherapy + surgery	Median survival (months)	29	19 (NS)
3. Coppin et al. 1996[65]			
1. Cisplatin	No. of patients	62	60
2. Cystectomy	Median survival (months)	32	36 (NS)
3. Martinez-Pineiro et al. 1995[66]			

Figure 46.14 Adjuvant studies in muscle-invasive bladder cancer using single-agent chemotherapy. NS, not significant.

addition of chemotherapy to radiotherapy or surgery has not been excluded, any such benefit must be small. The international collaborative study (Fig. 46.15), by far the largest, has excluded a 3-year survival advantage of more than 11%. The increase in median survival seen in this study – 6.5 months – is of a similar order to the difference in survival seen in metastatic disease between high- and low-intensity chemotherapy[57,59]. As only a small minority of patients in the international collaborative study received chemotherapy on relapse, the result is consistent with the hypothesis that chemotherapy temporarily delays disease progression and almost never makes the difference between cure and failure.

RECENT DEVELOPMENTS

The chemotherapy that has become standard over the last 15 years has failed to make an important impact on the survival of patients with muscle-invasive bladder cancer. This is disappointing considering the successes with adjuvant chemotherapy seen in breast, colon, and cervical cancers – diseases like bladder cancer where chemotherapy is only moderately successful in metastatic disease. Are there more potent treatments that might succeed where cisplatin, methotrexate and vinblastine (CMV) has failed?

Accelerated M-VAC

The use of granulocyte and granulocyte–macrophage colony stimulating factors (G-CSF and GM-CSF) accelerates the return of these white cell components to normal levels following chemotherapy. This often allows chemotherapy cycles to be repeated at short intervals, so increasing the intensity of the treatment. In the case of M-VAC an early study using GM-CSF was not successful at increasing intensity or reducing toxicity[72]. Using G-CSF however it has been possible to increase the intensity of the Adriamycin and cisplatin components by 140% and

50% respectively[73], though probably not beyond three cycles[74]. A large randomized study comparing a similar accelerated schedule with standard M-VAC is being carried out in metastatic disease. An early report demonstrated the reduction in toxicity with the accelerated schedule. The benefit was not just to hematologic indices with a reduction of febrile episodes, but also in the episodes of oral mucositis[75]. Whether an improvement in efficacy will be seen must await study completion.

Taxanes

Both paclitaxel[76] and docetaxel[77] have single-agent activity on previously untreated bladder cancer. For Paclitaxel a response rate of 42% in 26 patients[76] has led to the drug's inclusion in combinations with carboplatin or cisplatin. These have produced response rates in the 40–55% range[78]. The activity of the taxanes in disease previously treated with the established anticancer drugs is only modest[79,80].

The toxicity of the taxanes includes peripheral neuropathy, hair loss, and myelosuppression. Because of the risk of allergic responses, patients are premedicated with high doses of steroids.

Gemcitabine

The antimetabolite gemcitabine also appears to be active in previously untreated metastatic bladder with appreciable response rates, not only against previously untreated metastatic disease[81,82] but against patients who had received prior platinum-containing chemotherapy[83]. The toxicity of gemcitabine is generally mild and largely confined to the hematologic system. In combination with cisplatin the hematologic toxicity can be severe, though response rates of between 41% and 59% have been seen[78].

Both gemcitabine and the taxanes can be given to patients with impaired renal function which is frequently seen in a transitional cell carcinoma population. In both cases large randomized studies are in progress comparing the toxicity and efficacy of such

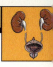
Adjuvant studies in muscle invasive bladder cancer using combination chemotherapy			
1. Chemotherapy used 2. Definitive radical treatment 3. Reference		Chemotherapy arm	Control arm
1. Cisplatin 70mg/m² + doxorubicin ×2 cycles 2. Radiotherapy followed by cystectomy 3. Malmstrom et al. 1996[67]	No. of patients	151	160
	Survival at 5 years (%)	59	51 ($p=0.1$)
1. Cisplatin, methotrexate, vinblastine ×3 cycles 2. After cystectomy 3. Freiha F et al. 1996[68]	No. of patients	25	25
	Median time to relapse (months)	37	12 ($p=0.01$)
	Median survival (months)	63	36 ($p=0.32$)
1. Cisplatin, methotrexate, vinblastine ×2 cycles (prior to) 2. Radiotherapy + concurrent cisplatin + cystectomy 3. Shipley W Y et al. 1998[69]	No. of patients	61	62
	Median survival (%)	48	49 (NS)
1. Carboplatin, methotrexate, vinblastine ×2 cycles 2. Cystectomy 3. Abel-Enein H et al. 1997[70]	No. of patients	94	100
	5-year disease-free survival (%)	62	42 ($p=0.013$)
1. Cisplatin, methotrexate, vinblastine ×3 cycles 2. Radiotherapy or cystectomy 3. International collaboration 1999[71]	No. patients	491	485
	Median time to relapse (months)	20	16.5 ($p=0.01$)
	Median survival (months)	44	37.5 ($p=0.075$)

Figure 46.15 Adjuvant studies in muscle-invasive bladder cancer using combination chemotherapy.

combinations with those of M-VAC. If the toxicity is found to be reduced for equivalent efficacy this would be welcome news to patients with metastatic and locally recurrent transitional cell carcinoma. An early report suggests that this has been achieved for gemcitabine[83b]. Only if the efficacy of the new developments described above is considerably increased is there likely to be a chance of improving the cure rate in locally advanced bladder cancer.

CHEMOTHERAPY IN UROLOGY: KIDNEY CANCER

Michael G Leahy

KEY POINTS

- 60% of patients die from systemic disease.
- No systemic therapy yet has a proven role in prolonging survival.
- Interpretation of research data is complicated by wide variation in natural history of the disease.
- Biological therapies appear to show useful activity in this disease.
- Patients should be referred to centers running clinical trials.

INTRODUCTION

As a curative procedure for kidney cancer, surgery is intrinsically limited by the fact that this tumor is characterized by early metastatic spread and late clinical presentation. Thus, a third or more of patients have clinically detectable metastases at presentation and even among patients with clinically localized disease at diagnosis half of these will relapse and die of metastases or local recurrence within 5 years of radical nephrectomy. At best, then, surgery may offer a cure to about a third of patients (Fig. 46.16).

There are two approaches to reduce the failure rate of surgery in this condition: improve early detection and devise systemic therapies that are effective for systemic disease. The latter is the subject of this section. A broad definition of the term 'chemotherapy' will be used, including all systemic anticancer therapies including cytotoxic chemotherapy, hormonal therapy, biologic therapy, immunotherapy, and the newer generation of novel agents including retinoids and angiogenesis inhibitors.

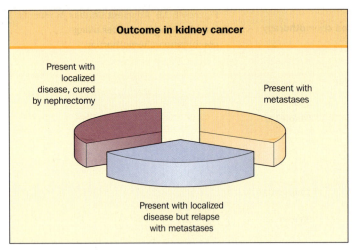

Outcome in kidney cancer

Present with localized disease, cured by nephrectomy

Present with metastases

Present with localized disease but relapse with metastases

Figure 46.16 Outcome in kidney cancer.

As in other cancers, systemic therapies may be considered in two situations. Adjuvant therapy attempts to reduce the risk of subsequent recurrence or relapse after definitive local therapy. In the case of patients with known metastatic disease, systemic therapy may palliate symptoms, prolong survival, or, potentially, eradicate the disease. These situations are clearly quite distinct but, of course, both rely on the effectiveness of the systemic therapies.

This chapter will review the various systemic therapies that have been tried in the treatment of kidney cancer. None of these yet are supported by sufficient evidence to warrant considering them as standard therapy. On the other hand there is a wealth of

data on these agents (Fig. 46.17), some quite encouraging, which can be confusing to interpret. This section will also therefore try to highlight some of the difficulties in interpretation of these data.

Natural history of metastatic kidney cancer

The management of patients with kidney cancer must be considered in the context of its unique natural history[84]. There is a wide variation in the progression of this disease in different patients. The median survival after developing metastases is about 12 months. However, unlike other common adult epithelial malignancies, which are usually inexorably progressive without treatment, some patients present with metastases many years after nephrectomy for their primary tumor, and may undergo periods of quite prolonged stable disease lasting months or even years when their metastases do not progress. Spontaneous regression of metastases, though rare, is well documented, sometimes apparently related to the resection of the primary[85]. With this natural history in mind, it may be difficult to attribute an effect to a medical intervention (Fig. 46.18). Sometimes efforts have been made to document (by CT scan for example) that the disease is progressing before starting a patient on systemic therapy in order to be more certain that responses are due to the intervention. However, this has not been a universally adopted approach.

Endpoints of therapy

The effectiveness of a systemic therapy can be measured in several ways. The ideal endpoint is a prolongation of survival, hopefully of useful, productive, active, life. Thus, both quantity and

\multicolumn{8}{c}{**Summary of response rates for systemic therapy for kidney cancer**}
Regimen	Schedule	No. of patients	RCT	CR (%)	PR (%)	Overall response rate (%)	Comment
MPA			No	? 0		<5	Effect on survival unknown
IFN	Various	767	Yes	14 (1.8)	76 (10)	12	Duration of response 6–12 months; 12% improvement in 1 year survival
IL-2	Total	1712	No	65 (3.8)	197 (11.5)	15.4	Duration of response 12–24 months but median not reached for CRs. Possible effect on survival but needs RCT
	i.v.b.	733		38 (5.2)	83 (11.3)	16.5	
	c.i.v.	789		21 (2.7)	86 (10.9)	13.5	
	s.c.	190		6 (3.2)	28 (14.7)	18.6	
IL-2 + IFN	Total	1411	Yes	62 (4.4)	229 (16.2)	20.6	No evidence of benefit over single agent
	s.c.	675		34 (5.0)	109 (16.1)	21.2	
	c.i.v.	556		19 (3.4)	92 (16.6)	20.0	
	i.v.b.	180		9 (5.0)	28 (15.6)	20.5	
IL-2 + IFN + 5FU	s.c. IL-2, s.c. IFN, i.v. 5FU	139	No	16 (11.5)	40 (28.7)	40	Effect on survival and duration of response unknown
IL-2 + LAK	Total	461	Yes	29 (6.3)	68 (14.8)	21.0	No evidence of benefit over IL-2
	c.i.v.	245		9 (4.0)	29 (11.8)	16.3	
	i.v.b.	216		20 (9.3)	39 (18.1)	27.3	
IL-2 + TIL		34	No		4 (11)	11	
ALT		45	Yes	0	8/39	21	Survival increased by 2.5 times in one study

Figure 46.17 Summary of response rates for systemic therapy for kidney cancer. 5FU, 5-fluorouracil; ALT, autolymphocyte transfusion; c.i.v., continous intravenous; CR, complete response; IFN, interferons; IL-2, interleukin-2; i.v., intravenous; i.v.b., intravenous bolus; LAK, lymphokine-activated killer; MPA, medrotyprogesterone acetate; RCT, randomized control trial; s.c., subcutaneous; TIL, tumor infiltrating lymphocytes; PR, partial response. (Adapted from references at the end of this section.)

quality of life are important. Both of these are difficult to measure, however. In view of the wide variation in natural history of the tumor, there is the potential for (inadvertent) selection bias in uncontrolled clinical series. This may explain the much better results obtained in early clinical trials of new agents, which are not reproduced in later studies. Randomized controlled studies are required but even these may be confounded for assessment of survival by the treatment patients receive after the study period. Instead of attempting to measure survival, therefore, it is more common for researchers to measure response to therapy (i.e. shrinkage of tumor deposits). Standard definitions have been developed by the World Health Organisation (WHO) to allow better comparison of studies but it should be remembered that these are secondary measures of efficacy. It is assumed, but rarely proved, that response to therapy translates into a survival benefit. The quoting of 'stabilization of disease' is particularly questionable in this disease unless compared with a randomly selected control group.

Specific anticancer systemic therapy represents only a part of the care for a patient with metastatic kidney cancer. Palliation of symptoms is a priority and may include surgical, radiotherapeutic, pharmacologic, or nursing intervention.

The multidisciplinary team in the care of a patient with metastatic kidney cancer includes:

- surgeon,
- radiation oncologist,
- medical oncologist,
- specialist nurse oncologist, and
- palliative care team,

all to liaise with the primary care doctor.

Skilful best supportive care may in itself improve survival and may be another reason why patients involved in intensive trials with a high degree of medical and nursing input fare better than 'historical controls' not included in trials. Ideally all patients should have the benefit of management by clinicians skilled in cancer medicine whether they receive systemic therapy or not.

REVIEW OF CLINICAL TRIALS IN SYSTEMIC THERAPIES FOR KIDNEY CANCER

Cytotoxic chemotherapy

Kidney cancer is generally considered to be resistant to most cytotoxic agents. Motzer and Vogelzang reviewed the results of 155 trials that studied the effects of 80 different agents in patients with metastatic kidney cancer published between 1975 and 1994. In all, only 143 patients out of 3,951 showed responses[86]. None of the agents produced a response in more than 20% of patients. Combinations of cytotoxic agents have

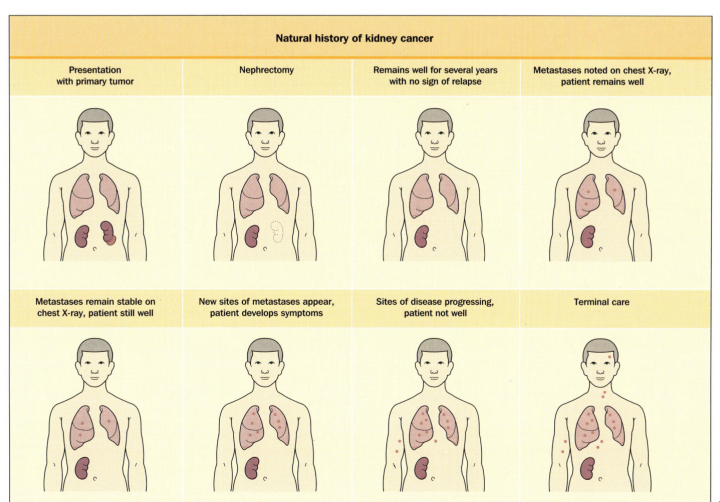

Figure 46.18 Natural history of kidney cancer. A typical time line for a patient with kidney cancer. Question: When should systemic therapy be given therapy?

not been found to be more effective and often resulted in worse toxicity. Among the newer cytotoxics, suramin, methyl-GAG and melphalan, vinorelbine, gemcitabine, and taxol have all been the subject of clinical trials but appear to show no substantial activity. Of all these agents only vinblastine and perhaps 5-fluorouracil (5FU) have shown sufficient activity to warrant further investigation.

The reason for the failure of cytotoxic chemotherapy in kidney cancer is not known. Most cytotoxic agents target cell division and the cells may only be sensitive during a part of the cell cycle. On this basis, infusional regimens have been tried to maximize exposure of the cells to the cytotoxic agent during critical points of the cell cycle. 5FU has been particularly investigated, although with little improved efficacy. Active cellular depletion of cytotoxic agents is well described and may be caused by a calcium-dependent transmembrane glycoprotein called P-glycoprotein, the product of the *MDR1* gene (multidrug resistance) (Fig. 46.19). Kidney cancer cells frequently express high levels of P-glycoprotein. However, attempts to overcome chemoresistance in kidney cancer by modulating the effect of P-glycoprotein (for instance with calcium channel blockers or cyclosporin) have so far not improved the response rates to the cytotoxics used. It would appear, therefore, that there are multiple mechanisms for chemoresistance in kidney cancer.

Hormone therapy

The use of hormones in the treatment of kidney cancer predates the work on cytotoxic chemotherapy and followed the observation in the early 1950s that estrogens could induce kidney cancers in Syrian hamsters and that their growth could be inhibited by progestagens. As a result, medroxyprogesterone acetate (MPA) became the standard for the treatment of patients with metastatic kidney cancer[87]. This therapy has the advantage that it has relatively few side effects, often improving appetite and energy levels. A response rate of 5–10% is reported in a number of studies but there are no data on the effect of MPA on survival. In the absence of any other more effective treatment, many patients are still treated with MPA today. In a postal survey in the UK, MPA was the most frequently quoted systemic therapy used by urologists and oncologists for patients with metastatic kidney cancer and was therefore selected as the control arm for the UK Medical Research Council's (MRC) first large randomized controlled trial (RCT) in kidney cancer: RE01 (see below)[88]. Other hormonal therapies such as the antiestrogen tamoxifen have also been tried with no better results than MPA and usually without the palliative benefit offered by that drug. A modestly sized RCT of adjuvant MPA for kidney cancer showed no reduction in the risk of relapse after nephrectomy in the treated arm[89].

Bio-/immunotherapy
Rationale

The interest in biologic therapy in the treatment of kidney cancer stems from the hypothesis that host immunologic factors are responsible for the features of the natural history of this tumor described above, namely the periods of prolonged stable disease and the occasional spontaneous regression of metastases. The contribution of immunologic mechanisms in malignant conditions remains incompletely understood. However, in vitro

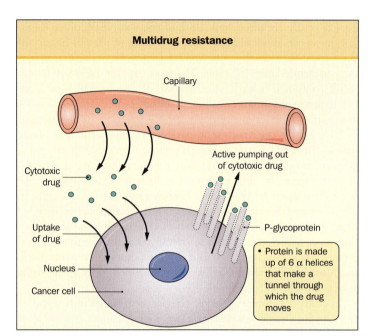

Figure 46.19 Multidrug resistance. P-glycoprotein pumps cytotoxic agents out of a cell.

experiments have clearly shown that cytotoxic T lymphocytes have the ability to detect and kill cancer cells. Kidney tumors are invariably infiltrated by populations of such cells, so-called tumor infiltrating lymphocytes (TILs). The development of progressive cancer may to some extent be caused by a failure or an overwhelming of this normal physiologic function of the immune system and thus a patient may benefit from interventions that enhance the immunologic response to their cancer.

Biologic response modifiers (BRMs)

There are a number of agents that enhance or activate T-lymphocyte cytotoxicity in a nonspecific way. These include levamisole, coumarin, cimetidine, bacille Calmette-Guérin (BCG), and (more recently) *Mycobacterium vaccae*. These agents have been associated with responses in some patients but as yet their role remains experimental. More specific ways of enhancing the immunologic response in patients with kidney cancer include the use of specific cytokines, known to be important in normal immunologic response. In particular, interferons and interleukins are now available in pharmacologic doses thanks to recombinant technology. Adoptive immunotherapy refers to the technique of transferring immunologically competent cells (or other reagents) to the patient that can mediate antitumor effects, either directly or indirectly.

Interferons

α-, β-, and γ-interferons (IFN) are a family of naturally occurring cytokines. They have a number of actions, including the upregulation of class I HLA molecules on the cell surface. These cell surface molecules present antigens to the immune system and therefore this may be their mechanism of action as a treatment for kidney cancer, in effect making the cancer cells a better target for cytotoxic T lymphocytes (CTLs) by enhancing the presentation of tumor specific antigens (Fig. 46.20). However,

Immunotherapy mechanism of action

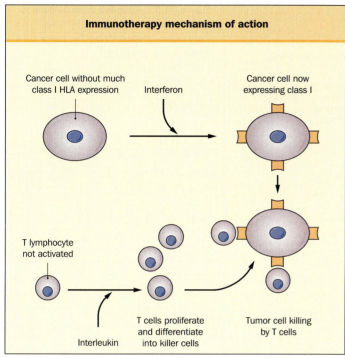

Figure 46.20 Immunotherapy mechanism of action. Interferon causes cancer cells to express more HLA class I on their cell surface and thus become better targets for T lymphocytes, and interleukin-2 causes T lymphocytes to proliferate and develop into LAK cells with enhanced cancer-cell-killing ability.

other mechanisms may also be important. The majority of studies have concentrated on interferon alpha. A range of doses has been investigated and there is limited data that support an intermediate dose of 5–10MU/m^2 i.m. or s.c. 3–5 times a week. The side effects include flu-like symptoms of fever, rigors, and sweats, which usually start about 2 hours after each injection, subside after about 2 hours and can be offset by premedication with acetaminophen (paracetamol). The following day there may be myalgia; flitting arthralgia; fatigue, anorexia, diarrhea, or constipation. With prolonged use there is frequently a reduction in these physical symptoms but some patients complain of depression of mood. In some patients myelosuppression may occur and treatment with interferon may exacerbate hypertension, angina, and renal insufficiency. Treatment can be continued for a year or even longer if successful. The estimated response rate to interferon alpha from various uncontrolled studies is about 15% and some durable complete remissions have been observed. No improvement in survival was noted in a small ($n = 60$) RCT of IFN-α versus MPA or in a larger RCT of 197 patients treated with IFN-γ or placebo[90,91]. However, early reports from the MRC's trial RE01 with 350 patients randomized between IFN-α or MPA show a 28% reduction in the risk of death in the IFN arm and a 12% improvement in survival at 1 year or a median improvement in survival of 2.5 months[92]. This modest improvement of survival appears confirmed in another RCT of vinblastine alone versus vinblastine with IFN-α[93]. No improvement in relapse-free survival has been noted in a RCT of adjuvant interferon after nephrectomy[94].

As a result of these studies many would now consider IFN an appropriate therapy for selected patients with metastatic kidney cancer. However, the improvement in survival is modest and toxicity can be significant.

Interleukin-2

Another cytokine, interleukin-2 (IL-2), stimulates T lymphocytes to proliferate and also to differentiate into cells that demonstrate enhanced cancer-cell-killing ability [lymphokine activated killer cells (LAK); Fig. 46.20]. Initially, interleukin-2 (IL-2) was given as an i.v. bolus (i.v.b.) at maximum tolerated doses. This led to severe toxicity and drug-related deaths in some patients. In particular, a capillary leak syndrome was described. This is associated with peripheral edema, pulmonary edema, renal failure, cardiac dysfunction, and cerebral edema. Vasopressor therapy for hypotension and intensive care may be required. This limited the use of IL-2. Subsequently however, a continuous i.v. infusion schedule (c.i.v.), which led to lower peak blood levels and finally a low-dose subcutaneous regimen (s.c.) using a 10th of the previous dosage were developed. These are associated with much lower incidence of side effects, even allowing outpatient administration. The US Food and Drug Administration (FDA) approved aldesleukin (a human recombinant IL-2) for the treatment of metastatic kidney cancer on the basis of combined experience in uncontrolled trials of the high-dose i.v. regimen pioneered by Rosenberg at the National cancer Institute (NCI) (latest update[95]). Whether this regimen is really more efficacious than others and, even if it is, whether it is sufficiently more efficacious to warrant the much higher toxicity, cost, inconvenience, and associated risk of death is hotly contested by the proponents of the various regimens[84].

In a recent comparison of 327 patients treated with c.i.v. IL-2 with matched historical controls treated with various cytotoxic agents from the Eastern Co-operative Oncology Group (ECOG) database, an apparent survival advantage was found to be associated with IL-2 treatment[103]. While not as rigorous as a randomized trial, this study lends support to the use of IL-2 but the authors recommend formal testing of efficacy by RCT.

Interleukin-2 + interferon combinations

The proposed actions of the two cytokines should lead to synergism. This has been confirmed by animal experiments. Combination schedules have therefore been developed[97]. However, no definite conclusion has yet been reached as to whether this approach translates into a clinically significant benefit.

In a reasonably sized RCT ($n = 128$) of tamoxifen versus IL-2 + IFN + tamoxifen in Sweden[98], no difference was found between the survival of the two groups. This study used a s.c. regimen for the IL-2. Tamoxifen was chosen as the control arm as it has been reported to show some limited activity in kidney cancer, has low toxicity, and may potentiate the activity of IL-2.

In the French multicenter CRECY study, 425 patients were randomized in a three-arm trial between i.v. IL-2, s.c. IFN-α or both[99]. Response rates were low in all three arms but significantly better for the combination therapy than either agent alone (6.5% versus 7.5% versus 18.6%, $p = 0.01$). However, despite this there was no difference in overall survival between the three arms.

Adoptive immunotherapy

LAK cell therapy	TIL cell therapy	Autolymphocyte therapy
1. Peripheral blood harvesting (leukapheresis)	1. Tumor removed from patient and sent to lab	1. Leukapharesis
2. T-cells are separated and incubated in tissue culture flasks with IL-2	2. Tissue prepared by mincing and digestion	2. Co-culture with mitogen/tumor extract
3. T-cells proliferate and differentiate into LAK cells	3. Tissue cultures with IL-2	3. Re-infusion
4. LAK cells are re-infused to the patient leading to tumor cell kill	4. TIL cell population expands, tumor cells eventually die	
	5. Expanded TIL cells re-infused to the patient	

LAK

ALT

Lymphocytes + tumor + IL-2 + mitogen

Re-infusion

Leukapheresis

Tumor

IL-2

Lymphocytes   IL-2

Tissue culture

TIL

Drips

Drips

Re-infuse

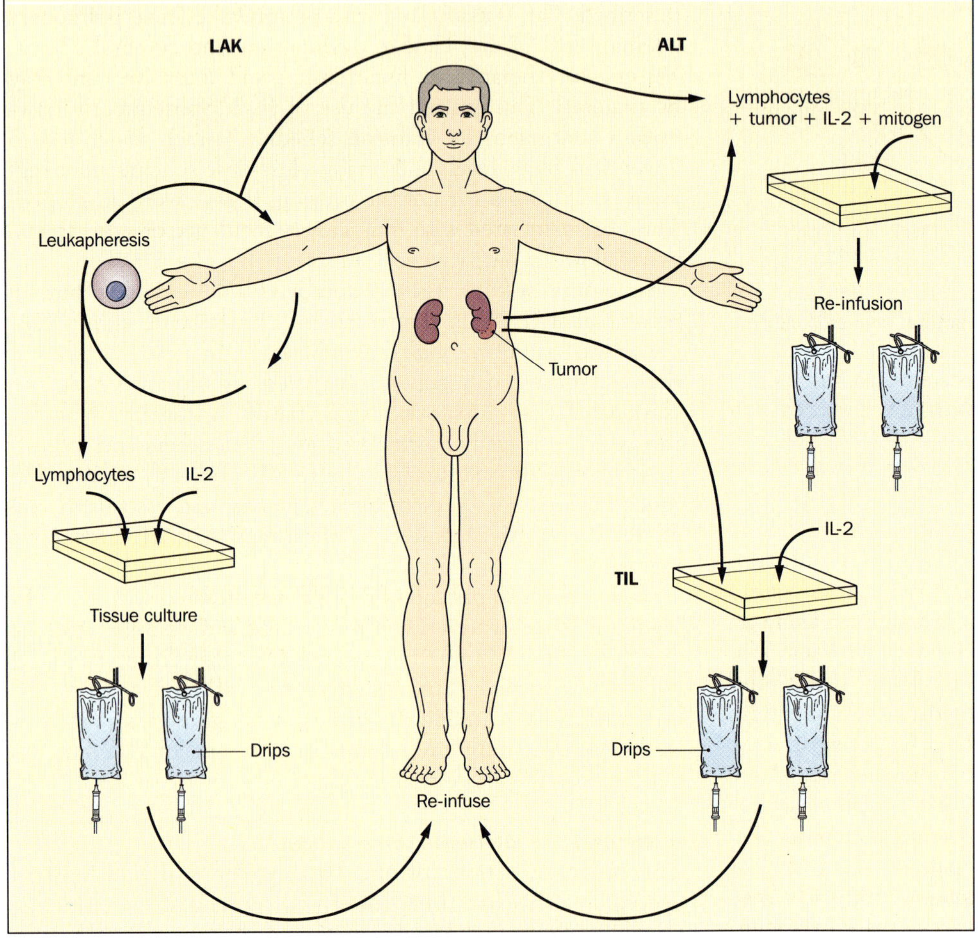

Figure 46.21 Adoptive immunotherapy.
ALT, autolymphocyte transfusion; LAK, lymphokine-activated killer; TIL, tumor infiltrating lymphocytes.

These well conducted studies suggest that combination therapy may increase the response rate but that this does not translate into a survival benefit. Whether a response to therapy is associated with an improvement in quality of life has not been assessed and the combination treatment is associated with considerable toxicity.

Adoptive immunotherapy

The use of BRMs and cytokines for therapy relies on the patient's own immune system to perform the necessary cell kill. Adoptive immunotherapy attempts to enhance this response by directly delivering to the patient an activated immunologic reagent such as a cellular population. The simplest method of doing this is to harvest peripheral blood (unactivated) lymphocytes and

incubate them with IL-2 in tissue culture. This leads to an expansion of the T lymphocyte population and differentiation as lymphokine activated killer cells (LAK cells). LAK cells recognize and kill cancer cells. Once expanded sufficiently, the cells are then re-infused to the patient (Fig. 46.21). This technology is highly labor intensive and not without its risks to the patients, who may require intensive care after reinfusion as a result of margination of many of the LAK cells in the lungs. Furthermore, the activation of the lymphocytes is not specific to the tumor.

The technique has been further developed for some patients where the laboratory can have access to the primary tumor at the time of nephrectomy (or in some cases a metastatic deposit). In these cases, it has been possible to expand the lymphocyte population that infiltrates the tumor (so called tumor infiltrating lymphocytes or TILs) and co-culture them with the tumor cells and IL-2. The advantage of this approach is that the TILs may be more specific for the antigens expressed on the malignant cells. The cells are expanded and reinfused to the patient (Fig. 46.21). Autolymphocyte transfusion (ALT) is a form of adoptive immunotherapy in which cytotoxic lymphocytes are harvested from a patient's peripheral blood, activated, and then reinfused. Activation can be attempted in a number of ways, including incubation with a mitogenic antibody, a variety of cytokines, or even an extract of the patient's own tumor, if it is available (Fig. 46.21).

Despite interesting and encouraging work in animal models and in individual patients, the efficacy of adoptive immunotherapy for metastatic kidney cancer in humans has been difficult to demonstrate. For example, a RCT of LAK + IL-2 versus IL-2 alone showed no significant difference in survival[100]. However, in a modestly sized RCT (90 patients) of ALT versus cimetidine, a clear survival advantage was found in the ALT treated group[101], although no complete remissions were observed. Further studies of these techniques are under way.

Immunochemotherapy

In view of the lack of response to cytotoxic chemotherapy described above, it has been somewhat surprising and exciting to find that dramatically improved response rates can be achieved by combining cytotoxic chemotherapy with immunotherapy. In a program developed mainly in Europe, patients are given an 8-week regimen consisting of s.c. IL-2, IFN and 5FU. By careful patient selection and encouraging patients to repeat this rather debilitating therapy while response is evident, 48% of 35 patients responded in a recent published series[102]. These results have been in part confirmed by an RCT of the three-drug combination against tamoxifen[103] but in comparison of the three-drug regimen against IL-2 and IFN no significant difference in response rate was noted[104]. Not all centers using this regimen have been able to reproduce these high response rates.

Predictors of response to therapy

The selection of patients who are more likely to respond to therapy, while it can make uncontrolled trials very difficult to interpret, would be of immense clinical value if it was reliable and reproducible. Specific molecular markers have not yet been found that fulfill these criteria. Clinical indices have some value but are really of insufficient specificity and sensitivity to be very useful. Of many criteria that have been examined, general well-being as measured by standard performance scores has been the one to frequently predict prognosis[105]. This includes survival after nephrectomy and survival after treatment with IL-2. However, as with many apparent predictors of prognosis and response to therapy in cancer medicine, this may merely be due to a lead time effect – i.e. by selecting patient with a worse performance score one may simply be selecting a population of

The ideal patient for biological therapy

Nephrectomized some time in the past (primary tumor removed, delay in developing metastases)

Feels generally well, good performance score, no other co-morbid conditions

Lung metastases the only site of relapse, multiple small-volume deposits

Figure 46.22 The ideal patient for biological therapy.

patients in whom the cancer has progressed further – it is not surprising, then, that their survival is shorter whatever intervention is performed. There is some data to suggest that patients who develop metastases some time after their nephrectomy, have small-volume lung metastases only, and are otherwise generally well are the most likely to respond to biologic therapies (Fig. 46.22). Certainly, very few patients with bone metastases have been reported as responding to IFN but, on the other hand, responses at all sites including bone have been seen with IL-2 therapy.

Novel agents

Until relatively recently, the search for new effective treatments for cancer was restricted to developing new cytotoxic agents. This is now no longer the case, with a variety of new classes of agents being researched that act in completely different ways. These include cytodifferentiating agents, which push the tumor cells to develop a less malignant phenotype, angiogenesis inhibitors, which restrict tumor growth by preventing the development of tumor blood supply, metalloproteinase inhibitors, which inhibit metastasis, and gene therapy. Thus, despite the disappointing results with cytotoxic chemotherapy in kidney cancer referred to above, the expanding armament of novel agents means that cytotoxics are a component of diminishing importance. Since many of these agents have relatively minor and nonoverlapping toxicity, the potential for combination therapy is great. This presents some hope for the future but also a significant problem in devising effective research strategies.

CONCLUSIONS

The systemic therapy for kidney cancer remains a research issue with no treatment sufficiently effective to warrant to be considered standard therapy. However, a number of approaches, particularly immunotherapy and perhaps combination immunochemotherapy are successful in some patients. The development of effective therapies for the future will depend on well-designed randomized controlled trials. Ideally, urologic surgeons should develop collaborative relationships with research departments of oncology and patients should be encouraged to consider entry to clinical trials as part of their multidisciplinary care.

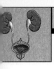

REFERENCES

Chemotherapy in urology: testis cancer

1. Bosl GJ, Motzer RJ. Testicular germ cell cancer. New Engl J Med. 1997;337:242.
2. IGCCC G. A prognostic factor based staging system for metastatic germ cell cancers. J Clin Oncol. 1997;15(2):594–603.
3. Bajorin D, Mazumdar M, Meyers M, et al. Metastatic germ cell tumours: modelling for response to chemotherapy. J Clin Oncol. 1998;16(2):707–15.
4. Oliver R, Ong J, Blandy J, Altman D. Testis conservation studies in germ cell cancer justified by improved primary chemotherapy response and reduced delay 1978–1994. Br J Urol. 1996;78:119–24.
5. Oliver RTD, Leahy M, Ong J. Combined seminoma/non-seminoma should be considered as intermediate grade germ cell cancer (GCC). Eur J Cancer. 1995;31A:1392–4.
6. Petersen PM, Skakkebaek NE, Vistisen K, Rorth M, Giwercman A. Semen quality and reproductive hormones before orchiectomy in men with testicular cancer. J Clin Oncol. 1999;17(3):941–7.
7. Mead GM, Stenning SP, Cullen MH, et al. The Second Medical Research Study of prognostic factors in nonseminomatous germ cell tumours. J Clin. Oncol. 1992;10(1):85–94.
8. Tsetis D, Sharma A, Easty M, Brown I, Oliver R, Chan O. Potential of limited d21 post chemotherapy in predicting need for post chemotherapy surgery in nonseminomatous testicular germ cell cancer. Urol Int. 1996;61:22–6.
9. Williams SD, Birch R, Einhorn LH, Irwin L, Greco F, Loehrer P. Treatment of disseminated germ-cell tumors with Cisplatin, Bleomycin, and either Vinblastine or Etoposide. New Engl J Med. 1987;316(23):1435–40.
10. Oliver R. Future trials in Germ Cell Malignancy (GCM) of the testis. Eur J Surg Oncol. 1997;23:117–122.
11. Shamash J, Oliver R, Ong J, et al. 60% salvage rate for germ cell tumours using sequential m-BOP, surgery and ifosfamide based chemotherapy. Ann Oncol. 1999;10:1–8.
12. Beyer J, Kingreen D, Krause M. Long term survival of patients with recurrent or refractory germ cell tumours after high dose chemotherapy. Cancer 1997;79:1605–10.
13. Ravi R, Ong J, Oliver RTD, Badenoch DF, Fowler CG, Hendry WF. Surgery as salvage therapy in chemotherapy resistant nonseminomatous germ cell tumours. Br J Urol. 1998;81(6):884–8.
14. Lange P, Hekmat K, Bosl G, Kennedy B, Fraley E. Accelerated growth of testicular cancer after cytoreductive surgery. Cancer. 1980;45(6):1498–1506.
15. Nicholls C, Catalano P, Crawford E, Vogelzang N, Einhorn L, Loehrer P. Randomized comparison of cisplatin and etoposide either bleomycin or ifosfamide in treatment of disseminated germ cell tumours: An Eastern Cooperative Oncology Group, Southwest Oncology Group, and Cancer and Leukamia Group B Study. J Clin Oncol. 1998;4:1287–93.
16. Bokemeyer C, Harstrick A, Metzner B, et al. Sequential high dose VIP-chemotherapy plus peripheral stem cell (PBSC) support for advanced germ cell cancer. Ann Oncol. 1996;7(Suppl. 5):55 abst 259.
17. Boshoff CB, Begent RHJ, Oliver RTD, et al. Secondary tumours following etoposide containing therapy for germ cell cancer. Ann Oncol. 1995;6(1):35–40.
18. Travis L, Rochelle E, Curtis H, Per H, Hollowaty E. Risk of second malignant neoplasms among long term survivors of testicular cancer. J Nat Cancer Inst. 1997;89:1429–39.
19. Lampe H, Horwich A, Norman A, Nicholls J, Dearnaley DP. Fertility after chemotherapy for testicular germ cell cancers. J Clin Oncol. 1997;15(1):239–45.
20. Stenning S, Parkinson MC, Fisher C, et al. Postchemotherapy residual masses in germ cell tumour patients. Cancer. 1998;83:1409–19.
21. Pizzocaro G, Nicolai N, Salvoni R. Comparison between clinical and pathological staging in low stage non seminomatous germ cell testicular tumors. J Urol. 1992;148:76.
22. Oliver RTD, Hope-Stone HF, Blandy JP. Justification of the use of surveillance in the management of stage 1 germ cell tumours of the testis. Br J Urol. 1983;55:760–763.
23. Donohue JP, Thornhill JA, Foster RS, Rowland RG, Bihrle R. Primary retroperitoneal lymph node dissection in a clinical stage A non-seminomatous germ cell testis cancer. Review of the Indiana University experience 1965–1989. Br J Urol. 1993;71:326–35.
24. Oliver R. Epidemiology of testis cancer. In: Comprehensive textbook of genito-urinary oncology 1999.
25. Petersen PM, Skakkebaek NE, Giwercman A. Gonadal function in men with testicular cancer: biological and clinical aspects. Apmis. 1998;106(1):24–34; discussion 34–6.
26. Nargund V, Oliver R, Ong J, Sohaib S, Reznek R, Badenoch D. Chemotherapy ± partial orchidectomy for testis conservation in patients with germ cell cancer (GCC): is it safe, is it justified? Eur Urol. 1999; submitted.
27. Heidenreich A, Holtl W, Albrecht W, Pont J, Engelmann UH. Testis-preserving surgery in bilateral testicular germ cell tumours. Br J Urol. 1997;79(2):253–7.
28. Friedman M. Supervoltage Roentgen therapy at Walter Reed General Hospital. Surg Clin North Am. 1944;24(6):1424–32.
29. Zagars G. Stage I testicular seminoma following orchidectomy – to treat or not to treat? Eur J Cancer. 1993;29A:1923–4.
30. Horwich A, Oliver R, Fossa S, Wilkinson P, Mead G, Stenning S. A randomised MRC trial comparing single agent carboplatin with the combination of etoposide and cisplatin in patients with advanced metastatic seminoma. Proc Am Soc Clin Oncol. 1996: 15: abst 668, 1996.
31. Oliver R, Edmonds P, Ong J, Ostrowski M, Jackson A. Pilot studies of 2 and 1 course carboplatin as adjuvant for Stage I seminoma: should it be tested in a randomized trial against radiotherapy? Int J Radiation Oncol Biol Phys. 1994;29(1):3–8.
32. Nouri A, Oliver R. Tetraploid arrest with over expressed non-mutated p53 in germ cell cancers. Relevance to their chemosensitivity and possible application in non germ cell cancers. Int J Oncol. 1997;11:1167–71.
33. Williams SD, Stablein DM, Einhorn LH, et al. Immediate adjuvant chemotherapy versus observation with treatment at relapse in pathological stage II testicular cancer. New Engl J Med. 1987;317:1433.
34. Wettlaufer JN, Feiner AS, Robinson WA. Vincristine, cisplatin and bleomycin with surgery in the management of advanced metastatic non seminomatous testis tumours. Cancer. 1984;53:203–9.
35. Horwich A, Brada M, Nicholls J, et al. Intensive induction chemotherapy for poor risk non-seminomatous germ cell tumours. Eur J Cancer Clin Oncol. 1989;25:177–84.
36. Lewis CR, Fossa SD, Mead G, et al. BOP/VIP – A new platinum-intensive chemotherapy regimen for poor prognosis germ cell tumours. Ann Oncol. 1991;2(3):203–11.
37. Horwich A, Dearnaley D, Norman A, Nicholls J, Hendry W. Accelerated chemotherapy for poor-prognosis germ-cell tumors. Eur J Cancer. 1994;30a:1607–11.
38. Horwich A, Mason M, Fossa S, et al. Accelerated induction chemotherapy (C-BOP-BEP) for poor and intermediate prognosis metastatic germ cell tumors (GCT). Proc Am Soc Clin Oncol. 1997;16:319 abst 1137.
39. Amato R, Finn L, Logosthetis C, et al. Preliminary results of alternating sequential combination chemotherapy (CHT) for the treatment of high volume nonseminomatous germ cell tumor (HVNSGCT). Proc Am Soc Clin Oncol. 1996;15(243):abst 608.
40. Motzer R, Mazumdar M, Bajorin D, Bosl G, Lyn P, Vlamis V. High-dose carboplatin, etoposide, and cyclophosphamide with autologous bone marrow transplantation in first line therapy for patients with poor risk germ cell tumours. J Clin Oncol. 1997;15:2546–52.
41. Kaye S, Mead G, Fossa S, et al. Intensive induction-sequential chemotherapy with BOP/VIP-B compared with treatment of metastatic nonseminomatous germ cell tumour. J Clin Oncol. 1998;16:692–701.

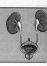

42. Rorth M, Jacobsen G, Maase Hdvd, et al. Surveillance alone verses radiotherapy after orchidectomy for clinical stage 1 nonseminomatous testicular cancer. J Clin Oncol. 1991;9:1543–48.

43. Skinner D, Scardino P. Relevance of biochemical tumor markers and lymphadenectomy in management of non-seminomatous testis tumors: current prospective. J Urol. 1980;123(3):378–82.

44. Ekman E, Edsmyr F. Chemotherapy in non-seminomatous testicular tumours stage 1. Br J Urol. 1981;53:184–7.

45. Sandeman T, Yang C. Results of adjuvant chemotherapy for low stage nonseminomatous germ cell tumors of the testis with vascular invasion. Cancer. 1988;62:1471–5.

46. Cullen M, Stenning S, Parkinson M, et al. Short-course adjuvant chemotherapy in high risk stage I nonseminomatous germ cell tumours of the testis: a Medical Research Council report. J Clin Oncol. 1996;14:1106–13.

47. Pont J, Holtl W, Kosak D, et al. Risk adapted treatment choice in stage 1 nonseminomatous testicular germ cell cancer by regarding vascular invasion in the primary tumour: a prospective trial. J Clin Oncol. 1990;8:16–20.

48. Studer U, Fey M, Calderoni A, Kraft R, Mazzucchelli L, Sonntag R. Adjuvant chemotherapy after orchidectomy in high-risk patients with clinical stage 1 non-seminomatous testicular cancer. Eur Urol. 1993;23(4):444–9.

49. Ravi R, Ong J, Oliver RTD. Long term follow up surveillance versus adjuvant chemotherapy treated stage 1 non-seminoma patients. J Urol. 1998;159(Proc AUA):abst 180.

50. Dearnaley D, Fossa S, Kaye S, et al. Adjuvant bleomycin, vincristine and cisplatin for high risk clinical stage 1 nonseminomatous germ cell tumors – a Medical Research Council pilot study. Proc Am Soc Clin Oncol. 1998;17(1189):309.

Systemic chemotherapy and bladder cancer

51. Yagoda A. Chemotherapy of urothelial tract tumours. Cancer. 1987;60(Suppl.):574–85.

52. Sternberg CN, Yagoda A, Scher HI, et al. Preliminary results of M-VAC (methotrexate, vinblastine, doxorubicin and cisplatin) for transitional cell carcinoma of the urothelium. J Urol. 1985;133:403–7.

53. Oliver RTD, Kwok HK, Highman WJ, Waxman J. Methotrexate, cisplatin and carboplatin as single agents and in combination for metastatic bladder cancer. Br J Urol. 1986;58:31–5.

54. Carmichael J, Cornbleet MA, McDougal RH, et al. Cisplatin and methotrexate in the treatment of transitional cell carcinoma of the urinary tract. Br J Urol. 1985;57:299–302.

55. Harker WG, Meyers SJ, Frieha FS, et al. Cisplatin, methotrexate and vinblastine (CMV): an effective chemotherapy regimen for metastatic transitional cell carcinoma of the urinary tract – a Northern California Oncology Group Study. J Clin Oncol. 1985;3:1463–70.

56. Tannock I, Gospodarowicz M, Connolly J, Jewett M. M-VAC (Methotrexate, Vinblastine, Doxorubicin and Cisplatin) chemotherapy for transitional cell carcinoma: the Princess Margaret Hospital Experience. J Urol. 1989;142:289–92.

57. Saxman SB, Propert KJ, Einhorn LH, et al. Long-term follow up of phase II intergroup study of cisplatin alone or in combination with methotrexate, vinblastine and doxorubicin in patients with metastatic urothelial carcinoma: a co-operative group study. J Clin Oncol. 1997;15:2564-9.

58. Logothetis CJ, Dexeus FH, Finn L, et al. A prospective randomised trial comparing M-VAC and CISCA chemotherapy for patients with metastatic urothelial tumours. J Clin Oncol. 1990;8:1050–5.

59. Mead GM, Russell M, Clark P, et al. A randomised trial comparing methotrexate and vinblastine with cisplatin, methotrexate and vinblastine in advanced transitional cell carcinoma: results and a report on prognostic factors – a Medical Research Council study. Br J Cancer. 1998;78:1067–75.

60. Scher HI, Yagoda A, Herr HW, et al. Neo-adjuvant M-VAC (methotrexate, vinblastine, doxorubicin and cisplatin): effect on the primary bladder lesion. J Urol. 1988;139:470–4.

61. Splinter TAW, Denis L, Scher HI, Schroder FH, Dalesio O. Neo-adjuvant chemotherapy for locally advanced bladder cancer. In: Murphy GP, Khoury S, eds. Therapeutic progress in urological cancers. New York: Alan R Liss; 1989:525–531.

62. Fossa SD, Harland SJ, Kaye SB, et al. Initial combination chemotherapy with cisplatin, methotrexate, vinblastine in locally advanced transitional cell carcinoma – response rate and pitfalls. Br J Urol. 1992;70:161–8.

63. Shearer RJ, Chilvers CED, Bloom HJG, et al. Adjuvant chemotherapy in T3 carcinoma of the bladder – a prospective trial: preliminary report. Br J Urol. 1988;62:558–64.

64. Wallace DMA, Raghavan D, Kelly KA, et al. Neo-adjuvant (pre-emptive) cisplatin therapy in invasive transitional cell carcinoma of the bladder. Br J Urol. 1991;67:608–15.

65. Coppin CML, Gospodarawicz MK, James K, et al. Improved local control of invasive bladder cancer by concurrent cisplatin and pre-operative or definitive radiation. J Clin Oncol. 1996;14:2901–7.

66. Martinez-Pineiro JA, Gonzalez-Martin M, Arocena F, et al. Neo-adjuvant cisplatin chemotherapy before radical cystectomy in invasive transitional cell carcinoma of bladder: a prospective randomised phase III study. J Urol. 1995;153:964–73.

67. Malmstrom PU, Rintala E, Wahlqvist R, et al. Five year follow up of a prospective trial of radical cystectomy and neo-adjuvant chemotherapy: Nordic Cystectomy Trial. J Urol. 1996;155:1903–6.

68. Freiha F, Reese J, Torti FM and Scher HI. Randomised trial of radical cystectomy versus radical cystectomy plus cisplatin, vinblastine and methotrexate chemotherapy for muscle invasive bladder cancer. J Urol. 1996;155:495–500.

69. Shipley WU, Winter KA, Kaufman DS, et al. An RTOG phase III trial (#89–03) of neo-adjuvant chemotherapy in patients with invasive bladder cancer treated with selected bladder preservation by combined radiation therapy and chemotherapy. Proc ASCO. 1998;17:abst 1197.

70. Abol-Enein H, El-Makresh M, El-Baz M, et al. Neo-adjuvant chemotherapy in the treatment of invasive transitional bladder cancer: a controlled prospective randomised study. Br J Urol. 1997;79(Suppl. 4):43(abst 174).

71. International Collaboration of Trialists. Neo-adjuvant cisplatin, methotrexate and vinblastine chemotherapy for muscle-invasive bladder cancer: a randomised controlled trial. Lancet. 1999;354:533–40.

72. Logothetis CJ, Finn LD, Smith T, et al. Escalated M-VAC with or without recombinant human granulocyte-macrophage colony-stimulating factor for the initial treatment of advanced malignant urothelial tumours: results of a randomised trial. J Clin Oncol. 1995;13:2272–7.

73. Seidman AD, Scher HI, Gabrilove JL, et al. Dose intensification of M-VAC with recombinant granulocyte colony-stimulating factor as initial therapy in advanced urothelial cancer. J Clin Oncol. 1993;11:404–14.

74. Moore MJ, Iscoe N, Tannock IF. A phase II study of methotrexate, vinblastine, doxorubicin and cisplatin + recombinant granulocyte-macrophage colony-stimulating factors in patients with advanced transitional cell carcinoma. J Urol. 1993;150:1131–4.

75. Sternberg CN, De Mulder P, Fossa S, et al. Interim toxicity analysis of a randomised trial in advanced urothelial tract tumors of high-dose intensity M-VAC chemotherapy and recombinant granulocyte colony-stimulating factor (G-CSF) versus classic M-VAC chemotherapy (EORTC 30924). Proc ASCO. 1997;16:1140 (abstr).

76. Roth B, Dreicer R, Einhorn LH, et al. Significant activity of paclitaxel in advanced transitional cell carcinoma of the urothelium: a phase II trial of the Eastern Co-operative Oncology Group. J Clin Oncol. 1994;12:2264–10.

77. Dimopoulos MA, Deliveliotis C, Moulopoulos LA, et al. Treatment of patients with metastatic urothelial carcinoma and impaired renal function with single agent docetaxel. Urology. 1998;52:56–60.

78. Vogelzang NJ, Stadler WM. Gemcitabine and other new chemotherapeutic agents for the treatment of metastatic bladder cancer. Urology. 1999;53:243–50.

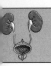

79. Papamichael D, Gallagher CJ, Oliver RT, et al. Phase II study of paclitaxel in pre-treated patients with locally advanced/metastatic cancer of the bladder and ureter. Br J Cancer. 1997;75:606–7.

80. McCaffrey JA, Hilton S, Mazumda RM, et al. Phase II trial of docetaxel in patients with advanced or metastatic transitional-cell carcinoma. J Clin Oncol. 1997;15:1853–7.

81. Moore MJ, Tannock IF, Ernst DS, et al. Gemcitabine: a promising new agent in the treatment of advanced urothelial cancer. J Clin Oncol. 1997;15:3441–5.

82. Stadler WM, Kuzel TM, Roth B, et al. Phase II study of single agent Gemcitabine in previously untreated patients with metastatic urothelial cancer. J Clin Oncol. 1997;15:3394–8.

83a. Lorunno V, Pollera CF, Antimi M, et al. A phase II study of Gemcitabine in patients with transitional cell carcinoma of the urinary tract previously treated with platinum. Italian Co-operative Group on Bladder Cancer. Eur J Cancer. 1998;34:1208–12.

83b. von der Maase H, Hansen SW, Roberts JT, et al. Gemcitabine and cisplatin (GC) versus methotrexate, vinblastine, adriamycin and cisplatin (MVAC) in advanced or metastatic transitional cell carcinoma of the urothelium: a large randomized multicenter, multinational phase III study. Proc. Am. Soc. Clin. Oncol. 2000:19:abst 1293.

Chemotherapy in urology: kidney cancer

84. Bukowski RM. Natural history and therapy of metastatic renal cell carcinoma: the role of interleukin-2. Cancer. 1997; 80(7): 1198–220.

85. Oliver RT, Nethersell AB, Bottomley JM. Unexplained spontaneous regression and alpha-interferon as treatment for metastatic renal carcinoma. Br J Urol. 1989;63(2):128–31.

86. Motzer RJ, Vogelzang NJ. Chemotherapy for renal cell carcinoma. In: Raghavan D, Scher HJ, Leibel SA, Lange PH, eds. Principles and practice of genitourinary oncology. Philadelphia: Lippincott-Raven; 1997:885–96.

87. Bloom HJ. Hormone-induced and spontaneous regression of metastatic renal cancer. Cancer. 1973;32(5):1066–71.

88. Fayers PM, Cook PA, Machin D, et al. On the development of the Medical Research Council trial of alpha-interferon in metastatic renal carcinoma. Urological Working Party Renal Carcinoma Subgroup. Stat Med. 1994;13(21):2249–60.

89. Pizzocaro G, Piva L, Salvioni R, Di Fronzo G, Ronchi E, Miodini P. Adjuvant medroxyprogesterone acetate and steroid hormone receptors in category M0 renal cell carcinoma. An interim report of a prospective randomized study. J Urol. 1986;135(1):18–21.

90. Steineck G, et al. Recombinant leukocyte interferon alpha-2a and medroxyprogesterone in advanced renal cell carcinoma. A randomized trial. Acta Oncol. 1990;29(2):155–62.

91. Gleave ME, et al. Interferon gamma-1b compared with placebo in metastatic renal-cell carcinoma. Canadian Urologic Oncology Group. N Engl J Med. 1998;338(18):1265–71.

92. MRC Renal Cancer Collaborators. Interferon-alpha and survival in metastatic renal carcinoma: early results of a randomised controlled trial. Medical Research Council Renal Cancer Collaborators. Lancet. 1999;353(9146):14–7.

93. Pyrhonen S, Salminen E, Lehtonen T. Recombinant interferon alpha-2A with vinblastine vs vinblastine alone in advanced renal cell carcinoma: a Phase III study. Proc ASCO. 1996;15:614 (abstr).

94. Pizzocaro G, Piva L, Costa A, Silvestrini R. Adjuvant interferon (IFN) to radical nephrectomy in Robson's stages II and III renal cell cancer (RCC), a multicentre randomized study with some biological evaluations. Proc ASCO. 1997;16:318a (abstract 1132).

95. Fyfe G, Fisher RI, Rosenberg SA, Sznol M, Parkinson DR, Louie AC. Results of treatment of 255 patients with metastatic renal cell carcinoma who received high-dose recombinant interleukin-2 therapy. J Clin Oncol. 1995;13(3):688–96.

96. Jones M, Philip T, Palmer P, et al. The impact of interleukin-2 on survival in renal cancer: a multivariate analysis. Cancer Biother. 1993;8(4):275–88.

97. Holdener EE, Emmons RP, Brunda M, Evans L, Levitt D. Interferon-alpha and interleukin-2 in the treatment of renal cell cancer. Prog Clin Biol Res. 1990;348:61–9.

98. Henriksson R, Nilsson S, Colleen S, et al. Survival in renal cell carcinoma – a randomized evaluation of tamoxifen vs interleukin 2, alpha-interferon (leucocyte) and tamoxifen. Br J Cancer. 1998;77(8):1311–7.

99. Negrier S, et al. Recombinant human interleukin-2, recombinant human interferon alfa-2a, or both in metastatic renal-cell carcinoma. Groupe Francais d'Immunotherapie. N Engl J Med. 1998;338(18):1272–8.

100. Rosenberg SA. Karnofsky Memorial Lecture. The immunotherapy and gene therapy of cancer. J Clin Oncol. 1992;0(2):180–99.

101. Osband ME, Lavin PT, Babayan RK, et al. Effect of autolymphocyte therapy on survival and quality of life in patients with metastatic renal-cell carcinoma. Lancet. 1990;335(8696):994–8.

102. Atzpodien J, Kirchner H, Hanninen EL, Deckert M, Fenner M, Poliwoda H. Interleukin-2 in combination with interferon-alpha and 5-fluorouracil for metastatic renal cell cancer. Eur J Cancer. 1993;29A(Suppl. 5):S6–8.

103. Atzpodien J, Kirchner H, Franzke A, et al. Results of a randomised clinical trial comparing SC interleukin-2, SC alpha-2a-interferon, and IV bolus 5-fluorouracil against oral tamoxifen in progressive metastatic renal cell carcinoma patients. Proc ASCO. 1997;16:326a (abstract 1164).

104. Negrier S, et al. Randomized study of interleukin-2(IL2) and interferon (IFN) with or without 5-FU (FUCY study) in metastatic renal cell carcinoma (MRCC). Proc ASCO. 1997;16:326a (abstract 1161).

105. Sene AP, Hunt L, McMahon RF, Carroll RN. Renal carcinoma in patients undergoing nephrectomy: analysis of survival and prognostic factors. Br J Urol. 1992;70(2):125–34.

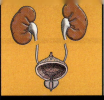

Chapter 47

Pathology Review

Norman L Reeve, Richard J Hale, and Lorna J McWilliam

This chapter is not intended to be a comprehensive review of uropathology. Other specialized books will meet that need (see references). The histology slides presented here are intended to illustrate common or interesting conditions that might be encountered in any busy urologic practice and that,

we hope, provide a flavor of this fascinating area of pathology. All sections apart from Figure 47.37 are stained using a routine hematoxylin and eosin method. Figure 47.37 is stained using an immunoperoxidase technique.

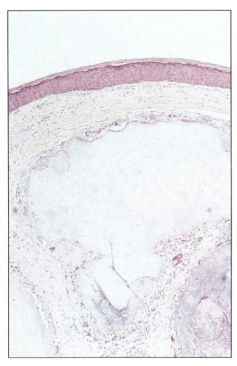

Figure 47.1 Scrotal calcinosis. Within the dermis, areas of foreign body giant cell reaction are present at the margins of a previously calcified dermal nodule (decalcified section).

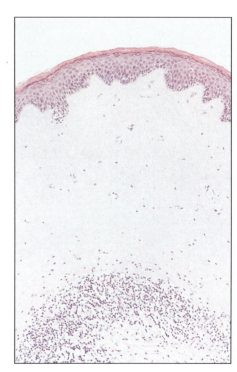

Figure 47.2 Balanitis xerotica obliterans. The overlying epidermis shows mild hyperkeratosis. The upper dermis contains a band-like area of pale, homogenous eosinophilic tissue. Deep to this there is a predominately lymphocytic infiltrate.

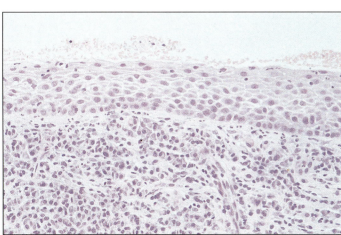

Figure 47.3 Balanitis circumscripta plasmacellularis (plasma cell balanitis: Zoon's balanitis). The overlying epidermis shows mild reactive changes. The subjacent dermis contains a dense chronic inflammatory cell infiltrate consisting predominantly of plasma cells.

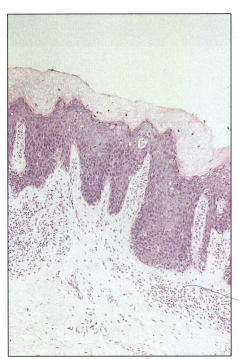

Figure 47.4 Squamous cell carcinoma-in-situ. This penile skin biopsy shows marked atypia with frequent mitotic figures within an acanthotic and hyperkeratotic epidermis. The changes are present throughout the full thickness of the epithelium. No dermal invasion is present.

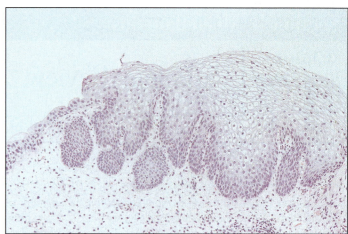

Figure 47.7 Squamous metaplasia. This bladder biopsy from the trigone shows a transition from urothelium to stratified nonkeratinizing squamous epithelium of vaginal type. No significant cellular atypia is present.

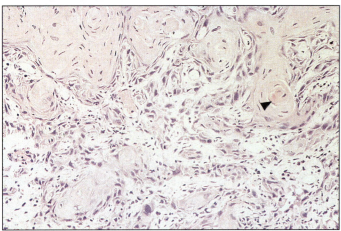

Figure 47.5 Invasive squamous cell carcinoma. A well-differentiated squamous cell carcinoma of the penis with tongues of epithelium infiltrating the dermis. Keratinization is apparent (arrowhead).

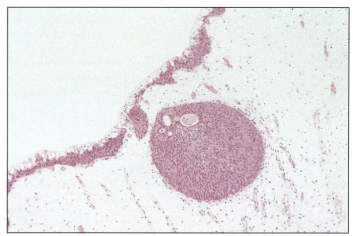

Figure 47.8 Von Brunn's nest. The lamina propria contains a rounded nest of transitional cells that appears to be separate from the overlying urothelium.

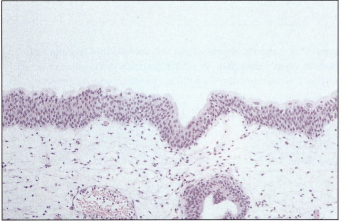

Figure 47.6 Normal bladder. The surface urothelium is up to six cells thick. The superficial layer is composed of 'umbrella' cells, which contain slightly larger nuclei. The underlying cells are smaller and regular, containing ovoid nuclei. Nucleoli are inconspicuous throughout.

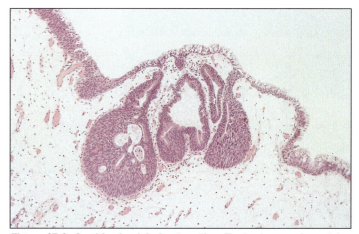

Figure 47.9 Cystitis glandularis et cystica. The lamina propria contains several rounded nests of transitional cells that show cystic dilatation; some of these are lined by tall columnar epithelium.

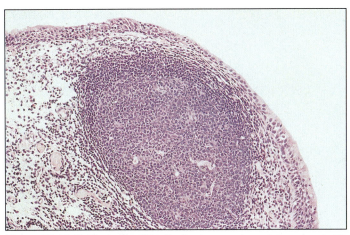

Figure 47.10 Follicular cystitis. The lamina propria contains a lymphoid follicle with a prominent germinal center. The overlying urothelium is elevated and mildly attenuated.

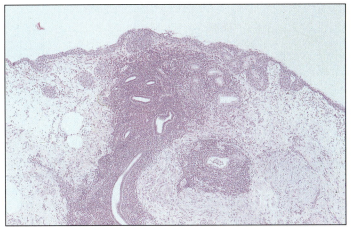

Figure 47.11 Endometriosis. The bladder wall contains foci of endometriosis composed of glandular structures surrounded by endometrial-type stroma.

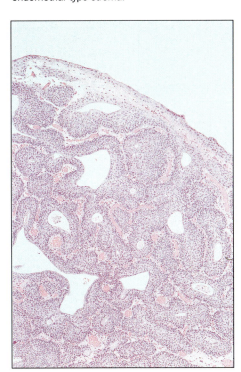

Figure 47.12 Inverted papilloma. This polypoidal lesion consists of anastomosing trabeculae and islands of transitional cells within the lamina propria. Some of these islands contain cystic spaces. The overlying urothelium is attenuated.

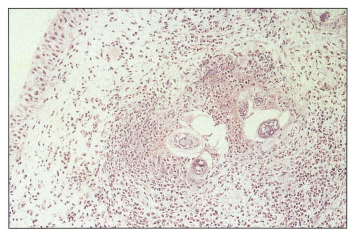

Figure 47.13 Schistosomiasis. This bladder biopsy contains scattered schistosomal ova with terminal spines. These have elicited a florid inflammatory reaction including numerous eosinophils.

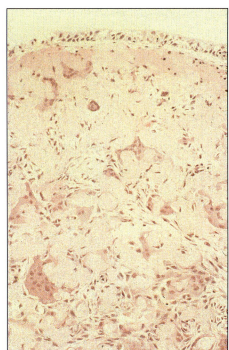

Figure 47.14 Amyloidosis. Masses of acellular pale eosinophilic material are present within the lamina propria, which has elicited a florid foreign body giant cell reaction. The diagnosis was confirmed using a Congo red stain.

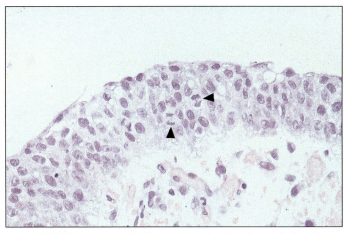

Figure 47.15 Transitional cell carcinoma in situ. The urothelium is slightly thickened and the transitional cells show severe atypia and prominent mitotic figures are present (arrowheads). No invasive tumor is present.

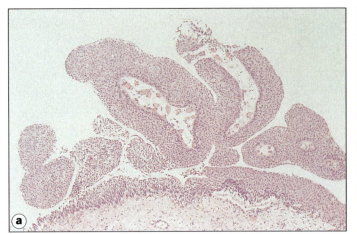

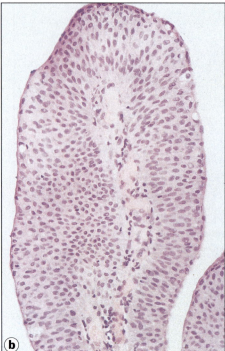

Figure 47.16 Papillary transitional cell carcinoma, low grade.
(a) A papillary transitional cell carcinoma of the bladder, which has a relatively regular growth pattern. (b) The urothelium covering the papillae is thickened and shows only mild nuclear pleomorphism. There is no stromal invasion.

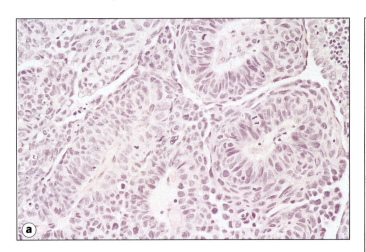

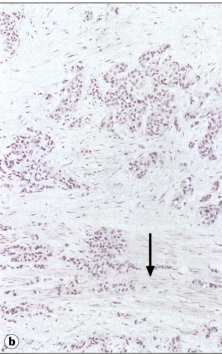

Figure 47.17 Transitional cell carcinoma, high grade.
(a) This tumor has a more solid growth pattern and shows marked atypia with scattered mitoses. (b) Tumor is seen infiltrating into the lamina propria and muscularis propria (arrow).

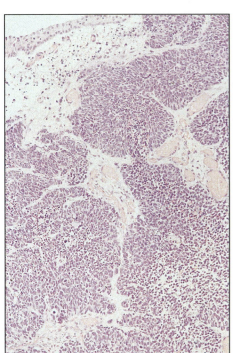

Figure 47.18 Small cell carcinoma. The bladder wall can be seen to be infiltrated by loosely cohesive sheets of small nuclei with scanty cytoplasm and with scattered mitotic figures. The tumor cells were positive for chromogranin, a marker of neuroendocrine differentiation.

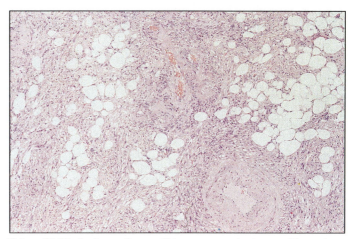

Figure 47.21 Angiomyolipoma. This uncommon benign renal tumor is composed of a mixture of spindly smooth muscle cells, mature adipocytes, and prominent, thick-walled blood vessels.

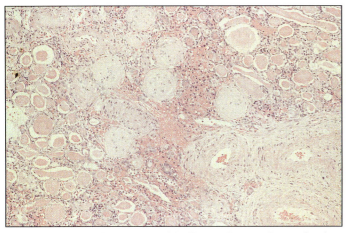

Figure 47.19 Chronic pyelonephritis. The renal cortex shows sclerotic glomeruli, atrophic tubules containing eosinophilic casts ('tubular thyroidization'), interstitial fibrosis, and thick-walled blood vessels.

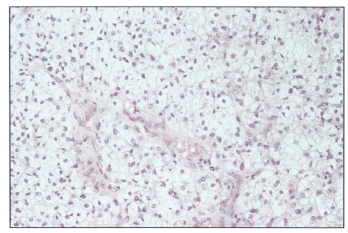

Figure 47.22 Renal cell carcinoma (hypernephroma). A typical clear cell carcinoma composed of sheets of clear cells with moderate nuclear atypia and a delicate vascular supporting stroma.

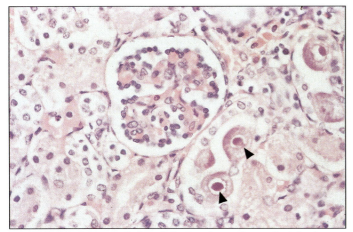

Figure 47.20 Cytomegalovirus infection. Large, intensely stained purple viral inclusions are seen (arrowheads) in tubular epithelial cells adjacent to a normal glomerulus in this neonatal kidney.

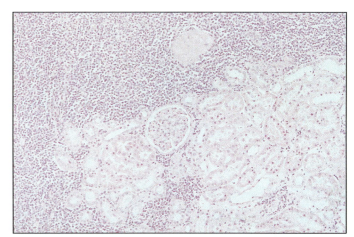

Figure 47.23 Non-Hodgkin's lymphoma. The upper half of this field of renal cortex is diffusely infiltrated by sheets of monotonous lymphoid cells of a low-grade B-cell non-Hodgkin's lymphoma. This is a relatively rare occurrence but quite different in appearance from epithelial neoplasms of the kidney.

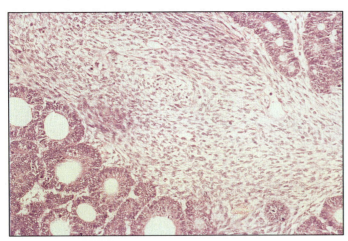

Figure 47.24 Wilms tumor. This is an example of a biphasic tumor with a primitive spindle-celled stroma in the central area and surrounding glandular epithelial elements.

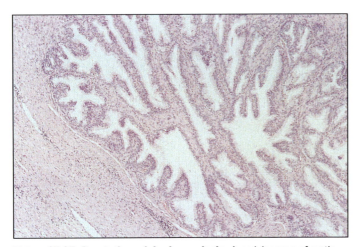

Figure 47.25 Prostatic nodular hyperplasia. A nodular area of cystic glandular hyperplasia with a circumscribed outline.

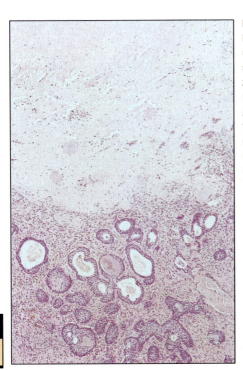

Figure 47.26 Prostatic infarct. The upper half of the field shows an acellular zone of infarction. The lower part consists of glandular prostatic tissue showing basal cell hyperplasia and squamous metaplasia (see Fig. 47.27).

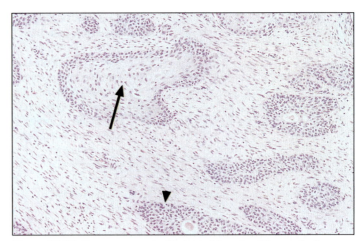

Figure 47.27 Squamous metaplasia and basal cell hyperplasia. This shows glandular prostatic tissue with squamous metaplasia (arrow) and basal cell hyperplasia (arrowhead), in the glandular components (see Fig. 47.26).

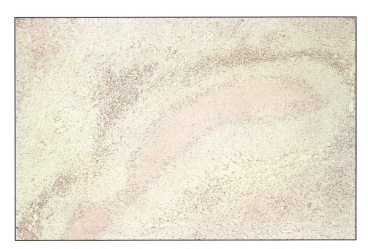

Figure 47.28 Postoperative necrotizing granuloma. This is prostate with a necrotizing palisaded granuloma (centrally situated) occurring after previous prostatic surgery (transurethral resection of the prostate).

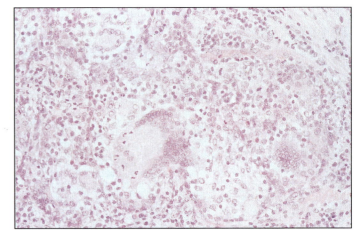

Figure 47.29 Granulomatous prostatitis. This is prostate showing granulomatous inflammation involving glandular tissue with epithelioid histiocytes and multinucleate giant cells.

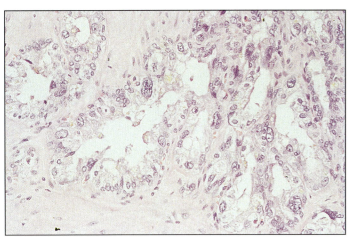

Figure 47.30 Normal seminal vesicle. The bizarre cellular features of the glandular lining cells can cause confusion with neoplasia in small prostatic biopsies. The cells typically also contain brown/yellow lipofuscin pigment in the cytoplasm.

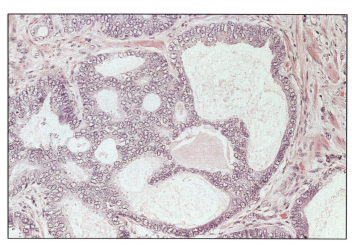

Figure 47.32 High-grade prostatic intraepithelial neoplasia. A large duct with an atypical cribriform pattern of proliferating cells with large nuclei and prominent nucleoli.

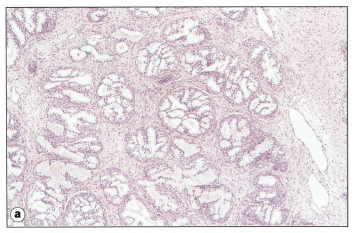

Figure 47.31 Prostatic cribriform hyperplasia. This variant of benign hyperplasia is characterized by the proliferation of glands with a cribriform pattern that should not be mistaken for prostatic intraepithelial neoplasia

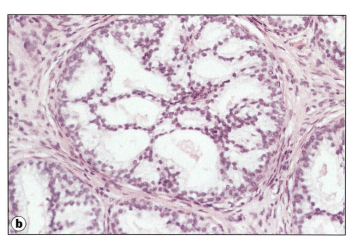

(see Fig. 47.32). The cells have abundant cytoplasm and regular small nuclei without atypical features.

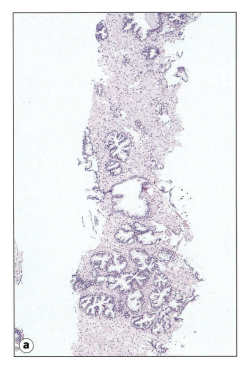

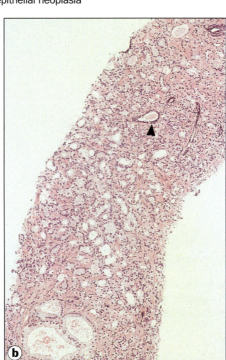

Figure 47.33 Prostatic needle biopsies. (a) Normal biopsy with irregular shaped glands clearly separated by stroma. (b) Prostatic adenocarcinoma with closely packed small fairly uniform glands surrounding occasional residual normal glands (arrowhead).

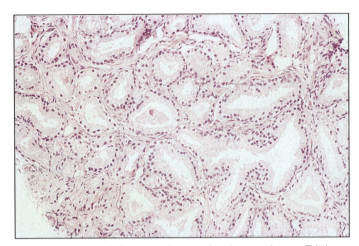

Figure 47.34 Well-differentiated prostatic adenocarcinoma. This is a medium-power view from a case of Gleason grade 3+2 adenocarcinoma containing closely packed, well-defined glands with minimal cytologic atypia.

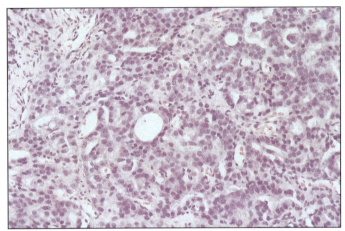

Figure 47.35 Moderately to poorly differentiated prostatic adenocarcinoma. This is a medium-power view from a case of Gleason grade 4+5 adenocarcinoma with poorly formed glandular spaces, marked nuclear atypia, and prominent nucleoli.

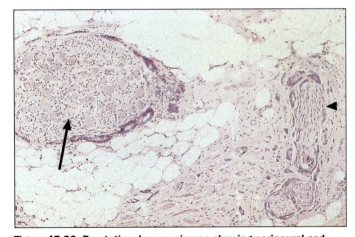

Figure 47.36 Prostatic adenocarcinoma showing perineural and periganglionic invasion. Malignant glands surround a ganglion (arrow) and several nerves (arrowhead) in peripheral tissue from a radical prostatectomy.

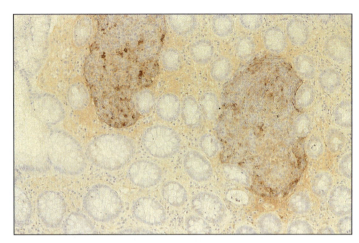

Figure 47.37 Prostatic specific-antigen (PSA) staining. A case of metastatic prostatic adenocarcinoma in colonic mucosa stained for PSA. The brown stain reveals positive groups of tumor cells. PSA can be useful to help determine the origin of metastatic carcinoma.

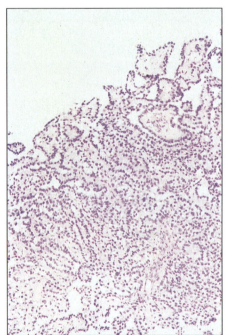

Figure 47.38 Urethral nephrogenic metaplasia. This biopsy from a papillary lesion has the tubulopapillary pattern of this benign process, which is more commonly seen in the bladder.

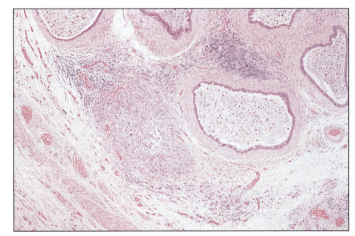

Figure 47.39 Epididymal sperm granuloma. There is granulomatous inflammation of the epididymis adjacent to intact, dilated epididymal tubules. A similar reaction frequently occurs around the vas deferens following vasectomy.

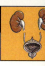

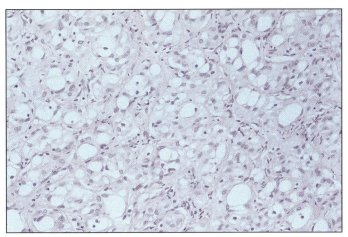

Figure 47.40 Adenomatoid tumor. In this example the cells have a prominent 'signet ring' pattern. This is a benign tumor believed to be of mesothelial origin.

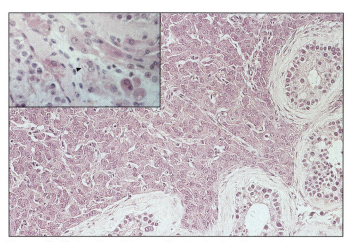

Figure 47.43 Leydig cell tumor. Sheets of cells with abundant eosinophilic cytoplasm from a well-defined nodule in the testis. Compare cells with normal Leydig cells in the inset where a rare Reinke crystalloid is seen (arrowhead).

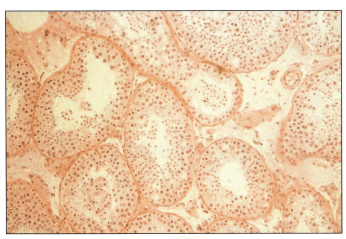

Figure 47.41 Normal testis. Some tubules show active spermatogenesis. Occasional Leydig cells are seen. Fixation with Bouin's fluid, which preserves tubular structure, is useful when assessing potential fertility.

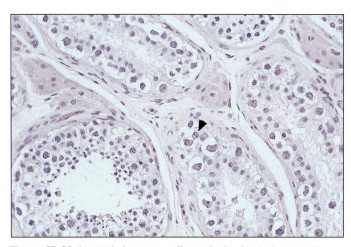

Figure 47.44 Intratubular germ cell neoplasia. Atypical germ cells (arrowhead) are seen lining these seminiferous tubules from a case of testicular seminoma.

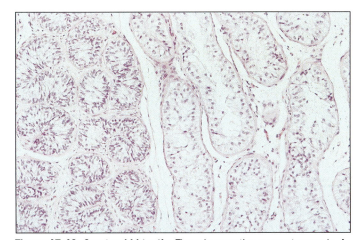

Figure 47.42 Cryptorchid testis. There is no active spermatogenesis. A frequent finding is the presence of clusters of tubules showing Sertoli cell hyperplasia (congeries of Sertoli) as seen on the left.

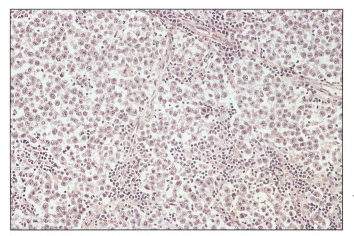

Figure 47.45 Testicular seminoma. This is a classic seminoma with sheets of malignant germ cells separated by fibrous septa containing abundant lymphocytes. Cells typically have clear (glycogen-rich) cytoplasm and contain prominent nucleoli.

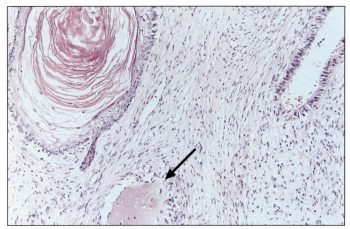

Figure 47.46 Mature teratoma (teratoma differentiated). The differentiated structures in this example include keratinizing squamous epithelium (top left), glandular epithelium (top right), and osteoid (arrow).

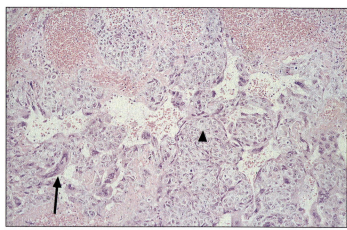

Figure 47.48 Choriocarcinoma (malignant teratoma trophoblastic). This region of tumor resembles placental trophoblastic tissue with syncytiotrophoblastic (arrow) and cytotrophoblastic (arrowhead) cells in a hemorrhagic nodule.

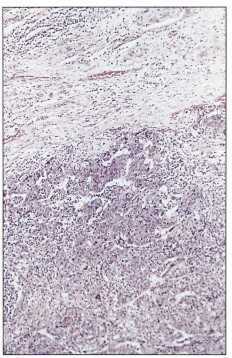

Figure 47.47 Embryonal carcinoma (malignant teratoma undifferentiated). There is a solid proliferation of highly pleomorphic, primitive epithelial cells.

REFERENCES

1. Bernstein J, Churg J. Urinary tract pathology: An illustrated practical guide to diagnosis. New York: Raven Press; 1992.

2. Bostwick DG, Dundore PA. Biopsy pathology of the prostate. Biopsy Pathology Series 20. London: Chapman & Hall; 1997.

3. Bostwick DG, Eble JN. Urologic surgical pathology. St Louis: Mosby; 1997.

4. Foster CS, Bostwick DG. Pathology of the prostate. Major problems in pathology 34. Philadelphia: WB Saunders; 1998.

5. Murphy WM. Urological pathology, 2nd ed. Philadelphia: WB Saunders; 1997.

6. Peterson RO. Urologic pathology, 2nd ed. Philadelphia: JB Lippincott; 1992.

Index

Entries in italic refer to figures.

A

abdominal wall defects, 29, 203
abdominal wall development, 21
ABH antigen markers, bladder cancer progression, 383
Abrams–Griffiths pressure–flow nomogram, 77, *78*
absorptive hypercalciuria, 314, *314*
   dietary calcium restriction, 316
   pharmacologic therapy, 323–4
   type I, 314, 323–4
   type II, 314, 324
accelerated M-VAC chemotherapy, 680
acetohydroxamic acid, 325, 326
acetylcholine
   detrusor neuromuscular transmission, 70–1
   metabolism, 63, *63*
   penile erection, 600
   ureter receptors, 63, 64
   see also cholinergic innervation
acetylcholinesterase, 63
acid–base balance, renal regulation, 56, *57*
acidosis, 263
   acute renal failure, 266, 267
   chronic renal failure, 269
acontractile bladder, congenital cord lesions, 514
action potential
   bladder contraction, 71
   ureter, 59–60, *59*
activin, 587
adenocarcinoma, bladder, 376
adenomatoid tumor, *699*
adenosine, 93
adhesins, 297, *298*
adoptive immunotherapy, 686–7, *686*
adrenal adenoma, 183
adrenal androgen inhibitors, 419–20
adrenal gland anatomy, 33, *34*
adrenal hyperplasia, congenital, 27, 234, 236, 593
   clinical features, 236
   diagnosis, 236–7
   gender reassignment, 237–8, 240
   management, 238, *238*
   prognosis, 241
   salt-losing crisis, 237
   surgery
      feminizing genitoplasty, 239–40, *239, 240, 241*
      vaginal replacement, 240–1
adrenalectomy, laparoscopic, 183
adriamycin see doxorubicin
age associations
   benign prostate hypertrophy, 451

bladder cancer, 364
   erectile dysfunction, 602
   incontinence, 477
   urinary tract infection, 301
AIDS patients, indinavir calculi, 98, 319
ALARA principle, 134
alcohol intake, erectile dysfunction, 602
aldosterone
   potassium regulation, 56
   tubular sodium transport, 55
   see also renin–angiotensin–aldosterone system
alexandrite laser therapy, 654
alfuzosin, 467
allopurinol, 324, 326
alpha decay, 132
alpha-adrenergic agonists, 484
alpha-adrenoreceptors
   bladder neck/proximal urethra, 484
   prostate, 467
   ureter, 63, 64, *64*
alpha-blockers
   benign prostate hypertrophy, 11, 462–3, 466–7
   combined drug treatments, 468
   mode of action, 467
   nonbacterial prostatitis, 308
   priapism, 619
   side effects, 462–3, 467
   spinal/bladder voiding pathway activity, 467
   uroselectivity, 467
alpha-calcidol, 269
alpha-fetoprotein serum level
   normal infant, *230*
   testicular tumors, 229, 431, 675
alpha-interferon
   renal cell carcinoma, 355, 685
   toxicity, 355, *355*
alpha-mercaptopropionylglycine, 325, 326
alpha-naphthylamine, 374
5-α reductase, 26, 210, 587
   isoenzymes, 467
   prostate androgen metabolism, 417
5-α reductase deficiency, 28, 239
   type 2, 467
5-α reductase inhibitors
   advanced/late prostate cancer, 416
   benign prostate hypertrophy, 11, 462, 463
Alport's syndrome, 275
alprostadil
   intracavernous injection, 618
   transurethral therapy, 609, *609*
alveolar rhabdomyosarcoma, 227

Alzheimer's disease, 601
ambiguous genitalia, 26, 235, *236*, 467
   mixed gonadal dysgenesis, 235
   newborn, 236, *238*
      examination, 236–8
      management algorithm, *238*
   XY gonadal dysgenesis, 235
   see also intersex states
ambulatory cystometry, 75–6, *76*
amino acids, renal tubular handling, 51
4-aminobiphenyl, 363
aminoglutethamide, 419
5-aminolevulinic acid (5-ALA) fluorescence, 370, 656
aminosalicylic acid, 4
amitriptyline, 480, 502
ammonia, renal tubular handling, 51, 56
ammoniogenic coma, 529
ampicillin, 307
ampulla, 17
amyloidosis, *693*
anabolic steroids, 593
analgesia, acute stone episode, 322
analgesic nephropathy, 263
anastomotic urethroplasty, 579
Anderson–Hynes pyeloplasty, 345, *345*
androgen deficiency, erectile dysfunction, 601
   replacement therapy, 608, *608*
androgen deprivation therapy, prostate cancer, 415–16, *418*
   early versus delayed, *417*, 418
   intermittent androgen suppression, 418–19
   maximum androgen blockade (MAB), 417–18
   neoadjuvant therapy, 415
androgen insensitivity, 28, 239, *239*
anemia
   bladder cancer, 376
   chronic renal failure, 269
   late prostate cancer, 421–2
anesthesia
   extracorporeal shock wave lithotripsy, 627–8, *628, 629*
   historical aspects, 8
angiogenesis inhibitors, 420
angiography, 88–9, *88*
   computed tomography, 103, *103*
   erectile dysfunction, 605, *606*
   post-renal transplantation renal artery stenosis, 289, *292*
   renal cell carcinoma, 352–3
angiomyolipoma, 348, *695*
   computed tomography, 101

magnetic resonance imaging, 111, *112*
renal artery embolization, 156
ultrasound, 107
angiostatin, 384
angiotensin II
   glomerular arteriolar tone, 50
   tubular sodium transport, 54
angiotensin receptor antagonists, 268
angiotensin-converting enzyme (ACE) inhibitor renography, 144, *145*
angiotensin-converting enzyme (ACE) inhibitors, 261
   accelerated hypertension, 270
   chronic renal failure, 268
   renal allograft toxicity, 283
antegrade endopyelotomy, 345
antegrade pyelography, 151–2
   post-renal transplantation ureteric obstruction, 286, *286*
anterior colporrhaphy, 484, 549
antiandrogen therapy, 403
   benign prostate hypertrophy, 468
   prostate cancer
      advanced/late, 416
      hormone refractory, 419
antibiotics
   acute interstitial nephritis, 263
   acute pyelonephritis, 303, *303*, *304*
   bowel tissue urinary tract reconstructions, 523
   emphysematous pyelonephritis, 304
   Fournier's gangrene, 309
   historical aspects, 4
   malacoplakia, 306
   perinephric abscess, 307
   renal transplantation surgery, 280
   urinary tract infection, 300–2
      bacterial resistance, 296
      cystitis, 300–1
      prophylaxis, 302–3
   vesicoureteral reflux management, 254
   xanthogranulomatous pyelonephritis, 306
antiCD3 monoclonal antibody, 280, 286
antiestrogen therapy, 419–20
antiglomerular basement membrane disease
   post-transplantation recurrence, 277
   renal transplantation, 275–6
antihistamines, 503
antihypertensives, 270
   patients with renal impairment, 270, *270*

701

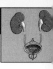

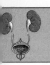

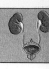

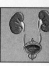

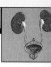

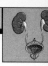

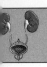

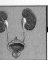

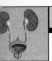

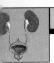